Operative Surgery
and Management

Operative Surgery and Management

Third edition

Edited by

G. Keen MS FRCS

Consultant Cardiothoracic Surgeon, Emeritus
Bristol Royal Infirmary, UK

J. Farndon BSc MD FRCS

Professor of Surgery,
University of Bristol;
Consultant Surgeon,
Bristol Royal Infirmary, UK

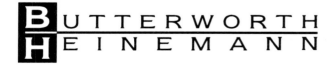
BUTTERWORTH
HEINEMANN

Butterworth-Heinemann Ltd
Linacre House, Jordan Hill, Oxford OX2 8DP

A member of the Reed Elsevier group

OXFORD LONDON BOSTON
MUNICH NEW DELHI SINGAPORE SYDNEY
TOKYO TORONTO WELLINGTON

First published 1981
Second edition 1987
Third edition 1994

British Library Cataloguing in Publication Data
Operative Surgery and Management.—
3Rev.ed
  I. Keen, G. II. Farndon, John R.
  617.91

ISBN 0 7506 1377 7

Library of Congress Cataloging in Publication Data
Operative surgery and management/edited by G. Keen, J. Farndon. –
  3rd ed.
  p. cm.
  Includes bibliographical references and index.
  ISBN 0 7506 1377 7
  1. Surgery, Operative. 2. Surgery. I. Keen, G. II. Farndon, J.
  [DNLM: 1. Surgery, Operative. WO 500 0605]
  RD32, 06   93–5474
  617–dc20   CIP

Typeset by Bath Typesetting Ltd
Printed and bound in Great Britain by the Bath Press, Avon

Contents

Perfusion techniques in cardiac surgery

Amputations and prostheses

Contributors

D. Alderson MD FRCS
Consultant Senior Lecturer in Surgery
Department of Surgery
Bristol Royal Infirmary
Bristol, UK

J. D. Atwell FRCS
Consultant Paediatric Surgeon
Wessex Regional Centre for Paediatric Surgery
Southampton

J. S. Bailey BA FRCS
Consultant Cardiothoracic Surgeon
Groby Road Hospital
Leicester, UK

R. N. Baird ChM FRCS
Consultant Surgeon
Bristol Royal Infirmary
Bristol, UK

D. C. C. Bartolo FRCS
Consultant Surgeon
Department of Surgery
The Royal Infirmary
Edinburgh, UK

M. J. M. Black FRCS
Consultant Plastic Surgeon
Royal Victoria Infirmary
Newcastle-upon-Tyne, UK

K. Burnand MS FRCS
Assistant Director
Surgical Unit
St Thomas' Hospital
London, UK

Sir Roy Calne MA FRS FRCS
Professor of Surgery
University of Cambridge; and
Honorary Consultant Surgeon
Addenbrooke's Hospital
Cambridge, UK

J. A. S. Carruth FRCS
Consultant Otolaryngologist and
Senior Lecturer in Otolaryngology
Southampton University and
University Hospitals, UK

C. Charlton MS FRCS
Consultant Urologist
Royal United Hospital
Bath, UK; and
Member Court of Examiners of RCS

D. A. Cooley MD
Surgeon in Chief
Texas Heart Institute
Houston, Texas, USA

M. J. Cooper MS FRCS
Consultant Surgeon
Royal Devon and Exeter Hospital (Wonford)
Exeter, UK

B. R. Davidson MB ChB
Consultant Surgeon
Royal Free Hospital
London, UK

H. B. Devlin MA MD MCh FRCS FRCS(I) FRCS(Ed) FACS
Consultant Surgeon
North Tees General Hospital; and
Lecturer in Clinical Surgery
University of Newcastle-upon-Tyne, UK

N. E. Dudley FRCS
Consultant Surgeon
John Radcliffe Hospital
Oxford, UK

P. Durdey MS FRCS
Senior Lecturer and Consultant Surgeon
Department of Surgery
Bristol Royal Infirmary
Bristol, UK

H. Espiner MB(NZ) ChM FRCS
Consultant Surgeon
Bristol Royal Infirmary
Bristol, UK

J. R. Farndon MD FRCS
Professor of Surgery
University of Bristol; and
Consultant Surgeon
Bristol Royal Infirmary, UK

R. C. L. Feneley MCh FRCS
Consultant Urologist
Southmead General Hospital
Bristol, UK

C. G. Fowler BSc FRCS
Consultant Urologist
The London Hospital
London, UK

F. Glassow FRCS FRCS(C)
Formerly Associate Surgeon
Shouldice Hospital
Thornhill
Ontario, Canada;
Hunterian Professor
Royal College of Surgeons of England

H. B. Griffith FRCS FRCP (deceased)
Consultant Neurosurgeon
Frenchay Hospital
Bristol, UK

H. C. Grillo MD
Chief of General Thoracic Surgery
Massachusetts General Hospital
Boston, USA; and
Professor of Surgery
Harvard Medical School
USA

N. A. Habib ChM FRCS(Ed)
Consultant Senior Lecturer
The Royal Postgraduate Medical School
Hammersmith Hospital
London, UK

R. W. Hiles FRCS
Consultant Plastic Surgeon
Frenchay Hospital
Bristol, UK

M. Horrocks MS FRCS
Professor of Surgery
The Royal United Hospital
Bath, UK

P. W. J. Houghton FRCS
Consultant Surgeon
Torbay, UK

R. Hurt FRCS
Consultant Thoracic Surgeon (retired)
St. Bartholomew's Hospital
London, UK

J. A. Hutter BSc FRCS
Consultant Cardiac Surgeon
Bristol Royal Infirmary
Bristol, UK

K. Jeyasingham MB ChM FRCS FRCS (Ed)
Consultant Thoracic Surgeon
Frenchay Hospital
Bristol; and
Honorary Clinical Lecturer in Surgery
University of Bristol, UK

G. Keen MS FRCS
Consultant Cardiothoracic Surgeon, Emeritus
Bristol Royal Infirmary
Bristol, UK

D. J. Leaper MD ChM FRCS FRCS(Ed)
Consultant Senior Lecturer
University Department of Surgery
Southmead Hospital
Bristol, UK

J. Lendrum MA FRCS
Consultant Plastic and Reconstructive Surgeon
Withington Hospital
Manchester, UK

T. W. Lennard MD FRCS
Senior Lecturer
Department of Surgery
University of Newcastle-upon-Tyne, UK; and
Consultant Surgeon
The Royal Victoria Infirmary
Newcastle-upon-Tyne, UK

G. N. Lumb FRCS
Honorary Consultant Urologist
Musgrove Park Hospital
Taunton, UK

D. McCoy FRCS FRCS(Ed) FRCOG
Consultant Obstetrician and Gynaecologist
Southmead Hospital
Bristol, UK

M. McGee-Collett FRACS
Consultant Neurosurgeon
Royal Prince Alfred Hospital
Sydney
Australia

J. A. Massey MD FRCS
Consultant Urologist
St Helens & Knowsley Hospitals Trust
Merseyside, UK

D. B. Mathias FRCS
Consultant ENT Surgeon
Freeman Hospital
Newcastle-upon-Tyne, UK

D. J. Mathison MD
Associate Professor of Surgery
Harvard Medical School, USA; and
Associate Surgeon
Massachusetts General Hospital
Boston, USA

J. P. Neoptolemos MD FRCS
Reader in Surgery and Honorary Consultant Surgeon
Department of Surgery
Dudley Road Hospital
Birmingham, UK

S. Nicholson MB BS
Consultant Surgeon
Weston General Hospital
Weston-super-Mare, UK

D. A. Ott MD
Associate Surgeon
Texas Heart Institute; and
Clinical Assistant Professor of Surgery
University of Texas Medical School
Houston, Texas, USA

J. N. Rawlinson FRCS
Staff Doctor in Accident and Emergency
Bristol Royal Infirmary
Bristol, UK

G. J. Reul, Jr MD
Associate Chief of Surgery
Texas Heart Institute; and
Clinical Associate Professor of Surgery
University of Texas Medical School
Houston, Texas, USA

K. P. Robinson MS FRCS
Consultant Surgeon
Westminster Hospital and Queen Mary's Hospital
Roehampton, London, UK; and
Director
Regional Limb Surgery Unit

J. W. Ross FDSRCS(Eng)
Consultant Oral and Maxillo-Facial Surgeon
Bristol Royal Infirmary and Frenchay Hospital
Bristol, UK

R. T. Routledge FRCS
Consultant Plastic Surgeon
United Bristol Hospitals
Frenchay Hospital and South West
Regional Hospital Board
Bristol, UK

S. D. Scott MS FRCS
Lecturer in Surgery
University Surgical Unit
Southampton General Hospital
Southampton, UK

D. Skinner MD
President of New York Hospital; and
Professor of Surgery
New York Hospital–Cornell University Medical Center
New York, USA

P. J. B. Smith ChM FRCS
Consultant Urological Surgeon
Bristol Royal Infirmary
Bristol, UK

I. Taylor MD ChM FRCS
Professor of Surgery
University College London
London, UK

J. Terblanche ChM FRCS FCS(SA)
Professor and Chairman
Department of Surgery
University of Cape Town and Groote Schuur Hospital
Cape Town, South Africa; and
Co-Director
Medical Research Council Liver Research Centre
University of Cape Town
Cape Town, South Africa

D. A. Tolley FRCS FRCS(Ed)
Consultant Urologist
Lothian Health Board; and
Director
The Scottish Lithotriptor Centre
Western General Hospital
Edinburgh, UK

P. L. G. Townsend BSc FRCS(C) FRCS
Consultant Plastic and Reconstructive Surgeon
Frenchay Hospital
Bristol, UK

J. Wallwork FRCS(Ed)
Consultant Cardiothoracic Surgeon
Papworth Hospital
Cambridge, UK

A. J. Webb MB ChM FRCS FIAC
Consultant Surgeon
Bristol Royal Infirmary
Bristol, UK

G. Westbury OBE FRCS FRCP
Professor of Surgery, Emeritus
Royal Marsden Hospital
London, UK

R. C. N. Williamson MA MD MChir FRCS
Professor of Surgery
Department of Surgery
The Royal Postgraduate Medical School
University of London; and
Director of Surgery
Hammersmith Hospital
London, UK

J. D. Wisheart BSc MCh FRCS
Consultant Cardiothoracic Surgeon
Department of Surgery
Bristol Royal Infirmary
Bristol, UK

Preface

It has been a great pleasure to cooperate in this edition and the incoming editor acknowledges the original insight of Gerald Keen in introducing the concept of surgical management into a standard textbook of surgery. Surgical complications and operative shortcomings are fully discussed with a view to their rectification and future avoidance.

It is our intention to continue to produce a reference text on operative techniques and strategy and we remain resolute in the belief that a thorough understanding of the principles of operative surgery is essential for the trainee and practising surgeon. There has been a revolution in surgical practice and the widespread use of stapling devices, laparoscopic, thoracoscopic and endoscopic procedures has inevitably demanded that surgeons acquire these techniques. Despite the obvious advantage of short hospital stay, increased patient comfort and earlier return to work, these newer methods produce their own serious problems which will require solution by conventional surgery and experienced surgeons.

The original artwork has been complemented by many new illustrations by Peter Cox. We are ever grateful to the publishing staff of Butterworth-Heinemann for their patience and support during the production of this edition.

G. KEEN

J. R. FARNDON

1993

Introduction

1

Suture material and the healing of surgical wounds

D. J. Leaper

We have records which show that wound suture and management was practised in Assyrian, Egyptian and Indian cultures, implying that the surgeons of the time had a workable understanding of healing. Sutures and threads and tape closures were all in use. By the time of the Greek and Roman civilizations, quite sophisticated techniques were described in Hippocratic and Galenic teachings which involved ligation of blood vessels and wound drainage. The most esoteric suture material was probably the use of a soldier ant's jaws to hold wound edges together (and is possibly still in use in isolated South American cultures), a technique used today as Michel clips or disposable skin stapler units. Catgut and silk soon became the mainstay sutures (and still are in their worldwide use) but are rapidly giving way to synthetic polymers of absorbable and non-absorbable type which are tailor-made for their use in specific operations.

Suture materials

Wound closure fails because the suture material used may be inappropriate for its purpose, because knots slip following inadequate technique, or because tissues tear when there are local (such as infection) or systemic (such as hypovolaemic poor tissue perfusion) adverse factors.

The number of suture materials now in common use is legion. The more popular ones are shown in Table 1.1, with a classification into natural or synthetic, absorbable or non-absorbable categories. The ideal suture does not exist, but we want to leave the smallest possible bulk of material which will retain its integrity with an adequate tensile strength (if the suture is to remain indefinitely, as in vascular surgery). When the suture can be allowed to completely absorb, once its function to hold tissues together is completed until healing, it must do so without exciting an excessive tissue reaction and predisposition to infection or wound failure (as in gastrointestinal surgery). Some sutures can be removed once tissue is healed (as in skin). Suture material needs to be easily sterilized and modern materials are packaged in disposable units which can be gamma-irradiated on a bulk basis. Some absorbable sutures may be damaged by this process and exposure to ethylene oxide gas is an alternative. Recourse to autoclaving is unnecessary as it may denature all but the non-absorbable polymers and metallic materials.

Catgut

Derived from the collagenous component of sheep gut, catgut is presented as a monofilament twist suture. Chromic acid tanning has the effect of delaying absorption, but can disrupt quickly (within a few days) in an infected wound. Catgut loses its strength when wet and its knots can become loosened by swelling. It is highly irritant in tissues and may predispose to infection in contaminated wounds with an associated, highly variable resorption and integrity. Consequently it has been recognized that it is inappropriate for deep layer closure of the abdominal wall because of a high rate of burst abdomen. Catgut is still highly popular because of its good handling and knot-tying, for bowel anastomosis and for tying of ligatures.

Silk

This material is presented as a twist or braid which facilitates knotting and handling. A silicone coat does not prevent its biodegradability and irritant nature in tissues. It acts as a foreign body, and should not be used in contaminated wounds as its presence exponentially decreases the size of a bacterial inoculum which is sufficient to cause an infection. The braid allows capillarity and migration of bacteria. On skin the unacceptable 'herring-bone' scar related to multiple suture abscesses may follow its use. Like cotton and linen (other braided materials), it has its adherents for tying ligatures, but is being replaced in many surgeons' practices by the polymeric absorbables which handle as well.

Metal clips and monofilament wire

Both these materials are safe in contaminated wounds and have a high tensile strength. Monofilament wire has been popular for closing fascial wounds and tendons but is difficult to tie. The Shouldice Clinic, has reported a very successful use in inguinal hernia repair. Metal does fatigue and can break, and a laparotomy made through an old wound closed with metal can be difficult. Clips and staples have met with

Table 1.1 Classification and examples of modern sutures

Natural		Synthetic	
Absorbable	Non-absorbable	Absorbable	Non-absorbable
Plain catgut	Silk	Polyglycolic acid (Dexon)	Polyamide (nylon)
Chromic catgut	Cotton, linen	Polyglactin (Vicryl)	Polyester (Dacron)
	Stainless steel wire	Polydioxanone (PDS)	Polypropylene (prolene)
		Polyglyconate (Maxon)	Polytetrafluoroethylene (PTFE)
			Polyester (Novafil)

success, but are an expensive alternative when disposable units are used.

Synthetic polymeric absorbables

These sutures are replacing catgut, as their resorption rates are predictable and they are less irritant in tissues. Braided filaments (Dexon and Vicryl) and monofilaments (PDS and Maxon) are available. Some have a long tissue integrity (PDS retains half of its strength in tissues at 4 weeks) and may be used for fascial closure, but there is no convincing evidence that they are as safe as non-absorbable sutures. Further trials are required to assess whether wound infections or chronic knot sutures are reduced. Those sutures with a shorter tissue integrity excite more tissue reaction but can be used for subcuticular skin closure to avoid the need for suture removal. Braided materials are ideal for tying ligatures.

Synthetic polymeric non-absorbables

These materials are extruded polymers presented as monofilaments or braids. The latter may be coated for easier handling and knotting. Nylon is biodegradable and should not be used for vascular surgery. Its modulus of elasticity and structural 'memory' gives poor knot security. Without adequate antimicrobial prophylaxis, nylon knots tend to be the nidus for infection and chronic suture sinuses. Polypropylene, polyester or polytetrafluoroethylene (PTFE) monofilaments are appropriate for vascular surgery.

All the synthetic materials in this group excite little or no tissue reaction and are ideal for use in contaminated wounds and have a high tensile strength which allows fine sutures to be used. Braided forms are useful in hernia repair. Coating reduces tissue drag but diminishes knot security. As meshes or sponges they may be used for larger defects, incisional hernia repairs or in rectal prolapse operations. Monofilament subcuticular sutures (which need removal) give acceptable cosmetic scars.

Tape

Tape closures for skin, whether for primary or secondary closure, or as an adjunct to or later replacement for suture closure, are probably underused. They are associated with a minimal tissue response and a low wound infection rate.

Suture size and needles

The modern polymeric sutures have a high tensile strength, particularly the non-absorbables, which allows the least bulk of material to be used. Size 1 or 0 material is needed for fascial abdominal wall deep layer closure to resist high intra-abdominal pressures. Large 1 cm mass bites 1 cm apart reduce the risk of wound failure which may be related to poor tissue in the abdominal wall. A ratio of suture length to wound length of 1:4 has been calculated to offer adequate security. In vascular surgery, when a graft is used the suture (2/0 to 5/0) must retain its tensile strength indefinitely, whereas in bowel, a simple waterproof apposition with no great strength is required (2/0 or 3/0). In microvascular surgery, sizes as fine as 10/0 are required. Knots should employ a surgical, square reef-knot and three throws of double, single and double knots are secure. In vascular surgery, as many as five or six throws may be considered necessary.

Modern sutures are swaged onto needles without an eye to avoid tissue drag. The needles are made of high-quality stainless steel to avoid corrosion and are easily sterilizable. Needle points are round bodied with a taper point, for easy passage through soft tissues such as bowel or peritoneum, or with a cutting edge (conventional, reverse or side-cutting) to pass through tough tissue. Needle bodies are contoured to allow a firm grip in a needle holder. Double-needled sutures may be used in vascular and intestinal surgery.

Recommendations for closure

Abdominal closure

Layered closure, following the lateral paramedian incision, or mass closure for other incisions using a 0 or 1 monofilament non-absorbable polymer (nylon or prolene), should have no burst abdomens and a low incisional rate (<5%). Tissue bites should be 1 cm from the edge and 1 cm apart, preferably with continuous closure to avoid too many knots. The 5/8 Moynihan hand needle facilitates mass closure. The use of polymeric absorbables (PDS or Maxon) is an alternative, but further proof of their safety is required. Catgut is not acceptable. In these days of AIDS, hand needles may need to be discarded.

Intestinal anastomosis

An inverting technique, particularly in colon, using 2/0 or 3/0 material, is acceptable with one- or two-layer, continuous or interrupted sutures. All materials have been used, but the author prefers Vicryl and PDS to catgut or silk. A minority of surgeons use polymeric non-absorbables with equally good results. Stapling with metal allows speed and may make some procedures easier and safer. Paradoxically, end-to-end staplers give an everting anastomosis which is safe.

Vascular anastomosis

Continuous fine polymeric non-absorbables are essential. Prolene is the most secure and widely used: 2/0 at aortic level, 4/0 at inguinal and 6/0 in the popliteal fossa or below.

Skin closure

Subcuticular closures allow cosmetic results and there is no evidence of increased infection rates following contaminated (non-military) surgery. Continuous non-absorbables such as prolene (which need removal) or absorbables (such as Dexon, Vicryl or PDS which do not) are equally acceptable. Tapes and staples are also associated with acceptable cosmetic results and low infection rates, but silk is unacceptable.

Healing of surgical wounds

Following an incision there is an arrest of haemorrhage which is mediated through vascular spasm and the formation of thrombin, through the clotting cascades, fibrin and platelet aggregation, which follow tissue damage, exposure of collagen and an imbalance of intimal prostacyclin and platelet thromboxane. Following trauma there is release of kinins, prostaglandins and activation of complement, which, together with release of chemo-attractants and growth hormones, initiate the acute inflammatory response.

Healing in epithelia

Epithelial defects close by a combination of epithelialization at the wound edge and wound contraction which is mediated by myofibroblasts (discussed below). In a moist wound environment these processes are enhanced and a plethora of new dressings has appeared on the market to supply this need, for wounds healing either by primary or secondary intention. Transparent polyurethane adhesive drapes, originally introduced as incise drapes, are particularly popular for this use. Epithelia heal by regeneration (as can the liver), but connective tissues heal by repair.

Healing in connective tissues

The acute inflammatory phase immediately following wounding was referred to as the 'lag' phase, when a wound had no inherent strength. White cells become activated and marginate in adjacent capillaries before diapedesis into the wound space. Within hours, neutrophils and lymphocytes allow local host defences to develop with release of opsonins, lymphokines and oxygen-free radicals. The wound exudate which accompanies this has been called the 'oedema of injury'. Within 24–48 hours, circulating monocytes become transformed as macrophages and divitalized tissues and bacteria are removed by ingestion. There next follows the preparation and proliferation phases of healing, during which time mesenchymal cells are transformed into dividing fibroblasts and myofibroblasts, and endothelial buds begin to grow into the wound from the damaged capillaries. The latter canalize and form new capillary loops (angiogenesis) which bring oxygen and nutrients to the wound. It is during this period (4–5 days after wounding) that wound strength begins to be acquired, with the laying down and polymerization of the triple helix protein, collagen. The module of macrophage, fibroblast and angiogenesis is directed through many complex interrelations by the macrophage.

The hypoxic dead space of the wound is the stimulus for macrophage activity. Normal tissue oxygenation is between 10 and 20 mmHg and macrophages and fibroblasts can be identified along a gradient; macrophages < 10 mmHg tissue Po_2 and fibroblasts 10–20 mmHg. When repair is nearing completion, tissue oxygenation – through angiogenesis – reaches normal values and the release of mediators and growth factors is repressed. It is in this final cicatrization phase that there is maturation of collagen with crosslinking and orientation of fibres, and rapid acquisition of tensile strength. Final scar strength in skin is reached within 10–14 days. In the gastrointestinal tract, tensile strength is acquired more quickly in a sound anastomosis, particularly in stomach and small bowel, and approaches pre-wounding strength. In the abdominal wall, however, final tensile strength does not exceed 70% of pre-wounding strength and takes up to 3 months to be acquired. Second wounds made through a recent wound in the abdominal wall heal more quickly.

Sutured wounds heal by primary intention. Open wounds heal by secondary intention and, when granulation tissue is mature and there is no evidence of infection, they can be closed by delayed primary or later secondary suture. Wounds which are large but shallow can be skin grafted. If wounds are allowed to heal by secondary intention they do so by epithelialization and contraction. The latter is effected by myofibroblasts which were initially recognized on electron microscopy to be associated with contractile protein. These cells can be cultured on a collagen lattice, and contraction effected by them can be directly observed. Further proof of wound contraction can be seen when equidistant radial tattoos are made around an open wound. When healing is complete the proximal tattoos become more distantly placed from the distal tattoos.

Wound contraction is distinct from aberrations of scar formation, hypertrophic or keloid scar or contracture, which are related to racial factors, infection or burns. Delayed wound healing, relating to granulating wounds, may result in excessive fibrosis which in a hollow viscus causes stricture formation.

During the healing process in connective tissues there is a balance of formation of new collagen and lysis of old, during the remodelling phase. This is particularly precarious in colon where bacterial collagenases also add to lysis, which may lead to anastomotic leak. Other factors contribute also, such as ischaemia and obstruction, which makes primary anastomoses hazardous in affected patients. Even if healing occurs without leakage there may be a degree of healing by secondary intention, which can lead to stricture formation.

Factors affecting healing

In general terms, local and systemic factors should be considered. The single most important factor is tissue perfusion at the site of the wound. Local factors which impair perfusion are part of established surgical ritual but are difficult to measure. These include the excellence of surgical technique in which tissues are handled gently, without overuse of diathermy and avoidance of tension, strangulation of tissue by ligatures or suturing, and avoidance of collections of body fluids. Poor perfusion related to systemic factors (shock), hypovolaemia, sepsis or cardiopulmonary failure are more easily quantifiable and correctable.

Other adverse factors include old age and being of male sex, but these, like many other factors, are interrelated to presenting diseases and can rarely be shown to be univariate on regression analysis. Poor nutrition, measured as recent >20% weight loss or by anthropomorphic indices (mid-arm circumference, subcapsular fat and serum albumin, for example) has been related to poor healing, but there is a closer relation to the development of sepsis which is itself a major determinant of wound healing. Zinc and vitamins A and C deficiencies are probably unrelated to surgical practice in Western civilizations. Other factors such as steroids, radiotherapy and chemotherapy, and metabolic diseases (uraemia, diabetes and jaundice), can all affect fibroblast function in the early phases of collagen synthesis.

Further reading

Barbul, A., Pines, E., Caldwell, M. and Hunt, T. K. (eds) (1988) *Growth Factors and Other Aspects of Wound Healing*, Alan Liss, New York

Bucknall, T. E. and Ellis, H. (eds) (1984) *Wound Healing for Surgeons*, Baillière Tindall, Eastbourne, UK

Cassie, A. B. (1987) Suture material and the healing of surgical wounds. In *Operative Surgery and Management*, 2nd edn (ed. G. Keen), Wright, Bristol, UK

Hunt, T. K. (ed.) (1980) *Wound Healing and Wound Infection*, Appleton-Century-Crofts, New York

Irvin, T. T. (1981) *Wound Healing. Principles and Practice*, Chapman and Hall, London

Leaper, D. J. (1986) The wound healing process. In *Advances in Wound Management* (eds T. D. Turner, R. J. Schmidt and K. G. Harding), Wiley, Chichester, UK

Leaper, D. J. (1992) Local effects of trauma and wound healing. In *Ian Aird's Companion to Surgical Studies* (eds K. G. Burnand and A. E. Young), Churchill Livingstone, Edinburgh

Leaper, D. J. and Foster, M. E. (1989) Wound healing and abdominal wound closure. In *Progress in Surgery*, Vol. 3 (ed. I. Taylor), Churchill Livingstone, Edinburgh

2
Mechanical stapling in surgery

D. Alderson

History

Numerous devices for closing abdominal wounds and creating gastrointestinal anastomoses were developed throughout the nineteenth century. The first instrument to be put to practical use, however, was demonstrated in 1908 by the Hungarian surgeon, Humer Hültl. It took about two hours to assemble, but incorporated three features that still exist in many current stapling devices: steel wire as the staple material, staple placement in double staggered rows and a B-shaped configuration when the staples close. The first stapler to enjoy widespread popularity was introduced by another Hungarian surgeon, Aladar von Petz, in 1924. It weighed over 3 kg, was cumbersome to prepare and use but provided the basis on which other staplers would be developed. In 1934, Friedrich introduced the first stapling device to feature a replaceable preloaded cartridge, but it was not until the 1940s, when the USSR established a programme to develop surgical stapling instruments at The Scientific Research Institute for Experimental Surgical Apparatus and Instruments in Moscow, that problems such as tissue thickness, healing, choice of metals, instrument design and applications outside the gastrointestinal tract began to be tackled methodically. The first staplers to be used in the USA in the 1960s were licensed from Russian patents. Thereafter American manufacturers were largely responsible for the development of stapling technology to the present day. Importantly, instruments became simpler and lighter, with the majority of moving parts contained in a disposable preloaded cartridge. In recent years, titanium staples have replaced stainless steel, being stronger and producing less artefact on computerized tomograms.

Basic designs

There are basically three different types of instrument used to create gastrointestinal anastomoses or close viscera. These are linear staplers, linear cutting instruments and intraluminal staplers. Stapling devices exist for the closure of skin and for the closure and division of blood vessels, but these are not discussed further in this chapter. In addition, a number of ancillary devices are available (e.g. instruments to place purse-strings) which are described later. Instrument manufacturers produce disposable cartridges to fit a re-usable shell and completely disposable devices. Staplers are manufactured with different staple heights designed for varying tissue thickness (Auto Suture) or the facility for adjusting the width of the closed staples (Ethicon).

Staple configuration

All internal staplers join tissue with B-shaped metallic staples (Figure 2.1). When the instrument is fired, the open legs of the staple are driven through the tissue and formed into a B shape by a corresponding anvil indentation. Staple placement in a staggered double row provides effective tissue closure. Small vessels can still pass through the openings, in and between staples, so that the tissue between the staple line and cut edge remains viable. Bleeding can therefore occur through a perfectly adequate staple line which may require cautery or suture control.

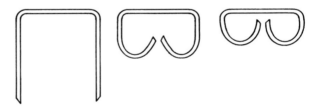

Figure 2.1 Open and closed shape of staples used to approximate internal tissues

Linear staplers

These instruments produce a linear everting (mucosa-to-mucosa) double line of staggered staples (Figure 2.2). They are commonly used to close internal organs prior to transection, or to close the common opening after an anastomosis has been created with a linear cutting stapler. These staplers are widely used for sealing pulmonary parenchyma prior to incision or excision. A variety of staple line lengths are available. An important design feature is that there is a retaining pin which prevents tissue from being squeezed out when the jaws are closed.

Linear cutting staplers

These instruments place two double staggered rows of staples and, in the same operation, divide the tissue between the two pairs of staggered rows or can be

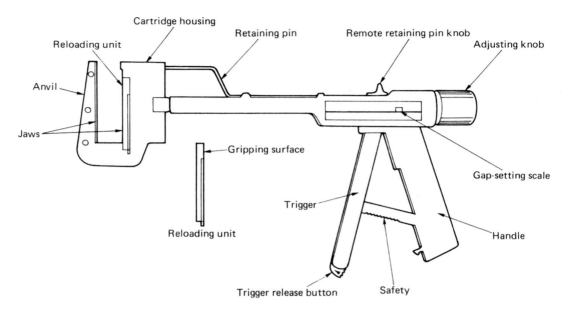

Figure 2.2 Linear stapler

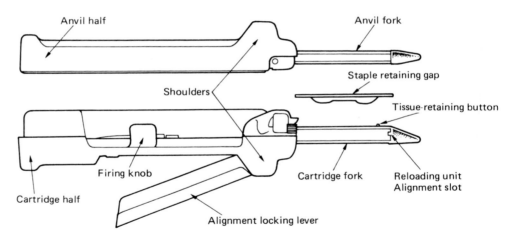

Figure 2.3 Linear cutting stapler

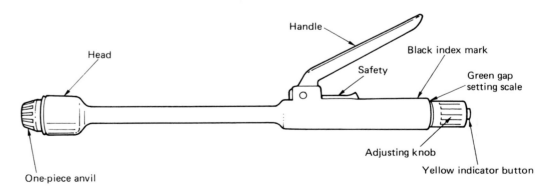

Figure 2.4 Intraluminal stapler

supplied without a knife to create a four-rowed staple line (Figure 2.3). The device is commonly used to transect organs and to create side-to-side and functional end-to-end anastomoses.

Since there is no tissue-retaining pin, the operator must be certain that all tissue to be divided is within the staple-bearing portion of the jaws. Mesentery and omentum must not be in the suture line as their vessels will not be controlled. Anastomoses created by these devices are inverted with mucosa-to-mucosa apposition. Small vessels can still pass through and between the staples so that such anastomosis should always be inspected and significant bleeding points dealt with.

Intraluminal staplers

These produce a circular double staggered row of staples and are employed for the creation of end-to-end inverted anastomoses (Figure 2.4). As the instrument is fired, the staples are driven through the tissue and simultaneously a circular knife cuts a uniform stoma in the joined tissue. The instruments are available with a variety of head diameters appropriate to the organ lumen and are straight or curved. As with linear cutting staplers, it is important that bowel only, and not mesentery, is included within the head and the anvil.

Anastomotic techniques

Virtually all hollow viscera can be resected and anastomosed using a variety of stapling instruments. The majority of procedures are, however, based on a number of common instrument combinations which are then applied to individual operations.

End-to-end anastomosis

Functional end-to-end anastomosis can be created in three ways: the closed technique; the one-stage technique; and the intraluminal technique.

Closed technique

After transecting the mesentery and creating windows adjacent to the proposed transection sites, an opened linear cutter is placed across the bowel from either the mesenteric or the antimesenteric border. The instrument is closed and fired by pushing the firing knob forward, while holding the instrument body still. A double staggered staple line is placed on both the specimen and patient side, and simultaneously a knife transects the bowel between the two double staple lines. The instrument is then reloaded and the procedure performed at the other resection site. A simple alternative here, is to place a crushing clamp across the bowel at the resection site and place a linear stapler across the bowel on the patient side, push the

retaining pin into place and fire the instrument, after releasing the safety catch. The bowel can then be transected with a scalpel, using the side of the stapling anvil as a guide. The anastomosis is then created by a single application of a linear cutting stapler. To obtain perfect apposition between the two bowel loops, stay sutures should be inserted as shown in Figure 2.5. After excising the antimesenteric corners of the staple line closures on both bowel limbs, one fork of a linear cutting instrument of appropriate length is introduced into each bowel lumen, the instrument halves joined together and then fired. This type of anastomotic staple line should always be carefully inspected internally for haemostasis. The common opening is then closed with a linear stapler, after distracting the edges of the previous linear closures and aligning the tissue edges of the common opening using either clamps or traction sutures (Figure 2.6).

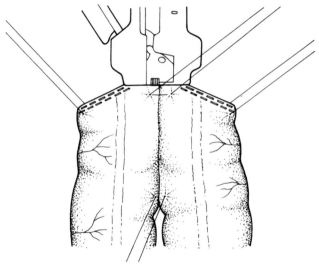

Figure 2.5 Stay sutures to ensure proper apposition of bowel loops

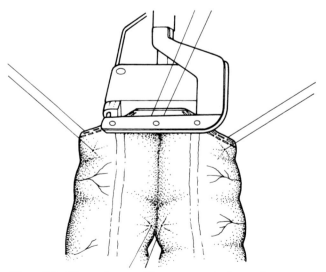

Figure 2.6 Linear closure of the common staple opening

One-stage technique

After preparing the proposed segment for resection along with its mesentery, the anastomosis is created with a single application of a linear stapler. A crushing clamp is placed across both bowel loops at the transition between viable and non-viable tissue. Small openings are then made in the proximal and distal limbs of the bowel to be anastomosed and one fork of a linear cutter inserted into each lumen. Again, the placement of a traction suture, to keep the loops in perfect apposition, is useful. The instrument is fired to create the anastomosis and when the stapler is removed the now common opening can be closed with a single application of a linear stapler as above. The bowel to be resected is then cut off using the instrument edge as a guide to transect the redundant bowel loop (Figure 2.7).

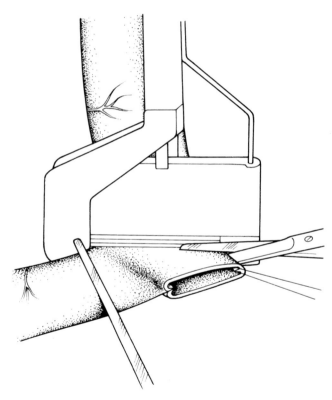

Figure 2.7 Simultaneous closure of the common staple opening and removal of the specimen by the one-stage technique

Intraluminal technique

This technique uses an intraluminal stapler alone or in combination with other stapling instruments. The most common use is in performance of low anterior resection for carcinoma of the rectum, but can be used in the performance of right hemicolectomy or oesophagectomy.

Bowel is resected and segments to be anastomosed are prepared between non-crushing intestinal clamps.

It is necessary then to dissect back the mesentery beyond the proximal and distal points of transection for 2 cm. Purse-string sutures are placed on each end of the transected bowel using a 2/0 monofilament suture. This can be done using one of the instrument manufacturers' purse-string devices or the purse-string suture can be inserted by hand when a true purse-string or a whip stitch can be used. With either technique, the tissue cuff must include all layers of the bowel wall and should not exceed 2.5 mm, in order to avoid incorporating excessive tissue within the closed instrument. In low anterior resection the instrument is introduced via the anus. For oesophagectomy or hemicolectomy, an opening is made on an antimesenteric border, large enough to admit the instrument anvil and staple head. An appropriately sized intraluminal stapler (sizers are available), with the anvil and staple head in the closed position, is inserted into the gut lumen through this opening until the anvil protrudes through the open end of the gut. The instrument is then opened by turning the adjusting knob to expose the centre rod. The purse-string suture is then snugged down securely against the centre rod and cut just above the knot. To facilitate the insertion of the anvil into the other end of the bowel, triangulation or quadrantic stay sutures should be inserted, and, when fully introduced, the purse-string suture is tied snugly around the centre rod (Figure 2.8). After properly aligning the bowel segments to be anastomosed, the instrument is closed and fired. In doing so, staples are driven through the tissue and formed against the anvil, while at the same time a knife blade advances to cut a uniform stoma between the proximal and distal bowel segments. To remove the intraluminal stapler, it is opened slightly by turning the adjusting knob approximately three-quarters of a turn and rotating the instrument through 180° to ensure that there is no trapped tissue. The anastomotic staple line can then be manoeuvred over the lip of the anvil by hand or with the aid of a traction suture.

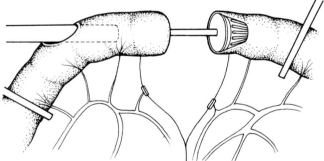

Figure 2.8 Intraluminal stapling using two purse-string sutures

Intraluminal staplers are also supplied with a detachable centre rod/anvil assembly. This instrument is particularly useful in colonic reanastomosis following Hartmann's operation (see below).

Side-to-side anastomosis

This is widely used in the creation of enteroenterostomy or gastroenterostomy and is achieved with a single application of a linear cutter and one application of a linear stapler. Using traction sutures, bowel segments should be aligned side by side along their antimesenteric borders. A small opening is made into the lumen of both bowel loops and one fork of a linear cutter inserted into each loop, closed and fired. After inspection of the anastomosis line for haemostasis, the common opening is closed using a linear stapler. Redundant tissue protruding through the jaws of the stapler can be removed after firing, with a scalpel or heavy scissors, prior to removing the stapler.

Roux-en-Y anastomosis

All of the techniques above involve either single staple lines or intersections between two staple lines. There are, however, occasions where three staple lines can potentially meet, the most common of which is in the creation of a Roux-en-Y anastomosis. The proximal jejunum is stapled and transected using an appropriate linear cutting instrument. This duodenojejunal limb is then matched to the jejunal limb 45 cm from the transected end. The Y anastomosis is again created with a linear cutting instrument between the antimesenteric sides of the bowel, as shown (Figure 2.9). It now becomes necessary to close this common opening after removal of the linear cutter, using a linear stapler. Traction sutures or clamps are used to align the tissue edges in an inverted manner and it is important to offset the anastomosis staple lines, created by the linear cutting instrument, to avoid an intersection between three staple lines (Figure 2.10). Appropriate placement of traction sutures allows this, so that when the opened jaws of the linear stapler are approximated they incorporate all tissue layers and intersect both anastomotic staple lines.

Problems with gastrointestinal stapling

Numerous studies have indicated that, when performed correctly, stapled anastomoses are as safe and effective as those created by sutures.

Certain principles, which apply to sutured anastomoses, apply equally well to those created by staples. It is vital that structures to be joined should have an adequate blood supply and that gross sepsis is avoided. Tissues which are not fit to be sewn should not be stapled. There are, however, specific problems identifiable with the use of staplers, which need to be avoided.

Tissue thickness and staple height

If the tissue to be stapled is too thick for the staple

height selected, then serosal cracking will occur when the instrument is closed and fired. This most commonly occurs in staple closure of a thick-walled stomach. It is necessary to oversew such a staple line with a continuous suture.

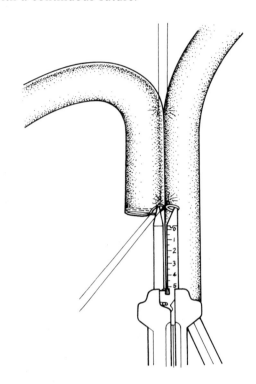

Figure 2.9 Creation of a Y anastomosis

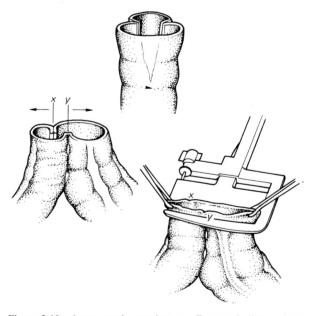

Figure 2.10 Anastomotic rotation to offset staple lines prior to linear closure

Staple line bleeding

Every staple line should always be checked for bleeding and controlled appropriately. Gastric staple lines are probably the commonest sites of this problem.

Mechanical failure

Mechanical failure is extremely rare and is virtually unheard of with disposable instruments, unless they are dropped and damaged. The anvil of a reusable shell, however, can be damaged so that the staples are not formed into a complete B configuration. Such instruments should be returned to the manufacturer.

Linear tension

Linear tension on any anastomosis increases the risk of disruption, but this is theoretically greater for stapled anastomoses because the diameter of each staple is less than that of a suture, allowing tissue to be lacerated as tension is applied. It is particularly important, when creating oesophagogastric or low colorectal anastomoses, to be certain that stomach or colon has been thoroughly mobilized to ensure that no tension is applied to the staple line.

Leakage from intersecting staple lines

Firing a stapler through another staple line does not necessarily create problems, but it is not reliable through two staple lines and should be avoided. A simple example of this is in closing the common opening following the creation of a functional end-to-end anastomosis with a linear cutting instrument. In Figure 2.10, the points x and y should not be placed opposite each other, but the bowel should be rotated slightly to offset these points for linear closure.

Purse-string problems

It is important to make sure that all layers of bowel wall are included in such a stitch and it should not extend more than 2.5 mm back from the cut edge. A true purse-string is actually preferable to the more commonly used whip stitch because when the viscus has a thick wall or is larger than normal, then no matter how tightly tied, it may be impossible to get the tissue snug around the centre rod of the instrument. A simple method to overcome this is to insert one or two mattress sutures, as shown in Figure 2.11.

Common general surgical applications

Most intra-abdominal procedures on the viscera can be performed using staple combinations, but only those which are commonly performed and which are either simpler or faster than their hand-sutured counterparts will be described. A number of pro-

cedures can only be performed with stapling devices, such as vertical banded gastroplasty and stapled transection for oesophageal varices.

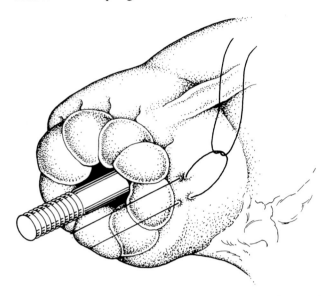

Figure 2.11 Use of a mattress suture to obtain a snug fit around the centre rod

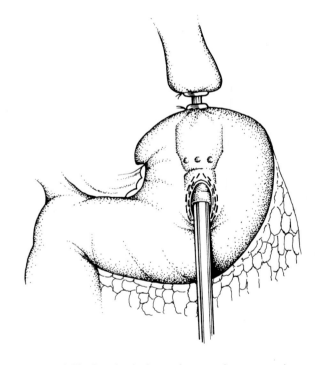

Figure 2.12 Intraluminal oesophagogastric anastomosis

Oesophageal procedures

Prospective studies indicate that the results are identical to those obtained by hand suturing. The most widely used method uses the intraluminal stapler with a removable head, introduced through a gastrotomy. The spiked centre rod is pushed out through the stomach wall, about 3–4 cm away from the line of stapled gastric closure or through the end of this staple line. The head of the instrument is introduced separately into the oesophagus, the purse-string tied down around the centre rod snugly, and the two parts of the instrument mated together and fired in the usual fashion (Figure 2.12). An equally effective method creates the anastomosis with a linear cutting stapler as shown in Figure 2.13 and closes the common opening with two applications of a linear stapler.

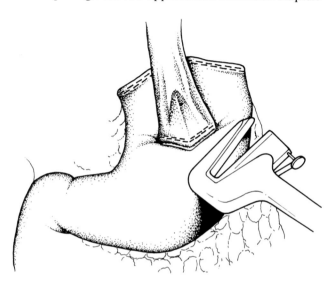

Figure 2.13 Oesophagogastric anastomosis using a linear cutting instrument with linear staple closure.

Transection of oesophageal varices

The intraluminal stapler is introduced via a gastrotomy in the closed position and then opened so that the centre rod straddles the oesophagogastric junction. A ligature is then tied tightly around the oesophagus, immediately above the gastro-oesophageal junction. It is essential to ensure that the stitch is tied tightly around the centre rod to ensure that transection occurs circumferentially (Figure 2.14).

Gastric procedures

Partial gastrectomy

Billroth II gastrectomy is accomplished very rapidly when stapled. The duodenum and proximal gastric resection site are closed with linear staplers. After removal of the specimen a linear cutting stapler is inserted through a small gastric opening and one in an adjacent small bowel loop to create the anastomosis, leaving a common opening to be closed with a further application of a linear stapler (Figure 2.15). Billroth I gastrectomy can be conveniently carried out using an intraluminal stapler after closing the stomach with a linear stapler. The intraluminal stapler is introduced through a small gastrostomy on the anterior surface of the stomach, with the head of the instrument removed. The spiked centre rod is pushed out through the posterior wall of the stomach. The duodenum receives a purse-string and the anvil of the instrument is inserted into the head of the duodenum and the purse-string tied snugly around the centre rod. The instrument is fired in the usual fashion and the gastrotomy closed with a linear stapler (Figure 2.16).

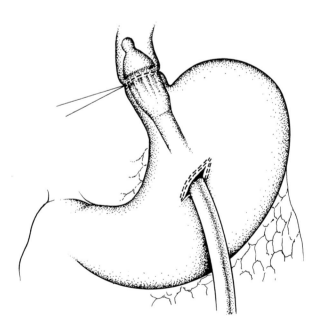

Figure 2.14 Transection of oesophageal varices using an intraluminal stapler

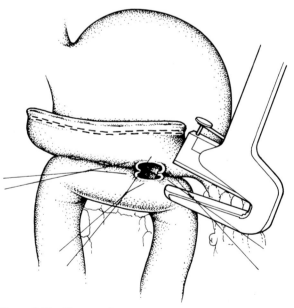

Figure 2.15 Closure of the common opening after Billroth II gastrectomy. Note the placement of stay sutures

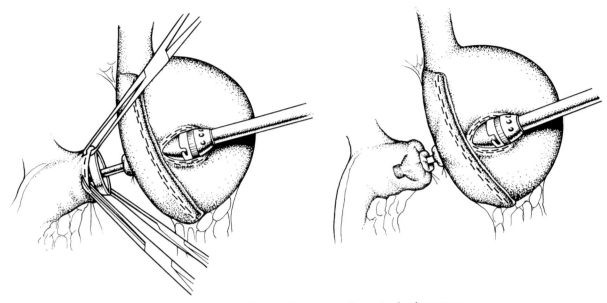

Figure 2.16 Billroth I gastrectomy using an intraluminal stapler to create the gastroduodenostomy

Vertical banded gastroplasty

Vertical banded gastroplasty is an effective surgical procedure for morbid obesity. The important steps in the performance of this procedure are the creation of a gastric window, using a spiked intraluminal stapler to pierce the anterior and posterior walls of the stomach, and firing the intraluminal stapler to cut out a disc of stomach. A special four-rowed linear stapler is then inserted through this window to create a vertical staple line up to the left side of the gastro-oesophageal junction. The pouch outlet is conventionally restricted with a strip of polypropylene mesh (Figure 2.17).

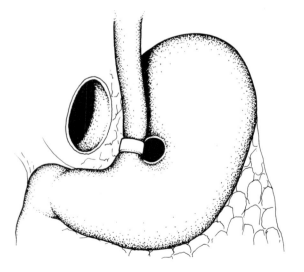

Figure 2.17 Vertical banded gastroplasty

Intestinal procedures

The operation which has probably attracted more interest than any other is low anterior resection for carcinoma of the rectum. Staplers facilitate restoration of intestinal continuity after the Hartmann procedure.

Anterior resection

Low anterior resection is performed using an intraluminal stapler with purse-strings of the ends for anastomosis, or by using the 'fire-through' or double-stapling technique in which the rectal stump is transected with a linear stapler and the spiked centre rod of an intraluminal stapler pushed up through the rectum close to this transverse closure, obviating the need for the lower purse-string which can be difficult to insert (Figure 2.18). The same fire-through approach is used when restoring continuity after Hartmann's operation.

Shortly after the introduction of stapled low anterior resection, there were fears that the procedure was associated with an increased risk of local recurrence compared with hand-sutured anastomoses. To some extent this reflected the lower level and hence narrower pelvis at which the stapled anastomosis could be performed. With appropriate patient selection and strict adherence to the principles of mesorectal and wide lateral excision there are no particular problems inherent in the use of staplers regarding local recurrence. There are, however, certain technical difficulties. Anastomotic strictures seem more common after stapling than hand suturing. This appears to be a function of the diameter of the intraluminal

luminal staplers make this easier. An alternative is to insert a rigid sigmoidoscope and pass a rubber catheter down through a small incision in the apex of the rectum to be retrieved and pulled down to the anus. This can then be fitted over the centre rod and used to pull the intraluminal stapler safely to the top of the rectum.

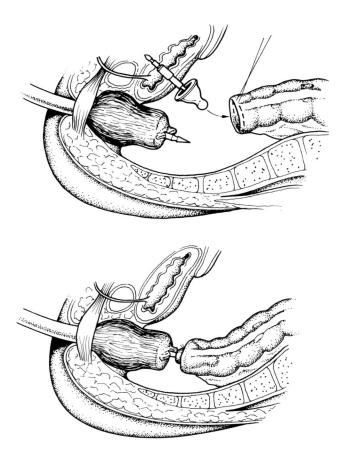

Figure 2.18 Low colorectal anastomosis using the 'fire-through' technique

stapler, and the widest diameter staple head which can be accommodated should be chosen. It is rare to have a problem with the rectum, but the colon, particularly the sigmoid, may split when a large head is introduced. The easiest solution is to ensure that the full left colon is mobilized so that the proximal resection site can be in the transverse colon if required. As in the rectum, there are usually no particular difficulties in accommodating a 31 mm stapler in the transverse colon. Some surgeons test such anastomoses using air insufflation under water or intrarectal povidone-iodine to look for air or fluid leaks so that these can be corrected or the procedure converted to a Hartmann operation. In any event, such low rectal anastomoses should be protected by a loop ileostomy.

There are two specific problems related to secondary restoration of continuity. In female patients, when the rectal stump is very short great care should be taken to ensure that the spike exits the apex of the rectal stump posteriorly. There is a very real risk of incorporating part of the vaginal wall in the closure if the spike exits anteriorly when the instrument is subsequently closed. Conversely, when the rectal stump is long and close to the pelvic brim it may be difficult to negotiate the rectum blindly. Curved intra-

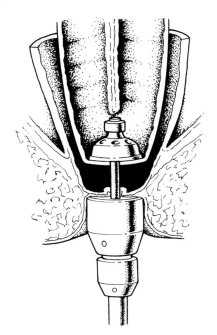

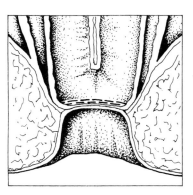

Figure 2.19 J pouch construction with an intraluminal stapler

Restorative proctocolectomy

Restorative proctocolectomy using a J or W configuration ileal pouch can be facilitated by stapling. In the creation of a J pouch, the terminal ileum is closed and transected with a linear cutting stapler and the rectal stump closed immediately above the anorectal ring, using a linear stapler. This can sometimes be facilitated by using a linear stapler with an articulating head to ensure that this closure does not leave an unduly long rectal segment. The J pouch is created by looping the distal 30–40 cm of ileum and approximating the antimesenteric borders to form a J-shaped loop with 15–20 cm limbs. A linear cutting stapler is inserted through a small stab wound in the apex of this loop, closed and fired to create an opening between the two approximated loops. This manoeuvre is repeated until pouch construction is complete. Care should be taken to incorporate the end staples of the previous application, to ensure continuity of the staple lines. An intraluminal stapler with a detachable centre rod/anvil assembly is inserted through the anus with the anvil removed and the spiked centre rod is pushed up through the linear staple closure. The anvil is inserted through the ileal stab and the purse-string there tightened around the centre rod. The two parts of the intraluminal stapler are approximated, closed and fired in the usual fashion (Figure 2.19). A majority of surgeons protect this complex staple closure with a covering loop ileostomy.

Laparoscopic stapling

The widespread enthusiasm for minimally-invasive surgery via laparoscopes has led to the development of laparoscopic stapling. Simple clip applicating devices required little modification from their conventional counterparts. A linear cutting stapler (Endo GIA, Auto-Suture) (Figure 2.20) represents the first laparoscopic device which can be used for the same range of functions as linear cutting staplers during open procedures. This has already resulted in the performance of laparoscopic bowel resections and reanastomosis such as right hemicolectomy. There can be little doubt that there will be enormous technical development over the next few years to increase the number of procedures which can be effectively performed via the laparoscope and this will involve the development of novel stapling devices.

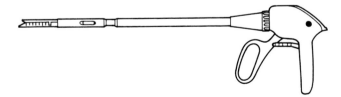

Figure 2.20 Laparoscopic linear cutting stapler

Further reading

Chung, R. S. (1987) Blood flow in colonic anastomoses: effect of stapling and suturing. *Ann. Surg.*, **206**, 335–339

Davies, A. H., Bartolo, D. C. C., Richards, A. E. M., Johnson, C. D. and Mortensen, N. J. McC. (1988) Intraoperative air testing: an audit on rectal anastomosis. *Ann. R. Coll. Surg. Engl.*, **70**, 345–347

Dorsey, J. S., Esses, S., Goldberg, M. and Stone, R. (1980) Esophago-gastrectomy using the autosuture EEA surgical stapling instrument. *Ann. Thorac. Surg.*, **30**, 308–312

Fok, M., Ah-Chong, A. K., Ching, S. W. K. and Wong, J. (1991) Comparison of a single layer continuous hand sewn method and circular stapling in 580 oesophageal anastomoses. *Br. J. Surg.*, **78**, 342–345

Kennedy, H. L., Langevin, J. M., Goldberg, S. M. *et al.* (1985) Recurrence following stapled coloproctostomy for carcinomas of the mid portion of rectum. *Surg. Gynecol. Obstet.*, **160**, 513–516

Kmiot, W. A. and Keighley, M. R. B. (1989) Totally stapled abdominal restorative proctocolectomy. *Br. J. Surg.*, **76**, 961–964

Ravitch, M. M. (1985) Intersecting staple lines in intestinal anastomoses. *Surgery*, **97**, 8–15

Ravitch, M. M. and Steichen, F. M. (eds) (1984) Stapling techniques. In *Surgical Clinics of North America*, Vol. 64, W. B. Saunders, Pennsylvania

Seufert, R. M., Schmidt-Matthiesen, A. and Beyer, A. (1990) Total gastrectomy and oesophago-junostomy – a prospective randomised trial of hand sutured versus mechanically stapled anastomoses. *Br. J. Surg.*, **77**, 50–52

Spence, R. A. J. and Johnson, G. W. (1985) Results in one hundred consecutive patients with stapled oesophageal transection for varices. *Surg. Gynecol. Obstet.*, **160**, 323–329

Varma, J. S., Chan, A. C. W., Li, M. K. W. and Li, A. K. C. (1990) Low anterior resection of the rectum using a double stapling technique. *Br. J. Surg.*, **77**, 888–890

Waxman, B. P. (1983) Large bowel anastomoses II. The circular staplers. *Br. J. Surg.*, **70**, 64–67

West of Scotland and Highland Anastomosis Study Group (1991) Suturing or stapling in gastrointestinal surgery: a prospective randomised study. *Br. J. Surg.*, **78**, 337–341

Wong, J., Cheung, H., Lui, R., Fan, Y. W., Smith, A. and Siu, K. F. (1987) Oesophago-gastric anastomosis performed with a stapler: the occurrence of leakage in suture. *Surgery*, **101**, 408–415

3

The use and hazards of surgical diathermy

G. N. Lumb

Surgeons tend to take the availability of diathermy for granted, but surgical diathermy as we know it today is the result of many years of research into the effects of heat production by the use of high-frequency alternating currents. The frequencies lie in the range of 500 kHz to 3 MHz; that is to say, they are produced by equipment similar to a simplified version of older radio transmitters.

Usage

The therapeutic use of diathermy began in the first decade of the twentieth century and is now almost universal for surgical technique. To avoid the potential hazards in the use of surgical diathermy some understanding of the mechanism by which the current is produced is mandatory. Planned instruction of surgeons, nurses and operating department assistants is very necessary, since there are medicolegal implications from imprecise use. The final responsibility for use of the diathermy machine lies in the hands of the operating surgeon, no matter to whom he may delegate part of the setting up of the apparatus.

Use of diathermy is for three main functions: cutting, coagulation and fulguration (Figure 3.1). These functions are produced by a variety of generators, familiar to those who work in operating theatres.

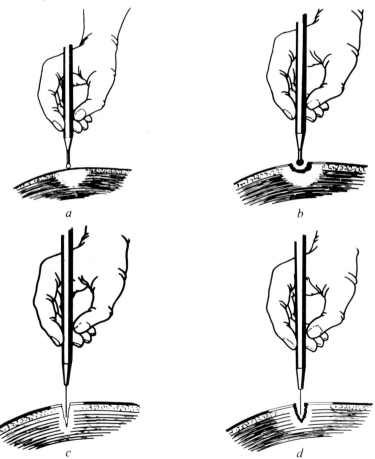

Figure 3.1 A diagrammatic comparison of the three major surgical effects of diathermy. *a*, Coagulation – haemostasis with only a small amount of tissue damage. *b*, Fulguration – haemostasis with charring and deep-tissue necrosis. *c*, Cutting with a valve or transistorized oscillator, which shows minimal surrounding tissue damage. *d*, Cutting with a 'blended' current which gives a moderate degree of surrounding tissue coagulation

They may vary from the early spark-gap machine (remembered for its excellent coagulation) through valve machines (a few still in use) to transistorized and solid-state machines. Solid-state technology has brought to these machines the means to imitate the excellent coagulation of the spark-gap machine, combined with the smooth cutting of the valve machine, in one complex circuit. It is possible also to blend these in such a way that the desired function is achieved without increasing the total power input to the patient. Some surgeons prefer to cut freely, and coagulate separately, whereas others use a heavily blended 'coagulation with cutting' setting which seals the edges of tissues dissected, albeit with more eschar. It must be remembered that the second method can result in cell destruction as much as 0.5 cm from the cut edge. Either way is acceptable provided that implications to wound healing are taken into consideration.

Power

Power output of the machine and the power required for the necessary function are the essential key to correct understanding of the safe use of diathermy generators. This power is passed through the patient by suitably designed electrodes. The essential difference between diathermy and electrocautery is the power used, and the fact that with diathermy the patient forms part of the current-carrying circuit (Figure 3.2). This applied power produces heat in the patient's body, graduated throughout the entire path between the electrodes.

Electrodes

The heat developed in this way will be in inverse proportion to the size of the applying electrodes; thus their design is the key to efficient results. The smaller we make the electrode for the surgeon, the greater the heat that will develop. Appropriately, point, wire, loop and ball electrodes have been manufactured and designated the 'active' electrode.

Equally, the 'plate' – the 'indifferent' or 'passive' electrode – is made large in order to dissipate the heat generated beneath it as speedily as possible, and avoid a thermoelectric burn. The normal dissipation of heat is by the circulation and this is no exception, which is why the plate area should be large enough to bring it into contact with as large an area of skin as practicable, and with a good blood supply underneath. In children this is even more important because of their generally smaller surface area, and it may be practical in infants to attach the return circuit (plate) clips to the foil often used to wrap infants for preservation of body heat.

Because the power output has to be absorbed between the function required, and the rest dissipated throughout the body in the path between the electrodes, it is necessary to limit the power output of the machines. This has been agreed by the International Electrotechnical Commission and a maximum output of 400 W advised; but this power is rarely necessary and it is as well to limit the power to 100 W when using the diathermy on infants or children. All reasonable functions required should be possible at these levels, provided that proper servicing and maintenance is done on the machine. At this power even the

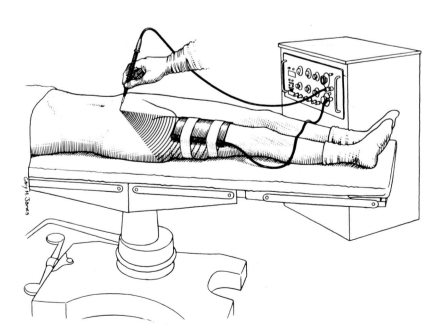

Figure 3.2 Diagrammatic representation of the passage of a diathermy current through the body from a diathermy machine, via the active electrode to the large metal plate electrode

most demanding function of all, i.e. underfluid cutting as in transurethral resection of the prostate, is amply covered at middle settings of the power control.

Utilization

The choice of electrodes must be the surgeon's responsibility, and he will require those suitable for the operation to be performed, but it is also his responsibility to control the application of the diathermy current. The foot switch or finger switch should always be the medicolegal responsibility of the operating surgeon. It is considered reasonable to delegate the setting up of the machine and application of the plate electrode to nursing or technical staff, provided that they have been properly trained in details of application, and the surgeon should assure himself that this has been done.

The dial settings on machines unfortunately vary from one manufacturer to another, so the more recent calibration of some machines in wattage of power output is a boon. Arbitrary dial numbers may vary from machine to machine, but measured wattage is the same whatever make of machine is used. Typical wattage settings will be from 25 to 50 W for 'coagulation', and from 100 to 250 W for 'cutting'. It is very rarely necessary to exceed these levels for even the most demanding surgery.

Blending the current is useful to some surgeons and was achieved in the older machines by a simple mixing of the outputs from each part of the twin circuits. This of course resulted in much larger power, being the summation of the two outputs. In today's solid-state and transistorized machines the blending can be produced by internal modification of the waveform and an output equivalent to the single circuit can be the result. The effect of blending is to produce coagulation of the smaller vessels simultaneously with the cut.

Earthing

Many of the hazards and problems with diathermy have arisen because the requirement for safety from the mains supply in the UK necessitated all equipment with metal parts and cases to be connected to an earthed point, usually in the form of three-pin plug. As a result of this, the return path of the diathermy current to the plate electrode was also earthed. This meant that the diathermy could continue to operate in the absence of a plate connection, since the return current could choose any path back to the machine via earthed equipment otherwise connected to the patient, or even via equipment used to reduce antistatic potentials. If the contact between these and the patient was small, then a reduced area very similar to the 'active' electrode may occur and the result would be equal heat development with a probable thermo-

electric burn. Metal stirrups, anaesthetic screens and an exposed part of the operating table have all been implicated (Figure 3.3).

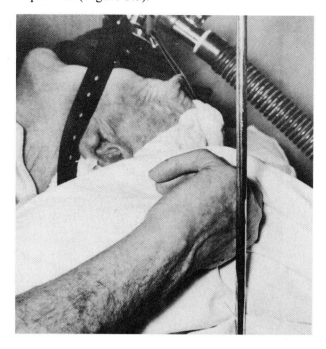

Figure 3.3 Patient's hand in contact with the bar of the anaesthetic screen

The problem of increasing attachment of other apparatus – electrocardiographs, respiratory monitors and other electronic devices – led to the development of earth-free or floating-earth machines. These machines will fail to operate if the indifferent electrode (plate) is not attached to the patient, with increased safety protection against thermoelectric burns. A false sense of security may result from this if the plate electrode is allowed to come into contact with any metal object also in contact with the patient, or into contact with the machine (Figure 3.4). It does not necessarily need to be good electrical contact, since capacitative coupling can be sufficient to allow activation of the machine as far as the active electrode is concerned.

Monitoring

In order to avoid the major factors responsible for thermoelectric burns it is necessary to introduce suitable warnings for the surgeon. These take the form of 'noise' to show that the machine is actively working and to draw attention to the connection of the indifferent electrode and any failing mechanical connection to the patient.

The early spark-gap machines made an unmistakable noise on operation of the foot control, but the valve and solid-state machines are silent. Sometimes operation is by finger switch or foot control(s) that

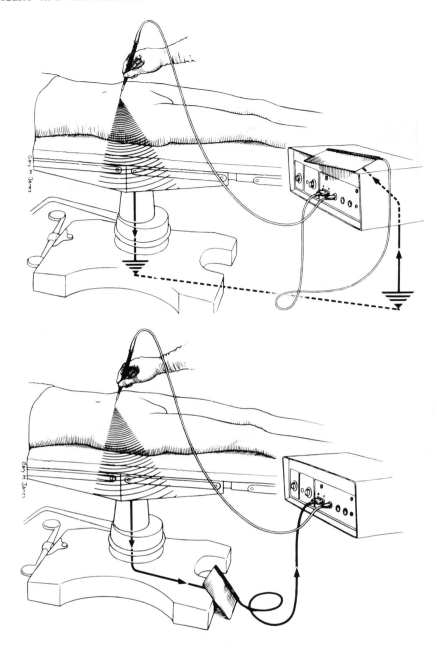

Figure 3.4 Return path of diathermy current to earth, resulting from the indifferent electrode being left on the top of the diathermy cabinet in an isolated circuit, or on the pedestal of the operating table

are more sensitive in their function, and accidental activation of the machine may be disastrous should the assistant leave his or her foot on the pedal, unless a warning noise is introduced. It has also been known for foot switches to become jammed in the 'on' position wedged under the edge of the operating table (Figure 3.5). It is necessary to have some warning bleep or buzz to show activation of the machine, and this is accepted by the British Standards Institution code of practice as being essential. The problem is that noise is not an acceptable option in many opera-

ting theatres, but provided that there is a control that can reduce the monitor's sound without complete inaudibility, this should be accepted. It should be an acceptable hum or buzz audible above the extraneous noise of any routine operating theatre.

The monitoring of the indifferent electrode should be louder and indeed should also inactivate the power output of the machine if electrical continuity in the plate electrode's cable is interrupted. There are many types of plate electrode: simple aluminium foil, thin stainless steel foil, armoured studding, foil with foil connecting cable, foil with accessory clip connector, and foil with self-adhesive surround. Any of these varieties may be modified with a contact conductive jelly. With the latter it is essential that the contact cream is still moist and the manufacturer's directions strictly carried out.

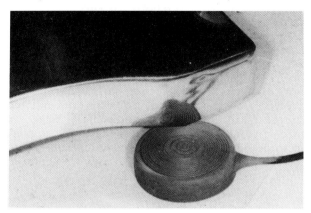

Figure 3.5 The foot switch pedal jammed under the pedestal of the operating table

Siting the plate electrode

There are certain factors that are important in the use of the plate electrode to ensure its correct application. First, it must be smooth and make even contact with the patient's skin. *Very* hairy areas should be shaved and the patient should have been warned about this in the 'consent to operation' procedure. Secondly, it should be ensured that contact cream and 'gel'-type plates are not used where pressure on them may increase drying out, e.g. under the buttocks. Dry foil plates are acceptable here, but it is not an ideal situation. The old lead plate wrapped in towelling soaked in concentrated saline should be abandoned, as it is difficult to monitor and use. Foil, as used to wrap babies in order to preserve heat, is monitored with a twin lead with separated clips.

There is a possibility, particularly with older generators, of building up potentials away from the site of operation. These stray currents may seek a return via earthed apparatus. This is rare in floating-earth machines but still possible, whereas it was common in the earthed plate machines. Because of this, diathermy should be operated in such a way that the current path does not cross the cardiac axes. This means that in operations on the head and neck it is better to site the plate on one or other upper arm or behind the right shoulder blade and out of the path of any electrocardiograph electrodes (Figure 3.6.).

Indications for surgical diathermy

All the foregoing description applies to what is termed 'monopolar diathermy', in which the patient's

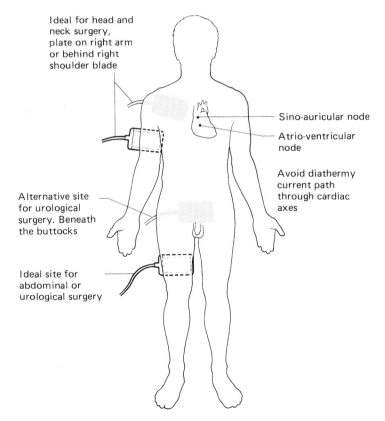

Ideal for head and neck surgery, plate on right arm or behind right shoulder blade

Sino-auricular node

Atrio-ventricular node

Avoid diathermy current path through cardiac axes

Alternative site for urological surgery. Beneath the buttocks

Ideal site for abdominal or urological surgery

Figure 3.6 Sites of choice for diathermy plate electrode

body forms part of the current-carrying circuit. On the other hand, in 'bipolar diathermy' the current path is integral within the surgeon's electrode and its connection to the generator. This latter has advantageous application in many circumstances, but the electrodes used tend to be more cumbersome.

Whichever method is appropriate there is no doubt that diathermy is the method of choice for haemostasis of smaller vessels and for dissection of tissues in at least 90% of operative procedures. In electrodissection it must be remembered that the margin of cell destruction extends beyond the site of the cut and that this will only show some hours subsequently. It is therefore wise to leave a slightly greater margin in anastomoses where the tissues have been divided by diathermy rather than with the knife. In excising tumours this may give a safer cellular margin of excision.

Diathermy in endoscopy

Operating through endoscopes is where diathermy reaches its full potential. It is possible to perform many operations through a wide variety of endoscopes. The cystoscope, proctoscope and sigmoidoscope started the field, but now operations are performed via gastroscopes, colonoscopes, laparoscopes, arthroscopes and resectoscopes. In performing these operations, either electrically inert fluid or non-explosive gas is needed to fill the selected cavity. Where the possibility exists that the fluid used might enter the circulatory system, that fluid must be isotonic as well, compatible with the elements of the blood and non-toxic.

Diathermy will not function beneath a pool of blood or through a bladderful of conducting saline. This is why in resection of the prostate or bladder neoplasms the fluid used is usually 1.1% glycine, an amino acid. It is non-conducting and almost isotonic if absorbed into the circulation. Like many other substances, if absorbed in large quantities into the circulation it can cause haemodilution, particularly of the sodium ion. It may also have possible toxic effects in large quantity, and these aspects contribute to what is known as the transurethral resection of prostate (TUR) syndrome. In laparoscopy, carbon dioxide or pure nitrogen is usually used to produce the artificial 'pneumoperitoneum'. It may also be wise to use a similar procedure in colonoscopy or sigmoidoscopy to displace any air, since methane and other colonic gases are flammable in the presence of air.

Bipolar diathermy

There are scarcely any contraindications to the use of diathermy in open surgical procedures, but in certain circumstances a 'channelling' effect can occur. This arises where there is only a single end vessel supplying the part, or where there is a series of very small vessels. If the organ supplied in this way is held away

from the body, for example the testis during an operation for hydrocele using diathermy, then the current will be channelled through the narrow part of one small artery (and vein). The result from the intensity of the current at the narrowing may be to thrombose the main blood supply with subsequent gangrene of the testis (Figure 3.7.). This effect can be obviated by use of a saline-soaked pad on the thigh close to the diathermy plate and resting the organ on it. Much safer, however, is the use of bipolar diathermy, where the entire current is integral within the forceps or electrode. Bipolar diathermy is the safest form of diathermy where any such channelling is involved, and can be used with care (and not too excessively) in operations on the penis or finger. In these circumstances there is no need for a plate electrode on the patient. Bipolar diathermy is undoubtedly the safest diathermy to use for operations in the paediatric or neonatal case.

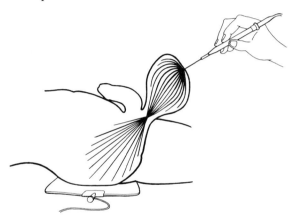

Figure 3.7 The channelling effect which can concentrate sufficient heat to thrombose vessels in a narrow pedicle, such as in the cord when diathermy is applied to the testis

Pacemakers and other implants

There is no contraindication now to operations being performed using diathermy when the patient has a modern pacemaker *in situ*. Earlier pacemakers controlled by an inductance field were reported as being damaged by diathermy, but now many prostatectomies have been carried out safely by ensuring that the plate and active electrodes are kept well away from the region of the pacemaker itself. It is important always to seek the prior advice of the cardiologist in any operation that may need diathermy.

Implants such as metal plates and screws pose no real hazard, although old filigrees and some of the modern urethral meshwork prostheses may be damaged if touched with an activated diathermy electrode. Also the surrounding tissues may be coagulated. This can be a problem in some endoscopic work such as ureteric meatotomy, where the stone has been brought successfully to the orifice and then impacted. If the diathermy electrode touches the fine wire of a Dormia stone dislodger while activated, it may well divide the wire structure with disastrous results.

Safety in diathermy

Safety in diathermy means the avoidance of the complications of surgical diathermy. Because of the very nature of its components, the surgeon has to consider the effects of heat production including flammability. He must also think of the physics of conductivity of high-frequency current within the body, and about the control and safety of the apparatus used to produce the desired surgical result.

Flammable solvents are used for many standard skin preparation solutions. Arrangements must be made to allow time for the fluid to evaporate, for any pool to be mopped up thoroughly, and any vapour allowed to clear. 'Pooling' in body cavities such as the vagina has been the subject of litigation, when the vapour from the flammable solution used has ignited at the time of diathermy cautery of the cervix.

Thermoelectric burns can result from heat production at stray contacts with metal objects, or with defective cables (Figure 3.8), in particular with those machines that have an earthed plate circuit and allowing alternative return paths to earth. This is less likely to occur in isolated plate circuit machines, now more commonly in use, but many theatres have both sorts of machine, and it has not been unknown in the event of failure of a modern machine for an older one to be substituted. It is still important to observe the precautions of avoiding contact with metal arm rests, leg rests and perineal tray attachments, etc.

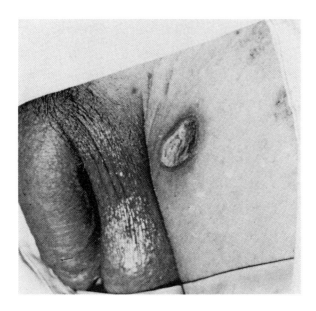

Figure 3.8 A deep diathermy burn, resulting from an exposed junction of an active electrode lead

Another cause for thermoelectric burns is the use of an improperly applied plate electrode so that it makes an inadequately small area of contact. Drying out of the contact solution or gel may also cause areas of poor contact and areas of very good contact. The latter will carry all the current and with prolonged use the heat generated may be enough to cause a burn.

Not all burns associated with the plate electrode are thermoelectric. The aluminium foil used for the plate and the risky combination of a mercury-containing skin preparation (e.g. Mercurochrome) will result if the two come into combination in a chemical reaction displacing the mercury from its salts – a reaction associated with intense heat and a chemical burn.

Anaesthetics

The avoidance of flammable gases has almost entirely become a matter of routine by anaesthetists, but there is still an obligation on the part of the surgeon to consult with his anaesthetist on the safe use of diathermy; and on the part of the anaesthetist, where operations are routinely performed with diathermy, to advise where it may not be safely used.

A code for safety

1. Full training in understanding, setting up, safe use, and the effects of diathermy, for doctors, nurses and operating department assistants.

2. Delegation of setting up to appropriately trained personnel, but no delegation of operation of the machine. The operating surgeon must always retain control of the activation of the diathermy machine to avoid accidental activation.

3. Failure checks:

(a) Machine still active (indicator light on). Check active lead first. Repeated sterilization often causes separation of the cable within the insulation 2–3 cm from either moulded connector (it can be checked with a sharp tug). The plate lead failure should produce a response from the monitor device and so is checked in second place.

(b) Machine inactive (indicator light off). Check wall socket, mains fuse, machine fuses and, in some machines, the circuit breaker button. If all normal, a service engineer is needed.

(c) Weak output – the most dangerous fault. If (a) and (b) prove normal, try a different machine. *Never* turn up the power to compensate if the machine was previously working properly, as this is one of the most frequent causes of burns. Check also in endoscopy that a conducting solution for irrigation has not been given by mistake.

4. The foregoing indicates how important is the servicing of the machine. If a medical electronics department is available, then technical advice regarding purchase and servicing of machines can readily be

sought. Otherwise it may be more economical to negotiate a service contract with the manufacturer, as the technicalities of these machines are very different from ordinary electrical work.

In summary, diathermy is used in the vast majority of surgical procedures nowadays, and it behoves all staff to make its use as safe as possible. Because it is so universal there is increased risk of litigation. This situation can easily be avoided by all surgeons having a working knowledge of its use, and insisting on proper training for all grades of staff associated with diathermy.

Illustrations

Figures 3.1–3.3., 3.5, 3.7 and 3.8 are taken from Mitchell, J. P., Lumb, G. N. and Dobbie, A. K. (1978). *A Handbook of Surgical Diathermy*, 2nd edn, Bristol, Wright.

Figure 3.4 is taken from Mitchell, J. P. (1984). *Endoscopic Operative Urology*, Bristol, Wright.

Further reading

This chapter deals only with the use of diathermy in general, but for specific applications in certain specialties the reader is referred to the following literature:

Mitchell, J. P. (1984) Surgical diathermy in urological endoscopy. In *Endoscopic Operative Urology*, Bristol, Wright, Chap. 6

Mitchell, J. P., Lumb, G. N. and Dobbie, A. K. (1978) *A Handbook of Surgical Diathermy*, 2nd edn, with chapters by Harris, P. and Smart, G. E., Bristol, Wright

Lumb, G. N. (1990) Surgical diathermy in urological practice. In *Scientific Foundations of Urology*, 3rd edn (eds G. D. Chisholm and W. R. Fair), Heinemann Medical Books, Oxford, Chap. 78

4

Lasers in medicine and surgery

J. A. S. Carruth

Introduction

Albert Einstein described the basic physics of the laser in 1917, but it was not until 1960 that the first was produced by T. H. Mainman using a synthetic ruby as the lasing medium. Since that time a very large number of lasers have been developed with a vast range of scientific, industrial, medical and, indeed, military uses. This range is now so great that many have said that when the age in which we live is finally named it will not be known as the atomic or space age but the age of the laser.

In the past decade, lasers have been used increasingly in almost all medical and surgical disciplines, but despite this increase in usage the words of Leon Goldman – one of the fathers of laser surgery – must never be forgotten: 'If you don't need the laser don't use it'. A laser should only be used when it can be proved conclusively that it can perform a particular medical or surgical task better than established conventional techniques which are almost invariably less technically complex and far less expensive.

Almost any surgical procedure could be performed by using a laser or a combination of lasers, but in the clinical part of this chapter an attempt will be made to show not only that lasers can be used in the performance of a particular clinical procedure but also why they should be used and the advantages which they offer to the doctor, the patient and to those who finance health care.

The laser

The word 'laser' is derived from the acronym – light amplification by stimulated emission of radiation – but it is important to state that in this context the radiation refers to non-ionizing light radiation and there is no 'radiation hazard' with any surgical or medical laser in use at present. A laser produces coherent light which is an intense beam of pure non-diverging monochromatic light in which all the light waves are of the same length and travel in step and in the same direction.

The major component of each laser is the laser tube which contains the lasing medium which, in most medical lasers, is a gas. At each end of the tube is a mirror, one of which is partially reflective to allow passage of the laser beam, and the lasing medium is excited electrically or by another high-powered light source. This excitation produces a population inversion of excited/non-excited particles which normally has a large excess in the non-excited state. An excited particle will decay to the low-energy ground state with the release of a photon – a quantum of radiant energy or light particle. If this photon strikes another excited particle of the lasing medium it 'stimulates it to emit' an identical photon, and in a population of excited particles of the lasing medium it is easy to envisage a series of collisions producing an increasing number of identical photons. The photons produced by these collisions are released in all directions, but within a fraction of a second one will be released in the axis of the laser tube and, by reflection back into the lasing medium from the mirrors, there is a rapid build up of light energy within the laser tube – the cascade effect – and the coherent light so produced is then emitted through the partially reflective mirror.

The name of each laser is derived from the lasing medium and this also determines the wavelength of coherent light produced by the laser. The wavelength of laser light determines the effect of the beam on body tissues and that, in turn, defines the clinical role of that laser. As each laser produces essentially one wavelength, each laser has one main clinical role and to change roles one must necessarily change the laser.

The effects of the laser beam on body tissues are also dependent on the rate of delivery of the laser energy to the tissues. The pulsed neodymium YAG laser, for example, is used to destroy opaque bodies within the eye and the energy is delivered in nanosecond (1/1 000 000 000 of a second) pulses which raise the temperature of a point in the eye to that of the sun and this causes explosive disruption of the intraocular opaque body such as an opaque posterior lens capsule after a cataract has been removed. However, the extreme short pulse prevents damage beyond and adjacent to the focal points of the beam.

Medical lasers

Carbon dioxide

The carbon dioxide (CO_2) laser produces far infrared coherent light at a wavelength of 10 600 nm which is absorbed by water and, therefore, by the soft tissues of the body which contain 70–90% water.

Intracellular water absorbs the energy and is

boiled, causing a thousand-fold expansion within the cell and destroying the cell by instantaneous vaporization at the relatively low temperature of 100°C. The explosive disruption of the cell releases cell contents into the beam where they are carbonized and fall as 'carbon soot' around the laser wound. It had been stated that the particles released in this way do not contain viable material, but recent work has thrown doubt on this basic assumption and it is now suggested that in the vaporization of viral lesions there may be viable viral particles within the vapour.

With this 'instantaneous low-temperature vaporization' of cells there is minimal spread of heat to adjacent normal tissues and it has been shown, both in theory and experimentally, that if a 'short sharp' dissection technique is used with a high power and short exposure the thermal damage to tissues adjacent to the laser wound is reduced to a minimum. In addition, there is no 'shock impact' when the beam strikes the tissues and these features mean that precise surgery can be performed very close to vital structures, particularly within the central nervous system.

As a result of the minimal damage to adjacent normal tissues, healing is not complicated by oedema and is relatively rapid and pain free. It has also been shown experimentally that there is less contracture of a mucosal wound cut by this laser than of one cut by conventional techniques.

The CO_2 laser is used as a 'high-precision, bloodless light scalpel' and is of particular value in mucosal surgery – ENT and gynaecology – and in surgery to the central nervous system where it provides true 'no touch' surgery. In mucosal surgery, tissue destruction is immediate – an advantage over cryosurgery – and dissection is relatively bloodless as the beam seals vessels of up to 0.5 mm in diameter and also seals lymphatics, possibly reducing the spread of malignant cells via this route.

A majority of the work with the CO_2 laser is carried out under the operating microscope or colposcope which provide a well-illuminated magnified view of the operative field. Within this operative field the working beam is aimed by a coaxial, low-powered visible laser controlled by a micromanipulator on the laser delivery head. Tissue destruction can be precisely controlled by selecting an appropriate 'spot size' and power of the beam giving a power density (W/cm^2) appropriate to the tissues and the required speed of dissection. Further control of tissue removal can be achieved by selecting the exposure time of the beam on the tissues. As the beam does not denature the tissues through which it is passing and as there is neither blood nor instruments in the wound, the progress of dissection can be followed with great accuracy under the microscope. The only instrument needed is for suction at the point of surgery to remove the vapour produced by tissue destruction both for visual access and to prevent the vapour from causing thermal damage to the normal structures. This lack of instruments in the wound is of great value where access is limited in, for example, paediatric laryngology.

A wide range of CO_2 lasers are now available, including truly portable machines, giving this laser great versatility and multidisciplinary usage.

Argon

This laser produces blue/green coherent light at wavelengths 488 and 514 nanometres which will pass through clear and colourless structures without absorption and without causing thermal damage. The beam is then absorbed by structures which are pigmented or blood-containing and it is possible, therefore, to treat relatively deep-seated lesions through overlaying clear normal tissues. This laser is used primarily for coagulating both normal and abnormal blood vessels, but at higher power levels relatively imprecise and slow thermal tissue destruction may be performed. The energy of this laser can be transmitted by a flexible fibre, and for work in dermatology a handpiece is used commonly with a spot size of 1 mm diameter. When used in ophthalmology for retinal photocoagulation and in ENT for surgery to the middle ear, the work is carried out under an operating microscope using a spot size measured in microns and aiming is provided by an attenuated beam positioned by a micromanipulator on the laser/microscope attachment. All microscopes are fitted with an automatic shutter which closes just before the beam fires, to protect the eyes of the surgeon. For work on the aerodigestive tract the beam is transmitted by a fibre introduced through the biopsy channel of a flexible fibreoptic endoscope.

In the coagulation of blood vessels a precisely localized lesion of the vessel can be created by delivering an exactly calculated dose of energy without any mechanical contact with the vessel and there is no spread of thermal or electrical energy to adjacent structures.

Neodymium YAG

The neodymium YAG (Nd YAG) laser produces near infrared coherent light at a wavelength of 1060 nm which is deeply absorbed in tissues without colour or tissue specificity. This laser has largely replaced the argon laser for a majority of work on the aerodigestive tract, both for the removal of obstructing tumour and also the control of bleeding vessels in upper gastrointestinal ulcers.

At high power levels thermal tissue destruction can be performed with, in many cases, better haemostasis than can be achieved with the CO_2 laser. In addition, in the control of bleeding vessels, in particular in the upper gastrointestinal tract, the beam is not absorbed by blood but by perivascular fibrous tissue causing perivascular contraction and subsequent fibrosis, allowing larger vessels to be controlled than with the 'blood-absorbed' argon laser.

However, with the deeper penetration of the beam into the tissues there is a significant risk of thermal damage to adjacent structures even beyond the organ which is being treated. It has been shown histologically that when a tumour is removed with this laser there are three layers of damage: first, a layer which is vaporized; secondly, a layer of damage which will slough; and thirdly, a layer of damage to cells which are replaced by fibrous tissue, but without loss of physical integrity. Thus, in the treatment of tumours of a hollow viscus there is a minimal risk of perforation.

The beam can be transmitted via a flexible fibre and tissue removal may be by a 'contact' or 'non-contact' technique. The delivery fibre may be coupled to a 'sapphire scalpel' and a large amount of work has been carried out in the performance of soft-tissue resection using this combination. In addition, the delivery fibre may be coupled to a contact tip and is now widely used to carry out haemostasis during 'laser-assisted' cholecystectomy and other intra-abdominal laparoscopic procedures. A number of contact tips are also being evaluated for percutaneous transluminal angioplasty.

The pulsed Nd YAG laser is being evaluated in angioplasty and, using nanosecond pulses, it is widely used in ophthalmology to destroy, by explosive disruption, opaque structures within the eye.

Krypton

This laser is used in ophthalmology similarly to the argon laser for retinal photocoagulation.

Ruby

Much of the early medical research work on lasers was carried out with the pulsed ruby laser, but it is now rarely used except in the treatment of some pigmented skin lesions and in the removal of blue- and black-coloured tattoos.

Dye

A dye laser may be 'pumped' by either an argon or a copper vapour laser, and by dye selection each laser may be tuned over a significant range of the visible spectrum. These dye lasers are utilized in the photoactivation of intratumour haematoporphyrin derivative for the destruction of malignant tumours by the technique of photodynamic therapy and they are also being researched for the destruction of intradermal blood vessels. The flashlamp pumped pulsed dye laser appears, at present, to be the laser of choice for the destruction of intradermal blood vessels in the treatment of portwine stain birthmarks, particularly in children. Using different parameters the pulsed dye laser may also be used to destroy stones within the urinary and biliary tracts.

Gold vapour

This pulsed laser produces red light at the appropriate wavelengths for activation of haematoporphyrin derivative for photodynamic therapy.

Excimer

The name of this laser is taken from 'excited dimer' and the lasing medium is composed of substances which can only exist in the excited state such as argon fluoride. These violet/ultraviolet lasers can remove tissue by molecular disruption and not by thermal means and much research is in progress at present in reshaping the cornea to correct refractive errors with this laser. Excimer lasers are also being widely researched in angioplasty.

Safety

It must be shown that safe lasers are being used in an entirely safe manner by fully trained medical personnel in appropriate medical and surgical situations.

Although the lasers used in medicine and surgery are much less powerful than many used in science and industry, all those used therapeutically are in the highest power class and their use 'requires extreme caution'. In Britain the safe use of medical lasers is controlled by the Health and Safety at Work Act, The British Standards Code BS 4803 and the Guidance on the Safe Use of Lasers in Medical Practice produced by the Department of Health and Social Security. All codes insist on the appointment of a local laser safety officer who will produce local codes of safe practice for each laser in each clinical situation. Work is in progress at present, under a European Community Concerted Action Programme on medical laser development, on the development of a code of safe practice for use within the EEC. In addition, guidance will be provided on 'minimal required training standards' for medical and surgical practitioners working with lasers, as at present these training standards have not been defined.

The eyes of the patient and of operating theatre personnel are particularly at risk with all therapeutic lasers. It is vital that appropriate and carefully fixed eye protection is provided for the patient and that all in the operating theatre wear appropriate laser-proof eye wear as defined in the various codes of safe practice. When working with the CO_2 laser, the eyes of the surgeon are protected by the optics of the microscope; and when the argon laser is used with a microscope or slit lamp, shutters are provided, as described above, which close when the laser is activated. With the Nd YAG laser a filter is incorporated into the endoscope. However, for all other medical and surgical laser usage the surgeon must also wear laser-proof eye wear appropriate to the laser being used.

There are certain other specific hazards, such as anaesthetic tube ignition, when the CO_2 laser is used in laryngology, and the anaesthetist must be familiar with this problem and must use one of a number of laser-proof techniques.

Clinical use of lasers in medicine and surgery

This review of the use of lasers in medicine and surgery must, of necessity, be brief. Although all the statements made are supported by references these are not included in the text, but a guide to further reading is provided at the end of the chapter.

Cardiovascular

Percutaneous transluminal angioplasty using one of a variety of laser techniques is in routine clinical use in a large number of centres worldwide for the disobliteration of obstructed limb arteries. The laser may be used to heat a hot metal tip which creates the primary channel through the obstruction and this channel is then widened by conventional balloon angioplasty to provide an adequate lumen. Both continuous wave and pulsed lasers are being evaluated for the removal of atheroma using a variety of 'contact' tips. In the 2 mm 'smart laser' fibre there are 11 separate fibres each of which first analyses the target within the vessel as atheroma thrombus or vessel wall, and the laser is activated down that particular fibre when a pathological target is identified, allowing the fibre to pass through the obstruction under computer guidance. However, with all laser techniques it appears necessary to use balloon angioplasty to ensure an adequate lumen after the laser has created the initial channel.

A large amount of research and early clinical work is in progress on laser angioplasty within the coronary arteries. Recent evidence has shown that a laser technique is at least as effective and as safe as conventional balloon angioplasty and it would appear certain that dramatic progress can be expected in this field in the near future.

An alternative approach to the revascularization of the heart is to create multiple perforations of the myocardium into the ventricle using a high-powered CO_2 laser. Twenty channels per square centimetre are created, the outer end is sealed and it has been shown that these channels remain patent and become endothelialized, allowing blood to diffuse directly into the ventricular muscle. Animal work has confirmed that these channels can support the myocardium after the coronory arteries have been tied and some early clinical studies have been carried out which show that this technique is effective.

Intracardiac laser surgery can be used to relieve some forms of valvular stenosis and laser irradiation may be used to cause shortening of chordae tendinae to relieve valvular incompetence. A laser may also be used to carry out procedures on the conducting mechanisms of the heart.

Chest medicine

Many patients with 'untreatable' carcinoma of the bronchus die in extreme distress with obstruction of one of the main air passages by tumour. Both the Nd YAG and CO_2 lasers have been used to provide palliation of these patients by the removal of the obstructing tumour. The Nd YAG laser can be used via a flexible fibreoptic bronchoscope and appears to provide better haemostasis, whereas the CO_2 laser must be used with a rigid bronchoscope. Palliation can only be provided in patients with obstruction of the trachea and main bronchi, and in practice much of the work with the Nd YAG laser is also carried down a rigid scope which allows better suction and the removal of necrotic tumour fragments by forceps.

Photodynamic therapy offers enormous potential for the treatment of early cases of carcinoma of the bronchus when these can be diagnosed and studies are in progress to compare the palliation of advanced lesions by this technique with the palliation obtained using the Nd YAG laser.

Dermatology

The CO_2 laser may be used to cut the skin, but with no particular advantages over a scalpel except in patients with a haemorrhagic tendency and in the removal of multiple lesions such as warts or condylomata acuminata. For the past decade the argon laser has been the treatment of choice for the hitherto untreatable portwine stain. The blue/green beam passes through the clear epidermis without significant absorption and without causing irreversible thermal damage and is then absorbed by the blood in the network of abnormal capillaries in the outer dermis, causing thermal damage and thrombosis. It has been shown histologically that the thrombosed vessels are replaced, over a period of months, by colourless fibrous tissue with a marked reduction in the colour of the birthmark, but the epidermis should return to normal. There is, however, a low incidence of atrophic or hypertrophic scarring which should not exceed 2%.

Over the decade it has been shown clearly that the argon laser is only of value in older patients with mature birthmarks of the face and it has been of little value in the treatment of children. However, within the past few years several new laser-based techniques have been introduced for the treatment of portwine stains and other vascular malformations of the skin. New lasers include copper vapour, dye and frequency doubled YAG and the copper vapour and continuous dye lasers may be used either with a handpiece under microscopic control to erase individual vessels. The pulsed tunable dye laser appears to be of particular value in the treatment of children. This laser produces light at 585 nm with a pulse duration of 450 µs and this appears to cause an explosive disruption of the large number of normal capillaries which comprise an immature birthmark, and there appears to be almost no risk of scarring even in very young patients.

Almost all the work carried out to date has been performed using a handpiece, but a number of computer-controlled automatic systems have recently been introduced and these allow treatment to be performed with a much higher degree of precision and with a much better reproducibility.

Gastroenterology

The mortality from upper gastrointestinal haemorrhage remains high in those patients who continue to bleed and in those who rebleed. A number of uncontrolled and controlled trials have been performed to show the value of the argon and Nd YAG lasers in the control of the acute bleed and in the prevention of rebleeding, and it appears that the Nd YAG laser will prove to be the better in this field. Laser energy is delivered by a quartz fibre introduced via the biopsy channel of a flexible endoscope and the acute bleed can be controlled in 70–100% of cases, but only one series has claimed that the laser can control bleeding from oesophageal varices. One of the most valuable predictive signs for rebleeding is a visible vessel in the ulcer crater and, if these are treated by laser photocoagulation, a significant reduction in the incidence of rebleeding can be achieved. A reduction in mortality has also been reported in several series.

The Nd YAG laser can be used to provide palliation by removing obstructing oesophageal carcinoma to relieve dysphagia, and series are in progress to compare palliation by this means with that achieved by the insertion of an indwelling prosthesis.

Patients with inoperable rectal carcinoma suffer major distress from obstructing and bleeding tumour. Significant palliation can be achieved by removing this with the Nd YAG laser and troublesome bleeding can be controlled in a majority of cases.

General surgery

There is an increasing interest in 'minimally invasive surgery' and the Nd YAG laser forms a valuable part of the surgeon's armamentarium in the performance of various laparoscopic intra-abdominal procedures such as cholecystectomy. This is also widely used, attached to a contact sapphire scalpel, for the performance of a wide range of soft-tissue resections and for a number of intra-abdominal procedures.

Using a laser fibre implanted into solid tumours, successful treatment by hyperthermia has been carried out on both hepatic and pancreatic tumours.

The pulsed dye laser is also of value in the performance of lithotripsy and can be used for the destruction of both urinary and biliary stones.

Gynaecology

With the greater understanding of the natural history of premalignant conditions of the cervix, there has been an increasing tendency to treat these lesions by local destruction under the microscopic control of the operating colposcope. To destroy these lesions with the electrocautery requires a general anaesthetic and although cryotherapy can be performed without anaesthesia, many believe that the tissue removal lacks precision. Precise vaporization of appropriate cervical lesions can be performed using the CO_2 laser with excellent results, and a large majority of women can tolerate the technique without anaesthetic. Postoperative complications and bleeding are minimal and as there is no scarring of the cervical canal the women are able to have children. If the lesion necessitates a cone biopsy, it has been shown that this can be performed using the CO_2 laser with advantages over the conventional 'cold knife' technique. In the performance of pelvic reconstructional surgery for infertility, the lack of tissue reaction with the CO_2 laser offers potential advantages over conventional microsurgical techniques.

Through the laparoscope, the laser may be used to destroy areas of endometriosis within the abdominal cavity. Via a hysterescope, the Nd YAG laser may be used to ablate the endometrium in the treatment of menorrhagia, and where this has been used the number of hysterectomies has fallen dramatically. However, it must be stated that although this technique was developed using a laser, several electrosurgical techniques are now more widely used as these are both quicker and cheaper.

Neurosurgery

Lasers offer the neurosurgeon true 'no touch surgery' and surgery can safely be performed adjacent to vital areas of the central nervous system without the risk of mechanical or thermal injury. The CO_2 laser can be used to perform precise incisions into the brain and spinal cord, and after the opening of a tumour with this laser the bulk of the tumour is removed either with the Nd YAG laser or ultrasonic aspirator and the CO_2 laser is again used to vaporize the capsule. A three-dimensional computer model of a tumour may be made and the tumour removed stereotactically with the CO_2 laser, and access for the laser beam can be provided by a very narrow channel through silent areas of the brain. This laser may also be used to create precise lesions of the spinal cord for the control of pain. The argon and Nd YAG lasers are being evaluated for the photocoagulation of both normal and abnormal vessels within the central nervous system and some exciting research work is in progress on the control of aneurysms and vascular malformations. Several lasers are being investigated for the performance of sutureless microvascular anastomosis in the performance of revascularization procedures within the cranial cavity.

Photodynamic therapy offers great promise in the treatment of malignant brain tumours. A number of series have been carried out in which the tumour is removed surgically and the tumour bed photo-irradiated after injection of the sensitizer, and some very exciting early results have been achieved.

Ophthalmology

This was the first speciality in which lasers were used and remains in the forefront of laser usage. One of the main causes of blindness in the Western world is diabetic retinopathy with bleeding from new vessels which develop in front of the retina. The argon and krypton lasers are used to perform photocoagulation to destroy areas of avascular retina which are thought to be the stimulus to new vessel growth, and it has been shown in a large number of series that the prognosis for the preservation of sight has been dramatically improved. Laser photocoagulation may also be used to create chorioretinal adhesions around a retinal tear to prevent detachment.

The argon laser may be used to reduce the abnormal intraocular pressure in acute closed-angled glaucoma by creating a hole in the iris and also in chronic simple glaucoma by trabeculectomy, improving the drainage through the trabecular network.

The pulsed Nd YAG laser, using extremely short nanosecond pulses, creates precise lesions within the eye to remove opaque intraocular structures such as the posterior lens capsule after the removal of a cataract.

The excimer laser has been evaluated for reshaping the cornea to correct refractive errors. A majority of refractive errors may be corrected in this way: the shape of the patient's cornea and the shape it should be are programmed into a computer and the excimer laser, which removes tissue non-thermally by molecular disruption, is then used to create the new shape of the cornea. This technique has been extensively researched and several clinical studies are in progress.

Otolaryngology

All the features of tissue removal by the CO_2 laser make it of the very greatest value in surgery to the larynx, particularly in children. The ability to remove tissue with precision, no bleeding, no postoperative oedema and reduced scar formation with contracture are unique to this modality. The CO_2 laser is, therefore, the treatment of choice for a wide range of benign conditions of the larynx, in particular laryngeal papillomatosis in which the larynx, usually in children, becomes filled with frond-like viral warts which recur after removal. These patients require scores of procedures both to keep the airway open and to maintain the voice. Control of disease may be achieved by laser removal followed by one of the

antiviral agents, but there is evidence to show that recurrence can be expected when the medication is stopped.

The CO_2 laser can be used to treat endoscopically certain cases of laryngeal stenosis, and laser resection of early carcinomas of the larynx has been shown to produce equal 'cure rates' to those achieved by radiotherapy and more radical surgery.

Lesions of the mouth and tongue may be removed with precision and excellent healing, and it appears that there may be some reduction in postoperative morbidity. The Nd YAG laser with a contact scalpel may also be used with benefit in the performance of intra-oral resections.

The use of the argon laser under the operating microscope to perform delicate surgery to the middle ear is being evaluated, as is its role in the removal of posterior cranial fossa tumours.

Urology

After electrosurgical resection of malignant tumours of the bladder there is a relatively high rate of recurrence which is thought to be due both to the multifocal nature of the tumour and the possibility that viable tumour fragments are released during the resection and become implanted in the dome of the bladder. The Nd YAG laser can be used via a cystoscope without the need for a general anaesthetic, and by using an Albarren bridge the laser fibre can be directed into all parts of the bladder. In the destruction of a tumour first, tissue is coagulated around the base to prevent lymphatic spread and then the exophytic part of the tumour is destroyed without releasing viable fragments. Tumour within the bladder wall is then removed without risk of perforation.

Laser lithotripsy using a pulsed dye laser is now an accepted alternative to extracorporeal lithotripsy. Delivery fibres can be introduced via the ureter and some excellent results have been reported.

The CO_2 laser may be used to treat superficial lesions of the external genitalia and a number of lasers are being researched for the treatment of urethral stricture.

Photodynamic therapy is already providing a viable alternative therapy for superficial malignant disease of the bladder when conventional therapy has failed and in a large number of centres worldwide whole bladder photo-irradiation is resulting in long-term 'cures'. If the total light dose is controlled, then bladder wall damage with severe urinary symptoms is reduced to a minimum, as this was a significant problem in early series.

Photodynamic therapy

This technique represents a new and exciting approach to treatment of many forms of localized malignant disease. For ideal photodynamic therapy, a patient with a malignant tumour is given a photosensitive drug which is selectively absorbed by or retained by malignant tissue giving, after a period of time, a high tumour/normal tissue ratio. The intra-tumour photosensitive drug is then activated by a wavelength of laser light which penetrates deeply into the tissues causing destruction of the malignant tumour with sparing of surrounding normal tissues.

This ideal remains some way off, but already some exciting results have been obtained using the drug/light combination of haematoporphyrin derivative and red light at a wavelength of 630 nm.

Areas of particular interest mentioned above include the treatment of carcinoma of bronchus, where it has been shown from Japan that early lesions can be treated for cure and palliation can be achieved by the removal of obstructing tumour from the main air passages.

In the treatment of carcinoma in situ of the bladder, a large number of patients have been treated by this technique when conventional therapy has failed with long-term control. With careful dosimetry of the total light dose, significant damage to the muscle of the bladder wall can be avoided and this reduces to a minimum the severe urinary symptoms which were common in early series.

This technique appears to be particularly promising in the treatment of malignant brain tumours where the bed is treated following the surgical removal of the tumour. A number of studies are in progress with some very exciting preliminary results. A wide range of other tumours have been treated and the technique may also be of value in the management of viral lesions and of atheroma.

A large amount of research is in progress in the development of new drug/light combinations and it appears certain that as these are introduced photodynamic therapy will realize its full potential.

Conclusions

The first laser was produced in 1960 and we are only at the beginning of the 'laser age'. Lasers are now widely used in a large number of medical and surgical disciplines, with proven advantages over conventional techniques, and further exciting developments can be anticipated.

Further reading

Abela, G. S. (ed.) (1990) *Lasers in Cardiovascular Medicine and Surgery: Fundamentals and Techniques*, Nijhoff, Boston

Baggish, M. S. (ed.) (1985) *Basic and Advanced Laser Surgery in Gynaecology*, Appleton-Century-Crofts, Norwalk, Conn.

Biamino, G. and Muller, G. J. (eds). (1988) *Advances in Laser Medicine I,* Ecomed, Landsberg, Germany

Carruth, J. A. S. and McKenzie, A. (1986) *Medical Lasers, Science and Clinical Practice*, Hilger, Boston

Ciba Foundation (1989) *Photosensitizing Compounds: Their Chemistry, Biology and Clinical Use*, Ciba Foundation Symposium 146, Wiley-Interscience, New York

Dover, J., Arndt, K. *et al.* (1990) *Illustrated Cutaneous Laser Surgery: A Practitioner's Guide*, Appleton and Lange, Norwalk, Conn.

European Community Medical Laser Concerted Action Programme (1989) *Proceedings of the First Plenary Workshop on Safety and Laser Tissue Interaction*, Berlin, November 1988, Baillière Tindall, London

Gitter, K. and Schatz, H. (1989) *Laser Photocoagulation of Retinal Disease*, Pacific Medical Press, St. Louis

Hofstetter, A. G. (ed.) (1989) *Lasers in Gastroenterology. International Experiences and Trends*, Georg Thieme Verlag, Stuttgart

Isner, J. M. and Clarke, R. H. K. (1989) *Cardiovascular Laser Therapy*, Raven Press, New York

Joffe, S. N. and Oguro, Y. (eds) (1988) *Advances in Nd: YAG Laser Surgery*, Springer Verlag, New York

Martellucci, S. and Chester, A. N. (eds) (1985) *Laser Photobiology and Photomedicine*, Plenum Press, New York

Shapshay, S. M. (ed.) (1987) *Endoscopic Laser Surgery Handbook*, Marcel Dekker, New York

Smith, J., Stein, B. and Benson, R. (eds) (1989) *Lasers In Urologic Surgery*, 2nd edn, Yearbook Medical Publishers, Chicago

Trelles, M. A. (ed.) (1990) European Community Medical Laser Concerted Action Programme, Second Plenary Workshop, Tarragona, Spain

Abdominal wall and gastroenterology

5
Abdominal access and closure

S. D. Scott and I. Taylor

Introduction

Access to the abdominal cavity has been improved gradually, partly due to the improvements in wound closure, suture materials and control of sepsis, which allow the surgeon to feel much more confident about opening the abdomen. The age-old adage 'big mistakes are made through small incisions' is nowhere more appropriate than in abdominal surgery. With modern suture materials and techniques, understanding of delayed primary closure and better postoperative pain control, the modern surgeon need have no fear of making a hole big enough to allow adequate access and worrying that the end result may be less than ideal cosmetically. The concept of the mini-laparotomy or laparoscopic surgical techniques, the conflict of interest between the surgeon's need for adequate exposure and the patient's desire for minimal, cosmetically acceptable scarring results in a controversial surgical debate.

Adequate exposure is essential for safety and trainees must feel free to make incisions appropriate to their level of experience, without the worry of adverse criticism from chief or patient. Much can be done to improve the cosmetic effect and ease of access by careful planning of the surgical incision.

A number of important anatomical considerations should be noted:

1. In a *vertical incision* the amount of lateral retraction is closely related to the length of the incision. This is of importance in pelvic surgery, e.g. anterior resection where a long vertical incision to above the umbilicus is essential if lateral retraction is to be sufficient to enable access to the lower rectum.
2. Generally speaking, *muscle-splitting incisions* are less likely to result in incisional hernia than muscle-cutting ones.
3. For *upper abdominal incisions* the xiphocostal angle should be considered. In a patient with a very narrow angle, subcostal and midline incisions may require reconsideration and modification.
4. In general, better results are obtained if the *skin incision* is equal to or preferably greater than that of the fascia or peritoneum. If the skin incision is smaller than the underlying incision the subsequent closure of the angles of the incision is compromised.

Retractors

The length of an incision should take account of the amount and experience of available assistants, since a good assistant greatly facilitates any operation and allows a more modest incision. Self-retaining retractors such as the Goligher (for upper abdominal surgery) or the Codman ring retractor will greatly ease the exposure for the single-handed surgeon. Adequate muscle relaxation makes a vast difference to the ease of operating and particularly for closing the wound.

Incision of abdominal wall

Surgeons vary enormously in their preference for skin preparation. It is generally agreed that adequate shaving is necessary. It is a mistake not to remove all hair up to the nipples in upper abdominal surgery and well down over the pubis and both groins for lower abdominal incisions. Improper shaving resulting in multiple abrasions and incomplete removal of the hair must be avoided. The abdominal wall should be cleaned (iodine preparations are very popular) and the sterile drapes should be positioned to enable adequate access. Adhesive plastic drapes are popular for certain procedures, but the skin must be carefully dried prior to application. Drapes should not interfere with possible extensions of either end of the incision.

At the time of incision the abdominal wall is a flaccid structure and is best stretched between the fingers of the surgeon's left and the assistant's right hand. The skin and subcutaneous tissue are incised and haemostasis obtained with diathermy. Gauze swabs should be compressed against the wound. Following the knife skin incision, diathermy for the remainder of the wound has been advocated but no real benefit has been demonstrated. Laser incision confirms no advantage and is slower, expensive and not generally available. The scalpel remains the simplest and most effective tool!

Wound protection is controversial. If the gastrointestinal tract is opened or peritoneal sepsis is present, then wound protection is sensible. Wound protectors mounted on flexible plastic rings can be used to isolate the entire wound. Towels, soaked in antiseptics, e.g. iodine, are a simpler method of isolating the wound edges and are probably as effective.

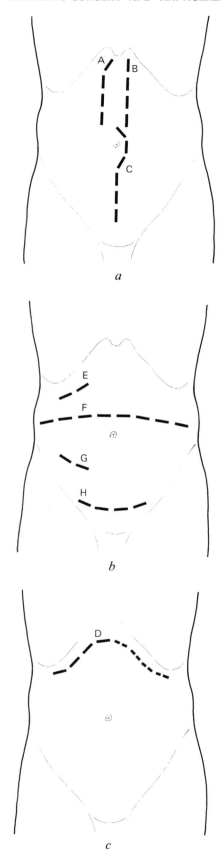

If wound drainage is considered necessary at the end of the procedure, it is probably best done by inserting suction drains through separate stab incisions.

Types of incision

Appropriate access is critical to abdominal surgery. Experience frequently dictates the decision, but the incisions described below are common (Figure 5.1).

Midline incision

This type (Figure 5.2) involves incision of the linea alba in the line of the skin incision to expose the 'bulging' extraperitoneal fat and peritoneum. The fibres from both rectus sheaths can be seen decussating in the midline and exposure and closure are easier if the flat of the knife's belly is used to push back the subcutaneous fat to clear about 1 cm of the fascial layer.

In cutting through the linea the extraperitoneal fat is seen and swept laterally by blunt dissection. There are a few small vessels which require coagulation. The peritoneum is then exposed, picked up and incised. In an infra-umbilical incision the parietal peritoneum moves away posteriorly over the dome of the bladder and care must be taken to avoid damage.

The incision can be extended by skirting to the right or left of the umbilicus. The xiphoid is best cut with a heavy pair of scissors rather than bypassed, since incisions into or near the xiphoid area are notoriously painful. The skin incision can be extended down as far as the mons pubis but not into it.

Paramedian incision

This incision gives slightly better access to one or other side of the abdomen than a midline incision. It is claimed that it is a more secure closure because the rectus acts as a buttress. Late hernia should be reduced in incidence by a sound rectus interposition. The disadvantage of a paramedian incision is that it takes longer and is slightly more laborious to make.

The technique is the same in the upper and lower abdomen (Figure 5.3). The rectus sheath is incised through the whole length of the wound. If the rectus is displaced, the sheath is picked up on the median side and held vertically in the tips of fine forceps. The tendinous intersections are adherent to and blend with the layer and are freed by sharp dissection. There

Figure 5.1 *a*, Common vertical abdominal incisions. A, Right paramedian with Mayo–Robson extension. B, Left paramedian. C, Midline skirting the umbilicus. *b*, Transverse incisions. E, Modified Kocher's for gallbladder surgery. F, Transverse para-umbilical. G, Lanz. H, Pfannenstiel. *c*, Marginal incisions. D, Half or full rooftop

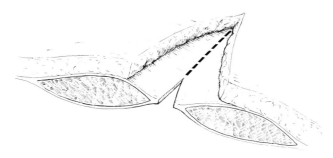

Figure 5.2 Line of incision for midline exposure

are vessels at these intersections which must be coagulated. Once the linea alba is reached the plane is bloodless and the muscle belly is separated round onto its posterior aspect. In the upper abdomen it is not usual to encounter any further bleeding, but in lower incisions the inferior epigastric vessels course upwards lateromedially to cross the linea semicircularis.

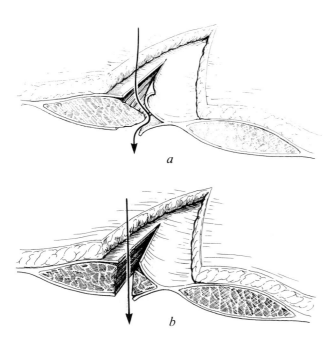

Figure 5.3 Rectus displacement (*a*) and rectus splitting (*b*) in a paramedian incision

Alternatively, the rectus muscle can be split longitudinally, approximately 1 cm from its medial border. This is quicker than rectus displacement. Bleeding is encountered from vessels in the muscular belly, but can be controlled easily by coagulation or with fine ligatures.

The posterior rectus sheath and its fused underlying peritoneum are picked up with two clips and incised with a knife blade held horizontally. In a patient who has not had a previous laparotomy there is very little danger of injury to a viscus because the

moment a hole has been made, air rushes in and gut moves away from the inner aspect of the parietal peritoneum. Palpation of the 'tented' peritoneum should be performed to ensure absence of underlying bowel. The small incision is then enlarged upwards and downwards with scissors. Towards the xyphoid, the right or left aspects of the falciform ligament are encountered. To aid exposure it may be desirable to ligate and divide the ligament which in addition to the obliterated umbilical vein usually contains a small terminal branch of the internal mammary artery. The peritoneum can then be incised upwards as far as the cupola of the diaphragm. Below the umbilicus the parietal peritoneum in the midline spreads out over the bladder and care must be taken to identify the peritoneum exactly. It is important, particularly when operating in the pelvis through a lower abdominal incision, to have the bladder emptied by catheter.

The lateral paramedian incision is merely an exaggeration of the conventional incision in which the anterior and posterior sheaths are incised in their lateral thirds, so increasing the buttress effect of the muscle (Figure 5.4)

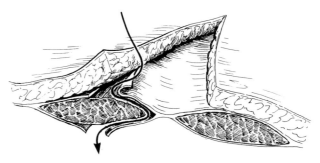

Figure 5.4 Path of dissection in a lateral paramedian incision

Kocher's incision

This incision is frequently used for biliary surgery on the right or splenic surgery on the left. It has the advantage of running parallel to the edge of the liver, so allowing this organ to be retracted uniformly upwards and to the right in order to expose the gallbladder. Its major disadvantage is that its exact direction depends on the obliquity of the costal margin and in patients with a very narrow angle the line intersects the midline acutely. This may prove a problem if vertical abdominal incisions are subsequently required. It may be difficult to carry out a thorough exploration of the abdomen through this incision. If pathology is found in the lower abdomen it is difficult to deal with unless a further incision is made.

The skin incision is made approximately 2 cm below the costal margin and parallel to it. The medial end extends to the midline. The incision then divides the rectus sheath. The rectus muscle itself is divided by cutting diathermy and the vessels in the posterior aspect of the rectus sheath are separately ligated or diathermized. The posterior muscles are divided in the same line across the external oblique aponeurosis, but in the line of the internal oblique. Every effort should be made to preserve the nerves which are visualized laterally in the wound.

If the position of the gallbladder is marked on the skin preoperatively, a mini-laparotomy incision can be performed transversely directly over the gallbladder. This '5 cm cholecystectomy incision' enables early patient mobility and discharge.

Rooftop incision

This is a transverse incision with a slightly complex upwards appearance and is suitable for patients with a wide costal angle. It is an ideal incision for liver surgery, particularly when major liver resection is required. It provides ideal exposure for the hepatic veins and the hiatus. The incision passes through all layers of the abdominal wall in the same line and divides both recti transversely. In the midline it is necessary for the falciform ligament to be ligated and divided, and by keeping the ligatures on the falciform ligament this can act as a useful retractor of the upper and lower margins of the wound.

Transverse incisions

A transverse muscle-cutting incision can be used for a variety of intra-abdominal operative procedures. Transverse incisions may be made either on the right or left side of the abdomen or indeed as a long transverse incision above or below the umbilicus. Such incisions are useful for aortic surgery and provide excellent exposure when dealing with a ruptured aortic aneurysm.

With transverse incisions the skin edges tend to be in the direction of Langer's lines and fall together easily and heal with the minimum of scarring. It is often possible to leave the skin layer of a transverse incision unsutured (particularly useful if infection is present) and be confident of a good cosmetic closure in due course. Transverse incisions are frequently said to be less painful in the postoperative phase and can be useful in upper abdominal surgery if the patient is known to have respiratory disease which may compromise postoperative healing.

Grid-iron incision

See Chapter 6.

Pfannenstiel's incision

This incision is used frequently in gynaecological and urological surgery, but is not often indicated in general surgery. It provides sufficient exposure for most pelvic procedures on the uterus and adnexa and gives excellent cosmetic results. It is very unusual for this incision to result in early or late disruption and hernia

formation. An incision is made in the suprapubic crease just below the hairline. The flaps are dissected upwards and downwards to expose the rectus sheath. The anterior rectus sheaths are divided in the same line and this cut may be extended laterally if more exposure is required. The sheath is reflected upwards. There are occasional vessels on the undersurface which require coagulation. The recti are separated in the midline and retracted laterally. The retroperitoneal tissues are split as far as it is judged appropriate superiorly and down to the pubic symphysis. There is no posterior rectus sheath at this level and extraperitoneal fat and peritoneum are encountered and are opened vertically.

Wound closure

Successful healing by first intention should occur in all laparotomy wounds. Healing relies upon the laying down of scar tissue protein, collagen and optimal conditions. Adequate use of sutures and technique to prevent wound disruption by increased abdominal pressure, due to ileus or coughing, and the avoidance of infection are the two main priorities.

Wounds heal after the initial inflammatory phase by the deposition and orientation of fibrous tissue which is initially rapid but is not complete in a fascial layer until at least 8–10 months have elapsed. It can therefore be argued that it is necessary to 'support' wound apposition for at least that length of time. It would then follow that in the abdominal wall nonabsorbable sutures should always be used. During the first 2–3 weeks, sutures do ensure mechanical support against destructive forces and are critical to the prevention of early wound dehiscence.

Certain factors delay healing in the abdominal wall. The primary cause of abdominal wound failure (burst abdomen) is related to the choice of suture and technique of closure. The cause of incisional hernias is less clear but likely to be associated with secondary factors which are not necessarily surgeon related. Infection is probably the greatest inhibitor of wound healing and nutrition has a role to play. A large wound haematoma prevents the collagen fibres binding together and delays healing and predisposes to infection. Critical attention to haemostasis is essential for good wound healing.

Infection has a variable effect on the dissolution rate of absorbable sutures. Tryptic digestion of catgut is markedly accelerated and this partly accounts for the bad results obtained from this material with abdominal wall closure. Synthetic absorbables are relatively unaffected by the presence of sepsis.

Organisms can lodge in the interstices of braided material and produce an intractable infection which will not subside until the suture is removed or extruded. It is equally apparent that infected wounds which contain monofilament non-absorbables heal even with the sutures *in situ*. Some wounds closed with monofilament can produce small sinuses many years after closure.

Suture materials for abdominal wall wound closure

The most commonly used materials are shown in Table 1.1 (page 4). Monofilament synthetic sutures are more popular because there is a smaller risk of wound infection following their use. There is probably no advantage in closing fat dead space with catgut. There is a marked tissue reaction to catgut, made worse when there has been contamination following open viscus operations. Braided materials risk the migration of bacteria along their length in the wound by capillary action.

Technique of abdominal wall closure

Proper and careful closure of the abdominal wall is essential. The incision should be closed in such a way that healing becomes sound and the complications of infection, undue pain and abdominal disruption should be reduced. The abdominal wall functions as a dynamic corset and in respiration, defaecation and micturition it is subject to more destructive forces than any other part of the body. Additional pressure increasing intra-abdominal disruptive forces (coughing and straining) provides extra distracting tension on a laparotomy wound. Wound closure must have sufficient strength to withstand these forces and keep edges opposed until, in the fullness of time, intrinsic strength is restored. Sutures must be inserted in such a manner that they do not cut out but grip the tissues in a most advantageous way.

Wound failures (burst abdomens or incisional hernias) can be due to poor technique; for example, broken sutures, knot slippage or the suture cutting out. A discharge of serosanguinous fluid in the early postoperative period heralds failure of the wound. Peritoneal discharge is appearing and if this 'pink sign' occurs the wound should be resutured, rather than packed. This usually occurs between the sixth and tenth postoperative day. Incisional hernia appearing within weeks or months of the operation usually represents a covert dehiscence where the skin was the only layer to heal. Later incisional hernias probably result from wound sepsis and most clinical reviews estimate an incidence of 5–10%

To reduce the force per unit area at the suture/ tissue interface, big bites of relatively coarse material are required to ensure that sutures are placed outside the biochemically active lytic zone. Number 1 metric gauge inserted at least 1 cm back from the wound edge is suitable. It should penetrate all fascial and muscular layers of the abdominal wall, which are usually about 1 cm thick. The peritoneal layer is probably unimportant and the exact anatomical apposition of each layer probably does not allow an adequately large bite to be taken to remove the risk to underlying viscera. Abdominal wounds probably

lengthen during postoperative abdominal distension and suture length to length of wound should be in a ratio of over 4:1. This should prevent wound failure. Small bites taken in a ratio of less than 2.5:1 place wounds at risk.

In layered closure it has been traditional to close the peritoneum with catgut or dexon and the anterior muscular and aponeurotic layers with a stronger material such as absorbable polydioxanone or nylon.

Mass closure

Mass closure (Figure 5.5) may be used in all abdominal incisions except those made by splitting muscles along different lines, for example, gridiron incision for appendicectomy. There are now many clinical trials which testify to the success of mass closure with an acceptably low risk of wound failure. Mass closure should take all layers of the musculo-aponeurotic abdominal wall with at least 1 cm bites placed 1 cm apart. The sutures can be placed either continuously or interrupted and there does not appear to be any suggestion that one is more effective than the other. The advantage of a continuous suture is speed. Those who support interrupted closure believe it to be intrinsically more secure.

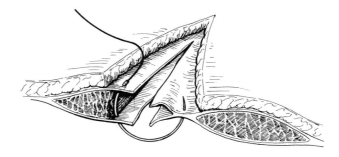

Figure 5.5 Taking large bites in mass closure (From Dudley, 1983, by permission)

A large 5/8 hand needle facilitates mass closure, and the peritoneal layer as previously mentioned does not need to be incorporated. The different types of suture material are given in Table 1.1. It is important that the skin is sutured separately. The viscera can be protected by the operator's non-dominant hand while taking a wide bite. A simple over and over technique using continuous mass suture is probably the most popular method. Tension sutures inserted prior to closing all layers or after posterior layering closure may be added to give additional security. This security is hypothetical! Tension sutures are cosmetically unacceptable, make siting of stomas difficult, and increase postoperative pain.

Skin closure

Skin closure will depend on the preference of the

individual surgeon. Vertical mattress sutures produce eversion of the skin edges and are preferred by some surgeons, particularly for transverse wounds. Monofilament sutures are generally preferred and subcuticular sutures are becoming increasingly popular. A continuous suture technique is usual, and absorbable or non-absorbable materials may be used. The non-absorbable polypropylene suture is easy to insert since it glides smoothly through the tissue, can be anchored at an appropriate tension with beads and metal collars at each end of the wound and is easily withdrawn when the wound no longer requires suture support.

Steel clips were a vogue for closing skin but are used less commonly for abdominal closure than at other sites. Recent evidence suggests that a subcuticular closure is less prone to wound infection and is particularly useful in vascular surgery with compromised ischaemic tissues.

Delayed primary closure

A wound which has been heavily contaminated can be left open so conditions for bacterial growth are unfavourable; for example, following surgery for generalized faecal or purulent peritonitis. If the wound is 'clean' after 3–4 days, it may be closed without delay. If the wound is dirty, it can heal by secondary intention or be closed formally when it is clean. Subsequent closure of the abdominal wall is made in the usual manner.

In patients who may require repeated re-exploration of the abdomen and free drainage of purulent peritoneal exudate, the technique of leaving the abdomen completely open or suturing a sheet of polypropylene mesh has been developed. The use of a zip-fastener incorporated in the mesh enables relaparotomy as required.

Acknowledgement

The authors freely acknowledge the contribution made by Professor Hugh Dudley in the original writing of this chapter which facilitated and eased their subsequent update and rewrite.

Reference

Dudley, H. A. (1983) *Rob and Smith's Operative Surgery: Alimentary Tract and Abdominal Wall*, Vol. 1, 4th edn, Butterworths, London

6

Hernias of the abdominal wall and pelvis, incisional hernias and parastomal herniation

H. B. Devlin and S. Nicholson

This chapter deals with the common abdominal wall hernias (excluding groin herniation) and some of the rarer varieties including lumbar, obturator and Spigelian and considers the important problem of incisional herniation and hernias related to intestinal and urinary stomas.

Umbilical hernia in infants and children

Minor degrees of umbilical hernias are present in many neonates, but most can be expected to resolve spontaneously. It is reported to be more common among Negro than white European children (James, 1982). The incidence among newborn in the UK who subsequently require surgery has been estimated to be less that 3 per 1000 live births (Devlin, 1988).

The hernia forms a small protrusion through the umbilical cicatrix which becomes more prominent when the child strains or cries. It contains a small peritoneal sac with a narrow neck through the linea alba. These hernias rarely become irreducible or strangulate, but they are a source of concern to the parents. All undergo spontaneous reduction in size as the child grows and very few persist beyond puberty. Unusually large hernias, those with a neck diameter greater than 1.5 cm and those failing to regress before school age, should be repaired.

If surgery is required, the recommended method is the Mayo operation. The umbilical cicatrix should always be preserved. Children with umbilical hernias should be treated as day cases (see Chapter 8).

A curved transverse incision is made below the umbilicus. The umbilical cicatrix is dissected upwards on a flap to face the hernial sac. It is often possible to reduce the contents of an infantile umbilical hernia without enlarging the opening in the linea alba, but if required transverse incisions are made into the rectus sheath.

A double-breasting repair (Mayo) is performed as in adults, but using a metric 3 polydioxanone (PDS) suture.

Adult umbilical hernia

These hernias occur with equal frequency in both sexes. They occur much less commonly than inguinal hernias, with an incidence of approximately 5 per 100 000 per year (Devlin, 1982). Umbilical hernia is uncommon before the age of 40 except as a complication of cirrhotic or malignant ascites or continuous ambulatory peritoneal dialysis (CAPD), the hernia being a consequence of raised intra-abdominal pressure. The hernia is always progressive and may attain a huge size.

Umbilical hernias usually contain omentum, sometimes transverse colon and occasionally small intestine and even stomach. The coverings of the hernia – skin, superficial fascia, rectus sheath, transversalis fascia and peritoneum – may become very thin and excoriated, leading to ulceration. Gangrene may occur over more dependent parts.

The neck is narrow in comparison to the size of the hernia and the contents usually adhere to each other, to the peritoneum of the fundus and in particular to the omentum. As a consequence, umbilical hernias are often irreducible.

Clinical features

Most patients seek treatment because of the painful protrusion at the umbilicus. Irreducibility is not an absolute indication for surgery and other risk factors such as ischaemic heart disease, obesity and diabetes should be evaluated. As far as possible these factors should be controlled prior to elective surgery which is usually recommended. Strangulation and obstruction are common complications and urgent surgery, after careful resuscitation, is required. In these circumstances, surgery is associated with high mortality.

The repair of massive hernias may result in respiratory and circulatory problems. The return of abdominal contents for which there is no intraperitoneal accommodation causes a marked elevation of intra-abdominal pressure, interfering with blood flow through abdominal veins, particularly the iliac veins and inferior vena cava, and with diaphragmatic movement. In these circumstances the induction of a pneumoperitoneum preoperatively may be used to enlarge the peritoneal cavity and render subsequent reduction of the hernial contents easier (Cauldirouis et al., 1990)

The operation

The method which has stood the test of time was first

described by William Mayo in 1898 (Mayo, 1901). The operation is best performed under general anaesthesia with full muscle relaxation. In smaller hernias, a semilunar incision is made beneath the umbilical cicatrix which is raised on the superior skin flap and mobilized off the hernia. In large hernias with distension, excoriation or ulceration of the overlying skin, the umbilical cicatrix is best excised by marking two semilunar incisions around the hernia (Figure 6.1). The incisions meet lateral to the bulge of the hernia and can be enlarged as far laterally as necessary to give adequate exposure. The hernia is separated from the subcutaneous tissues until the neck is identified. The anterior rectus sheath is cleared of subcutaneous fat for a radius of 3 cm around the neck of the hernia.

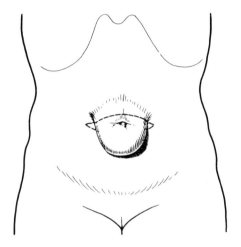

Figure 6.1 Two semilunar incisions are made around the hernia

The sac is opened near its neck where adhesions are least likely to be present and protruding bowel is returned. Omentum may sometimes be excised to lessen the volume of contents to be reduced. The whole sac along with any adherent overlying skin is excised. The opening in the abdominal wall is then enlarged laterally on either side for about 4 cm, taking care not to injure the epigastric vessels as the posterior rectus sheath is divided (Figure 6.2).

The repair is performed using strong non-absorbable suture material (metric 4 polypropylene or metric 3.5 nylon) on atraumatic needles. Interrupted sutures are placed through all layers of the upper flap from the outside 2–3 cm from the margin. The suture then picks up all layers of the lower flap, again about 2–3 cm from its margin, before being passed back through the upper flap from inside to out. When all these mattress sutures have been placed they are tied firmly down to bring the upper flap in front of the lower flap (Figure 6.3). The repair is completed by suturing the lower free edge of the upper flap to the front of the lower flap with a continuous suture of the same material used in the first part of the repair.

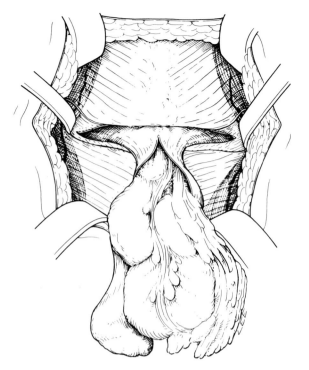

Figure 6.2 The deficit in the abdominal wall is enlarged laterally for 4 cm on either side; the rectus muscles are retracted to make this possible

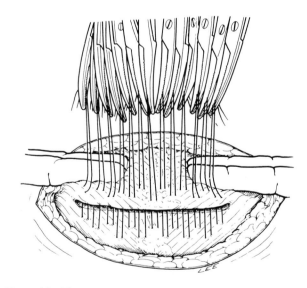

Figure 6.3 The sutures in the upper flap are all placed. The upper flap is now 'railroaded' down onto the lower flap

The subcutaneous tissues are closed with interrupted absorbable synthetic sutures after careful haemostasis. Closed suction drains are employed if the hernia was large or if bowel was resected, and prophylactic peroperative antibiotics are given to cover intestinal Gram-negative and anaerobic organisms. The skin is closed with a subcuticular suture of PDS.

Epigastric hernia

Epigastric hernia may occur in older children and adults. It is due to a protrusion of extraperitoneal fat between the decussating fibres of the linea alba. It usually occurs in the midline between the xiphisternum and umbilicus, but may occasionally protrude laterally into the rectus sheath. These hernias are usually small, but if large may develop a peritoneal sac.

Epigastric hernias may give rise to symptoms out of all proportion to their size which may mimic symptoms of other gastrointestinal disorders such as peptic ulceration or cholelithiasis. In symptomatic patients these conditions should be excluded by endoscopy and ultrasound before epigastric hernia repair. Excision of the hernial sac and repair of the defect in the linea alba are curative. This can be performed under general or local anaesthesia with lignocaine or bupivacaine as a day-case procedure. A Mayo-type repair is the most suitable method, using polypropylene sutures in adults or PDS in children. A transverse skin incision gives the best cosmetic result.

Obturator hernia

First described in 1724 by Arnaud de Ronsil, this condition still carries a high operative mortality because of diagnostic difficulties in an elderly population. It is six times more common in women than men and three times more common over the age of 50. Right-sided hernias are twice as common as those on the left. It is more frequent in Chinese than European or Negro people. The usual patient is an elderly woman who has recently lost weight rapidly and it should be particularly suspected if there is a history of recurrent small bowel obstruction (Craig, 1962).

The hernia is a protrusion of peritoneum through the obturator canal, a fibro-osseous channel between the obturator groove of the lower surface of the superior pubic ramus and the upper border of the obturator membrane which separates the obturator internus and externus muscles. This channel transmits the obturator nerve and vessels (Figure 6.4). Fifty per cent of hernias present with groin discomfort and pain or paraesthesiae radiating to the knee, caused by pressure on the adjacent nerve.

Emerging from the obturator canal the hernia comes into contact with the deep surface of the pectineus. It then protrudes forwards between pectineus and adductor longus to enter the femoral triangle where it can be mistaken for a femoral hernia.

The sac usually contains small intestine, rarely caecum or sigmoid colon, or ovary and fallopian tube. A partial enterocele (Richter's hernia) is often found, the rigid margins of the obturator membrane making early strangulation inevitable. The hernia often does not present until strangulation occurs and

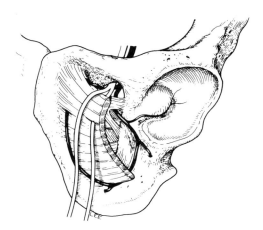

Figure 6.4   The obturator canal transmits the obturator vessels and nerve

even then the cause of the strangulation may not be obvious until after the abdomen has been explored. A telltale sign is an area of bruising over the hernia sac in the thigh (Devlin, 1988). Vaginal examination confirms the diagnosis, a tender mass being felt in the obturator region (Figure 6.5). Rectal examination is unhelpful because the obturator foramen is not palpable per rectum.

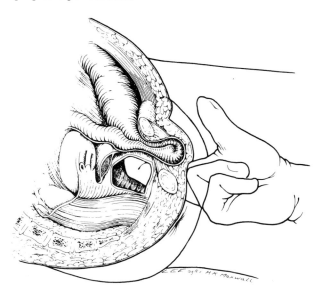

Figure 6.5   Obturator hernia is palpable on vaginal examination

Resuscitation should be carried out preoperatively if the hernia is strangulated, the bladder catheterized and prophylactic antibiotics given. The abdomen is explored through a lower paramedian incision under general anaesthesia with muscle relaxation.

If the hernia cannot be reduced by gentle traction, the constricting ring should be stretched with the index finger. If this is still not sufficient the contents may be aspirated through a long needle or the obturator membrane divided, taking care not to injure the obturator neurovascular bundle which lies posterolaterally, by making the incision in an upward and medial direction. Once the hernia has been reduced the viability of the contents are inspected and non-viable bowel resected. The sac of the hernia is invaginated, transfixed and excised. Usually the defect is small and no formal repair is used. If the defect is large an extraperitoneal patch of mesh can be placed and the peritoneum closed over it.

An alternative approach to an obturator hernia, useful if a diagnosis is made preoperatively, is the extraperitoneal approach as used for femoral or recurrent inguinal hernias. Again, repair with mesh placed in the extraperitoneal plane is recommended.

Semilunar line (Spigelian) hernia

Named after Adriaan van Spieghel, 1578–1625, who described the semilunar line, Spigelian hernias occur through slit-like defects in the anterior abdominal wall adjacent to the semilunar line at the lateral edge of the rectus muscle. Herniation is rare cephalad to the umbilicus. Below the umbilicus the rectus sheath is deficient and Spigelian hernias occur most commonly in this region.

The hernial ring is a defect in the transversus aponeurosis. The sac is often interparietal (interstitial) passing through the transversus and internal oblique aponeuroses and then spreading out beneath the intact external oblique aponeurosis or lying in the rectus sheath alongside the rectus muscle.

Spigelian hernias are most frequent in middle-aged adults and more common in women than men (1.5:1). The incidence has been estimated to be about 0.1% of all abdominal hernias (Stuckej *et al.*, 1973). They often cause diagnostic confusion, but where the diagnosis is suspected scanning of the abdominal wall with ultrasound is recommended (Spangen, 1984). The clinical features include a lump which aches more as the day goes on and disappears when the patient lies down in bed. The pain in the lump is exacerbated by raising the arm on the ipsilateral side above the head. The hernia may contain small or large bowel or omentum. Richter's type strangulation is reported, the sharp fascial margins of the aperture causing early pressure necrosis. For this reason, operation is advised for all cases.

General anaesthesia is preferred, but local infiltration anaesthesia can be used. An oblique incision is made directly over the hernia and the aponeuroses split in the line of their fibres to gain access to the sac. The sac is opened, the contents reduced and the neck transfixed or closed with a purse-string suture according to size. Redundant sac is excised. The deep and then the superficial layers of aponeurosis are separately closed with continuous polypropylene sutures (Figure 6.6). Alternatively, an overlapping Mayo-

type repair can be used. Closed suction drainage should be used.

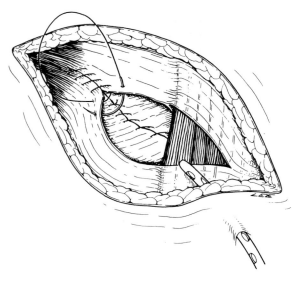

Figure 6.6 The deep and then the superficial layers of aponeurosis are separately closed with continuous sutures of polypropylene. A suction drain is always used.

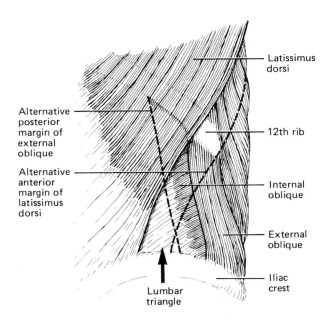

Figure 6.7 The boundaries of the lumbar triangle. The attachments of the external oblique muscle and latissimus dorsi to the iliac crest are variable, hence the dimensions of the lumbar triangle and the possibility of herniation vary

Lumbar hernia

This variety may be either congenital or acquired, following renal surgery, lumbar abscess or paralysis of the lateral lumbar muscles as a result of poliomyelitis or spina bifida. 'Congenital' lumbar hernias occur through two anatomical points of weakness in the lumbar region: (a) the lumbar triangle of Petit, bounded inferiorly by the iliac crest, posteriorly by the latissimus dorsi and anteriorly by the external oblique muscles (Figure 6.7); and (b) the superior (quadrilateral) lumbar space, bounded by the twelfth rib, lower border of serratus posterior inferior, anterior border of erector spinae and the internal oblique.

The neck of the hernia is usually wide and the sac, which is usually reducible, may contain right or left colon or omentum. If the defect is small and in healthy tissues it may be repaired directly with polypropylene sutures. A large hernia, particularly where the surrounding tissues are poor, requires repair using a prosthetic mesh placed in the extraperitoneal plane.

Gluteal and sciatic hernia

Gluteal hernias protrude through the greater sciatic notch; sciatic hernias pass through the lesser sciatic notch. Both are extremely rare and are only discovered during the course of a laparotomy performed for the relief of intestinal obstruction of unknown cause. Rarely, a palpable swelling, tenderness in the buttock or pain referred along the sciatic nerve may suggest the diagnosis.

At laparotomy through a lower paramedian incision, the distended loop of intestine is traced down to its entry in the sciatic opening which, in the female, is situated behind the broad ligament. Gentle traction on the gut will usually reduce the strangulation. The sac is inverted, if possible, transfixed and excised.

Pelvic hernia

These hernias may occur as a late complication of vaginal hysterectomy or, more commonly, after abdominoperineal resection of the rectum.

A 'false' pelvic hernia is the protrusion of peritoneum which may accompany a cystocele, rectocele or rectal prolapse. This is a variety of sliding hernia. A 'true' pelvic or vaginal hernia or hernia of the pouch of Douglas may occur spontaneously in the multiparous woman or, more commonly, as a result of trauma of childbirth. The hernia protrudes into the posterior vaginal wall and vulva and may be differentiated from a rectocele by a synchronous vaginal and rectal examination. A 'lateral' pelvic hernia occurs through a gap in the line of origin of the levator ani from the obturator fascia – a persistent hiatus of Schwalbe. Such a hernia may appear in the ischiorectal fossa or labium majora (pudendal hernia).

Internal hernia

Several varieties have been described and are all rare. They present as recurrent vomiting or acute small

bowel obstruction rapidly progressing to strangulation. In the case of chronic symptoms, the diagnosis can be made by small bowel contrast radiology but in the acute presentation the diagnosis is only made at laparotomy.

They occur into:

1. The lesser sac through either the foramen of Winslow, a congenital defect in the transverse mesocolon or postoperatively alongside the loops of a posterior gastroenterostomy or retrocolic gastrectomy. Strangulation of the afferent loop in these hernias can be confused with acute pancreatitis.
2. Paraduodenal fossae, often associated with anomalies of midgut rotation. In a left paraduodenal hernia the neck of the hernia is formed by the peritoneal fold containing the inferior mesenteric vein and ascending branch of the left colic artery. In the inferior duodenal hernia (Treitz) the neck is formed by the transverse peritoneal fold which runs from the duodenojejunal flexure. The mesentericoparietal hernia (Waldeyer) enters the sac from the left behind the mesentery with the third part of the duodenum above and the superior mesenteric artery in front. Retroduodenal hernias pass from right to left behind the ascending fourth part of the duodenum.
3. Mesenteric defects in the distal ileum, which may be multiple and usually present as small bowel obstruction. Reduction and simple closure of the defect is all that is required.
4. Paracaecal fossa, the best known of which lies behind the 'bloodless' fold of Treves.
5. Intersigmoid space – a potential sac between the two limbs of the sigmoid colon.
6. The rectovesical space. Such supravesical hernias are usually associated with recent weight loss and occur more frequently in males. The neck is a triangular space bounded by the median umbilical ligament (obliterated urachus), lateral umbilical ligament (obliterated umbilical artery) and the reflection of peritoneum onto the fundus of the bladder. They present with small bowel obstruction.
7. Defects in the broad ligament as a complication of gynaecological operations in elderly women where the tubes and ovaries have been preserved.

Management

When the sac is large necked, reduction is no problem and strangulation is rare. Sacs with a narrow neck generally have important structures in their margins which cannot be divided, e.g. the portal structures at the foramen of Winslow. If the hernia is strangulated and irreducible, the distended bowel should have its contents aspirated through a needle prior to reduction. Simple closure of the neck prevents recurrence.

Table 6.1 Incisional hernia: initial operative procedures

Procedure	Akman (1962) Total no., 500 patients (%)	Ponka (1980) Total no., 794 patients (%)	Devlin (1982) Total no., 214 patients (%)
Hysterectomy and other gynaecological interventions	18.6	34	19
Cholecystectomy and biliary tract operations	9.6	21	11
Appendicectomy	43.8	16	16
Colorectal operations*	7.6	9	9
Gastric operations	4.2	11	30
Caesarean section	4.2	2	12

* Colorectal operations are not defined separately by Akman: the figure quoted is the sum of 'laparotomy other than specified' and 'non-specified (i.e. non-urological and non-gynaecological) pelvic operations'.

Incisional hernia

The increasing incidence of incisional hernia is probably an indication of more frequent abdominal surgical intervention. With the introduction of high-quality suture materials this problem is nearly always a failure of surgical technique. It can be defined as 'a bulge visible and palpable when the patient is standing, often requiring support or repair' (Leaper *et al.*, 1977) and is a diffuse extrusion of peritoneum and abdominal contents through a weak scar following an abdominal operation or penetrating wound.

The incidence is difficult to define accurately since asymptomatic patients are not referred, but may be as high as 6% at 5 years and 12% at 10 years. Incisional hernias occur slightly more frequently in males that females (55:45) (Ellis *et al.*, 1983; Mudge and Hughes, 1985). There is little doubt that the number of incisional hernias coming to operation is lower than their overall incidence. More than half can be expected to appear later than 1 year after the initial operation, by which time most patients have been discharged from follow-up in routine clinical practice. Some operations have a notorious reputation, for instance gynaecological and gastric procedures, but a high incidence has been reported after appendicectomy, particularly in earlier series (Table 6.1).

Aetiology of incisional hernia

Risk factors for the development of incisional herniation can be broadly divided into two groups: technical failure by the surgeon and tissue failure by the patient.

Technical factors

1. Postoperative haematoma, necrosis and sepsis. Sixty per cent of patients developing an incisional hernia within the first year after surgery have had significant wound infection. Devitalized tissue in wounds and wound haematoma both predispose to sepsis.
2. Faulty closure technique. The use of absorbable suture materials for the closure of abdominal aponeuroses must be avoided. Catgut alone is totally unacceptable. Newer absorbable polymers such as polyglactin 910 (Vicryl) and polyglycolic acid (Dexon) are less good than non-absorbable sutures. Early results with the longer life polymer polydioxanone (PDS) appear promising, but the characteristics of wound healing and suture degradation would suggest, at least in theory, that even these new polymers are unsuitable (see Chapter 8).

   The taking of too small bites and failure of the surgical knot are important technical factors. An adequate length of suture material compared with the length of the wound must be used. This latter point reflects the depth of 'bites' taken and the distance between them: the deeper the bites and the closer they are together the longer the length of suture material which will be used (Jenkins, 1976).
3. Placement of drains or stomas in wounds. Particularly notorious are capillary drains, as these allow potentially infected fluids to drain around them, thus infecting the wound. Ponka (1980) records that of 126 patients with herniation through a subcostal incision for biliary surgery, all had had drains delivered through the wound at the time of the initial operation. Intestinal stomas placed within the main wound invariably lead to wound infection with its attendant risk of subsequent herniation.
4. Choice of incision. Midline incisions are at greater risk than paramedian incisions (Ausobsky *et al.*, 1985) (Table 6.2). The revival of interest in the 'lateral paramedian' incision with its considerably lower risk of wound failure should decrease the incidence of incisional herniation (Donaldson *et al.*, 1982).

Table 6.2 Site of incisional hernias

Site	Akman (1962) n = 500 (%)	Ponka (1980) n = 794 (%)
Midline		
lower abdomen	33	26
upper abdomen	5.4	16
Subcostal: right and left	–	16
Paramedian: right and left	9.6	11
Transverse and muscle-splitting right lower quadrant: McBurney, etc.	21	9
Peristomal	–	4
Vertical:		
right upper quadrant	–	4
right lower quadrant	–	3
Vertical: midline xiphoid to pubis	–	11

Tissue factors

1. Age is an important factor and incisional hernias are infrequent under the age of 40 years.
2. Immunosuppression. Any factor or disease which reduces the efficacy of the immune response increases the risk of incisional herniation. Diabetes mellitus is an important cause, as between 0.5% and 1% of the population is affected. Jaundice, renal failure and treatment with corticosteroids also impair wound healing and predispose to herniation.
3. Obesity is an important risk factor both for the occurrence of the original incisional hernia and for the likelihood of recurrence of the hernia after repair (Pitkin, 1976; Bucknall *et al.*, 1982). The obese, elderly diabetic is at particular risk.
4. Malignant disease. Many factors contribute to poor wound healing in patients with malignancy, increasing their risk of incisional herniation. Malnutrition, hypoalbuminaemia, anaemia and advanced age are all associated with gastrointestinal and gynaecological malignancies.
5. Late development of incisional hernia is unrelated to the original suture used for wound closure; it appears to be a collagen failure (Mudge and Hughes, 1985). A satisfactory explanation of why mature collagen should yield to form a hernia so long after healing has occurred is not available, although the concept of metastatic emphysema may offer an explanation (Cannon and Read, 1981)

Indications for surgery

Small, asymptomatic bulges in elderly patients do not require repair. Symptoms of discomfort and pain or recurrent colic when episodes of subacute intestinal obstruction occur are the main indications for surgical referral. Many patients request repair for cosmetic reasons. Irreducibility and a narrow-necked hernia are indications for more urgent surgery, whereas obstruction and strangulation are an absolute indication.

Contraindications to elective surgery

These include extreme obesity, which makes operation difficult and increases the risk of recurrence, as well as thromboembolic and cardiorespiratory complications. Continuing deep sepsis in the wound should be treated before a definitive attempt at repair is made. This will often entail removal of foreign material inserted at previous repair attempts. On occasions, the skin wound will need to be left open and allowed to heal by granulation. Only when the wound has been without deep sepsis for some months should repair surgery be undertaken. The skin also should be in good condition before the definitive repair and this may necessitate vigorous preoperative treatment of skin infections and intertrigo beneath large incisional hernias.

Principles of repair

1. Reconstitution of the normal anatomy. The linea alba must be repaired in midline hernias, and in local hernias a layer-by-layer closure is required.
2. Repair of only tendinous, aponeurotic or fascial structures. *In situ* darning over the defect without adequate mobilization gives a 100% recurrence rate (Harding *et al.*, 1983).
3. Only non-absorbable suture materials must be used.
4. Use deep bites at not more than 5 mm intervals to achieve a ratio of suture length to wound length of not less than 4:1 (Jenkins, 1980).
5. Reduction of weight prior to surgery in obese patients.
6. Minimal handling of viscera to prevent postoperative abdominal distension caused by adynamic ileus.

7. Improvement in respiratory status preoperatively by stopping smoking, and giving physiotherapy to clear bronchial secretion to reduce postoperative coughing.
8. Meticulous aseptic technique.

Incisional hernias following appendicectomy are reported in all series (Table 6.1). Severe postoperative wound sepsis, the placement of drains through the wound and destruction of the rectus sheath when the wound is extended medially to improve exposure are aetiological factors. These hernias are difficult to repair, as they occur through the muscle fibres, and unless an adequate overlap can be constructed they often recur. When the tissues are inadequate a prosthetic mesh should be used to reinforce the external oblique aponeurosis. Management of giant incisional hernia is often compromised by obesity, intrahernial adhesions and contraction in the volume of the abdominal cavity. Forceful replacement of viscera into an adequate abdominal cavity can lead to ileus, pulmonary restriction and cardiac embarrassment. In such cases the establishment of a progressive pneumoperitoneum with nitrous oxide prior to operation greatly facilitates the hernia repair. Insufflation is carried out either through a Verres needle inserted under local anaesthetic or through a peritoneal catheter left in place for the duration of the treatment. Between 1000 ml and 1500 ml nitrous oxide is introduced at each session (48 h apart) over a 1–2-week period (Cauldirouis *et al.*, 1990). The end point is judged by the tension of the abdominal wall, which should feel as tight as a drum, especially in the flanks.

Choice of technique

Several operative techniques are available and the choice depends on the size of the hernia and the presenting symptoms. The sac and its fibrous margins should be examined with the patient standing and supine and with the abdomen relaxed and tensed (Figure 6.8). In some hernias, particularly upper midline ones, the margins of the defect close together on movement and the contraction of the abdominal wall will then hold the sac reduced. If the margins close when the patient tenses the muscle, an 'anatomical' repair is appropriate. If a defect remains when the muscles are tensed, a prosthesis should be inserted. Prostheses may be placed superficial to the muscles or deep to them in the extraperitoneal plane. This latter, the 'French operation', has considerable advantages.

The operation

The patient is placed supine on the operating table and general anaesthesia with full muscle relaxation is employed for larger hernias. In patients with large hernias and poor respiratory reserve, postoperative pain control in the first 48–72 h is ideally achieved using thoracic epidural anaesthesia.

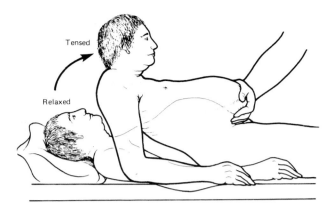

Figure 6.8 Examination of an incisional hernia. The anatomy of the sac must be known. The patient is examined laid and relaxed, and with the muscles tensed. Do the margins of the sac close or open during activity? Is there a tissue defect?

Redundant skin and scar tissue are separated from the underlying sac and excised. Care is needed to prevent damage to the hernia contents which may be adherent over wide areas of the inside of the sac. The edge of the abdominal wall defect is carefully defined and an elliptical incision made around the defect where scar tissue merges with the abdominal wall aponeurosis (Figure 6.9).

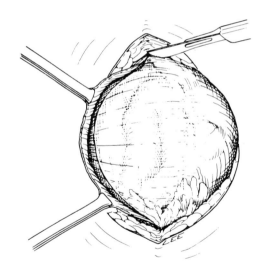

Figure 6.9 The peritoneal sac is defined at its neck; this clearly identifies the aponeurotic defect

When there has been no history of intestinal obstruction and where the sac is large, diffuse and pendulous but the margins of the defect can be approximated, the keel repair is ideal, in which case the sac is not opened. When the sac needs to be opened and explored, this is performed close to its neck to avoid damage to the contents which are usually most adherent at the fundus of the sac. Viable bowel is freed and returned to the peritoneal cavity. If the sac is closely adherent to bowel, particularly the large bowel, no attempt should be made to dissect it free. Devitalized small bowel can be resected with primary anastomosis. Strangulated colon should be resected, the proximal end brought out as a colostomy and the distal end as a mucous fistula, both well away from the main wound. Peroperative antibiotic prophylaxis should be given. Omentum of doubtful viability is excised. Following excision of the redundant portion of the sac the peritoneum is closed with a continuous absorbable polymer. A closed suction drain is placed down to this layer.

Keel operation

The unopened peritoneal sac is gradually inverted with a series of continuous sutures of absorbable polymer, taking great care not to puncture adherent underlying bowel. Further layers are inserted until the fibro-aponeurotic margins of the defect are approximated (Figure 6.10). A closed suction drain is placed along this suture line. The fibro-aponeurotic layer is now sutured over the drain as in the layer-by-layer closure.

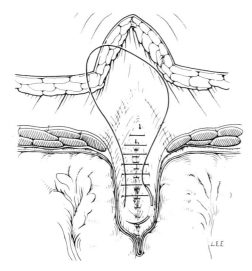

Figure 6.10 The keel operation, stage 2

Closure of aponeurotic layer

This technique is applicable only when the edges of the defect can be approximated. It is used in the keel operation and the layer-by-layer closure after the redundant sac has been excised and the peritoneum closed. The edge of the defect must be dissected until normal aponeurosis and not scar tissue is identified. Then the full thickness of the margins are approximated using a mass closure technique.

Monofilament non-absorbable suture (polypropylene or steel) is started at each end of the defect taking big bites (2.5 cm from edge) with short intervals (0.5 cm) (Figure 6.11). At least two layers of sutures are inserted and when completed the defect in the aponeurosis should resemble a very closely meshed darn

(Figure 6.12). A further suction drain is placed to this layer and meticulous haemostasis obtained in the subcutaneous tissues before closing the fat with interrupted absorbable sutures. The skin is closed with subcuticular PDS.

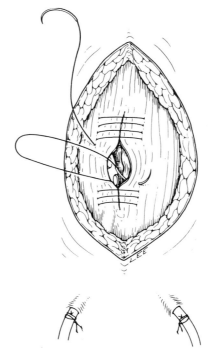

Figure 6.11 Closure of the aponeurosis, suturing from each end simultaneously to distribute the load. Notice the drains

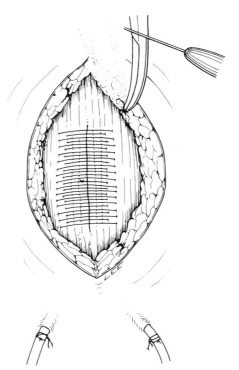

Figure 6.12 When completed, this type of darn repair needs checking for meticulous haemostasis

Postoperatively, early active mobilization is encouraged. In the keel operation or the layer-by-layer closure if there has been little handling of the intestine, nasogastric tubes and intravenous drips should not be necessary. Suction drains should be removed after 24–48 h.

Prosthetic mesh repair – extramuscular onlay technique

This technique is recommended for larger hernias where a large tissue defect can be demonstrated. The sac is handled either by excision or imbrication, as in the keel operation. The prosthesis (polypropylene mesh or expanded PTFE) is used to repair the defect in the anterior rectus sheath (Figure 6.13). The prosthesis should be sufficiently large to overlap the defect by at least 4 cm laterally and 2 cm at each end. The prosthesis is sutured to the anterior rectus sheath with multiple non-absorbable sutures. An alternative technique of inserting the prosthesis is to suture the mesh in two halves to each side of the defect with continuous polypropylene sutures (Figure 6.14). The defect is then closed by suturing the medial edge of each half of the mesh together (Figure 6.15).

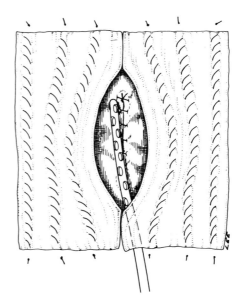

Figure 6.14 Fine suction drainage is always used

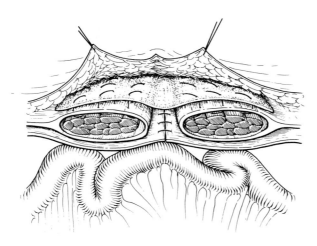

Figure 6.13 Repair using a mesh onlay

Prosthetic mesh repair – the French operation

The principle is to place a very large layer of prosthesis in the extraperitoneal plane, between the peritoneum and the parietal muscles. The mesh is held in position by the intra-abdominal pressure and the parieties, like ham in a sandwich. The mesh must extend laterally at least to the anterior axillary line, down into the pelvis to cover the myofascial orifices in the groin (inguinal and femoral) and sufficiently cephalid to overlap the margins of any hernia defect by 4 cm. The hernia is approached and the margins of the sac dissected away from the fibrous ring in the muscle defect. The extraperitoneal plane is then developed in each direction and down into the pelvis. A

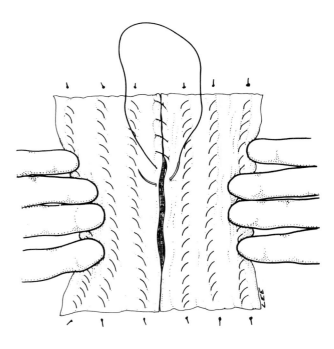

Figure 6.15 The two halves of the mesh are sutured together at the correct tension

large piece of mesh is cut with a lower V-shaped margin to go to the pelvis and an upper V-shaped margin to overlap the defect – a 'double chevron' (Figure 6.16). A series of stab wounds is made on either side of the abdomen and through these sutures are passed into the prosthesis. For a major defect 4–6 sutures are needed on either side of the abdomen. The sutures are held loose at this stage. Sutures are placed in the pelvis to the pectineal line. When all the sutures

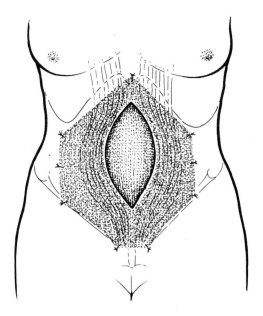

Figure 6.16 A large piece of mesh is cut so that it overlaps the margins of the defect by at least 2 cm, or over 3 cm if possible – the larger the overlap the better. The mesh should be cut with a chevron shape to go down into the pelvis behind the pubis and inguinal ligaments, and above with an inverted chevron so that it fits up to the costal margin

are positioned the mesh is slid into place and the sutures tied to hold it in position (Figures 6.17A and 6.17B). Suction drains are placed through puncture wounds to prevent any accumulation in the extraperitoneal layer. If there is a big defect, the margins of it are fixed to the prosthesis. Finally, the abdomen and all the skin wounds are closed (Stoppa, 1987; Wantz, 1989, 1991).

Results of incisional hernia repair

In the largest series, the Shouldice Clinic reports excellent results using a layered stainless steel wire technique with a 1.6% recurrence rate (Ackman, 1962), but others have reported recurrence rates as high as 46% using keel or mass closure techniques (George and Ellis, 1986). Recurrence rates with prosthetic mesh replacement are superior (10%) (Usher, 1979) and perhaps surgeons in the UK should use this technique more frequently.

Parastomal hernia

Parastomal hernias complicate at least 10% of colostomies and ileostomies (Burgess *et al.*, 1984; Lubbers and Devlin, 1984) and the incidence of para-ileal conduit hernias is similar in urological practice. The problem is greater in patients with transverse loop colostomies, 20% of whom develop hernial complication (Devlin, 1988). The presence of a large protru-

sion related to a stoma may necessitate repair irrespective of hernial complications because it may make the stoma impossible to manage.

The risk of stomal herniation is reduced if the stoma is brought out through the rectus muscle and greatest when brought out laterally through the fleshy flank muscles. The worst parastomal hernias occur when the stoma is brought out through the laparotomy incision.

Four anatomical varieties of stomal hernia are described:

1. Interstitial – the hernial sac lies within the layers of the abdominal wall and distorts the stoma which becomes asymmetrical. The vascular supply of the stoma may be compromised.
2. Subcutaneous – the hernial sac lies alongside the stoma and protrudes into the subcutaneous space. This is the commonest form of paracolostomy hernia.
3. Intrastomal – a problem only of spout ileostomies, the sac entering the potential space between the emergent and the everted layer of the stoma.
4. Perstomal or prolapse – this can affect all stomas, but transverse loop colostomies are the most notorious, prolapsing three times more frequently than any other stoma. A prolapsed stoma contains hernial sac within itself but other viscera, especially the small intestine, can enter the sac and become strangulated.

Careful placement of stomas and the correction of nutritional problems prior to elective surgery will help reduce the incidence of stomal herniation. Prior to

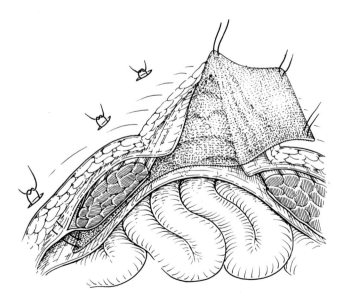

Figure 6.17A A series of tiny stab wounds is made 2 cm or more from the margins of the defect. Sutures are passed through each stab wound, through the full thickness of the abdominal wall and through the mesh. The lowermost sutures should pick up the pectineal ligament and the mesh. The sutures are held in clips and not tied until all the sutures are in position

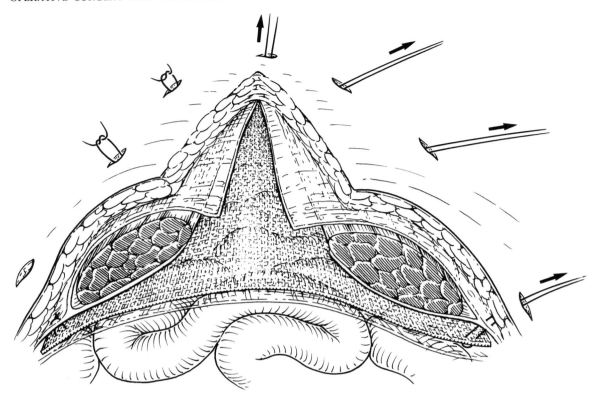

Figure 6.17B When all the sutures are in position and held in clips the mesh is slid into position in the extraperitoneal plane deep to the musculo-aponeurotic layer of the abdominal wall. The sutures are then tied securely using robust non-slip knots. The stab wounds are then closed with subcuticular strands

repair, the anatomy of stomal hernias must be determined by examination of the patient recumbent and relaxed, and with the muscles tensed and erect. Alternative stoma sites should be chosen and marked preoperatively in case relocation of the stoma is needed.

Indications and contraindications to surgery

Absolute indications include intestinal obstruction related to a stomal hernia and perforation of a paracolostomy hernia occurring during colostomy irrigation. Relative indications include problems with stoma management, especially leakage around colostomies and ileostomies. Contraindications include problems with general health such as poor cardiac or respiratory reserve as well as morbid obesity.

Operative technique

Three methods are described: (a) local repair operation; (b) prosthetic repair; and (c) relocation of stoma.

Local repair operation

This cannot be recommended as the recurrence rate is very high. This is because it usually involves suturing fleshy muscle layers rather than aponeurotic structures.

Prosthetic repair

An adherent wound drape is used to occlude the stoma and restrict contamination. Prophylactic antibodies should be given peroperatively. An L-shaped incision is made through the original incision then laterally above and around the stoma (Figure 6.18). The sac is identified, opened and its contents reduced. The aponeurotic defect is closed with non-absorbable sutures. The prosthetic mesh can be inserted into either the extraperitoneal or the extraparietal plane. The mesh should extend 3 cm outside the margins of the aponeurotic defect, with a cuff surrounding the emergent stoma preventing subsequent prolapse (Figure 6.19). If there is excess skin around the stoma the aperture can be reduced using the 'Mercedes Benz' operation (Figure 6.20). The wound is closed over suction drains as described previously.

Relocation of stoma

If doubt exists about the condition of the abdominal wall at the original stoma site or if the cause of the obstructive symptoms is considered to be intra-abdominal rather than related to the stomal hernia, the choice of procedure is relocation of the stoma.

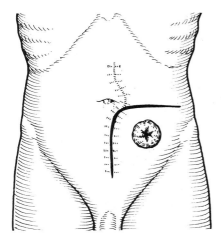

Figure 6.18 An L-shaped incision is made; this allows the stoma to be raised on a flap

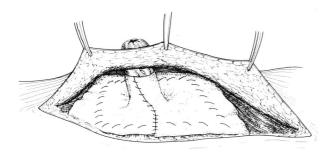

Figure 6.19 The mesh surrounds the stoma and is fixed by quilting sutures to the underlying external oblique aponeurosis

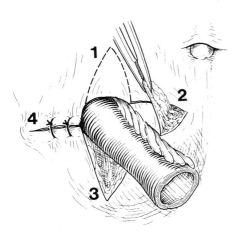

Figure 6.20 'Mercedes Benz' operation to reduce the skin aperture around a stoma

The new stoma site should be very carefully planned. The original stoma is mobilized using a circumstomal incision leaving a narrow cuff of skin attached. The stoma is straightened out, an everted ileostomy being uneverted and then closed with a continuous circular suture of polypropylene taking small bites of the skin at the margin of the stoma. A second, inverting layer of sutures can be used if there is doubt as to the competence of the first closure layer. The stoma is cleansed with an antimicrobial solution.

The incision around the stoma is deepened and the hernial sac identified and dissected free. The hernial contents are checked for viability and returned to the peritoneal cavity. The sac is excised and closed. If the aponeurotic defect is large, the abdomen can be explored through it to facilitate relocation of the stoma. If the aponeurotic defect is small, a separate laparotomy incision will be required. A very adequate length of intestine must be mobilized to allow construction of the new stoma without tension. The new stoma is now constructed in standard fashion. The original aponeurotic defect is closed with metric 3 polypropylene and the wound closed over suction drainage as described previously. Some degree of postoperative ileus followed by hyperactivity of the stoma usually necessitates intravenous fluid replacement for 24–72 h.

Conclusions

Stoma relocation is the most successful method but the most traumatic. It is recommended for the young ileostomate. A more conservative attitude is advised with the elderly colostomate.

References

Ackman, P. C. (1962) A study of 500 incisional hernias. *J. Int. Coll. Surg.*, **37**, 125–142

Ausobsky, J. R., Evans, M. and Pollock, A. V. (1985) Does mass closure of midline laparotomies stand the test of time? A random controlled clinical trial. *Ann. Roy. Coll. Surg. Engl.*, **67**, 159–161

Bucknall, T. E., Cox, P. J. and Ellis, H. (1982) Burst abdomen and incisional hernia: a prospective study of 1129 major laparotomies. *Br. Med. J.*, **284**, 931–933

Burgess, P., Matthew, V. V. and Devlin, H. B. (1984) A review of terminal colostomy complications following abdominoperineal resection for carcinoma. *Br. J. Surg.*, **71**, 1004 (Abstract)

Cannon, D. J. and Read, R. C. (1981) Metastatic emphysema. A mechanism for acquiring inguinal herniation. *Ann. Surg.*, **194**, 270–276

Cauldirouis, M. W., Romano, M., Bozza, F., Pluchinotta, A. M. *et al.* (1990) Pneumoperitoneum in giant incision hernias: a study of 41 patients. *Br. J. Surg.*, **77**, 306–307

Craig, R. D. P. (1962) Strangulated obturator hernia. *Br. J. Surg.*, **49**, 426–428

Devlin, H. B. (1982) Hernia. In *Recent Advances in Surgery II* (ed. R. G. C. Russell), Churchill Livingstone, Edinburgh

Devlin, H. B. (1988) *Management of Abdominal Hernias*, Butterworths, London

Donaldson, D. R., Hegarty, J. H., Brennan, T. G., Guillou, P. J. *et al.* (1982). The lateral paramedian incision – experience with 850 cases. *Br. J. Surg.*, **69**, 630–632

Ellis, H., Gajraj, H. and George, C. D. (1983) Incisional hernias: when do they occur? *Br. J. Surg.*, **70**, 290–321

George, C. D. and Ellis, H. (1986) The results of incisional hernia repair: a twelve year review. *Ann. Roy. Coll. Surg. Engl.*, **68**, 185–187

Harding, K. G., Mudge, M., Leinster, S. J. and Hughes, L. E. (1983) Late development of incision hernia: an unrecognized problem. *Br. Med. J.*, **286**, 519–520

James, T. (1982) Umbilical hernia in Xhosa infants and children. *J. Roy. Soc. Med.*, **75**, 537–541

Jenkins, T. P. N. (1976) The burst abdominal wound: a mechanical approach. *Br. J. Surg.*, **63**, 873–876

Jenkins, T. P. N. (1980) Incisional hernia repair: a mechanical approach. *Br. J. Surg.*, **67**, 335–336

Leaper, D. J., Pollock, A. V. and Evans, M. (1977) Abdominal wound closure: a trial of nylon, polyglycolic acid and steel sutures. *Br. J. Surg.*, **64**, 603–606

Lubbers, E. J. C. and Devlin, H. B. (1984) The complications of a permanent ileostomy. Poster, 8th World Congress of Collegium International Chirurgiae Digestivae, Amsterdam; 11–14 September

Mayo, W. J. (1901) An operation for the radical cure of umbilical hernia. *Ann. Surg.*, **31**, 276–280

Mudge, M. and Hughes, L. E. (1985) Incision hernia, a ten year prospective study of incidence and attitudes. *Br. J. Surg.*, **72**, 70–71

Pitkin, R. M. (1976) Abdominal hysterectomy in obese women. *Surg. Gynec. Obstet.*, **142**, 532–536

Ponka, J. L. (1980) *Hernias of the Abdominal Wall*, W. B. Saunders, Philadelphia

Spangen, L. (1984) Spigelian hernia. *Surg. Clin. North. Am.*, **64**, 351–366

Stoppa, R. (1987) Hernia of the abdominal wall. In *Surgery of the Abdominal Wall* (ed. J. P. Chevrel), Springer Verlag, New York

Stuckej, A. J., Lutjko, G. D. and Tivarovskij, V. I. (1973) Hernias of the Spigeli line. *Tsitologiia*, **15**, 10–13

Usher, F. C. (1979) New technique for repairing incision hernias with Marlex mesh. *Am. J. Surg.*, **138**, 740–741

Wantz, G. E. (1989) Giant prosthetic reinforcement of the visceral sac. *Surg. Gynecol. Obstet.*, **169**, 408–417

Wantz, G. E. (1991) Incisional hernioplasty with Mersilene. *Surg. Gynecol. Obstet.*, **172**, 129–137

7

Inguinal hernia repair by the Shouldice method

F. Glassow

Hernia repair is the most common operation in men. The recent upsurge in interest is motivated both by a genuine concern by all surgeons in improving results and by an increasing appreciation of the important socioeconomic implications of the operation.

In a 33-year association at the Shouldice Clinic, the author has performed more than 20 000 inguinal hernia repairs, of which more than 2500 were recurrent repairs. In the first 5 or 6 years the technique of the repair was being developed by the late Dr E. E. Shouldice. It has now become standardized.

Only elective inguinal repairs are considered here. There are many different operations for the repair of inguinal hernia, each with its own followers, and the operation here is a modified Bassini. At every operation the internal ring is routinely strengthened, as is the posterior inguinal wall, using a multilayered technique to achieve this. The recurrence rates recorded have remained consistently around 1% for many years. However, an operation can be considered truly successful only when other surgeons around the world achieve comparable results using the same technique (Table 7.1)

Table 7.1 Inguinal herniorrhaphies (Shouldice repairs).

Name of surgeon	No. of repairs	No. of recurrences	% of recurrences
Barwell (UK)	2572	38	1.5
Berliner (USA)	1084	12	1.1
Devlin (UK)	787	7	0.9
Dunn (USA)	3665	40	1.1
Shearburn (USA)	953	7	0.7
Wantz (USA)	5477	78	1.4
Total	14538	182	1.3

Preoperative assessment

All medical conditions are carefully assessed and priorities judged. Many patients are in the older age groups so that cardiac, pulmonary and prostatic problems are common. Obesity is common, and these patients are encouraged to lose excess weight slowly before operation at a rate of about 0.5 to 1 kg a week. The operation is scheduled accordingly. Age in itself is no bar to operation, and 10% of patients were over 70 years old. Older patients do just as well as the younger age groups and their recurrence rates are no different.

Anaesthesia

The use of local anaesthesia (Glassow, 1984a) is gradually increasing everywhere. Ambulatory surgery (Glassow, 1984b) or day-care surgery becomes ever more important from a socioeconomic viewpoint, especially combined with local anaesthesia.

A local anaesthetic is used in more than 95% of cases. A general anaesthetic is used only for children less than 12 years of age, for a few of the patients who have multirecurrent hernias and, very rarely, for a very apprehensive patient.

A local anaesthetic is preferred for many reasons. It avoids the risks of general anaesthesia, and in some poor-risk and elderly patients it is the anaesthetic of choice. In Third World countries where first-class anaesthesia is less available it is ideal. Induction is quicker and the interval between operations in the operating theatres is lessened. It imposes a gentle technique on the surgeon because the patient is only interested in a painless operation at this stage. The surgeon is less likely to use tension with the repair. A conscious patient can be asked to cough to identify an evasive hernia or to test a repair. Patients can walk out of the operating theatre which boosts their morale preoperatively and subsequently has a great impact on their short hospital stay. They are ambulant throughout. Many patients specifically request local anaesthesia, and almost without exception, including those who previously had had a general or a spinal anaesthetic, state after operation that they prefer local anaesthesia. Immediate postoperative complications are fewer with the questionable exception of the degree of discomfort experienced in the first 24 hours. Catheterization is eliminated (Nicholls, 1977; Makuria et al., 1982; Teasdale et al., 1982; Hashemi and Middleton, 1983).

A number of local anaesthetic agents are employed. Our experience is limited almost entirely to the use of 2% procaine hydrochloride without adrenaline, but more recently I have been using 1% and 1.5% for the over-70 age group.

Premedication commences $1\frac{1}{2}$ h preoperatively with oral administration of 10–20 mg valium. Twenty minutes preoperatively, 50–75 mg meperidine hydrochloride are given intramuscularly. A maximum of 150 ml of local anaesthetic solution may be used; 80–100 ml is initially injected as a subcutaneous regional infiltration in the line of the inguinal canal. A further 10–20 ml is used beneath the external oblique aponeurosis and a third injection of a similar amount is given around the internal ring, avoiding the inferior epigastric vessels. This volume of local has been used many thousands of times without adverse effects, given the adequate premedication cover described.

Operative technique (Glassow, 1984c)

Skin incision

Immediately after the subcutaneous local has been given the incision is made in the line of the inguinal canal. It is straight or slightly convex downwards. Pfannenstiel incisions are not used. A scar from a previous repair may require excision.

Cremaster muscle

This structure is often ignored in descriptions of technique. It is identified surrounding the spermatic cord once the external oblique has been divided in the line of the inguinal canal. It is divided longitudinally along the cord so defining and mobilizing two separate leaves – one lateral, one medial. The lateral one is more bulky containing the cremasteric vessels, in its base, and the genital branch of the genitofemoral nerve. Once the cord is isolated and retracted laterally, the third injection of local is given at the internal ring.

Internal ring

All inguinal hernia repairs have two main components. The first is the dissection at the internal ring, the second the dissection of the posterior inguinal wall. This ritual attitude is very helpful when confronted by a very large primary hernia or by a difficult recurrent hernia. Scrotal hernias are usually indirect. The rare direct ones are recognized by the lateral position of the inferior epigastric vessels. The attenuated posterior wall of the inguinal canal covers the true peritoneal sac in these rare cases.

High ligation of the indirect sac is standard practice and standard teaching, yet I do not regard it as vitally important (Glassow, 1965). I regard the complete freeing of the indirect sac from its fascial investments at the internal ring to be of equal or even greater importance. If this freeing is really complete, whether the sac is ligated high or low, the remaining ligated stump will retract out of sight within the internal ring. If the freeing is inadequate, the stump remains adherent at the internal ring and remains a potential hazard. The most obvious justification for this manoeuvre is that the recurrence rate achieved for primary indirect inguinal hernia repair is 1%. Utilizing these same principles, the treatment of sliding indirect inguinal hernia is an extension of this argument, and converts a difficult operation into an easy one. Once identified, the sliding hernia is simply freed completely at the internal ring and reduced within it without further treatment, even when large. The recurrence rate for sliding indirect hernia repair so achieved is also 1%, and indeed few of these recurrences were sliding themselves (Ryan, 1956). Sliding hernias are nearly always indirect and left-sided, usually in men who are overweight and more than 50 years old. At this stage careful examination at the internal ring will detect the rare unsuspected interstitial hernia.

In the absence of an indirect inguinal hernia a peritoneal protrusion must be routinely identified on the cord at the internal ring where it appears as a small whitish convex crescent. This eliminates the risk of missing an indirect hernia in cases in which the surgeon's attention may already be focused on an obvious direct inguinal hernia. The combination of an indirect and direct hernia is encountered in 8% of men.

The two cremasteric leaves are now excised. This important step clearly demonstrates the whole posterior inguinal wall. If omitted, a direct hernia may be missed.

Posterior inguinal wall and the transversalis lamina

The dissection and treatment of this layer constitute the second main component of any inguinal hernia operation and are of vital importance. Primary indirect hernia is twice as common as primary direct, yet recurrent indirect is less common than recurrent direct. This finding reflects the importance of the quality of the repair. Many direct inguinal recurrences may be iatrogenic. Some of mine were.

The repair performed here and described in detail later is based on an oblique linear division of the transversalis with subsequent overlap of the two leaves so obtained, both leaves being considered important. In the Cooper ligament repair (McVay, 1965; Halverson and McVay, 1970; Glassow, 1976a) the lower part of the transversalis, which is equivalent to the lower leaf just described, is not utilized because it is not attached to the inguinal ligament (Glassow, 1976b).

Bilateral repairs

One patient in 10 has a bilateral hernia on admission. Using local anaesthesia the repairs are staged 48 h apart for several good reasons. A simultaneous bilateral repair would double the volume of local anaesthetic used. The timing of the second repair may be altered, for example in patients who have bilateral recurrent hernia or unilateral testicular atrophy, or in an elderly patient in whom the first repair was difficult, or in an extremely obese or tense individual. Occasionally, the patient decides on delay.

The external pudendal vessels should be preserved on one side at least to minimize prepuceal oedema.

Recurrence rates in simultaneous bilateral repairs are slightly higher, and tension may be a factor.

Testis

Orchidectomy is rarely performed and it is usually possible to preserve the testis even in patients who have multirecurrent hernias. The patient who has a recurrent hernia is warned of the risks and a consent form for orchidectomy should be obtained in most cases. Testicular atrophy postoperatively is uncommon but, in recurrences where records are unavailable, the cord may lie subcutaneously and easily be damaged.

Patients of all ages welcome this conserving attitude.

Suture materials

Monofilament stainless steel wire gauge no. 34 is the suture material preferred. Occasionally no. 32 is needed for greater strength. Many surgeons use other non-absorbable sutures achieving excellent results. Absorbable sutures are unsatisfactory and their use is condemned. A continuous suture technique is used and is considered important because it distributes tension evenly. I have repaired many direct inguinal recurrences in patients in whom individual non-absorbable sutures were visible on either side of the neck of the hernia. It was considered that such ligatures were either inadequately placed or tied with uneven tension.

I have not used mesh. It is rarely needed. In many recurrent repairs I had to remove it. Nevertheless it is used successfully by many surgeons (Usher, 1978). Bellis (1969) has a huge series including more than 3000 mesh repairs. Since 1983 it has been used here 249 times for difficult recurrent inguinal or inguino-femoral repairs. (Statistics kindly supplied by Dr D. R. J. Welsh.)

Posterior inguinal wall

Examination and principles of repair (Glassow, 1976a, 1976c)

The assessment of the strength of the posterior inguinal wall is fundamental. This is accomplished first by inspection and then by testing its strength using a finger inserted at the internal ring deep to the trans-

versalis plane. A direct inguinal hernia is obvious or will be demonstrated by this manoeuvre. In some cases only a weakness is present, but in either case a standard repair is applicable. The opening in the transversalis already made at the internal ring (Figure 7.1) is extended medially towards the pubic bone over the centre of the direct hernia which is freed. If the transversalis is strong medially it may be left undivided, but attenuated excess transversalis may require excision. Firm transversalis of satisfactory quality can always be found even in the presence of a large direct or a recurrent direct hernia. A funicular direct sac is excised, although the more common diffuse direct sac is simply reduced.

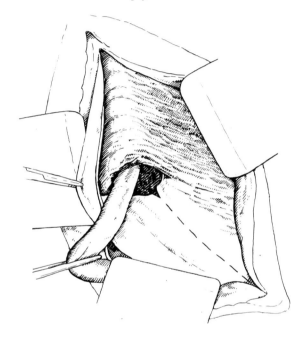

Figure 7.1 Intended line of incision of transversalis lamina

The lower leaf of the divided transversalis should be wider than the upper (Figure 7.2). In the subsequent repair it is carried upwards and medially beneath the upper leaf which is then brought downwards over it. This overlap is further strengthened by another immediately superficial to it bringing muscular structures medially to the inguinal ligament laterally.

Technique of repair

In the reconstruction of the posterior wall four continuous lines of gauge no. 34 stainless steel wire are inserted using only two separate sutures, each being responsible for two lines. The first line starts medially at the pubic bone (Figure 7.3) where it attaches the free edge of the lower transversalis flap to the posterior aspect of the lateral edge of the rectus, easily identified as a white border inserting onto the pubic

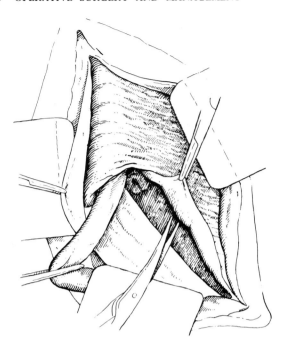

Figure 7.2 Division of transversalis lamina

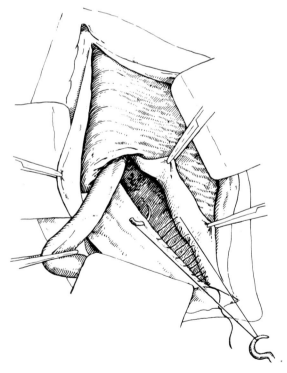

Figure 7.3 First line of sutures

bone. The suture should start as far medially as possible and be tied without tension. The entire free edge is now attached under the upper flap. After one or two small bites on the rectus it picks up the deep

surface of the transversus and internal oblique as it travels laterally. Just medial to the internal ring the upper lateral ligated cremasteric stump is included in this first line, taking small bites without tension. At the internal ring the inferior epigastric vessels are avoided. After completion of this line of sutures, it can be seen that quite a firm barrier has already been established and the defect or weakness eliminated. The suture is reversed and continues medially as the second line (Figure 7.4). This brings the upper flap of divided transversalis downwards and laterally to the shelving surface of Poupart's ligament until it reaches the pubic bone again, where it is tied. This overlap strengthens the first layer and is particularly effective in the occasional case in which the first layer is of poor quality.

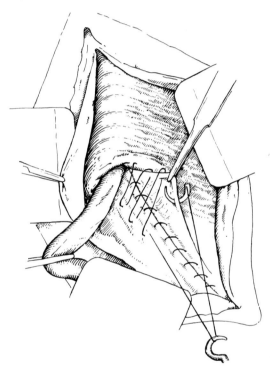

Figure 7.4 Second line of sutures

The third line (second suture) commences at the internal ring. Travelling medially (Figure 7.5) it reinforces the subjacent lines, bringing the internal oblique and transversus lying medially to the deep surface of the inguinal ligament laterally. At the pubic bone it is reversed and travels laterally again utilizing the same structures. At the internal ring it is tied.

The repair should be performed without tension and relaxing incisions are never used. The spermatic cord should slide easily into the internal ring and the cord veins should not be engorged. The cord is replaced deep to the external oblique. The subcutaneous plane is separately closed eliminating dead space. Michel's skin clips are used.

Typically a primary inguinal repair takes about 40 min. A once recurrent repair might take 80 min, whereas a more difficult multirecurrent repair takes 2 or 3 h.

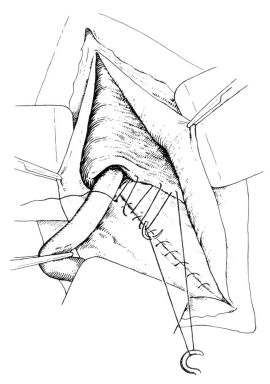

Figure 7.5 Third line of sutures

Length of hospital stay and economics
(Devlin *et al.*, 1977)

Medical care costs continue to rise rapidly everywhere. Following surgery very early discharge from hospital is possible, consistent with an early return to work and good long-term results (Adler, 1977). A period off work of longer than 4 weeks is rarely authorized. A greater combined effort on the part of both surgeon and general practitioner would help to shorten longer periods allowed elsewhere. Patients may remain in hospital for 2 or 3 days because many live far away and earlier travel is inconvenient. In 1972 the average hospital stay in one large centre in Britain was 10 days, but these periods are now very much shorter. One study showed that patients who were ambulant early (Glassow, 1984b) did better in all respects than those kept in bed for longer periods (Palumbo and Sharpe, 1971). Many operations are now performed on an outpatient or day-care basis (Farquharson, 1955; Bellis, 1969, 1975; Ruckley, 1978; Goulbourne and Ruckley, 1979).

Hernias in women

Groin hernias are approximately 25 times less common in women. While the inguinal to femoral ratio is 40:1 in men and only 3:1 in women, nevertheless inguinal hernia is also more frequent in women (Glassow, 1963). However, in women a primary inguinal hernia is almost always indirect. Primary direct hernia is very rare because the posterior inguinal wall is strong (Glassow, 1973). This is a good reason for performing a low operation for repair of a primary femoral hernia in women. However, recurrent direct inguinal hernia in women is more common than recurrent indirect suggesting an iatrogenic aetiology.

Follow-up

With the very large and ever-increasing number of repairs performed, follow-up becomes increasingly more difficult, burdensome and expensive. Completely adequate long-term follow-up of very large series is impossible for a number of reasons, including shifting population, loss through death and indifference to correspondence. The argument that the patient who is lost to the follow-up may be the one who has a recurrence is unanswerable, but unlikely. All the evidence we can muster is to the contrary.

Of all recurrent hernias which followed a repair here, 50% had developed at the end of 5 years, and 75% at the end of 10 years, which indicates a minimum follow-up period of 10 years. If such rates are plotted graphically it is possible to predict eventual long-term recurrence rates if the rates for a shorter period are known (Figure 7.6).

Recurrences

The main criterion of success in any series of inguinal hernia repairs is the recurrence rate. In 1977 a *British Medical Journal* Editorial quoted the recurrence rates for indirect hernias at 5–10%, for direct hernias 15–20% and for recurrent inguinal hernias 30% (Editorial, 1977). A surgeon should aim at 1% for repair of primary inguinal hernia, whether indirect or direct (Kirk, 1983).

Table 7.2 Primary inguinal herniorrhaphies, 1954–1986 (personal series).

Type of primary hernia	No. of repairs	No of recurrences	% of recurrences
Indirect	11359	81	0.7
Direct	5403	58	1.1
Combined indirect and direct	1077	7	0.6
Total	17839	146	0.8

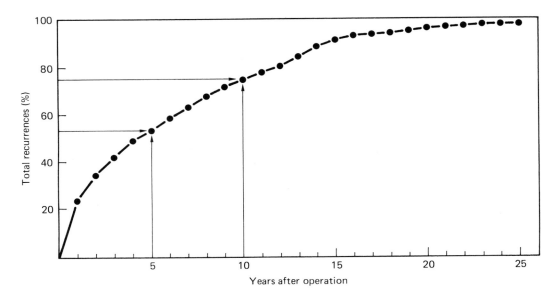

Figure 7.6 Inguinal hernia repair by the Shouldice method

Table 7.3 Recurrent inguinal herniorrhaphies, 1954–1986 (personal series).

Type of recurrent hernia	No of recurrences	No of re-recurrences	% of re-recurrences
Indirect	1108	25	2.3
Direct	1538	46	3.0
Total	2646	71	2.7

Table 7.4 Primary inguinal herniorrhaphies, 1954–1980 (followed to 1990; personal series).

Type of primary hernia	No of repairs	No of recurrences	% of recurrences
Indirect	9099	97	1.1
Direct	4865	64	1.3
Combined indirect and direct	946	5	0.5
Total	14910	166	1.1

Table 7.5 Recurrent inguinal herniorrhaphies, 1954–1980 (followed to 1990; personal series).

Type of recurrent hernia	No of recurrences	No of re-recurrences	% of re-recurrences
Indirect	1060	28	2.6
Direct	1390	64	4.6
Total	2450	92	3.8

Tables 7.2 and 7.3 represent my personal recurrence rates in a favourable light, since no 'allowance' has been made for recent repairs. Tables 7.4 and 7.5 represent cases followed up for at least 10 years, representing more accurately my true recurrence rates (see Figure 7.6). Table 7.1 (page 55) represents the experience of other surgeons using this technique.

Discussion

It has been customary to give a general anaesthetic when repairing an inguinal hernia. It is hoped that this review has demonstrated how successfully such patients can be managed using local anaesthesia. Its indication and advantages have been intentionally described in detail in the hope that it may eventually become the anaesthetic of choice.

Emphasis is laid on the detailed appreciation of the anatomy of the inguinal canal, in particular the internal ring and the transversalis lamina. The technique used here has been carefully described and it is hoped that other surgeons may be persuaded of its efficacy. In our hands it has resulted in a short hospital stay, early return to a normal lifestyle and a recurrence rate of approximately 1% for repair of primary inguinal hernia.

Conclusion

In 1971, Professor L. M. Zimmerman (Zimmerman, 1968) of Chicago wrote: 'The larger the series the more valuable are the figures offered and the percentage of patients returning for the follow up is also of great significance...'. Moreover, 'Hernia surgery demands meticulous technique, gentle handling of tissues, free anatomical exposure, accurate approximation of sutured structures, avoidance of tension and utilization of fine atraumatic needles and suture materials. The disregard of any of these attributes of good surgery will be reflected in a higher recurrence rate. With the same method the results will vary with the skill of the surgeon.'

I leave the most telling comments to the very end of this presentation because he put them more eloquently than I am able to do. Wakeley (1940) said: '... that so little interest is taken in the care of a hernia is a pity. The various operations are usually regarded as of minor importance and to be undertaken by a house surgeon, being beneath the dignity of a surgeon. A surgeon can do more for the community by operating on hernia cases and seeing that his recurrence rate is low than he can by operating on cases of malignant disease.'

Illustrations

Figures 7.1–7.5 were previously published in Nyhus, L. M. and Condon, R. E. (eds) (1978) *Hernia*, 2nd edn, Lippincott, Philadephia, and have been modified.

References

Adler, M. W. (1977) Randomised controlled trial of early discharge for inguinal hernia and varicose veins. *Ann. R. Coll. Surg. Engl.*, **59**, 251–254.

Bellis, C. J. (1969) Immediate unrestricted activity after inguinal herniorrhaphy – 9727 personal cases with specific reference to local anaesthesia and polyester fiber mesh. *Int. Surg.*, **52**, 107–112

Bellis, C. J. (1975) 16069 inguinal herniorrhaphies using local anaesthesia with one day hospitalisation and unrestricted activity. *Int. Surg.*, **60**, 37–39

Devlin, H. B., Russell, I. T., Muller D. *et al.* (1977) Short-stay surgery for inguinal hernia. Clinical outcome of the Shouldice operation. *Lancet* **1**, 847–849

Editorial (1977) Activity and recurrent hernia. *Br. Med. J.*, **275**, 3–4

Farquharson, E. L. (1955) Early ambulation with special reference to herniorrhaphy as outpatient procedure. *Lancet*, **2**, 517–519

Glasgow, F. (1963) Inguinal hernia in the female. *Surg. Gynecol. Obstet.*, **116**, 701–704.

Glasgow, F. (1965) High ligation of the sac in indirect inguinal hernia. *Am. J. Surg.*, **109**, 460–463

Glasgow, F. (1973) An evaluation of the strength of the posterior wall of the inguinal canal in women. *Br. J. Surg.*, **60**, 342–344

Glasgow, F. (1976a) Inguinal hernia repair: a comparison of the Shouldice and Cooper ligament repair of the posterior inguinal wall. *Am. J. Surg.*, **131**, 306–311

Glasgow, F. (1976b) Short-stay surgery (Shouldice technique) for repair of inguinal hernia. *Ann. R. Coll. Surg. Engl.*, **58**, 133–139

Glasgow, F. (1976c) The Shouldice repair of inguinal hernia. In *Controversy in Surgery* (eds R. L. Varco and J. P. Delaney), W. B. Saunders, Philadelphia, pp. 375–387

Glasgow, F. (1984a) Inguinal hernia repair using local anaesthesia. *Ann. R. Coll. Surg. Engl.*, **66**, 382–387

Glasgow, F. (1984b) Ambulatory repair. *Contemp. Surg.*, **24**, 107–130

Glasgow, F. (1984c) The Shouldice repair. In *Mastery of Surgery* (eds L. M. Nyhus and R. I. Baker), Little, Brown, Boston, pp. 1268–1273

Goulborne, L. A. and Ruckley, C. V. (1979) Operations for hernia and varicose veins in a day-bed unit. *Br. Med. J.*, **2**, 712–714

Halverson, K. and McVay, C. B. (1970) Inguinal and femoral hernioplasty: a 22-year study of the authors' methods. *Arch. Surg.*, **101**, 127–135

Hashemi, K. and Middleton, M. D. (1983) Subcutaneous bupivacaine for postoperative analgesia after herniorrhaphy. *Ann. R. Coll. Surg. Engl.*, **65**, 38–39

Kirk, P. M. (1983) Which inguinal hernia repair? *Br. Med. J.*, **287**, 4–5

McVay, C. B. (1965) Inguinal and femoral hernioplasty. *Surgery*, **57**, 615–625

Makuria, T., Alexander-Williams, J. and Keighley, M. R. B. (1982) Comparison between general and local anaesthesia for groin hernias. *Ann. R. Coll. Surg. Engl.*, **64**, 238–242

Nicholls J. C. (1977) Necessity into choice: an appraisal of inguinal herniorrhaphy under local anaesthesia. *Ann. R. Coll. Surg. Engl.*, **59**, 124–127

Palumbo, L. T. and Sharpe, W. S. (1971) Primary inguinal hernioplasty in the adult. *Surg. Clin. North Am.*, **48**, 143–154

Ruckley, C. V. (1978) Day case and short stay surgery for hernia. *Br. J. Surg.*, **65**, 1–4

Ryan, E. A. (1956) Analysis of 313 consecutive cases of indirect sliding inguinal hernias. *Surg. Gynecol. Obstet.*, **102**, 45–48

Teasdale, C., McCrum, A., Williams, N. B. *et al.* (1982) A randomised controlled trial to compare local with general anaesthesia for short-stay inguinal repair. *Ann. R. Coll. Surg. Engl.*, **64**, 238–242.

Usher, F. C. (1978) Hernia repair with Marlex mesh. In *Hernia*, 2nd edn (eds L. M. Nyhus and R. E. Condon), Lippincott, Philadelphia, pp. 561–580

Wakeley C. P. G. (1940) Treatment of certain types of external herniae. *Lancet* **1**, 822–826.

Zimmerman L. M. (1968) The use of prosthetic materials in the repairs of hernias. *Surg. Clin. North Am.*, **48**, 143–154.

8

Groin hernias and their complications

H. B. Devlin and S. Nicholson

Anatomy

A clear understanding of the anatomy of the lower anterior abdominal wall is the key to successful surgery for groin hernias and the surgeon should be aware of the anatomical variants. The surgeon requires a three-dimensional view of the abdominal wall, from the cutaneous aspect looking in and from the internal aspects of the abdominal wall. This internal or 'inside out' view is essential to the understanding of surgery for inguinal, femoral and recurrent groin hernias.

The external oblique

The outermost musculo-aponeurotic layer of the lower abdominal wall is the external oblique. The muscle fibres arise by eight digitations from the outer surface of the lower eight ribs and fan downwards and medially from their upper origins and continue anteriorly as the external oblique aponeurosis, but more vertically from the lower origins to insert into the anterior external lip of the iliac crest.

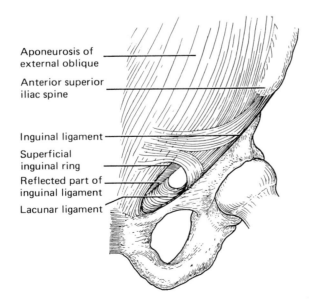

Aponeurosis of external oblique

Anterior superior iliac spine

Inguinal ligament

Superficial inguinal ring

Reflected part of inguinal ligament

Lacunar ligament

Figure 8.1 The inguinal ligament is the lower margin of the external oblique muscle. Medially it is attached like a fan to the iliopectineal line (Cooper's ligament) and the tubercle of the pubis

Superiorly the external oblique aponeurosis is relatively thin, but inferiorly it is very strong and along its lower margin it forms the inguinal ligament (Poupart) which is attached superolaterally to the anterior superior iliac spine and inferomedially to the pubic tubercle. Just above the pubis a triangular defect in the aponeurosis – the superficial inguinal ring – allows passage of the spermatic cord in the male from the inguinal canal to the scrotum. The cleft of the superficial ring is confined to the medial half of the inguinal canal in 80% of individuals, but occasionally its lateral extent may extend close to the anterior superior iliac spine. Medially the inguinal ligament continues as the triangular lacunar ligament (Gimbernat) which fuses with the pectineal ligament (Cooper) on the superior pubic ramus (Figure 8.1).

The reflected part of the inguinal ligament (Colles) is a broad band of thin fibres which arise from the pubic crest and the medial end of the iliopectineal line and pass anterosuperiorly behind the superior crus of the superficial inguinal ring to the linea alba.

The internal oblique

Deep to the external oblique muscle and aponeurosis lies the internal oblique. The muscle arises from the lateral half of the abdominal surface of the inguinal ligament, the intermediate line on the anterior two-thirds of the iliac crest and the lumbodorsal fascia. The fibres pass in an upward and medial direction and end in a strong aponeurosis. The lower fibres, from their origin from the inguinal ligament, arch medially and downwards, passing with the lowest fibres of the transversus muscle in front of the rectus muscle as a component of the anterior rectus sheath, and insert on the pubic crest and iliopectineal line behind the lacunar ligament and reflected part of the inguinal ligament.

Like the external oblique, the anatomy of the internal oblique is variable. Its origin may commence at the deep inguinal ring or at a variable distance lateral to it. It may insert either into the pubic crest and tubercle or into the lateral margin of the rectus sheath a variable distance above the pubis. This leads to important variations in the contribution of the internal oblique to the 'defences' of the inguinal canal. There are important racial differences in the anatomy of the inguinal region which account for differences in the epidemiology of inguinal hernia (see later).

The spermatic cord passes through or adjacent to the medial margin of the internal oblique muscle. Laterally the cord lies deep to the fleshy muscular fibres and acquires a coat of cremaster muscle as it emerges from the medial border of the internal oblique. The fibres of the internal oblique follow a transverse or oblique direction and medial to the cord convert to an aponeurosis which continues to the insertion. There is considerable variation in both the medial and inferior extent of the muscle fibres, which extend to the inferior margin in only 2% of cases; in 75% the extent is a centimetre or more above the margin, and in 20% there is a broad aponeurotic leaf superior to the spermatic cord. Similarly the fleshy muscle extends as far as the emergent cord in 20%, medial to the cord but not to the rectus margin in 75% and medial to the lateral margin of the rectus in only 2%. Direct inguinal herniation is most frequently found when the internal oblique muscle is replaced by a flimsy aponeurosis in the roof of the inguinal canal (Anson *et al.*, 1960)

The transversus abdominis

The transversus abdominis is the deepest of the three abdominal muscle layers, arising from the iliopsoas fascia along the internal lip of the anterior two-thirds of the iliac crest. Anteriorly, the muscle fibres end in a strong aponeurosis which inserts into the linea alba, the pubic crest and the iliopectineal line. The fibres run transversely, but in the lower abdomen they curve downward and medially to form an arch over the inguinal canal. The insertion of the transversus aponeurosis is broader than that of the internal oblique, extending further along the iliopectineal line. The transversus is more aponeurotic and less muscular than either of the oblique muscles, fleshy muscle covering the upper part of the inguinal region in only 67% of cases. Fleshy fibres are found in the lowermost fibres arching over the inguinal canal in only 14% of cases. Fleshy muscle fibres extend medially to the deep epigastric vessels in less than 30% of cases.

The lower border of the transverse aponeurosis is called the 'arch', above which is a strong aponeurotic sheet with no spaces between its fibres. Below the arch the posterior wall of the inguinal canal is closed only by transversalis fascia. It is through this potentially weak area that direct herniation can occur.

The lowermost fibres of the transversus and internal oblique aponeuroses sometimes fuse to form the conjoint tendon. In these cases the transversus contributes 80% of the conjoint tendon. The conjoint tendon lies lateral to the rectus muscle and immediately deep to the superficial inguinal ring, and the spermatic cord, or round ligament, lies anterior to it as it passes through the superficial ring.

The conjoint tendon is another very variable anatomical structure and is absent as a discrete structure in up to 20% of individuals. It may be absent or only slightly developed, it may be replaced by a lateral

extension of the rectus origin, or it may extend laterally to the deep inguinal ring so that no interval exists between the lower border of the transversus and the inguinal ligament (Figure 8.2). If there is full attachment of the conjoint tendon to the iliopectineal line, the posterior wall of the inguinal canal is completely reinforced by aponeurosis. If this attachment is absent or incomplete, there is the potential to develop a direct or a large indirect hernia.

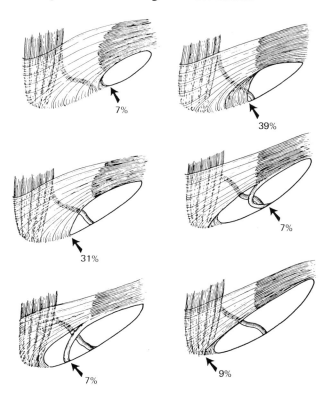

8.2   The extent of the tendon of transversus abdominis contributes to the posterior wall of the inguinal canal. The arrows indicate the lateralmost extension of the tendon in the percentages of subjects (From Anson, Morgan and McVay, 1960, by permission)

The transversalis fascia

Deep to the transversus aponeurosis lies the transversalis fascia, extending from the rib cage above to the pelvis below and continuous from side to side. In the upper abdominal wall the transversalis fascia is thin but inferiorly, especially in the iliofemoral region, it is thicker with specialized folds and bands. The deep inguinal ring is an opening in the fascia just above the mid-point of the inguinal ligament and just lateral to the deep epigastric vessels. On its medial margin the fascia condenses into a U-shaped sling, supporting the emergent cord in its concavity, and the two limbs extending superiorly and laterally to be suspended from the posterior aspect of the transversus muscle. This sling lies at or just above the lower border of the transversus arch. During coughing or straining the transversus muscle contracts, pulling the pillars of the deep ring together and drawing the entire sling upwards and laterally. This inguinal 'shutter' mechanism increases the obliquity of exit of the spermatic cord and provides protection from forces tending to cause an indirect hernia (Lytle, 1970). In the adult with an obliterated processus vaginalis, a flat lid of peritoneum covers the ring internally since the spermatic vessels and vas deferens lie extraperitoneally.

The lower border of the fascia transversalis condenses into the iliopubic tract which extends from the anterior superior iliac spine laterally to the pubis medially lying on a slightly deeper plane to the inguinal ligament, which becomes clear at operation. The iliopubic tract thus forms the inferior margin of the defect in the fascia transversalis in both an indirect and direct inguinal hernia and is anterior to the peritoneal sac of a femoral hernia (Figure 8.3).

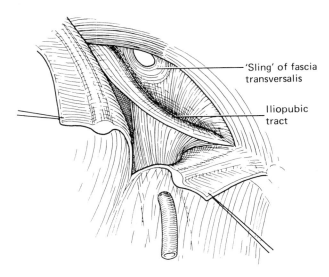

Figure 8.3 Dissected further anteriorly, if the inguinal ligament is divided, the fascia transversalis can be seen to be continuous with the femoral sheath. The thickening at the junction of fascia transversalis with the femoral sheath is the iliopubic tract. The internal oblique muscle, which arises from the lateral inguinal ligament, acts as a shutter or 'lid' on the deep inguinal ring

Superior to the iliopubic tract the fascia transversalis extends over the posterior wall of the inguinal canal up to and behind the transversus arch with which it merges. Medial to the deep ring and deep to the fascia transversalis lying in the extraperitoneal fat, the deep epigastric vessels pass upward and medially to the deep aspect of the rectus muscle. This forms a triangular area medial to the deep epigastric vessels, lateral to the rectus muscle and above the inguinal ligament known as Hesselbach's triangle. It is through this area that a direct inguinal hernia protrudes or more exactly through the transversalis fascia above the iliopubic tract, the medial limb of the fascia transversalis sling laterally and the transversus arch superiorly. At operation the iliopubic tract, the deep ring and the 'white line' of the transversus arch

are easily identifiable if the transversalis fascia is adequately dissected. Identification of these features is an essential prerequisite for adequate inguinal hernia repair (Condon, 1971).

Behind the inguinal ligament the transversalis fascia descends into the thigh as a funnel-like sheath around the femoral vessels as far as the fossa ovalis in the deep fascia of the thigh. This arrangement leaves a small 'space' medial to the femoral vein which normally contains some fat, a lymph node (Cloquet's) and some lymphatics. This space, bounded medially by the lacunar ligament, posteriorly by the iliopectineal ligament, anteriorly by the inguinal ligament and iliopubic tract and laterally by the femoral vein, becomes expanded in femoral herniation.

Hernial sacs are composed of peritoneum and contain intra-abdominal viscera. A loose layer of extraperitoneal fat lies between the peritoneum and fascia transversalis. As the hernia protrudes through the musculo-aponeurotic layers of the abdominal wall, it carries this layer of extraperitoneal fat with it. The extraperitoneal plane is important in the surgical approach to both inguinal and femoral hernias.

The spermatic cord

The spermatic cord is composed of: (a) arteries – testicular, cremasteric and artery of the vas deferens; (b) veins – testicular, forming the pampiniform plexus; (c) lymphatics – draining to the para-aortic nodes; (d) nerves – genital branch of the genito-femoral nerve and autonomic nerves; (e) the vas deferens; and (f) the processus vaginalis.

As it emerges through the abdominal wall the cord receives investments from each layer – the internal spermatic fascia from the fascia transversalis, the cremasteric muscle from the internal oblique and, most superficially, the external spermatic fascia from the external oblique as it passes through the superficial inguinal ring. Each of these fascial layers must be opened to reveal the processus vaginalis or the sac of an indirect hernia. Until birth the processus vaginalis, although minute, remains as an uninterrupted diverticulum from the peritoneal cavity to the testis where it spreads out as the tunica vaginalis. It closes soon after birth in most males, but may persist into adult life when a hernia or hydrocele may complicate peritoneal dialysis in patients with chronic renal failure or ascites in cardiac, malignant or cirrhotic liver disease (Issac, 1961). An indirect inguinal hernia progressively dilates this remnant diverticulum of the parietal peritoneum.

The inguinal canal

The inguinal canal is an oblique space passing between the musculo-aponeurotic layers of the abdominal wall to transmit the spermatic cord from the retroperitoneum to the scrotum. It commences internally at the deep inguinal ring and passes anterior to the fascia transversalis and deep epigastric vessels and deep to the external oblique aponeurosis. Inferiorly lie the iliopubic tract of the fascia transversalis and the inguinal ligament. Superiorly the transversus arch curves forward and downward and medially the posterior wall is variably reinforced by the conjoint tendon. The key to direct herniation is the anatomy of the transversus/conjoint arch and to indirect herniation the inguinal 'shutter' mechanism and constriction of the fascia transversalis at the deep inguinal ring.

Aetiology and epidemiology of primary hernias in adults

Inguinal hernias are the commonest of all abdominal wall hernias and occur in all races. The male to female ratio varies between 10:1 and 12:1 in different series. The ratio of indirect to direct also varies between races; 65% of inguinal hernias in adult European males, for instance, are indirect. In parts of Africa as many as 89% are indirect. The African pelvis is more oblique and has a lower arch than the European pelvis. This 'lowness' of the pubis is associated with a narrower origin of the internal oblique muscle from the lateral inguinal ligament. This reduces the effectiveness of the inguinal shutter and leaves the deep ring relatively unprotected, predisposing to indirect herniation. The incidence of inguinal hernia varies widely, but in the UK it is approximately 100/100 000 males per year. In parts of Africa the incidence is much greater, for example reaching 30% in the adult male population of the Island of Pemba, off the Zanzibar coast.

Direct herniation is associated with smoking and with aortic aneurysm. A collagen defect has been identified in these individuals characterized by disorganized collagen fibrils in aponeuroses, a raised leucocyte count, raised serum α_1 antitrypsin and delayed and deficient aponeurotic healing. The term 'metastatic emphysema' has been used to describe this phenomenon (Cannon and Read, 1981).

Femoral hernias are less frequent than inguinal, accounting for only 10% of all groin hernias in adults. The sex distribution varies between reported series: most find that the femoral hernia is commoner in females, with a ratio of between 2.5:1 and 8:1. In females, however, inguinal hernias occur as frequently as femoral hernias.

Types and definitions of groin hernias

Indirect (oblique) inguinal hernia

The indirect inguinal hernial sac is the remains of part or the whole of the processus vaginalis. The sac, therefore, is congenital, even though the hernia may often not appear until late in adult life. It is considered congenital because of the following:

1. Its anatomical relations are the same as those of the processus vaginalis.
2. An empty sac in this position is often found at other operations when there is no actual hernia and 15–30% of men have a patent processus in autopsy studies (Hughson, 1925).
3. In childhood, simple removal of the sac is curative and in infants with inguinal hernia the contralateral processus is patent in 60%, while 10–20% have a contralateral hernia
4. In childhood commonly and occasionally in adults it is associated with other abnormalities of the embryological development of the inguinal canal such as imperfectly descended testis.
5. In patients with ascites of any aetiology or on continuous ambulatory peritoneal dialysis (CAPD) at all ages it can fill with fluid and become apparent.

The primary defect in indirect inguinal hernia, therefore, is failure of the processus vaginalis to obliterate completely. Before the hernia becomes apparent, there must be a failure of the mechanism which protects the deep inguinal ring – the inguinal shutter. In complete scrotal hernia the sac extends through the deep ring, inguinal canal and superficial ring to reach the scrotum (or labium majus in the female). If there is a complete vaginal sac, the testis lies in the fundus of it. Hernias limited to the canal are termed incomplete (bubonocele). An *interstitial hernia* occurs between the layers of the abdominal wall and is associated with ectopic testes in 60% of patients.

Direct inguinal hernia

The sac lies behind the cord medial to the deep epigastric vessels. The hernia passes directly forward through the defect in the posterior wall of the canal where the fascia transversalis is unprotected by the conjoint tendon or transversus aponeurosis. Only rarely does the hernia follow the cord down into the scrotum. It is prominent when the patient coughs or stands and disappears when he is recumbent. Primary direct hernias are almost unknown in women.

Femoral hernia

In the UK, femoral hernia is $2\frac{1}{2}$ times commoner in females than in males, although in females indirect inguinal hernia is as common as femoral hernia. As with inguinal hernia there is considerable geographic variation in the incidence of femoral hernia. Rare in native Africans, it is postulated that chronic foot infections leading to repeated inflammation of the inguinal lymphatics, involving Cloquet's node, produce fibrosis in the femoral canal (Wosornu, 1974).

The hernial sac is considered to be acquired and

has never been demonstrated at autopsy on a new-born infant. The hernia commonly arises later in life, most frequently in multiparous females. Nurses are said to be prone to femoral herniation. Weight loss predisposes to femoral herniation in both sexes. Male patients with femoral hernias have frequently undergone an inguinal hernia repair (Glassow, 1971) and 10% of femoral hernias follow a previous operation for inguinal hernia. Femoral hernias are more frequent on the right side than the left side (2:1) and are bilateral in 5%.

The aetiology of femoral hernia, in contrast to indirect inguinal hernia, is ill-understood. They occur more commonly in females than in males because: (a) The angle between the inguinal ligament and the superior pubic ramus is wider in the female; (b) enlargement of fat in the femoral canal in middle-aged females stretches the femoral sheath, predisposing to herniation later in life if weight is lost; and (c) stretching of the fascia transversalis with the increased intra-abdominal pressure during pregnancy may predispose to herniation, but this of course fails to explain why direct inguinal hernias are almost unknown in women.

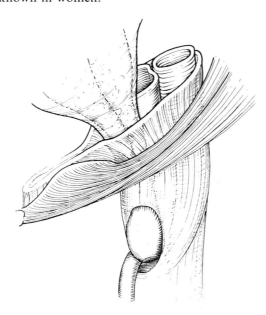

Figure 8.4 Anatomy of a femoral sheath. The hernial sac progresses down the femoral sheath 'funnel' to present in the thigh. In the thigh, the fundus of the hernia carries the attenuated cribriform fascia before it

A femoral hernia emerges through the potential space medial to the femoral vein below and lateral to the inguinal ligament. The sac lies initially within the femoral sheath and becomes superficial after passing through the fossa ovalis in the deep fascia of the thigh (Figure 8.4). It may then bend upwards over the inguinal ligament, leading to diagnostic confusion. The neck of a femoral hernia always lies below the medial end of the inguinal ligament, lateral to the pubic tubercle. The neck of an inguinal hernia, on the contrary, lies above the inguinal ligament, medial to the pubic tubercle. An inguinal hernia may be reduced by backward and lateral pressure, whereas a femoral hernia, if it is reducible at all, must be reduced directly downwards then backwards and upwards.

Differential diagnosis of groin swellings

This depends on demonstrating the clinical features of a hernia – a lump of varying size with a cough (expansile) impulse. Hernias are often reducible, whereas other lumps are not. Femoral hernias, however, are rarely reducible and often do not have a cough impulse – a soft swelling with a cough impulse exiting from the fossa ovalis on standing and which can be pushed back in place is much more likely to be a saphena varix than a femoral hernia. It is usually possible to differentiate between a femoral and an inguinal hernia, but even experts find this difficult on occasions and some 10% of femoral hernias may be misdiagnosed as inguinal (Glassow, 1966). Differentiating between direct and indirect inguinal hernias on clinical grounds is almost impossible and since the operative approach is identical, preoperative differentiation is irrelevant.

Other groin swellings which may lead to diagnostic difficulty include:

1. Hydroceles of the canal of Nuck – come and go, transilluminate and can be manipulated in the long axis of the cord. When this is done, the testis moves too. The testis does not move when a hernia is reduced.
2. Ectopic/undescended testis – always fully examine the scrotum in a patient with a suspected hernia.
3. Cord lipomata – soft and lobulated without a cough impulse.
4. Inguinal lymphadenopathy – generally multiple and lie both sides of the femoral vessels.
5. Psoas abscess – may transmit a cough impulse but is usually lateral to the femoral vessels. There will usually be signs and symptoms of retroperitoneal, gastrointestinal or spinal pathology.
6. Iliofemoral aneurysm – rhythmic expansile pulsation, bruit or thrill.

Clinical examination remains the mainstay of the diagnosis of groin hernias. Persistent intermittent groin pain in obese women is difficult to diagnose and in these cases ultrasound may demonstrate an impalpable hernia (Spangen et al., 1988). Occasionally elderly patients will present with intestinal obstruction and a groin hernia may be impalpable and remain undiagnosed until laparotomy – dilated intestine and fluid levels, however, may be visible on plain abdominal X-rays. Other useful but rarely used imaging techniques include herniography, performed by injecting water-soluble contrast into the peritoneal cavity. This may be useful in the diagnosis of hernias in infants and to evaluate obscure groin and pelvic pain in adults. Computed tomography (CT) scanning does not have sufficient resolution to show small hernia defects but does delineate abdominal wall and soft-tissue tumours, as does scanning by magnetic resonance imaging (MRI).

An intravenous urogram in a small child will show the common hernias of the bladder ('bladder ears') sliding into indirect inguinal hernias, but is not performed routinely for this purpose alone. Sliding hernias of the bladder also occur in adults with outflow obstruction and in the femoral sacs of females. An important rarity is the ureter in the wall of a large femoral hernia.

Complications of hernia

Irreducibility, obstruction and strangulation

The constricting agent is the neck of the peritoneal sac which is often fibrosed and rigid where it traverses the defect in the abdominal wall. In the case of indirect inguinal hernia this is in the fascia transversalis at the deep inguinal ring. The formation of an indirect hernia in an adult is a gradual process involving failure of the shutter mechanism and a stretching of the deep ring with opening of the processus vaginalis. As a result the constricting ring at the neck of the hernia is relatively wide and the risk of obstruction/strangulation in the lifetime of an indirect inguinal hernia is low – estimated at about 4% (Koontz, 1963). In direct hernia the defect is still within the fascia transversalis, but because this medial space is wider obstruction or strangulation rarely occurs.

The constriction ring of a femoral hernia is, in contrast, rigid due to fibrosis of the peritoneum of the neck of the sac where the peritoneum abuts on the inguinal ligament anteriorly, the lacunar ligament medially and the pectineal ligament posteriorly. The femoral vein laterally is rarely obstructed in strangulated femoral hernia, confirming that the constriction is in the wall of the sac rather than by the adjacent structures. In British practice, over 40% of femoral hernias present as emergencies with strangulation or obstruction (Nicholson et al., 1990).

In babies and infants, who do not yet have an oblique inguinal canal, the constricting agent is the rigid aponeurotic margin of the superficial inguinal ring. Obstruction is more common in these inguinal hernias after a period of irreducibility, but sedation and nursing with slight head-down tilt usually allows reduction and emergency operation is rarely needed. Since the risk of repeated attacks is relatively high, however, these hernias should be repaired on the next available operating list.

Due to the anatomical attachment of the base of the small bowel mesentery, strangulated bowel is twice as frequent in right-sided hernias.

Taxis, reductio-en-masse

A firm but gentle attempt can be made to reduce an obstructed/strangulated hernia but the risks are considerable:

1. Rupture of intestine at the neck of the hernia.
2. Return of devitalized intestine to the abdomen.
3. Reductio-en-masse of the whole sac and strangulated contents. The patient may have done this himself and then present some days later with the signs of strangulation and/or peritonitis.
4. Stricture following relief of strangulation by taxis (intestinal stenosis of Garré). This is often a double stricture of both the afferent and efferent loops. The patient develops diarrhoea and malaena and the signs of progressive obstruction a few days after reduction of the hernia.

Maydl's hernia, afferent loop strangulation, Richter's and Littré's hernia

Maydl's hernia is a complication of large hernial sacs, especially right-sided scrotal hernias in Africans, when a double loop (W) of small intestine lies in the same sac. The intermediate loop is strangulated within the main abdominal cavity at the peritoneal ring between the afferent and efferent loops. Perforation leads to generalized peritonitis. Afferent loop strangulation is a complication of large inguinal scrotal hernias in Africans who have a long pendulous caecum. The caecum is incarcerated in the hernial sac; a loop of small bowel passes behind the ascending colon and is strangulated to the right of the colon. Laparotomy is required to reduce the hernia.

Richter's hernia (partial enterocele) occurs when only the antimesenteric margin of the intestine becomes strangulated. Intestinal obstruction is incomplete, but increasing toxaemia occurs as the intestinal wall becomes devitalized. This type of hernia most commonly occurs in femoral, obturator and small incisional hernias (Figure 8.5). The appendix is not uncommonly seen in an inguinal or femoral hernial sac and may become strangulated, behaving clinically like a Richter's partial enterocele (Cronin and Ellis, 1959). In Littré's hernia the sac contains a strangulated Meckel's diverticulum, and spontaneous resolution has been recorded following formation of a local fistula.

Involvement in disease of the peritoneal cavity

The peritoneal lining of a hernial sac may become involved in any disease affecting the general peritoneal cavity. Abdominal carcinomata can involve a hernial sac by transperitoneal seeding or by direct invasion of an incarcerated viscus, e.g. colon. If ascites or thickening of the sac are found unexpectedly, then the fluid should be examined cytologically and the sac histologically. Routine histological examination of hernial sacs is not advised since the pick-up

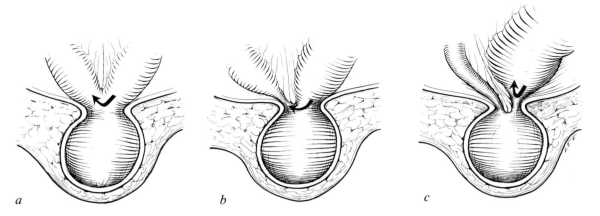

a   *b*   *c*

Figure 8.5 Richter's hernia (partial enterocele). The antimesenteric circumference of the bowel is first held by the rigid neck of the hernial sac, usually a femoral or obturator hernia. The situation is progressive: from (*a*) partial involvement of the bowel circumference without obstruction, to (*b*) subacute obstruction, to (*c*) complete obstruction and strangulation of the incarcerated bowel

rate of occult malignancy is exceedingly rare. If intra-abdominal malignancy is suspected it may be possible to perform a 'mini-laparotomy' through the sac. Embarking on major abdominal surgery without a tissue diagnosis in an ill-prepared patient is not recommended. The usual primary site is colon, stomach or ovary.

Hernial sacs may become involved in primary mesothelioma which must be distinguished from the reactive mesothelial hyperplasia encountered in infancy (Brenner *et al.*, 1981). Endometriosis sometimes occurs in the hernial sacs of menstruating women, but is most common in incisional hernias after Caesarean section or gynaecological operation.

Generalized peritonitis from whatever cause can lead to pus filling hernial sacs which become inflamed and tender leading to diagnostic difficulty (Cronin and Ellis, 1959). Acute appendicitis in inguinal, femoral and umbilical hernias has been described (Thomas *et al.*, 1982).

Sliding hernia – hernia-en-glissade

In this variant, part of the circumference of the hernial sac is formed by the wall of a viscus such as the caecum or sigmoid colon which are in part retroperitoneal structures. Sliding hernias are more common at the extremes of life; in children, bladder may be found in the medial wall and, in girls, the ovaries and fallopian tubes. In elderly adults large, long-standing hernias may contain considerable lengths of sigmoid colon or caecum (Figure 8.6).

The repair of these large hernias follows the same principles as any other indirect inguinal hernia, except that there is often little excess sac to excise. The hernia is completely mobilized away from the spermatic cord and reduced back into the abdominal cavity. The fascia transversalis is then repaired in front of the hernia and a new deep ring constructed snugly around the cord to prevent recurrence.

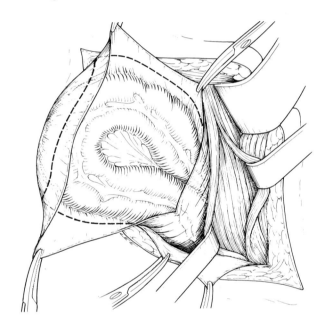

Figure 8.6 Sliding hernia. The sigmoid loop of colon in a left inguinal hernia. These hernias are sometimes very difficult to reduce and close. A muscle-splitting incision 5 cm or so above and parallel to the inguinal ligament can facilitate mobilization. The hernia is delivered through the higher incision, excess sac is trimmed away and the sac closed. Care with the colon and its blood supply is needed. The repair of the defect is described elsewhere

Herniation of the female genitalia – pregnancy

Care must be taken when operating on hernias in baby girls to avoid damage to the fallopian tubes or ovaries. In older women, sliding hernias of the ovary and tubes are not infrequent in femoral, inguinal and obturator hernias. The uterus is a rare finding in a hernial sac, but pregnancy in irreducible umbilical and inguinal hernias is well recorded.

Testicular complications

Ischaemia or infarction of the testis may occur in infants with irreducible/obstructed inguinal hernias. If emergency operation must be performed, care should be taken to dissect the vessels off the sac and to ensure that at completion the testis is down in the scrotum. If possible the testis should not be mobilized from the scrotal bed at all, as this will reduce the risk of postoperative testicular ischaemia. The ischaemic testis will feel hard and swollen postoperatively, but should be left because many will recover at least endocrine function and be cosmetically useful later in life.

General principles of hernia management

Patients about to undergo hernia repair should be fully prepared. Attention to and correction if possible of other conditions is crucial to minimizing morbidity and mortality; this is especially true in neonates and the elderly (Buck *et al.*, 1987).

The mortality of elective groin hernia repair is almost zero at all ages. This has been achieved because of attention to the cardiopulmonary state of the patient, with correction of hypertension and cardiac failure, stabilization of angina and optimization of respiratory function. Preoperative care of patients with diabetes mellitus has contributed to the reduction in mortality of elective surgery. In patients with obstructed or strangulated hernias, mortality increases with age: at 60 years it is 3%, at 70 years 6%, rising to 12% at 80 years.

The mortality of strangulated hernia is almost entirely due to haemodynamic respiratory and renal disease. Elderly patients have impaired renal function and low cardiorespiratory reserve. A period of intestinal obstruction leads to significant losses of extracellular and intravascular fluid, with concomitant changes in electrolyte balance. Adequate time should be spent preoperatively attempting to correct these. Patients should have good intravenous access and normal saline (with added potassium if required) should be infused and the efficacy of resuscitation monitored by regular measurements of pulse, arterial blood pressure and urine output. In frail patients or the very young, serum urea and electrolytes should be checked at the start of the process and preoperatively to ensure adequate resuscitation.

Following *resuscitation*, the principles of operative management are *reduction* of the hernia and *repair* of the defect.

Haemostasis

Careful haemostasis and gentle handling of the tissues will minimize haematoma formation and the risk of sepsis. Diathermy is employed for small vessels, taking great care close to the cord. Larger vessels should be ligated with absorbable, synthetic sutures. Chromic catgut is not recommended because of adverse effects on wound healing. It initially provokes a slow inflammatory response, but this increases at about 10 days with the appearance of foreign body giant cells, after which tensile strength fails rapidly.

Closed suction drains should be employed if extensive dissection has been used, as in the repair of a large, long-standing, sliding hernia.

Sepsis is the great hazard of hernia repair, particularly when non-absorbable material is used as in the repair of all adult groin hernias. The skin is carefully prepared with an antiseptic solution such as chlorhexidine or povidone-iodine and the operation site covered with transparent, sterile, adherent film, which is not removed until the skin is closed. Interrupted skin sutures should not be used as they may introduce bacteria into the wound. Skin closure with a buried, absorbable subcuticular suture or by sterile adhesive tapes is recommended. Postoperative wound infection increases the risk of hernia recurrence by a factor of four (Glassow, 1964; Devlin *et al.*, 1986). Prophylactic antibiotics are not normally recommended for elective hernia repair, but for patients with obstructed/strangulated hernias these should be used. An appropriate choice would be a penicillin or aminoglycoside and metronidazole or cephalosporin combination.

Wound healing and sutures

The function of the suture material used to repair the hernia defect is to appose the aponeurotic structures until fibroblast activity has laid down new collagen fibrils of sufficient tensile strength to prevent breakdown of the repair.

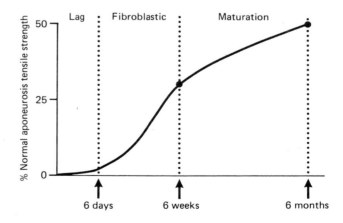

Figure 8.7 Phases of wound healing. During the initial lag phase the wound is quiescent and during the fibroblastic phase wound strength increases rapidly over a few days; however, it is in the third, maturation, phase that significant and permanent strength gain occurs

Optimal results are not obtained unless aponeurosis or fascia is incised prior to suturing; incised wounds heal faster and are ultimately stronger than invaginated or infolded aponeurotic or fascial wounds. Continuous suturing produces better results than interrupted sutures, since it distributes the load more evenly and requires less suture than all the knots in interrupted suturing. Severe protein malnutrition, prolonged hypovolaemia, vitamin C deficiency and tissue hypoxia are factors which may impair wound healing (Devlin, 1988). Figure 8.7 gives the phases of wound healing – the lag, fibroblastic and maturation phases.

The process of collagen synthesis and maturation does not reach completion until a year or more after hernia repair. Absorbable sutures, whether natural or synthetic, do not persist long enough for adequate structural integrity to be restored (Figure 8.8).

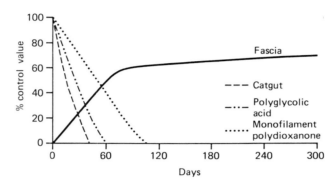

Figure 8.8 Relationship of wound strength gain to the rate of wound healing in aponeurotic wounds. Absorbable sutures do not survive long enough to ensure wound stability. Polydioxanone occupies an intermediate position between the traditional catgut and the absorbable polymers on the one hand and the non-absorbables on the other

Although modern synthetic, absorbable sutures such as polydioxanone would appear, in theory, to be adequate, any impairment of wound healing such as sepsis or factors discussed above would result in inadequate fascial healing before suture dissolution, risking increased recurrence rates. The use of these sutures cannot, therefore, be recommended.

The ideal suture material should be chemically and biologically inert, easily sterilizable and not likely to 'hold' sepsis, flexible and not prone to physical change or hardening in the body, and strong enough to perform its function until complete healing of the aponeurotic/fascial wound has occurred and then disappear.

Such a material does not exist, but modern polymer chemistry has provided close compromises. Stainless steel wire provides the best tensile strength and knot security of all available materials, but it is difficult to handle and therefore not recommended for routine use. Monofilament nylon or polypropylene offer the best compromise of tensile strength, knot security and handling characteristics (Herman, 1974). Many abdo-

minal hernias occur through parietal defects too large to close by simple suture coaptation. Prosthetic materials are required and should have similar characteristics to the 'ideal' suture material. In addition, the prosthesis should remain inert and strong for the whole lifetime of the patient. It should be easy to cut to size and fit into the body. Monofilament knitted polypropylene (Marlex mesh) is a popular and proven prosthesis. Another is expanded polytetrafluoroethylene (PTFE) which has long been available as a vascular prosthesis, now available in sheets of various sizes. Matching PTFE sutures are available which are flexible, knot easily and lack 'memory'. As a general principle, the prosthesis should be sutured in place with identical material.

The operations

Inguinal hernia in babies and children

Inguinal hernia is the commonest indication for surgery in early life. The incidence in male children is just over 4% and the male to female ratio is 9:1. Ten per cent require emergency admission because of incarcerated or strangulated hernias (Devlin, 1988). The incidence is increased with low birth weight and prematurity – up to 30% in infants of birth weight 1000 g or less. The greatest risk is in the first 3 months of life. The probability of incarceration is 1 in 4 for all inguinal hernias in male children aged under 1 year, but progression to strangulation is rare. Infantile inguinal hernias should be repaired electively as soon as practicable. An experienced paediatric surgeon can readily undertake the operation no matter how young the child.

The inguinal canal does not develop its obliquity until 11–12 years of age; before this, simple herniotomy suffices to repair an indirect inguinal hernia. Great care must be taken to avoid damage to the testicular blood supply and to give a cosmetically acceptable scar. There can be little justification for the 'occasional' operator.

Children with inguinal hernias are ideally treated as day-case patients. This requires good hospital organization and hospital to community communication. The mother or parent should accompany the child to hospital and take him or her home after recovery. Adequate facilities should be available for the parents.

Day-case surgery in young children is best performed between 10.00 a.m. and 3.00 p.m., giving the mother and child adequate time to get from home to hospital. Hypoglycaemia and dehydration are a problem if children are starved unnecessarily. These physiological problems can be prevented by giving the child a normal morning feed and then a preoperative drink of maltose and metoclopramide, and by operating as early after the morning feed as is safe (Atwell *et al.*, 1973). Operation should always be completed before 3.00 p.m. to ensure that the child is fully recovered from anaesthesia before being sent home.

General anaesthesia is employed and the patient placed supine on the operating table with light cotton blankets over the chest and upper abdomen and over the lower limbs to prevent heat loss. Drapes are applied so that the groin area and scrotum are exposed throughout the operation.

A skin-crease incision about 2 cm long and 1 cm above the external inguinal ring is made (Figure 8.9). The superficial fatty subcutaneous tissue is incised until a fascial layer is encountered. This is the membranous layer of the superficial fascia (Scarpa's) which is well defined in infants. This is incised and the dissection deepened to the cord as it emerges from the superficial ring. The cord is recognized by the interlacing pink bundles of the cremaster muscle. The cremasteric fibres are gently parted to reveal the bluish grey peritoneal sac on the superomedial aspect of the cord. Separation of the sac from the cord structures usually requires a little sharp dissection to divide the internal spermatic fascia (Figure 8.10). If the sac is complete (extending to the scrotum), the distal sac is not dissected out. The sac is divided and the distal end left open. The sac is dissected proximally and the neck to the parietal peritoneum identified. Care is needed to ensure that the sac is empty before transfixing at the deep ring and that the vas is not still attached to it, or that it is not a sliding hernia of the ovary and fallopian tube in a girl. An absorbable polymer such as metric 3 braided polyglactin 910 or polyglycolic acid is used. The excess sac is excised (Figure 8.11). Care is taken to close the subcutaneous tissue to obliterate any 'dead' space and the skin is closed with a clear absorbable monofilament suture such as polydioxanone or with adhesive strips. Skin sutures requiring removal should be avoided. At the completion of the operation the surgeon must check that the testis lies in the scrotum – a testis left high will become held by postoperative adhesions, leading to an iatrogenic ectopic testis.

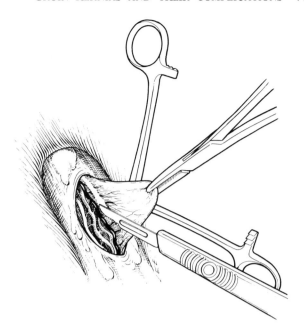

Figure 8.10 The sac being separated from the cord structures. A gentle stroke with a sharp scalpel will divide the internal spermatic fascia, opening up a plane between the sac and the cord structures

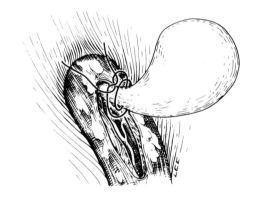

Figure 8.11 The sac is closed with a transfixion ligature

Wound infection is uncommon after repair of infantile inguinal hernias. The problem of testicular ischaemia has been discussed previously. This complication is minimized by not mobilizing the testis from its scrotal bed. Division of the vas deferens may occur, but the incidence is difficult to quantify. Fragments of vas deferens were found in 5 of 313 infantile hernial sacs (1.6%) examined histologically (Weiner, 1962). If the vas is damaged and recognized, immediate repair should be performed.

Inguinal hernia repair in adults

Repair of an inguinal hernia does not constitute a major operation. There should be little manipulation

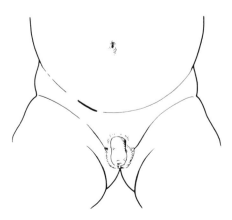

Figure 8.9 A 1.5 cm long incision is made just above and medial to the external inguinal ring

of viscera, no haemodynamic hazard and no metabolic consequences. The risk of sepsis is low after elective repair and the use of antibiotic prophylaxis is unnecessary. Elective repair should be advised for most patients.

The low risk of strangulation and the relatively high frequency of inguinal hernia in adults (5–8% of elderly male population) make hernia repair an unnecessary treatment in an asymptomatic elderly male with a spontaneously reducible inguinal hernia. An active, elderly man with a symptomatic hernia, on the other hand, should be offered surgery. A truss rarely controls an inguinal hernia satisfactorily and may lead to further weakening of the inguinal canal with prolonged usage.

The history of inguinal hernia repair in adults is long and many of the essential elements of successful repair were used over 100 years ago by Bassini (1890). He realized that the essential defect in both indirect and direct inguinal hernia was a failure of the transversalis fascia/transversus lamina of the lower abdominal wall and that repair and reinforcement of these layers should result in cure. Bassini always divided and repaired the transversalis fascia – a fact overlooked by many contemporary surgeons (Catterina, 1934).

Reinforcement of the inguinal canal by darning between the conjoint tendon and the inguinal ligament is an old concept. Several different materials have been employed, e.g. kangaroo tendon, human fascia lata, floss silk and wire, but long-term results were poor. The monofilament nylon darn was popularized by Moloney in Oxford who reported no recurrences at 2 years' follow-up of 400 hernia repairs (Moloney et al., 1948). His technique, however, was meticulous, with careful dissection and suturing of the fascia transversalis at the deep ring. Subsequently this part of the operation has been omitted and the most recent report of a darn technique gives a cumulative recurrence rate greater than 10% at 5 years (Lifschutz and Juler, 1986). In modern surgical practice the best results have been obtained using techniques which concentrate on the faulty layer – the fascia transversalis. Three such techniques are described: The Shouldice operation (Glassow, 1976), the McVay–Cooper ligament operation (McVay and Chapp, 1958) and the French extraperitoneal mesh operation (Stoppa et al., 1982).

Shouldice operation

Earle Shouldice and his co-workers in Toronto stressed good anatomical technique and thus reduced the recurrence rate at the Shouldice Clinic from 6.5% in the mid-1940s to 0.1% in the early 1950s (Shouldice, 1953). The main principles of the Shouldice operation are:

1. Reconstitution of the normal anatomy with particular attention to the transversalis fascia –

attenuated fascia transversalis is excised and this lamina is reconstructed using an overlapping or double-breasting technique.
2. Assessment of all possible hernia sites – direct, indirect and femoral – so as to avoid the 'missed' hernia.
3. Suture only of tendinous, aponeurotic or fascial structures and never fleshy muscle.
4. The use of monofilament, non-absorbable suture materials.

The Shouldice repair and its variations have produced uniformly excellent results in the hands of numerous surgeons worldwide (see Table 7.1, page 55). In the classical Shouldice operation, a repair is fashioned with three double-breasted suture lines (see Chapter 7). Based on experience of a large number of repairs performed under local anaesthesia, Barwell in the UK realized the importance of the deepest row of sutures in the transversalis fascia and in his technique the fascia transversalis/transversus arch is sutured to the iliopubic tract from medial to the deep ring laterally, and then the transversus lamina/conjoint tendon is sutured from the deep ring laterally to medial using one continuous suture. In over 1200 indirect inguinal hernia repairs performed since 1977 there have been only 5 recurrences (0.4%) (N. J. Barwell, personal communication).

The Shouldice technique achieves a strong, durable repair under very low tension, and relaxing incisions in the rectus sheath are not needed. Because the fascia transversalis is reconstituted to form a new deep ring around the emergent cord, division of the cord and/or orchidectomy are never needed, even for repair of recurrent hernias. A detailed account of the Shouldice operation is given in Chapter 7.

McVay–Cooper's ligament operation

This is an alternative to the Shouldice operation. The repair of the transversalis lamina is made by mobilizing the transversus arch/transversalis fascia which, after making a generous relaxing incision in the anterior rectus sheath medially, is sutured to the iliopectineal (Cooper's) ligament medially and to the anterior femoral sheath and iliopubic tract more laterally using a continuous monofilament, non-absorbable suture (Figure 8.12). The direct and indirect inguinal and the femoral regions are reinforced by a stout layer of fascia transversalis and adherent transversus muscle and this technique is recommended for the dual repair of an inguinal and femoral hernia (Isaac, 1961). Recurrence rates of 1.3% at a median follow-up of over 6 years have been reported, equalling the results of the Shouldice technique (Rutledge, 1980).

In both the Shouldice and McVay techniques the hernial sac or remnant is placed behind the repair and the deep inguinal ring reconstituted. Both these techniques are, therefore, ideally suited for repair of

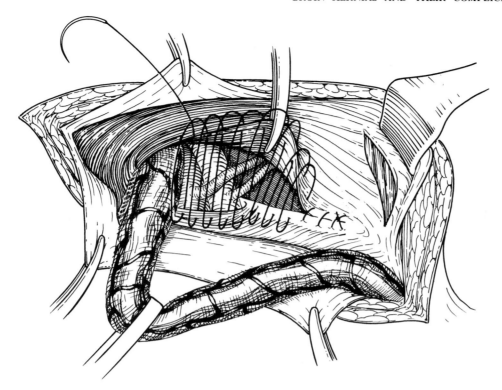

Figure 8.12 The McVay–Cooper ligament hernia repair opens the relaxing incision in the anterior rectus sheath (internal oblique and transversus tendons) and sutures the upper flap of transversalis fascia, transversus and internus to the inguinal and pectineal ligaments

sliding hernias, this variety giving rise to no extra technical difficulty.

The French extraperitoneal mesh operation

See section on recurrent groin hernia (page 75).

Femoral hernia

A femoral hernia is rarely large and may be difficult to detect in an obese patient. It is not usually reducible and a palpable cough impulse is infrequent. The femoral hernial sac usually only contains omentum and if it contains bowel it is only a small knuckle. A Richter's hernia is more common at this site than at any other and occurs more often on the right.

Early elective operation should always be advised because femoral hernias have a high risk of obstruction. Elective operation carries a low morbidity and almost zero mortality, even in elderly patients. Emergency operation with obstruction or strangulation carries a much greater risk even when preceded by the most careful resuscitation (Nicholson *et al.*, 1990).

As with all other lower abdominal hernias the primary defect is a weakness in the transversalis fascia and overlying parieties which allow a peritoneal protrusion to occur. The principles of femoral hernia repair involve removal of the sac, repair of the fascia

transversalis and reinforcement by aponeurosis (or prosthetic mesh). Three approaches to femoral hernia repair are described; although there are several variations of each of these basic operations, the 'complete' surgeon should have each in his repertoire:

1. The abdominal, suprapubic, retroperitoneal, preperitoneal or *extraperitoneal* operation (eponyms: Cheatle, Henry, McEvedy – McEvedy, 1950).
2. The inguinal or 'high' (eponyms: Annandale, Lothiessen or Moschcowitz – Moschcowitz, 1907).
3. The crural or 'low' (eponyms: Bassini or Lockwood – Lockwood, 1893).

The extraperitoneal approach is elegant but unfamiliar to many surgeons and the most useful for a strangulated hernia. The inguinal approach enables femoral and inguinal hernias to be repaired simultaneously, but it is crucial that a careful inguinal repair is made to prevent an inguinal hernia recurrence. The crural operation is easy to do, without much tissue trauma, and is best reserved for elective situations. If it is used in an emergency where gut resection is needed, a standard laparotomy incision is necessary to deal with the devitalized bowel or omentum.

The crural or 'low' approach

This can be performed under general anaesthetic or

with local anaesthetic infiltration. The patient is positioned supine with slight (15°) head-down tilt as for inguinal hernia repair. Many femoral hernias have a sliding component of bladder in the medial wall of the sac and, therefore, preoperative catheterization of the bladder is a sensible precaution.

A skin incision about 6 cm long is made over the hernia and parallel to the inguinal ligament, and the subcutaneous fat separated down to the coverings of the hernial sac. The fundus of the sac often lies over the inguinal ligament. The fascial layers are cleared off the sac by blunt dissection. Once the neck of the sac has been cleared of fat and fascia, the boundaries of the femoral canal will be visible. Care must be taken to prevent damage to the femoral vein which is covered in a quite opaque fascial sheath.

The sac is then opened on its lateral side (to prevent bladder injury). Any contents can now be gently freed, adhesions divided and the contents reduced back into the peritoneal cavity. The sac is then transfixed at its neck using an absorbable polymer suture and excised.

The repair is fashioned by apposing the inguinal and pectineal ligaments with a single figure-of-eight suture of metric 3 polypropylene on a J-shaped needle, taking the first bite through the pectineal ligament close to the femoral vein. The next bite picks up the inguinal ligament and iliopubic tract of fascia transversalis, then back down to the pectineal ligament and finally back to inguinal ligament–iliopubic tract. The knot is tied medially so as to avoid damage to the femoral vein (Figure 8.13).

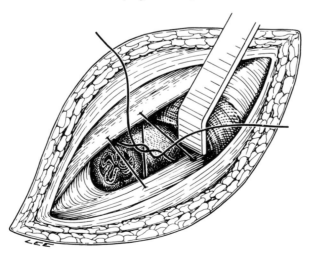

Figure 8.13 The knot is tied deeply at the medial side away from the femoral vein

Since the repair at this stage consists of two tendinous structures apposed under tension, it is advisable to reinforce it with a further aponeurotic patch which is not under tension. This is readily achieved by raising a flap of fascia off the pectineus muscle which

is then sutured with continuous metric 3 polypropylene to the external oblique aponeurosis to cover the initial repair of the femoral canal (Figure 8.14).

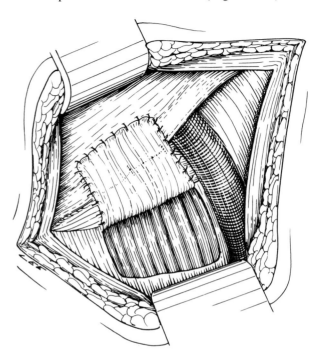

Figure 8.14 The flap of pectineus fascia sutured over the femoral canal

The inguinal or 'high' approach

The inguinal canal is exposed and opened as for repair of an inguinal hernia and the fascia transversalis opened in the same way to access the femoral canal from above. The extraperitoneal fat on the neck of the femoral hernia can be identified and removed by blunt dissection. The sac can now either be delivered above the inguinal ligament or opened below and its contents reduced. The neck of the sac is then transfixed and ligated. The repair is then fashioned by apposing the pectineal ligament and the iliopubic tract–inguinal ligament, but in this operation the sutures are placed from above with a clear view of the structures. The inguinal canal is then repaired using the Shouldice technique, taking care to reinforce the femoral repair with the overlapped fascia transversalis at the medial part of the canal.

In women with a broad pelvis, it is recommended that the medial repair is reinforced by suturing the transversus arch/conjoint tendon/transversalis fascia lamina down to the pectineal ligament, as in the McVay–Cooper ligament repair.

The inguinal operation is not recommended for routine use because it is more difficult and time consuming to perform and because it disrupts an otherwise normal inguinal canal. Failure to repair the inguinal canal exposes the patient to the risk of a direct inguinal hernia subsequently.

The extraperitoneal operation

More than any other procedure in hernia surgery this illustrates the genius of an expert surgical anatomist exploiting fascial plane dissection at its most elegant. Henry's extraperitoneal approach to the anterior pelvis gives excellent exposure of both femoral canals simultaneously, but it is not an operation for the novice.

The patient is positioned supine and the bladder catheterized. A Pfannenstiel incision with a suprapubic side-to-side opening of the anterior rectus sheath and separation of the rectus muscles gives comparable exposure and a much more cosmetic scar than the classical vertical midline incision. The space between the peritoneum and abdominal wall muscles is opened by blunt dissection to approach the femoral canal on either side. The femoral canal is repaired in the same way as in the inguinal operation and the abdominal wall closed in layers.

In the UK, the extraperitoneal approach is most popular when the hernia is strangulated and the 'low' operation for elective procedures, in most series these operations being employed in approximately equal numbers. In a typical UK series the overall recurrence rate for the extraperitoneal operation was 12.5%, for the crural operation, 4.5%, but over 30% for the inguinal operation (Wheeler, 1975). In a more recent study from Stockton-on-Tees (1976–1987), 145 patients underwent femoral hernia repair: 63 presented as emergencies with obstruction or strangulation and 82 had elective repair. Five patients suffered a recurrence (3.4%), with zero recurrence after 29 extraperitoneal operations, 3 recurrences following 35 inguinal operations (8.6%) and 2 recurrences following 82 low operations (2.4%) (Nicholson et al., 1990). When the inguinal approach is used electively and combined with a Shouldice repair of the inguinal canal, an impressively low recurrence rate of under 2% is recorded (Glasgow, 1966).

The recurrent groin hernia

Recurrent hernia is defined as any weakness of the operation area necessitating a further operation or the provision of a truss. In modern practice, using a scrupulous technique and synthetic, monofilament, non-absorbable suture material to perform a transversalis lamina repair, recurrence rates at 5 years should be less than 2% (Glasgow, 1984). After surgery, 30% of recurrences will be apparent at 2 years, 60% by 5 years and 90% by 10 years. When inguinal hernias recur, 55% of the recurrences are indirect and these tend to occur early, 45% are direct (late) and 5% are femoral in type.

Recurrence is related to the experience of the surgeon, technical failure at the original operation, sepsis, haematoma, inept tight suturing and 'missed' hernia. It is important that every possible hernia site, indirect, direct and femoral, must be inspected at every operation for groin hernia. Division of the transversalis fascia and careful dissection of the cord, give the best possible view of all hernia sites. To repair the direct hernia, overlooking the indirect sac, and have the patient to return in 3 months with an indirect 'recurrence' is a poor advertisement for the surgeon's skill!

The repair of a recurrent groin hernia is a technically demanding task and should not be performed by or delegated to an inexperienced surgeon. If it is a first-time recurrence an anterior approach is recommended. Each anatomical layer must be carefully dissected and great care taken not to divide any of the cord structures and risk testicular ischaemia. In the case of inguinal hernia, it is likely that the original repair was not performed using a transversalis fascia type of repair and, therefore, this is likely to be 'virgin' territory. Using the Shouldice technique to repair recurrent inguinal hernias, Glasgow (1984) reports a recurrence rate as low as 3.1%.

If the hernia has recurred on multiple previous occasions or if it was associated with much sepsis or scarring, or when a major tissue defect exists, the extraperitoneal approach with prosthetic reinforcement of the fascia transversalis lamina is the operation of choice. Division of the spermatic cord to repair a recurrent inguinal hernia is never necessary.

The extraperitoneal prosthetic repair: the French operation

The Amiens (France) group of surgeons have devised an ingenious operation for groin hernias, ideal for the multirecurrent hernia, allowing incision through virgin extraperitoneal tissue. Since the spermatic cord does not have to be dissected, the risk of testicular infarction is reduced (Stoppa et al., 1982). Recurrent direct hernias are often bilateral and this operation allows bilateral hernias to be repaired at one operation (Read, 1979). Although the dissection is more extensive, there is less postoperative pain and immobility than with the anterior operation. The disadvantages include the need for general anaesthesia with muscle relaxation to enable access to both sides of the lower pelvis. An experienced assistant is essential to display the tissues by retraction.

Attention to aseptic technique and careful haemostasis are essential factors in minimizing the risk of sepsis. A soft PTFE patch (Goretex) or polypropylene mesh (Marlex) are recommended prostheses and both of these are resistant to sepsis. If sepsis does occur it will resolve without removal of the prosthesis. Postoperatively, oedema of the lower flap and genitalia is a common problem and although this is sometimes considerable it can always be expected to resolve spontaneously.

THE OPERATION

An indwelling catheter is advisable, as an empty bladder is essential to allow adequate exposure of the anterior pelvis. The patient is positioned supine with 15° of head-down tilt. The skin incision and initial exposure are identical to the extraperitoneal (Henry) operation for femoral hernia, with a Pfannenstiel incision providing the best cosmesis. Where there has been extensive scarring in the groin from previous surgery, a lower midline incision may be preferable.

The extraperitoneal plane behind the pubis down to the anterior prostatic capsule is developed by a combination of sharp and blunt dissections. The plane is extended laterally behind the pubis and obturator internus muscles. At this stage the hernial sacs must be identified. The neck of an indirect sac is separated from the cord as it leaves the extraperitoneal space to enter the inguinal canal at the deep ring. Small indirect sacs can usually be milked back, the contents reduced and the sacs transfixed and ligated so that the stump is closed off flush with the peritoneum. In the case of a large inguinoscrotal hernia, complete mobilization of the sac should not be attempted. A proximal 2–3 cm of the sac should be milked back into the extraperitoneal space and divided and sutured flush with the parietal peritoneum once the sac has been emptied. Any attempt to fully mobilize the distal sacs will only lead to extensive bruising and haematoma in the scrotum. Direct inguinal and femoral sacs are usually easily reduced and excised.

The testicular vessels and vas running on the peritoneum posteriorly are mobilized away from the peritoneum for 4–5 cm, allowing the cord structures to be placed against the parieties and the prosthesis positioned between them and the peritoneum, so that the entire groin hernia area, the femoral, the direct and indirect inguinal areas are closed by the mesh (Figure 8.15).

The prosthesis should be cut like a chevron and needs to be large enough to reach from one anterior superior iliac spine to the other, down behind the pubis and pubic rami on either side and at least 3 cm above the lower margin of the conjoint tendon.

The lower edge of the prosthesis is eased down into the pelvis using long artery forceps. The prosthesis is secured to the pectineal ligament close to the femoral vein on either side with a single suture of the same composition. Further sutures are placed medially and when the position of the mesh is seen to be satisfactory the sutures are tied.

Laterally the mesh is secured to the deep surface of the inguinal ligament with care, to avoid damage to the cord or femoral nerve. Closure of the deep inguinal ring and parietalization of the cord is now complete. Finally, the prosthesis is sutured to the conjoint/transversus arch with two interrupted sutures on each side.

The wound is closed in layers with metric 2 polypropylene to the linea alba, picking up the prosthesis in the midline (Figure 8.16). Closed suction drains are routinely placed in the extraperitoneal space. Subcutaneous tissue and skin are closed as for the inguinal operation.

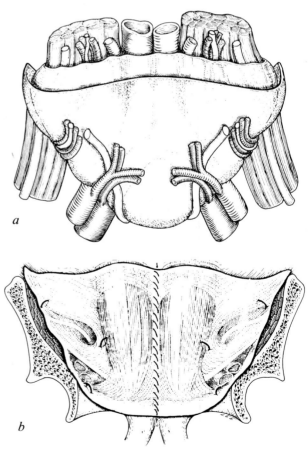

a

b

Figure 8.16 (*a,b*) The completed operation: the mesh lies in the extraperitoneal layer and completely encloses the anterior pelvic peritoneum

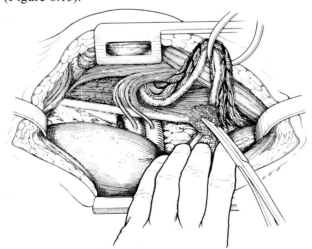

Figure 8.15 The testicular vessels and the vas are mobilized for 4 or 5 cm from the deep ring. These structures are then spread out, 'parietalized', prior to insertion of the mesh

Early mobilization is encouraged and the urinary catheter and drains removed after 24–48 h. In the event of a pyrexia above 38.5°C in the first week postoperatively, blood cultures are taken and parenteral antibiotics started, altering these if necessary once sensitivities are known. Since there is no opening of the peritoneum or manipulation of viscera, ileus is not a problem. If it occurs, particularly if associated with a mild fever, a haematoma in the extraperitoneal space is likely.

Unilateral extraperitoneal prosthetic repair for recurrent hernia

This alternative approach for the repair of the difficult unilateral recurrent hernia, where the contralateral side is sound, was pioneered by Wantz of New York (G. E. Wantz, personal communication) and is really a modification of the Amiène operation. The prosthesis is placed in the extraperitoneal space through a horizontal incision just above the anterior superior iliac spine (Figure 8.17). The sac is milked back from the defect, as already described, and the cord parietalized. Again the prosthesis is placed down into the pelvis to overlap from within the inguinal and femoral regions and to guard against recurrence. The prosthesis is fixed to the back of the pelvis, the pectineal ligament and the abdominal wall laterally (Figure 8.18). A prosthesis of either expanded PTFE or polypropylene mesh is again recommended.

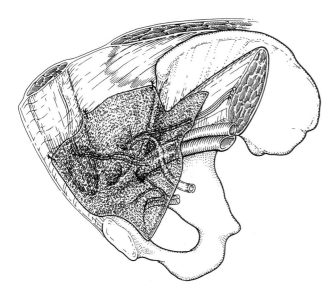

Figure 8.17 A horizontal incision is made in the lower abdomen above the inguinal region. The incision is deepened through the external oblique muscle, the rectus is retracted medially and the extraperitoneal space opened. This space is then developed by blunt dissection. The hernial sac is milked back from the defect in the inguinal canal. The testicular vessels and the vas are dissected and cleared for some 4 cm about the deep ring to allow the prosthesis to be introduced

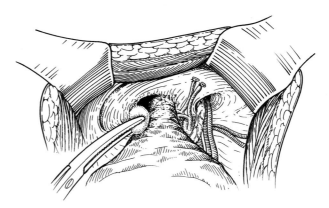

Figure 8.18 The prosthesis is introduced extraperitoneally anterior to the peritoneum and hernial sac, and deep to the parietes. The testicular vessels and vas are 'hooked' over the edge of the prosthesis or placed in a small slot in its margin. The prosthesis must overlap the defect widely. It is held in place by a few nonabsorbable sutures to the pectineal ligament, and the abdominal wall laterally

Conclusions

1. Recurrent inguinal hernia occurs after 10% of primary repairs performed by non-specialists.
2. An important factor in groin hernia recurrence is the 'missed' hernia, and it is crucial to check the direct, indirect and femoral sites during every groin hernia repair.
3. Repair of a recurrent groin hernia is a task for an expert. Even in the best hands, 5–10% of recurrent inguinal hernias will recur again.
4. The extraperitoneal approach with mesh reinforcement of the transversalis fascia is recommended for repair of the multirecurrent hernia.

Complications of hernia repair

Sinus formation is uncommon with modern monofilament sutures, but was a problem when braided sutures were used.

Ischaemic orchitis and testicular atrophy

The testis receives its major blood supply from the testicular artery which joins the spermatic cord at the deep inguinal ring. The cord receives an additional supply from the cremasteric artery and the artery of the vas deferens. These three arteries form an anastomosis in the cord proximal to the testis. Between the superficial inguinal ring and the neck of the scrotum the cord receives an additional supply from the superficial and deep pudendal arteries. All these arteries anastomose freely with each other, and if any one is damaged as the cord is dissected in the canal the anastomosis should be adequate to secure viability of the testicle. It is important to preserve all the testicular blood supply consistent with making an adequate repair of the fascia transversalis. To preserve the distal anastomosis, the testicle should *never* be mobilized from the scrotum and the superficial dissection should *never* extend medial to or inferior to the pubic tubercle. If an indirect sac extends down beyond the pubic spine it should not be dissected but be divided, and the distal portion left open and *in situ*. Previous scrotal surgery, for instance a hydrocele operation or vasectomy, may have damaged the testicular blood supply and will increase the hazard. The venous drainage of the testis will be preserved if the testis is left undisturbed in the scrotum even if the pampiniform plexus is damaged. Thrombosis of the testicular veins may complicate inguinal hernia repair and lead to transient scrotal and testicular oedema, but provided the scrotal venous anastomoses are intact, this settles spontaneously. Damage to the testicular lymphatics in the cord can precipitate a postoperative hydrocele – another reason for not dissecting out the distal sac.

Avascular inflammation may complicate inguinal hernia surgery in infants, children and adults and affects up to 10% of strangulated infantile inguinal hernias due to pressure on the cord vessels by the rigid margins of the external ring. After reduction of the hernia or herniotomy, the testis remains firm and tender, but it will usually recover although there may be some degree of testicular atrophy.

In adults, the ischaemic orchitis syndrome commences 3–4 days postoperatively, with swelling and tenderness of the cord as it emerges from the superficial ring. The testis becomes tender and painful. There may also be a transient leucocytosis and low-grade fever. Half the cases will resolve spontaneously, but in the other half progressive testicular atrophy ensues, taking up to 12 months to become established.

The Shouldice Clinic reports an incidence of 1% in 28 760 primary repairs (Glassow, 1984), but the incidence has been reported as low as 0.1% (Wantz, 1982; Devlin, 1988). When recurrent hernias are repaired, the incidence of testicular atrophy may be as high as 5% when the anterior approach is employed – one argument for employing the extraperitoneal approach which does not disturb the vital scrotal/pudendal anastomosis. Testicular ischaemia and atrophy is an unfortunate complication which may result in litigation. Provided the points listed are adhered to, it should be rare.

Injury to the vas deferens

This should be a rare complication of primary inguinal hernia repair in adults and should never happen during inguinal herniotomy in children. The vas is at greater risk when recurrent hernias are repaired, particularly if an anterior approach is used to repair a multirecurrent hernia. If recognized, vas transection should be repaired immediately with interrupted fine polypropylene sutures, using magnification to ensure accurate end-to-end apposition.

Hydrocele

This complicates 1% of Shouldice repairs, but is lax and resolves spontaneously. Conservative management is recommended, but if troublesome a once-off sterile aspiration allows resolution.

Genital oedema

This is common, but settles spontaneously within 72 hours. It may be more extensive after extraperitoneal mesh repair for bilateral recurrent hernias. Reassurance and scrotal support is all that is required, as it always settles spontaneously.

Impotence

This is transient and there is no organic cause. It will usually resolve.

Nerve injury

During inguinal hernia repair, the iliohypogastric, ilio-inguinal and genitofemoral nerves are all at risk. Nearly all patients will have some numbness below and medial to the incision postoperatively. The ilio-inguinal nerve is most at risk when the external oblique aponeurosis is first opened to isolate the spermatic cord. The iliohypogastric nerve lying above the canal is most vulnerable if a relaxing incision is needed in the anterior rectus sheath. Division of only one nerve causes little if any permanent disturbance because of the degree of overlap in their sensory functions. The motor function of the genitofemoral nerve is effectively lost by dissection and division of the cremaster muscle. Any initial postoperative numbness almost always resolves in a few months. It is preferable to divide the minor sensory nerves than risk entrapment in a non-absorbable suture line, with resultant postoperative paraesthesia.

The femoral nerve is at risk during the extraperitoneal mesh operation for recurrent hernias and it is important to identify the femoral nerve during this operation. Sutures through the fascia transversalis lateral to the cord during the anterior approach are dangerous and are never required if a Shouldice-type repair is used.

Persistent postoperative pain

This may result from nerve entrapment or neuroma formation and should respond to ablation by phenol injection. Persistent pain at the pubic tubercle may result from osteitis and if protracted a plain radiograph should be taken. If this is normal, injection with a local anaesthetic/corticosteroid combination may help.

Femoral vein compression

This may complicate either a femoral hernia repair or

a McVay–Cooper ligament repair of an inguinal hernia if sutures are placed too far laterally. It presents as oedema of the leg and in rare cases a pulmonary embolism. The vein can also be torn by carelessly placed sutures. Removal of the suture and firm pressure usually stems the venous leak.

Urinary retention

This is found in as many as 30% of male patients immediately after groin hernia repair. If simple methods such as mobilization and upright posture do not resolve the problem, a once-only catheterization is advised before the bladder becomes too distended. In older men, a history of bladder outflow obstruction should be ascertained before elective hernia repair. If present, this is preferably assessed and treated first.

Visceral injury

Structures in the wall of a sliding hernia are particularly at risk if an attempt is made to dissect them away to make a complete sac. The viscus most commonly at risk is the bladder. If inadvertently opened the bladder is closed with absorbable sutures and an indwelling catheter left in place for 7 days. If it is necessary to open a narrow-necked direct inguinal sac, it should be opened laterally, as with a femoral hernia, to avoid bladder injury.

Air embolism

Cirrhotic patients with ascites may develop inguinal herniation. Surgical repair is recommended, as these hernias can become irreducible and strangulate. If these patients have had a peritoneovenous shunt inserted previously, introduction of air into the peritoneal cavity during an inguinal hernia repair can put them at risk of air embolism. This can be prevented by clamping the shunt with a small bulldog clamp below the clavicle before operation and injecting the venous side of the shunt with heparin to prevent blockage. The infraclavicular incision is closed, leaving the clamp *in situ*. The abdomen is X-rayed daily following the hernia repair and the clamp removed when all the air has been absorbed.

Deep vein thrombosis and pulmonary embolism

This is a rare occurrence following elective hernia repair and early ambulation. The Stockton experience is of one non-fatal pulmonary embolism in the 10 years 1970–80, an incidence of less than 1 in 1500 elective cases (Devlin, 1988).

Mortality from hernia repair

The mortality following elective groin hernia repair is very low in all reported series; the Shouldice Clinic,

for instance, had a mortality rate of 0.05% in 1969 (Iles, 1969). There were no deaths in the 1500 cases from Stockton-on-Tees in the 1970s. In contrast, strangulated groin hernia carries a considerable mortality today. The Confidential Enquiry into Perioperative Deaths (CEPOD) in the UK estimated that approximately 7.5% of adults with strangulated groin hernia had a fatal outcome (Buck *et al.*, 1987).

In the Northern region of the UK the overall mortality figure for the 10 years 1973–82 inclusive was 5.9%, but this was age-dependent, rising from 1% in the under 60s to 11% in the over 80s (Devlin, 1988) (Table 8.1).

Table 8.1 Outcome after operation for strangulated inguinal and femoral hernias: Northern Region, UK, 1973–82*

Age	Outcome		Total	Death rate
	Discharged alive	Dead		
<60	870	9	879	0.010
60–64	216	6	222	0.027
65–69	331	15	346	0.043
70–74	408	28	436	0.064
75–79	449	39	488	0.080
80–84	387	48	435	0.110
85+	400	47	447	0.105
Total	3061	192	3253	0.059

* The test statistic $\chi^2 = 85.087$ is highly significant ($P < 0.001$ on 6 d.f.). The conclusion is that there is a highly significant association between outcome and age.

General conclusion

Groin hernias demand specialist care if optimal results are to be obtained. The occasional operator produces less than optimal results. Outmoded techniques should be abandoned and new techniques subjected to careful scientific appraisal in properly conducted trials. A surgeon who cannot achieve a recurrence rate of around 1% should re-evaluate his technique. Recurrent hernias, in particular, are a task for the expert, and the surgeon without a specialist interest should not attempt to 'repair his own recurrences'.

'No disease of the human body, belonging to the province of the surgeon, requires in its treatment a greater combination of accurate anatomical knowledge with surgical skill, than hernia in all its varieties.' (Sir Astley Cooper, 1804)

'Hernia surgery demands meticulous technique, gentle handling of tissues, free anatomical exposure, accurate approximation of sutured structures, avoidance of tension and utilization of fine atraumatic needles and suture materials. The disregard of any of these attributes of good surgery will be reflected in a high recurrence rate. With the same method the results will vary with the skill employed by the surgeon.' (L. M. Zimmerman, 1971)

References

Anson, B. J., Morgan, E. H. and McVay, C. B. (1960) Surgical anatomy of the inguinal region based upon a study of 500 body halves. *Surg. Gynecol. Obstet.*, **III**, 707–725

Atwell, J. D., Boon, J. M. S., Dewar, A. K. and Freeman, N. V. (1973) Paediatric day case surgery. *Lancet*, **2**, 895–897

Bassini, E. (1890) Uebar die Behandlung des Leistenbruches. *Arch. Klin. Chir.*, **40**, 429–476

Brenner, J., Sordillo, P. P. and Magill, G. B. (1981) An unusual presentation of malignant mesothelioma. The incidental findings of tumours in the hernia sac during hernioplasty. *J. Surg. Oncol.*, **18**, 159–161.

Buck, N., Devlin, H. B. and Lunn, J. N. (1987) *Report of a Confidential Enquiry into Perioperative Deaths*, Nuffield Provincial Hospitals Trust and King's Fund, London

Cannon, D. J. and Read, R. C. (1981) Metastatic emphysema – a mechanism for acquiring inguinal herniation. *Ann. Surg.*, **194**, 270–276

Catterina, A. (1934) *Bassini's Operation*, Lewis, London

Condon, R. E. (1971) Surgical anatomy of the transversus abdominis and transversalis fascia. *Ann. Surg.*, **173**, 1–5

Cronin, K. and Ellis, H. (1959) Pus collections in hernial sacs. *Br. J. Surg.*, **46**, 364–367

Devlin, H. B. (1988) *Management of Abdominal Hernias*, Butterworths, London

Devlin, H. B., Gillen, P. H. A., Waxman, B. P. and MacNay, R. A. (1986) Short stay surgery for inguinal hernia; experience of the Shouldice operation 1970–1982. *Br. J. Surg.*, **73**, 123–124

Glassow, F. (1964) Is perioperative wound infection following simple inguinal herniorrhaphy a predisposing cause of recurrent hernia? *Can. Med. Ass. J.*, **91**, 870–871

Glassow, F. (1966) Femoral hernia: review of 1143 consecutive repairs. *Ann. Surg.*, **163**, 227–232

Glassow, F. (1971) Femoral hernia in men. *Am. J. Surg.*, **121**, 637–640

Glassow, F. (1976) Short stay surgery (Shouldice technique) for repair of inguinal hernia. *Ann. Roy. Coll. Surg. Eng.*, **58**, 133–139

Glassow, F. (1984) Inguinal hernia repair using local anaesthesia. *Ann. Roy. Coll. Surg. Eng.*, **66**, 382–387

Herman, R. E. (1974) Abdominal wound closure using a new polypropylene monofilament suture. *Surg. Gynecol. Obstet.*, **138**, 84–86

Hughson, W. (1925) The persistent or preformed sac in relation to oblique inguinal hernia. *Surg. Gynecol. Obstet.*, **41**, 610–614

Iles, J. D. H. (1969) Mortality from elective hernia repair. *J. Abdom. Surg.*, May, 87–95

Isaac, R. E. (1961) Inguinal hernia and the ilio-pectineal line. *Br. J. Surg.*, **49**, 204–208

Koontz, A. R. (1963) *Hernia*, Appleton-Century-Crofts, New York

Lifschutz, H. and Juler, G. L. (1986) The inguinal drain. *Arch. Surg.*, **121**, 717–719

Lockwood, C. B. (1893) The radical cure of femoral and inguinal hernia. *Lancet*, **2**, 1297–1302

Lytle, W. J. (1970) The deep inguinal ring, development, function and repair. *Br. J. Surg.*, **57**, 531–536

McEvedy, P. G. (1950) Femoral hernia. *Ann. Roy. Coll. Surg. Eng.*, **7**, 484–496

McVay, C. B. and Chapp, J. D. (1958) Inguinal and femoral hernioplasty. *Ann. Surg.*, **148**, 499–512

Moloney, G. E., Gill, W. G. and Barclay, R. C. (1948) Operations for hernia – technique of nylon darn. *Lancet*, **2**, 45–48

Moschcowitz, A. V. (1907) Femoral hernia: a new operation for radical cure. *New York J. Med.*, 396–400

Nicholson, S., Keane, T. E. and Devlin, H. B. (1990) Femoral hernia: an avoidable source of surgical mortality. *Br. J. Surg.*, **77**, 307–308

Read, R. C. (1979) Bilaterality and the prosthetic repair of large recurrent inguinal hernias. *Am. J. Surg.*, **138**, 788–793

Rutledge, R. H. (1980) Cooper's ligament repair for adult groin hernias. *Surgery*, **87**, 601–610

Shouldice, E. E. (1953) The treatment of hernia. *Ontario Med. Rev.*, 1–14

Spangen, L., Andersson, R. and Olisson, L. (1988) *Ann. Surg.*, **54**, 574

Stoppa, R., Warlaumont, C. R., Verhaeghe, P. J., Odimba, B. K. F. E. and Henry, X. (1982) Comment pourquoi quand utiliser les prostheses de tulle de Dacron pour traiter les hernies et les eventrations. *Chirurgie*, **108**, 570–575

Thomas, W. E. G., Vowles, K. D. L. and Williamson, R. C. N. (1982) Appendicitis in external herniae. *Ann. Roy. Coll. Surg. Eng.*, **64**, 121–122

Wantz, G. E. (1982) Testicular atrophy as a risk of inguinal hernioplasty. *Surg. Gynecol. Obstet.*, **154**, 570–571

Weiner, D. O. (1962) Bilateral exploration in inguinal hernia in juvenile patients. *Surgery*, **51**, 393–406

Wheeler, M. H. (1975) Femoral hernia: analysis of the results of surgical treatment. *Proc. Roy. Soc. Med.*, **68**, 177–178

Wosornu, L. (1974) External herniae: femoral hernia. *Trop. Doct.*, **4**, 59–63

9

Oesophageal and gastric carcinoma

K. Jeyasingham

The majority of malignant neoplasms of the oeso-phagus and stomach are epithelial in origin. Oeso-phageal tumours arise predominantly from the squa-mous lining of the mucosa, whereas gastric tumours arise from the columnar and glandular lining of the gastric mucosa. There is, however, an increasing inci-dence of a glandular carcinoma in the lower oesoph-agus arising from metaplastic columnar epithelium which will need special consideration.

Surgical anatomy

The *oesophagus* is a midline hollow viscus commenc-ing at the cricopharyngeal sphincter at the level of the 6th cervical vertebra (C6), entering the chest at the level of the suprasternal notch, traversing the poster-ior mediastinum and entering the abdomen through the oesophageal hiatus in the diaphragm to join the stomach at the cardia. During this course through three regions of the body it bears a close relationship to the trachea and pericardium in front, and the vertebral column posteriorly. It bears a close relation-ship to the vagus and its branches in its entire length and is not too distant from either pleural cavity during its thoracic course. For all practical purposes

it is devoid of a serosal covering, but like other organs it does have a fascia propria.

The *blood supply* of the oesophagus is derived from the aorta and its major branches, directly as oeso-phageal branches or in common with branches to adjacent organs such as the pulmonary hilum, trachea and thyroid gland. The *venous drainage* is through tributaries draining into the azygos and hemi-azygos systems in the chest and via the thyroid veins in the neck and gastric veins in the upper abdomen.

The *lymphatics* of the oesophagus (Figure 9.1) are distributed predominantly in the form of a submuco-sal plexus and a para-oesophageal plexus. Both plex-uses receive lymph from all parts of the respective

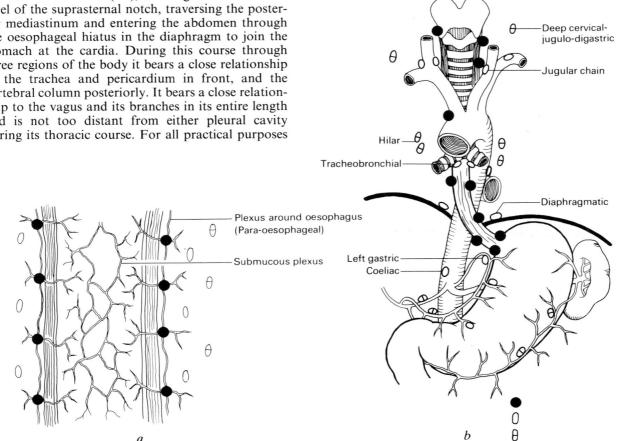

Figure 9.1 *a*, Lymphatic drainage of the oesophageal wall. *b*, Distribution of lymph nodes in relation to regional drainage from the oesophagus

layers of the oesophageal wall. The plexuses communicate with each other through penetrating vessels which traverse the longitudinal and circular muscle walls. The para-oesophageal plexus drains into para-oesophageal lymph nodes which are situated on the surface of the oesophagus, and also into peri-oeso-phageal lymph nodes situated in close proximity to the oesophagus. Lymphatics also drain from the peri-oesophageal nodes to the lateral oesophageal nodes, or directly from the para- to the lateral oesophageal nodes, skipping the peri-oesophageal group (Japanese Society for Esophageal Disorders, 1976) (Table 9.1).

Table 9.1   Lymph nodes of the oesophagus

Para-oesophageal nodes (on the wall of the oesophagus)	Cervical Upper thoracic Middle thoracic Lower thoracic
Peri-oesophageal nodes (in immediate apposition to the oesophagus)	Deep cervical Supraclavicular Paratracheal Subcarinal Para-aortic Diaphragmatic Left gastric Lesser curvature Coeliac
Lateral oesophageal nodes (located lateral to the oesophagus)	Posterior triangle of neck Hilar Superior pancreatico-duodenal and pyloro-duodenal Hepatic Greater curvature

Regionalization of the oesophagus has been adopted as an arbitrary mechanism of describing the exact location of the pathology in the organ. The cervical oesophagus commences at the cricopharyn-geal sphincter and ends at the level of the sternal notch anteriorly and the lower border of the 2nd dorsal vertebra posteriorly. The upper thoracic oesophagus ends at the level of the aortic arch, azygos vein and tracheal bifurcation, while the middle thoracic oesophagus ends at the level of the inferior pulmonary vein. For practical purposes the upper and middle thoracic are together described as 'thoracic' oesophagus, whereas the lower portion together with the abdominal portion of the oesophagus are called the 'lower' oesophagus. The importance of such regionalization becomes more evident when appropriate surgical procedures are planned for lesions situated at levels of the oesophagus (Figure 9.2).

The stomach is a hollow viscus situated in the upper abdomen under cover of the left dome of the diaphragm and protected to a great extent by the costal margin of the chest cage. It bears a close relationship to the left lobe of the liver and the spleen and pancreas. Unlike the oesophagus it has a serosal covering over 90% of its surface, the walls of which contain three distinct muscle layers. Like the oeso-phagus, the stomach is arbitrarily divided into three regions – upper (cardiac and fundus), middle (body) and lower (pyloric) (Figure 9.3).

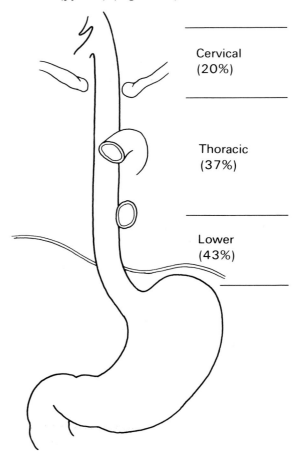

Figure 9.2   Regionalization of the oesophagus and the approximate distribution of carcinoma by region

The blood supply of the stomach is received through branches of the left and right gastric arteries, branches of the gastro-epiploic arteries, and short gastric branches of the splenic artery. It is thus clear that the stomach receives all its arterial blood directly or indirectly from all three major divisions of the artery of the foregut – the coeliac axis. The venous drainage from the stomach reaches the portal veins via the right and the left gastric veins and the splenic veins. The lymphatics of the stomach are also disposed in the submucosal and subserosal plexuses with intercommunication but, unlike in the oesophagus, the lymph nodes draining the stomach are distributed along the lesser and greater curvatures in the first tier of drainage, while the second tier of drainage is situated around the main arterial branches – the left gastric, splenic and gastro-epiploic. The third tier of nodes is located in a suprapancreatic position and around the superior mesenteric artery. Para-aortic and hepatic hilar nodes would constitute the fourth tier of nodes (Soga *et al.*, 1979) (Table 9.2).

Table 9.2 Gastric nodes – N status denoting involvement by tumour

N1 First tier or perigastric	Lesser curve } of same	
	Greater curve } segment	
N2 Second tier	Left gastric	
	Splenic hilum	
	Left gastro-epiploic } body and	
	Oesophagogastric } fundus	
N3 Third tier	Suprapancreatic	
	Superior mesenteric	
N4 Fourth tier	Para-aortic and pre-aortic	
	Hepatic hilum	

TNM classification

The TNM classification of oesophageal and gastric malignant neoplasms has been considerably modified and yet relatively simplified by the Union Internationale Contre le Cancer (UICC, 1990). The regionalization of the oesophagus has been made in such a manner as to follow the International Classification of Diseases (ICD) coding, thereby retaining the concept of cervical, upper thoracic, mid-thoracic and lower thoracic subsites. The stomach likewise would be divided into upper, middle and lower subsites. These subsites would then be conceptually adjacent organs for purposes of primary tumour (T) stratification as given below.

Oesophageal carcinoma – T (Figure 9.3)

TX Primary tumour cannot be assessed
T0 No evidence of primary tumour
Tis Carcinoma in situ
T1 Tumour invades lamina propria or submucosa
T2 Tumour invades muscularis propria
T3 Tumour invades adventitia
T4 Tumour invades adjacent structures or subsites

Gastric carcinoma – T (Figure 9.3)

TX Primary tumour cannot be assessed
T0 No evidence of primary tumour
Tis Carcinoma in situ
T1 Tumour invades lamina propria or submucosa
T2 Tumour invades muscularis propria or subserosa
T3 Tumour invades serosa but not adjacent structures
T4 Tumour invades adjacent structures or subsites

N staging for oesophageal carcinoma

This depends on the quantification of the nodal spread and is as follows:

NX Regional lymph nodes cannot be assessed
N0 No regional lymph node metastases
N1 Regional lymph nodes involved

For the cervical oesophagus the regional nodes are those in the neck, including the supraclavicular nodes. For the intrathoracic oesophagus the mediastinal and perigastric, excluding the coeliac nodes, form the regional nodes. Involvement of lymph nodes outside the regional nodes on the current UICC classification constitutes M1 status (distant metastasis).

N staging for gastric carcinoma

NX Regional nodes cannot be assessed
N0 No regional node metastases
N1 Metastases in perigastric nodes < 3 cm from the peripheral edge of the tumour
N2 Metastases in perigastric nodes > 3 cm from the end of the primary or in the second tier of nodes

Metastatic involvement of other intra-abdominal nodes such as the hepatoduodenal, retropancreatic, mesenteric or para-aortic is classified as distant metastases (M1).

M status for both oesophageal and gastric carcinoma

MX Presence of distant metastases not assessed
M0 No distant metastases
M1 Distant metastases proven

Pathology

By and large 90–98% of all oesophageal carcinomas are squamous (epidermoid) carcinomas. The higher the tumour, the more closely it approximates the 98% figure. About 1–9% of the tumours are adenocarcinomas, the likelihood of this being about 9% in the lower oesophagus (Gunnlaugsson *et al.*, 1970).

Adenocarcinoma occurring in the lower oesophagus is commonly due to a tumour of the cardia of the stomach spreading upwards, occasionally due to adenocarcinoma arising in a columnar-lined lower oesophagus, and only rarely due to a truly oesophageal adenocarcinoma arising in the mucous glands of the oesophageal lining.

In recent years the incidence of adenocarcinoma in the lower oesophagus has been seen to rise. The increasing incidence is not entirely due to an increase in carcinoma developing in dysplastic columnar-lined oesophagus. So far there is no evidence to link this rise to a popular trend towards treating gastro-oesophageal reflux disease with medical regimens for prolonged periods with acid-reducing drugs, thereby exposing the lower oesophagus to an alkaline refluxate. However, the systematic surveillance of patients with columnar-lined oesophagus with or without dysplasia is mandatory if cancerous changes in this form of lining are to be detected early in its evolution.

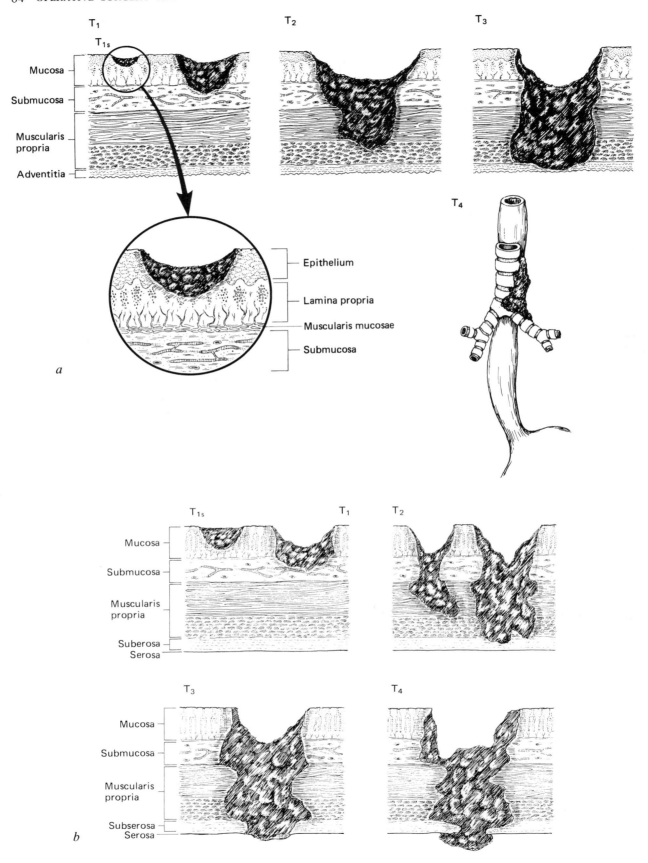

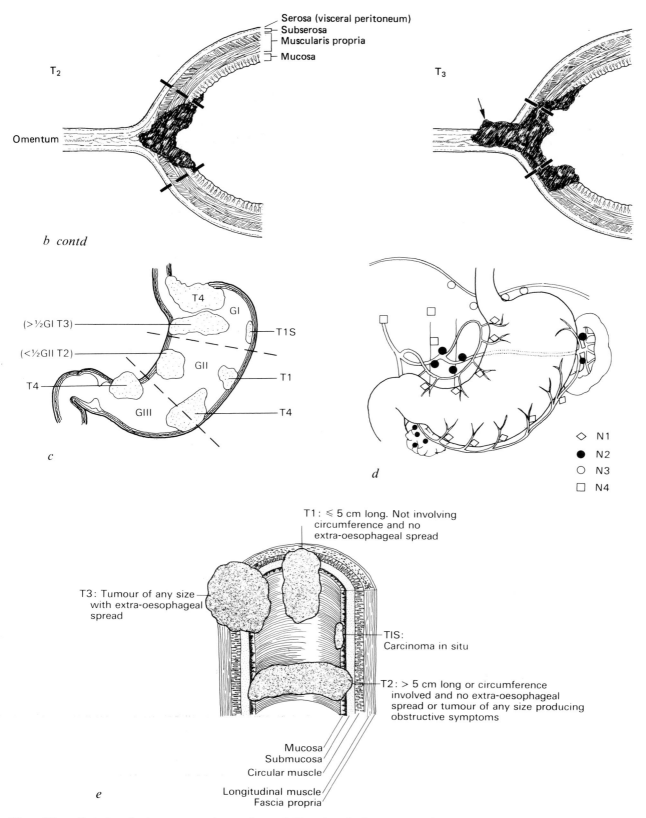

Figure 9.3 *a*, T staging of primary tumour in oesophagus. *b*, T staging of primary tumour in stomach. *c*, T staging of gastric carcinoma. The interrupted lines show the demarcation of the stomach into the upper middle and lower regions. *d*, Lymph nodal drainage of the stomach in staging by nodes. *e*, T staging of oesophageal carcinoma (UICC)

Primary malignant melanoma, mixed squamous and adenocarcinoma, muco-epidermoid carcinoma, adenoid cystic carcinoma and oat cell carcinoma and carcinosarcoma have all been reported in the oesophagus. Tumour spread is characterized by direct infiltration through all layers of the oesophageal wall and into the lumen of the oesophagus. Based on the speed of proliferation, nature of direct progression, extent of trauma and ulceration of the surface and the proportion of fibrous stroma in the tumour, it assumes one of several morphological descriptions (Table 9.3). As the oesophagus has no serosal layer, direct spread into the adjacent organs occurs early. Depending on the location of the tumour, the larynx, trachea, aorta and great vessels, azygos vein, pleura, pericardium, diaphragm and stomach are involved early in the direct spread of the tumour.

Table 9.3 Carcinoma of the oesophagus

Types of lesion

Ulcerative with undermined edges
Constrictive
Scirrhous infiltration
Diffuse-superficial
Polypoidal and necrotic
Rolled edge ulcer
Adenocarcinoma of Barrett's ulcer

Lymphatic spread occurs in different directions based on the flow of lymph in the submucosal plexus in a longitudinal or transverse manner and through penetrating lymphatics to the para-oesophageal lymphatic plexus. Tumour cell aggregates trapped in the submucosal lymphatics produce 'skip lesions'. These have been noted as far as 8 cm away from the outer edge of the primary tumour – an aspect that needs important consideration in deciding the upper limit of transection of the oesophagus (Burgess *et al.*, 1951; Miller, 1962). The para-oesophageal plexus in turn drains into lymph nodes situated in para-oesophageal groups, peri-oesophageal groups and in lateral oesophageal situations. Spread through the bloodstream occurs late in oesophageal carcinoma and is often a terminal feature.

Gastric carcinoma is glandular in origin, but depending on the rate of proliferation and extent of stromal tissue it may again take on one of several morphological forms (Table 9.4).

Table 9.4 Gastric carcinoma

Types of lesion

Polypoidal
Plaque like
Ulcerative and ulcerocancer
Infiltrating
Linitis plastica

Based on a histopathological typing, Järvi and Lauren devised a classification of gastric carcinoma into diffuse (D), intestinal (I) and other (O) (Lauren, 1965). Depending on the degree of advancement of the tumour one can also identify three phases of the same malignant process: early gastric carcinoma, early simulating advanced gastric carcinoma and advanced gastric carcinoma. Early gastric cancer has been defined by the Japanese Society for Gastroenterological Endoscopy as a lesion confined to the mucosa or submucosa with or without nodal metastases. Advanced gastric cancer shows deep invasion, serosal involvement, invasion of adjacent organs, extensive nodal metastases and spread to distant organs. The early simulating advanced gastric cancer, as the name implies, is an advanced gastric cancer masquerading as an early lesion.

Because of the continuity of the oesophagus with the stomach, adenocarcinoma of the cardia often directly involves the lower oesophagus but the presence of the serosa delays direct spread into adjacent organs in the abdomen quite significantly. Lymphatic spread to regional nodes occurs early, whereas submucosal spread of tumour does not appear to occur to the same extent as occurs in oesophageal carcinoma. The occurrence of subserosal nodules some distance from the outer limit of the primary tumour is, however, not uncommon. Bloodstream spread is again a feature of late disease. Extension of tumour from the pylorus into the duodenum does occur, although a form of mucosal block appears to be exercised at the submucosal plane where the pylorus ends and the duodenum begins. It is not uncommon, however, to find direct infiltration of the first part of the duodenum by tumour of the pyloric antrum.

Clinical features

In the early stages, both oesophageal and gastric carcinomas are asymptomatic. The earliest symptom of oesophageal carcinoma is, however, painless dysphagia. Dysphagia is initially experienced with solids, and it gradually progresses, with short periods of remission, to dysphagia with liquids. Occasionally a patient presents with total dysphagia due to impaction of food at the neoplastic lesion. If painless dysphagia progresses to a stage of painful dysphagia, one should suspect direct spread of tumour into the mediastinal structures. Progressive weight loss accompanies increasing dysphagia and is not necessarily due to extensive disease, a fact that needs to be borne in mind before denying surgical treatment to an emaciated patient. Blood loss in the form of haematemesis or melaena is not a common symptom, and anaemia is not a regular feature. Nausea and vomiting, cough, hoarseness, hiccups and halitosis are symptoms suggestive of oesophageal carcinoma. Excessive salivation is often a sign of obstructive pathology, and retrosternal oppression and shortness of breath may also accompany oesophageal carcinoma. Occurrence of cough induced by food would suggest recurrent laryngeal palsy or malignant tracheo-oesophageal fistula.

Physical examination, if it produces a positive sign, almost invariably indicates extensive disease. Palpable nodes in the neck or para-aortic area, hepatomegaly and pleural effusions are all features of late stages of the disease.

The clinical features of gastric carcinoma are even less specific than those of oesophageal carcinoma. Dysphagia, nausea, vomiting, anaemia, dyspepsia, anorexia, gaseous eructations with halitosis, are some of the symptoms noted in patients with gastric carcinoma. Persistent epigastric pain, unabated by food, is an important symptom which when present should draw a suspicion of gastric carcinoma. Melaena and haematemesis in the absence of an ulcer history should suggest a possible malignant cause. The physical presence of lymph nodal enlargement, hepatomegaly, ascites, abdominal mass and jaundice are all features of late disease.

Investigation of oesophageal and gastric carcinoma

The purpose of investigation in these diseases is manifold:

1. Diagnostic.
2. Assessment of extent of disease.
3. Assessment of physical status of patient.
4. Grading of symptoms – dysphagia.
5. Grading of performance status.
6. Grading of nutritional status.
7. Pathological staging of disease.

Radiology

Radiological screening of the patient is undertaken initially with liquid contrast medium with cine or video recording or with serial exposure. The examination is carried from the buccal cavity through to the small bowel. This is then followed by double-contrast radiography, especially if the initial examination has not produced an obvious extensive lesion. Double-contrast radiography has in recent years contributed immensely to the detection of small lesions of the oesophagus and stomach, especially of the plaque-like and polypoidal varieties without any obstruction. When a lesion has been demonstrated on contrast radiography, in those centres where facilities are available for computed tomography the procedure is being increasingly employed to assess the length, the extent of infiltration of the organ, involvement of adjacent organs including the liver, and lymph node enlargement. The addition of a contrast medium to computed tomography adds a further dimension to the examination.

Azygography by the injection of a soluble contrast medium into the marrow of a rib on each side of the chest had been suggested as a useful investigation to detect extra-oesophageal spread, in the days prior to computed tomography, but has failed to gain popularity. Similarly, lymphangiography has no place, currently, in the investigation of oesophageal or gastric carcinoma.

Magnetic resonance imaging is being increasingly employed as an additional technique for evaluation of the tumour. However, it may have very few advantages over and above computed tomographic scanning and transluminal endo-ultrasonography.

Upper gastrointestinal endoscopy

This is the one investigation that has revolutionized the diagnosis, early detection and assessment of neoplasms of the oesophagus and stomach. A full and thorough examination of the entire pharynx, oesophagus, stomach and duodenum is carried out with full documentation of the appearances, both normal and abnormal. Suspicious areas are systematically biopsied and brushed. The size, extent and fixity of the tumour are assessed. The use of *intra vitam staining* of the mucosa to highlight suspicious plaques is a recent innovation (Monnier *et al.*, 1985). The flexible slimline endoscopes have also enabled clinicians to look back at the cardia and fundus to pick up lesions that could easily have been missed otherwise.

Transluminal endo-ultrasonography (EUS)

Endo-ultrasonographic equipment has undergone such extensive refinement that ultrasonography of the oesophagus can define five echodense layers and pick out any abnormalities in these areas. Early detection by screening of the high-risk population and staging of the primary tumour, as well as identification of enlarged lymph nodes, are some of the advantages that have resulted from the development of this technique.

Bronchoscopy

In carcinoma of the cervical and thoracic oesophagus, examination of the tracheobronchial tree is an essential prerequisite, in order to detect compression, infiltration and invasion with or without tracheo-oesophageal fistulation.

Haematological assessment

This is carried out to detect anaemia, alterations in the blood picture, estimate the serum protein, and estimate the liver function tests, with special reference to the liver enzymes. Any alteration of the alkaline phosphatase, alanine transaminase and the aspartate transaminase to above normal levels would be highly suggestive of liver metastases in the presence of neoplasia, but could equally well be due to alcoholic liver damage in patients with oesophageal carcinoma.

Perfusion scan of the liver and bone is undertaken if the alkaline phosphatase has been known to be abnormal, but in the presence of a normal value the investigation could be immediately waived. Ultrasonography of the liver is an alternative procedure. In the presence of symptoms suggestive of brain metastases, a computed tomography scan of the head would be justified.

Mediastinoscopy and laparoscopy or mini-laparotomy are all investigations that could be appropriately employed if exploration with a view to resection is a contraindication.

Assessment of metastases

Computed tomographic scanning, laparoscopy and abdominal ultrasound have been assessed prospectively to evaluate their sensitivity, specificity and accuracy in detecting intra-abdominal metastases in patients with oesophageal and gastric cancer (Watt et al., 1989). Laparoscopy was significantly more sensitive than either ultrasound or computed tomographic scanning in the detection of hepatic metastases and only laparoscopy was able to identify (and therefore histologically confirm) peritoneal metastases.

Early detection of oesophageal and gastric carcinoma

The incidence of carcinoma of the upper gastrointestinal tract varies according to the region of the world under consideration. The routine screening of a whole population for detecting early carcinoma of the upper gastrointestinal tract is justified in parts of the world where there is a high incidence of oesophageal and gastric carcinoma such as the Orient. In the Western world, with the exception of parts of France, the incidence is such that routine screening of the general population is not an economic proposition. There are, however, groups of the population who would appear to be at high risk of developing oesophageal carcinoma and others for gastric carcinoma (Table 9.5).

Grading of dysphagia

It is only by proper documentation of the pretreatment grading of symptoms that one could assess the usefulness of any form of treatment, be it palliative or curative in intent. Such a grading scheme is seen in Table 9.6 which indicates inability to eat different types of food.

Grading performance

This could be achieved either according to the World Health Organization grading from 0 to 4 or on the

Karnofsky scale from 9 to 0 under three groups, A, B and C. They are both non-specific systems for assessment of performance status for each individual patient and can be usefully employed in routine follow-up for assessment of each patient after treatment (against his or her own norm).

Table 9.5 High-risk population for oesophageal and gastric carcinoma

Oesophageal carcinoma
1. Heavy alcohol drinkers who also smoke
2. Patients with a long history of dyspepsia with oesophagitis
3. Patients with columnar-lined oesophagus
4. Patients with achalasia cardia with or without surgical treatment
5. Patients with corrosive strictures treated conservatively
6. Patients with scleroderma
7. Patients with long-standing diverticula not treated surgically
8. Patients with Plummer–Vinson syndrome
9. Patients with hyperkeratosis (tylosis)

Gastric carcinoma
1. Achlorhydric patients
2. Patients with pernicious anaemia
3. Patients with polypoid adenomas
4. Patients with chronic atrophic gastritis (alcoholic patients)
5. Patients who have undergone previous gastrectomy
6. Patients with Ménétrièr's disease

Table 9.6 Grades of dysphagia

0 Normal
1 Intermittent dysphagia to solids
2 Inability to eat solids
3 Inability to eat minced food
4 Inability to eat puréed food
5 Inability to drink liquids (or saliva)

Grading of nutritional state

Patients with carcinoma of the oesophagus and of the stomach are progressively depleted of their nutritional requirements, which are reflected in the blood chemistry, total body compartment and in the cellular components of the blood. Apart from the deprivation of intake of nutrients, and the increasing demands of malignant cachexia, these patients often have impaired liver function from long-standing alcohol and tobacco abuse. The ability of any modality of treatment to correct the nutritional state of the patient is an important factor to be taken into consideration in the choice of the appropriate treatment.

Cardiological and respiratory assessment

Assessment of the cardiac and respiratory reserve of

the patient has to be made both in the grading of the performance status as well as in the evaluation of his or her suitability to any specific modality of treatment. The presence of respiratory problems or of cardiac decompensation, while temporarily excluding surgical resection, may be a total contraindication for chemotherapy or radiotherapy. The pretreatment preparation of the patient should be aimed at controlling any cardiac decompensation by suitable therapy, and respiratory problems have to be adequately treated before a decision is made as to suitability or otherwise for surgical intervention.

Pathological staging of disease

Although pretreatment investigations can greatly assist in assessing the extent of local and distant metastases, the final and conclusive procedure is documenting the exact extent of the primary lesion and of neighbouring structures. Without exploration, all pretreatment staging is arbitrary. Non-exploratory treatment based on such staging is not comparable with post-exploratory treatment based on pathological staging of disease achieved by full assessment of the tumour, lymph nodes and neighbouring structures. Therefore randomized trials of non-surgical modalities such as radiotherapy and chemotherapy against surgical resection based on pretreatment staging are already loaded unfavourably to surgery. Imaging techniques of staging of disease should *ipso facto* involve considerable numbers of invasive and time-consuming investigations, all of which could be far more expensive and demanding to the patient than surgical exploration, which, when feasible, almost always leads to a therapeutic procedure of a palliative or curative nature, with the added advantage of operative staging.

Whichever TNM system one adopts, it is essential that each entity is precisely defined and that peroperative sampling be carried out in a prospective fashion (Table 9.7).

Table 9.7 Objectives of staging

Assessment of tumour extent	T
Nodal assessment	N
Distant metastases	M
Histological type	H
Allocation of region–site	S

Treatment of oesophageal carcinoma

Oesophageal carcinoma often presents at a stage when obstructive symptoms have been present for an average of 5 months, and tumour in existence several more months. The disease has now spread not only into the lumen and wall of the organ but also beyond the fascia propria and probably to distant lymph nodes and organs. Treatment at this stage, therefore, is unlikely to be productive in terms of long-term survival, but to the patient suffering from progressive dysphagia, loss of weight and increasing retrosternal discomfort, any treatment that alleviates these, and in doing so prolongs life, is likely to bring comfort, provided that the treatment can be applied with a low morbidity and mortality, and does not occupy a great proportion of what life expectancy remains. Oesophageal carcinoma, at least in the Western hemisphere, is a disease of the elderly except in certain high-risk groups mentioned earlier (page 88). Surprisingly, elderly patients do tolerate surgical intervention well, but not radiotherapeutic or chemotherapeutic regimens, both of which carry far more debilitating systemic effects for much longer periods.

In recent years, with the widespread use of routine endoscopy of the upper gastrointestinal tract by an increasing number of endoscopists, for symptoms non-specific to oesophageal carcinoma, and with the development of routine screening endoscopy at regular intervals in high-risk populations, aided by brush cytology, lavage cytology or biopsy of suspicious areas highlighted by toluidine blue, it is likely that oesophageal carcinoma will be increasingly detected early in the disease, and the pessimism apparent in most reviews of the therapy of this disease will yield to a much healthier attitude towards it.

At present several modalities of treatment are available to the clinician dealing with this disease: (a) chemotherapy; (b) radiotherapy; (c) surgery; (d) endoscopic procedures.

Any one or a combination of such modalities may have to be employed in the management of each patient. The treatment has to be tailored to the needs of the patient, not vice versa. While randomized clinical trials of a multi-centred nature are essential for progress when new therapeutic vistas open up, the mature clinician managing the oesophageal cancer patient has to exercise judgement in the choice of an appropriate modality or combination of modalities in the first instance, and at later periods institute one or other of the modalities during the remaining lifetime of the patient, if the need arises.

Chemotherapy

Single-agent chemotherapy and combination chemotherapy have both been evaluated. Among the drugs that have been studied are bleomycin, 5-fluorouracil, doxorubicin (Adriamycin), methotrexate, Cyclophosphamide, vindesine, cisplatin and mitomycin. Single-agent activity and combination therapy have only produced a response rate ranging from 15% to 35% and a median duration of response only in weeks, and almost unmodified survival (Gisselbrecht *et al.*, 1983). Currently popular regimens are based on the synergism between Adriamycin and 5-fluorouracil or between Adriamycin and cisplatin.

Pretreatment investigations, with the known toxicity of some of these drugs, should include a chest radiograph, creatinine clearance, serum bilirubin, full blood picture and an excretion pyelogram. The administration of cisplatin should be preceded by forced diuresis with mannitol.

Examples of combination chemotherapy are set out below:

Regimen I   Forced diuresis prior to cisplatin with mannitol 25 g in 1000 ml of 50% dextrose in N/2 saline with 30 mg KCl.
Cisplatin 100 mg/m^2 on day 1 every 3 weeks.
5 Fu 1000 mg/m^2 in 2000 ml of 50% dextrose in N/2 saline over 24 h as an infusion on 4 days every 3 weeks.

Regimen II   5 Fu 1000 mg/m^2 per day in one injection of 120 ml of fluid with cisplatin 100 mg/m^2 with forced diuresis every 3 weeks.

Regimen III   5 Fu 600 mg/m^2 on day 1 and day 8.
Adriamycin 30 mg/m^2 on day 1.
Cisplatin 75 mg/m^2 on day 1 with forced diuresis and hydration.

Each course is repeated every 4 weeks.

Chemotherapeutic regimens are constantly changing, and varying response rates are being claimed by different investigators using different combinations. Although sporadic claims of complete response are recorded, no claims for cure have been made. In the context of the knowledge of histological confirmation of the presence of tumour cells at the time of resection after three cycles of chemotherapy, its role as a single-modality treatment can only be palliative. However, as a combination modality it has a role as a pre-surgery adjuvant with or without post-resection therapy based on whether there are widespread microscopic deposits at the time of resection.

A recent working party of the Medical Research Council (UK) on oesophageal cancer has formulated a randomized controlled clinical trial of surgery with or without preoperative chemotherapy in the treatment of resectable cancer of the oesophagus (Medical Research Council, 1992). The schema for randomization and treatment is as shown in Figure 9.4. The drug regimen on this trial contains:

Cisplatin 80 mg/m^2 in 1 litre of 0.9% saline over 4 h.
Fluorouracil 1 g/m^2 per day as a continuous infusion over 96 h.
Each day the daily dose is added to a 1 litre bag of 5% dextrose and infused over 24 h.

This regimen requires that the patient be protected by adequate hydration before, during and after the cisplatin infusion to ensure a good diuresis.

Recruitment to the trial commenced in January 1992 and the results will need to be evaluated over the next few years.

Radiation therapy

This modality has been a more popular form of palliation since the early 1960s when the results of surgical resection in extensive disease were proving to be poor. Relief of dysphagia is achieved for some considerable duration of time, as most patients remain ambulant throughout the therapy until terminal disease and death. Since the publication of the Edinburgh results for patients treated in a 20-year period from 1948 to 1968 (Pearson, 1975) the curative potential of radiotherapy has been extensively explored. The Edinburgh results of that period have never been reproduced either in the same city or elsewhere, by Pearson or by others. Furthermore, palliation of dysphagia may not occur for several weeks after treatment has been completed. Stricture and tracheo-oesophageal fistulation rate is relatively high. Therefore, its place as a single-modality curative therapy is suspect.

Pre-resection irradiation has been applied with a view to local tumour shrinkage after preliminary laparotomy to exclude metastases (Guernsey *et al.*, 1969; Groves and Rodriguez-Antunez, 1973) or after exclusion bypass of tumour, and staged resection. No significant improvement was achieved in any of these studies compared with surgical resection alone. In some of the more recently reported studies the deterioration and drop-off rate has been so high that results have been disappointing.

Radiotherapy as a single-modality treatment has, however, an important place in the treatment of hypopharyngeal (postcricoid) carcinoma where the response rate and cure rate have been high compared with those for other sites, especially taking into consideration the fact that the patient still has a voice, albeit a hoarse one, and is able to swallow satisfactorily. Some examples of dosage of irradiation with cobalt beam are given below.

Palliative

A total dose of between 3000 and 5000 rad is usually administered on a daily dose of 200 rad 5 times a week, for 3 weeks. The higher the total palliative dose, the longer the survival of the patient and the duration of symptomatic relief, but this may be a reflection of the general condition of the patient at the commencement of treatment and the ability of the patient to tolerate a higher dosage.

Curative

A total dose of 5000–6600 rad is divided into 20 fractions over 4–6 weeks through a portal of approximately 8 × 15 cm. The tumour margin is cleared by approximately 6 cm and if necessary by a separate portal for lymph nodal involvement not covered in the same field.

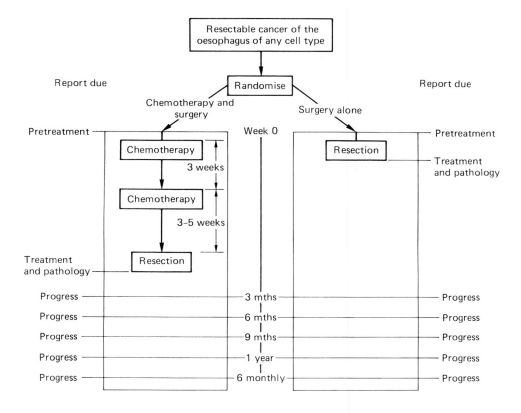

Figure 9.4 Preoperative chemotherapy for cancer of the oesophagus – trial outline

Preoperative irradiation

Dosage is limited to 2000–3000 rad in divided doses over 5–6 days, followed by an interval of 10–14 days before proceeding to resection.

Palliative irradiation to bony metastases

The total dose required for relief of pain is all that is necessary for control of symptoms of bony metastases occurring late after definitive treatment of the primary. Total dosage may vary from 600 to 1000 rad administered over 3–5 days.

Surgery

This modality has been the treatment of choice in the palliation of symptoms of oesophageal carcinoma since Torek's first oesophagectomy in 1913. In the 1960s and early 1970s there was a swing to other forms of therapy based on statistical data of 5-year survivals, and operative mortality and morbidity achieved from cumulative figures of several publications. The hopes raised by claims for radiotherapy or chemotherapy as a curative modality were therefore explored and are still being explored as a single modality, or more rationally as an adjuvant to surgery. Examples of such adjuvant or multi-modality treatment are:

1. Preoperative radiotherapy and surgery.
2. Preoperative chemotherapy and surgery.
3. Preoperative chemotherapy followed by surgery and then by postoperative radiotherapy.
4. Preoperative radiotherapy and then surgery followed by postoperative radiotherapy.

The morbidity and mortality of oesophageal resections vary according to the experience and expertise of the team managing the patient. With proper assessment and preoperative preparation of patients, resectability rates of 80–90% can be achieved, especially with increasing awareness and screening of high-risk populations. Morbidity and mortality of exploration are dependent on the preoperative preparation of the patients. Perioperative mortality rates of less than 5% are being constantly achieved by teams dealing with substantial numbers of patients. Although the temptation does exist for every surgeon to take on this very demanding surgery, there is no place for the occasional oesophagectomist. One has to be a member of a team constantly dealing with oesophageal problems, both benign and malignant, to be able to achieve and guarantee the low mortality and morbidity of oesophageal surgery. Long-term survival with surgical resection can only follow early detection, and with stage I disease 5-year survivals of 80% have been achieved (Nakayama and Kinoshita, 1975). The pessimistic attitude towards surgical treatment is based on the wrong assumption that because high mortality and morbidity are a rule with several smaller series, a few specialized teams dealing with the problem cannot improve on the results.

The objectives of surgery are:

1. To remove the oesophageal carcinoma, if resectable.
2. To reconstruct the upper gastrointestinal tract in one stage.
3. To bypass the tumour if found irresectable at exploration.
4. If preoperatively assessed as inoperable, or the patient found unsuited to major surgical resection, to establish a satisfactory oesophageal lumen for feeding purposes, by
    (a) dilatation of the tumour alone;
    (b) endoscopic intubation – pulsion intubation;
    (c) operative intubation – traction intubation;
    (d) endoscopic diathermy fulguration;
    (e) endoscopic laser coagulation;
    (f) brachy therapy by endoscopic insertion of after loading remote-controlled 'Selectron' probes.
5. When other modalities of treatment have previously been employed and the patient has obstructive symptoms warranting surgical intervention, relief by pulsion or traction intubation.
6. When a complication such as fistulation has occurred following radiotherapy, to bypass the malignant or radionecrotic tracheo-oesophageal fistula with total exclusion of the fistula-bearing segment of mid-oesophagus from the rest of the upper gastrointestinal tract.

Curative surgical resection of oesophageal carcinoma is based on the concept that if all neoplastic tissue can be removed, then resection and reconstruction should lead to a substantial 5-year survival provided that the operative mortality is low and the life expectancy of the patient is not short. Provided that the tumour is contained within the fascia propria of the oesophagus, and submucosal spread has not occurred far, radical removal of the oesophagus by total or subtotal oesophagectomy with radical clearance of the lymph nodes draining the organ is a justifiable procedure. Some justification can also be applied to efforts to improve the cure rate by proceeding to an extended radical procedure if the tumour has invaded the peri-oesophageal tissues and local nodes in a fit, young adult. However, the same arguments would be untenable in the elderly patient in whom a shortened chance of survival should be preferred to the high morbidity and mortality that would ensue with an extended radical procedure.

Preoperative preparation of the patient

This is aimed at correction of any anaemia, attention to septic teeth, improvement of the cardiac and respiratory status, and correction of nutritional deficiencies. Although some nutrition can be maintained by the oral route, most patients require correction of hypo-albuminaemia, dehydration and electrolyte disturbances. The need for parenteral hyperalimentation over a short term has to be carefully weighed against the insertion of a thin nasogastric feeding tube past the neoplasm. There is increasing evidence to suggest that whichever route is employed, the impact on the serological and corpuscular components of blood may not be significantly different (Brister *et al.*, 1984). In those patients who have failed to show satisfactory improvement, it may be necessary to construct a feeding jejunostomy either before or at the time of surgery in order to continue hyperalimentation via the enteral route (Figure 9.5).

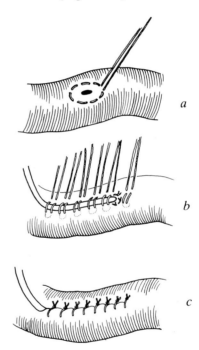

Figure 9.5 Technique of construction of feeding jejunostomy for hyperalimentation pre- and postoperatively. *a*, Purse-string suture jejunostomy. *b*, Tunnelling of the small-bore tube. *c*, Final appearance

Choice of surgical procedure

In oesophageal carcinoma this is dependent on the tumour location, the extent of spread and the objectives of the surgical intervention.

CARCINOMA OF THE HYPOPHARYNX AND
CERVICAL OESOPHAGUS –
LARYNGOPHARYNGO-OESOPHAGECTOMY

Resection here is achieved by removal of the larynx, lower pharynx, cervical trachea, one or both lobes of the thyroid gland and oesophagus. If the tumour is located in the hypopharynx only (postcricoid) the thoracic oesophagus can be conserved and a free graft of jejunum can be transferred by microvascular anastomosis of the jejunal vessels to the superior thyroid artery and internal jugular vein (Figure 9.6). If tumour has extended on to the lower part of the cervical oesophagus, a total laryngopharyngo-oesophagectomy and gastric pull-up with immediate pharyngo-gastric reconstruction is the treatment of choice (Figure 9.7).

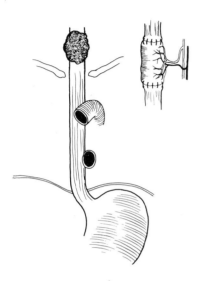

Figure 9.6 Area of resection in postcricoid tumour prior to free jejunal autograft

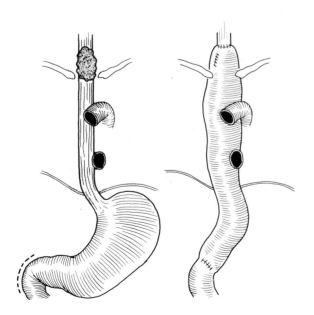

Figure 9.7 Extent of resection when postcricoid tumour extends lower, needing total oesophagectomy with gastric pull-up

If the stomach has been rendered unsuitable by previous surgery, then a long segment of right or left hemicolon is brought up through the posterior mediastinum or retrosternally, to be anastomosed to the pharynx. As an alternative to the gastric pull-up the reversed (Figure 9.8) *gastric tube* can be used, but except in the hands of a few it is often complicated by problems associated with suture line dehiscence. The operation of laryngopharyngo-oesophagectomy can be undertaken by one surgical team or by two teams operating simultaneously, performing the removal of the cervical tumour while the other mobilizes the stomach, colon or jejunum as the case may be. Microvascular techniques for free pedicle graft, being a well-established specialty procedure, would demand the services of a team constantly involved in small vessel surgery.

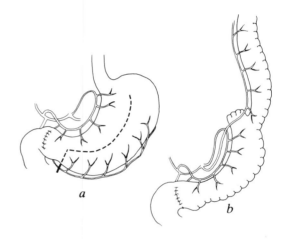

Figure 9.8 *a*, Mobilization of the stomach retaining the blood supply derived from the left and right gastric arteries, and the anastomosis between the short gastric and gastro-epiploic arteries. Line of resection shown by interrupted line. *b*, Tube of greater curve after the Heimlich–Gavrileau fashion

CARCINOMA OF THE THORACIC OESOPHAGUS

This is resected by total or subtotal oesophagectomy with cervical oesophagogastric anastomosis via a laparotomy, right thoracotomy and cervical incision in one operation (McKeown, 1972), often erroneously described as a three-stage procedure. The procedure can be performed by the same operating team starting with a laparotomy, and having mobilized the stomach, closing the abdomen, turning the patient on the left side and performing a right postero-lateral thoracotomy to free the tumour and resecting the tumour-bearing segment of oesophagus, before anchoring the oesophageal remnant to the pulled-up stomach and closing the chest with drainage. The patient is then turned on his or her back once again for dissection of the cervical oesophagus and completion of a total oesophagectomy and anastomosis to the stomach pulled up into the neck. The entire

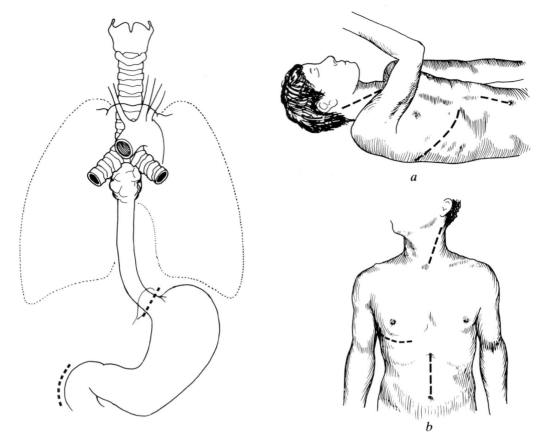

Figure 9.9 Total oesophagectomy via a triple approach. *a*, Laparotomy, right posterolateral thoracotomy and right cervical approach requiring two turnings of the patient for the three incisions. *b*, Laparotomy, right anterolateral thoracotomy and left cervical exposure for synchronous surgery by two teams with the patient in the same supine position

procedure can also be performed with the patient on his or her back right through the operation via a laparotomy, right anterolateral thoracotomy and a cervical exposure, in which case either one or two teams could be operating at any one moment with considerable reduction in the time required (Royston and Dowling, 1976) (Figure 9.9).

If the tumour is located in an area where clearance of tumour can be achieved with a 10 cm margin above the upper limit of tumour and the oesophagus transected in the chest, then a subtotal oesophagectomy and intrathoracic oesophagogastric anastomosis is performed high up in the apex of the chest (Franklin, 1942; Lewis, 1946). The operation is commenced with the patient on his or her back via a laparotomy for mobilization of the stomach, followed by closure of the abdomen and the patient being positioned in the left lateral decubitus for the right posterolateral thoracotomy.

CARCINOMA OF THE LOWER OESOPHAGUS

This is resected via a left thoracotomy, mobilization of the stomach through the diaphragm, mobilization

of the tumour-bearing oesophagus both below and above the aortic arch with transection of the oesophagus in the apex of the chest for an intrathoracic oesophagogastric anastomosis in a supra-aortic level, the stomach remnant being positioned either in the posterior mediastinum, medial to the aortic arch, or in the pleural cavity lateral to the aortic arch (Figure 9.10).

PALLIATIVE RESECTION

Where carcinoma of the lower oesophagus is being resected purely as a palliative excision without any attempt at clearance of lymph nodal territory, a right thoracotomy and oesophagectomy can be performed without opening the abdomen, but by mobilizing the stomach through the oesophageal hiatus (Belsey and Hiebert, 1974).

In recent years, the procedure first described by Grey Turner (1936) for mobilization of the oesophageal carcinoma (and subsequently employed by Ong and Lee, 1960, and Le Quesne and Ranger, 1966, for freeing the normal oesophagus for a gastric pullup without opening the chest) has been rejuvenated

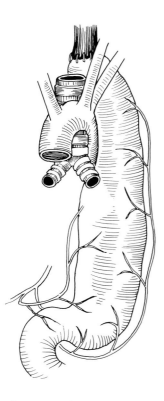

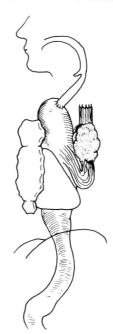

Figure 9.10 A supra-aortic oesophagogastric anastomosis after resection of a lower oesophageal carcinoma via a left thoracotomy.

by Orringer (Orringer and Sloan, 1978; Orringer and Orringer, 1983; Kron *et al.*, 1984; Orringer, 1984; Finley *et al.*, 1985) in an almost single-handed fashion with the transhiatal oesophagectomy without thoracotomy. While enabling removal of the tumour, the procedure contravenes almost all the principles of radical surgery for malignancy, especially if spread has occurred beyond the submucosal and muscle layers of the oesophagus. Furthermore, it contributes little to the knowledge of proper pathological staging of the tumour at the time of the surgery. Despite these drawbacks one has to concede that the procedure will have a place in the techniques available for removal of an oesophageal tumour if the operator is reluctant to enter the chest cavity, as was the case in Grey Turner's time. It may also gain application in the future as an appropriate procedure in the resection of carcinoma in situ (CIS) of the oesophagus.

Irresectable tumour of the oesophagus ascertained at the time of exploration can be appropriately bypassed depending on the stage at which irresectability is determined. The oesophagus is transected well clear of the tumour. The lower oesophageal remnant may be stapled and closed. The fundus of the stomach is then pulled up to reach the upper cut end of the oesophagus to which it is anastomosed in an end-to-side manner (Figure 9.11).

A malignant or radionecrotic tracheo-oesophageal fistula is a life-threatening complication, and even if the patient has only a short time left, the choking

Figure 9.11 Palliative end-to-side oesophagogastric bypass of mid-oesophageal tumour found irresectable after mobilization of the stomach and exploration of the chest

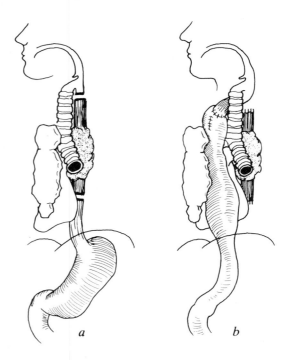

Figure 9.12 Retrosternal bypass of irresectable oesophageal tumour with oesophagotracheal fistula – by total disconnection and oesophagogastric anastomosis in the neck.

associated with saliva and food entering the tracheo-bronchial tree can be alleviated by a retrosternal bypass of the oesophagus with the stomach anastomosed to the transected cervical oesophagus, having

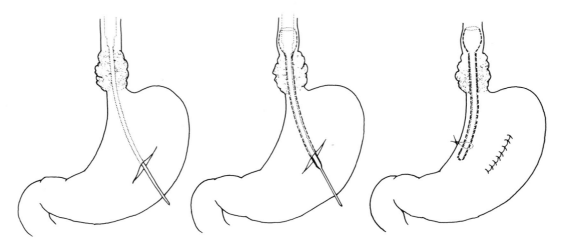

Figure 9.13 Operative insertion of a Celestin tube by the traction method – for an irresectable carcinoma of the cardia or of the lower oesophagus with obstructive symptoms.

excluded the thoracic part of the oesophagus from the rest of the alimentary tract (Orringer and Sloan, 1975). Surgery of this nature should be preceded by a thorough preparation of the chest with physiotherapy, etc., to overcome the effects of spillage into the tracheobronchial tree (Figure 9.12).

Palliation of inoperable patients with oesophageal tumour by intubation (Souttar, 1924; Mousseau *et al.*, 1956; Celestin, 1959) is effective if the tumour is located low in the chest. The higher the location of the tumour, the less satisfactory is the outcome of intubation, because of the proximity of the funnel of the tube to the glottic inlet. Operative intubation is performed by a laparotomy and gastrotomy with the traction technique described by Mousseau and Barbin for tumour of the cardia (Mousseau *et al.*, 1956) and subsequently improved by Celestin (1959) for oesophageal and cardiac tumours (Figure 9.13).

Pulsion intubation. This was originally described by Souttar for mid-oesophageal tumour where the tube was introduced via the rigid oesophagoscope. Current techniques of pulsion intubation enable the placement of the funnelled tube over an introducer or mandril after passing a guide wire through the tumour and dilating it with bougies of the Eder–Puestow or the Celestin variety. Endoscopic intubation of oesophageal carcinoma has enabled patients who would otherwise have been unsuitable for general anaesthesia to receive palliation (Figure 9.14). Intermittent dilatation of neoplastic stricture of the oesophagus has been known to produce palliation of dysphagia for variable intervals of time, and can be resorted to if intubation is not tolerated or has been complicated by problems with the need for removal of the tube.

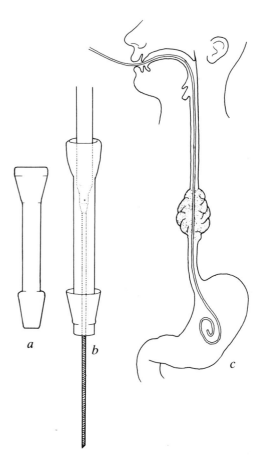

Figure 9.14 Two types of prosthetic tubes suitable for pulsion insertion endoscopically over a guide wire. *a*, Atkinson tube. *b*, Celestin tube. *c*, Diagram showing a guide wire passing through an endoscopically dilated tumour.

Endoscopic photocoagulation (laser fulguration). This is gaining popularity as a preferred form of enlarging the lumen of the oesophagus to palliate symptoms where the tumour is irresectable (Mc-Caughan *et al.*, 1984) (Figure 9.15). There is an ever increasing experience with this form of palliation and on current reports the success rate is variable. Full benefit is seen within a few days, but regrowth of tumour and recurrence of dysphagia will require further visits to a laser centre for frequent treatments. Such treatment can be carried out on a day-case basis at 4–6-week intervals.

Palliation of oesophageal carcinoma may require a combination of modalities, such as laser photocoagulation followed by dilatation and endoscopic insertion of pulsion tubes when frequency of laser treatments necessitates intubation. The concept of recanalization by photocoagulation followed by endoluminal brachy therapy seems exciting and is being pursued in some centres. The outcome of such combination of modalities needs further evaluation.

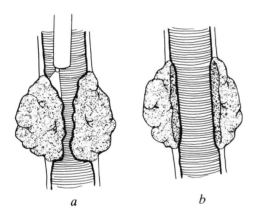

Figure 9.15 Endoscopic photocoagulation of oesophageal tumour that is not resectable. *a*, Before. *b*, After. Note that the lumen is re-established but most of the tumour is still there.

Treatment of gastric carcinoma

With the declining incidence and increasing pick-up of early gastric cancer, surgery offers the best chance of long-term survival in this disease. Overall resectability rates of nearly 80% can be achieved with surgical exploration (Yan and Brooks, 1985), with an overall operative mortality of less than 5%. With curative radical resection in stage I disease, 5-year survivals of 80% have been achieved. If irresectability has been established after exploration, traction intubation or bypass surgery can be resorted to as palliation of symptoms if dysphagia is a major one, as happens with tumour of the cardia. Radiotherapy and chemotherapy may still have a role to play in the palliation of symptoms of the primary disease or of metastases (Gunderson, 1976; Moertel, 1978; Yan and Brooks, 1985).

Principles in the choice of the surgical procedure
(Jeyasingham *et al.*, 1967; Jeyasingham, 1978)

As with carcinoma of the oesophagus, the choice of the procedure depends on the location and extent of tumour and the objectives of the surgical intervention.

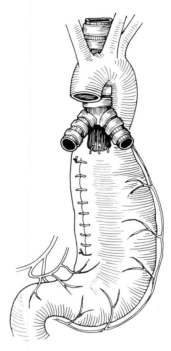

Figure 9.16 A subaortic oesophagogastric anastomosis for carcinoma of the cardiac end of the stomach.

Curative radical resection

This is aimed at total removal of all demonstrable tumour with the lymphatic field of drainage from the tumour, with an adequate margin of normal tissue. With carcinoma of the cardia, this would necessarily involve removal of the lower oesophagus, almost the entire lesser curve, a considerable proportion of the greater curve and omentum, spleen, tail of pancreas, with the lymph nodes in the subcarinal, paraoesophageal, diaphragmatic, left gastric and coeliac areas and in the splenic hilum (Figure 9.16). A margin of diaphragm at the hiatus would have to be removed in continuity with the tumour. An extended radical procedure aimed at a curative resection of tumour of the cardia would involve a total gastrectomy in addition to the rest of the field described (Jeyasingham *et al.*, 1967). For tumours of the body of the stomach, curative resection would involve a total gastrectomy removal of all omentum in addition to all the areas described above (Figure 9.17). A radical procedure in tumours of the pylorus should incorporate a subtotal gastrectomy with removal of all the omentum and lymph nodes in the regional drainage of this area

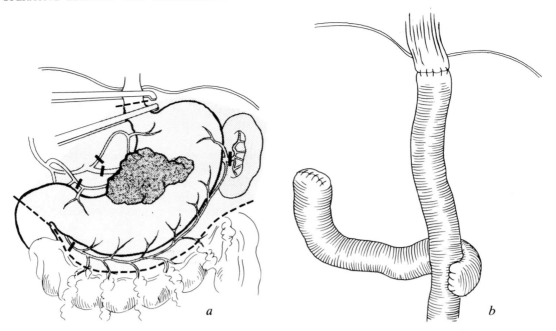

Figure 9.17 *a*, Extent of resection in a radical total gastrectomy for carcinoma of the body of the stomach. *b*, Roux-en-Y reconstruction below the diaphragm if sufficient clearance can be obtained above the upper limit of tumour. If the tumour extends to within 10 cm of the diaphragm, a transthoracic approach with a subaortic anastomosis should be undertaken

(Figure 9.18). An extended radical procedure here would involve a total gastrectomy, splenectomy and removal of pancreas as a whole with the first part of the duodenum. However, such a procedure would carry a formidable mortality and morbidity and would not be justified. Radical dissection is therefore limited to the spleen and body and tail of pancreas, and dissection of the pancreaticoduodenal nodes in addition to nodes in the coeliac and hepatic regions.

Palliative oesophagogastric resection (Figures 9.19 and 9.20)

This is aimed at removal of tumour with reconstruction of the upper alimentary tract with the knowledge that disease has spread to adjacent organs or the third and fourth tiers of lymph nodes. In tumour of the cardia, resection is achieved with subaortic oesophagogastrostomy. With tumour of the body, a total gastrectomy is justified provided that the line of

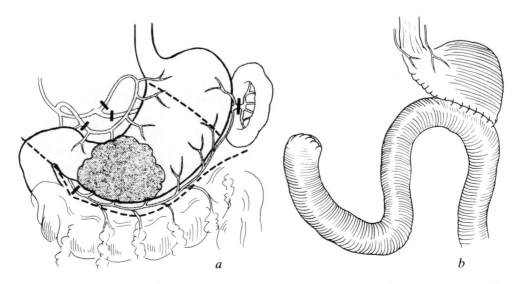

Figure 9.18   Distal subtotal gastrectomy (*a*) and a Billroth II reconstruction (*b*) for a carcinoma of the pyloric antrum. The stippled area indicates the extent of resection in an extended radical procedure which should include the spleen and body and tail of pancreas

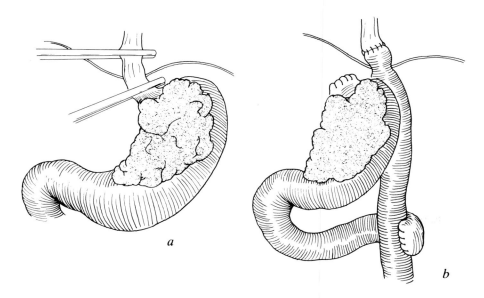

Figure 9.19 Palliative bypass of carcinoma of the body or cardiac end of stomach by intrathoracic oesophagojejunal anastomosis and Roux-en-Y biliary diversion

section does not go through macroscopic residual tumour. In tumours of the pylorus, palliative resection is achieved with a distal subtotal gastrectomy and a Billroth II gastrojejunal anastomosis or with a defunctioning posterior gastroenterostomy. The involvement of adjacent organs such as the pancreas, transverse colon or the left lobe of the liver should not deter from a palliative resection provided that these areas can be resected without leaving obvious tumour behind.

If, on exploration, a tumour is deemed irresectable and if obstructive symptoms have been present, a *traction intubation* is done before closing the abdomen. If, however, dysphagia has not been a major symptom, biopsy of the tumour and sampling of the regional nodes are all that are performed at this stage. In patients who are considered unsuitable for surgical exploration, if dysphagia is a major problem endoscopic intubation or photocoagulation can be performed without recourse to a general anaesthetic. Except in the tumour of the cardia, the results of such pulsion intubation are on the whole unsatisfactory.

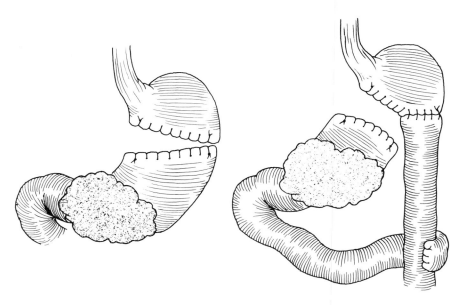

Figure 9.20 Exclusion–diversion operation for an irresectable carcinoma of the pyloric antrum with obstructive symptoms

Operative surgical technique in specific procedures in the management of oesophageal and gastric carcinoma

1. Mobilization of the tumour-bearing cervical oesophagus in the operation of radical pharyngolaryngo-oesophagectomy

With the patient in a supine position, anaesthetized with a standard endotracheal anaesthesia, a sandbag is placed under the chest between the scapulas, the neck being extended and the chin facing directly upwards. An incision is made obliquely on either side along the anterior border of each sternomastoid and joined in the skin crease with a curved transverse incision 2 cm above the sternal notch (Figure 9.21). The incision is deepened through the platysma and flaps are elevated upwards, outwards and downwards. In order to facilitate elevation of the flaps over the posterior triangle of the neck, two short incisions are placed from the outer limits of the transverse portion extending to the anterior borders of the trapezius muscles on each side. Dissection of all the deep cervical chain of lymph nodes is completed, but both internal jugular veins are preserved, and both sternomastoid muscles are preserved (Figure 9.22). The thyroid gland is mobilized with the trachea and larynx by control of the superior and inferior thyroid arteries and the thyroid veins. If the tumour is not extensive on one or the other side, the thyroid lobe of that side is preserved. If both lobes of the thyroid are removed, the parathyroids are identified and at least two of them are implanted into a muscle bed in one of the sternomastoids. The trachea is now partially divided above the sternal notch and the anterior wall of the lower end attached to the skin edge here. An armoured endotracheal tube with a cuff is now passed into the lower end of the trachea in place of the

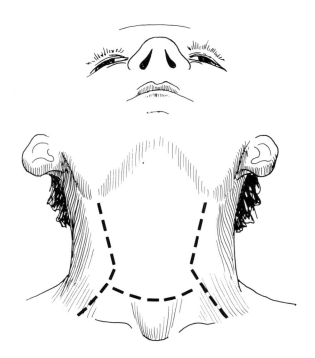

Figure 9.21 Cervical incision in the operation of laryngo-pharyngo-oesophagectomy for postcricoid carcinoma

previously sited endotracheal tube which is removed in readiness. Having gained control of the ventilation via the armoured tube, the posterior wall of the trachea is disconnected totally.

The hyoid bone is detached from its muscle anchorage to expose the epiglottis. The mucosa of the pharynx above the epiglottis is incised and stripped upwards and the incision is continued laterally to detach the lateral walls of the pharynx and finally the posterior wall is transected. The pharynx and larynx are then stripped off the prevertebral fascia down to

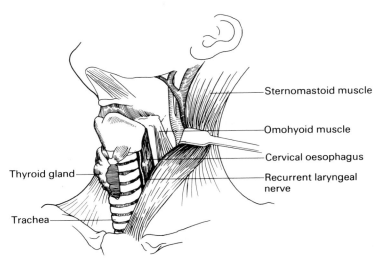

Figure 9.22 Cervical exposure to show the more relevant anatomical structures during mobilization of the cervical oesophagus

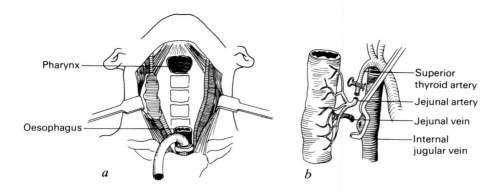

Figure 9.23 *a*, Field of surgery after removal of postcricoid carcinoma. *b*, Free jejunal autograft ready for interposition, with vascular anastomosis to local vessels in the neck

the thoracic inlet with the tumour-bearing portion of cervical oesophagus. If the cervical oesophagus is being replaced by a pedicled free graft of jejunum, it is transected at the thoracic inlet level (Figure 9.23). If on the other hand a gastric pull-up (Figure 9.24) is planned, the entire viscus is covered in a pack and the operation field is covered with a sterile towel to await the next step in the procedure.

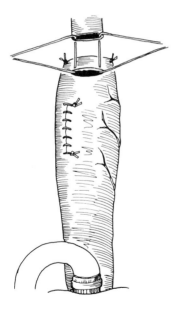

Figure 9.24 Pharyngogastric reconstruction after laryngopharyngo-oesophagectomy

2. Mobilization of the normal stomach via a laparotomy for gastric pull-up in the neck with concomitant removal of the normal oesophagus

This procedure is common to others such as mobilization of the stomach for transhiatal blunt oesophagectomy and substernal defunctioning bypass of mid-oesophageal neoplasm with or without tracheo-oeso-

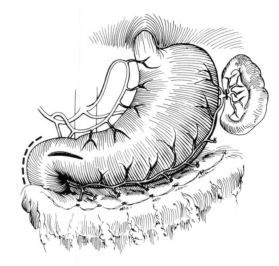

Figure 9.25 Mobilization of the stomach via an upper abdominal incision in readiness for a gastric pull-up into the chest and as far up as the pharynx. Note the pyloroplasty incision and the Kocherization of the duodenum

phageal fistula. The abdomen is entered through a midline upper abdominal incision from xiphisternum to the umbilicus. If necessary the xiphoid cartilage is removed. The left triangular ligament of the liver is divided and the left lobe of the liver is gently retracted to the right. The stomach has to be mobilized with the minimum of handling of the organ, retaining the maximum amount of vascularity at the end of the procedure, and yet in such a manner as to enable the operator to position the fundus of the stomach at the level of the pharynx. The right gastric artery and the right gastro-epiploic artery are the only source of blood supply, but every attempt is made to preserve the collaterals at the termination of these vessels where they meet branches of the left gastric and left gastro-epiploic vessels. The epiploic branches of the gastro-epiploic arcade are divided commencing at a convenient point near the midline and proceeding towards the pylorus. Special care is taken here to

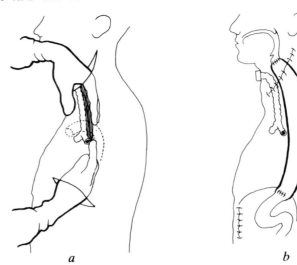

Figure 9.26 Blunt oesophagectomy without thoracotomy. *a*, Diagrammatic representation of the bimanual dissection of the oesophagus from above and from below. *b*, The stomach pulled up into the neck and anastomosed to the pharynx in the operation of laryngopharyngo-oesophagectomy

preserve the gastro-epiploic vein which parts company from the artery to reach the groove between the neck and the uncinate process of the pancreas. The division of the omentum is then carried to the left towards the splenic hilum where special attention is paid to divide the vessels close to the spleen, thereby preserving every possible collateral channel that may carry some blood to the short gastric arteries. Ligation of the left gastric vessels is carried out close to the take-off before the bifurcation of the vessel, again preserving collateral channels (Figure 9.25).

Extensive mobilization of the duodenum is achieved by Kocherization and dissection of the first and second parts from the posterior abdominal wall, freeing under these to reach the vena cava and aorta. The stomach is now freed from the subdiaphragmatic peritoneum and the oesophagus is freed from the hiatus. Dissection is carried upwards around the lower oesophagus. The hiatal margins are dilated with, if necessary, an anteriorly placed releasing incision to facilitate the next step in the procedure.

3. Dissection of the normal oesophagus without a thoracotomy

This technique (Figure 9.26) is common to the gastric pull-up with removal of a normal oesophagus, as well as for blunt oesophagectomy without thoracotomy for palliative blind resection of neoplasia of the thoracic oesophagus. Blind finger dissection is done upwards, keeping close to the oesophagus as much as possible. Small oesophageal arterial branches are torn with the dissecting finger, but can be controlled with firm packing at a later stage. The cervical operator simultaneously dissects downwards, carefully avoiding the recurrent laryngeal nerve and avoiding

damage to the back of the trachea. As the thoracic inlet is small, most of the dissection has to be done from below and it will be necessary for the abdominal operator to pass an entire fist into the posterior mediastinum to reach the carina and back of the trachea from below. By gentle traction from above, and supportive assistance from below, the stomach is pulled up through the posterior mediastinum, bringing the duodenum and pancreas towards the midline in the epigastrium. The pylorus comes to be near the hiatus or above it. A pyloromyotomy or pyloroplasty has therefore to be completed prior to closure of the abdomen if any abnormality of this area is noted at this stage.

The recent development of *video-assisted endoscopic surgery* has led to the development of laparoscopic mobilization of the stomach, endoscopic mobilization of the thoracic oesophagus and cervical pullthrough with a cervical anastomosis without the need for a laparotomy or thoracotomy. Although mobilization of advanced gastric cancer and oesophageal cancer are not best suited for this form of endoscopic blunt oesophagectomy, it may certainly prove to be the operation of the future once these neoplasms come to be diagnosed in T1 N0 stages.

4. Pharyngogastric anastomosis after gastric pull-up

The stomach is pulled up and the cardia is transected, stapled and oversewn with suture material. The highest point in the gastric fundus is now anchored to the anterior longitudinal ligament almost at the level of the atlas vertebra, and an end-to-side pharyngogastric anastomosis is completed. A nasogastric tube is introduced via the nose and left in the intrathoracic portion of the stomach.

The skin flaps are now approximated and the posterior wall of the trachea is finally anchored to the skin edges before closing the platysma and skin, with a Redivac drain in the neck.

5. Mobilization of the stomach via a midline incision in the first phase of a total or subtotal oesophagectomy

This is carried out in exactly the same manner as in procedure 2 above, except in so far as paying special attention to the lymph nodal clearance from the left gastric and coeliac areas.

6. Right thoracotomy and mobilization of a tumour-bearing thoracic or lower oesophagus, as part of a Lewis–Franklin procedure or as part of a triple procedure to carry out a total oesophagectomy

The patient is placed in a left lateral position and the chest entered through the 5th intercostal space. The lung is carefully retracted forwards. The azygos vein is dissected, ligated flush with the superior vena cava anteriorly and also posteriorly over the dorsal vertebral bodies without disturbing the intercostal veins. The intervening horizontal portion of the azygos vein is detached and left attached to the oesophagus. The pleura over the dorsal spine is incised longitudinally over the entire length of the chest cavity. Dissection is now commenced between the oesophagus and aorta posteriorly, and between the oesophagus and spine above the aortic arch. The oesophageal tumour is mobilized with a clear margin of the healthy tissue by keeping the dissection close to the aortic wall. Dissection is then continued between the oesophagus and trachea superiorly, and behind the right main bronchus and pericardium in the lower part. Once the oesophagus is encircled above the tumour, a sling is passed round it to enable easier dissection to free the tumour-bearing segment. All lymph nodes in the subcarinal and hilar areas are included with the perioesophageal tissues. Similarly, in the lower chest the pulmonary ligament is divided close to the lung and dissection is carried into the oesophageal hiatus (Figure 9.27). Once the dissection of the entire length of the thoracic oesophagus has been completed, and then only, gentle traction is applied to deliver the stomach into the chest, ensuring that the organ does not undergo any rotation on its own axis. Dissection of the apex of the chest is now continued so as to free the cervical oesophagus from below.

7. Subtotal oesophagectomy with a thoracic anastomosis

Once the mobilization of the oesophagus has been completed through the right chest, the stomach is transected obliquely at the cardia including a short length of the lesser curve, in order to remove some of the paracardiac lymph nodes with the oesophagus.

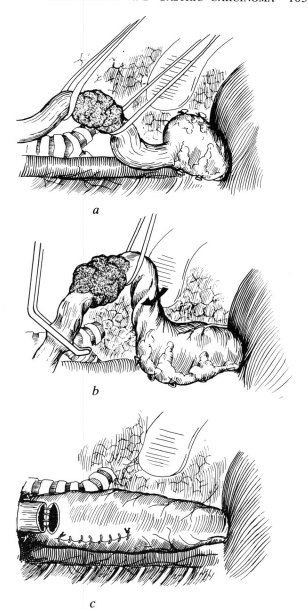

a

b

c

Figure 9.27 Mobilization of the thoracic oesophagus via a right posterolateral thoracotomy for oesophagectomy and intrathoracic oesophagogastric anastomosis. *a*, Step-by-step mobilization of stomach through the oesophageal hiatus without a laparotomy – as a purely palliative procedure. *b*, Delivery of a previously mobilized stomach into the chest by a pull-up technique. *c*, Stomach anchored to the apex of the mediastinum in readiness for end-to-side oesophagogastric anastomosis

The stomach remnant is stapled and oversewn. The fundus is then gently pulled up to the apex of the chest where it is anchored to the prevertebral tissues, making sure that the transection suture line is to the right and the fundus to the left. The oesophagus is transected with a clear 10 cm margin of normal oesophagus above the tumour, and an end-to-side anastomosis is completed, making an opening on the anterior surface of the stomach at a convenient point below the apex of the fundus. A nasogastric tube is then positioned into the intrathoracic stomach.

8. 'Total' oesophagectomy with a cervical anastomosis

The mobilized oesophagus and stomach are left intact and the chest closed with drainage. The patient is then turned over on to his or her back and the right side of the neck is exposed via an incision placed in the posterior triangle 2 cm above the clavicle. As an alternative procedure, the stomach can be transected in the chest as in procedure 7 above, stapled and oversewn, and the oesophagus transected in the apex of the chest with a clear margin of normal oesophagus and anchored to the fundus at the uppermost point of its curvature with two or three anchoring sutures. This would then enable the oesophagus to be delivered into the neck at a later stage with the fundus of the stomach attached to it. The incision in the neck is retracted backwards and the middle thyroid vein may require ligation at this level. The carotid and jugular vessels are retracted laterally. The oesophagus is identified and the recurrent laryngeal nerve is carefully preserved alongside the trachea. Having dissected the oesophagus a sling is passed around it, and with gentle traction the oesophagus with the attached stomach is pulled up into the neck and if the cardia has not already been transected this is carried out now, followed by transection of the oesophagus at an appropriate length. Having performed a 'total' oesophagectomy, the remnant of the oesophagus is now anastomosed in an end-to-side fashion to the fundus of the stomach and the entire area is allowed to drop gently back into the mediastinum with a nasogastric tube in position. The incision in the neck is then closed without drainage.

9. Mobilization of tumour-bearing lower oesophagus for supra-aortic oesophagogastric anastomosis for a lower oesophageal tumour via a left thoracotomy (also applicable for cervical anastomosis)

With the patient placed in a right lateral position an incision is made over the 7th rib on the left side and the chest entered through the bed of the resected 7th rib and a divided portion of the back end of the 6th rib. As an alternative, the chest may be entered through the 6th interspace with portions of the 6th and 7th ribs being excised posteriorly. The lung is retracted forwards after division of the pulmonary ligament close to the lung attachment, retaining all the lymph nodes in this ligament with the oesophagus. An incision is placed in the pleura overlying the descending aorta and dissection commenced above the hiatus in a subadventitial plane of the aorta, continued upwards controlling each of the oesophageal branches from the descending aorta by liga-

tion and division. Dissection is then carried to a subaortic level where temporarily dissection is discontinued. An incision is then made anterior to the oesophagus in the sulcus between the pericardium and oesophagus, and with blunt dissection all the tissues around the oesophagus are separated from the fibrous pericardium, entering the right pleural cavity in order to retain all the peri-oesophageal tissues within the field of dissection. The downward dissection is continued to reach the diaphragm where all pericardiac fat is removed with the oesophageal segment. Dissection upwards is continued behind the pulmonary hilum, taking all the subcarinal lymph nodes and any visible hilar lymph nodes that may be situated posteriorly. The back of the bronchus and the pulmonary artery are bared. The inferior pulmonary vein covered by the pericardium is also cleaned thoroughly. At the level of the aortic arch the right and left vagi are disconnected distal to the left recurrent laryngeal nerve. In order to dissect the oesophagus above the aortic arch, a second incision may have to be placed in the 4th interspace with division of the back end of the 5th rib. If dissection, however, is carried out through the previously made 6th interspace exposure, then adequate separation of the ribs can be achieved by mere division of the back end of the 5th rib and 5th and 6th intercostal bundles, and retracting the rib cage further.

Having passed a sling around the oesophagus above the tumour, an incision is made in a longitudinal manner in the pleura above the aortic arch. The superior intercostal vein is doubly ligated anteriorly and posteriorly and divided between these ligatures. The oesophagus is identified. A finger is passed from below the aortic arch to dissect around the aortic arch close to the media, but taking great care not to traumatize the recurrent laryngeal nerve. The oesophagus is then cleared from under the aortic arch by careful blunt dissection, preserving the azygos vein on the right and ensuring that the back wall of the trachea is not damaged. Having carried the blunt dissection to a supra-aortic level, the supra-aortic oesophagus is encircled with a sling of rubber and dissection is then carried through under direct vision to the apex of the chest. Special care is exercised not to damage the thoracic duct. If a supra-aortic intrathoracic anastomosis is contemplated, the dissection comes to a close at this stage. Mobilization of stomach through an incision in the diaphragm is then commenced as for tumour of the cardia.

10. Mobilization of the oesophagus and stomach for carcinoma of the cardia in the operation of oesophagogastrectomy for carcinoma with a subaortic anastomosis (Figure 9.28)

Having mobilized the oesophagus as for a lower oesophageal carcinoma, ensuring that dissection around the oesophagus is carried out in a subadventi-

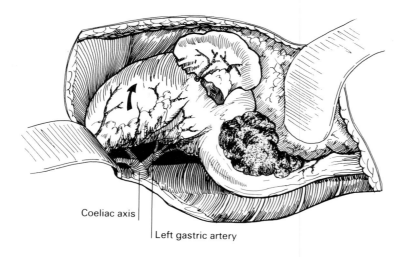

Coeliac axis

Left gastric artery

Figure 9.28 Mobilization of the oesophagus and stomach for a carcinoma of the cardia via a left thoracotomy in preparation for a subaortic anastomosis. The stomach and spleen with the tail of the pancreas have been rotated forwards to expose the coeliac axis and its main branches.

tial plane of the aorta, the hiatus is defined. The diaphragm is then incised in a radiate fashion, taking the incision in the diaphragm to the hiatus where a cuff of diaphragmatic muscle is excised with the oesophagogastric junction, controlling phrenic branches of the aorta on either side and inserting two stay sutures at the anterior ends of the divided hiatus for later reconstruction. If, however, a peripheral detachment is carried through which gives adequate exposure for mobilization of the entire stomach right out of the duodenum, an incision is made from under the sternum, carried through to a point on the diaphragm under the costal margin close to the apex of the spleen. Mobilization is then commenced at the splenic flexure of the colon taking the gastrocolic omentum along its avascular attachment to the colon all the way along the transverse colon, detaching the lieno-renal ligament, freeing the posterior aspect of the splenic hilum, controlling the splenic vessels and taking with the spleen the tail of the pancreas by cross-clamping the pancreas and dividing between the clamps, suturing the pancreas with interrupted non-absorbable sutures, reflecting the spleen forwards to carry the dissection upwards, controlling the short gastric vessels and reaching the diaphragmatic hiatus to expose the descending aorta at the point where it passes through the median arcuate ligament. At this stage the gastrohepatic omentum is detached close to the liver, controlling the communicating branch between the left hepatic artery and the left gastric artery. Having rotated the stomach and oesophagus forwards the pancreas is retracted downwards and the left gastric artery and coeliac axis are exposed, dissecting away all the lymph nodes in this area towards the stomach and controlling the left gastric artery after identifying the hepatic branch of the coeliac

axis, so that this vessel is not damaged. The dissection in the gastrocolic omentum is now carried through towards the gastro-epiploic arcade to reach it at a convenient point chosen well clear of the tumour in the stomach, allowing approximately 10 cm of clear stomach. The stomach is then transected, taking almost the entire lesser curve after dissociating the right gastric anastomosis with the branches of the left gastric artery on the lesser curve and dividing the gastro-epiploic arcade at a chosen point. The transected stomach is stapled and oversewn, and attention is now directed towards the oesophagus which has been mobilized up to the subaortic level behind the pulmonary hilum in a manner similar to that in procedure 8 above.

A non-crushing clamp is applied at a point chosen with a clear margin of at least 10 cm of oesophagus above the tumour and the oesophagus is then transected below this clamp. The stomach is pulled up through the hiatus or the divided hiatus to be brought up into the chest, ensuring that there is no rotation of the organ in its long axis. The pylorus is inspected at this stage and if there is any abnormality a pyloroplasty or pyloromyotomy is carried out. The oesophagus is then anastomosed in an end-to-side fashion to the gastric remnant and a Ryle's tube is positioned in the intrathoracic part of the stomach. The diaphragm is repaired, reconstructing the hiatus around the gastric remnant. No attempt is made to anchor the stomach remnant to the margins of the hiatus, but the stomach is anchored to the parietal pleura with a few interrupted sutures along its length in the chest. The left chest can then be closed with drainage and as the right pleura has been opened, that too is drained with a separate tube inserted between the stomach remnant and the back of the pericardium.

11. Mobilization of the oesophagus and stomach via the right chest and oesophageal hiatus for palliative resection of tumour in the thoracic or lower oesophagus

The procedure for entering the chest and mobilizing the oesophagus is exactly as was described for the Lewis–Franklin operation (procedure 6 above), but having divided the pulmonary ligament the dissection is carried down to reach the oesophageal hiatus where the margins of the hiatus are defined first, and entry into the peritoneal cavity is established initially in an anteromedial position avoiding damage to the ascending branch of the left gastric artery. The index finger is then passed into the peritoneal cavity and the left gastric artery is hooked up with the finger to be delivered into the hiatus where it is controlled with a clamp, divided between clamps, and ligated. Upward pull on the oesophagus and stomach with the sling now delivers branches of the short gastric vessels which are dealt with in a similar fashion. Sequential division of the remaining short gastric branches delivers more and more of the greater curvature to bring the gastro-epiploic arcade into view. From thence onwards the epiploic branches of the gastro-epiploic arcade are systematically divided until almost the entire length of the stomach is delivered into the chest. Delivery of the stomach into the chest is facilitated by dilatation of the hiatus using the index finger of each hand to stretch the muscular fibres. The gastrohepatic omentum is also divided during the course of the delivery of the stomach. The pylorus comes to lie almost at the level of the hiatus or just below it, but the exposure would be totally inadequate to carry out a pyloroplasty if it was required. However, it is possible by digital invagination of the stomach to achieve sufficient dilatation of the pyloric sphincter, provided there is no fibrous scarring in the area.

It is worth noting that this procedure does not enable a thorough dissection of the lymph nodes along the lesser curve of the stomach, nor the collection of nodes around the coeliac and left gastric artery that are frequently involved by tumour in the lower or thoracic oesophagus. It is a purely palliative procedure. Having delivered a sufficient length of stomach, a tube of greater curve with the vascular arcade of the gastro-epiploic vessels is fashioned sufficient to enable an end-to-side oesophagogastric anastomosis after resection of the oesophagus with a clear 10 cm margin above the tumour. With this technique, no difficulty is encountered in bringing the fundus of the stomach or end of the gastric tube to a level high enough for apical intrathoracic anastomosis or a cervical anastomosis if that was required.

12. Mobilization of the tumour-bearing stomach in proximal subtotal gastrectomy with oesophagogastric anastomosis via a left thoracolaparotomy

This procedure is carried out through a left-sided thoracolapartotomy incision of which the anterior end is completed first with an opportunity to explore the abdomen before completing the rest of the incision. An initial exploratory laparotomy would reveal if a radical procedure was feasible or whether some form of palliative procedure would be justified. The incision is placed over the level of the 8th rib and carried across the costal margin towards the umbilicus. The abdominal part of this incision is deepened through to the peritoneum and exploration of the upper abdomen is undertaken through this part of the incision. Having ascertained resectability, the incision is carried through into the chest where the chest cavity is entered through the bed of the resected 8th rib and continuity of the operative field is achieved by detaching the periphery of the diaphragm from its costal attachment.

Mobilization of the stomach is commenced by detaching the colonic attachment of the gastrocolic omentum along its avascular plane all the way from the splenic flexure to the hepatic flexure. The entire omentum is detached and retracted upwards with the stomach, dissection then being continued upwards towards the splenic hilum where the splenic vessels are dissected and divided between ligatures, the tail of the pancreas clamped and divided between clamps to be included in the field of dissection, the pancreas being controlled with interrupted non-absorbable sutures. Having detached the spleen, tail of pancreas and stomach from the posterior abdominal wall, the cardia is mobilized with a cuff of diaphragm around the oesophagogastric junction; the gastrohepatic omentum is detached controlling the gastric branch of the hepatic artery which communicates with the left gastric artery. The entire stomach and spleen are rotated forwards and upwards to expose the coeliac axis and left gastric artery after retraction of the pancreas downwards. A thorough dissection of the lymphatic drainage reaching the coeliac lymph nodes is carried out to remove all visible tissue of a lymphatic nature. The dissection is further carried towards the pylorus where the pancreaticoduodenal lymph nodes are removed for histological examination. A tube of greater curve is now constructed, retaining the gastro-epiploic arcade but removing the weight of the omentum by ligation and division of the epiploic branches of the arcade over the extent of the omental detachment followed by transection of the stomach with a full 10 cm clearance of normal healthy stomach from the lower edge of the tumour, taking the entire lesser curve and reconstructing the tube in two layers either by sutures or by stapling, and oversewing the stapled line. The entire mass of viscus detached is now wrapped in a gauze pack and swung upwards, without axial rotation, oesophageal dissection having been performed earlier as in mobilization of the lower oesophagus. A clamp is applied approximately 10 cm away from the upper margin of the tumour of the stomach. The oesophagus is then transected and an end-to-side oesophagogastric anastomosis is completed after pulling the tube of stomach up into the chest through the hiatus. This having been achieved, a Ryle's tube is now positioned in the stomach remnant; the diaphragm is reattached to the costal margin ensuring total isolation of the abdominal from the pleural cavity. The entire incision is then closed with drainage of the chest cavity, ensuring layer-by-layer closure of each of the two portions.

13. Distal subtotal gastrectomy with Billroth II gastrojejunal anastomosis for tumour of the pylorus

A midline upper abdominal incision is made with the patient lying supine. The incision may have to be extended below the level of the umbilicus on one or other side of this structure. Initial exploratory laparotomy is performed to ensure resectability and extent of resection required for control of tumour. A subtotal gastrectomy for tumour of the pylorus would not include resection of the spleen and tail of pancreas. However, if an extended radical subtotal gastrectomy is anticipated, then mobilization of the spleen and tail of pancreas is required for adequate clearance of lymph nodes in that area. The left lobe of the liver is retracted after division of its triangular ligament. Mobilization of the entire gastrocolic omentum is achieved by detachment of the omentum from the transverse colon, the mobilization being continued towards the greater curve of the stomach, detaching the anastomosis between the left and right gastro-epiploic arcades at a point estimated to be well clear of the tumour. The gastrohepatic omentum is detached close to the liver to expose the coeliac axis with its main branches. A thorough clearance of the lymph nodes in this area is achieved before identifying the three individual branches and ligating the left gastric artery close to its origin. The dissection is now concentrated on the first part of the duodenum to free the posterior aspect of the duodenum to gain an adequate margin of the first part of the duodenum away from the outermost border of the tumour. The gastro-epiploic arcade is then divided close to its origin from the gastroduodenal artery. The duodenum is transected well clear of the tumour and closed either by stapling or by suture in two layers. The stomach is then transected obliquely, extending the line of resection upwards towards the lesser curve so as to take almost all the left gastric lymph nodal distribution. The transection line is partially closed towards the lesser curve end and a Billroth II type gastrojejunal anastomosis is completed in a retrocolic fashion. As an alternative a Roux-en-Y anastomosis is achieved with the vertical limb looped on itself to enable an end-to-side gastrojejunal anastomosis and add to the reservoir of the stomach remnant.

An extended radical subtotal gastrectomy would include the splenic hilum, tail of pancreas and the involved lymph nodes in that area as part of the region of resected tissues.

14. Total gastrectomy and Roux-en-Y anastomosis for a tumour of the body of the stomach

The procedure as for distal subtotal gastrectomy is carried out with disarticulation of the xiphoid cartilage of the sternum for adequate exposure. The left triangular ligament of the liver is divided and retracted as before. Dissection is carried out to free the oesophagus in its intra-abdominal course, carrying the dissection around the oesophagus and into the gastrohepatic omentum. Dissection is then commenced again at the attachment of the gastrocolic omentum to the transverse colon from which it is totally detached, dissection being continued across its attachment and splenic flexure into the posterior abdomen where the lienorenal ligament is divided and the spleen and tail of pancreas are dissected away from their bed. Control of the pancreas by double clamping and division is achieved to remove the tail and body of the pancreas with the spleen and splenic vessels. The stomach is retracted away from the liver upwards and to the left to expose the coeliac axis and left gastric artery which are dealt with in a similar fashion to the previous operation. The gastrocolic vessels are divided at their point of origin from the gastroduodenal, and the right gastric artery controlled close to the first part of the duodenum. Having done this, sufficient mobilization of the first part of the duodenum is achieved to enable transection of this structure with an adequate margin of normal tissue, the duodenum then being stapled and oversewn or sutured in two layers. The stomach is retracted downwards, dissection continued up to the hiatus to free a length of intrathoracic oesophagus which is delivered into the abdomen. Transection of the oesophagus is achieved with a clamp controlling the oesophagus and the entire mass of viscera is removed. The jejunum is now mobilized to create a Roux-en-Y anastomosis or a looped Roux-en-Y anastomosis as in the previous section. Closure of the abdomen in both procedures is achieved with drainage of the duodenal stump area.

15. Techniques of oesophagogastric anastomosis

The ideal anastomosis is end to side with a clear-cut end of the oesophagus joined to a definitive opening made on the stomach remnant, well clear of any suture lines. The strength of such anastomosis depends on the one hand on the oesophageal mucosa and submucosa, and on the other hand on the gastric seromuscular coat. The gastric mucosa is fragile and tends to bleed on handling, while the oesophageal muscle coats tend to tear if grasped with a pair of forceps. Handling of these structures has therefore to be done with extreme care so as not to cause any damage. The success of any oesophagogastric resection is dependent on the integrity of the anastomotic sites involved in the reconstruction. Breakdown of anastomosis may occur early due to technical faults,

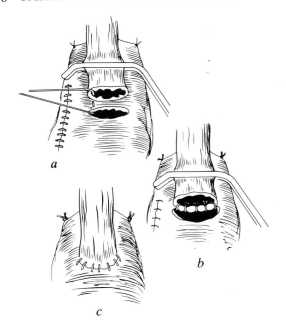

Figure 9.29 Author's own preferred anastomotic technique: end to side, interrupted, all coats sutured using no. 38 stainless steel gauge wire mounted on an atraumatic needle

and late as a result of poor tissues, inadequate vascularity and inadequate healing.

A single layer of interrupted sutures inserted meticulously at 3 mm intervals, with the material passing through all coats of each viscus and the knots tied on the lumen, is the technique preferred by the author (Figure 9.29). Stainless steel wire of no. 38 gauge mounted on an atraumatic needle is the author's choice for the suture material. The posterior layer is completed first, the two corners are rounded in turn

and then the anterior layer is completed. The last stitch on the anterior layer is tied with a knot to the exterior. A three-layered ink-welling technique (Figure 9.30) can be used with interrupted non-absorbable sutures such as polyester or Prolene, while the original technique described by Sweet (1945, 1950) is still the most popular. Anastomotic stapling guns can also be used to achieve a two-layered stapled anastomosis. In the hands of the occasional oesophageal surgeon, this instrument has contributed to a safer operation, at some compromise to the gentle handling of tissues (Figure 9.31).

16. Pyloroplasty

As to whether a pyloroplasty should be routinely performed after transection of the oesophagus is a question that has vexed more than one generation of surgeons. If the pylorus appears scarred from previous disease, a pyloroplasty is performed routinely. If the pylorus is healthy, the golden rule that the author has adopted is as follows: if the greater part of the stomach is preserved in the reconstruction then pyloroplasty is done routinely, especially if the pylorus comes to lie at the hiatus level or above it. This avoids an embarrassing manoeuvre if the pyloroplasty was not performed initially and came to be necessary in the long-term post-resection follow-up. If, however, a greater part of the stomach is removed and only a tube of stomach is retained, then a pyloroplasty is not performed as hypotonicity and delayed emptying of the gastric remnant are rarely noticed. In these patients the pylorus is usually situated well below the hiatus at the end of the operation, and is easily exposed if a pyloromyotomy should be required at a later date.

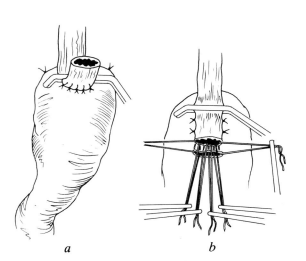

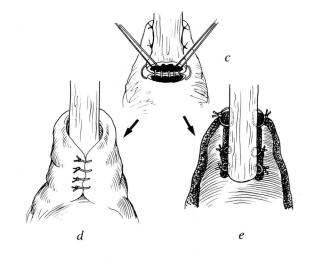

Figure 9.30 Anti-reflux techniques in oesophagogastric anastomosis. *a–c*, Stages in an end-to-side anastomosis with a 5 cm length of oesophagus anchored to the anterior surface of the stomach at three levels. *d*, Total 'fundoplication' wrap of stomach remnant around the oesophagus in the Nissen fashion. *e*, 'Ink-welling' of the oesophagus into the stomach in the Ottosen–Søndergaard fashion

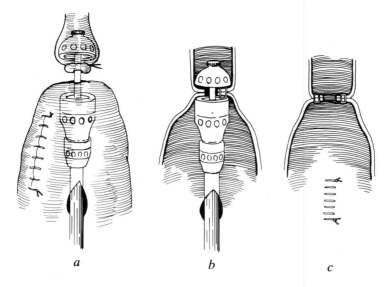

Figure 9.31 Diagrammatic representation of an oesophagogastric anastomosis achieved with a stapling device

Routine postoperative management

1. Nasogastric decompression is continued for 48 h, and if the gastric aspirate or jejunal aspirate shows signs of receding, the tube is removed after that interval of time.

2. 'Nil by mouth' is the rule for 24 h after surgery and then 30 ml of water are allowed every hour for the next 24 h. On the 3rd postoperative day, 60 ml are allowed every hour, increasing by 30 ml each day until free fluids are established after 5 days from surgery.

3. Parenteral nutrition is maintained with only crystalloids being allowed in the first 24 h after surgery. A central venous line is maintained for the purposes of parenteral nutrition and once the postoperative circulatory state has been stabilized for 24 h, total parenteral nutrition is established until such time as the patient is taking free fluids orally. Prolonged total parenteral nutrition has not been found necessary unless a complication has supervened.

4. By the end of the 1st week the patient is permitted sloppy food by mouth and by the 8th day boiled fish and minced meat are permitted.

5. The intercostal tubes are removed once oral fluids have been commenced and drainage has ceased, and lungs fully expanded. In the event of the slightest suspicion of a 'leak', at least one intercostal tube is retained until the false alarm has passed on.

6. Systemic antibiotics are commenced on the morning of the operation and continued for 5 days, as a prophylactic measure.

7. Subcutaneous low-dose heparin is administered routinely for 5 days or until the patient is fully mobile.

8. Chest physiotherapy is commenced in the recovery room, and continued 4-hourly for the first 3 days, and then twice daily throughout the patient's hospital stay.

9. The chest is monitored daily with erect radiographs to ensure full expansion of the lungs and no accumulation of any fluid within the pleural cavities.

10. The need for routine intermittent positive pressure ventilation varies according to the practice of the individual department, but is not employed by the author.

11. A pre-discharge barium meal screening is performed on the 10th to the 12th day after surgery.

12. From the time the patient is extubated, he or she is nursed on an inclined bed of approximately 15° with wooden blocks under the head end of the bed, to prevent inhalation of refluxed gastric or intestinal contents. Prior to discharge the patient is instructed that this should be followed for life, if the oesophagogastric junction has been resected in the course of the surgery.

13. Instructions are given on the need to restrict the quantity of each meal, the need to avoid unnecessary stooping, bending or heavy lifting, and the need to stay upright for at least 3–4 h after meals, before retiring to bed. Patients are advised against 'nightcaps'.

Complications following oesophagogastric resection

Complications of oesophagogastric surgery in malignant disease fall into two broad groups. The first group consists of complications that are common to any major surgical procedure in a relatively older age group, and are best avoided by proper preoperative evaluation of the suitability of the patient and by adopting active prophylactic measures to counteract the predisposing factors.

Respiratory complications constitute by far the largest proportion of this group. In a recent analysis nearly 50% of the complications in a personal series fell into this category. The pain that accompanies an incision, be it abdominal or thoracic, is the biggest contributory factor to impaired breathing, atelectasis of parts of the lung leading to bronchopneumonia and respiratory failure. Added to this is the element of impaired diaphragmatic movements due to incisions placed on the diaphragm. The extensive dissection of mediastinal lymph nodes, and especially of the bilateral pulmonary hilar and subcarinal lymph nodes, results in a compromise to the lymphatic drainage of the pulmonary alveoli, leading to parenchymal fluid retention which seeps from the interalveolar membrane into the alveoli – resulting in a form of acute pulmonary oedema. All these factors are at their peak in the first 72 h after surgery.

Adequate measures for pain relief, such as epidural analgesia, proper choice of incisions, both on the skin and on the diaphragm, fluid restriction in the first 24–48 h after surgery, and prophylactic systemic antibiotics, all play their respective roles in avoiding such complications. The use of a short period of synchronized intermittent mandatory ventilation (SIMV) in the routine postoperative management of these patients is aimed at reducing such factors to a bare minimum, while chest physiotherapy is by far the most important preventive measure.

Thrombo-embolic complications are not uncommon in malignant disease and in the elderly age groups. Prolonged preoperative stay in bed and long-term parenteral nutrition predispose to this complication. Prophylactic low-dose heparin, early ambulation and active physiotherapy to limbs help in preventing these problems. In the event of a thrombo-embolic complication setting in, routine therapeutic anticoagulation with heparin in the first instance and warfarin in the long term becomes imperative.

Myocardial ischaemia and congestive cardiac failure are again complications specific to the age group we are dealing with in this disease. Both during and after surgery every precaution is taken not to cause a significant degree of hypoxia, or of hypotension. In the event of the complication showing up in the postoperative period, specific medical therapy is instituted.

Cerebrovascular episodes, like the above, are specific to the age group and are precipitated by hypoxia and hypotension. Treatment of a cerebrovascular catastrophe in a patient who has had a major resection can prove to be futile, but has to be persevered with and the routine postoperative management modified accordingly to ensure adequate respiratory and nutritional support.

Haemorrhage is relatively uncommon, and although the blood loss during operation can range from 250 ml to 1500 ml, acute *primary* haemorrhage from any of the major vessels is not common. The largest amount of peroperative blood loss occurs when an advanced tumour is being mobilized from its bed, when adjacent venous and arterial structures can present a problem. *Secondary* haemorrhage is relatively rare despite the prophylactic low-dose anticoagulation regimen, but can occur in the event of mediastinal infection from a specific complication such as an anastomotic leak.

Wound infection. Despite the severity of the procedure and the time taken, wound infections are relatively rare. Peroperative antibiotic prophylaxis in addition to meticulous aseptic technique can reduce this to an insignificant factor.

The second group of complications following oesophagogastric operations are specific to the procedure, the most significant of which is: *leakage from the anastomotic area* and from the *gastric resection line*. If this occurs within the first 24 h and if the patient's general condition is good, the patient should be returned to the operating room for correction of a technical fault on the part of the surgeon. If, however, the patient's condition or the extent of disease was such that further operative intervention is likely to be detrimental, then conservative measures such as oesophagogastric decompression, drainage of the chest and therapeutic antibiotic regimens for Gram-positive and Gram-negative organisms should be commenced early, while nutritional requirements are maintained by the parenteral route.

Delayed breakdown of anastomosis or suture lines are usually attributable to ischaemic factors, or to sepsis, and are best treated conservatively in the above manner. Contrast radiography to localize the leakage site and determine the extent of destruction should precede surgical intervention.

Recurrent laryngeal palsy has begun to occur in recent years with oesophageal resections, due to the current vogue for cervical oesophagogastric anastomosis. It is often unilateral and may well be transient. The use of a mini-tracheostomy as a routine with these operations has minimized the inhalational problems that accompany this complication. Recurrent laryngeal palsy is, however, extremely rare when the anastomosis is constructed in the apex of the chest via the thoracotomy route for subtotal oesophagectomy.

Chylothorax – mobilization of advanced oesophageal tumours, whether through a thoracotomy or through a transhiatal route, is fraught with danger to the chylous duct which is often drawn into the perineoplastic tissues. The duct can often be identified and protected during dissection, but occasionally a chylothorax shows up in the second week after surgery when the patient has just commenced oral intake, especially of fat-containing nutrients. By now the chest drains have been removed as have any intravenous feeding lines. In these situations, immediate measures have to be taken to institute total parenteral nutrition, chest drainage, and then to regulate the fat intake by the oral route by manipulating the medium-chain triglyceride content of the oral diet. If, despite instituting these measures, the accumulation and drainage of chylous fluid continues, pleuroperitoneal shunting may have to be resorted to and, if that fails, open exploration of the chest and ligation of the thoracic duct at the cut ends may be mandatory. An immediate pre-exploratory intake of cream helps to locate the leaking cut ends.

Delayed complications specific to this form of surgery are encountered as shown below.

Pyloric stasis, occurring either in the short or long term, may require smooth muscle-relaxant drugs or prokinetic drugs for the gastric detrusor. In approximately 10–15%, endoscopic balloon dilatation or open pyloroplasty may have to be resorted to.

Acid or alkaline reflux is more prone to occur if the anastomosis is below the level of the aortic arch and is said to be rare with cervical anastomosis. Pyloric stasis predisposes to acid reflux, whereas pyloromyotomy or pyloroplasty both predispose to alkaline reflux; therefore, proper endoscopic and radiological evaluation of the entire upper gastrointestinal tract is essential prior to any oesophageal resectional procedure in order to minimize these complications.

Anastomotic stenosis is a delayed complication following any form of anastomotic ischaemia or healing of leakage, and needs to be addressed early in the follow-up period following routine postoperative radiological contrast studies. In the event of a stenosis being anticipated, the patient should be reviewed within 6–8 weeks of discharge from hospital and endoscoped with a view to endoscopic dilatation of the anastomosis. The incidence of anastomotic stenosis is higher with cervical anastomosis compared with intrathoracic anastomosis, and with stapled anastomosis compared with hand-sewn anastomosis.

'*Dumping*' after oesophagogastric reconstruction is a not uncommon problem in patients for about 12–18 months after the operation, but is usually self-rectified by dietary regulation.

Iatrogenic diaphragmatic herniation can occur through the diaphragmatic hiatus or through any incisions that may have been placed in the diaphragm. The complication usually presents with chronic symptoms and is more dramatic to the investigator than to the patient, but it will need surgical correction as an elective procedure at an early date in order to prevent the more dramatic incarceration or strangulation of herniated bowel. Often the approach for this complication is a thoracolaparotomy, as it enables adequate visualization of the upper abdomen and lower chest for mobilization by freeing the unavoidable adhesions after the previous surgery.

References

Belsey, R. and Hiebert, C. A. (1974) An exclusive right thoracic approach for carcinoma of the middle third of the oesophagus. *Ann. Thorac. Surg.*, **18**, 1–15

Brister, S. J., Chiu, R. L. J., Brom, R. A. *et al.* (1984) Clinical impact of intravenous hyper-alimentation on esophageal carcinoma: is it worthwhile? *Ann. Thorac. Surg.*, **38**, 617–621

Burgess, H. M., Baggenstoss, A. H., Moersch, H. J. *et al.* (1951) Carcinoma of the esophagus: clinicopathologic study. *Surg. Clin. North Am.*, **31**, 965

Celestin, L. R. (1959) Permanent intubation in inoperable cancer of the oesophagus and cardia – a new tube. *Ann. R. Coll. Surg. Eng.*, **25**, 165–170

Finley, R. J., Grace, M. and Duff, J. H. (1985) Esophagectomy without thoracotomy for carcinoma of the cardia and lower part of the oesophagus. *Surg. Gynecol. Obstet.*, **160**, 49–56

Franklin, R. H. (1942) Two cases of successful removal of the thoracic oesophagus for carcinoma. *Br. J. Surg.*, **30**, 141–146

Gisselbrecht, C., Calvo, F., Mignot, C. *et al.* (1983) Fluro-uracil (F) Adriamycin (A) and Cisplatin (P) FAP. Combination chemotherapy of advanced esophageal carcinoma. *Cancer*, **52**, 974–977

Groves, L. K. and Rodriguez Antunez, A. (1973) Treatment of carcinoma of the esophagus and gastric cardia with concentrated pre-operative irradiation followed by early operation. *Ann. Thorac. Surg.*, **15**, 333–338

Guernsey, J. M., Doggett, R. L., Mason, G. R. *et al.* (1969) Combined treatment of cancer of the esophagus. *Am. J. Surg.*, **117**, 157–161

Gunderson, L. L. (1976) Radiation therapy; results and future. In *Clincis in Gastroenterology*. Vol. 5, W. B. Saunders, London, pp. 743–776

Gunnlaugsson, G. H., Wychulis, A. R., Roland, C. *et al.* (1970) Analysis of the records of 1,657 patients with carcinoma of the esophagus and cardia of the stomach. *Surg. Gynecol. Obstet.*, **130**, 997–1005

Japanese Society for Esophageal Disorders (1976) Guidelines for the clinical and pathologic studies for carcinoma of the esophagus. *Jap. J. Surg.*, **6**, 79–86

Jeyasingham, K. (1978) Clinica e terapia del carcinoma esofageo. In *Dal Bollettino delle Scienze Mediche* (eds A. Franchini *et al.*), Organo Della Societa E Scuola Medica Chirurgica Di Bologna.

Jeyasingham, K., Beligaswatte, A. M. L. and Sandrasegara, F. A. (1967) Carcinoma involving the oesophagus. *Ceyl. Med. J.*, **12**, 187–201

Kron, I. L., Cantrell, M. D., Johns, M. E. *et al.* (1984) Computerised axial tomography of the oesophagus to determine suitability for blunt oesophagectomy. *Ann. Surg.*, **200**, 173–174

Lauren, P. (1965). The two main types of gastric carcinoma: diffuse and so-called intestinal-type carcinoma. *Acta Pathol. Microbiol. Immunol. Scand.*, **64**, 31–49

Le Quesne, L. P. and Ranger, D. (1966) Pharyngo-laryngectomy with immediate pharyngo-gastric anastomosis. *Br. J. Surg.*, **53**, 105–109

Lewis, I. (1946) The surgical treatment of carcinoma of the oesophagus with special reference to a new operation for growth of the middle third. *Br. J. Surg.*, **34**, 18–31

McCaughan, J. S., Hicks, W., Laufman, L. *et al.* (1984) Palliation of esophageal malignancy with photoradiation therapy. *Cancer*, **54**, 2905–2910

McKeown, K. C. (1972) Trends in oesophageal resection for carcinoma. *Ann. R. Coll. Surg. Engl.*, **51**, 213–218

Medical Research Council (1992) *Pre-operative Chemotherapy for Cancer of the Oesophagus*, MRC, Cambridge

Miller, C. (1962) Carcinoma of the thoracic oesophagus and cardia. A review of 405 cases. *Br. J. Surg.*, **49**, 507–522

Moertel, C. G. (1978) Chemotherapy in gastro-intestinal cancer. In *Clinics in Gastroenterology*, Vol. 5, W. B. Saunders, London, pp. 777–793

Monnier, P., Savary, M. and Anani, P. (1985) Endoscopic morphology of 'early' esophageal carcinoma. In *Esophageal Disorders: Pathophysiology and Therapy* (eds T. R. De Meester and D. B. Skinner), Raven Press, New York, pp. 333–346

Mousseau, M., le Forestier, J., Barbin, J. *et al.* (1956) Place de l'intubation a demeure dans le traitement palliative du cancer de l'esophagi. *Arch. Mal. Appar. Digest.*, **45**, 208–216

Nakayama, K. and Kinoshita, Y. (1975) Surgical treatment combined with pre-operative concentrated irradiation. Current concepts in cancer. Esophagus – treatment localized and advanced. *JAMA*, **227**, 178–181

Ong, G. B. and Lee, T. C. (1960) Pharyngogastric anastomosis after oesophago-pharyngectomy for carcinoma of the hypopharynx and cervical oesophagus. *Br. J. Surg.*, **48**, 193

Orringer, M. B. (1984) Transhiatal oesophagectomy without thoracotomy for carcinoma of the thoracic esophagus. *Ann. Surg.*, **200**, 282–288

Orringer, M. B. and Orringer, J. S. (1983) Transhiatal oesophagectomy without thoracotomy – a dangerous operation? *J. Thorac. Cardiovasc. Surg.*, **85**, 72–80

Orringer, M. B. and Sloan, H. (1975) Substernal gastric bypass of the excluded thoracic oesophagus for palliation of oesophageal carcinoma. *J. Thorac. Cardiovasc. Surg.*, **70**, 836–851

Orringer, M. B. and Sloan, H. (1978) Oesophagectomy without thoracotomy. *J. Thorac. Cardiovasc. Surg.*, **76**, 643–654

Pearson, J. G. (1975) Value of radiation therapy. Current concepts in cancer. Esophagus – treatment. *JAMA*, **227**, 181–183

Royston, C. M. S. and Dowling, B. L. (1976) A combined synchronous technique for the McKeown three-phase oesophagectomy. *Br. J. Surg.*, **63**, 122–124

Soga, J., Kobayashi, K., Saito, J. *et al.* (1979) The role of lymphadenectomy in curative surgery for gastric cancer. *World J. Surg.*, **3**, 701–708

Souttar, H. S. (1924) Method of intubating the oesophagus for malignant stricture. *Br. Med. J.*, **1**, 782–783

Sweet, R. H. (1945) Transthoracic gastrectomy and esophagectomy for carcinoma of the stomach and esophagus. *Clinics*, **3**, 1288

Sweet, R. H. (1950) *Thoracic Surgery*, W. B. Saunders, Philadelphia, pp. 271–279

Turner, G. G. (1936) Carcinoma of the oesophagus – the question of its treatment by surgery. *Lancet*, **1**, 130

Union Internationale Contre le Cancer. (1990) *TNM Atlas*, Springer-Verlag, Heidelberg

Watt, I., Stewart, I., Anderson, D. *et al.* (1989) Laparoscopy, ultrasound and computed tomography in cancer of the oesophagus and gastric cardia: a prospective comparison for detecting intra-abdominal metastases. *Br. J. Surg.*, **76**, 1036–1039

Yan, C. J. and Brooks, J. R. (1985) Surgical management of gastric adenocarcinoma. *Am. J. Surg.*, **149**, 771–774

Further reading

Preoperative evaluation

Duignan, C. G., McEntee, G. P., O'Connell, D. J. *et al.* (1987) The role of CT in the management of carcinoma of the oesophagus and cardia. *Ann. Roy. Coll. Surg. Eng.*, **69**, 286–288

Watt, I., Stewart, I., Anderson D. *et al.* (1989) Laparoscopy, ultrasound and computed tomography in cancer of the oesophagus and gastric cardia: a prospective comparison for detecting intra-abdominal metastases. *Br. J. Surg.*, **76**, 1036–1039

Early gastric cancer

Ballantyne, K. D., Morris, D. L., Jones, J. A. *et al.* (1987) Accuracy of identification of early gastric cancer. *Br. J. Surg.*, **74**, 618–619

Bringaze III, W. L., Chappuis, C. W., Cohn, I. Jr. *et al.* (1986) Early gastric cancer 21-year experience. *Ann. Surg.*, **204**, 2

De Dombal, F.T., Price, A.B., Thompson, H. *et al.* (1990) The British Society of Gastroenterology early gastric cancer/dysplasia survey: an interim report. *Gut*, **31**, 115–120

Endo, M., Ide, H., Yoshino, K. *et al.* (1986) Diagnosis and treatment of early esophageal cancer. In *Diseases of the Esophagus* (eds J. R. Sievert and A. H. Hölscher), Springer-Verlag, Heidelberg, pp. 375–380

Hisamichi, S. (1989) Screening for gastric cancer. *World J. Surg.*, **13**, 31–37

Lawrence, M. and Shiu, M. H. (1991) Early gastric cancer. *Ann. Surg.*, **34**, 327–334

Misumi, A., Harada, K. and Murakami, A. (1989) Early diagnosis of esophageal cancer. *Ann. Surg.*, **210**(6), 732–739

Nabeya, K., Hanaoka, T. and Onozawa, K. (1986) New measures for early detection of carcinoma of the esophagus. In *Diseases of the Esophagus* (eds J. R. Sievert and A. H. Hölscher), Springer-Verlag, Heidelberg, pp. 105–108

Surgery for oesophageal cancer

Lu, Y. K., Li, Y. M. and Gu, Y. Z. (1987) Cancer of esophagus and esophagogastric junction: analysis of results of 1,025 resections after 5 to 20 years. *Ann. Thorac. Surg.*, **43**, 176–181

Mannell, A. and Becker, P. J. (1991) Evaluation of the results of oesophagectomy for oeosphageal cancer. *Br. J. Surg.*, **78**, 36–40

Mannell, A., Becker, P. J. and Nissenbaum, M. (1988) Bypass surgery for unresectable oesophageal cancer: early and late results in 124 cases. *Br. J. Surg.*, **75**, 283–286

Mathisen, D. J., Grillo, H. C., and Wilkins, E. W. (1988) Transthoracic esophagectomy: a safe approach to carcinoma of the esophagus. *Ann. Thorac. Surg.*, **45**, 137–143

Muller, J. M., Erasmi, H., Stelzner, M. *et al.* (1990) Surgical therapy of oesophageal carcinoma. *Br. J. Surg.*, **77**, 845–857

Surgery for gastric ulcer

Irvin, T. T. and Bridger, J. E. (1988) Gastric cancer: an audit of 122 consecutive cases and the results of R1 gastrectomy. *Br. J. Surg.*, **75**, 106–109

Noguchi, Y, Imada, T., Matsumoto, A. *et al.* (1989) Radical surgery for gastric ulcer – a review of the Japanese experience. *Cancer*, **64**, 2053–2062

Ovaska, J., Kruuna, O., Saario, I. *et al.* (1989) Surgical treatment of gastric carcinoma. *Am. J. Surg.*, **158**, 467–471

Paterson, I. M., Easton, D. F. and Corbishley, C. M. (1987) Changing distribution of adenocarcinoma of the stomach. *Br. J. Surg.*, **74**, 481–482

Multiple modality treatment

Allum, W. H., Hallissey, M. T., Kelly, K. A. *et al.* (1989) Adjuvant chemotherapy in operable gastric cancer. *Lancet*, **i**, 571–574

Hilgenberg, A. D., Carey, R. W. and Wilkins, E. W. (1988) Preoperative chemotherapy, surgical resection, and selective postoperative therapy for squamous cell carcinoma of the esophagus. *Ann. Thorac. Surg.*, **45**, 357–363

Medical Research Council (1992) *Preoperative Chemotherapy for Cancer of the Oesophagus*, MRC, Cambridge

Orringer, M. B., Forastiere, A. and Perez-Tamayo, C. (1990) Chemotherapy and radiation therapy before transhiatal esophagectomy for esophageal carcinoma. *Ann. Thorac. Surg.*, **49**, 348–355

Wolfe, W. G., Burton, G. V. and Seigler, H. F. (1989) Early results with combined modality therapy for carcinoma of the esophagus. *Ann. Surg.*, **205**(5), 563–571

10

Replacement of the oesophagus

D. Alderson, M. J. M. Black and D. B. Mathias

Introduction

Lesions requiring oesophageal replacement

The oesophagus may need replacing for benign and malignant conditions. In the former group this includes: congenital lesions such as oesophageal atresia, inflammatory lesions producing strictures secondary to gastro-oesophageal reflux or chemical burns, benign tumours and trauma.

Primary malignant lesions of the oesophagus, particularly carcinoma and those carcinomas of the cardia which spread submucosally up the oesophagus, are the important malignant lesions requiring oesophageal replacement.

The choice of oesophageal substitute is influenced by the location and length of oesophagus removed. Stomach, jejunum and colon can all be used as conduits. In reaching a decision about which to use, the comments made by Belsey (1965) are worth repeating (see also Belsey, 1983):

1. The morbidity and mortality risks of the operation must be acceptable.
2. It must be possible to excise the obstructive lesion as radically as necessary and reconstruct the oesophagus in one stage.
3. Sufficient viscus must be available to replace the entire oesophagus when necessary.
4. The method should be applicable to infants and children as well as adults.
5. The relief of the patient's dysphagia must be complete and lasting.

The use of stomach as an oesophageal substitute

History

In 1920, Kirschner developed a bypass procedure in which the mobilized stomach was brought up subcutaneously for anastomosis with the cervical oesophagus. In 1933, Oshawa described resection of the cardia and an oesophagogastric anastomosis. The first transpleural resection of the oesophagus with oesophagogastric anastomosis was described in 1938 by Adams and Phemister.

Higher oesophageal resections required greater mobilization of the stomach, resulting in the classical operations associated with oesophagogastric anastomosis. These are: the abdominal and right thoracic approach described by Lewis; the three-stage oesophagectomy described by McKeown; and the transhiatal techniques of Ong and Lee (Lewis, 1946; Ong and Lee, 1960; McKeown, 1972).

Indications

The stomach is the preferred substitute for most malignant lesions arising in the oesophagus and for those lesions arising at the gastro-oesophageal junction, where the lesser curvature and left gastric pedicle can be resected in continuity with oesophagus. Provided that full mobilization of the stomach is not hindered by previous gastric surgery or removal of part of the stomach, then, based upon its right gastro-epiploic and right gastric arteries, the fundus will reach high into the neck. Further lengthening of the stomach can be achieved using the reversed gastric tube technique described below, particularly for pharyngogastric anastomoses. Gastric substitution is also the procedure of choice when the oesophagus either cannot or need not be removed, when the conduit is located substernally, e.g. for unresectable carcinoma, or for tracheo-oesophageal fistula, whenever non-operative methods have failed. The stomach is also the preferred conduit when the entire oesophagus is removed for benign disease, such as Chagasic mega oesophagus or other severe primary motility disturbances resistant to other forms of therapy.

Preoperative selection and management

With malignant oesophageal neoplasms, correct patient selection for surgery is vital and is discussed elsewhere. The type of gastric substitute and its location are discussed below. Specific preoperative preparation of the stomach is unnecessary, except that the surgeon should be aware of any past history of peptic ulcer disease which might compromise gastric mobilization or which might have produced pyloric scarring. It is important, therefore, that a careful endoscopic examination of the stomach is carried out, to assess these features and to have a careful appraisal of the extent of intragastric involvement by tumours arising at the gastro-oesophageal junction. In patients where the tumour is unequivocally gastric in origin, laparoscopy should be undertaken prior to resective surgery, since extensive gastric involvement by a tumour apparently arising from

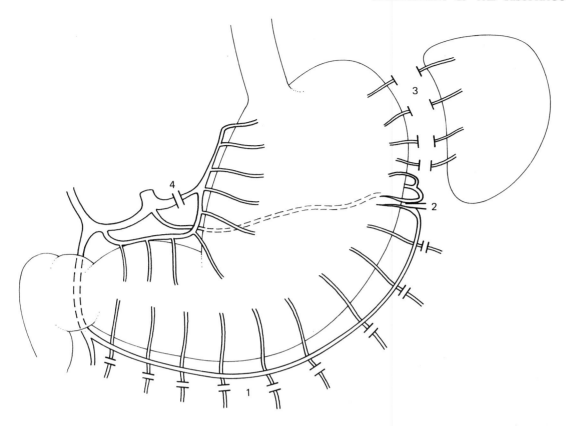

Figure 10.1 Sites for gastric vascular ligation. 1, Omental vessels outside the right gastro-epiploic arcade. 2, Left gastro-epiploic. 3, Short gastrics. 4, Left gastric

the gastro-oesophageal junction merits an appropriate gastric resection. There is little evidence that preoperative radiotherapy or chemotherapy significantly damages the stomach to render it unsuitable as the conduit.

Irrespective of the conduit chosen, a number of general preoperative measures are indicated. Severe malnutrition should be addressed either by oral feeding or fine-bore tube feeding; if this cannot be achieved, total parenteral nutrition should be administered. Dehydration and anaemia should be corrected. A significant proportion of patients with neoplasia, and many of those with major motor disturbances in the oesophagus, will be at risk of aspiration pneumonia, and vigorous physiotherapy may help to improve pulmonary function preoperatively. Some surgeons routinely digitalize patients because of the frequency of cardiac irregularities during oesophagectomy. There is no real evidence that this is necessary.

Techniques

The stomach may be routed through the oesophageal bed, substernally or even subcutaneously, although the latter is hardly ever used today. Bringing the stomach through the oesophageal bed to the neck usually poses no technical difficulties in delivering the fundus through the thoracic inlet. This is not always the case, however, with substernal placements, when it may be necessary to resect the medial end of the clavicle and upper corner of the manubrium on the same side, to avoid compression of the stomach at this point. The technical details of this latter procedure are well described by Orringer (1988).

Gastric tube lengthening is easily achieved using the method described by Gavriliu (1988), which employs a greater curvature tube based on the right gastro-epiploic artery and is rapidly performed with multiple applications of a linear cutting stapler. Such a manoeuvre will extend the length of gastric tube, enabling it to reach the pharynx if required.

There are, irrespective of the route chosen for the stomach, a number of technical points that are common to all operations, the most important of which is meticulous preparation of the gastric blood supply (Figure 10.1). This is ideally based on the right gastro-epiploic and right gastric vessels, with complete preservation of the greater curvature arcade. In dividing the short gastric vessels, it is important that the stomach wall proper is not included in the ligatures. It is imperative that when the operation is being carried out for cancer the left gastric lymph node pedicle is taken completely and this implies division of the left gastric artery at its origin, without damage to either the splenic or hepatic arteries. This subsequently enables the lesser curvature and cardia to be resected in continuity with the oesophagus, but preserving gastric length through retention of the fundus. The second critical area is mobilization of the duodenum, which needs to be extensive, requiring the exposure of 7–10 cm of inferior vena cava. Correct vascular and duodenal mobilization will enable the pylorus to reach comfortably to the oesophageal hiatus.

It is difficult to pass the gastric tube comfortably through an undilated hiatus, and anterior division of the crura and the tendinous part of the diaphragm should be carried out to enable the conduit to pass freely. There is considerable debate about the value of pyloroplasty. Despite the fact that the stomach is totally vagotomized, there is no real evidence that a gastric drainage procedure confers benefit in patients who do not have objective evidence of disease at the pylorus (Hölscher, 1988).

Postoperative management

Two points are specific to the use of stomach as the replacement viscus. These are: (a) the prevention of gastric distension; and (b) the prevention of aspiration.

Prevention of gastric distension

The stomach usually takes a few days to regain its ability to empty gas and fluids. A nasogastric tube may be placed for the early postoperative period, but many oesophageal surgeons do not use nasogastric tubes routinely and do not perceive this as a significant problem. Because of the associated risk of aspiration, there seem to be at least theoretical reasons why gastric distension should be prevented.

Prevention of aspiration

Pulmonary aspiration is a complication which is almost unique to oesophagectomy because free reflux occurs into the oesophageal substitute in the absence of a lower oesophageal sphincter. The risk can be partly reduced by making use of gravity and preventing gastric distension. An important factor, however, which increases the risk of aspiration, is temporary or permanent damage to the recurrent laryngeal nerves, either in the thorax or during a dissection of the cervical oesophagus. Gastric stasis, in combination with recurrent laryngeal nerve injury, must be avoided at all costs.

Complications

The stomach has an excellent blood supply and ischaemic necrosis is rare. Leak rates from oesophagogastric anastomoses in recent surgical series are of the order of 5–10%. Subsequent mortality, however, is still high, but is less when the anastomosis is in the neck. This usually results in a salivary fistula rather than mediastinitis.

The principal late complications are related to reflux and anastomotic stenosis. Clearly, all patients with an oesophagogastric anastomosis, irrespective of level, have the potential for reflux. Patients with low (infra-aortic) anastomoses have the highest incidence of symptomatic reflux and as the anastomosis is created at a higher level, so the incidence of reflux, as determined both radiologically and endoscopically, falls. This presumably accounts for the lower incidence of anastomotic stenosis with supra-aortic or cervical anastomoses (Borst et al., 1978).

The use of jejunum as an oesophageal substitute

History

Replacement of the oesophagus with jejunum was first proposed in 1904 by Wüllstein and was first successfully performed by Roux in 1907. Jejunum is ideally suited to segmental replacement of the oesophagus. Replacement of the lower oesophagus is accomplished using either a Roux-en-Y technique or by segmental interposition. Replacement of the upper oesophagus is accomplished by microvascular free jejunal transfer. Although it is possible to create a long loop for replacement of the entire thoracic oesophagus, the jejunum should be considered the third choice conduit behind stomach and colon and would therefore be chosen in only a minority of patients, where the other two organs were not suitable for mobilization.

Replacement of the lower oesophagus with jejunum

Indications

1. In conjunction with total gastrectomy in which a short segment of lower oesophagus is removed.
2. As a salvage procedure for patients with benign oesophageal strictures which have failed to respond to endoscopic therapies and failed surgery.
3. As a short-circuit procedure to bypass inoperable lesions at the oesophagogastric junction.

Preoperative selection and management

There are no specific measures necessary to deal with the small bowel preoperatively, other than to identify patients who are known to have small bowel disease. As with gastric substitution, all of the general points regarding preoperative patient management apply. Some authors have advocated the use of oral antibiotics as a preoperative measure, but this is unnecessary and of no proven value.

Techniques

The technical details described in the original articles by Roux in 1907, and by Allison and DeSilva (1953), have never been bettered. Usually an appropriate loop is identified in the upper jejunum within the first 10 cm after the duodenal-jejunal flexure. At this point there is a typical jejunal vascular pattern of arterial arcades supplied at intervals by larger primary jejunal arteries (Figure 10.2). The veins and arteries are close together but bifurcate at different levels, making separate division of the veins and arteries essential. Identification of the jejunal vasculature is facilitated by transillumination, and an appropriate length of jejunum is selected from the proposed site of proximal transection. From this proposed point of transection, the peritoneum is incised towards the root of the mesentery, dividing the first primary artery and vein with considerable care to avoid damage to branches at this point. Similar primary branches are then divided within the mesentery to create a loop of the desired length. It is important to realize, in the creation of a jejunal loop, that it is the length of the free edge of mesentery which will determine the length of the loop created, rather than the length of the jejunum itself. The latter is usually longer than the mesentery and will therefore have a tendency to become redundant. An ideal Roux loop is created when it will reach to the point of anastomosis without tension in its mesentery and without surplus length in a straight line. Doubt regarding the adequacy of blood supply within such a loop can be minimized by the temporary application of bulldog clamps across jejunal vessels, to be certain that they can be safely divided without compromise to the loop. Division of the bowel with modern stapling instruments, and the restoration of intestinal continuity with staplers, considerably hastens the preparation of this type of conduit.

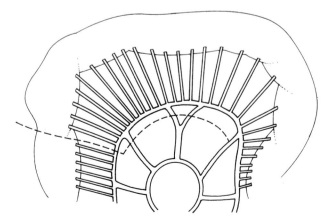

Figure 10.2 Creation of a jejunal Roux loop. Note that the length of jejunum is greater than the length of its mesentery

Postoperative management

Nasojejunal intubation is not really necessary following a Roux-en-Y anastomosis when the stomach is absent and is probably unnecessary after short interposition for benign stricture. Contrast radiology of the anastomosis is not essential, and in patients who are clinically well, oral fluids can be reintroduced as soon as the ileus resolves. The more frequent use of modern catheter systems for distal enteral feeding, which can be inserted at the time of primary surgery, is recommended in patients where there may be a delay in the restoration of conventional oral feeding.

Complications

Necrosis of the jejunum is unusual and largely related to the length of the Roux loop which the surgeon wishes to create. This is principally a function of compression, stretching or twisting of the vascular pedicle of the graft, usually leading to venous congestion and thrombosis, rather than an arterial defect. Because of the way in which this occurs, it tends to be an early complication within the first few days and is recognized by profound tachycardia and usually an associated leucocytosis. As the conduit becomes progressively ischaemic, so there are increasing signs of mediastinal and pleural contamination. Contrast radiology will not always demonstrate this event adequately, until the viscus ruptures or there is dehiscence of the anastomosis. A clinical suspicion of necrosis is an indication for prompt reoperation after resuscitation. The situation is managed by removal of the conduit, drainage of the oesophagus and the provision of a distal gastrostomy for feeding. When the patient has recovered, an alternative conduit should be used, with reconstruction of an anastomosis at a different site.

Anastomotic leakage usually occurs at the upper anastomosis of an interposition and is rare after a standard Roux-en-Y reconstruction. Small radiological leaks may never be symptomatic and will heal spontaneously. Significant leaks are clinically recognizable by symptoms of mediastinitis, pain, tachycardia and dyspnoea. The presence of air and fluid in the pleural cavity or in the mediastinum on a chest X-ray are virtually diagnostic, and if doubt remains a radio-opaque swallow will confirm frank leakage. The situation is rarely recognized at such an early stage that local repair is feasible and this practice should not be encouraged. A range of alternative strategies has been proposed. Of these, only two seem to merit real consideration; a 're-do' anastomosis, ensuring that there is no local contamination and that this can be done in a tension-free manner with adequate blood supply to both ends; or an exclusion procedure, diverting the oesophageal contents by cervical oesophagostomy and the introduction of distal enteral feeding by catheter jejunostomy.

Anastomotic stenosis is rare and may reflect a small

leak or a degree of ischaemia. This can usually be dealt with by endoscopic dilatation. The other important cause of stenosis is tumour recurrence which can be extremely difficult to deal with, particularly if marked angulation should occur between the oesophagus and jejunum.

Reflux is not usually a problem because the stomach has been removed. With jejunal interposition, however, provided that an adequate length of intra-abdominal jejunum of about 10 cm is created, then symptomatic reflux is also infrequent. Pain is a late postoperative complication which occasionally occurs in patients with a jejunal interposition, especially post-prandially. Its exact cause is not well understood, but may relate to gastric distension.

Technique of microvascular free jejunal transfer for reconstruction of the pharynx and cervical oesophagus

Reconstruction of the continuity of the upper alimentary tract may be accomplished by a variety of operative procedures. Microvascular free jejunal transfer, gastric pull-ups and tubed myocutaneous island flaps are the most commonly used techniques. Microvascular free colon, ileum and gastric antral grafts have all been described and pedicle colon transplant may be used when circumstances dictate.

History

Extirpative surgery has been described previously, but the use of local skin flaps, as advocated by Wookey in 1942, represented the first realistic reconstructive procedure. Variations of this technique were used until the early 1960s when gastric pull-up procedures and subcutaneous pedicle colon transplants replaced the previous multi-stage operations. In 1975, Bakamjian described the use of the deltopectoral flap as a two-stage procedure, which became very popular. The use of tubed myocutaneous island flaps, based on pectoralis major, latissimus dorsi and trapezius muscles has largely superseded the deltopectoral flap technique in the past decade. Seidenberg and Hurwith (1959) reported the first clinical use of free jejunal graft. The technique became established by the early 1980s and has gained in popularity with the concomitant advances in microvascular surgery. The technique is ideally carried out using a team approach with specialist head and neck, microvascular and abdominal surgeons.

Indications

Free jejunal transfer may be indicated in the following situations:

1. After pharyngolaryngectomy performed for carcinoma of the hypopharynx, post-cricoid oesophagus and cervical oesophagus.
2. After pharyngectomy and upper cervical oesophagectomy with preservation of the larynx in early post-cricoid carcinoma confined to the posterior wall.
3. Following recurrence of carcinoma in the pharynx after laryngectomy.
4. In the rare instance of benign stricture caused by trauma or chemical burns of the cervical oesophagus.
5. For partial non-circumferential repair of the pharynx.

The operation may be performed with or without radical neck dissection, as part of the primary treatment programme including radiotherapy, or as palliative surgery following recurrence after radiotherapy.

Preoperative selection and management

Patients presenting with a history of peripheral vascular disease, with or without thrombotic episodes, are not ideal candidates for microvascular anastomosis. Previous major abdominal surgery does not preclude the technique, but may increase the morbidity, and consideration should be given to the use of alternative reconstructive techniques.

Patients who have undergone previous radiotherapy to the neck should be carefully evaluated to ensure that recipient vessels may be found outside the fields of treatment. Once the patient is selected as a suitable candidate for surgery, routine preoperative investigations should include chest X-ray, barium swallow and CT scanning. It is of vital importance to assess the lower margin of the tumour accurately with respect to its relationship to the thoracic inlet. In cases requiring total thyroidectomy, both thyroid function tests and estimation of ionized calcium should be carried out.

Preoperative radiotherapy may be given, but it is best limited to the area of pharynx and oesophagus to be resected. Adjuvant chemotherapy has been used. No anticoagulant therapy is required, but prophylactic antibiotics are given routinely. Preoperative bowel preparation is unnecessary.

Technique

A U-shaped incision is preferred, extended in cases requiring block dissection of cervical lymph nodes. Extirpative surgery is carried out according to the site of the lesion to be excised. In the case of carcinoma, adequate margins should be achieved below and above the tumour, as para-pharyngeal spread is common.

It is preferable to site the tracheostomy in a separate incision. During the course of surgery, one or other superior thyroid artery should be selected as the recipient artery, care being taken to avoid damage and to retain as long a trunk as possible. An external jugular vein should be selected on the same side as the artery and divided high in the neck. The vein should be dissected out for several inches to allow scope for anastomosis without tension to the pedicle. Other branches of the external carotid artery may be used and both transverse cervical and suprascapular vessels can be considered if branches of the carotid have been exposed to radiotherapy. Should the external jugular vein be unsuitable, venous anastomosis can be accomplished by an end-to-side anastomosis with the internal jugular vein. Stay sutures should be inserted in the oesophagus below the tumour prior to transection of the oesophagus, to prevent retraction of the oesophageal stump into the thoracic inlet.

In patients in which an adequate clearance below the tumour cannot be achieved through a cervical incision, consideration may be given to removal of part or all of the manubrium or to sternal splitting. Recipient vessels are prepared after the specimen has been removed. As the extirpative phase of this operation is nearing completion, the abdominal phase can begin.

The abdomen is opened through an upper midline incision. Proximal jejunum is selected and its mesenteric vessels examined by translumination and palpation. The aim is to select a suitable length of jejunum supplied by a single good-sized branch of the superior mesenteric artery and drained by an accompanying single vein (Figure 10.3). The arteries are usually 3 mm in diameter and the veins 4 mm. A marker suture or clip is applied proximally to ensure later placement of the transplant in an isoperistaltic direction in the neck. Once the neck recipient vessels are prepared, the jejunal segment is removed and immediately transferred to the neck. Ischaemic time may be limited by carefully inserting an anastomotic staple gun into the jejunal segment prior to severance of the blood supply in the abdomen.

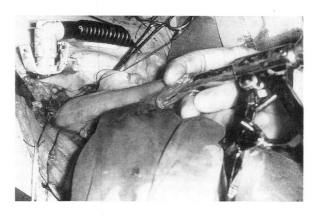

Figure 10.4 Anastomotic staple gun fixation to the oesophageal stump prior to microvascular anastomosis

The first step in the neck is then to staple the transplant into the oesophageal stump, after careful orientation to place the vessels ideally for anastomosis. Stability of the transplant is thereby provided and inadvertent traction on the vascular anastomosis during this step avoided (Figure 10.4).

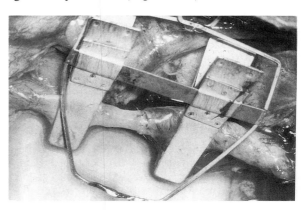

Figure 10.5 Completed microvascular anastomosis of the superior thyroid artery to the jejunal artery

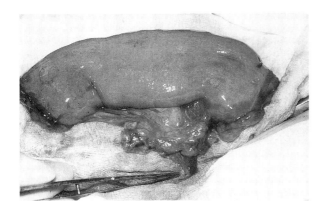

Figure 10.3 Isolated upper jejunal segment supplied by a single branch of the superior mesenteric artery and drained by a single accompanying vein. Note the clip marking the proximal end of segment

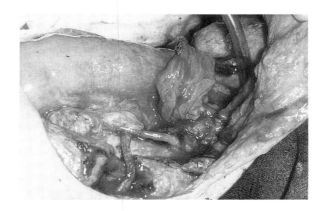

Figure 10.6 The revascularized jejunal transplant. The major thyroid artery and the external jugular vein are anastomosed to the mesenteric vessels

The microvascular anastomoses are undertaken in standard fashion with the operating microscope, using 10/0 nylon interrupted sutures (Figure 10.5). Care must be taken to avoid compression, kinking or tension on the vessels which may be introduced at the time of wound closure. When the external jugular vein is pedicled across an intact sternomastoid muscle, it has been found helpful to partially cut the muscle to let the vein sit in a groove without any tension (Figure 10.6).

The upper anastomosis to the pharyngeal stump is carried out after revascularization and observation of peristaltic movement in the transposed jejunum. This limits the ischaemic time to a minimum. A sterile nasogastric feeding tube is carefully passed by the anaesthetist and threaded through the anastomosis by the surgeon.

At the donor site, end-to-end bowel continuity is restored and the abdomen closed. By using a team approach, this part of the procedure can be carried out simultaneously with the microvascular anastomosis.

After achieving careful haemostasis, drains are inserted on both sides of the neck through separate stab incisions, without suction. The wound is closed in layers.

Postoperative assessment

In the immediate postoperative phase, tracheostomy tapes should be avoided to prevent compression of the venous drainage. The tube is secured by adhesive tape or sutures.

Direct monitoring is not usually employed, but Katsaros (1985) has described a possible technique. Invasive monitoring probes are currently under evaluation. Viability of the jejunal segment can often be evaluated by compression of the tongue and direct inspection. The duration of nasogastric tube aspiration and intravenous fluid therapy is partially dictated by the duration of ileus and status of the intra-abdominal anastomosis. Swallowing of fluids is permitted at about 7 days (Figure 10.7).

In patients requiring total thyroidectomy, serum calcium should be carefully monitored and intravenous calcium gluconate given in the immediate postoperative phase. This should be continued until maintenance therapy can be achieved via the nasogastric tube.

Radiotherapy has been used postoperatively, but care should be taken to avoid irradiation of the transposed jejunum.

Complications

1. *Failure of vascular anastomosis*. This has been observed, but is very unusual in the hands of experienced microvascular surgeons and when proper selection of patients has taken place.
2. *Failure of bowel anastomosis*. With modern

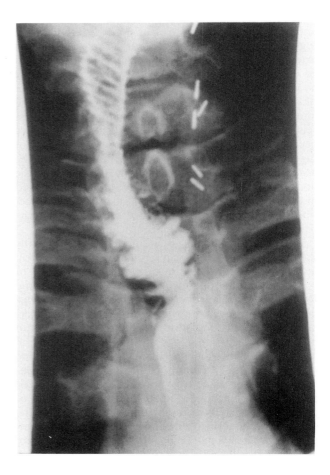

Figure 10.7 X-ray contrast swallow, at 7 days, showing the jejunal transplant in the neck

staplers, it is most unusual to have any problems with leakage at the oesophagojejunal anastomosis. Leaks at the pharyngojejunal anastomosis are more common, but seldom give rise to long-term difficulties. They are usually self-limiting.
3. *Swallowing*. Patients often experience a slowing down of the initial phase of swallowing, and in thin patients peristalsis can be observed in the jejunal segment, which obviously limits the speed of swallowing. Stenosis is rare, but has been observed at the jejuno-oesophageal junction in a long-term survivor. Should this occur, dilatation is best accomplished using a flexible fibreoptic endoscope to pass a guide wire, over which is introduced a graduated dilator. Rigid endoscopy is to be discouraged because of the danger of damaging the jejunum.
4. *Speech*. Good non-laryngeal speech is seldom developed following jejunal transfer, but some patients do develop useful voice. The authors have no experience in the use of voice prostheses in this procedure, but there may be scope for the use of such appliances in future developments.
5. *Aspiration pneumonia*, as a result of the secretory

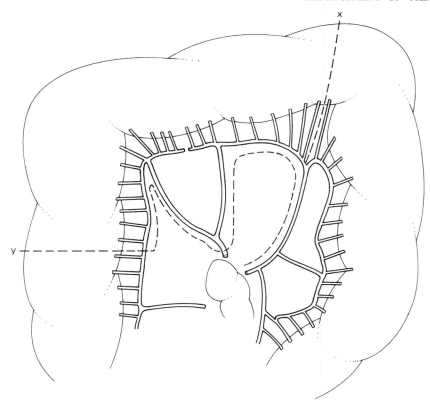

Figure 10.8 Colon transposition based on the ascending branch of the left colic artery; x and y indicate sites of bowel transection

activity of the jejunum, has been reported by Sasaki (1980). He used patches for smaller defects without tracheostomy in 7 cases. Reuther (1984), using only patches, stated that the secretions actually helped those patients with post-irradiation xerostomia.

The use of colon as an oesophageal substitute

History

The use of long segments of colon, either for replacement or bypass of all or part of the thoracic oesophagus, was introduced independently by Kelling (1911) and Vulliet (1911).

Indication

The principal indication for the use of a colonic conduit is for cancer, particularly those tumours close to the gastro-oesophageal junction, which necessitate both an extensive oesophageal as well as gastric resection. The colon is also the preferred substitute after previous failed oesophageal surgery following caustic injury and occasionally for advanced motility disorders where stomach is not available. Colon interposition is the appropriate procedure for infants with oesophageal atresia.

Preoperative selection and management

The general points made in relation to assessment of the patient's disease, which pertain for other conduits, apply equally well but there are specific measures which are essential for the appropriate use of a segment of colon. A barium enema or a colonoscopy should be performed to ensure that the colon is disease free. The author agrees with DeMeester and colleagues that preoperative mesenteric angiography provides important information in adult patients about the nature of the colonic blood supply. The most important aspect here, is the area between the right and left branches of the middle colic artery, where the marginal vessel may be deficient, and particular attention should be directed towards this area on the angiogram. There is continued controversy regarding the need for colonic cleansing. Most surgeons find an empty colon easier to deal with. There is little evidence that mechanical cleansing of the colon is necessary but antibiotic prophylaxis is essential.

Technique

The right, transverse or left colon may be employed for oesophageal replacement or bypass. The segment selected depends largely upon the configuration of the blood vessels. The majority of surgeons seem to prefer the left or transverse colon, based upon the ascending branch of the left colic artery because the blood supply is more consistently favourable and an adequate length of colon can usually be easily prepared (Figure 10.8). Both substernal and oesophageal bed routes can be used. The same constraints for stomach are important for colon when a substernal route is used. There are excellent complete technical descriptions for the use of various segments of colon by Belsey (1965), DeMeester (1988) and Postlethwaite (1988). A number of technical points, however, are common to most of the operations. Adequate colonic mobilization is essential beyond the area of the conduit, to ensure that a series of tension-free anastomoses can be created. The tethering artery, for instance the ascending branch of the left colic artery for a left/transverse colon interposition, should allow the bowel at this point to reach to the xiphisternum. The colon should be marked with a stitch on the antimesenteric border directly opposite this point, which will indicate the subsequent point of distal resection. Careful preparation of the blood supply is vital, and proposed points of vascular division should be temporarily occluded with bulldog clamps to test the adequacy of both the arterial input and the venous outflow. Only the local end-arteries to the colon, at its proposed points of transection, should be divided at an early stage, retaining the colon in continuity for as long as possible. Once it is determined that the blood supply is adequate, then the proximal colon should be divided and, after anastomosis to the oesophagus, placed on sufficient stretch to prevent redundancy within the chest or in the substernal area. The colon should then be anchored in its straightened position by sutures to the left crural margin of the hiatus, although not circumferentially. At the distal end of the colonic resection, it is important not to damage the marginal artery, to preserve additional blood supply to and from the distal colon.

Postoperative management

Numerous series have indicated that colonic interposition can be performed with a mortality of around 5%, although it may be higher in series where many of the patients have carcinoma. The most common complication is necrosis of the conduit and, as with jejunal interposition, this is largely related to kinking, twisting or compression of the blood supply and venous thrombosis. The intraperitoneal anastomoses used to obtain restoration of intestinal continuity rarely fail, but if they do, peritonitis will result. Leakage of the anastomosis between oesophagus and colon in the neck is the most frequent non-fatal complication and may occur in as many as 25% of patients. An impaired blood supply is the usual cause of anastomotic failure at this level. The same principles of management which apply for necrosis of the conduit or anastomotic leakage with jejunal interposition are employed.

There are two late complications related to colon interposition. The first is anastomotic stricture, which is thought to develop in about 10% of patients in the cervical region and is probably a consequence of minor anastomotic leakage. The second relates to long-term swallowing ability, which can be problematic when the intrathoracic colon is redundant. This tends to present with minor symptoms such as fullness after eating or the sensation of hold-up with swallowing. In general, however, the long-term results in terms of meal capacity and swallowing ability indicate that colon is a durable conduit with a good functional outcome.

References

Adams, W. and Phemister, D. B. (1938) Carcinoma of the lower thoracic esophagus. Report of a successful resection and esophago-gastrostomy. *J. Thoracic Surg.*, **7**, 621

Allison, P. R. and DeSilva, L. T. (1953) The Roux loop. *Br. J. Surg.*, **41**, 173

Belsey, R. (1983) Reconstruction of the oesophagus. *Ann. R. Coll. Surg. Engl.*, **63**, 360

Belsey, R. H. R. *et al.* (1965) Reconstruction of the esophagus with left colon. *J. Thorac. Cardiovasc. Surg.*, **49**, 33

Borst, H. G. *et al.* (1978) Anastomotic leakage, stenosis and reflux after oesophageal replacement. *Wld J. Surg.*, **2**, 861

DeMeester, T. R. (1988) Indications, surgical technique and long-term functional results of colon interposition or bypass. *Ann. Surg.*, **208**, 460

Gavriliu, D. (1988) Replacement of the oesophagus by a gastric tube. In *Surgery of the Oesophagus* (ed. C. G. Jamieson), Churchill Livingstone, Edinburgh, p. 765

Hölscher, A. H. (1988) Function of the intra-thoracic stomach as esophageal replacement. *Wld J. Surg.*, **12**, 835

Katsaros, J. (1985) Monitoring free vascularized jejunum grafts. *Br. J. Plast. Surg.*, **38**, 220–222

Kelling, G. (1911) Oesophago-plastik mit hilfe des querkolon. *Zentbl. Chir.*, **38**, 1209

Kirschner, M. B. (1920) Ein neves verfahren der oesophagoplastik. *Arch. Klin. Chir.*, **144**, 606

Lewis, L. (1946) The surgical treatment of carcinoma of the oesophagus with special reference to a new operation for growths of the middle third. *Br. J. Surg.*, **34**, 18

McKeown, K. C. (1972) Trends in oesophageal resection for carcinoma, with special reference to total oesophagectomy. *Ann. R. Coll. Surg. Engl.*, **51**, 213

Ong, G. B. and Lee, T. C. (1960) Pharyngo-gastric anastomosis after oesophago-pharyngectomy for carcinoma of the hypopharynx and cervical oesophagus. *Br. J. Surg.*, **48**, 193

Orringer, M. B. (1988) Sub-sternal gastric bypass of the oesophagus. In *Surgery of the Oesophagus* (ed. C. G. Jamieson), Churchill Livingstone, Edinburgh, p. 739

Oshawa, R. (1933) Surgery of the oesophagus. *Jap. Chir.*, **10**, 604

Postlethwaite, R. W. (1988) Oesophageal bypass using the colon. In *Surgery of the Oesophagus* (ed. C. G. Jamieson), Churchill Livingstone, Edinburgh, p. 727

Reuther, J. F. (1984) Reconstruction of large defects in the oropharynx with a revascularized intestinal graft: an experimental and clinical report. *Plast. Reconstr. Surg.*, **73**, 345

Sasaki, T. M. (1980) Free jejunal graft reconstruction after extensive head and neck surgery. *Am. J. Surg.*, **139**, 650

Seidenberg, B. and Hurwith, A. J. (1959) Immediate reconstruction of the cervical oesophagus by a revascularized isolated jejunal segment. *Ann. Surg.*, **149**, 162

Vulliet, T. H. (1911) De'l oesophago-plastikie et des diverses modifications. *Sem. Méd.*, **31**, 529

11

Neuromuscular disorders of the oesophagus

G. Keen

The passage of food into the oesophagus depends on a well-coordinated oropharyngeal mechanism, and similarly the propulsion of food through the lower sphincter into the stomach is accomplished very satisfactorily if there is well-coordinated peristaltic activity. Disorders of motility and coordination of muscle contraction may affect the entrance of the oesophagus, the exit of the oesophagus, a localized segment or the whole of the oesophagus. The conditions to be discussed are:

1. Pharyngeal diverticulum.
2. Achalasia of the cardia.
3. Oesophageal diverticulum.
4. Diffuse spasm of the oesophagus.

Pharyngeal diverticulum

Surgical anatomy

This is a false diverticulum consisting of the thick mucosal layer of the oesophagus lined by stratified squamous epithelium but with no external muscle coat. It herniates through a weak point posteriorly, the Kilian–Jamison dehiscence, which is situated between the inferior pharyngeal constrictor muscle above and the cricopharyngeus muscle below (Figure 11.1). The cause of this condition is unknown but its occurrence in patients over the age of 50 years and rarely in younger people suggests that it is an acquired rather than a congenital condition. However, the constant site of origin of the diverticulum just between the cricopharyngeus muscle and the inferior constrictor pharynx suggests the possibility of an anatomical weak point in the muscular layers as well as some distal obstructive role of the cricopharyngeal sphincter.

The diverticulum is initially small and protrudes either to the left or to the right side, but with increase in size it becomes central. Because of the recurrent pressures involved, and the constant distension of the sac with food, there is rapid increase in size. Its neck overhangs the cricopharyngeus and the sac falls between the oesophagus and the vertebral column, compressing and deflecting the oesophagus anteriorly. Obstruction to swallowing follows and since the mouth of the diverticulum is above the cricopharyngeus, spontaneous emptying is often associated with aspiration into the bronchial tree in addition to regurgitation into the mouth. The chief complications are therefore nutritional and respiratory. Squamous-celled carcinoma may rarely develop within the diverticulum. This condition is premalignant for much the same reason as is achalasia of the cardia, which is the persistent exposure of the mucosa to stagnant food carcinogens.

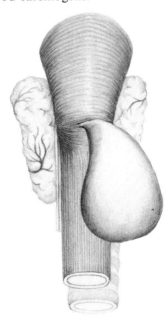

Figure 11.1 Surgical anatomy of pharyngeal diverticulum

Oesophagoscopy is dangerous in this condition. It is good practice that oesophagoscopy, with the rigid or flexible instrument, should never be undertaken without excellent barium studies showing the whole of the oesophagus including the cervical portion. Neglect of this advice is the cause of occasional perforation of the pharyngeal pouch, for the oesophagoscope will tend to enter the pouch rather than pass into the oesophagus. When a pouch is not suspected, perforation is then inevitable and will be followed by the most serious complications of continuing leakage into the mediastinum, and mediastinitis. This hazard may be reduced when the flexible fibreoptic instrument is used.

The operation

The two important and separate aims of operation

are attention to the pouch and division of the crico-pharyngeus muscle.

Position of the patient

The patient lies on his or her back with the head rotated to the right, the left arm by the side and a small pillow behind and between the shoulder blades. An incision 10 cm long in the line of the anterior border of the sternomastoid muscle, and with its centre at the level of the cricoid cartilage, is ideal for this operation (Figure 11.2). The platysma muscle is incised, as is the deep fascia. The sternomastoid muscle is then retracted posteriorly with the carotid sheath and internal jugular vein. The thyroid gland is retracted anteriorly together with the larynx, and with swab dissection the sac is identified. It should then be cleaned down to the muscular neck, and to facilitate this procedure the pouch may be grasped with light tissue forceps. Care should be taken not to mistake the thyroid gland for the pharyngeal diverticulum. With the sac cleaned, the decision is made whether or not to excise it. Small pouches may be left undisturbed. Large pouches require excision and those of a size between these two extremes may be suspended (Figure 11.3).

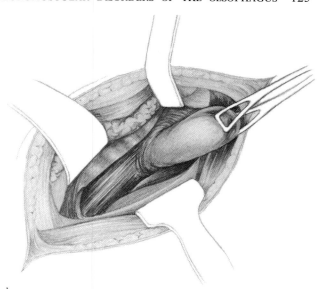

Figure 11.3 Mobilization and cleaning of pharyngeal diverticulum. The transverse and constricting muscle distal to the diverticulum is well shown

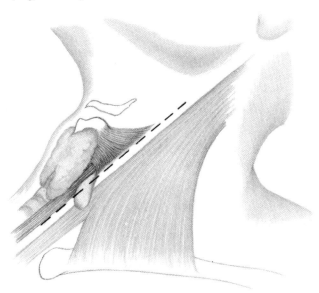

Figure 11.2 Operative approach for excision of pharyngeal diverticulum

Excision of the sac

It is wise at this stage for the anaesthetist to introduce a no. 30 Fr. gauge gum elastic or plastic bougie into the oesophagus to avoid surgical narrowing at this level, and when the bougie is in place the sac is excised. This may be undertaken either as an open procedure or over a vascular clamp, but in any event the sac must not be excised so enthusiastically that

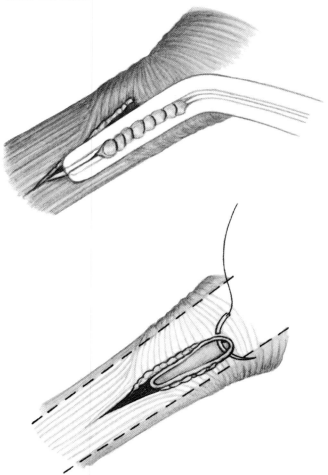

Figure 11.4 Pharyngeal diverticulum. Closure of the mouth of the excised diverticulum may be undertaken with or without an occluding clamp, but it is important that this closure is undertaken over a large intra-oesophageal bougie to prevent narrowing

closure can be completed only by narrowing the oesophagus. Closure is undertaken using fine interrupted catgut sutures to the mucosa with a further row of fine interrupted Mersilene sutures to the muscle (Figure 11.4).

Closure is also most elegantly and safely achieved by using the stapler.

Diverticulopexy

Moderate-sized pouches need not be excised, for if cricopharyngeal myomotomy is adequately undertaken the suspended pouch will drain well. The dissected pouch is drawn up posteriorly to the pharynx and tacked by a series of interrupted fine sutures to the prevertebral fascia (Figure 11.5).

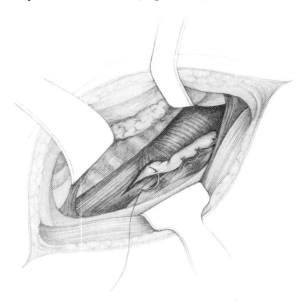

Figure 11.5 Small pharyngeal diverticula may be sutured to the prevertebral fascia

Cricopharyngeal myomotomy

This is probably the most important part of the operation and for many patients pharyngeal diverticulectomy is unnecessary. Certainly no matter how thoroughly the pouch is removed, failure to deal with the cricopharyngeus muscle will result either in early postoperative fistula formation or in late recurrence of the pouch, together with its symptoms. A curved artery forceps is gently insinuated between the oesophageal mucosa and the cricopharyngeus muscle and passed slowly distally, opening and closing the instrument carefully (Figure 11.6). The muscle readily separates from the underlying mucosa and is then cut with scissors (Figure 11.7). It is advisable to cut this muscle for a length of at least 2 cm to ensure a satisfactory result. The platysma and skin are closed and a soft corrugated drain is passed down to the site of operation.

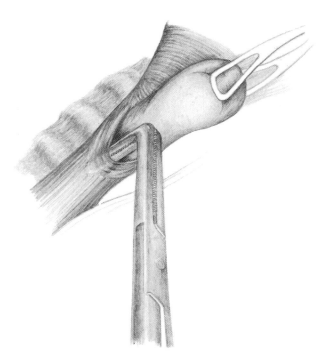

Figure 11.6 Pharyngeal diverticulum. Cricopharyngeal myomotomy

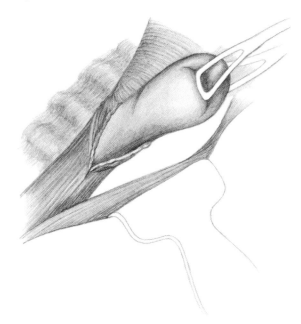

Figure 11.7 Cricopharyngeal myomotomy completed

Postoperative management

The patient is allowed fluids in small amounts on the 1st and 2nd postoperative days, progressing to soft foods from the 3rd day onwards. A normal diet is resumed by the 7th day.

Complications

A combination of inadequate suture of the neck of the pouch and inadequate attention to the cricopharyngeus muscle is the cause of fistula formation. Although these salivary fistulas rarely cause mediastinitis, and tend to close spontaneously, this complication may be attended by the later recurrence of symptoms and of the pouch. Should the fistula fail to close, it is likely that the distal spastic obstruction of the cricopharyngeus muscle will need attention. In the presence of induration and sepsis, approaching the cricopharyngeus muscle from the contralateral side should be considered.

Other operations have been practised for this condition, one of which, the peroral diathermy excision of the septum or common wall between the diverticulum and oesophagus, was popular among some surgical groups. The effect of this procedure is to divide the cricopharyngeus muscle posteriorly, but of course this does not deal with the sac, which if large and dependent will continue to compress the oesophagus. This procedure appears to have no advantage over the operation described above and certainly is not free of the risks of cervical cellulitis, mediastinitis and recurrence. It is not recommended and is considered obsolete.

Achalasia of the cardia

This disease is characterized by (a) poor or absent oesophageal peristalsis and (b) failure of relaxation of the lower end of the oesophagus.

Thus it is that any operation is usually palliative, for the disorder of motility cannot be overcome by surgery. Furthermore, the liability of up to 10% of these patients to carcinoma of the oesophagus, whether or not the achalasia is surgically treated, invites both careful operation and close long-term follow-up.

Preoperative investigations

Barium swallow

The oesophagus may be almost normal in size or gigantic with a large sigmoid loop at the lower end, and between these two extremes there are many variations. The poor motility of the oesophagus associated with tertiary contractions and failure of relaxation of the lower end of the oesophagus with delayed emptying are characteristic of the condition. Certain drugs such as octyl nitrite and Buscopan (hyoscine butylbromide) will relax the lower end of the oesophagus in this condition, and if administered during the course of radiological study will demonstrate relaxation and emptying, confirming the diagnosis.

Oesophagoscopy

This is a most important investigation and should be conducted with great care. The oesophagus in this condition often contains a good deal of fluid and decomposing food material which may be readily aspirated into the lungs during the induction of general anaesthesia for oesophagoscopy. For this reason it may be advisable to undertake oesophagoscopy under local anaesthesia supplemented by intravenous diazepam while the patient reclines in a dental chair. Aspiration of oesophageal contents should be conducted using a wide-bore suction catheter, many of the larger food particles requiring removal with biopsy forceps. It requires considerable patience to clear the oesophagus adequately, but this is essential to obtain a good view of the whole of the interior of the oesophagus. Failure to do so and thus obtain excellent visualization of the whole of the interior of the organ will possibly allow a carcinoma to be overlooked. It is indefensible to undertake an operation for achalasia of the cardia in the presence of an undiagnosed carcinoma of the oesophagus.

Oesophageal lavage during oesophagoscopy, if attempted at all, should be undertaken with very great care, for it is only too easy for fluid and decomposing food to find their way into the air passages.

Treatment

Regular dilatation by self-bouginage is mentioned only to be discarded as a modern treatment. This method was introduced early in this century when operative treatment was either not available or was extremely dangerous, and it would be difficult nowadays to select the patient able to undertake self-bouginage who was otherwise unfit for corrective surgery. Regular dilatation at oesophagoscopy is of such limited benefit that it is not recommended, and furthermore it is in these patients that the risk of eventual perforation of the oesophagus during dilatation is unacceptably high.

Treatment with the hydrostatic bag

The treatment of achalasia by rupture of the constricting muscular fibres, using Negus' modification of Tucker's bag, has in the past been used with varying degrees of success. In some hands, nearly two-thirds of the patients treated with a hydrostatic dilator have been reported to have good to excellent results over an average follow-up period of about 10 years. Although few deaths have been reported, there is good evidence that the complication rate is extremely high, and many patients have required surgical intervention because of inadvertent rupture of the distal oesophagus. While clearly a valuable form of treatment in some hands, this method is not without serious risk, and usually must be repeated to be effective. Hydrostatic dilatation was introduced as the natural successor to regular bouginage by the patient, and preceded the development of the safe, modern operation. With surgical procedures carrying minimal risk, forcible dilatation using the hydrostatic bag can no longer be seriously recommended as a method of treatment, although no doubt specialists in their use will continue to use these instruments for some time to come.

Operative treatment

Many historic operations to relieve achalasia have been described, which usually involved destruction of the lower oesophageal sphincter with disastrous results. Although initially successful in relieving dysphagia, these procedures were often complicated by the development of severe reflux oesophagitis, and further dysphagia from this cause. For this reason, apart from the operation described by Heller (1913), the majority of these procedures have been abandoned. Von Mikulicz, in 1904, described four patients in whom he had dilated the cardiac sphincter and lower 5 cm of the oesophagus by introducing his hand into the stomach and then inserting the fingers into the oesophagus, gradually dilating it until the sphincter was ruptured. After dilatation, the stomach was closed. This became a popular operation in the first quarter of the present century but it is open to many obvious criticisms, the main complication, frequently fatal, being rupture of the lower end of the oesophagus followed by mediastinitis or peritonitis. Furthermore, digital dilatation failed to relieve the obstruction in over 25% of the cases thus treated. It seems unlikely that this operation is practised today.

Oesophagogastrostomy, undertaken by side-to-side anastomosis between the dilated oesophagus and the fundus of the stomach, was also practised early in this century, but although dysphagia was readily relieved the resultant severe reflux oesophagitis proved such a serious drawback that this operation was also abandoned.

HELLER'S OPERATION (EXTRA MUCOUS OESOPHAGOCARDIOMYOMOTOMY)

This operation was first described in 1913 and Heller made two longitudinal incisions, an anterior and a posterior one, to ensure thorough division of all the constricting circular muscle fibres.

In 1923, Zaaiger modified this procedure, considering that an anteriorly placed incision through the coats of the oesophagus and stomach down to the mucous membrane was all that was needed to produce a cure.

Patients submitted to Heller's operation may be comparatively fit or in an extreme state of malnutrition and dehydration. Clearly this latter group of patients needs careful parenteral feeding and rehydration before an operation is contemplated, and in several instances of advanced wasting and dehydration the author has used preliminary feeding gastrostomy for several weeks to prepare the patient for operation.

The operation may be performed via the abdomen or using the transthoracic route. The transthoracic route has many advantages, not the least being the more ready access to the oesophagus and upper stomach, enabling the surgeon to undertake a more careful and complete oesophagomyomotomy. There is less likelihood of perforating the oesophageal mucosa via the thoracic approach than when using the more difficult exposure from the abdomen. Furthermore, the hiatus is more readily repaired following myomotomy from above than below.

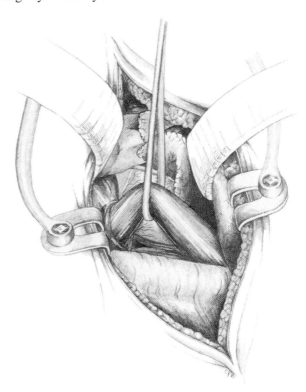

Figure 11.8   Mobilization of oesophagus in achalasia of the cardia

The right lateral position is used with the left chest uppermost. The skin incision is made along the line of the 7th rib and reaches almost to the costal margin. The chest is opened through the bed of the 7th rib and, following retraction of the lung forwards and the diaphragm downwards, the oesophagus is mobilized from the hiatus as high as the inferior pulmonary vein and encircled with a rubber catheter (Figure 11.8). Although the oesophagus in many patients looks remarkably normal, it is usual that distal to the oesophageal dilatation the organ is very narrowed and the muscle is very thickened. The aim of myomotomy is to incise both the longitudinal and circular muscles of the oesophagus along its lower 10 cm, completely dividing the hypertrophied musculature above the pathological constriction itself, allowing the mucosa to bulge freely through the incision, and it is important to avoid perforation of the mucosa (Figure 11.9). It was formerly routine practice to divide the muscle over the upper 2 or 3 cm of the stomach in addition to dividing the oesophageal muscle, with a resulting 8–10 cm length of oesophageal and gastric mucosa, pouting through the incision. More recently, however, it is held that dividing the gastric muscle is both unnecessary and illogical, for there seems to be no reason for the gastric muscle to hypertrophy and there is also no evidence that the neuromuscular incoordination involves gastric muscle. The mobilization of the hiatus and the disruption of the phreno-oesophageal ligament made necessary by such an extended myotomy may in some patients produce gastro-oesophageal reflux.

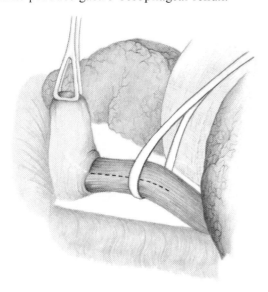

Figure 11.9 Achalasia of the cardia, oesophageal incision. It is not considered necessary to continue this incision over the stomach; the constricting element terminates at the cardia

It is fortunate that the muscle layers of the oesophagus are separated from the submucous layer by a well-defined space which is amenable to blunt dissection and separation. The oesophagus is supported by the index finger and an incision is made longitudinally into the oesophageal mucosa using a scalpel or blunt-ended scissors until the oesophageal mucosa pouts into view. Either side of the mucosa, the muscle is then gently grasped using tissue forceps. A right-angled vascular clamp is then insinuated distally between the muscle layers and the mucosa, gently opening and closing the instrument, and when the muscle is readily separated from the mucosa it is then incised (Figure 11.10). The instrument is again introduced and the procedure repeated down to the cardia.

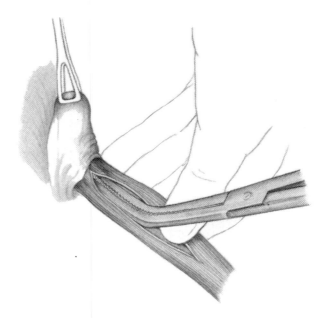

Figure 11.10 Achalasia of the cardia. Blunt dissection separating the two muscle layers from the mucosa prior to extramucous oesophagomyomotomy

Although the muscle is readily separated from the mucosa of the oesophagus, it unfortunately becomes much more adherent at the cardia and over the stomach, and great care is required for it is in this situation that perforation of the mucous membrane is liable to occur. While dividing the muscle, numerous small blood vessels in the muscular and submucous venous plexus will be divided and these will produce a certain amount of bleeding. The majority of this will cease with patient pressure using a swab, although some of these vessels may require ligation. Diathermy should be avoided in this area, lest the mucosa is inadvertently coagulated with the danger of later necrosis and fistula formation.

Following the completed myotomy the site of operation should be very carefully inspected for residual undivided constricting circular fibres, for if overlooked these will eventually hypertrophy and cause further symptoms and recurrence of the condition (Figure 11.11). Accidental perforation of the mucosa of the stomach or the oesophagus during this operation is a serious mishap. The mucosa is of the consistency of thin parchment and perforations are extremely difficult to repair using even the finest suture material. Nevertheless, attempts must be made to close these perforations. In the unhappy event of a small perforation becoming considerably larger during an attempt at closure, the consequences must be assessed realistically, for clearly the fistula cannot be left to heal of its own accord. Resuture of the muscle layer over the perforation would, of course, vitiate the operation. In these circumstances it might be necessary to consider oesophagogastrectomy with

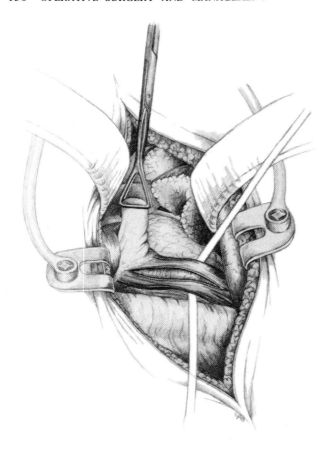

Figure 11.11 Achalasia of the cardia. The bulging mucosa protrudes through the completed myomotomy

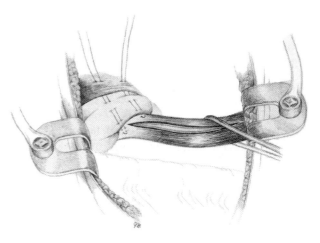

Figure 11.12 Achalasia of the cardia. Should the hiatus be disturbed during this operation, repair of the hiatus should be undertaken

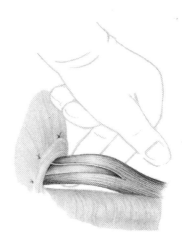

Figure 11.13 Completed Heller's operation showing reduction and repair of cardia

oesophagogastric anastomosis at the level of the aortic arch, or short-segment colon replacement.

During myomotomy it is possible that associated manipulations at the cardia may result in the patient developing symptoms of gastro-oesophageal reflux with possible oesophagitis and stricture formation. Since it is impossible to predict which patients will develop gastro-oesophageal reflux following Heller's operation, it is the practice of some surgeons to perform an anti-reflux manoeuvre following the myomotomy (Figures 11.12 and 11.13).

Complications. The important immediate complication, that of fistula formation, should be avoided if perforations of the mucosa are noted and dealt with at the time of operation. Should a fistula develop postoperatively, the safest method of dealing with this is to undertake immediate oesophagogastrectomy.

Late dysphagia. Dysphagia may recur from immediately postoperatively to more than 20 years following Heller's operation, and is due to one of three causes:

1. *Failure to relieve achalasia.* This is caused by the persistence of a few circular fibres that were not divided at the original operation. These few fibres

hypertrophy over the years and will produce early or late recurrence. The diagnosis is made at barium meal examination when the typical appearance of achalasia of the cardia is again seen. The treatment of the condition is a further myomotomy, where the offending fibres are identified and divided.

2. *Peptic stricture due to reflux oesophagitis.* The occurrence of late dysphagia due to peptic stricture of the oesophagus was more commonly noted in the past, following Heller's operation, than it is now that the operation is associated with an anti-reflux operation. These strictures are usually unresponsive to dilatation and often require surgical treatment, usually oesophagogastrectomy or colon interposition.

3. *Carcinoma of the oesophagus.* Achalasia of the cardia is a premalignant condition. It is presum-

ably due to the prolonged overexposure of the oesophageal mucosa to carcinogenic agents in food, which remain in the oesophagus with slow transit time. The development of dysphagia due to carcinoma of the oesophagus associated with achalasia of the cardia, either before myomotomy or after operation, is of very serious significance. These patients are accustomed to dysphagia and do not complain until the dysphagia is almost complete. In view of the large oesophagus, the carcinoma will have grown to a very large size before dysphagia is an important symptom, and it is almost invariably found that once diagnosed these tumours are inoperable.

Surgical management of very advanced achalasia of the cardia

When the oesophagus is very dilated and the lower end is a sigmoid sump, it is clear that Heller's operation is unlikely to drain the oesophagus adequately. In these patients consideration should be given to the operation of oesophagogastrectomy, excising the lower third of the oesophagus and the upper two-thirds of the stomach, and anastomosing the stomach to the oesophagus at the level of the aortic arch. An alternative procedure is to resect the oesophagus and to perform retrosternal gastric replacement with neck anastomosis.

Abdominal approach to achalasia of the cardia

Although the author considers the thoracic approach a superior and safer approach for the performance of Heller's operation, some gastroenterological surgeons continue to favour the abdominal approach.

Through a left upper paramedian incision or a midline incision above the umbilicus, the cardia and lower oesophagus may be readily identified, although excellent retraction and good relaxation anaesthesia are necessary. The left triangular ligament of the liver is divided, following which the peritoneum over the intra-abdominal oesophagus is incised, enabling a tape to be passed round the lower oesophagus. Using blunt and sharp dissection the lower 5–8 cm of the oesophagus can then be drawn into the abdomen. Care is taken to avoid damaging the anterior or left vagus nerve, and the procedure for extramucous oesophagogastric myotomy is identical to that when using the thoracic approach. In view of the difficulty of access via the abdomen, it is important to ensure that the oesophageal mucosa has not been perforated during this procedure and it is advisable to undertake an anti-reflux operation.

Oesophageal diverticulum

False diverticula may occur anywhere in the oesophagus and give rise to a variety of symptoms, including dysphagia, haematemesis and retrosternal pain. These diverticula are often associated with hypermotility of the oesophagus, the diverticulum being as it were a mucosal blow-out above a spastic area of musculature.

Surgical treatment

It is dangerous to excise the diverticulum without attention to the spastic muscle at its neck, and such diverticula should be treated similarly to pharyngeal diverticula. The small diverticulum need not be excised, the operation being limited to an extensive extramucous oesophagomyomotomy below the diverticulum (Figure 11.14). However, some of these diverticula are extremely large, reaching down almost to the diaphragm – so called 'epiphrenic diverticula' – and in these patients excision is inevitable. Nevertheless, very great care must be taken in closing the neck of the diverticulum and ensuring an adequate oesophagomyomotomy distally, for in the presence of residual obstruction the suture line will possibly give way with most serious consequences.

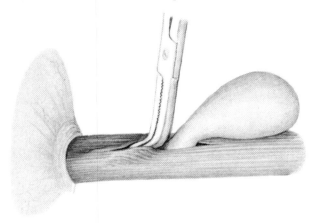

Figure 11.14 Oesophageal diverticulum. Extramucous separation of oesophageal muscle

Diffuse spasm of the oesophagus

Hypermotility of the oesophagus or diffuse oesophageal spasm is often associated with hypertension of the lower oesophageal sphincter, and this condition may be associated with oesophageal diverticula. In these patients, oesophageal motility studies demonstrate high-amplitude non-peristaltic contractions of the body of the oesophagus in response to swallowing, and pressures at the lower sphincter may be normal or elevated. The condition does not appear to be related to achalasia of the cardia. Pain is a more prominent symptom than is dysphagia, being typically substernal and often radiating through to the back, the neck or even into the arms, suggesting

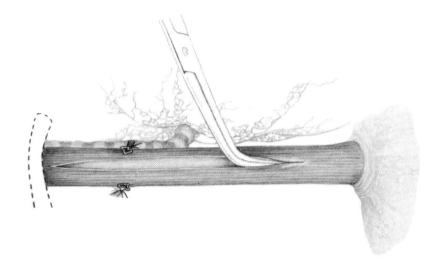

Figure 11.15 Diffuse oesophageal spasm. Extensive extramucous oesophagomyomotomy

angina pectoris. The pain may be spontaneous or produced by eating. Oesophageal radiography will usually show advanced spasm of the whole oesophagus, the so-called 'corkscrew' oesophagus. In selected patients, extramucous oesophagomyomotomy of the whole oesophagus sometimes produces relief of symptoms, but the condition seems less amenable to good surgical relief than does achalasia of the cardia. Following myomotomy it may be wise to complete the operation with an anti-reflux procedure, as in the modified Heller's operation, to prevent gastro-oesophageal reflux and late stricture formation. Operation is best undertaken through the right side of the chest, when division of the azygos vein will expose the oesophagus from the thoracic inlet to the cardia (Figure 11.15).

It is important in patients with diffuse oesophageal spasm to ascertain that their symptoms are not due to the irritation caused by gastro-oesophageal reflux, for in these patients repair of the hiatus hernia should cure the oesophageal symptoms.

References

Heller, E. (1913) Extramuköse Cardioplastic beim chronischen Cardiospasmus mit Dilatation des Oesophagus. *Mitt. Grenzgeb. Med. Chir.*, **27**, 141–149.

von Mikulicz, J. (1904) *Dtsch. Med. Wochenschr.* Jan–Feb.

Further reading

Belsey, R. (1966) Functional disease of the oesophagus. *J. Thorac. Cardiovasc. Surg.*, **52**, 164–188

Browne, D. C. and McHardy, G. (1939) A new instrument for use in oesophagospasm. *JAMA*, **113**, 1963–1964

Castell, D. O. (1976) Achalasia and diffuse esophageal spasm *Archs. Intern. Med.*, **136**, 571–579

Cohen, S. (1987) Esophageal motility disorders and their response to calcium channel antagonists. *Gastroenterology*, **93**, 301–303

DeMeester, T. R., Wang, C. I., Wernly, J. A., Pellegrini, C. A. *et al.* (1980) Technique, indications and clinical use of 24 hour esophageal pH monitoring. *J. Thorac. Cardiovasc. Surg.*, **79**, 656–667

Dohlman, G. and Mattsson, O. (1959). The role of the cricopharyngeal muscle in cases of hypopharyngeal diverticula: a cineroentgenographic study. *Am. J. Roentgenol Rad. Ther. Nucl. Med.*, **81**, 561–569

Ellis, F. H., Jr, Code, C. F. and Olsen, A. M. (1960) Long oesophagomyotomy for diffuse spasm of oesophagus and hypertensive gastroesophageal sphincter. *Surgery*, **48**, 155–168

Ellis, F. H., Jr, and Olsen, A. M. (1969) Achalasia of the oesophagus: major problems. In *Clinics in Surgery*, Vol. 9, Saunders, Philadelphia, p. 221

Ellis, F. H., Jr, Schlegal, J. F., Lynch, V. P. *et al.* (1969) Cricopharyngeal myotomy for pharyngo-oesophageal diverticulum. *Ann. Surg.*, **170**, 340–349

Kurlander, D. T., Raskin, H. F., Kirsner, J. B. *et al.* (1963) Therapeutic value of the pneumatic dilator in achalasia of the oesophagus: long term results in 62 living patients. *Gastroenterology*, **45**, 604–613

Moersch, H. J. and Camp, J. D. (1934) Diffuse spasm of the lower part of the oesophagus. *Ann. Otol. Rhinol. Laryngol.*, **43**, 1165–1173

Negus, V. E. (1950) Pharyngeal diverticula: observations on their evolution and treatment. *Br. J. Surg.*, **38**, 129–146

Payne, W. S. and Clagett, O. T. (1965) Pharyngeal and oesophageal diverticula. *Curr. Probl. Surg.*, April, 1–31

Payne, W. S., Ellis, F. H., Jr and Olsen, A. M. (1960) Achalasia of the oesophagus: a follow-up study of patients undergoing oesophagomyotomy. *Arch. Surg.*, **81**, 411–417

Payne, W. S., Ellis, F. H. Jr and Olsen, A. M. (1961) Treatment of cardiospasm (achalasia of the oesophagus) in children. *Surgery*, **50**, 731–735

Vantrappen, G. and Hellemans, J. (1976) Diffuse muscle spasm of the oesophagus and the hypertensive lower oesophageal sphincter. *Clin. Gastroenterol.*, **5**, 59–72

Vantrappen, G., Janssens, J., Hellemans, J. and Coremans, G. (1979) Achalasia, diffuse esophageal spasm, and related motility disorders. *Gastroenterology*, **76**, 450–457

Vinson, P. P. (1934) Diverticula of the thoracic portion of the oesophagus: report of 42 cases. *Arch. Otolaryngol.*, **19**, 508–513

Wychulis, A. R., Gunnlaugsson, G. H. and Clagett, O. T. (1969) Carcinoma occurring in pharyngoesophageal diverticulum: report of three cases. *Surgery*, **66**, 976–979

12

Peptic ulcer: resection procedures and highly selective vagotomy

P. W. J. Houghton

Introduction

The incidence of peptic ulcer disease is continuing to fall (Langman, 1988) along with the number of operations carried out for the disease. With the introduction of the H_2 antagonists and more recently the H^+-K^+-ATPase blocking agent (Omeprazole), acid secretion can now be much better medically controlled. Further advances, with the increasing understanding of the role of *Helicobacter pylori*, also allow the disease to be treated with antibacterial triple therapy regimens (Moss and Calam, 1992).

Although failure of medical treatment is still an indication for surgery, by far the majority of operations now carried out are for the complications of peptic ulcer disease. There is evidence to suggest that although the incidence of perforation and bleeding has also declined, this appears to be limited to the younger age group. In the elderly, there has been an increase in the mortality of these complications and this is almost certainly due to the widespread prescription of non-steroidal anti-inflammatory drugs (NSAIDs) (Langman, 1988).

The other major change which has occurred in the past few years is the introduction of laparoscopic surgery for peptic ulcer disease. This is a rapidly advancing field and at the present time operations have been carried out both in experimental animals (Voeller *et al.*, 1991) and in humans (Mouret *et al.*, 1990). This is an area which will become increasingly important in the future, but despite this there will still be a need for the surgeon to remain familiar with the operations to be discussed in this chapter.

Gastric ulcer

Gastric ulcers are strongly related to the presence of gastritis (Gear *et al.*, 1971), which may be caused by *H. pylori* infection, NSAIDs or pyloric reflux in different patients. Aetiological theories of gastric ulceration currently focus on damage to the mucous layer and changes in the gastric mucosal hydrophobicity (Spychal *et al.*, 1990) which might be caused by the organism itself or by the inflammation that it produces (Younan *et al.*, 1982; Sidebotham and Baron, 1990).

Approximately 85% of chronic gastric ulcers are found on or close to the lesser curve, the great majority being closer to the incisura angularis than the cardia: 12% are found in the antrum, 2% of these in the pyloric canal. Only 3% of chronic gastric ulcers are found at the cardia. The greater curvature of the stomach, fundus and anterior and posterior walls are the site of only 5% of benign gastric ulcers.

Diagnosis

Diagnosis of a gastric ulcer will depend on a complete medical history, clinical examination and upper gastrointestinal tract endoscopy. All patients with a suspected gastric ulcer should be endoscoped and the ulcer should be biopsied, preferably at four sites at least, to exclude malignancy.

Indications for operation

1. Relative

(a) Failure of medical treatment.
(b) Recurrent gastric ulceration.
(c) Combined gastric and duodenal ulceration.
(d) Haemorrhage.

Having established that the gastric ulcer is benign, the patient will initially be treated medically and most ulcers will heal. There is no universal agreement on how many times a patient with a recurrence of gastric ulcer should be treated medically before being submitted to surgery.

2. Absolute

(a) Perforation.
(b) Suspicion of malignancy which cannot be excluded by endoscopy and biopsy.
(c) Anatomical organic deformity of the stomach owing to stenosing ulceration.

These complications and their management are discussed later in the chapter.

Preoperative management of gastric surgery patients

General

A full medical history and clinical examination are necessary to exclude disease in other systems. Elderly patients should have a full cardiovascular assessment with a baseline preoperative ECG. Chest X-ray, full blood count, urea and electrolytes are also useful information prior to embarking on major surgery. If there is any history of liver disease or abnormal bleeding tendencies, in addition to the full blood count, a platelet count, prothrombin time and liver function tests should be performed. Sputum retention is common after upper abdominal surgery and post-operative physiotherapy is required in most patients, especially those who are smokers.

Specific measures

Gastric operations are associated with a high incidence of wound sepsis which is related to the underlying pathology. Most infections occurring after gastrointestinal surgery are caused by dissemination of organisms present in the lumen of the gastrointestinal tract at the time of operation (Gatehouse *et al.*, 1978). Prophylactic antibiotics should be used in all cases; a cephalosporin and metronidazole are a good combination. Depending on the contamination, this should be either as a single dose or three doses in a heavily contaminated case. The antibiotics should be given with the induction of anaesthesia. Low-dose subcutaneous heparin (5000 u 12-hourly) should be used as prophylaxis against deep venous thrombosis and pulmonary embolus in patients over 50 years of age and in the obese. The first dose is given preoperatively and is continued until the patient is ambulatory. In high-risk patients, such as those with previous deep vein thrombosis, compression stockings should also be used.

Incision and exposure in gastric surgery

The patient is placed in the supine position with the table tilted so that the head is slightly raised. A vertical upper abdominal midline incision is used, and the incision should be made from the xiphisternum to the umbilicus. This incision is excellent for virtually all gastric surgery. Transverse or oblique incisions do not allow adequate exposure near the oesophageal hiatus in all patients. The midline incision is superior to the paramedian incision, first with regard to speed of entry which may be important, e.g. in cases of haemorrhage, and, secondly, closure of the abdomen is more secure as there is one good, firm fibrous layer for stitching as opposed to two rather flimsy fascial layers. The midline incision also gives a better cosmetic appearance.

Having opened the abdomen, a retractor may be inserted to aid the initial careful laparotomy which must be carried out before starting any intra-abdominal procedure. Having confirmed the presence of the peptic ulcer, some surgeons favour the insertion of a self-retaining retractor.

Choice of operation for benign gastric ulcer

1. Billroth-I gastrectomy or Polya gastrectomy.
2. Truncal vagotomy and drainage plus biopsy or resection of the ulcer.

3. Highly selective vagotomy plus biopsy or resection of the ulcer.

Partial gastrectomy was for many years the most commonly performed operation for benign gastric ulcer. It had the advantage of removing at the same time the ulcer, the pylorus and the antrum. Thus the pathological lesion plus all the susceptible mucosa, as well as the site of the most favoured aetiological factors, are eliminated. Unfortunately, while this procedure has the advantage of giving a very low incidence of recurrent disease, the disadvantages are the mortality attached to a major procedure, and the problems associated with rapid gastric emptying. After gastric resection for gastric ulcer, the gastric remnant may be anastomosed to the duodenum or the jejunum. With a lesser curve gastric ulcer, the gastric remnant can with safety be anastomosed to the duodenum. With a pre-pyloric ulcer or a combined gastric and duodenal ulcer, the acid secretion is often too high and it is important to use a gastrojejunal anastomosis because the Billroth-I gastrectomy would be associated with a high incidence of recurrent ulceration. In general, it may be said that approximately 70% of gastric ulcers may be resected with a Billroth-I gastrectomy, in some cases coupled with a Pauchet manoeuvre.

Vagotomy is now used increasingly in the treatment of gastric ulcer, but until recently the results have been somewhat inferior to those of partial gastrectomy. The recurrence rate of gastric ulceration after vagotomy and pyloroplasty alone has been 5–13% and is similar after highly selective vagotomy. For this reason, in most centres partial gastrectomy has held pride of place in treatment with recurrence rates of 0–5%. There are, however, as previously mentioned, other post-gastrectomy symptoms occurring after Billroth-I procedures, although fewer than after gastrojejunostomy (Polya) anastomosis. Many of the postprandial symptoms are attributed to lack of control of gastric emptying. The operative mortality of partial gastrectomy may be low in specialized units, but the accepted world mortality is of the order of 2% and may reach 4–5%. In contrast, the mortality of vagotomy is about 1% and is even lower after HSV (0.3%) (Johnston, 1975). Vagotomy may be preferred to gastrectomy in selected patients with gastric ulcer, namely poor-risk patients, some patients with an ulcer high on the lesser curve in whom gastrectomy would be difficult and hazardous, and in many patients with a bleeding gastric ulcer. If vagotomy is used, multiple biopsies should be taken or the ulcer excised completely to establish that it is benign.

Operative technique
1. Billroth-I gastrectomy

If the site of the gastric ulcer is not obvious and difficult to locate by palpation, a small suture may be placed into the serosal surface of the stomach over its superior border so that the mobilization can be performed without constant reference back to the site of the ulcer by palpation. If, however, the ulcer is adherent to the liver or pancreas, and is pinched off, this may leave a hole in the stomach which can be temporarily closed with a few stitches. The granulating base of the ulcer is left alone.

The stomach is initially mobilized at the greater curve by making an opening through an avascular area of the gastrocolic omentum. This hole is enlarged laterally in both directions by clamping, dividing and ligating the gastrocolic omentum on the colic side of the gastro-epiploic arch (Figure 12.1).

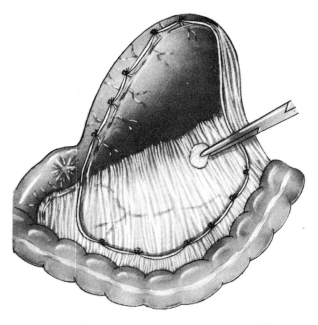

Figure 12.1   Billroth-I partial gastrectomy. Initial mobilization of greater curvature of the stomach with preservation of the gastro-epiploic arch

The transverse mesocolon is very closely applied to the back of the stomach and it is very easy to damage the middle colic artery unless the mesocolon is identified and pushed downwards away from the site of dissection as soon as the initial hole in the gastrocolic omentum is made. To the right, the dissection is taken to the inferior border of the pylorus, the main right gastro-epiploic vessels being ligated in this region. To the left, the site of resection on the greater curve of the stomach is estimated and the vessels are divided up to this level. For 2 cm above and below this position the vessels are individually ligated on the greater curve of the stomach as opposed to outside the gastro-epiploic arch. The right gastric vessels are then identified on the superior border of the duodenum running to the left in the free edge of the lesser omentum and are divided between artery forceps and ligated.

The filamentous lesser omentum is divided proximally, feeling for and preserving an accessory hepatic

artery if it is present. The lesser curve is then cleared over a 1 cm length, 2 cm proximal to the upper edge of the ulcer. This necessitates dividing the descending branches of the left gastric artery and its accompanying veins, plus the nerve of Latarjet. This is best done by inserting a pair of blunt dissecting forceps through the lesser omentum directly onto the wall of the stomach. The tissue is then divided between double ties placed with the aid of an aneurysm needle. The duodenum may now be divided just distal to the pylorus. A Payr clamp may be used on the stomach and the duodenum may be held in a Lang–Stevenson or similar clamp. The pyloric end of the stomach is held and a further Payr clamp is applied at right angles to the greater curve approximately halfway along the greater curve. Prior to placing this clamp, the Ryle's tube, if present in the stomach, should be withdrawn into the fundus so that it will not be caught in the clamps. A Lang–Stevenson clamp is then applied parallel and just proximal to the Payr clamp. The stomach is divided halfway across between the clamps (Figure 12.2). A curved Parker–Kerr clamp is arranged to grasp the stomach from the tip of the Lang–Stevenson clamp and curving up to cross the lesser curve of the stomach about 1 cm above the ulcer. A second Parker–Kerr clamp is applied just distally and the stomach divided between these two clamps, thus removing the antrum and a piece of lesser curve, including the ulcer.

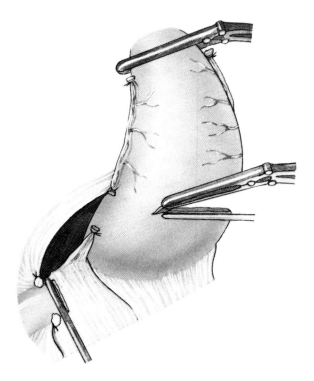

Figure 12.2   Billroth-I partial gastrectomy. Partial division of stomach between clamps, prior to application of Parker–Kerr clamps to reconstruct the 'lesser curve'

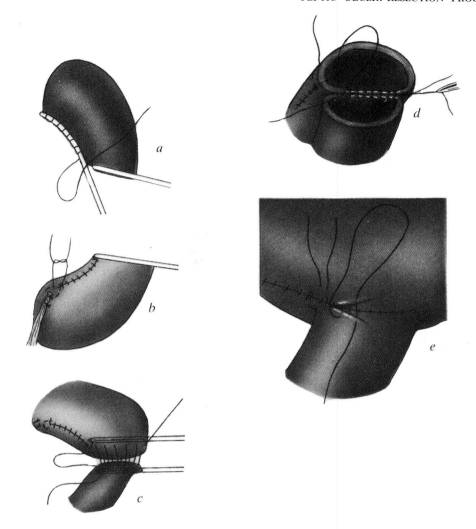

Figure 12.3 Billroth-I partial gastrectomy. *a*, The gastric remnant is held by a Lang–Stevenson clamp (across the segment for duodenal anastomosis) and a Parker–Kerr clamp (over the newly fashioned lesser curve). *b*, The newly formed lesser curve is closed with a final continuous seromuscular suture, taking particular care to invert fully at the proximal end. *c*, The stomach and duodenum are approximated and a continuous posterior seromuscular suture is inserted, beginning at the greater curve. *d*, The duodenal and gastric clamps are removed and a continuous all-layers suture is inserted posteriorly and carried anteriorly to complete the anastomosis. *e*, The completed operation to show careful inversion at the junction of lesser curve and duodenal closure

The new 'lesser curve' of stomach will be formed from the stomach in the Parker–Kerr clamp and this may be closed with an over-and-over 2/0 absorbable atraumatic suture. Catgut or one of the more modern absorbable sutures may be used. This suture is tightened as the clamp is released and withdrawn. The first layer of sutures may be invaginated by a second seromuscular 2/0 suture.

The distal part of the stomach included in the Lang–Stevenson clamp is then approximated to the duodenum held in a similar clamp. If there is any tension, the duodenum may be mobilized by a Kocher manoeuvre. This initial posterior seromuscular Lembert suture is of 2/0 absorbable material and is best inserted with the clamps held a few centimetres apart, starting from the greater curve and working up to the lesser curve side of the stomach, and then the suture is tightened (Figure 12.3c). The clamps are then removed. The posterior wall of the stomach and duodenum are then sutured with an all-layers 2/0 absorbable suture, again working from the greater to lesser curve aspect (Figure 12.3d). Great care is taken at the upper border where the other suture line is encountered. Good inversion is required and this may be best provided by one or two Connell sutures. The suture line is then completed across the anterior wall of the stomach and duodenum by an over-and-over inverting suture. The original posterior seromuscular suture is then completed across the front of the stomach and duodenum. An extra absorbable suture may help to support the critical angle and obviate any leak (Figure 12.3e).

On completion of the anastomosis a systematic check of the abdomen should be made, having checked that the anastomosis is patent. The spleen should be checked for damage, the omental ties should be dry and the colon should be a good colour if the middle colic artery has not been damaged.

Sometimes a benign ulcer may be encountered on the posterior wall of the stomach rather than on the lesser curve. The technique described above can still be performed by rotating the walls of the stomach so that the ulcer comes to lie at one edge. This edge is then held with a tissue forceps and the clamps are then applied from the other side in the manner already described and illustrated.

At the conclusion of the operation, a Ryle's tube is positioned in the stomach and the midline incision is closed in one layer with a continuous monofilament nylon suture, taking at least a 1 cm depth of tissue with 1 cm between the stitches (Jenkins, 1976; Pollock et al., 1979). The skin is closed with a continuous subcuticular absorbable or non-absorbable suture. No drain is necessary.

POSTOPERATIVE COMPLICATIONS

(a) Immediate. Haemorrhage may occur from faulty haemostasis at the suture line in the stomach and in particular from the region of the refashioned lesser curve. Fresh blood in variable quantities will be aspirated up the Ryle's tube.

When haemorrhage does occur from the gastric anastomosis it often stops spontaneously, and sedation of the patient coupled with some gentle gastric lavage may be all that is required. If the haemorrhage continues and the patient begins to show signs of decompensation despite blood transfusion, it may be necessary to take the patient back to theatre and to partially dismantle the anastomosis to find the bleeding point. Intraperitoneal haemorrhage may occur within the first 24 h from unidentified damage to the spleen or the slipping of an omental tie. Bleeding from a damaged spleen is occasionally attributed to injudicious retraction. The damage usually results from vigorous traction on the greater curve of the stomach and adjacent transverse colon, tearing one of the small omental adhesions from the lower pole of the spleen. Under these circumstances, further surgical intervention is required but splenorrhaphy rather than splenectomy should be attempted if possible (Cooper and Williamson, 1984).

(b) Delay in gastric emptying. There is always some postoperative oedema at the suture line and if the gastric mucosa is initially thickened there may be a delay in gastric emptying beyond the usual 3–4 days. Large quantities of bile-free gastric aspirate will be obtained. With patience, this problem will usually resolve and in the meantime the electrolyte content in the gastric aspirate should be estimated and the appropriate fluid given as an intravenous supplement. Failure to be able to take a normal diet after 5 days will require intravenous hyperalimentation. If a finger and thumb can be approximated across the stoma at the end of the operation, drainage will always eventually occur.

(c) Leakage from the suture line. This may occur after a few days and is usually from the critical angle, i.e. the junction of the lesser curve closure and the gastroduodenal anastomosis. The patient may suddenly complain of upper abdominal pain or alternatively the general condition may insidiously deteriorate with equivocal abdominal signs. A straight radiograph is usually not very helpful because free gas is always present at this stage, but a Gastrografin swallow may confirm the diagnosis. Reoperation is required with excision of the necrotic tissue and conversion to a gastrojejunal anastomosis with closure of the duodenal stump. This complication carries a high mortality, partly because of delay in diagnosis.

REMOTE COMPLICATIONS

(a) Recurrent ulceration. The incidence varies from 0% to 5% in various series. The diagnosis is made by endoscopy as barium studies after gastric surgery are difficult. Endoscopy allows multiple biopsies to be taken. If malignancy can be excluded and if the stoma is patent, recurrent gastric ulceration may be treated by truncal or selective vagotomy rather than by further gastric resection.

(b) Postgastrectomy syndromes. Following gastroduodenal anastomoses, the complications of dumping and bilious vomiting are rare. Diarrhoea, either continuous or episodic, also seems to be less frequent after a Billroth-I than after a Polya gastrectomy.

(c) Deficiency states. Many patients after gastric operations may develop deficiencies of iron, vitamin B_{12}, folic acid and other minerals and vitamins essential for bone development. Such deficiencies often develop insidiously and may not present as an obvious clinical syndrome for many years after the original operation. For this reason, these deficiency states may escape detection until the patient is severely disabled.

Minor degrees of iron deficiency are extremely common after any gastric surgery. The cause of the iron deficiency is probably not due to diminution of the oral intake of iron, but to a combination of impaired absorption and minimal increases in iron losses following gastric surgery. The majority of patients with chronic iron deficiency will respond to simple oral treatment with iron compounds. Instructions to take 3 tablets of iron 1 day a week on a regular basis will usually obviate the development of iron-deficient anaemia.

Examination of patients 5 years after partial gastrectomy for peptic ulcer shows that between 15% and 60% of patients have low serum levels of B_{12}. This is the result of impaired absorption of vitamin B_{12} due to decreased production of intrinsic factor associated with gastric mucosal atrophy. Post-gastrectomy vitamin B_{12} deficiency may be followed by all the complications associated with vitamin B_{12} deficiency from whatever cause.

Folate acid deficiency may also be found after major gastric resection and may be present in 6–12% of patients if serum folic acid levels are estimated. Clinical manifestations of folic acid deficiency will take longer to become manifest.

(d) Metabolic bone disease. The detection and assessment of metabolic bone disease after gastric operations are more difficult than the assessment of haematological abnormalities. The two major metabolic bone diseases that have been studied are osteomalacia and osteoporosis. Osteomalacia is due to vitamin D deficiency and is probably rare, but may occur if there is a poor oral intake of fat-containing foods or if there is malabsorption due to steatorrhoea. If present, extra-oral vitamin D may be given. Osteoporosis is more difficult to assess, but where it occurs after gastric operations it is probably due to deficiency of calcium and protein. It appears that bones age earlier in patients after partial gastrectomy.

(e) Malignant change. The majority of post-gastrectomy patients have an abnormal mucosa when seen endoscopically. Some of these patients develop a mild or moderate dysplasia when the mucosa is examined histologically and it would seem that a proportion of these progress to a malignant change (Clark *et al.*, 1985). The reflux of bile acids into the gastric remnant may be an aetiological factor (Houghton *et al.*, 1986).

2. Vagotomy and drainage and highly selective vagotomy

These operations have obvious attractions in older, more poorly nourished patients and results would appear similar to resection procedures. The technique of these operations is described later in this chapter. When using these operations for the treatment of gastric ulcer, either biopsy or excision of the gastric ulcer must be performed. Preoperative biopsy of the ulcer may be obtained endoscopically and multiple biopsies are required. The ulcer is best excised by opening the stomach opposite the ulcer and excising the ulcer from the mucosal aspect, the defect being closed with absorbable sutures. Alternatively, the ulcer-bearing area may be excised from the serosal aspect.

Duodenal ulcer

Helicobacter pylori was first cultured in 1983 (Warren and Marshall, 1983), and was later found to occur in about 90% of patients with duodenal ulcer disease (Dooley and Cohen, 1988). It is now thought that both acid/pepsin and *H. pylori* probably reduce mucosal resistance, but the bacteria may also directly attack the epithelium.

Approximately 75–80% of chronic peptic ulcers are found in the duodenum. More than 90% of chronic duodenal ulcers are found in the first portion of the duodenum. In one postmortem series (Portis and Jaffe, 1938), 85% were found within the first 2 cm of the duodenum, 10% were within the next 3 cm, and the remaining 5% were below the first 5 cm and above the ampulla of Vater. Of those ulcers occurring in the first part of the duodenum, 85% are found on the posterior wall or to have extended from the posterior wall, and may subsequently completely encircle the duodenum. Multiple duodenal ulcers are said to occur in 10% of cases and are usually seen on both anterior and posterior walls. Gastric and duodenal ulceration may occur in the same patient.

Diagnosis

Initially a full history must be taken from the patient, coupled with a complete physical examination. The investigation of choice is an upper gastrointestinal endoscopy. Laboratory investigations have become less important. Gastric analysis is rarely performed, but the serum gastrin assay may be useful in the diagnosis of hypergastrinaemia, e.g. the Zollinger–Ellison syndrome.

Indications for operation

1. Relative

(a) Failure of medical treatment.
(b) Haemorrhage.

2. Absolute

(a) Perforation.
(b) Pyloric stenosis.

These conditions and their management are discussed later in this chapter.

Choice of operations for duodenal ulcer

1. Polya gastrectomy.
2. Truncal vagotomy and drainage.
3. Highly selective vagotomy.

The aim of any operation for duodenal ulcer is to try to reduce the excessive acid secretion and to do this as safely as possible, with the minimum of disturbance of the other normal functions of the stomach and duodenum. Acid secretion may be reduced surgically by vagotomy which will abolish the nervous secretion and will also reduce the antral release of gastrin.

Alternatively, antrectomy will abolish gastrin-dependent acid production by the remaining parietal cells, but they will still respond to nervous stimulation. Partial gastrectomy, however, will remove the gastrin-producing antrum and a variable number of parietal cells, depending on the extent of the gastrectomy.

When partial gastrectomy is used in the treatment of duodenal ulcer, it should involve a gastrojejunal anastomosis, as gastroduodenal anastomosis is associated with a 15% stomal ulcer rate. The Polya type of gastrectomy is an effective treatment of duodenal ulcer. The mortality rate is, however, higher than with vagotomy and drainage and highly selective vagotomy, and there are other consequences following extensive gastric resection, although the stomal ulceration rate is low.

Truncal vagotomy may reduce gastric secretion by up to 70% of maximum secretion, and thus in many duodenal ulcer patients acid secretion may be reduced to normal levels. Following the pioneer work of Dragstedt in the early 1940s, the operation was introduced, but it was soon found that unless coupled with a drainage procedure gastric stasis with foul flatulence and vomiting became an incapacitating problem. This complication having been resolved, the operation of truncal vagotomy and drainage was found to be a safe procedure with a lower mortality (0.6%) than gastrectomy. However, the recurrent ulceration rate was higher. Goligher found that the rate was twice as high. Other figures have varied from 1% to 15%, and this may be due to an incomplete vagotomy.

Heineke–Mikulicz pyloroplasty is the commonest drainage procedure that is performed with truncal vagotomy. A pyloroplasty has the theoretical advantage of preserving the continuity of the duodenal loop and hence the integrity of the various hormonal systems which act on the food as it passes. Occasionally, however, the duodenum may be so scarred as to render a pyloroplasty difficult and dangerous and then a gastroenterostomy is preferable. Tanner preferred an anterior juxtapyloric gastroenterostomy, but the classic operation is a posterior gastroenterostomy to the most dependent part of the stomach.

Vagotomy combined with antrectomy is a popular operation in the USA because it gives the most complete control of acid secretion. The stomal ulcer rate is the lowest of all procedures. However, the addition of a gastric resection brings the mortality nearer to that of partial gastrectomy, while in the survivors the morbidity is the sum of that of gastric resection and that resulting from vagotomy.

In 1948, bilateral selective vagotomy was described by Jackson, of Ann Arbor, and by Franksson, of Stockholm (Jackson, 1948; Franksson, 1948). This was a more logical procedure than truncal vagotomy because it spared the hepatic and coeliac branches of the vagus which supplied the extragastric viscera. Nevertheless, the whole of the stomach is denervated and the propulsive power of the antral musculature is weakened, hence a drainage procedure is required to avoid gastric stasis. Attempts by Burge in the late 1960s to carry out selective vagotomy without drainage in selected cases failed and were abandoned in favour of highly selective vagotomy.

Prospective randomized trials of truncal and selective vagotomy have shown that the latter leads to significantly fewer incomplete vagotomies and is followed by significantly less diarrhoea. Nevertheless, the overall Visick grading of selective vagotomy has not been significantly better than truncal vagotomy (Kennedy, 1973). Highly selective vagotomy (HSV) or parietal cell vagotomy was introduced into clinical practice in 1970 by Johnston and Wilkinson of Leeds and by Amdrup and Jensen of Copenhagen (Johnston and Wilkinson, 1970; Amdrup and Jensen, 1970). In contrast to other operations for duodenal ulcer, the motor nerve supply to the antrum and pyloric sphincter are left intact by the preservation of the nerves of Latarjet and the pyloric branch of the vagus. Vagal denervation is confined to the acid-secreting part of the stomach, the parietal cell mass (PCM). The antral 'mill', pyloric sphincter and duodenum are left intact, so that gastric emptying is well controlled and reflux of bile into the stomach is minimized. Experience with HSV has shown that the incidence of recurrent ulceration averages about 8% (range 3% to 30%), which is the same incidence as after truncal vagotomy with a drainage procedure, while side-effects such as 'dumping', diarrhoea and bilious vomiting are significantly less common after HSV than after either truncal vagotomy and drainage or partial gastrectomy.

The vagal denervation of the liver and biliary tract, pancreas and small intestine in the course of truncal vagotomy and drainage did not have any logical basis, but was condoned in the past because it did not seem to do any harm. It is now known, however, that section of the hepatic vagal fibres causes the gallbladder to dilate, alters the chemical composition of the bile and leads to a significant increase in the incidence of gallstones in the human (Rudick and Hutchinson, 1964; Parkin et al., 1973; Csendes et al., 1978). Likewise, section of the coeliac vagal branch, as in posterior truncal vagotomy, significantly impairs enzyme output from the pancreas in the human (Malagelada et al., 1974; MacGregor et al., 1977; Lavigne et al., 1979). HSV is now the operation of choice for patients with chronic duodenal ulcer uncomplicated by pyloric stenosis. Very rarely, in an unfit patient, truncal vagotomy and drainage should be performed. There is at present no established basis for the addition of antrectomy to vagotomy in patients who are found to have gross hypersecretion of acid (>45 mmol HCl/h) at the preoperative pentagastrin test.

1. Polya gastrectomy

Although this operation is now rarely performed for

duodenal ulcer, it is described in detail as the technique forms the basis of the operation for resection of the distal half of the stomach for neoplasm.

The initial mobilization of the stomach is carried out in exactly the same way as for Billroth-I gastrectomy, namely that an opening is made through the gastrocolic omentum in the region of the midline. The posterior wall of the stomach is then identified. This is often adherent to the transverse mesocolon and the latter is separated by pushing it in a downward direction to the right and to the left of the midline, ensuring that the middle colic vessels will not be injured. The gastrocolic omentum is then clamped, divided and ligated in sections on the colic side of the gastro-epiploic arch. If tied in this area, fewer vessels need division and tying than if performed flush on the wall of the greater curve of the stomach. To the right, this dissection is taken round to the pylorus. The main gastro-epiploic vessels are tied on the inferior border of the pylorus. To the left, the dissection is taken up in the direction of the spleen. When 50% of the greater curve of the stomach has been mobilized, the left main gastro-epiploic vessels are divided and the dissection is then taken right up onto the wall of the greater curve of the stomach. One or two of the short gastric vessels are then divided, leaving a 3 cm length of the greater curve of the stomach clean and ready for subsequent resection.

Attention is then turned to the duodenum once again. The right gastric vessels which are usually small are identified and isolated and tied as they run to the left in the lesser omentum just above the duodenal bulb. The filamentous omentum is then divided proximally, ensuring by palpation that an accessory hepatic artery, if present, is preserved. The duodenum is then divided between clamps. The first Payr clamp is placed across the duodenum just distal to the pylorus. The second Payr clamp may be placed across the pylorus or, if the tissue is thickened, a non-crushing clamp may be applied across the distal stomach. The important point is to ensure that no gastric antral mucosa remains attached to the duodenum.

The duodenal stump may be held up by the Payr clamp and inspected to ensure that it is sufficiently mobile to facilitate easy closure. Frequently, small additional blood vessels need to be ligated on the posterior wall or on the superior and inferior borders of the duodenum. These are divided flush on the wall of the duodenum to avoid damage to adjacent structures, such as the common bile duct and the gastroduodenal artery. Closure of the duodenal stump may be further facilitated by performing a Kocher manoeuvre. The stump may be closed by an initial over-and-over suture including the clamp, using a 2/0 atraumatic absorbable suture (Figure 12.4). As the clamp is eased out, the suture is gradually tightened; the suture line is then buried by inserting a purse-string suture of 2/0 absorbable suture. If there is sufficient tissue, a second purse-string suture will

provide a secure three-layer closure. The more difficult duodenal closure is discussed at the end of this section.

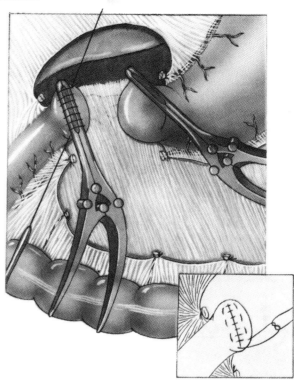

Figure 12.4 Polya partial gastrectomy. The duodenum has been divided between clamps and the first row of duodenal closure sutures has been placed over the clamp. (Insert shows purse-string seromuscular closure of the duodenal stump)

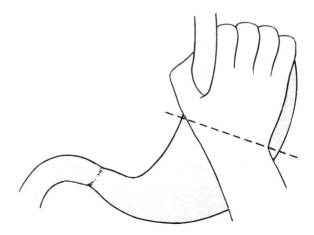

Figure 12.5 Polya partial gastrectomy. Author's technique for assessing size of gastric remnant

Modern stapling devices give excellent closure and may now be recommended for duodenal stump closure. The stomach is then inspected and the approximate level of resection is estimated. In the absence of pyloric or duodenal stenosis, a 60% resection of the stomach is necessary in duodenal ulcer and will be achieved by placing the right hand on the anterior wall of the stomach, curving the tips of the fingers over the fundus. A resection of the stomach at the level of the base of the thenar eminence of the thumb will give a reasonable gastric remnant (Figure 12.5). However, if the stomach is distended from preoperative obstruction and the same procedure is adopted, the gastric remnant which is left will shrink postoperatively and the patient will have an inadequate gastric reservoir, hence a larger gastric remnant must be left in these circumstances.

Having assessed the site of resection, the antrum of the stomach is held up, tensing the left gastric vessels as they run down close to the lesser curve of the stomach. These vessels are isolated at the level of the proposed resection, underrun and tied (Figure 12.6). The second suture may be added after clamping and dividing the vessels. It is important that the left gastric artery is divided on the stomach wall rather than at its origin from the coeliac axis on the posterior abdominal wall. If this is performed, the coeliac branch of the posterior vagus nerve may well be damaged. Having cleared the greater and lesser curves of the stomach at the level of the resection, the stomach is held up and one half of the Lane twin gastroenterostomy clamp is applied, making sure that the nasogastric tube in the stomach is drawn back into the fundus to avoid it being trapped in the clamp. The other half of the twin clamp is applied to the jejunum, the proximal end being about 5 cm from the duodenojejunal flexure. Before the clamp is applied, the surgeon should demonstrate to the first assistant that he or she has indeed isolated the proximal jejunum in his or her hand by demonstrating the duodenojejunal flexure and the proximity of the inferior mesenteric vein. In this way the appalling error of

an inadvertent gastro-ileostomy may be avoided. The jejunum is brought up in front of the transverse colon and the clamps united so that the proximal jejunum lies against the lesser curve and the efferent loop against the greater curve of the stomach (Figure 12.7).

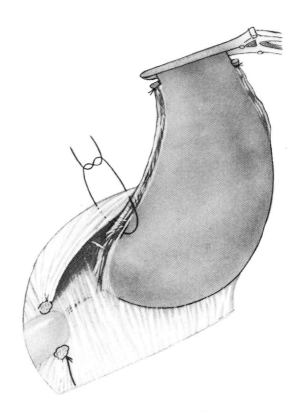

Figure 12.6 Polya partial gastrectomy. The left gastric vessels are secured and divided close to the stomach. If the left gastric artery is dissected and divided at its origin, the coeliac branch of the vagus nerve will be unnecessarily damaged

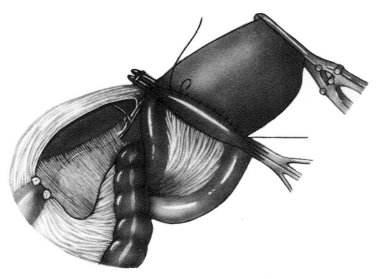

Figure 12.7 Polya partial gastrectomy. Application of Lane gastrojejunostomy clamps

The two-layered 2/0 absorbable suture anastomosis is started with a posterior seromuscular Lembert suture joining the adjacent stomach and jejunum. The stomach is then held up and a Payr clamp is applied from the lesser curve to about 5 cm from the greater curve and the stomach is crushed about 1 cm distal to the seromuscular suture. A non-crushing clamp is then applied to the stomach to prevent contamination, as the stomach is divided on the Payr clamp (Figure 12.8). The small piece of stomach between the tip of the clamp and the greater curve is cut with care so that the layer nearest to the jejunum is cut 1 cm distal to the posterior seromuscular suture and the other layer is cut in a curved fashion so that the centre is about 2 cm longer. This will facilitate fashioning of the anastomosis (Figure 12.9a).

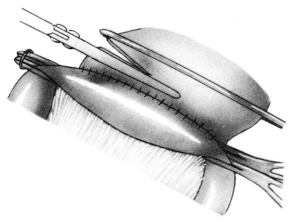

Figure 12.8 Polya partial gastrectomy. The posterior seromuscular suture has been inserted, following which a Payr clamp and a non-crushing clamp are applied to the stomach, and the stomach is divided distal to the Payr clamp

The segment of the stomach in the Payr clamp is then closed to form a valve. This may be achieved using an atraumatic suture and a sewing machine technique (Figure 12.9a). This achieved, a 5 cm hole is made through all coats of the jejunum with diathermy to correspond with the hole in the gastric remnant. The posterior layers are then united with an all-layers 2/0 absorbable suture, and the suture is then brought round onto the anterior layer, where it is continued as an over-and-over inverting haemostatic suture to complete the inner layer (Figure 12.9b,c). A Connell suture should not be used in this situation as it is not a haemostatic suture and any potential bleeding site will be masked by the clamps.

The Lane clamps are now unlocked, individually released and removed with care as the anastomosis is yet to be completed. This is achieved by continuing the original posterior seromuscular Lembert suture round and across the anterior gastric and jejunal walls back to the starting point. Having completed the anastomosis, it is inspected from the front and the back and any imperfections or bleeding points may be reinforced by an extra interrupted 2/0 suture.

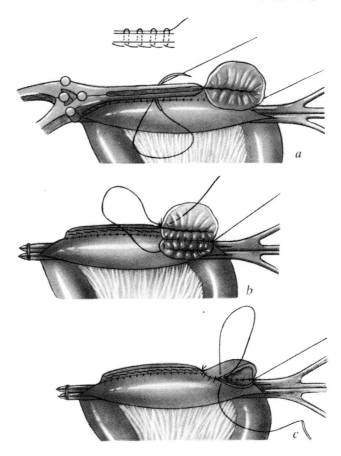

Figure 12.9 Polya partial gastrectomy. *a*, The segment of stomach held by the Payr clamp is closed to form a valve using a sewing machine technique (inset). The small piece of stomach between the tip of the clamp and the greater curve is cut with care so that the lip nearest to the jejunum is cut 1 cm distal to the posterior seromuscular suture and the other lip is cut in a curved fashion so that the centre is about 2 cm longer, facilitating fashioning of the anastomosis. *b*, *c*, A jejunal opening is created to correspond with the gastric stoma and these are anastomosed with an all-layers continuous suture

The anastomosis is checked with finger and thumb to make sure that it is patent. The transverse colon and omentum are then pulled over to the right so that the gastrojejunal anastomosis is sitting in front of the splenic flexure (Figure 12.10). There should be no tension on the 5 cm long afferent loop, but at the same time it lies snugly against the colon and the omentum plugs the gap, preventing all the interesting postoperative complications described by Stammers and Williams (1963).

Prior to closing the abdomen, a systematic check is carried out, working from left to right. The spleen is visualized to exclude a minor tear and any blood is aspirated from the subphrenic space. The front of the anastomosis is examined again, and after the posterior layer has been checked any blood is aspirated from the lesser sac. The position of the Ryle's tube is checked so that it is lying in the middle of the gastric

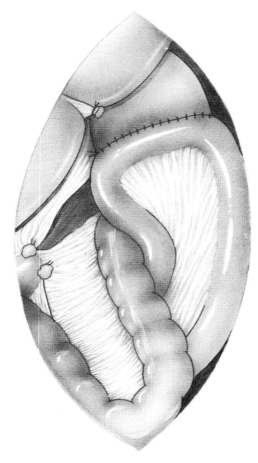

Figure 12.10 Polya partial gastrectomy. The completed antecolic operation shows the stoma lying comfortably in front of the splenic flexure

remnant. The omental ties in the colon and the colour of the omentum are checked. The latter may be slightly cyanosed if mobilization has been made outside the gastro-epiploic arch as described. This can be ignored; if omentum is grossly cyanosed it should be excised but this is only rarely necessary and usually in an obese patient. The pulsation of the middle colic artery and the colour of the transverse colon are also checked, as also is the duodenal stump. If the duodenal stump has been closed in three layers, as described, drainage is probably unnecessary. However, if the surgeon is relatively inexperienced or if the stump has been difficult to close, or if the closure has been in only one or two layers, drainage is mandatory. Either a tube or a Redivac drain can be used. Finally, any blood is aspirated from the hepatorenal pouch and from below the diaphragm on the right, and the abdomen is closed in one layer as previously described. The skin is then closed in a continuous subcutaneous fashion.

SPECIAL POINTS OF TECHNIQUE

There has been much controversy in the past as to whether or not the anastomosis should be fashioned in an antecolic or retrocolic manner. The original Polya gastrectomy as described was a retrocolic anastomosis, and some believe that this is the only way to obtain a short afferent loop. However, if the technique already described is used, a 5 cm afferent loop is all that is required. Tanner found no difference in the results of his antecolic and retrocolic operations and, since it is easier to construct and dismantle an antecolic anastomosis, the author strongly recommends the antecolic anastomosis when gastrectomy is performed.

The difficult duodenal stump is associated with a posterior penetrating ulcer eroding into the pancreas, and since these stumps are difficult to close, some would recommend that this situation is best treated by vagotomy rather than resection. However, if for some reason resection and closure of the duodenum are necessary, the following technique should be employed.

Having mobilized the antrum in the usual fashion, the stomach is pinched off the pancreas until the posterior ulcer crater is entered just distal to the pylorus (Figure 12.11a). The ulcer crater may be at least 1 cm across and this will mean that the duodenum will have already been divided, possibly one-third to halfway round its full circumference. The stomach is then completely separated from the duodenum by dividing the anterior wall just distal to the pylorus. One is then faced with the situation shown in Figure 12.11b. The posterior wall of the duodenum may be freed from the edge of the crater by inserting the index finger into the duodenum and by placing a Babcock tissue forceps on the edge of the duodenal mucosa. By slight traction on the tissue forceps and sharp dissection, the posterior wall of the duodenum may be mobilized off the pancreas. The plane of dissection lies close to the duodenal wall. There is often some oedema on the edge of the ulcer crater and this may facilitate the separation. The plane is often surprisingly avascular and by keeping close to the duodenal wall no damage will be done to the surrounding tissues, such as the common bile duct. When it has been possible to free a 1 cm length of posterior wall of the duodenum, closure may be effected with an economical Connell suture of 2/0 atraumatic absorbable suture (Figure 12.11c). A Kocher manoeuvre may then be carried out if the duodenal stump is not sufficiently mobile and the second layer of closure may be achieved by rolling the duodenum onto the ulcer crater and inserting a series of interrupted 2/0 absorbable sutures between the duodenal stump and the edge of the ulcer crater which is firm, fibrous tissue and holds the sutures well (Figure 12.11d). There is no fear of damage to the pancreas. In such a closure the duodenal stump must always be drained.

2. Truncal vagotomy

For any form of vagotomy an upper midline is the

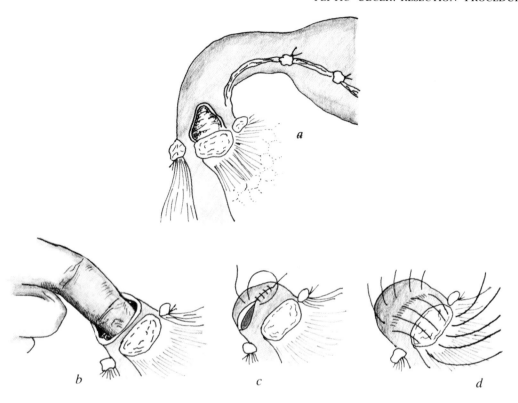

Figure 12.11 Closure of the difficult duodenal stump. *a*, The ulcer is pinched off the pancreas until the posterior ulcer crater is entered just distal to the pylorus. *b*, The stomach is completely separated from the duodenum by dividing the anterior wall just distal to the pylorus. Dissection between the opened duodenum and pancreas may be facilitated by placing the index finger into the duodenal stump. *c*, *d*, The duodenal stump is closed by the use of a Connell suture and rolling the duodenum onto the ulcer crater where it may be held in place using a series of interrupted catgut sutures between the duodenal stump and the edge of the crater. This latter tissue is firm and fibrous and holds the sutures well

incision of choice which is taken from the umbilicus and extended up over the xiphisternum. The exposure of the stomach and hiatus may be improved by inserting a sternal lifting retractor which hooks up under the xiphisternum and pulls it in an upwards cranial direction (Goligher, 1974). The left triangular ligament is divided (beware the inferior phrenic vein), and the left lobe of the liver is folded upon itself and tucked away to the right. In a more obese patient, a self-retaining retractor may be required.

PROCEDURE

The abdominal oesophagus is more easily identified if a Ryle's tube is already in place. The surgeon holds the body of the stomach and pulls it downwards while at the same time placing the index and middle fingers either side of the lower oesophagus. The peritoneum is divided transversely over the cardio-oesophageal junction. Beneath this layer there is a condensation of connective tissue called the 'phreno-oesophageal ligament'. This is picked up in forceps and lifted off the oesophagus and again excised in a transverse fashion. A pair of scissors may then be placed under this layer and if opened the surface of the oesophagus is exposed. The tips of the scissors can slip into the

posterior mediastinum. Failure to incise deliberately this fibrous layer ensures that the surgeon will be in the incorrect layer and makes subsequent dissection more difficult.

If the cardio-oesophageal junction of the stomach is grasped in the finger and thumb of the right hand and lightly pulled down, the anterior vagus is usually seen and can be palpated as a taut strand, usually towards the left border of the oesophagus. If elevated with a curved artery forceps, it can be seen dividing inferiorly into its hepatic and gastric branches. The nerve is divided between two artery forceps. The proximal part is dissected off the oesophagus and is tied as high as possible to avoid missing any branches. The lower end is also clamped and divided and the intervening section sent for histology. The anterior oesophagus is then gently palpated to exclude any other vagal nerve. Occasionally the anterior vagus does appear to be in two trunks. The lower oesophagus is then encircled with the right thumb and forefinger, and the tissue behind and medial to the oesophagus is palpated between finger and thumb. The right vagus is usually palpated about 1 cm behind and medial to the lower oesophagus and is often thicker than the anterior vagus. Once identified, the nerve may be lifted on an aneurysm needle and dissected both upwards and downwards, where it may be seen dividing into its coeliac and gastric branches. Again the nerve is clamped and divided and tied at its division into its principal branches. A final search is made to identify any other branches of the nerve that have been missed.

Haemostasis is then checked and the oesophagus and spleen inspected to make certain neither has been damaged in the course of the dissection. Finally, some advocate suturing the divided phreno-oesophageal ligament with two or three absorbable sutures in the hope that this might fix the stomach and reduce the chances of gastro-oesophageal reflux, which may occur after vagotomy. What is probably more important is a gentle handling of the oesophagus and the minimal amount of mobilization compatible with identification and ligation of the vagal trunks. The left lobe of the liver is then replaced and a pack is placed between the left lobe of the liver and the upper stomach. This is left in place until the drainage procedure has been completed and the area is once again checked for haemostasis.

The drainage procedure which is then performed is described below. The Ryle's tube is checked to make certain that it is in the correct position, lying in the antrum, and the abdomen is closed in layers in a routine fashion.

Drainage procedures

1. Heineke–Mikulicz pyloroplasty

If this procedure is performed through a midline incision, and in particular if the patient is fat, it may be facilitated by initially performing Kocher's mobilization of the duodenum. The position of the pylorus is identified by palpation and a longitudinal incision is made with the cutting diathermy, or scissors, starting on the gastric side of the pylorus. Having incised down to the mucosa and entered the lumen of the stomach, any gastric juice is aspirated and a pair of blunt dissecting forceps is inserted into the stomach and through the pylorus. The diathermy or scissors incision is continued through the pylorus by incising the tissue between the blades of the dissecting forceps. This will ensure that no inadvertent damage is done to the posterior wall of the stomach or duodenum. The total length of the incision should be about 6 cm, extending approximately 3.5 cm on the gastric side and 2.5 cm on the duodenal side of the pylorus. It should be midway between the greater and lesser curves of the stomach and superior and inferior borders of the duodenum.

The interior of the duodenum of the stomach is inspected and a finger is inserted down the duodenum to make sure that there is no distal, stenotic segment. A tissue forceps is then applied to both sides at the midpoint of the incision. The tissue forceps are separated and traction on the stomach is relaxed. The incision becomes transverse and the two layers are

sutured together to make a transverse incision line (Figure 12.12b).

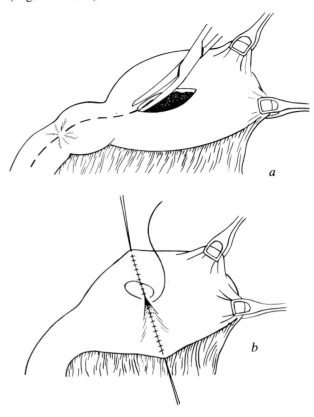

Figure 12.12 Heineke–Mikulicz pyloroplasty. *a*, The stomach and duodenum are opened by a longitudinal incision across the pylorus. *b*, The longitudinal incision is closed transversely in two layers

The technique of this closure is controversial. The traditional method is with a two-layer closure, which virtually eliminates the complication of leakage. The invaginated tissue does project into the lumen, but if done with all reasonable care this is never a problem and it certainly does not leave any permanent projection. If this technique is used an atraumatic 2/0 absorbable suture may be used for the initial all-coats layer, having previously ligated any previous individual bleeding vessels on the edge of the incision. The second layer is a continuous seromuscular Lembert suture, again of 2/0 absorbable material. On completion of the anastomosis, a finger and thumb are inserted on either side of the suture line to make sure that there is an adequate lumen through the anastomosis. Usually the tips of the thumb and two fingers may be passed through. The alternative technique is to use a one-layer closure, usually using a nonabsorbable material such as silk or linen. While this has proved safe in the hands of more experienced surgeons, in reported series in which this technique has been used there has usually been some morbidity and mortality from an occasional leak which may be reduced to a minimum by meticulous attention to detail.

2. Gastroenterostomy

If the duodenum is grossly scarred and access is difficult, the easier drainage procedure to perform is a gastroenterostomy. This may be either antecolic or retrocolic. The advantage of an anterior juxtapyloric gastroenterostomy is that the anastomosis is close to the obstructing lesion and the anastomosis is between the alkaline-secreting gastric antrum and the jejunal mucosa. The anastomosis is simple to perform and is also easy to dismantle. In general, drainage through such an anastomosis is very satisfactory. Occasionally, however, although technically perfect there is a delay in satisfactory emptying through the stoma. Hence, if immediate drainage is imperative it may be better to perform a posterior gastroenterostomy.

A. ANTERIOR JUXTAPYLORIC GASTROENTEROSTOMY

The anterior wall of the gastric antrum is grasped with one of the Lane twin gastroenterostomy clamps. The anterior wall of the stomach is clasped towards the greater curve aspect and if held in the hand one can ensure that the mucosa does not slip out of the grasp as the clamp is applied by the assistant. The omentum and transverse colon are lifted and the duodenojejunal flexure is identified. The other twin clamp is applied to the jejunum approximately 10–20 cm from the duodenojejunal flexure. The afferent loop should be as short as possible. The clamps are locked together so that the efferent loop of small gut is close to the pylorus. Before embarking on the anastomosis, one should check that there is no undue tension on the small bowel mesentery. The anastomosis is with two layers of 2/0 absorbable suture, the initial suture being a continuous seromuscular Lembert suture uniting the adjacent gastric and jejunal walls. This suture line is usually about 7 cm long. An opening is then made between the jejunum and the gastric antrum, which is slightly shorter than the posterior suture layer. This incision with diathermy is usually made 5 cm long. The adjacent gastric and jejunal walls are then united with a running all-layers absorbable suture. On the anterior wall, the layers are inverted using an over-and-over suture. A Connell suture must not be used in this situation because it is not haemostatic and any bleeding will be masked by the clamps. The inner suture having been completed, the clamps are removed and the posterior seromuscular suture is carried around the end and along the anterior walls to bury the all-layers suture.

B. POSTERIOR GASTROENTEROSTOMY

In this operation the jejunum is brought to the most dependent portion of the greater curve of the stomach. To do this, an initial opening is made in the gastrocolic omentum and the lesser sac is opened. The mesocolon is inspected and an incision made parallel and to the left of the middle colic vessels about 8 cm long. The duodenojejunal flexure is identified and a loop of proximal jejunum is brought up through the hole in the mesocolon. The one half of the Lane twin clamp is applied to a convenient part of the posterior wall of the stomach close to the greater curve. The two clamps are then locked together and the anastomosis is performed as with an anterior gastroenterostomy. On completion of this anastomosis, the margins of the mesocolic defect are sutured to the stomach to prevent any small gut prolapsing through this hole and causing an internal hernia (Figure 12.13).

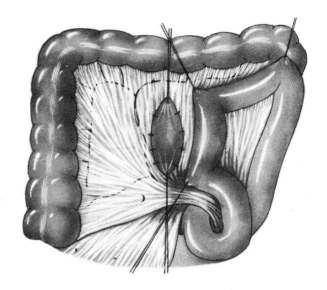

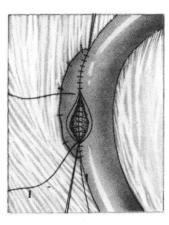

Figure 12.13 Gastroenterostomy. An incision is made in the mesocolon parallel and to the left of the middle colic vessels, following which a two-layer anastomosis is undertaken. In this diagram the Lane clamps are not shown and the anastomosis is undertaken from below for the sake of clarity, although the author accomplishes this procedure on the other side of the mesocolon by passing the jejunum through the defect

3. Highly selective vagotomy

Good access to the upper abdomen and to the oeso-phageal hiatus is essential. A midline incision is used, extending from the xiphoid process to 3–4 cm below the umbilicus. The xiphoid is not excised. The edges of the wound are retracted by a self-retaining retrac-tor. Access to the oesophagus is greatly improved if a metal hook is inserted under the xiphoid notch and strong traction exerted upwards toward the head of the operating table. This upward retraction of the rib cage is rendered more effective if the table is tilted about 15° head up, which has the additional advan-tage of causing the other viscera to fall away from the stomach and oesophagus. The left lobe of the liver is next mobilized to the right by division of the left triangular ligament (beware the inferior phrenic vein). Access to the oesophagus is now complete. The diagnosis of chronic duodenal ulceration is con-firmed, the stomach and oesophageal hiatus are assessed carefully, and a full laparotomy is carried out.

The next step is to mobilize the distal half of the greater curvature of the stomach by division of the gastrocolic omentum outside the gastro-epiploic arcades. The gastro-epiploic vessels are preserved so that interference with the stomach's blood supply will be kept to a minimum. Such mobilization of the greater curvature confers the advantage that the pos-terior nerve of Latarjet can then usually be seen, and this of course makes it easier to preserve. In addition, each of the major vessels entering the lesser curve on its posterior aspect can be ligated and divided pre-cisely, close to the stomach, while the nerve is kept in view. Another advantage of this approach is that the stomach, which itself is the main 'retractor' in HSV, is easier to grip and pull upon if part of the greater curvature has been mobilized.

The anterior vagal trunk enters the abdomen in front of the oesophagus and runs downwards and to the right, giving off one or more large anterior gastric branches. It leaves the oesophagus near the cardia, gives off the hepatic fibres, and then runs downwards in the lesser omentum parallel to the lesser curvature and 1–2 cm from it, as the anterior nerve of Latarjet. This important nerve lies immediately beneath the peritoneum. It accompanies the descending branch of the left gastric artery, and terminates just distal to the incisura angularis, 5–7 cm from the pylorus, by passing across onto the anterior aspect of the antral region of the stomach, usually in the form of two major terminal branches (Figure 12.14).

The posterior vagal trunk enters the abdomen behind or to the right of the oesophagus, gives off the large coeliac branch and a variable number of gastric branches, and then runs downwards in the posterior aspect of the lesser omentum as the posterior nerve of Latarjet. The course and distribution of this nerve to the posterior aspect of the stomach are similar to those of the anterior nerve of Latarjet to the anterior aspect. The anterior nerve of Latarjet is visible in

95% of patients and even in the most obese its terminal branches can be discerned. Likewise, the posterior nerve of Latarjet is usually visible when the lesser sac has been opened (Figure 12.15).

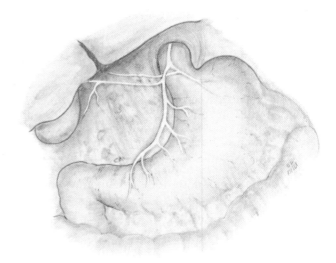

Figure 12.14 Distribution of the anterior vagal trunk is shown. Note hepatic fibres and main continuation of trunk, the anterior nerve of Latarjet reaching the antrum distal to the incisura about 6 cm from the pylorus

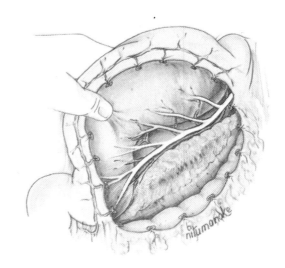

Figure 12.15 Greater curvature has been mobilized by division of gastrocolic omentum to show the posterior nerve of Latarjet, which terminates on the antrum distal to the incisura. The terminal Y fork of the nerve is preserved and all the other branches to the stomach are divided. Mobilization of the greater curvature is normally much less extensive than that illustrated. Note also that the gastro-epiploic arcades are carefully preserved

The first phase of the operation is to separate the lesser omentum, with its nerves of Latarjet, from the lesser curvature of the stomach between the incisura angularis and the cardia; and in the course of this dissection a delicate technique must be employed to avoid damage both to the muscular wall of the stomach and to the nerves of Latarjet. The second major phase of the operation involves thorough mobilization of the distal 5–6 cm of the oesophagus and clearance from it of all nerve fibres. The key questions are, first, how much of the distal stomach should be left innervated (i.e. where does the dissection begin on the lesser curvature), and secondly, how far proximally should the dissection be pursued on the oesophagus? While the answers cannot be absolutely precise, it may be stated as a rule of thumb that about 6 cm of stomach proximal to the pylorus should be left vagally innervated and that 6 cm of distal oesophagus should be cleared of all blood vessels and nerve fibres.

The anterior nerve of Latarjet is identified, and the position of its terminal branches noted. The nerve is rendered more obvious if the assistant exerts traction on the greater curvature. There is a 'crow's foot' arrangement of large veins (not of nerves) in the region of the incisura, and the major terminations of the nerve of Latarjet accompany the veins that form the 'toe' of the foot. The anterior part of the dissection begins just proximal to the point where these nerves pass across onto the musculature of the antral region. This point is usually 5–6 cm proximal to the pylorus. Hence, 5–7 cm of distal stomach are usually left innervated. Thus, one should identify the major nerves to the antrum and preserve them, rather than measure off an arbitrary length of the stomach and denervate the remainder.

The dissection begins at the chosen spot near the incisura on the anterior aspect of the stomach. The objective is to separate the lesser omentum from the lesser curvature between the incisura and the cardia by dividing all blood vessels and nerves that enter the lesser curvature from the lesser omentum. The blood vessels run in two distinct leashes, one of which passes to the anterior surface of the stomach and the other to the posterior surface. Each sizeable vessel is divided individually, and for this reason also it is an advantage to have secured access to the posterior aspect of the stomach.

The serosa overlying the vessels is divided by means of curved McIndoe's scissors, between the incisura and the cardia, along the line of the lesser curvature and well to the left of the nerves of Latarjet. The instruments can then be slid gently under the vessels, rather than having to be 'punched' forcibly through the serosa, which is surprisingly tough. Dissection begins near the incisura, about 2 cm proximal to the determined distal extremity of the dissection (this 2 cm segment is cleared at the end of the operation, because if it were divided at this stage the nerves of Latarjet would be at risk of injury by traction during the dissection). A curved haemostat, such as a Kilner or Roberts, is gently insinuated beneath each major vessel (Figure 12.16), a ligature is passed, seized by the jaws of the haemostat, drawn under the vessel and

the vessel is tied in continuity on the lesser omental side and then clamped close to the lesser curvature. The vessel is then divided (Figure 12.17). This method is felt to be preferable to the application of two haemostats and division of the vessel between them, because it ensures that the vessel cannot slip from a clamp and retract into the fat of the lesser omentum where it cannot be pursued and clamped for fear that the nerves of Latarjet will be damaged. In addition, a haemostat placed on the lesser omental side may inadvertently crush one of the nerves of Latarjet or, when lifted up, may tent up a nerve and cause it to be trapped in the ligature.

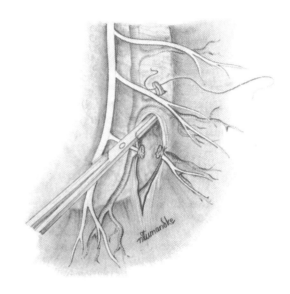

Figure 12.16 Dissection of anterior leaf of lesser omentum. Note that each major vessel is separately underrun and ligated in continuity

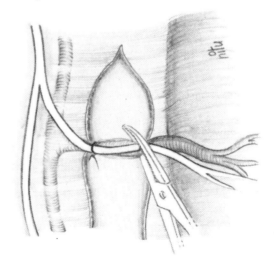

Figure 12.17 Vessel is ligated in continuity on lesser omental side and clamped on lesser curve side. A fine-pointed haemostat is used and great care is taken to avoid damage both to the nerve of Latarjet and to musculature of the lesser curvature

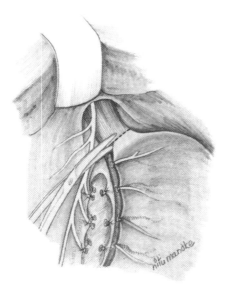

Figure 12.18 Anterior leaf of lesser omentum has been divided and serosa overlying oesophagogastric junction is being divided as far as the angle of His

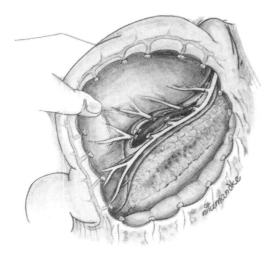

Figure 12.19 Division of posterior leaf of lesser omentum has begun, leaving about 5 cm of pre-pyloric stomach innervated. Demonstration of posterior nerve of Latarjet in this way helps to prevent damage to it

Each vessel should be ligated individually, because if large bites of tissue are taken the pedicle has a broad base and the ligature is more likely to slip when strong traction is exerted on the stomach during the oesophageal dissection. Loose areolar tissue between the blood vessels is clamped in a haemostat, coagulated with diathermy and then divided. The anterior leaf of the lesser omentum is divided in this way from near the incisura to the cardia and then to lay bare the anterior aspect of the oesophagus as far as the angle of His in like manner (Figure 12.18). Alternatively,

the entire oesophageal dissection may be left until later. The stomach is then turned over and the posterior leaf of the lesser omentum is dealt with similarly: the dissection begins at the incisura and is carried upwards to near the cardia (Figure 12.19). One then returns to the anterior aspect of the stomach and if a breakthrough has not yet been achieved between front and back this is now done and the few remaining vessels and nerves entering the lesser curvature are divided. Separation of the lesser omentum from the stomach between incisura and cardia in this way is relatively straightforward, and ensures that vagal fibres cannot possibly enter the stomach between these two points. Thus the vagotomy of the parietal cell mass can only be incomplete either distally, at the antral end or on the oesophagus.

If only 5–7 cm of distal stomach are left innervated, there is little likelihood of the vagotomy being incomplete distally, because Amdrup and Jensen (1970), who routinely mapped the extent of the antrum at the time of operation, found that the boundary between parietal cell mass and antrum lay 8 or 9 cm on average proximal to the pylorus and seldom extended more distally than 6 cm from the pylorus. Thus the problem of incomplete vagotomy is, for the most part, a problem of missed vagal fibres on the oesophagus.

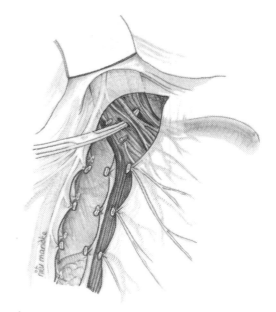

Figure 12.20 Small vessels and nerves running down the anterior surface of the oesophagus in the meso-oesophagus are gently lifted by haemostat, seized in the forceps and destroyed by diathermy or else ligated with fine thread

The next step is to expose the anterior surface of the oesophagus. The mobilized left lobe of the liver is drawn across to the right by means of a deep Kelly's retractor, and the serosa covering the oesophagogastric junction is divided with long curved scissors (see

Figure 12.18). Small vessels are picked up in Roberts forceps, lifted off the muscle layer and coagulated with diathermy (Figure 12.20). The Roberts forceps are then slipped gently across the surface of the lower oesophagus, on the muscle layer and beneath the larger vessels and the anterior gastric branches of the anterior vagal trunk. These are then ligated in continuity proximally, clamped distally and divided. Division of these tissues frees the anterior vagal trunk, which remains out of harm's way above and to the left of the operator's scissors. The angle of His, 3 cm or so of upper greater curvature and the areolar tissue to the left of the oesophagus are then cleared of fat and blood vessels (Figure 12.21).

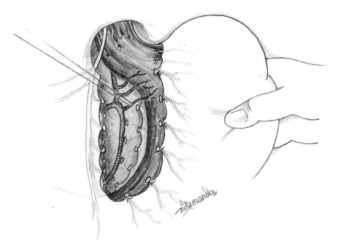

Figure 12.22 Division of vessels and nerves to cardia and posterior aspect of oesophagus. Note that the assistant pulls the stomach downwards and at the same time elevates it. The operator stays very close to the muscle of lesser curvature and oesophagus in order to avoid vagal trunks and hepatic and coeliac branches

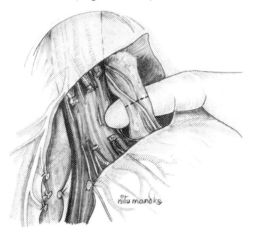

Figure 12.21 This step is often carried out at the same time as division of the anterior leaf of lesser omentum. The serosa to the left of the oesophagus is divided and then fatty areolar tissue to the left of the oesophagus, which contains nerve fibres, vessels and lymphatics, is lifted up with the right index finger. The angle of His and the adjacent oesophagus and fundus of stomach are thoroughly cleared and in this way small nerve fibres running to the proximal 3 cm of fundus ('criminal' nerves of Grassi) are eliminated

The next and most difficult step is to expose the posterior and right lateral aspects of the oesophagus. It is still too early to pass a sling or tube around the oesophagus. The assistant grasps the body of the stomach and pulls in both a distal and a vertical direction. The vessels and nerves entering the lower oesophagus and cardia are thus rendered taut and can be underrun, ligated in continuity and divided in the usual way (Figure 12.22). The dissection is kept very close to the wall of the upper stomach and lower oesophagus to avoid damage to the nerve trunks and to their coeliac and hepatic branches. The danger to these structures is not as great as might be feared, because division of the vessels and nerves along the lesser curvature has allowed them to be swept upwards and to the operator's left. As the dissection proceeds it becomes possible to pass a soft rubber tube around the oesophagus. Traction of this tube further facilitates access to the posterior aspect of the oesophagus. At this stage, a leash of vessels passing from the lesser omentum to the upper part of the

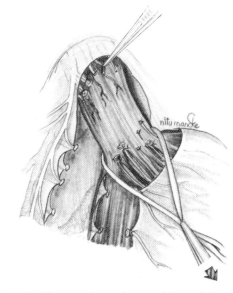

Figure 12.23 The oesophagus is now fully mobilized and the operator can exert strong but gentle traction on it, and can also rotate it in order to reach fibres running down the posterior aspect. Small blood vessels and nerve fibres are picked up by dissecting forceps or in the tip of a haemostat, coagulated and divided. This is a painstaking exercise and the whole oesophageal part of the dissection may take 30 min. None the less, this is where vagotomies are usually incomplete and the complete 'skeletonization' of the distal 5–6 cm of oesophagus in this way ensures that few of the postoperative insulin tests will be positive and that the incidence of recurrent ulceration will be low

greater curvature is encountered and divided. Finally, the rubber sling is withdrawn and the operator grasps the oesophagus in his right hand and draws it gently but firmly downwards (Figure 12.23). He should be able to pass three or four fingers behind the oesophagus at this stage. This manoeuvre invariably reveals many more vessels and nerve fibres entering the oesophagus, particularly on the right lateral and posterior aspects. These are painstakingly ligated or coagulated and divided with fine curved McIndoe's scissors. It is obviously important not to perforate the oesophagus, but this is unlikely to happen if both the vessels and the nerves are lifted clear of the oesophageal muscle before being coagulated.

The importance of spending a long time in ensuring that the vagotomy is complete on the oesophagus cannot be overemphasized. Postoperative insulin studies indicate that the distal extent of HSV vagally denervates the distal parietal cell mass in most patients (Johnston *et al.*, 1973). More proximally, there can be no doubt about the completeness of the vagotomy between the incisura and the cardia. It is on the oesophagus that HSV may be and indeed often is incomplete.

If there has been a good deal of oozing around the oesophagus, a fine suction drain is inserted which is withdrawn 1–2 days later. The linea alba is approximated with a running suture of monofilament nylon and the skin closed with a continuous subcutaneous suture.

4. Anterior seromyotomy and posterior truncal vagotomy

This operation was introduced in 1979 (Taylor *et al.*, 1982) as an alternative to HSV and the side effects of truncal vagotomy. A posterior vagotomy is performed and an anterior lesser curve seromyotomy preserving the anterior nerve of Latarjet. Side effects are less common than with truncal vagotomy, but the incidence of ulcer recurrence is as yet not established (Taylor *et al.*, 1990).

Suture material

In all the anastomoses described in this chapter, two layers of 2/0 absorbable suture have been used. This material seems to be very successful and the use of an outer layer of a non-absorbable suture, either as an interrupted or continuous layer, seems to be quite unnecessary. It has been suggested that the use of a non-absorbable suture may be the cause of recurrent ulceration. There is, however, little evidence of this and it may be that, as the ulcer enlarges, eroding through the wall of the bowel, if near an anastomosis, the suture material may eventually appear in the base of the ulcer. Chromic catgut may be used, but one of the more modern absorbable sutures may give a feeling of greater security.

Stapling devices have been available for some years to aid in the construction of a gastric anastomosis or to assist in closure of the duodenal stump. These instruments are of necessity expensive and with present financial constraints should be used with moderation. It is beyond the scope of this chapter to go into the details of constructing anastomoses with stapling devices.

Intraoperative tests for completeness of vagotomy

The usefulness of such tests is debatable. Burge's electrical stimulation test (Burge, 1964) records an increase in intragastric pressure if an intact vagal fibre is included within the electrode which is placed around the oesophagus. In Grassi's test (Grassi, 1971), a pH-recording electrode is introduced into the stomach, which is stimulated to secrete acid by the intravenous infusion of pentagastrin, If the entire gastric mucosa is found to be alkaline after vagotomy, the vagotomy is complete; conversely, the finding of an acid area indicates an incomplete vagotomy. Neither of these tests is now routinely performed.

Postoperative

Management following gastrectomy and vagotomy

General

The usual observations of vital functions are recorded in the recovery room. Initially, half-hourly pulse and blood pressure should be taken for the first 4 h and, after this, observations can be reduced to hourly for the next 8 hours. Effective relief of postoperative pain is essential so that early chest physiotherapy may be initiated.

Specific

1. The Ryle's tube is placed on free drainage and is in addition aspirated hourly for the first 12 h. After this, the tube is aspirated 4-hourly until removal. An accurate fluid chart recording all fluid input and output must be maintained. The Billroth-I anastomosis is smaller than a gastrojejunal anastomosis and it usually takes 3–4 days before it starts to drain. This is heralded by the appearance of bile in the gastric aspirate and a decrease in the volume of the aspirate, so that it becomes less than the input. The tube may then be removed. With a Polya gastrectomy the anastomosis is usually opened and is draining at 72 h, and this is usually so following a truncal vagotomy and drainage. After HSV, the Ryle's tube may be removed immediately or the following day.

2. Oral fluids in the volume of 25 ml hourly may be given from the first postoperative day. There is no point in increasing this volume until the stomach is emptying, as it is merely aspirated up the Ryle's tube and acts as a gastric lavage, removing more hydrogen and potassium ions. A standard intravenous regimen is given until sufficient fluid may be taken orally. Parenteral hyperalimentation is not as a rule required as the patients are usually taking sufficient calories orally by the 5th postoperative day.

It is important to convince all patients that they are capable of eating a normal diet prior to leaving hospital, otherwise they may continue to take a gastric diet indefinitely, the only restrictions being that where patients have had a gastrectomy or a vagotomy and drainage they should avoid eating citrus fruit (juice only) and nuts. This will avoid bolus obstructions developing due to a phytobezoar.

Complications of Polya gastrectomy and vagotomy

Immediate

Haemorrhage may occur following Polya gastrectomy from faulty haemostasis at the suture line. Fresh blood will be aspirated up the Ryle's tube in variable quantities. This problem may be prevented by meticulous attention to detail when constructing the gastrojejunal anastomosis. When stitching the inner layer, each suture must be approximately 3 mm apart and the suture must be followed down to make certain that it is evenly spaced and a steady tension must be maintained on the suture by the assistant. These points are particularly important if the gastrectomy is being constructed with the aid of gastrectomy clamps which will, of course, mask any potential bleeding until after they are removed. Haemorrhage may also occur from the suture line of a pyloroplasty or a gastroenterostomy associated with total or selective vagotomy. The length of the suture lines are, however, smaller and this reduces the chance of significant haemorrhage.

When haemorrhage does occur, it fortunately often stops spontaneously and no active measures are required. If haemorrhage does continue and the patient begins to show signs of decompensation despite blood transfusion, reoperation will be required. In the case of bleeding from a Polya anastomosis, the site of the bleeding may be identified through a small gastrotomy above the suture line and the bleeding point may be underrun from a gastroenterostomy, but in the case of a pyloroplasty it is probably best to dismantle the suture line from one end until the bleeding point is identified and ligated.

Delay in gastric emptying

This rarely occurs after a Polya gastrectomy because the stoma is larger than with a Billroth gastrectomy. Sometimes, however, one may get a false impression of delayed emptying because large quantities of fluid are aspirated up the Ryle's tube. At the same time, the patient says that he or she feels hungry and is having his or her bowels open. What has happened in these cases is that the Ryle's tube has slipped through the stoma into the efferent loop and the fluid that is being aspirated is a combination of gastric and pancreatic juice plus bile. The treatment is to remove the Ryle's tube and feed the patient.

Delay in gastric emptying following either truncal or selective vagotomy may occasionally be a problem, particularly if the patient has a preoperative pyloric stenosis. Under these circumstances, one may need to keep a Ryle's tube down until the gastric aspirate diminishes and the patient will require feeding parenterally. If the problem does not resolve within 10–14 days, re-exploration of the anastomosis may rarely be required. Approximately 0.5% of patients who have undergone HSV develop gastric retention and require the addition of a drainage procedure several months after the initial operation. This complication may be due to accidental damage of the nerves of Latarjet, cicatricial narrowing at the gastric outlet as the ulcer heals, or to other causes. The incidence of impaired gastric emptying is lower after HSV than after vagotomy combined with antrectomy (Dorricott et al., 1978).

Leakage from the gastrojejunal anastomosis

This is extremely uncommon after Polya gastrectomy, but may occasionally occur following a one-layer pyloroplasty. This will require reoperation and refashioning of the suture line.

Duodenal stump rupture or leakage may occur often on the 3rd postoperative day following Polya gastrectomy. Prevention of this problem is discussed earlier in this chapter. If a drain is present, the fluid escapes freely into the drainage bag and the patient's condition will remain stable and the problem may be treated conservatively. In the absence of a drain there will be flooding of the abdominal cavity with duodenal contents, mainly consisting of bile and pancreatic juice, which will lead to a rapid collapse. In the event of such a leak, the stump must be repaired and the rest of the anastomosis checked to make sure that there is no distal obstruction.

Small bowel obstruction secondary to internal hernia

Small bowel obstruction from adhesions may occur following any operation, but Stammers and Williams (1963) have described a number of cases of obstruction resulting from small bowel slipping behind the afferent and efferent loops of an antecolic gastrectomy. This problem may be prevented by the technique already described, using a short afferent loop. It may also complicate a retrocolic gastrectomy or gastrojejunostomy if the hole in the mesocolon is not closed around the anastomosis.

Dysphagia

This may be an occasional complication following either truncal or selective vagotomy and develops 7–10 days after the operation. The patient feels as if food sticks behind the lower sternum and has to be regurgitated. The problem often persists for 7–10 days and then improves. The aetiology of this self-limiting dysphagia is ill understood but may represent a neuropraxia affecting the lower gullet or the result of some oedema around the hiatus following the oesophageal mobilization.

Lesser curve necrosis

Complications specific to HSV are unusual. Oesophageal perforation may occur and 2–3% of patients require splenectomy because of operative trauma to the splenic capsule. Necrosis of the lesser curvature or fundus of the stomach occurs in approximately 1 in every 500 HSV operations, and caused death in 1 in 1000 (0.1%) (Johnston, 1975). In some cases it may be due to ischaemia, because the anastomotic network of blood vessels in the submucosa is much more sparse along the lesser curvature than in the anterior and posterior walls of the stomach. However, it seems likely that many cases of necrosis are also attributable to operative trauma to the gastric wall by diathermy, ligature or instrumental damage.

Remote complications

Recurrent ulceration

The mean incidence of recurrent ulceration following truncal vagotomy is about 7% (Koruth et al., 1990), but may be higher. Following HSV, recurrence rates of up to 30% have been reported, but two recent papers show late recurrence rates of about 15%. (Macintyre et al., 1990; Johnston et al., 1991). Polya gastrectomy has a mean incidence of approximately 3%, while vagotomy and antrectomy have the lowest incidence of recurrent ulceration of about 1%.

In cases of recurrent ulceration, particularly if they recur soon after the original operation, the possibility of a Zollinger–Ellison syndrome must be considered, which can be confirmed by serum gastrin assay. If the patient has previously had a Polya gastrectomy, the duodenal stump must be checked for retained gastric mucosa. If this is absent, the stomal ulceration may be treated by adding a vagotomy. On the other hand, where vagotomy has failed, there are usually dense adhesions around the hiatus and lesser curve and further surgery in this region is hazardous. Accordingly, gastric resection is usually performed to cure the recurrent ulceration. While in the past the treatment of recurrent ulceration has always been surgical, medical treatment is now the initial treatment of choice. Transthoracic vagotomy is another approach and this is now feasible laparoscopically.

Dumping

This syndrome, occurring 10–20 min after a meal, is associated with a feeling of fullness, weakness, sweating, palpitations, and sometimes even faintness. The syndrome is thought to be caused by rapid emptying of hypertonic food into the jejunum. This exerts an osmotic effect within the lumen of the gut, resulting in an outpouring of fluid into the gut. It is possible, however, that there may be a hormonal component contributing to the syndrome. This syndrome occurs most frequently after Polya gastrectomy (21%), but it may occur after any operation on the stomach in which a drainage procedure has been performed. It may therefore occur after a truncal or selective vagotomy. Humphrey et al. (1972) reported an incidence of 18% following truncal vagotomy and gastroenterostomy and 12% following truncal vagotomy and pyloroplasty.

Fortunately, the frequency and severity of the attacks of dumping seem to decrease in the months and years after operation, and dietary advice can be a help to patients. It should be suggested that they avoid sweet and starchy foods and should take their meals dry. A drink should be taken midway between meals. A relatively dry meal empties very much less rapidly from the stomach than does a fluid meal. Very rarely, if the symptoms are incapacitating and occur after a Polya gastrectomy, it may be possible to treat the patient by inserting a retroperistaltic loop between the gastric remnant and the duodenum. The results, however, as described by Alexander-Williams (1973), are not very encouraging.

Bilious vomiting

The typical history of patients with bilious vomiting is that shortly after a meal they begin to feel uncomfortably distended, become nauseated and then vomit a large quantity of pure bile. After vomiting, the symptoms are relieved. In some patients the symptoms are present when they wake in the morning, the nausea continuing until they vomit spontaneously or induce vomiting. This symptom may occur after any form of gastric surgery, but is particularly common after Polya gastrectomy and vagotomy and gastroenterostomy. Originally this syndrome was thought to be due to afferent loop constriction, but the evidence now points to the fact that it is the presence of bile in the gastric remnant which in some patients acts as an irritant and causes a gastritis and interferes with gastric emptying.

In order to cure this symptom it is necessary to prevent bile refluxing into the gastric remnant. In the case of Polya gastrectomy, this may be achieved by converting the gastrectomy to a Roux-en-Y or 'Roux 19' anastomosis (Tanner, 1951), ensuring that the bile enters 19 in (48 cm) below the gastric remnant. It is more rarely a problem after Billroth-I gastrectomy, but if so an isoperistaltic loop of jejunum may be placed between the gastric remnant and the duodenum, again preventing reflux of bile (Alexander-Williams, 1973).

Diarrhoea

Diarrhoea may occur after any gastric operation and may be either continuous or intermittent. Episodic diarrhoea is a common problem, particularly after operations associated with vagotomy. It may occur in 24% of patients following truncal vagotomy and drainage, but the incidence of severe diarrhoea is only 5%. The incidence of diarrhoea following selective vagotomy appears to be lower (18%) and is very low after HSV. In either case, symptoms become much less troublesome with the passage of time and they may be helped by avoiding milk products and wet sweet foods. Continuous diarrhoea is a less common problem and appears to occur with equal frequency after gastric resection or after vagotomy with drainage. In the more severe cases, investigation usually reveals a variable degree of steatorrhoea and this is due to pancreatic exocrine insufficiency. It certainly may be worth giving patients pancreatic replacement to see whether it is of any benefit. If the problem is intractable, the possibility of a reversed ileal loop might be considered. A rare but important cause of acute profuse diarrhoea is the development of gastrojejunocolic fistula due to stomal ulceration, and this is dealt with later in the chapter. Another rare cause is the Zollinger–Ellison syndrome, one feature of which may be diarrhoea. Finally, cases have been reported where the unfortunate patient has diarrhoea because the surgeon has inadvertently connected the gastric remnant to the ileum rather than to the jejunum. Once diagnosed, the remedy is obvious.

Deficiency states and metabolic bone disease

These may occur following Polya gastrectomy or vagotomy and are described earlier, under the section on Billroth-I gastrectomy.

Complications of peptic ulceration

The complications of peptic ulceration are now the main indication for surgery for this disease. The commonest complications are haemorrhage and perforation. Stenosis is also considered.

Haemorrhage

Bleeding from peptic ulceration is the most common cause of acute upper gastrointestinal tract haemorrhage. Most British series agree that around half the patients admitted have chronic peptic ulcers, duodenal ulcer outnumbering the gastric ulcer by 2 to 1. Before endoscopy, the incidence of bleeding from acute gastric erosions was assumed to be high. It now seems, however, to be less than previously supposed and most series in the UK report a frequency of less than 10%. Other common causes of upper gastrointestinal tract bleeding include evidence of oesophageal mucosal tears in the Mallory–Weiss syndrome (13%) and reflux oesophagitis (10%). Oesophageal varices are an infrequent cause of

haemorrhage in the UK and the majority of workers report an incidence of around 2%.

The role of drugs, especially NSAIDs, in the causation of acute upper gastrointestinal bleeding has now become a common problem (Langman, 1988). Aspirin and alcohol, either separately or together, may precipitate acute bleeding from the upper alimentary tract. The bleeding is usually from acute gastric erosions or sometimes from pre-existing chronic peptic ulcers. While there is no doubt that aspirin causes slight occult blood loss, in most individuals it probably only rarely produces major gastrointestinal bleeding. With the widespread use of NSAIDs, these have become the major culprit in the cause of peptic ulcers which may bleed (Cockel, 1987). Healing of the ulcers will occur when the drug is withdrawn. Contrary to the impression of most surgeons, there is no good evidence that corticosteroids in ordinary doses cause either peptic ulceration or gastrointestinal bleeding; these individuals are often taking other drugs that are known to precipitate bleeds such as the NSAIDs.

Management of the patient

When a patient presents with acute upper gastrointestinal tract bleeding, two questions have to be answered. First, how much blood has been lost, and secondly, where is the source of the bleeding?

1. BLOOD LOSS

An estimate of the blood loss may be made by taking a history, making an examination and by arranging some pathological investigations. With regard to history, haematemesis with melaena implies a considerably greater blood loss than melaena alone and the mortality is approximately twice as great. The volume of haematemesis can give some guide to the amount of blood loss, but the patient's assessment of the volume is usually inaccurate. Bleeding associated with a feeling of faintness suggests rapid significant loss. On examination, the obviously shocked patient with rapid pulse and low blood pressure has clearly lost several units of blood. When blood loss is less extreme, pulse rate, blood pressure and central venous pressure monitoring may be helpful in assessing the blood lost. It takes some hours for the blood to dilute and hence the haemoglobin level to fall after an acute bleed. However, if the bleeding is continued for some time, the haemoglobin level is a useful guide. A low haemoglobin level soon after an acute bleed suggests previous occult bleeding.

2. SOURCE OF BLEEDING

While the history may indicate the cause of bleeding, in over 30% of patients with peptic ulcer no symptoms relative to the cause of the bleeding are found. There are usually no physical findings likely to be helpful in the diagnosis of bleeding peptic ulcers, apart from possibly localized abdominal tenderness, but hyperactive bowel sounds may suggest rapid transit of blood through the gut.

3. INVESTIGATION

Ideally, these patients should be admitted to a centralized gastrointestinal unit supervised by both a medical and surgical team. Investigation of the haemorrhage is by endoscopy. A high diagnostic yield is obtained, particularly if endoscopy is carried out within 24 h of the admission. In patients with continued profuse haemorrhage, it may be difficult to detect the bleeding point because of the presence of blood clot in the stomach. If the bleeding is obviously profuse and continuous, surgery will be required, which when performed immediately after endoscopy may be complicated by the presence of large quantities of air in the small gut, making exposure and subsequent closure more difficult.

Treatment

Resuscitation is the most important initial part of management. An estimate of the blood loss must be obtained, and if the bleeding has been sufficient to bring the patient into hospital an intravenous infusion will be required. If clinical assessment suggests the blood volume to be depleted, then transfusion of blood should be started. Similarly, patients with a haemoglobin below 10 g per cent usually require transfusion. Blood volume studies have shown that the loss in patients with upper gastrointestinal tract bleeding tends to be more severe than is suspected clinically (Tudhope, 1958). In the more difficult cases, and particularly in elder patients, a central venous pressure line may be helpful in the initial assessment of the blood loss and also for guiding subsequent blood transfusion. It may also give early warning of further bleeds; fortunately 4 out of 5 patients stop bleeding spontaneously. It is important to recognize as early as possible patients with continuous or recurrent bleeding, since the mortality rate of those who rebleed is four times higher. Rebleeding may be detected indirectly from frequent measurements of pulse and blood pressure and by regular examination of postural changes in pulse, blood pressure and central venous pressure. An indwelling nasogastric tube to detect early rebleeding has been suggested by some workers, but the author has found this unhelpful as it frequently becomes blocked with clot and fails to drain and merely contributes to the patient's discomfort.

The traditional method of treatment in the past has consisted of small doses of opiates to sedate the patient, ice cubes to suck and regular ingestion of antacids. Recent studies have suggested that H_2 receptor antagonists are not effective in acute bleeding (Walt et al., 1992). Angiography may identify the bleeding point and allow a catheter to be introduced into the feeding vessel. Haemostasis may be attempted, either by infusing vasopressin or by occluding the vessel with emboli. More recent approaches have been via the endoscope. The injection of adrenaline or sclerotherapy in an attempt to arrest the bleeding (Steele et al., 1991) is being used in many centres as well as heater probe and laser coagulation (Sim et al., 1991).

SURGICAL INTERVENTION IN BLEEDING PEPTIC ULCER

The most common indication for surgical intervention is either continued heavy blood loss or recurrent haemorrhage. Jones et al. (1973) found that patients who suffered recurrent haemorrhage after admission had a fourfold increase in mortality rate, and they suggested that these patients should be submitted to early surgery in the hope of reducing this high mortality. Recent studies have shown a significant improvement in mortality by aggressive surgical intervention in high-risk patients (Morris et al., 1984; Wheatley and Dykes, 1990; Holman et al., 1990). The indications for surgical intervention recommended by these workers are: (a) exsanguinating haemorrhage or a spurting vessel at endoscopy; (b) in patients aged 60 or over – one rebleed, 4 units of blood for initial resuscitation, or 8 per 48 h during recovery; (c) in patients aged less than 60 – two rebleeds, 8 units for initial resuscitation or 12 per 48 h during recovery (Wheatley and Dykes, 1990). Using these criteria, the mortality rate has been brought down to 5%, despite a steadily ageing population.

Choice of operation for bleeding peptic ulcer

The aim of emergency surgery under these circumstances is to arrest the haemorrhage. Although important, a secondary consideration is the possibility of any sequelae as a result of the particular procedure. In the majority of cases the diagnosis will be made endoscopically preoperatively, but where this is not possible a gastrotomy or duodenotomy may be necessary to identify the site of bleeding.

Duodenal ulcer. With bleeding duodenal ulcer, the most frequently performed operation is underrunning of the ulcer with an atraumatic suture inserted as a Z stitch. One of the newer absorbable sutures should be used because these can guarantee retention of tensile strength until the ulcer has healed. The duodenotomy which has transgressed the pylorus is then closed as a Heineke–Mikulicz pyloroplasty and is followed by truncal vagotomy. This operation has the advantage over Polya gastrectomy of a much lower postoperative morbidity and mortality. Clark (1968) reported a postoperative mortality falling from 16% to 5% on changing his operation from partial gastrectomy to vagotomy and pyloroplasty. Schiller et al. (1970) reported a similar drop from 14.3%

for Polya gastrectomy to 5.5% with vagotomy and pyloroplasty. The recurrent bleeding rate is said to be no greater after vagotomy and pyloroplasty than after gastrectomy. Bleeding duodenal ulcers are almost invariably posterior penetrating ulcers, and when Polya gastrectomy was the routine operation the mobilization of the duodenum and the closure of the duodenal stump were more difficult than usual, and as a result of this there was an increased incidence of leakage from the duodenal stump which increased the postoperative morbidity and contributed to the mortality.

Control of the bleeding duodenal ulcer through a small duodenotomy, followed by highly selective vagotomy, may be used when the surgeon is experienced in the procedure and where the patient's condition is satisfactory. However, if the surgeon is relatively inexperienced in the technique, it is probably better to do a good truncal vagotomy in a reasonable time rather than a prolonged procedure with a possible incomplete highly selective vagotomy.

Gastric ulcer. Where the bleeding ulcer is in the distal half of the stomach, Billroth-I gastrectomy is still the most commonly performed operation, but this procedure carries a higher mortality than simple underrunning of the ulcer coupled with truncal vagotomy and pyloroplasty. Although sleeve resection of the lesser curve (Pauchet manoeuvre) will allow resection of a slightly higher gastric ulcer, it would seem that oversewing the ulcer with some form of vagotomy is advisable for the high bleeding gastric ulcer. Truncal vagotomy will be the more speedy procedure and will be necessary if the patient's condition is poor. However, Johnston has described the use of highly selective vagotomy under these circumstances. Clearly this could only be used by a surgeon who is skilled in the procedure which might well be more difficult under these circumstances because of the associated induration adjacent to the gastric ulcer. Once again, a complete truncal vagotomy may be preferable to an incomplete highly selective vagotomy. Local excision and vagotomy may also be carried out for the high gastric ulcer.

Perforation

The treatment of acute perforated ulcer in most hospitals is operative. Some surgeons use conservative treatment and Taylor (1951) described a series with a mortality of 9.6%. He recommended this treatment, however, only for those perforations where he considered there were good prospects of sealing off, such as the small duodenal perforation where there were signs of localization at the time they were first seen. He recommended that it should be instituted if some other factor such as heart or lung disease was present to contraindicate surgery. This may account for only 5% of all acute perforations.

The majority of perforations will be treated surgically and the procedure will depend, first, on whether the ulcer is acute or chronic, and, secondly, on the site of the ulcer.

In the case of duodenal perforation where there is no history of indigestion and at operation where there is no sign of chronicity, the correct treatment is simple closure of the perforation with an omental patch. With acute ulcer, 75% have good results, 25% relapse, and some may require further surgery. In the case of perforation of a chronic ulcer, the story is very different with approximately 80% developing recurrent ulceration and in the past over 50% requiring a second definitive procedure. Hence such patients should be treated by closure of the perforation combined with a definitive procedure, provided that they are fit enough to withstand a more lengthy procedure. This procedure should be either a truncal vagotomy and drainage or preferably a highly selective vagotomy if the surgeon performing the procedure has the necessary experience.

The mortality from perforation of a gastric ulcer is very much greater than that from duodenal ulcer when treated by simple suture, and most of these deaths are due to reperforation. This problem can be prevented by carrying out a definitive procedure in all cases of perforated gastric ulcer. With the advent of laparoscopic abdominal surgery, it is now possible to repair a perforated peptic ulcer either by suture or by a plug (Mouret *et al.*, 1990).

Pyloric stenosis and hour-glass contracture of the stomach

Pyloric stenosis

The term 'pyloric stenosis' is sometimes a misnomer, as the obstruction is often in the duodenum. A degree of narrowing is a common occurrence following the healing of a juxtapyloric or duodenal ulcer. This narrowing is not necessarily reflected by clinical symptoms of obstruction or radiological evidence of delayed emptying. This slight narrowing may be fully compensated by muscular hypertrophy of the stomach. The development of clinical symptoms of pyloric obstruction is often due to an exacerbation of the ulcer with increased narrowing from oedema in the presence of an already compromised lumen. The resultant gastric stasis may result in gross electrolyte disturbances in addition to weight loss.

The initial procedure in these patients is to improve their general condition by rehydration, and correction of their electrolyte and pH imbalance with appropriate intravenous infusions. The stomach is emptied each evening by the passage of a gastric tube. This has to be at least 32 Fr. gauge to remove some of the more solid material from the stomach. To pass this it may be necessary to spray the throat with Xylocaine (lignocaine) and to lay the patient flat and on his side to prevent aspiration of gastric contents. As the oedema resolves, the volume of gastric residue decreases and becomes clearer. The bacterial count in the stomach will decrease and the chance of any wound infection following subsequent surgery will be reduced. In the case of malignant pyloric obstruction, the gastric lavage makes no difference to the volume of gastric residue.

The surgical management of duodenal stenosis has changed over the years. Originally, partial gastrectomy was widely used. However, Ellis et al. (1966) reported the results of a series of cases treated by truncal vagotomy and drainage and showed that it was unnecessary to resect the distended stomach as it gradually returns to a normal size over the ensuing months. More recently, Johnston has shown that these cases may be treated by highly selective vagotomy, the duodenal drainage being improved by either a duodenoplasty, not traversing and damaging the pylorus, or alternatively dilating the pylorus and adjacent duodenum with Hegar's dilators through a gastrotomy in the antrum (Johnston et al., 1973). There have been reports of rupture of the duodenum following dilatation and there has now been a move away from this procedure.

Hour-glass deformity of the stomach

Large chronic gastric ulcers may cause marked distortion of the stomach. This initially may represent a degree of spasm but is replaced by fibrosis as the ulcer heals. The ultimate result of this process may be the division of the stomach into two parts by a narrow zone of fibrosis and often some residual ulceration. This deformity is known as the 'hour-glass stomach'. It tends to occur more frequently in women and the symptoms resemble pyloric stenosis. The diagnosis may be made by barium studies, but endoscopy will certainly be required to exclude malignancy. This is a rare surgical problem, but when it occurs the treatment of choice is gastrectomy which relieves the obstruction and also removes the cause of the gastric ulcer.

Chronic penetration of adjacent organs

Peptic ulcers as they enlarge may completely penetrate the wall of the stomach, duodenum or jejunum but may remain completely walled off from the peritoneal cavity by adhesions. Duodenal ulcer commonly penetrates into the pancreas and may rarely ultimately involve the common bile duct. Chronic gastric ulcers may penetrate the pancreas or the liver, while a stomal ulcer following partial gastrectomy may involve the chest wall or colon, causing severe pain or gastrojejunocolic fistula.

The management of the surgical problems presented has already been discussed, with the exception of gastrojejunocolic fistula. Preoperatively, patients may be emaciated following intractable diarrhoea and the consequent malabsorption. This may be improved by intravenous hyperalimentation and, while this is being achieved, endoscopy and biopsy may be carried out to exclude malignancy. If the ulcer is benign the possibility of a Zollinger–Ellison syndrome should be considered and serum gastrin studies will be required. If these results are normal, laparotomy will be necessary and the original gastric anastomosis will have to be dismantled and freed from the colon. If the hole in the colon is small, it may be oversewn. If large, local resection will be necessary. A fresh gastrojejunal anastomosis can be fashioned following resection of originally involved tissue. To avoid further peptic ulceration, a truncal or alternatively selective vagotomy should be added.

Ulcerogenic tumours of the pancreas (Zollinger–Ellison syndrome) (gastrinoma)

This syndrome was first described in 1955 and consists of a triad:

1. The presence of primary peptic ulceration in unusual locations, that is, in the second or third portions of the duodenum, upper jejunum or recurrent stomal ulcers following any gastric surgery short of total gastrectomy.
2. Marked gastric hypersecretion despite adequate or even intensive conventional or surgical therapy.
3. Identification of non-specific islet cell tumours of the pancreas.

The clinical syndrome may be that of severe diarrhoea or steatorrhoea, but the symptoms are ordinarily those of a fulminating ulcer, which is intractable to the usual treatment. The diagnosis may be suggested by barium studies showing huge mucosal folds with considerable fluid retention in the stomach. The duodenum tends to be enlarged and irregular in appearance, with one or more ulcers in an unusual location such as the second or third portion of the duodenum. Ulceration just beyond the ligament of Treitz is pathognomonic of an ulcerogenic tumour.

Barium studies after previous gastric resection may show multiple deep penetrating ulcers in the mesenteric border of the efferent loop rather than the usual marginal location. Gastric analyses are helpful, basal acid output > 15 mmol/h and the resting juice usually being in excess of 60% of the volume obtained following the augmented histamine study. The measurement of a serum gastrin level is now the mainstay of diagnosis (fasting level > 1000 pg/ml). Gastrinomas can occur sporadically or in combination with other endocrine tumours in a familiar setting, the so-called multiple endocrine neoplasia type I (MEN-I) syndrome. Hyperparathyroidism is the commonest endocrine abnormality in this setting (Farndon, 1990).

Approximately 70% of patients with ulcerogenic syndrome have multiple foci of gastrin-producing tumour and 60% of these are malignant. The tumours may be single or multiple and they may be very small or reasonably large. Seventy-five per cent will have metastases to either the liver or regional lymph nodes by the time of surgery. A small percentage of patients will have either diffuse islet cell hyperplasia (Polak *et al.*, 1972) or multiple benign adenomatosis. The majority of patients with Zollinger–Ellison syndrome, despite the fact that many are malignant, are now being treated medically with either H_2 antagonists or the H^+-K^+-ATPase blocking agent Omeprazole.

Surgical management

Once the diagnosis has been made, preoperative localization is usually undertaken. Selective arteriography, and CT scans, with or without contrast enhancement, will localize some tumours. Intraoperatively, real time ultrasound may also be used (Cromack *et al.*, 1987).

The management of this condition has changed in recent years. Prior to 1976 and the advent of H_2 receptor blocking drugs nearly all patients underwent total gastrectomy, thus removing the target organ from the excess of circulating gastrin. However, it is now possible to control the gastrin hypersecretion state pharmacologically and the role of total gastrectomy, lesser resection and even laparotomy has been reassessed (Mee *et al.*, 1983). Effective control of the hypersecretion has promoted a conservative approach in those patients whose investigations have failed to localize the primary tumour or where there is evidence of metastatic disease. While gastrinomas are slow growing and symptoms may be controlled pharmacologically, the only hope of cure is resection of an isolated tumour. Suitable patients are subjected to exploratory laparotomy and, unless a localized tumour is found and resected, truncal vagotomy and pyloroplasty are performed to assist in the subsequent control of acid hypersecretion. Subsequently, H_2 receptor antagonists or an H^+-K^+-ATPase blocking agent (Omeprazole) will provide good long-term medical control of continued hypersecretion of acid. Somatostatin analogue, SMS-201-995 or octreotide may also be used (Vinik, 1988). Total gastrectomy is reserved for patients in whom acid hypersecretion is not controlled pharmacologically. Chemotherapy is used when symptoms are due directly to the tumour and not to acid hypersecretion. 5-fluorouracil and streptozotocin have been helpful in producing relief of symptoms for over 12 months, but the long-term outlook is not known.

References

Alexander-Williams, J. (1973) Gastric reconstructive surgery. *Ann. R. Coll. Surg. Engl.*, **52**, 1–17

Amdrup, E. and Jensen, H.-E. (1970) Selective vagotomy of the parietal cell mass preserving innervation of the undrained antrum. *Gastroenterology*, **59**, 522–527

Burge, H. (1964) *Vagotomy*, Edward Arnold, London

Clark, C. G. (1968) Surgical aspects of gastrointestinal haemorrhage. *Postgrad. Med. J.*, **44**, 590–593

Clark, C. G., Fresini, A. and Gledhill, T. (1985) Cancer following gastric surgery. *Br. J. Surg.*, **72**, 591–594

Cockel, R. (1987) NSAIDs – should every prescription carry a Government Health Warning? *Gut*, **28**, 515–518

Cooper, M. J. and Williamson, R. C. N. (1984) Splenectomy: indications, hazards and alternatives. *Br. J. Surg.*, **71**, 173–180

Cromack, D. T., Norton, J. A., Sigel, B. *et al.* (1987) The use of high-resolution intraoperative ultrasound to localize gastrinomas: an initial report of a prospective study. *Wld J. Surg.*, **11**, 648–653

Csendes, A., Larach, J. and Godoy, M. (1978) Incidence of gallstone development after selective hepatic vagotomy. *Acta Chir. Scand.*, **144**, 289–291

Dooley, C. P. and Cohen, H. (1988) The clinical significance of *Campylobacter pylori*. *Ann. Intern. Med.*, **108**, 70–79

Dorricott, N. J., McNeish, A. R., Alexander-Williams, J. *et al.* (1978) Prospective randomized multi-centre trial of proximal gastric vagotomy or truncal vagotomy and antrectomy for chronic duodenal ulcer. *Br. J. Surg.*, **65**, 152–154

Ellis, H., Starer, F., Venables, C. *et al.* (1966) Clinical and radiological study of vagotomy and gastric drainage in the treatment of pyloric stenosis due to duodenal ulcer. *Gut*, **7**, 671–676

Farndon, J.R. (1990) Gastrin and gastrinomas. *Br. J. Surg.*, **77**, 1–2

Franksson, C. (1948) Selective abdominal vagotomy. *Acta Chir. Scand.*, **96**, 409

Gatehouse, D., Dimmock, F., Burdon, R. W. *et al.* (1978) Prediction of wound sepsis following gastric operations. *Br. J. Surg.*, **65**, 551–554

Gear, M. W. L., Truelove S. C. and Whitehead R. (1971) Gastric ulcer and gastritis. *Gut*, **12**, 639–645

Goligher, J. C. (1974) A technique for highly selective (parietal cell or proximal gastric) vagotomy for duodenal ulcer. *Br. J. Surg.*, **61**, 337–345

Grassi, G. (1971) A new test for complete nerve section during vagotomy. *Br. J. Surg.*, **58**, 187–189

Holman, R. A. E., Davis, M., Gough, K. R. *et al.* (1990) Value of a centralised approach in the management of haematemesis and melaena: experience in a district general hospital. *Gut*, **31**, 504–508

Houghton, P. W. J., Mortensen, N. J. McC, Thomas, W.E.G. *et al.* (1986) Intragastric bile acids and histological changes in gastric mucosa. *Br. J. Surg.*, **73**, 354–356

Humphrey, C. S., Johnston, D., Walker, B. E. *et al.* (1972) Incidence of dumping after truncal and selective vagotomy with pyloroplasty and HSV without drainage procedure. *Br. Med. J.*, **3**, 785–788

Jackson, R. G. (1948) Anatomic study of the vagus nerves. *Arch. Surg.*, **57**, 333

Jenkins, T. P. N. (1976) The burst abdominal wound, a mechanical approach. *Br. J. Surg.*, **63**, 873–876

Johnston, D. (1975) Operative mortality and post-operative morbidity of highly selective vagotomy. *Br. J. Surg.*, **62**, 160

Johnston, D., Lyndon, P. J., Smith, R. B. *et al.* (1973) Highly selective vagotomy without a drainage procedure in the treatment of haemorrhage, perforation and pyloric stenosis due to peptic ulcer. *Br. J. Surg.*, **60**, 790–797

Johnston, D. and Wilkinson, A. R. (1970) Highly selective vagotomy without drainage procedure in the treatment of duodenal ulcer. *Br. J. Surg.*, **57**, 289–296

Johnston, G. W., Spencer, E. F. A., Wilkinson, A. J. and Kennedy, T. L. (1991) Proximal gastric vagotomy: follow-up at 10–20 years. *Br. J. Surg.*, **78**, 20–23

Jones, P. F., Johnston, S. F., McEwan, A. B. *et al.* (1973) Further haemorrhage after admission to hospital for gastrointestinal haemorrhage. *Br. Med. J.*, **3**, 660–664

Kennedy, J. (1973) In *Vagotomy on Trial* (eds A. G. Cox and J. A. Williams), Heinemann, London, p.95

Koruth, N. M., Dua, K. S., Brunt, P. W. and Matheson, N. A. (1990) Comparison of highly selective vagotomy with truncal vagotomy and pyloroplasty: results at 8–15 years. *Br. J. Surg.*, **77**, 70–72

Langman, M. J. S. (1988) Ulcer complications and non-steroidal anti-inflammatory drugs. *Am. J. Surg.*, **84**, 15–19

Lavigne, M. E., Wiley, Z. D., Martin, P. *et al.* (1979) A study of gastric, pancreatic and biliary secretion and the rate of gastric emptying following parietal cell vagotomy. *Am. J. Surg.*, **138**, 644–651

MacGregor, I. L., Parent, J. and Meyer, J. H. (1977) Gastric emptying of liquid meals and pancreatic and biliary secretion after subtotal gastrectomy or truncal vagotomy and pyloroplasty in man. *Gastroenterology*, **72**, 195–205

Macintyre, I. M. C., Millar, A., Smith, A. N. and Small, W. P. (1990) Highly selective vagotomy 5–15 years on. *Br. J. Surg.*, **77**, 65–69

Malagelada, J. R., Go, V. L. W. and Summerskill, W. H. J. (1974) Altered pancreatic biliary function after vagotomy and pyloroplasy. *Gastroenterology*, **66**, 22–27

Mee, A. S., Ismail, S., Bornman, P. C. *et al.* (1983) Changing concepts in the presentation, diagnosis and management of the Zollinger–Ellison syndrome. *Q. J. Med.*, **52**, 256–267

Morris, D. L., Hawker, P. C., Brearley, S. *et al.* (1984) Optimal timing of operation for bleeding peptic ulcer: prospective randomised trial. *Br. Med. J.*, **288**, 1277–1280

Moss, S. and Calam, J. (1992) *Helicobacter pylori* and peptic ulcers: the present position. *Gut*, **33**, 289–292

Mouret, P., Francois, Y., Vignal, J. *et al.* (1990) Laparoscopic treatment of perforated peptic ulcer. *Br. J. Surg.*, **77**, 1006

Parkin, G. J. S., Smith, R. B. and Johnston, D. (1973) Gall bladder volume and contractility after truncal, selective and highly selective (parietal cell) vagotomy in man. *Ann. Surg.*, **178**, 581–586

Polak, J. M., Stagg, B. and Pearse, A. G. E. (1972) Two types of Z–E syndrome, immunofluorescent, cytochemical and ultrastructural studies of the antral and pancreatic gastric cells in different clinical states. *Gut*, **13**, 501

Pollock, A. V., Greenhall, M. J. and Evans, M. (1979) Single layer mass closure of major laparotomies by continuous suturing. *J. Roy. Soc. Med.*, **72**, 889–893

Portis, S. A. and Jaffe, R. H. (1938) A study of peptic ulcer based on necropsy records. *JAMA*, **110**, 6

Rudick, J. and Hutchinson, J. S. F. (1964) Effects of vagal nerve section on the biliary system. *Lancet*, **1**, 579–581

Schiller, K. F. R., Trulove, S. C. and Williams, D. C. (1970) Haematemesis and melaena with special reference to factors influencing outcome. *Br. Med. J.*, **2**, 7

Sidebotham, R. L. and Baron, J. H. (1990) Hypothesis: *Helicobacter pylori*, urease, mucus, and gastric ulcer. *Lancet*, **335**, 193–195

Sim, E., Tekant, Y., Kum, C. K. *et al.* (1991) Endoscopic management of bleeding peptic ulcer in Singapore: a multimodality approach. *J. Roy. Coll. Surg. Edinb.*, **36**, 388–391

Spychal, R. T., Goggin, P. M., Marrero, J. M. *et al.* (1990) Surface hydrophobicity of gastric mucosa in peptic ulcer disease. Relationship to gastritis and *Campylobacter pylori* infection. *Gastroenterology*, **98**, 1250–1254

Stammers, F. A. R. and Williams, J. A. (1963) *Partial Gastrectomy*, Butterworths, London, pp. 49–53.

Steele, R. J. C., Park, K. G. M. and Crofts, T. J. (1991) Adrenaline injection for endoscopic haemostasis in non-variceal upper gastrointestinal haemorrhage. *Br. J. Surg.*, **78**, 477–479.

Tanner, N. C. (1951) Operative methods in treatment of peptic ulcer. *Edinb. Med. J.*, **58**, 279

Taylor, H. (1951) Aspiration treatment of perforated ulcers. *Lancet*, **1**, 7

Taylor, T. V., Lythgoe, J. P., McFarland, J. B. *et al.* (1990) Anterior lesser curve seromyotomy and posterior truncal vagotomy versus truncal vagotomy and pyloroplasty in the treatment of chronic duodenal ulcer. *Br. J. Surg.*, **77**, 1007–1009

Taylor, T. V., MacLeod, D. A. D., Gunn, A. A. *et al.* (1982) Anterior lesser curve seromyotomy and posterior truncal vagotomy in the treatment of chronic duodenal ulcer. *Lancet*, **ii**, 846–848

Tudhope, G. R. (1958) Loss and replacement of red cells in patients with acute gastrointestinal haemorrhage. *Q. J. Med.*, **27**, 543–559.

Vinik, A. I., Tsai, S., Moattari, A. R. and Cheung, P. (1988) Somatostatin analogue (SMS-201-995) in patients with gastrinomas. *Surgery*, **104**, 834–842

Voeller, G. R., Pridgen, W. L. and Mangiante, E. C. (1991) Laparoscopic posterior truncal vagotomy and anterior seromyotomy: a porcine model. *J. Lap. Surg.*, **1**, 375–378

Walt, R. P., Cottrell, J., Mann, S. G. *et al.* (1992) Continuous intravenous famotidine for haemorrhage from peptic ulcer. *Lancet*, **ii**, 1058–1062

Warren, J. R. and Marshall, B. (1983) Unidentified curved bacilli on gastric epithelium in active chronic gastritis. *Lancet*, **i**, 1273–1275

Wheatley, K. E. and Dykes, P. W. (1990) Upper gastrointestinal bleeding – when to operate. *Postgrad. Med. J.*, **66**, 926–931

Younan, F., Pearson, J., Allen, A. *et al.* (1982) Changes in the structure of mucous gel on the mucosal surface of the stomach in association with peptic ulcer disease. *Gastroenterology*, **82**, 827–831

13

The pancreas

R. C. N. Williamson

Besides their intimate anatomical relationship, the exocrine and endocrine portions of the pancreas (Greek: 'all flesh') possess complementary functions in the digestion, absorption and metabolism of foodstuffs. The symptoms and signs of pancreatic disease may be slow to develop because of the relatively inaccessible position of the gland and its functional reserve; the ultimate effects tend to be wide ranging and severe. Trauma and acute inflammation can both cause extravasation of powerful digestive enzymes from the pancreas, with potentially devastating local and systemic sequelae. Chronic parenchymal destruction (often by alcohol) produces combined exocrine and endocrine impairment, and the combination of steatorrhoea and diabetes mellitus is reproduced by surgical excision of enough functioning pancreatic tissue. Usually advanced by the time of presentation, exocrine carcinoma tends to be rapidly lethal. Islet cell tumours, though rare, are increasingly recognized and give rise to a variety of fascinating clinical syndromes.

In this chapter, a brief outline of the anatomy of the pancreas is followed by a discussion of the various pathological processes that can affect the gland, including modern methods of diagnosis and treatment. Lastly, the common pancreatic operations are described. Since the surgery of the pancreas frequently involves that of neighbouring abdominal viscera, the relevant chapters on the stomach, biliary tree and spleen should also be consulted.

Surgical anatomy

The pancreas is draped against the posterior abdominal wall by the peritoneum bordering the lesser sac and, along its inferior border, by the root of the transverse mesocolon. The head of the gland lies snug in the duodenal loop. It is connected by a slight waist at the neck to the body and tail of the pancreas, which pass to the left and gradually upwards, tapering gently to end at the splenic hilum. The uncinate process (Latin: 'hooked') arises from the lower part of the head and projects to the left, behind the superior mesenteric vein and artery but in front of the inferior vena cava and aorta. Anteriorly the body of the pancreas is separated from the stomach by the lesser sac, and posteriorly the tail of the gland is related to the left kidney and adrenal. The common bile duct traverses the head of the pancreas in a groove that is palpable posteriorly.

The pancreatic head and duodenal loop share a common arterial supply (Figure 13.1) derived from the gastroduodenal and superior mesenteric arteries via the anterior and posterior pancreaticoduodenal arcades. The distal part of the gland receives blood from branches of the splenic artery, which pursues a sinuous course along its upper border. In about 25% of people, the right hepatic artery (or an accessory vessel) arises from the superior mesenteric artery and supplies the head of the pancreas. Venous drainage (Figure 13.2) is by corresponding veins entering the

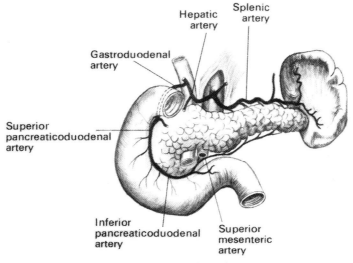

Figure 13.1 Arterial supply to the pancreas

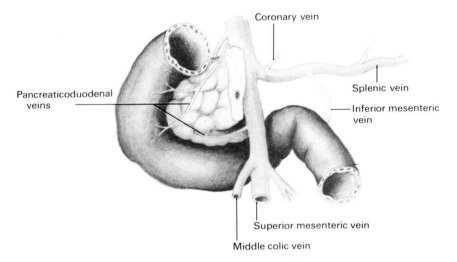

Figure 13.2 Venous drainage of the pancreas

superior mesenteric and splenic trunks; these unite to form the hepatic portal vein directly behind the neck of the pancreas. The gastric (coronary) vein usually joins the portal vein close to its origin, and the inferior mesenteric vein enters the terminal part of the splenic vein. Pancreatic lymphatics accompany the blood vessels and drain to nodes near the duodenum and pylorus and along the hepatic and splenic arteries; lymph then travels to the coeliac and superior mesenteric groups of lymph nodes.

Postganglionic sympathetic nerves and afferent fibres conveying pain sensation from the pancreas are relayed through the splanchnic nerves and coeliac plexus. Parasympathetic fibres from the vagus nerve provide a secretomotor supply to the exocrine gland and act in association with the duodenal hormones, secretin and cholecystokinin. Besides water and electrolytes (notably bicarbonate), alkaline pancreatic juice contains proteolytic and lipolytic enzymes as inactive zymogens as well as enzymes capable of splitting carbohydrate and nucleic acids.

During embryological development, dorsal and ventral pancreatic buds grow separately from opposite sides of the duodenum at the junction of the foregut and midgut; subsequently the gland retains a dual blood supply from foregut (coeliac) and midgut (superior mesenteric) arteries. The dorsal pancreas forms most of the adult gland apart from the lower part of the head and uncinate process, which arise from the ventral moiety. In association with the primitive bile duct, the ventral pancreas rotates around the duodenum and fuses with the dorsal outgrowth during the 7th week (Figure 13.3a). Following normal communication of the two ductal systems, the ventral pancreatic duct (of Wirsung) becomes dilated and acts as the final pathway for exocrine secretion from both the embryological parts of the gland (Figure 13.3b).

The common bile duct usually joins the duct of Wirsung as the two ducts pierce the medial wall of the descending limb of the duodenum, forming a short common channel (ampulla of Vater). The ampulla is surrounded by the circular muscle sphincter of Oddi and opens at the summit of a small papilla, lying 8–10 cm distal to the pylorus. Occasionally, the two ducts enter the duodenum separately at the apex of this (major) papilla. When present, a minor or accessory pancreatic papilla projects into the duodenum about 2 cm proximally and drains the terminal portion of the dorsal pancreatic duct (of Santorini).

The exocrine pancreas is a compound racemose gland. Acinar cells make up about 80% of the volume of the pancreas. Endocrine tissue is scattered throughout the pancreas in discrete islets of Langerhans, with a relative preponderance (about 70%) in the body and tail. Islet cells elaborate insulin, glucagon, pancreatic polypeptide (PP) and somatostatin. The four different cell types can be identified by their secretory granules.

Congenital pancreatic abnormalities

Annular pancreas

Incomplete rotation of the ventral pancreas causes the rare condition of annular pancreas, in which the second part of the duodenum is encircled by pancreatic tissue. If the ring is complete and tight, the condition presents in early neonatal life with persistent vomiting, usually of bile-stained material; other congenital anomalies are commonly associated. The classic appearance of a 'double bubble' on plain abdominal radiography is produced by gaseous distension of both the stomach and duodenal cap. Annular pancreas may not cause symptoms until adult life, when gastric outlet obstruction supervenes. Barium

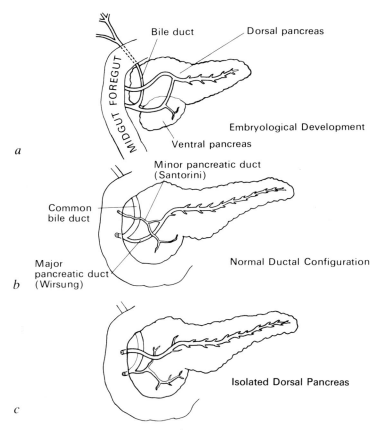

Figure 13.3 Embryological development of the pancreas. The gland develops from dorsal and ventral pancreatic buds which fuse during the 7th week of intra-uterine life (*a*). The normal adult configuration of the pancreatic ducts (*b*) includes a communication between the Wirsung and Santorini systems. In isolated dorsal pancreas or pancreas divisum (*c*) the two ductal systems remain entirely independent and the dorsal pancreas drains solely through the accessory papilla

meal and endoscopic examinations localize the site of obstruction to the second part of the duodenum. There may be associated pancreatitis or duodenal ulcer disease.

Since the annulus always contains a sizeable pancreatic duct, operative division of the ring has an unacceptable risk of pancreatic fistula. Moreover, the obstruction may not even be relieved, because the underlying duodenum is usually hypoplastic. Annular pancreas should therefore be circumvented by duodenoduodenostomy (where possible) or by duodenojejunostomy or retrocolic gastroenterostomy.

Ectopic (aberrant) pancreas

Islands of ectopic (aberrant) pancreas may occur in the wall of the small bowel at any point (including Meckel's diverticulum), but especially in the duodenum. These embryological rests are generally found within the submucosa and seldom give rise to symptoms.

Congenital pancreatic cysts

These are described later in this chapter (page 168).

Pancreatic ductal anomalies

Though common, these are of uncertain clinical relevance. The duct of Santorini and the accessory papilla may close or disappear during fetal life, leaving the major pancreatic ductal system to drain all the exocrine secretion. Alternatively, the duct of Wirsung may atrophy or remain very small, so that pancreatic juice escapes via the Santorini system. Virtual agenesis of either dorsal or ventral pancreas may even occur. Lastly, failure of fusion of the two ductal systems can result in the separate embryological components draining independently in the duodenum (Figure 13.3c). This anomaly of 'pancreas divisum'* is normally discovered at endoscopic retrograde choledochopancreatography† (ERCP).

* The term 'pancreas divisum' is slightly misleading, since it suggests physical separation of the two embryological moieties. 'Isolated dorsal pancreas' indicates that it is probably inadequate drainage of the body and tail that gives rise to symptoms.
† The pancreatogram obtained by cannulation of the major pancreatic papilla, as confirmed by the concomitant visualization of the biliary tree, is limited to the head and uncinate process. Cannulation of the minor papilla, though technically difficult, will establish the diagnosis.

Isolation of the dorsal pancreas from the major papilla should protect against gallstone pancreatitis. However, pancreas divisum may be commoner in patients with recurrent idiopathic pancreatitis. Perhaps the narrow duct of the dorsal pancreas is unable to cope with most of the pancreatic secretion, so that partial obstruction results. Endoscopic division of the accessory sphincter is technically demanding and may not provide lasting benefit. Transduodenal accessory sphincteroplasty may reduce the incidence of recurrent acute pancreatitis in such patients. The contribution of pancreas divisum to chronic abdominal pain and chronic pancreatitis is more controversial, although we have occasionally found periductal fibrosis in caudal pancreatectomy specimens in patients with no other cause for their symptoms.

Pancreatic trauma

Because the pancreas is placed deep within the upper adomen, it is well protected against moderate external forces, and pancreatic trauma constitutes only 1–3% of all abdominal injuries. As a corollary, the mortality rate is about 30%. Serious pancreatic injury is encountered among automobile drivers involved in road traffic accidents, in which the gland is compressed against the vertebral column by the impact of the steering wheel (Figure 13.4); seat belts should protect against this type of injury. Blunt trauma sufficient to disrupt the pancreas often damages adjacent viscera as well, and the resulting injuries, especially of major blood vessels, may prove lethal. Penetrating wounds of the pancreas almost always involve neighbouring organs in addition. Generally knife wounds carry a better prognosis than those caused by bullets or shot, and injuries from high-velocity missiles are lethal. The pancreas is at risk of operative trauma during splenectomy or occasionally gastrectomy (e.g. for penetrating ulcers), and pancreatitis is a recognized complication of endoscopic or surgical manoeuvres involving the sphincter of Oddi.

The prognosis and management of pancreatic injuries vary widely with the actual site of trauma to the gland. Injuries of the distal body or tail are usually the least severe, though they may be associated with damage to the spleen, stomach, diaphragm, left kidney or left colonic flexure. Trauma to the mid-pancreas (neck and proximal body) may be an isolated injury, typically a partial or complete fracture of the gland where it crosses the spine. There may be concomitant injuries of the liver, stomach, transverse colon or superior mesenteric vessels, however. Injuries of the pancreatic head are the most serious and the most difficult to manage. They often combine extensive destruction of the pancreas with duodenal trauma, which may also involve the bile duct and portal vein, liver, right kidney or right colonic flexure.

The clinical features of pancreatic trauma are

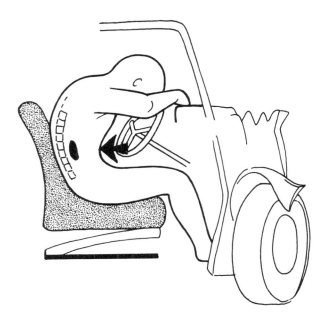

Figure 13.4 Pancreatic trauma. The common mechanism of injury

sometimes slow to develop; they include hypotension, an abdominal mass and evidence of peritonitis. Repeated estimations of serum amylase should be obtained, and high amylase contents may also be detected in fluid obtained by diagnostic peritoneal lavage. Following resuscitation of the patient, any suspected pancreatic injury requires early laparotomy and thorough exposure of the entire gland, together with the duodenum and duodenojejunal flexure. Haematomas in the duodenopancreatic region should always be explored. The principles of treatment include control of haemorrhage by ligation and suture, search for ductal damage and leakage of pancreatic juice, resection of devitalized tissue and extensive drainage. For lesions to the right of the midline, internal drainage of the injured area into a Roux loop of jejunum may be a safer option than pancreato-duodenectomy. Lesions to the left of the midline (including fracture of the neck of pancreas) are best treated by distal pancreatectomy, with or without splenectomy.

The late complications of pancreatic trauma are external pancreatic fistulas, sometimes accompanied by intestinal contents, and pseudocyst formation. Detectable by serial scanning with ultrasound or computed tomography (CT), traumatic cysts need early operative intervention because of the risk of haemorrhage, rupture or infection.

Acute pancreatitis

This term embraces a range of conditions that vary in severity from mild and transient oedema of the gland to widespread pancreatic necrosis. The overall mortality rate is at least 10%. The common presence of cholelithiasis* and the frequency with which small calculi can be recovered from the stools after an attack suggests that the passage of a small stone through the papilla may render the sphincteric mechanism incompetent, allowing duodenal reflux along the duct of Wirsung and thus intrapancreatic activation of the digestive enzymes.

Acute pancreatitis typically presents with epigastric pain of rapid onset, which radiates to the back and causes vomiting. Signs of peritonitis, often generalized in extent, may be accompanied by evidence of shock, dehydration, cyanosis or mild jaundice. Elevation of the serum amylase remains the single most valuable diagnostic test: levels usually exceed 1200 i.u./litre (600 Somogyi units/dl), and hyperamylasaemia of this degree is seldom seen in the absence of pancreatitis. Equally common, though non-specific, findings include an absolute neutrophilia and mild derangement of liver function tests. Blood gas analysis often reveals a surprisingly low arterial Po_2. Initial hypocalcaemia ($\times 8.0$ mmol/litre) denotes a severe attack, although later reductions in serum calcium reflect the fall in albumin concentration. Elevations in serum C-reactive protein reflect the severity of the disease. Analysis of peritoneal fluid obtained by paracentesis (with or without lavage) may confirm the severity of pancreatitis and help to exclude other causes of peritonitis, such as perforated peptic ulcer or gangrenous cholecystitis. Likewise, plain abdominal radiographs may be of value in the differential diagnosis, besides showing certain characteristic features of pancreatitis such as distension of the duodenal cap or a 'sentinel loop' of jejunum. Serial CT scanning is useful to monitor the extent and progress of the inflammatory process.

Management

Management of acute pancreatitis is hampered by the lack of any specific treatment for the disease and by difficulty in predicting the severity of the attack at the time of admission. The dominant requirement is rapid replacement of the large volumes of extracellular fluid sequestrated in the retroperitoneal pancreatic 'burn'. Several litres of intravenous fluid are often needed, including some units of plasma or plasma substitute; in these cases central venous pressure, haematocrit and serum urea and electrolytes must be carefully monitored. A nasogastric tube should be passed immediately to diminish upper alimentary secretion.

* In the UK, gallstones are present in over half the cases of acute pancreatitis, whereas in France and the USA alcoholism is commonly associated. Pancreatitis may follow abdominal trauma or operative procedures such as Polya gastrectomy, sphincterotomy and pancreatic biopsy. All series contain a proportion of 'idiopathic' cases, in which no definite aetiogical agent can be implicated.

Analgesia is best provided by parenteral administration of pethidine. Arterial hypoxaemia is countered by giving oxygen by face mask or, if necessary, by endotracheal intubation with assisted ventilation. Blood, calcium and vitamin supplements may be given intravenously. Antispasmodics are of doubtful value. Antibiotics are probably best reserved for septic complications. Steroids are contraindicated. H_2 receptor antagonists may prevent stress ulceration and bleeding in a seriously ill patient.

With supportive measures many cases of acute pancreatitis will resolve within 2–5 days, allowing a gradual return to oral feeding (with a low fat diet), but persisting ileus should be managed by intravenous hyperalimentation. Agents that diminish exocrine secretion (e.g. glucagon) or inhibit pancreatic enzymes (e.g. aprotinin) do not appear to ameliorate established pancreatitis, probably because of the invariable delay (mean about 24 h) between onset of symptoms and start of treatment. Somatostatin, free radical scavengers and plasmaphaeresis are other treatments of unproven value. Urgent endoscopic papillotomy may be beneficial in a severe attack of acute gallstone pancreatitis, but considerable technical expertise is required to avoid serious complications.

Peritoneal lavage has been recommended in the early treatment of severe pancreatitis or for subsequent pancreatic abscess. It is carried out through a dialysis catheter introduced into the pelvis via a small incision sited either in the midline below the umbilicus or in one or other iliac fossa, avoiding any previous scars. Catheter placement is performed under local anaesthetic, using strict aseptic precautions; alternatively, the catheter can be left *in situ* following diagnostic laparotomy. Peritoneal lavage is well tolerated and helps to counter initial hypovolaemia, but its therapeutic value is unproven. Postoperative lavage may be useful at a later stage following debridement of infected pancreatic necrosis.

Operative treatment

Operative treatment of acute pancreatitis may be diagnostic, therapeutic or prophylactic. Since serum amylase levels are not always diagnostic of pancreatitis, and hyperamylasaemia may accompany other upper abdominal catastrophes, laparotomy is mandatory if the diagnosis is in serious doubt (unless paracentesis resolves the issue). The findings in pancreatitis include bloodstained ascites, fat necrosis and marked peripancreatic and retroperitoneal oedema. It is safer to explore a case of acute pancreatitis than to treat a perforated gallbladder conservatively. Acute pancreatitis secondary to trauma always requires laparotomy.

There is no consensus regarding the best treatment of gallstones encountered at the time of diagnostic laparotomy. Cholecystectomy and choledocholithotomy are safe in the presence of mild or moderate pancreatitis. A calculus lodged at the ampulla is best disimpacted from above, since transduodenal sphincteroplasty can be technically difficult and represents a substantial escalation of the surgical attack. In the presence of haemorrhagic pancreatitis, operative procedures should be kept to a minimum, but cholecystectomy and T-tube drainage of the common bile duct may be necessary for cholangitis or biliary obstruction. Pancreatic debridement at this stage should be strictly avoided. Total or extended distal pancreatectomy is occasionally attempted in fulminating pancreatitis, but at least one-third of these patients die. The safety of an urgent endoscopic papillotomy requires further evaluation.

During the early convalescence from an attack the biliary tree should be thoroughly investigated for calculous disease (ultrasound scan, oral cholecystogram). If gallstones are confirmed, it is often wise to carry out cholecystectomy (and choledocholithotomy if necessary) during the same hospital admission to avoid the substantial risk of recurrent pancreatitis. In the absence of obvious gallstones or alcoholism, ERCP may be carried out, especially for recurrent pancreatitis, but this procedure should be delayed for 4–6 weeks after an acute attack.

Complications

There are many possible complications of acute pancreatitis. Chest infection, pleural effusion, venous thromboembolism, hypocalcaemia, diabetes mellitus, septicaemia and renal failure should be managed along standard lines. Pancreatic pseudocysts, which take several days to develop, are discussed later in this chapter (page 168). Gastrointestinal haemorrhage from acute peptic ulceration can be lethal and should be treated conservatively if possible, using cimetidine and blood transfusion. Rarely, prolonged duodenal ileus may necessitate gastroenterostomy.

Infected pancreatic necrosis (pancreatic abscess) is the commonest cause of death in patients who survive the acute phase of shock. Abscesses usually present in the 2nd or 3rd week of the disease with pyrexia, toxicity and a white cell count above 20×10^9/litre. Ultrasound and CT scanning will help to delineate the abscess, which is usually extensive and multilocular. Prompt external drainage should be undertaken. The retroperitoneum is opened widely, pancreatic slough is removed piecemeal, three or four wide-bore tube drains are inserted and broad-spectrum antibiotic therapy is begun. Postoperative irrigation of the abdominal cavity may be beneficial. If the patient survives, the resulting external pancreatic fistulas usually close spontaneously. Alternatively, the abdomen is left open without any attempt to close the wall (*laparostomy*). Moist packs are used to prevent evisceration and are changed daily in the intensive care unit. The abdomen can be inspected and further collections drained without the need for formal lapar-

otomy. In survivors the wound may heal by granulation; otherwise delayed closure is performed. The mortality rate of infected pancreatic necrosis varies between 20% and 50%. Death results from uncontrolled sepsis (with or without bleeding) and multiple organ failure.

Chronic pancreatitis

This disease most commonly affects middle-aged men who have a long history of alcohol abuse. Almost total destruction of the pancreas is compatible with minimal damage to the liver and vice versa. Sometimes the disease follows repeated attacks of acute pancreatitis or is idiopathic. Pain is the dominant symptom. It is situated deeply within the epigastrium, radiates to the back between the shoulderblades and is sometimes relieved by sitting bolt upright. It tends to be severe and unrelenting and causes loss of weight. Swelling of the pancreatic head, with or without pseudocyst formation, may cause cholestasis of varying degree. In addition, progressive glandular destruction causes exocrine and endocrine impairment, which may become clinically apparent (steatorrhoea, diabetes mellitus) or detectable only as abnormalities of measured faecal fat output and glucose tolerance. Rarer complications include pancreatic ascites following internal rupture of a cyst, duodenal stenosis and gastro-oesophageal varices resulting from splenic vein thrombosis.

The preoperative diagnosis of chronic pancreatitis relies on an appropriate clinical history (especially in an alcoholic), demonstration of exocrine insufficiency, the presence of calcification or cysts and pancreatographic evidence of a disordered ductal system.

The symptoms and signs of chronic pancreatitis can mimic those of pancreatic cancer, and the differential diagnosis of these two conditions (Table 13.1) is as important as it can be difficult. Moreover, the two often coexist, since ductal occlusion by tumour causes distal obstructive pancreatitis, and pancreatitis itself, like other chronic inflammatory conditions, may predispose to cancer. Both conditions cause enlargement and destruction of the pancreas, and operative differentiation can also be confusing. The appearance of the common bile duct may be a useful guide, however; in carcinoma of the head of pancreas the duct is green, thin walled and translucent, whereas in chronic pancreatitis it is generally white, thickened and opaque, because of recurrent cholangitis.

Intractable pain and obstructive jaundice are the usual indications for operative treatment in chronic pancreatitis, but the management of this 'benign' condition can be one of the most difficult problems in surgical practice. Addiction has developed not just to alcohol but often to the opiates used to obtain analgesia, and this complicates assessment of suitability for operation, ability to withstand major surgical pro-

Table 13.1 Investigations that help to differentiate between chronic pancreatitis and carcinoma of the pancreas

Diagnostic test	Common features	Chronic pancreatitis	Pancreatic cancer
Occult blood in stools	–	Usually negative	Often positive
Liver function tests	Obstructive jaundice (if head involved)	Obstruction often incomplete and fluctuates	Progressing unrelenting obstruction
Glucose tolerance test	Often diabetic	–	–
Analysis of duodenal juice	Findings often non-specific	Reductions in volume, bicarbonate and trypsin concentrations	Normal, or variable reductions
Plain abdominal X-ray	–	Pancreatic calcification in at least 50%	Usually normal, occasionally punctate calcification
Barium meal/hypotonic duodenography	Distortion of stomach, widening of duodenal loop	Flattening of medial duodenal wall	Invasion of duodenal wall
Cholangiography (percutaneous transhepatic or endoscopic retrograde)	Obstruction of common bile duct, if pancreatic head involved	Smooth, tapering stricture, often incomplete	Abrupt and complete cut-off
Ultrasonography/CT scan	Enlargement of pancreas	Swelling often diffuse, calcification, cysts	Swelling often discrete, local invasion, hepatic metastases
Pancreatography (endoscopic retrograde)	Abnormalities of ductal system	Areas of stenosis and dilatation, 'chain of lakes', side-branch ectasia, cysts, internal fistulas	Invasion of duodenal wall, sharp cut-off pancreatic duct, ductal dilatation behind tumour
Selective arteriography (coeliac, superior mesenteric)	Pancreatic tumours outlined	Tumours smooth and avascular (cysts), fewer vessels supplying pancreas	Vascularity normal or increased, irregular tumours, obstruction of portal vein, hepatic metastases
Biopsy (histology, cytology)	–	Benign pancreatic tissue fibrosis	Adenocarcinoma (if correct area sampled)

cedures and management of endocrine (and exocrine) insufficiency, created or aggravated by pancreatec-tomy. Major pancreatic resections should not be carried out on alcoholics who are continuing to drink, because of the serious risk of coma resulting from haphazard insulin medication after the patient has returned home. Splanchnicectomy, once performed as a definitive operation for pain, should be relegated to the role of an adjunctive procedure; similar benefit can often be obtained more readily by percutaneous coeliac plexus block. Transduodenal sphincteroplasty of the major pancreatic duct may relieve a localized stricture in the pancreatic head, but seldom provides adequate ductal decompression in generalized pan-creatitis. Injections of glue into the pancreatic duct and endoscopic insertion of stents are procedures of uncertain benefit. For practical purposes, therefore, the present choice of operation for chronic pan-creatitis lies between extensive ductal drainage and resection.

Despite the probability that peripancreatitis contributes to the pain, drainage of obstructed ducts alone often provides dramatic and persistent improvement in symptoms. Decompression of the oedematous parenchyma may contribute to a good result. This is the optimal procedure for generalized pancreatitis with ductal dilatation, and it avoids the pancreatic insufficiency implicit in major resections. Long-term decompression is best achieved by longi-tudinal pancreaticojejunostomy Roux-en-Y, after opening the duct widely throughout the strictured segment. Pancreatic calculi are removed and con-comitant cysts are opened into the ductal system or separately drained. The Puestow procedure of insert-ing the filleted pancreas into the end of a Roux loop conveys no obvious advantage and makes haemor-rhage less easy to control. End-to-side anastomoses between the transected pancreas and a Roux loop tend to close eventually, unless the duct is greatly enlarged. If the left side of the pancreas is grossly diseased, distal* pancreatectomy may be combined with drainage of the proximal duct, but the duct

* The term 'distal' is traditionally applied to that portion of the pancreas that lies to the left of the midline, although the 'distal' part of the pancreatic duct might be considered to be the terminal segment within the head of the gland. The terms 'left' and 'right' pancreas avoid this possible con-fusion, but are not in general usage.

should be opened for a short distance to increase the calibre of the pancreatico-intestinal communication.

Pancreatic resection is appropriate for those patients in whom either there is no ductal dilatation, or pancreatitis is essentially limited to one part of the gland, or previous drainage procedures have failed. Chronic inflammation of the left pancreas is readily treated by distal pancreatectomy, which normally includes splenectomy. Transection of the gland is carried out at the level of the portal vein or just to the right of this point, producing a 50–70% pancreatectomy; this procedure usually avoids overt impairment of endocrine or exocrine function. More extensive resections involving 80–95% of the gland (subtotal pancreatectomy) will inevitably aggravate pancreatic insufficiency without necessarily abolishing pain; proximal or even total pancreatectomy are usually better options. If the inflammatory process is limited to the head of the gland with relative sparing of the left pancreas, pancreatoduodenectomy is indicated. It is nearly always possible to preserve the pylorus and duodenal cap and avoid the distal hemigastrectomy of a conventional Whipple's operation. Erosive gastritis does not appear to be a complication of this type of conservative proximal pancreatectomy. Delayed gastric emptying is uncommon and the operation is less of a physiological insult.

Occasionally either severe and generalized pancreatitis or the failure of lesser operative procedures necessitate total pancreatoduodenectomy. Permanent diabetes and malabsorption are the inevitable sequelae* which require lifelong treatment, but in this type of patient they are usually present to a greater or lesser extent before operation. A good result can be anticipated in about 70% of patients surviving total pancreatectomy, but as in all types of operation for chronic pancreatitis the outlook is poor in those who continue to drink alcohol. As an alternative to total pancreatectomy in those with generalized disease but residual endocrine function, it may be possible to combine resection of the head with drainage of the duct in the body and tail.

Pancreatic cysts

These are traditionally classified as *true cysts*, which possess an epithelial lining, and *pseudocysts*, which do not. True cysts are congenital or neoplastic in origin, whereas pseudocysts occur in acute and chronic pancreatitis, trauma and sometimes carcinoma of the pancreas. The distinction becomes academic when true cysts are complicated by infection or haemorrhage that destroys the lining. It is of greater practical value to know whether a cyst is intrapancreatic or peripancreatic, and whether or not it communicates with the ductal system.

* Autotransplantation of islet tissue or the tail of pancreas is a potential method of avoiding diabetes that needs further evaluation.

Congenital pancreatic cysts are usually small, intrapancreatic and silent, but they sometimes enlarge or become infected later in life. Rarely the pancreas is the site of *polycystic disease*, usually in association with the liver and kidney. *Cystic fibrosis of the pancreas* (mucoviscidosis) presents either with meconium ileus in neonatal life, or with steatorrhoea and recurrent chest infection in infancy and childhood.

Cystadenoma, though rare, is one of the commoner benign tumours affecting the gland and usually presents as a painless epigastric mass. It has a marked female preponderance. Complete excision should be performed where practicable; otherwise the cyst remnant should be covered by a Roux loop of jejunum. There is a strong tendency towards malignant change, although histological differentiation from *cystadenocarcinoma* can be difficult. Malignant neoplastic cysts may be sensitive to radiotherapy or chemotherapy.

By far the commonest cysts arising in and around the pancreas are those that accompany pancreatitis or trauma. At least 10% of cases of *acute pancreatitis* produce encysted collections of fluid generally in the lesser sac but sometimes between the leaves of the lesser omentum or adjacent to the anterior surface of the gland. These (pseudo-) cysts cause pain, obstructive jaundice or an epigastric mass 1–2 weeks after admission, with renewed elevation in serum amylase levels. They can be detected by ultrasonography or CT at an earlier stage, but many smaller cysts resolve spontaneously. Larger cysts may cause vomiting by anterior displacement of the stomach, as confirmed on lateral radiographs taken during barium meal examination. Other complications include erosion into adjoining viscera, perforation into the peritoneal cavity (pancreatic ascites) or chest (pleural effusion), and infection (pancreatic abscess). All cysts that fail to resolve should be drained, either externally if they are acute and thin walled or internally if it is possible to wait until they are mature. Percutaneous aspiration under ultrasonic guidance is an acceptable alternative, particularly if drainage becomes necessary within 1 month of the attack of acute pancreatits. It is better to insert (percutaneously) a pigtail catheter than simply aspirate the fluid, which is likely to recur. Percutaneous cyst-gastrostomy and endoscopic cyst-gastrostomy are other new techniques.

The degenerative or retention cysts that arise in *chronic pancreatitis* are generally intrapancreatic and often communicate with the pancreatic ducts. Symptoms resemble those of the underlying disease. Cysts may be shown by pancreatic scans or ERCP, or by the operative finding of soft and fluctuant swellings in an otherwise hard and sclerotic gland. Besides confirming the presence of a cyst, needle aspiration permits introduction of contrast material to determine size, position and possible ductal communication. Treatment of the cyst must be combined with that of the associated pancreatitis. Localized disease may be suitable for resection, or cysts may be evacuated into the ductal system during pancreaticojejunostomy.

Discrete cysts within the head of the pancreas can be drained into the duodenum (page 177), although problems include damage to the bile duct and a lack of dependent drainage. Elsewhere in the gland, cysts may be treated by anastomosis to a Roux loop of jejunum. If drainage is performed (as opposed to resection), it is important to exclude a cystic neoplasm by biopsying the wall of the cyst.

Gastrointestinal haemorrhage is an uncommon but potentially lethal complication of a pancreatic pseudocyst, particularly in chronic alcoholic pancreatitis. The cyst enlarges and its contents digest the wall of neighbouring arteries, leading to pseudoaneurysms of the splenic or gastroduodenal arteries or their branches. These false aneurysms can rupture into the cyst (especially after internal drainage) or directly into the duodenum or pancreatic duct. Visceral angiography demonstrates the site of actual or potential bleeding. Elective resection of the cyst is the best option unless there is active bleeding, in which case transcatheter embolization with gelfoam is probably safer.

Pancreatic fistulas

Besides occurring as a delayed complication of trauma, *cutaneous fistulas* may follow biopsy and resection of the pancreas and pancreatico-intestinal anastomosis, as well as planned external drainage of cysts or abscesses. Pancreatic fistula is one of the commonest and most serious complications of pancreatoduodenectomy.

Pure pancreatic fistulas usually discharge no more than 300 ml of greyish fluid per day and cause little excoriation of the surrounding skin, because the digestive enzymes are not activated. The pancreatic origin of a suspected fistula can be confirmed by the high amylase content (> 5000 Somogyi units/100 ml) of the fluid. A fistulogram should be obtained and will often outline both the ductal system and any peripancreatic collection of fluid; alternatively ERCP may demonstrate the fistula.

Parenteral nutrition avoids the pancreatic stimulation that follows oral intake of food and counteracts the catabolic effect of protein loss. Most pure pancreatic fistulas close spontaneously with time, provided that there is adequate egress for any fluid collection and the underlying pancreatic disease is not too severe. Increasing pain or toxicity suggests the accumulation of infected fluid requiring proper drainage. If fluid loss is excessive or fails to diminish after prolonged conservative treatment, the fistula must be explored. Depending on the site of injury, either resection of the left pancreas or internal drainage of the leak into a Roux loop of jejunum will normally be appropriate.

The outpouring of dark or discoloured fluid rich in amylase indicates a *mixed* pancreatic fistula with concomitant leakage of bile or intestinal contents. Fluid losses and cutaneous inflammation are more severe, and there is a risk of secondary haemorrhage. Most of these patients require operation after a period of hyperalimentation.

Pancreatic ascites is an uncommon complication of chronic pancreatitis or trauma, in which progressive accumulation of fluid within the peritoneal cavity follows internal rupture of a communicating pancreatic cyst. Differentiation from ascites secondary to cirrhosis or carcinomatosis relies upon showing that the fluid obtained by paracentesis abdominis has a higher amylase content than serum. In some patients, pancreatic ascites will resolve with total parenteral nutrition. Endoscopic or operative pancreatography helps to localize the site of leakage from the duct, and treatment is again by distal pancreatectomy or pancreaticojejunostomy (Roux-en-Y).

Carcinoma of the pancreas

Already one of the commonest abdominal malignancies, pancreatic cancer is increasing in frequency. It is very seldom cured. Over 70% of carcinomas affect the head of the pancreas, and in these unrelenting jaundice and weight loss are the cardinal symptoms; abdominal and back pain are frequent but not invariable accompaniments. Vomiting suggests duodenal obstruction. Diabetes mellitus may develop *de novo* or deteriorate in an established diabetic. Besides progressive icterus, there may be hepatomegaly, a palpable gallbladder, an epigastric mass, ascites or thrombophlebitis migrans. Half the patients have occult gastrointestinal bleeding. Tumours of the body and tail are notoriously silent and may elude diagnosis during several months of malaise and vague abdominal pain.

Summarized in Table 13.1 (page 167) the diagnosis of pancreatic cancer rests on the demonstration of a solid pancreatic mass on scanning, radiological or endoscopic evidence of duodenal invasion, exclusion of common-duct stones in obstructive jaundice, obstruction of the pancreatic duct at ERCP and (unequivocally) detection of carcinoma cells after percutaneous needle biopsy, endoscopic aspiration of the duct or operative biopsy. Besides helping to discriminate from other causes of pancreatic enlargement, selective angiography delineates the arterial supply and venous drainage of the gland – valuable if resection is contemplated – and may demonstrate hepatic metastases.

Treatment

Surgery currently offers the only definitive prospect of cure in this disease, but macroscopically complete resection is feasible only for 10–20% of tumours of the head and very seldom for tumours of the body or tail. Moreover, major resection for cancer carries an appreciable mortality rate (5–20%), especially in jaundiced patients, and long-term survival thereafter is exceptional. Yet matters can only improve, as modern diagnostic techniques offer the chance of earlier detection and adjunctive cancer therapy improves. In experienced hands pancreatectomy remains the optimal procedure for pancreatic cancer. Resection is also indicated for other cancers in this region that cause obstructive jaundice, namely carcinoma of the ampulla, terminal bile duct and descending duodenum. These tumours are generally slow growing and carry a much better prognosis. Ampullary cancer is occasionally amenable to local excision, but adequate resection normally entails partial pancreatoduodenectomy.

The first step in any operation for pancreatic (or adjacent) cancer is to confirm the diagnosis, aided by frozen-section examination of tissue obtained by direct pancreatic biopsy or by sampling nodal or hepatic secondaries. In the absence of obvious metastases, the surgeon must next decide if the tumour is resectable, and this may involve a lengthy dissection. Adenocarcinomas of the left pancreas amenable to distal pancreatectomy are seldom encountered. Midline tumours of the gland usually involve the superior mesenteric artery and vein at an early stage. The common cancers of the head should be treated by pancreatectomy, unless there is encasement of the superior mesenteric pedicle, portal vein or aorta. Resection and grafting of major vascular structures or *en bloc* excision of involved adjacent viscera* (right kidney, transverse colon) are rarely indicated. In deeply jaundiced patients with resectable tumours, a two-stage procedure should be considered; the first stage is confined to the relief of the jaundice. Decompression of the obstructed biliary tree can be obtained by means of a transampullary stent inserted at ERCP or by percutaneous insertion of an endoprosthesis or even by a short preliminary operation. The complications of each procedure and the delay in resecting the cancer must be weighed against the increased safety of operating on an anicteric patient.

Resectable cancers of the head of the pancreas may be treated by either proximal or total pancreatoduodenectomy, and in either case preservation of the pylorus and duodenal cap should be considered. Partial resection of the gland usually prevents diabetes. The disadvantages are first that the pancreatico-intestinal anastomosis can be difficult to construct and thus may either leak or become occluded, and second that cancers may be multifocal or spread directly down the duct. In younger and fitter patients with tumours extending towards the pancreatic neck, and especially in those already diabetic, total pancreatectomy is probably the operation of choice. In older people with relatively normal glucose tolerance, or in those with a less favourable prognosis, the prospect of

* Radical resections of this kind are sometimes termed 'regional pancreatectomy'.

a modest gain in survival time is scarcely worth the extra misery of diabetes. Extensive lymphadenectomy increases operative time and morbidity without clearly improving prognosis.

In most cases of pancreatic carcinoma, resection is in any case impracticable, and efforts are directed towards obtaining a positive tissue diagnosis and palliating jaundice and pain. Biliary diversion is most easily achieved by fashioning a side-to-side anastomosis between the fundus of the dilated gallbladder and a loop of jejunum, but this is only appropriate if anticipated survival is very short (in which case non-operative stenting is a better option). Otherwise recurrent jaundice is likely to develop when the cancer spreads to involve the cystic duct, which often joins the common hepatic duct low down. It is generally better to create a retrocolic Roux loop for end-to-side choledochojejunostomy; the dilated bile duct makes for a simple anastomosis, especially after removal of the distended gallbladder. Complete transection of the bile duct with suture of the proximal end to the Roux loop has the theoretical advantage of being less liable to subsequent occlusion by submucosal spread of cancer than side-to-side anastomosis.

The possibility of late duodenal obstruction by direct invasion of the growth makes gastroenterostomy advisable in all but very advanced cases. One option is to use the top of the same Roux loop brought up for biliary anastomosis. H_2 receptor antagonists may be given postoperatively to prevent stomal ulceration and bleeding. Severe preoperative pain and evidence of marked pancreatitis distal to the cancer are indications to consider decompression of the obstructed pancreatic duct into the stomach or jejunum. Alternatively, intraoperative coeliac plexus block may give worthwhile relief of pain. It is doubtful whether postoperative radiotherapy (or chemotherapy) materially improves prognosis, but it may alleviate severe pain.

Preoperative and operative precautions

Since most operations on the pancreas are major undertakings, general preoperative precautions such as correction of anaemia and chest physiotherapy are especially important. Weight loss and malnutrition often complicate both pancreatic cancer and chronic pancreatitis. In obstructive jaundice, preoperative biliary decompression may be more effective than nutritional support in restoring a normal serum albumin.

Pancreatic function should be assessed in the first instance by excluding glycosuria and hyperglycaemia or obvious steatorrhoea. Any evidence of pancreatic insufficiency should be checked by performing a glucose tolerance test and exocrine function tests, while on a normal diet. 'Tubeless' tests of pancreatic exocrine function, such as the Pancreolauryl test, are well tolerated by the patient and can be performed before and after major operative procedures (especially pancreatectomy) for chronic pancreatitis. Psychiatric treatment may be valuable in patients with chronic pancreatitis who have problems of alcoholism or drug abuse.

As haemorrhage is sometimes unexpectedly severe during pancreatic surgery, cross-matched blood should always be available and monitoring of central venous pressure is wise. All major pancreatobiliary operations should be covered by prophylactic broad-spectrum antibiotics that are given parenterally, starting at the time of premedication.

Deeply jaundiced patients tolerate major operations poorly, though this is more often a serious problem in carcinoma of the head of the pancreas (or ampulla) than in chronic pancreatitis. If the serum bilirubin level exceeds 200 mmol/litre, biliary decompression should be considered as a prelude to pancreatectomy. A fine polythene cannula may be introduced into a dilated biliary radicle at the time of percutaneous transhepatic cholangiography (PTC) and left *in situ* thereafter; full antiseptic precautions must be observed and antibiotics are given. Problems of external drainage include catheter displacement, sepsis and electrolyte loss, so that it is important to replace the drainage catheter with a percutaneous endoprosthesis (across the stricture) within 2–3 days of decompression. Endoscopic insertion of a flanged tube across the biliary stricture is an alternative option that is particularly attractive for periampullary lesions; the risks of bleeding and acute pancreatitis are low when papillotomy and endoscopic stenting are performed by an experienced practitioner. Whichever route is employed, preoperative stenting will introduce infection into the obstructed biliary tree, which has usually been sterile up until that time. Some surgeons still prefer to carry out proximal pancreatoduodenectomy as a one-stage procedure unless there is evidence of cholangitis or renal impairment, or jaundice is particularly deep and prolonged. If non-operative stenting is unavailable, surgical decompression can be performed by means of cholecyst-jejunostomy, with resection 3–4 weeks later if the initial assessment has been favourable.

Operations on jaundiced patients may be complicated by renal failure, especially if anoxia or hypovolaemia supervenes. The risk of the hepatorenal syndrome developing can therefore be minimized by skilled anaesthetic technique, including full rehydration and administration of 40 g mannitol at the start of the operation. The patient is catheterized, and urinary output is monitored closely during the operation and for 24–48 h thereafter.

Lastly, obstructive jaundice is associated with an increased bleeding tendency owing to inadequate synthesis of prothrombin and other clotting factors. The prothrombin time should be corrected not only before operation but before any interventional procedure such as PTC or ERCP. Parenteral administration of vitamin K will usually suffice, but fresh frozen plasma should be considered if there is a severe coagulopathy.

Operative diagnosis of pancreatic disease

Exposure of the pancreas

Good access to this deeply placed organ is essential. Satisfactory exposure can be obtained through a long midline incision skirting the umbilicus, aided if necessary by the use of a sternal retractor. Just as good (and cosmetically often superior) is a bilateral subcostal incision or a curved transverse supra-umbilical incision that divides both recti and is convex upwards. Particular attention must be paid to the stomach and duodenal loop, liver, spleen and biliary tree before approaching the pancreas. Thorough mobilization of the duodenum (Figure 13.5) before insertion of the index finger through the epiploic

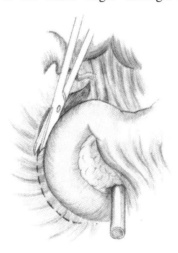

Figure 13.5 Mobilization of the head of the pancreas. The peritoneum is divided on the lateral aspect of the duodenal loop (Kocher's manoeuvre)

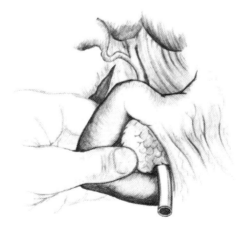

Figure 13.6 Palpation of the head of the pancreas. The surgeon's left index finger is inserted through the epiploic foramen after thorough mobilization of the duodenum

foramen facilitates palpation of the pancreatic head (and terminal bile duct), and its anterior surface can be directly inspected after clearing the overlying omentum (Figure 13.6). Examination of the rest of the gland requires entry into the lesser sac after ligation and partial division of the gastrocolic omentum outside the gastro-epiploic arcade (Figure 13.7). The filmy congenital adhesions passing from the front of the pancreas to the back of the stomach should then be separated. Incision of the peritoneum along the superior and inferior borders of the body of the pancreas allows the gland to be lifted forwards for systematic palpation throughout its extent.

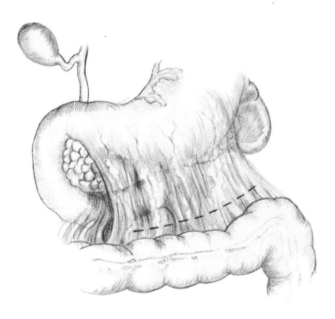

Figure 13.7 Entry into the lesser sac. Division of the greater omentum and elevation of the stomach from its bed afford exposure of the neck, body and tail of the pancreas

Pancreatic biopsy

Biopsy is generally carried out to exclude carcinoma, but sometimes to confirm the presence of chronic pancreatitis. Percutaneous fine-needle aspiration of the gland is increasingly performed to obtain a preoperative tissue diagnosis, usually during organ imaging. Cytological material can be obtained under direct vision at operation by fine-needle aspiration of any suspicious area of the gland. Direct pancreatic biopsy is usually superfluous if cancer can be confirmed by frozen-section examination of metastatic sites in the liver or adjacent lymph nodes. To obtain pancreatic tissue for histological examination requires either an incision into the gland or 'shave' biopsy of a superficial nodule or the use of a Tru-cut needle, which may be introduced transduodenally for lesions

in the head. Even needle biopsy may occasionally cause pancreatitis or a fistula, but the finer the needle the lower the likely risk; these potential complications make deep incision biopsies hazardous in the presence of ductal obstruction. If there is much leakage of pancreatic fluid following biopsy and if no further procedure is anticipated, it is wise to cover the biopsy site with a Roux-en-Y jejunostomy. In practice, however, multiple Tru-cut biopsies can generally be obtained without the need for such a precaution. Since chronic pancreatitis is difficult to differentiate from cancer (and frequently coexists), it is wise to submit biopsy material to immediate pathological examination before closing the abdomen.

Pancreatography

Satisfactory visualization of the pancreatic ducts helps to determine the best surgical procedure for chronic pancreatitis and, if ERCP is unavailable or unsuccessful, operative pancreatograms offer the only chance of obtaining this information (Figure 13.8). Even if prior endoscopic cannulation has outlined the ductal system, operative radiographs may clarify equivocal findings. Pancreatograms may be obtained by injection of water-soluble contrast (e.g. Omnipaque) from either end of the duct (depending on the operative approach). During transduodenal sphincteric surgery, for example, retrograde cannulation of the major (or minor) papilla is performed using a fine polythene cannula (Figure 13.9a). Care must be taken not to overdistend the small pancreatic ducts by injecting more than 2 ml of contrast in the first instance. If distal pancreatitis predominates, prograde cannulation after caudal resection will define the ductal anatomy of the residual pancreas (Figure 13.9b). Likewise, if proximal pancreatitis predominates, retrograde pancreatography after resection of the pancreatic head will delineate the distal ductal tree. This manoeuvre is particularly valuable when severe chronic pancreatitis in the head prevents complete preoperative ductography. If there is generalized inflammatory disease and a dilated ductal tree, the main duct may be felt as a softer area towards the upper surface of the sclerotic pancreas. Direct insertion of a needle into the duct will often permit introduction of contrast material in either direction (Figure 13.9c), i.e. ambigrade ductography. If the duct is impalpable or if needling fails to aspirate pancreatic juice, similar pancreatograms can be obtained by making a short vertical incision in the body of pancreas, deepening the incision to enter the main duct and inserting a T-tube. Distal pancreatectomy or drainage is usually necessary thereafter, so this technique is best avoided if possible. Lastly, any cysts in the region of the pancreas can be outlined radiologically after needle aspiration at the time of drainage. Operative cystography will demonstrate communications with the pancreatic ductal tree.

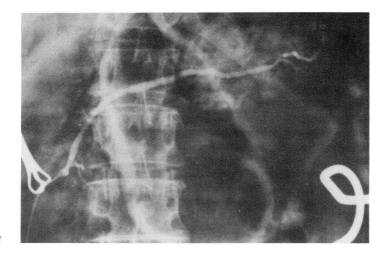

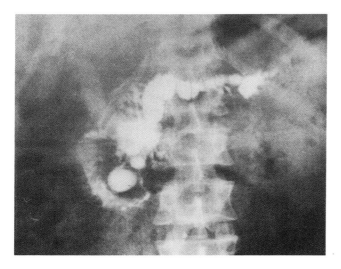

Figure 13.8 Operative pancreatography. *a.* A normal pancreatogram has been obtained by transduodenal cannulation of the major pancreatic papilla. The Babcock forceps have been applied to the papilla to prevent leakage of contrast into the duodenum. Slight overdistension of the ductal system has led to parenchymal filling in the distal pancreas. *b.* Gross ductal dilatation is shown after introduction of contrast via a needle inserted into the pancreatic duct in the body of the gland. The dilated duct was readily palpable in this 29-year-old man with a 10-year history of alcohol abuse. Associated pancreatic cysts are shown, and the biliary tree and duodenal loop are outlined by previous peroperative cholangiography. The patient was treated by longitudinal pancreaticojejunostomy and choledochojejunostomy to relieve his obstructive jaundice

Operations on the ampulla

Transduodenal sphincteroplasty

This operation is usually performed for calculi impacted in the transmural portion of the common bile duct or post-inflammatory stenosis in this region (papillitis). These conditions may be encountered during biliary surgery following acute pancreatitis. Sphincteroplasty allows direct inspection of the orifice of the major pancreatic duct, which can also be incised and sutured, if appropriate (*see below*). Biliary strictures caused by chronic pancreatitis, however, are usually too long to be dealt with by incision from below.

After mobilization of the duodenal loop (Kocher's manoeuvre), the papilla can be palpated on the medial wall of the descending duodenum. A longitudinal duodenotomy is made opposite this point. Identification of the papilla is easier in the presence of inflammation, calculus or tumour, and in these circumstances incision or biopsy of the papilla may be appropriate. Localization of a normal papilla is assisted by intravenous injection of secretin (1 unit/ kg), which rapidly produces an efflux of pancreatic juice from both pancreatic papillas (when present and

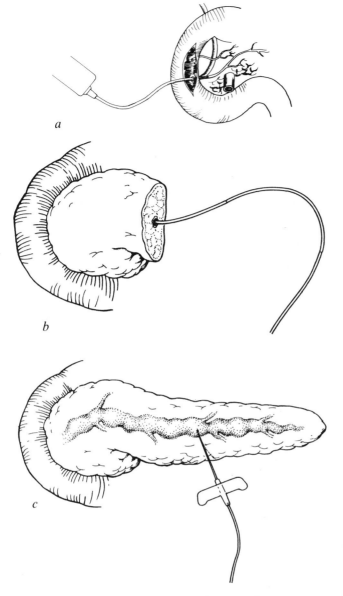

Figure 13.9 Three methods of obtaining operative pancreatograms. Retrograde visualization of the ductal tree may be achieved by transduodenal cannulation of the major pancreatic papilla (*a*). Prograde pancreatogram obtained by cannulation of the duct after distal pancreatectomy (*b*). A dilated pancreatic duct may be entered by direct needle puncture in the body of the gland (*c*)

patent). Alternatively, a soft polythene catheter (Jacques no. 8 Fr. gauge) may be passed through a supraduodenal choledochotomy down the bile duct and into the duodenum, aided by a small incision in the sphincter if the catheter is held up at this point. The tip of the catheter is amputated, a grooved hernia director is impacted into its lumen and the catheter is withdrawn from above until the director enters the lower common bile duct. The subsequent placement of 3/0 or 4/0 chromic catgut sutures through the mucosa of the papilla is assisted by the groove in the director. The first stay sutures are inserted and tied at 10 and 12 o'clock on the circumference of the papilla, and a short incision is made between them. Another two sutures inserted near the apex of this incision are then tied and held in haemostats, and the process is repeated until there is a generous communication (> 1.5 cm long) between the bile duct and the duodenal lumen. With this method of sphincteroplasty, haemorrhage is easily controlled and accurate mucosal coaptation can be achieved. The orifice of the major pancreatic duct can be seen on the lower lip of the papilla at about 5 o'clock. A polythene cannula (no. 4 or 5 Fr. gauge) can normally be inserted.

The duodenotomy is closed longitudinally in two layers, taking care not to narrow the lumen excessively when inserting the outer layer of sutures. The choledochotomy is closed with one layer of absorbable sutures. T-tube drainage is optional if a wide sphincteroplasty has been created, but it will permit postoperative radiological studies if desired. A drain is inserted before closure of the abdomen.

Apart from duodenal leakage, the most worrying complication of biliary sphincteroplasty is acute pancreatitis, but this should be avoidable if the pancreatic duct is identified and care is taken to avoid damaging its orifice during the insertion of sutures.

Pancreatic sphincteroplasty

The opening of the duct of Wirsung is routinely exposed during transduodenal (biliary) sphincteroplasty, though occasionally it can be seen to enter the duodenum independently of the bile duct. Scarring at and immediately behind this orifice is associated with generalized ductal dilatation in a few patients with chronic pancreatitis, for whom pancreatic or double sphincteroplasty is appropriate (synonyms: Wirsungoplasty, transampullary septectomy). This operation has also been advocated for certain patients with 'post-cholecystectomy syndrome', in whom injection of morphine/prostigmine reproduces symptoms and causes hyperamylasaemia (Nardi test). If the ductal orifice is stenosed, insertion of a lacrimal probe may permit cannulation and retrograde pancreatography. Stenosis is released by incising (or partly excising) the common septum between the terminal portions of the bile duct and pancreatic duct for a distance of 10 mm. The ductal mucosas are united with 5/0 chromic catgut or Vicryl sutures.

Sphincteroplasty of the minor (accessory) pancreatic duct (Santoriniplasty) may be carried out by a similar technique in patients with recurrent pancreatitis and an isolated dorsal pancreas. The orifice lies about 2 cm proximal to the major papilla. Identification is facilitated by intravenous secretin (*see above*) and the use of a magnifying lens.

Local excision of ampullary tumours

Although partial pancreatoduodenectomy is ordinarily the operation of choice for carcinoma of the ampulla, in elderly people with small tumours it may sometimes be appropriate simply to excise the tumour locally by a transduodenal approach. A circumferential incision around the ampulla is deepened through the duodenal wall, using a diathermy knife, and a short cone of tissue is excised including the ampulla. It is wise to check the completeness of excision by frozen-section examination of the specimen. The cut ends of the bile duct and pancreatic duct are then reattached to the duodenal mucosa, using interrupted sutures. In selected cases this procedure is well tolerated and may effect a cure.

Endoscopic papillotomy

Like any other operation this procedure should only be undertaken by an experienced practitioner. The patient is admitted to hospital. Carriage of hepatitis B antigen is excluded, together with anaemia and hypoprothrombinaemia. Since blood transfusion is occasionally required, appropriate arrangements should be made preoperatively. The patient is starved for 6 h, and endoscopy is performed with intravenous sedation (e.g. diazepam) and an agent to render the duodenum hypotonic (e.g. glucagon).

A side-viewing duodenoscope is passed through the pylorus and into the second part of the duodenum. The patient is rolled into the prone position, the papilla is identified with its covering fold of mucosa, and the instrument is rotated until the lens is 'face-on' to the papilla. The bile duct is cannulated in a retrograde fashion and cholangiograms are obtained, using a water-soluble contrast agent such as Conray 420. Retrograde pancreatography may also be performed. If papillotomy is indicated, a diathermy catheter is inserted into the bile duct and placed under traction, so that its wire abuts against the roof of the ampulla. Cutting diathermy is used to make a 10–15 mm incision at 11 o'clock, and haemostasis is achieved by means of the coagulation current. Calculi may be retrieved from the bile duct by a balloon catheter, but small stones will often pass spontaneously, either at the time or during the next few days. Complications of papillotomy include bleeding, duodenal perforation and acute pancreatitis; emergency laparotomy is occasionally required.

Pancreaticojejunostomy

This operation is normally reserved for patients with generalized chronic pancreatitis, ductal dilatation and at least some residual pancreatic function. With slight modifications the operation may be used to decompress the distended duct distal to an irresectable carcinoma, to cover any leakage of pancreatic juice following biopsy or trauma, or to provide internal drainage of a pancreatic fistula. The present description will be limited to longitudinal pancreaticojeju-

nostomy (Roux-en-Y), as performed for pancreatitis. If there are associated calculi in the gallbladder, cholecystectomy and operative cholangiography are performed. Obstruction of the common bile duct may be due either to concomitant ductal stones, which should be removed, or to chronic pancreatitis itself, in which case choledochojejunostomy may be required (see Figure 13.8).

Accurate knowledge of pancreatic ductal anatomy is an essential prerequisite for pancreaticojejunostomy. There should be little hesitation in carrying out operative pancreatography if ERCP has been inadequate. If needle aspiration successfully locates the dilated ductal tree, the needle should be left *in situ* while opening into the duct (Figure 13.10). Alternatively, a short vertical incision that partially traverses the body of the pancreas may be needed to demonstrate the position of an impalpable duct. In either case, one blade of a pair of angled scissors is inserted into the duct and the pancreas is opened along its axis in both directions. Stay sutures help to display the duct during the process of incision. Adequate division of all strictures may require the pancreatic duct to be laid widely open virtually throughout its extent. Haemorrhage is controlled by diathermy or suture ligation, and it is particularly important to secure the gastroduodenal artery as the ductal incision is carried into the head of the gland. All pancreatic calculi are removed. Small cysts can often be opened into the ductal tree. The spleen is left intact.

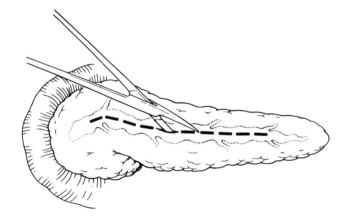

Figure 13.10 Pancreaticojejunostomy. After the dilated pancreatic duct has been located by needle aspiration, a short incision in the anterior surface of the gland is deepened into the ductal system. Thereafter, the duct may be opened widely in each direction

When the ductal dissection is complete, an appropriate segment of upper jejunum is selected for creation of a Roux loop. Transillumination of the mesentery reveals the disposition of the arterial supply, and two or three vascular arcades are divided to allow sufficient mobilization of the loop (Figure 13.11). The bowel is transected between clamps applied 15–30 cm beyond the ligament of Treitz, and the distal cut end is closed and invaginated and brought through a window made in the transverse mesocolon to the left or right of the middle colic vessels. To construct the retrocolic pancreaticojejunostomy, interrupted silk sutures are first inserted between the lower surface of the pancreas and the seromuscular layer of the Roux loop. The jejunum is then opened for a distance corresponding to the length of the previous pancreatic incision, and a running 2/0 Dexon or Vicryl suture is passed through all coats of the jejunum and the thickened pancreatic duct. Lastly, a layer of interrupted non-absorbable sutures is placed between the upper surface of the pancreas and the bowel. If the anastomosis is short or technically difficult, it may be splinted by a T-tube. The short limbs of the T lie in the pancreatic duct, and the long limb is brought through the anastomosis and out through the jejunum at several centimetres downstream, thence to the exterior via a stab incision in the overlying abdominal wall. In practice, a T-tube is only necessary when decompressing an obstructed pancreatic duct in patients with cancer of the pancreatic head. Intestinal continuity is then re-established by end-to-side jejunojejunostomy 30 cm below the pancreatic anastomosis (Figure 13.12). The mesocolic defect is sutured around the Roux loop. A drain is placed in the upper abdomen.

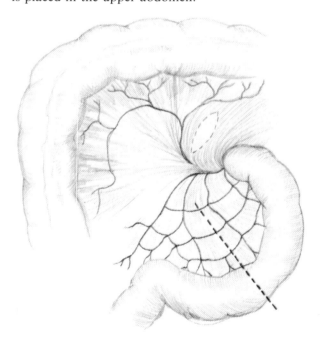

Figure 13.11 Creation of a Roux loop of jejunum. Following transection of the upper jejunum (see broken line), division of two to three vascular arcades provides sufficient mobilization for the loop to be brought through a mesocolic window for pancreatic anastomosis

The main postoperative complications are haemorrhage and anastomotic leakage, but these are generally avoidable with careful operative technique.

Exocrine and endocrine function are usually unaltered.

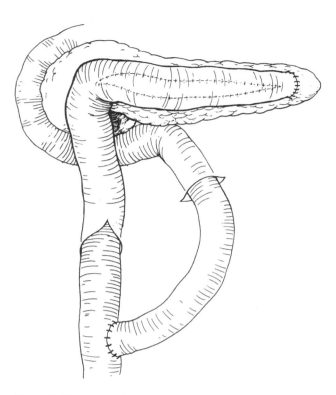

Figure 13.12 Pancreaticojejunostomy. Diagram to show the final anatomical arrangement

Internal drainage of pancreatic cysts

Cyst-gastrostomy

This operation (Figure 13.13) may be chosen for symptomatic collections of fluid in the lesser sac, provided that the posterior wall of the stomach is closely applied to the front of the (pseudo-)cyst and the gastrostomy can be sited low enough to provide dependent drainage. These criteria may partly be gauged by preoperative ultrasonography and CT scan, but they can be confirmed by peroperative cystography. After inspection of the upper abdomen and palpation of the fluctuant retrogastric swelling, a wide-bore needle is introduced through the great omentum and into the cyst. Some 30–50 ml of cyst fluid are withdrawn for bacteriological culture, cytological examination and amylase estimation. A similar quantity of contrast agent is instilled to show both the anatomical relationship of the cyst and the presence or absence of loculi. After longitudinal incision in the anterior wall of the body of the stomach, the edges of the gastrotomy are retracted to reveal the posterior wall, which is incised for 5 cm. This incision is deepened into the cyst and fluid contents are evacuated by suction. Digital exploration of the cyst cavity allows gentle division of trabeculas and removal of solid debris. The margin of the cyst-gastrostomy is oversewn with continuous Dexon or Vicryl sutures, and the anterior gastrotomy is resutured in two layers. The abdomen is closed with drainage.

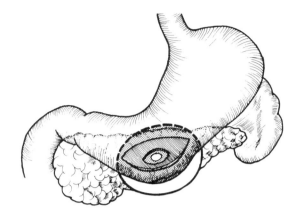

Figure 13.13 Pancreatic cyst-gastrostomy. Through an anterior gastrotomy, an incision in the posterior wall of the stomach will enter an adherent retrogastric (pseudo-)cyst

Cyst-duodenostomy

Small intrapancreatic cysts closely applied to the medial wall of the duodenum are sometimes suitable for direct drainage into the duodenal loop. If pancreatic imaging and operative findings suggest this possibility, a longitudinal duodenotomy is made and a needle is inserted into the cyst. Aspiration of bile is an indication not to proceed, but to drain the cyst into a Roux loop of jejunum instead. Cystography will delineate both the cavity itself and any communication with the pancreatic ductal system. If necessary, retrograde cholangiography via the papilla will outline the exact position of the bile duct. If cyst-duodenostomy is considered appropriate, the needle is left *in situ* and a stab incision is made alongside, through the duodenal wall and into the cyst. The margins of the opening are sutured as for cyst-gastrostomy. The duodenum is closed in two layers.

Cyst-jejunostomy

The use of a Roux loop of jejunum is the most flexible method for internal drainage of pancreatic cysts and should be performed when either of the foregoing operations is impracticable. It is contraindicated when the cyst wall is too thin to take sutures, however, as in the early peripancreatic collections that may complicate acute pancreatitis and require external drainage. After operative cystography, the cyst is opened near its lower pole and the contents are evacuated. Necrotic debris is usually encountered in addition to fluid. A Roux loop of jejunum is created as in pancreaticojejunostomy and is sutured directly to the cystotomy.

Whichever method of internal drainage is employed, postoperative complications include infection and reaccumulation of fluid, which may both be attributable to an inadequate stoma, and fistulization from a leaking anastomosis. Spontaneous haemorrhage into the cyst (before drainage) or the upper alimentary tract (after drainage) may arise from arterial pseudo-aneurysms. The bleeding, which may be catastrophic, is often extremely difficult to stop at operation, though insertion of a Foley catheter into the mouth of the vessel may apply sufficient tamponade to allow accurate suture ligation. If pseudo-aneurysms are shown on preoperative angiography, either the vessel should be ligated at operation or the cyst requires resection.

Distal pancreatic resection

Hemipancreatectomy

Diseases of the body and tail of the pancreas may be amenable to cure by appropriate distal resection, usually including splenectomy. Such conditions include chronic pancreatitis that is largely confined to the left pancreas, trauma, fistulas, tumours and cysts. Distal pancreatectomy and splenectomy may also be performed as part of a radical lymphatic clearance during gastrectomy for carcinoma of the stomach.

Splenectomy is usually the first step after examination of the pancreas. Division of the posterior layer of the lienorenal ligament allows the spleen to be mobilized into the wound for ligation and division of the short gastric vessels. If the spleen is torn during this manoeuvre, it should be removed after ligation of the splenic vessels at the hilum. Already partly mobilized with the spleen, the tail of the pancreas is further freed by dividing the peritoneum and underlying areolar tissue along its superior and inferior borders. As the dissection proceeds along the body of the pancreas, several small vessels must be secured by ligature or diathermy. The distal pancreas together with the spleen (if still attached) can now be lifted forwards and to the right, exposing the splenic vein coursing along its posterior surface. This vessel should be traced to its junction with first the inferior and then the superior mesenteric vein. The splenic artery is now dissected free and ligated just before it gains the superior border of the pancreas. The splenic vein is ligated immediately distal to the entry of the inferior mesenteric vein (Figure 13.14). The body of the pancreas can then be gently elevated from the portal vein and its main tributaries.

The disposition of the great veins provides the key to safe pancreatectomy. In chronic pancreatitis, periglandular inflammation and dense fibrosis often make the dissection difficult and potentially dangerous. In these circumstances the middle colic vein (see Figure 13.2) can be traced carefully downwards as a guide to the superior mesenteric and ultimately the portal vein.

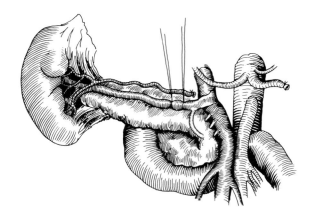

Figure 13.14 Distal pancreatectomy. The spleen and body of pancreas have been mobilized upwards and to the right, exposing their posterior surfaces. The splenic vein is now divided between ligatures immediately beyond the entry of the inferior mesenteric vein. The splenic artery has previously been secured

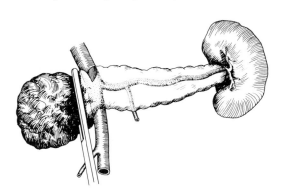

Figure 13.15 Distal pancreatectomy. Transection of the pancreas in front of the portal vein completes the removal of the distal half of the gland. A non-crushing intestinal clamp limits bleeding from the proximal stump

A suitable site should now be chosen for transection of the pancreas, usually where it crosses the portal vein (Figure 13.15). Stay sutures are inserted into the superior and inferior borders of the gland on either side of this point. A non-crushing intestinal clamp is applied across the neck of the pancreas, and the gland is divided by a scalpel to the left of the clamp, taking care to protect the subjacent portal vein. The distal pancreas and spleen are removed. Bleeding vessels are carefully oversewn with 3/0 silk sutures, and the clamp is removed to check haemostasis (Figure 13.16). Interrupted silk sutures are placed to close off the ends of the amputated stump of pancreas. The pancreatic duct should be indentified during closure of the stump and may be cannulated to allow pancreatography of the head.*A normal-calibre duct (2–3 mm) can best be closed with a silk transfixion stitch. A drain should be placed to the splenic bed.

* If operative radiographs are not required, transection of the pancreas may be performed using a gastrointestinal stapling gun.

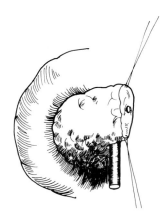

Figure 13.16 Distal pancreatectomy. The head and uncinate process are left *in situ* following division of the pancreas just to the left of the portal vein

If the duct is very dilated, it may be sensible to combine distal resection with a limited longitudinal pancreaticojejunostomy. The pancreatic duct is opened up for a few centimetres by incising the overlying glandular tissue. A Roux loop of jejunum is created for anastomosis to the spatulated duct, as previously described (pages 175–176).

The above description applies to the *prograde* or left-to-right dissection that is commonly practised in distal pancreatectomy. Dense inflammatory scarring and/or the presence of a pseudocyst will obliterate the tissue planes and necessitate the pancreas to be mobilized by sharp dissection. The splenic vessels can be very difficult to identify in such circumstances, and there is a risk of serious haemorrhage if the splenic vein is torn at or near its junction with the portal vein. Thus in patients with chronic pancreatitis it is often safer to commence the dissection by freeing the neck of pancreas from the portal vein (as described below under Whipple's operation) before mobilizing the spleen. Indeed, the pancreas can be transected through its neck, and the entire dissection can proceed in a *retrograde* or right-to-left direction (Figure 13.17), with early ligation of the splenic artery and vein. In particularly difficult cases, a combination of prograde and retrograde techniques may be safest.

Postoperative complications are relatively uncommon, after distal pancreatectomy, but include haemorrhage and infection in the splenic bed and sometimes a collection of pancreatic fluid which requires percutaneous aspiration under ultrasound control. High amylase levels can frequently be found in the drainage fluid, but an established pancreatic fistula develops in 10% or less of patients. Provided that there is no obstruction to the ductal system in the head of pancreas, the fistula should resolve spontaneously. Hemipancreatectomy will not seriously impair pancreatic endocrine (or exocrine) function if the residual gland is normal, but in chronic pancreatitis it may precipitate the need for insulin, so glucose tolerance should be reassessed postoperatively.

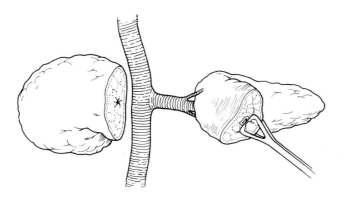

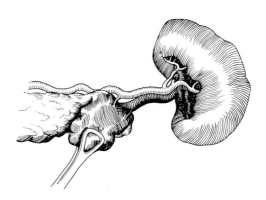

Figure 13.17 Right-to-left (retrograde) technique for distal pancreatectomy. The pancreas is divided in front of the portal vein, and the body and tail are mobilized towards the spleen. The plane of dissection is either between the splenic vessels and the pancreas (conservative resection) or deep to the splenic vessels, with ligation of the splenic artery and vein near their origin and termination (conventional resection – see text)

Figure 13.18 Conservative caudal pancreatectomy. The pancreatic tail has been elevated and displaced to the patient's right Several small branches of the splenic artery and vein need to be ligated and divided, but the parent trunks are preserved

Conservative caudal pancreatectomy

If the tail of the pancreas is relatively healthy, it can be dissected free from the splenic artery and vein and removed without the need for splenectomy and its attendant risks (see Chapter 14). This operation provides pancreatic tissue for histological examination and enables prograde pancreatography to be undertaken. It may therefore be of value in symptomatic patients with pancreas divisum or in those with suspected chronic pancreatitis but minimal changes on ERCP. It is also applicable for neuro-endocrine tumours and for selected cases of chronic pancreatitis with atrophy of the distal gland. The dissection can be tedious and bloody and is inappropriate in the presence of severe pancreatitis, especially if there is a pseudocyst or splenic vein thrombosis.

The pancreatic tail is approached through the lesser sac after ligation and division of the greater omentum. As in conventional distal pancreatectomy, the tail is mobilized by incising the peritoneum along its upper and lower borders. One or two retractors are placed within the lesser sac to displace the stomach and omentum. The tip of the pancreas is grasped by tissue forceps and elevated from its bed, taking care not to damage the subjacent splenic vein. The splenic vessels are closely applied to the posterior surface and may actually groove the gland. Several small arterial and venous branches need to be secured as they enter the pancreas (Figure 13.18). Once the correct plane is established and developed, the dissection proceeds more easily. Ultimately the pancreas is transected and closed in the standard manner, and a drain is placed within the lesser sac.

As with conventional distal pancreatectomy, it is often easier to carry out a conservative resection by retrograde dissection from right to left after preliminary mobilization and division of the pancreatic neck.

Subtotal pancreatectomy

This major operation is reserved for severe and generalized pancreatitis. It involves resection of 80–95% of the gland, leaving a rim of pancreatic tissue within the duodenal loop. The residual pancreas is seldom sufficient to maintain normal exocrine and endocrine function. Obstructive jaundice implies compression of the bile duct and is a contraindication to subtotal pancreatectomy.

The initial operative steps follow those of left hemipancreatectomy, but the dissection is often particularly laborious owing to peripancreatic fibrosis. The gland is elevated progressively from left to right and mobilization is continued well beyond the midline, with individual ligature of the many vessels that pass from the medial borders of the head and uncinate process to the portal and superior mesenteric veins. At this stage a bougie is introduced through a supraduodenal choledochotomy to allow accurate localization of the terminal bile duct. The duodenum is mobilized, the pancreatic head is grasped by a hand placed from behind and the gland is transected from front to back within the duodenal cavity, by means of a diathermy knife (Figure 13.19). The distal pancreas and spleen are removed. The remainder of the head is trimmed as required, preserving the bile duct and at least one (ideally both) of the superior and inferior pancreaticoduodenal arcades. If duodenal ischaemia develops, the operation must be converted into total pancreatoduodenectomy. The pancreatic duct is identified and closed by suture ligation as before. The incision in the common bile duct is sutured around a T-tube. The abdomen is closed with adequate drainage. During the recovery period, fluid balance and normoglycaemia must be maintained, and nasogastric intubation is required until the passage of flatus. Exocrine status is assessed on resumption of oral feeding.

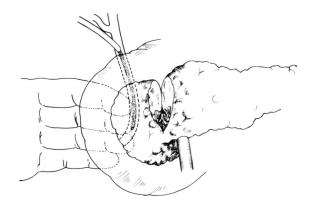

Figure 13.19 Subtotal pancreatectomy. The head of the pancreas is divided at a safe distance from the common bile duct, while the organ is firmly grasped by the surgeon's left hand. The position of the bile duct is confirmed by the introduction of a metal bougie via a supraduodenal choledochotomy. Further resection of the pancreatic head is performed to complete an 80–95% pancreatectomy, preserving a rim of glandular tissue within the duodenal loop to protect the pancreaticoduodenal arteries

Proximal pancreatic resection

Whipple's operation

Originally described by Dr Allen Whipple in 1935 for ampullary cancer, partial pancreatoduodenectomy is most commonly carried out for carcinoma of the head of the pancreas and is sometimes indicated for benign destructive disease of the proximal pancreas, as in trauma or chronic pancreatitis. It is the operation of choice for carcinomas of the ampulla, terminal bile duct and descending duodenum.

In operations for malignant disease, evidence of local invasion or metastases generally means that Whipple's operation should be abandoned in favour of palliative bypass. Preoperative tests including visceral angiography and CT scan will indicate the likelihood of resectability. In palliative operations, biopsies of the primary or secondary sites of tumour should always be taken to establish a tissue diagnosis (see page 172).

If the tumour mass is mobile and confined to the pancreatic head, an exploratory dissection is undertaken to assess resectability. After entry into the lesser sac, the superior mesenteric vein is traced to the inferior border of the neck of the pancreas. The duodenum is mobilized fully, and dissection within the free edge of the lesser omentum is undertaken to identify the (dilated) common bile duct, the hepatic artery with its right gastric and gastroduodenal branches and the portal vein, which lies posteriorly. The surgeon's left index finger is cautiously inserted alongside the portal vein from above and is introduced downwards behind the neck of pancreas (Figure 13.20). If this finger makes contact with the right index, which is gently insinuated along the superior mesenteric vein from below, the portal vein

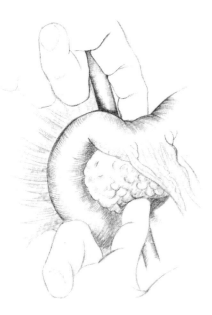

Figure 13.20 Partial pancreatoduodenectomy. If the neck of the pancreas can be freed from the anterior surface of the portal vein, resection of the tumour is normally feasible

is free of tumour anteriorly and resection is feasible.

Following ligation of the gastroduodenal artery close to its origin, four major structures require division: the order of dissection may be varied according to progress at different sites. Distal hemigastrectomy is performed by transecting the body of the stomach.* The supraduodenal bile duct is divided well above the tumour, and the gallbladder is removed. The neck of the pancreas is transected in front of the portal vein (Figure 13.21). The pancreatic duct is frequently dilated at this point. Several vessels running from the head and uncinate process to the portal and superior mesenteric veins now require careful individual ligation, together with the inferior pancreaticoduodenal vessels. After dividing the ligament of Treitz and the vessels that supply the duodenojejunal flexure, the resection is completed by transecting the upper jejunum at a convenient point. The operative specimen is removed, and the jejunum is advanced through the transverse mesocolon.

Occasionally the surgeon may find towards the end of the resection that the tumour extends very close to the portal vein. It may be possible to clear the involved tissue by gentle blunt dissection, but sometimes it is safer to leave a rim of pancreas (or tumour) to protect the great veins. Alternatively, a short segment of portal vein can be resected *en bloc*. Upward traction on the mesentery will usually allow vascular continuity to be restored by direct end-to-end anastomosis.

Several methods of reconstruction are possible. The author's preference is to start by joining the neck

* Truncal vagotomy and antrectomy are a reasonable alternative.

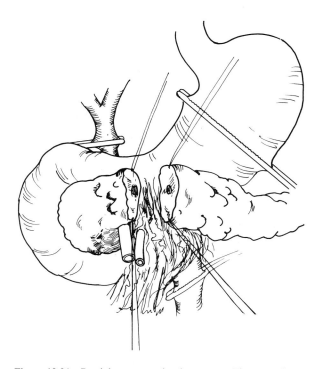

Figure 13.21 Partial pancreatoduodenectomy. The operative specimen is removed after transection of the stomach, bile duct, pancreas and upper jejunum

of pancreas to the upper end of jejunum (Figure 13.22). The two-layer *pancreatojejunostomy* is facilitated by mobilizing the posterior surface of the proximal body from off the splenic vein for 5 cm, carefully securing any venous branches leaving the gland. The end-to-end pancreatojejunostomy is carried out using two layers of interrupted 3/0 silk sutures. The first layer unites the cut surface of the pancreas and its duct to the full thickness of the jejunum. All the posterior sutures are placed before any one of them is tied. In elderly patients the pancreas is often friable, and the sutures must be tied with great care so as not to cut out. The jejunum is then invaginated for 1–2 cm to cover this anastomosis, and a second layer of sutures is placed between the seromuscular coat of the bowel and the pancreatic capsule. In practice, it is only possible to incorporate ductal mucosa in the inner layer of sutures if the duct is moderately dilated (>5 mm diameter). In the author's opinion, if the duct is unobstructed and small in calibre, it is better to abandon attempts to suture its mucosa and simply coapt the circumference of the pancreatic parenchyma to the full thickness of the jejunum. Ductal patency is maintained in such cases by a transanastomotic stent. An infant feeding tube (6 or 8 Fr) is passed down the pancreatic duct to the tail (with several side holes) and is anchored firmly to the duct with at least two absorbable sutures (3/0 Vicryl). The tube is brought out through the jejunum some 30 cm below the anastomosis and is then exteriorized (with suture of the jejunum to the abdominal wall at that

site). The tube must be in position before the pancreatojejunostomy is commenced. Postoperatively it is not removed for 10 days, although it can usually be clamped (with or without tubography) well before that time.

An alternative technique employs end-to-side pancreatojejunostomy (Figure 13.23). A circular disc of jejunal serosa and muscularis is excised, equal in size to the cut surface of the pancreatic neck. A tiny enterotomy is made in the centre of the denuded bowel. Direct mucosal apposition is achieved between jejunum and pancreatic duct, using a few interrupted 5/0 silk sutures. The pancreatic substance is sutured to the jejunal serosa, using 3/0 silk. If the pancreatic duct is narrow, the pancreatico-intestinal anastomosis may again be splinted by a fine cannula.

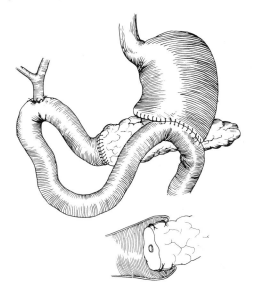

Figure 13.22 Partial pancreatoduodenectomy. A convenient method for reconstruction. The inset shows the completed pancreatico-intestinal anastomosis, with invagination of a short sleeve of jejunum to protect the inner row of sutures

For the *choledochojejunostomy* the bile duct is joined end-to-side to the jejunum, either above or below the pancreas, depending on the type of pancreatico-intestinal anastomosis chosen (Figures 13.22 and 13.23). Care must be taken to ensure that the length of the jejunal incision corresponds to the width of the bile duct (which is usually dilated). One layer of interrupted 3/0 catgut or Vicryl sutures is employed. It is easier to insert the entire posterior row of sutures before tying any individual stitch. This anastomosis can be splinted by a T-tube which is inserted through a separate incision in the bile duct; one limb of the T-tube is placed through the choledochojejunostomy. These splinting tubes are generally removed about 10 days after the operation.

Lastly, a side-to-side *gastroenterostomy* is created, as after Polya gastrectomy (see Chapter 12), either above or below the transverse mesocolon. The GIA stapler can be used at this stage. At least two drains are placed in the region of the pancreatic anastomosis before wound closure.

Besides the complications attendant upon any operation of this complexity, leakage may occur from any of the three or four suture lines, but especially the pancreaticojejunostomy. If a pancreatic fistula develops, one drain may be used for irrigation of sterile saline to prevent local haemorrhage, and parenteral nutrition is instituted. Gastrointestinal bleeding may follow stress ulceration, but this risk is lessened by adequate gastric resection and by intravenous administration of an H_2 receptor antagonist during the recovery period. Late obstruction of the pancreatic anastomosis may cause progressive exocrine atrophy, but Whipple's operation seldom aggravates diabetes mellitus appreciably.

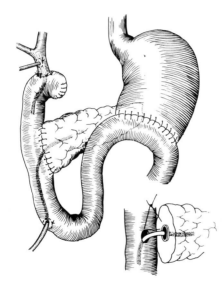

Figure 13.23 Partial pancreatoduodenectomy. An alternative method for reconstruction. Gastrojejunostomy may be carried out either above or below the transverse mesocolon. The inset shows construction of the pancreatico-intestinal anastomosis

Conservative proximal pancreatoduodenectomy

The conventional Whipple's resection includes a distal gastrectomy, partly to widen the lymph node clearance for cancer and partly to reduce gastric acidity and prevent bleeding stomal ulcers in the early postoperative period. In resecting the head of pancreas for inflammatory disease, a radical excision is unnecessary and erosive gastritis might be avoided by retaining the pylorus and preventing bile reflux. This is the basic concept of the pylorus-preserving proximal pancreatectomy introduced by Traverso and Longmire in 1978, and the results appear very satisfactory. The operation may also be appropriate not only for less invasive tumours such as ampullary cancer, but even for carcinoma of the head of pan-

creas. In the author's practice, pylorus-preserving proximal pancreatoduodenectomy (PPPP) has become the standard means of resecting the head of pancreas, and gastrectomy is reserved for those few patients with cancer abutting on the pylorus or concomitant peptic ulcer disease.

The key to success lies in maintaining an adequate blood supply to the pylorus and stump of proximal duodenum, which are retained in the body. The gastroduodenal artery can safely be ligated at its origin but the gastro-epiploic arcade should be carefully preserved by dividing the greater omentum at a distance from the greater curve of the stomach. If the inflammatory changes in and around the head of pancreas are very severe, it may be better to carry out Whipple's operation than to struggle to retain the duodenal cap and its vessels of supply. In favourable cases, however, the first part of duodenum can be dissected free of the pancreas, with ligation of the right gastro-epiploic artery and vein at the level of the pancreas. This dissection must proceed slowly in the presence of chronic inflammation but can usually be safely achieved. The bowel is transected 5–6 cm beyond the pylorus. The resection line should be carefully inspected to ensure that it is viable; it can be trimmed if necessary. Intestinal continuity is restored by end-to-side *duodenojejunostomy* (Figure 13.24), taking care not to narrow the channel. A small proportion of patients (ca. 10%) develop delayed gastric emptying in the early postoperative period and require prolonged nasogastric intubation. Stress ulceration is rare, and postoperative weight gain should be better than after a conventional resection incorporating gastrectomy.

Total pancreatoduodenectomy

Removal of the entire pancreas may be appropriate in a few cases of cancer or end-stage chronic pancreatitis, despite the permanent loss of function that ensues. The operation combines partial pancreatoduodenectomy with left hemipancreatectomy. The stomach and pylorus may again be preserved in benign disease (Figure 13.24). In the author's opinion, however, duodenum-preserving total pancreatectomy is an inappropriate procedure. In chronic pancreatitis, the dissection will ordinarily proceed from left to right, and the correct plane in front of the great veins is established as before. In carcinoma, metastatic disease and involvement of the portal vein are excluded before subsequent dissection is carried out away from the pancreatic neck in each direction. Reconstruction is simpler after total than after partial resection, because the difficult pancreatico-intestinal anastomosis is no longer required.

Insulin must be given postoperatively, the dose being altered according to blood and urinary sugar levels. Before discharge, patients are taught to manage their own diabetes. It is wise to allow patients to become hypoglycaemic once or twice, so that they can learn to recognize the warning symptoms. They should be instructed to take regular meals and to carry sugar with them at all times. Careful outpatient supervision of diabetes is mandatory during the early postoperative weeks. Pancreatic enzymes are given by mouth as soon as feeding is resumed. A low fat diet is advisable, and enzyme supplements are adjusted to prevent steatorrhoea.

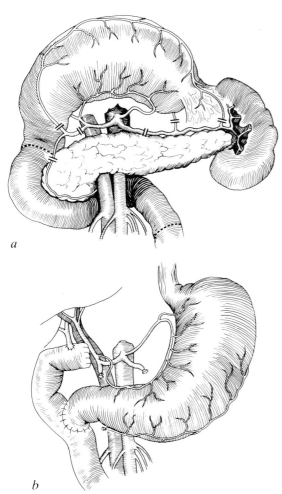

biliary diversion. After insertion of an Ochsner trocar and cannula into the fundus, the gallbladder is emptied by suction; if radiological visualization of the biliary tree is desired, contrast medium is instilled before evacuating all the bile. On withdrawal of the cannula the puncture site is grasped and sealed with Duval's forceps. A loop of upper jejunum is approximated to the gallbladder and short incisions are made in the adjoining viscera. A one-layer cholecysto-jejunostomy is fashioned using 2/0 chromic catgut sutures. Side-to-side jejunojejunostomy (entero-anastomosis) about 10 cm below this may limit entry of food into the biliary apparatus (Figure 13.25).

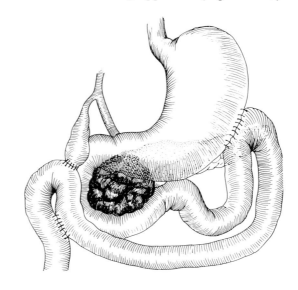

Figure 13.25 Bypass procedures for irresectable pancreatic cancer. An entero-anastomosis below the site of the cholecysto-jejunostomy may decrease the entry of food into the gallbladder. An antecolic gastroenterostomy circumvents present or future obstruction of the duodenum

Figure 13.24 Pylorus-preserving pancreatectomy. The duodenum is divided about 3 cm beyond the pylorus (*a*), and continuity is restored by end-to-side duodenojejunostomy (*b*). Total pancreatectomy is illustrated. Conservative proximal pancreatectomy can be performed by a similar technique but with preservation of the splenic artery and its branches and anastomosis of the distal pancreas to the upper jejunum

Bypass for pancreatic cancer

Cholecystojejunostomy

Subject to the caveats mentioned on page 170, a distended healthy gallbladder that communicates with the bile duct by a wide cystic duct entering well above the site of tumour can readily be used for

Choledochojejunostomy

Usually the above procedure is unsuitable, in which case jaundice should be relieved by end-to-side anastomosis between the transected common bile duct and a Roux loop of jejunum. The loop is brought up either behind or in front of the transverse colon and is closed at its end. The dilated bile duct is dissected free and opened transversely. Bile is evacuated, and the duct is divided completely below a bulldog clip or vascular clamp. The lower end is closed with catgut sutures, and the upper end is inserted into the Roux loop just below its apex, as after partial pancreato-duodenectomy. Intestinal continuity is restored as usual by end-to-side jejunojejunostomy about 30 cm downstream (Figure 13.26).

Other palliative procedures

Biopsies should always be taken (if at all possible) to confirm the tissue diagnosis (see page 172). Antecolic gastroenterostomy is carried out as for carcinoma of the stomach (see Chapter 12), in anticipation of duodenal invasion by tumour. Alternatively, side-to-side gastroenterostomy can be performed using the top of the Roux loop brought up for biliary anastomosis (Figure 13.26). To perform peroperative coeliac plexus block, 15–20 ml of 50% alcohol are injected into the retroperitoneal tissues surrounding the coeliac ganglion on either side of the aorta and the vena cava at the level of the diaphragmatic crura. Neurolytic agents must never be injected if blood is aspirated into the syringe. Careful wound closure and antibiotic cover are advisable during palliative operations for pancreatic cancer.

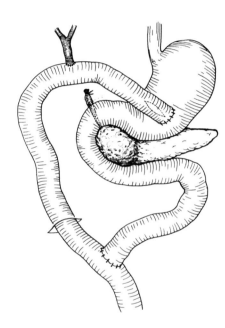

Figure 13.26 Bypass procedures for irresectable pancreatic cancer. The bile duct has been transected well above the tumour, and its upper end is anastomosed to a Roux loop of jejunum; the lower end is tied off. Cholecystectomy has been performed. Side-to-side anastomosis is created between the gastric antrum and the top of the Roux loop to permit duodenal bypass

An obstructed pancreatic duct may be drained into the Roux loop used for biliary diversion in a manner akin to pancreaticojejunostomy. A 2–3 cm longitudinal incision is made in the duct, and the anastomosis is splinted by a T-tube that is brought to the exterior. Alternatively, an intubated pancreaticogastrostomy is fashioned. The long limb of the T-tube is brought through the posterior wall of the stomach and then obliquely through the anterior gastric and abdominal walls. About 10 cm of the tube (containing a few side-holes) should be within the cavity of the stomach. A few sutures are used to approximate the small posterior gastrostomy to the margins of the pancreatic defect. The tube can usually be clamped at 5 days and removed at 10 days postoperatively.

Further reading

Braasch, J. W., Rossi, R. L., Watkins, E., Jr. *et al.* (1986) Pyloric and gastric preserving pancreatic resection. Experience with 87 patients. *Ann. Surg.*, **204**, 411–418

Bradley, E. L., III (1987) Long-term results of pancreatojejunostomy in patients with chronic pancreatitis. *Am. J. Surg.*, **153**, 207–213

Cooper, M. J. and Williamson, R. C. N. (1984) Drainage operations in chronic pancreatitis. *Br. J. Surg.*, **71**, 761–766

Cooper, M. J. and Williamson, R. C. N. (1985) Conservative pancreatectomy. *Br. J. Surg.*, **72**, 801–803

Cooper, M. J., Williamson, R. C. N., Benjamin, I. S. *et al.* (1987) Total pancreatectomy for chronic pancreatitis. *Br. J. Surg.*, **74**, 912–915

Corfield, A. P., Cooper, M. J. and Williamson, R. C. N. (1985) Acute pancreatitis: a lethal disease of increasing incidence. *Gut*, **26**, 724–729

Cotton, P. B. (1984) Endoscopic methods for relief of malignant obstructive jaundice. *World J. Surg.*, **8**, 854–861

Cotton, P. B. (1985). Pancreas divisum – curiosity or culprit? *Gastroenterology*, **89**, 1431–1435

Crist, D. W., Sitzmann, J. V. and Cameron, J. L. (1987) Improved hospital morbidity, mortality, and survival after the Whipple procedure. *Ann. Surg.*, **206**, 358–365

Desa, L. A. and Williamson, R. C. N. (1990) On-table pancreatography: importance in planning operative strategy. *Br. J. Surg.*, **77**, 1145–1150

Eckhauser, F. E., Strodel, W. E., Knol, J. A. *et al.* (1984) Near-total pancreatectomy for chronic pancreatitis. *Surgery*, **96**, 599–607

Fortner, J. G. (1984) Regional pancreatectomy for cancer of the pancreas, ampulla, and other related sites. Tumour staging and results. *Ann. Surg.*, **199**, 418–425

Gilchrist, B. F. and Trunkey, D. D. (1990) Injuries to the spleen and pancreas. In *Emergency Abdominal Surgery* (eds R. C. N. Williamson and M. J. Cooper), Churchill Livingstone, Edinburgh, pp. 36–51

Huizinga, W. K. J., Kalideen, J. M., Bryer, J. V. *et al.* (1984) Control of major haemorrhage associated with pancreatic pseudocyst by transcatheter arterial embolization. *Br. J. Surg.*, **71**, 133–136

Itani, K. M. F., Coleman, R. E., Akwari, O. E. *et al.* (1986) Pylorus-preserving pancreatoduodenectomy. A clinical and physiologic appraisal. *Ann. Surg.*, **204**, 655–664

Keighley, M. R. B., Moore, J. and Thompson, H. (1984) The place of fine needle aspiration cytology for the intraoperative diagnosis of pancreatic malignancy. *Ann. Roy. Coll. Surg. Engl.*, **66**, 405–408

Kivilaakso, E., Lempinen, M., Makelainen, A. *et al.* (1984) Pancreatic resection versus peritoneal lavation for acute fulminant pancreatitis. A randomised prospective study. *Ann. Surg.*, **199**, 426–431

Lambert, M. A., Linehan, I. P. and Russell, R. C. G. (1987) Duodenum-preserving total pancreatectomy for end stage chronic pancreatitis. *Br. J. Surg.*, **74**, 35–39

Longmire, W. P., Jr. (1984) The vicissitudes of pancreatic surgery. *Am. J. Surg.*, **147**, 17–24

Malt, R. A. (1983) Treatment of pancreatic cancer. *JAMA*, **250**, 1433–1437

Mayer, A. D., McMahon, M. J., Benson, E. A. *et al.* (1984) Operations upon the biliary tract in patients with acute pancreatitis: aims, indications and timing. *Ann. R. Coll. Surg. Engl.*, **66**, 179–183

Morrow, M., Hilaris, B. and Brennan, M. F. (1984) Comparison of conventional surgical resection, radioactive implantation, and bypass procedures for exocrine carcinoma of the pancreas 1975–1980. *Ann. Surg.*, **199**, 1–5

Nardi, G. L., Michelassi, F. and Zannini, P. (1983) Transduodenal sphincteroplasty. 5–25 year follow-up of 89 patients. *Ann. Surg.*, **198**, 453–461

Newell, K. A., Liu, T., Aranha, G. V. *et al.* (1990) Are cyst-gastrostomy and cyst-jejunostomy equivalent operations for pancreatic pseudocysts? *Surgery*, **108**, 635–640.

Poston, G. J. and Williamson, R. C. N. (1990). Surgical management of acute pancreatitis. *Br. J. Surg.*, **77**, 5–12

Sarr, M. G. and Cameron, J. L. (1984) Surgical palliation of unresectable carcinoma of the pancreas. *World J. Surg.*, **8**, 906–918

Shi, E. C., Yeo, B. W. and Ham, J. M. (1984) Pancreatic abscesses. *Br. J. Surg.*, **71**, 689–691

Thompson, M. H., Williamson, R. C. N. and Salmon, P. R. (1980) The clinical relevance of isolated ventral pancreas. *Br. J. Surg.*, **68**, 101–104

Traverso, L. W. and Longmire, W. P., Jr. (1978) Preservation of the pylorus during pancreaticoduodenectomy. *Surg. Gynecol. Obstet.*, **146**, 959–962

Trede, M. (1985) The surgical treatment of pancreatic carcinoma. *Surgery*, **97**, 28–35

van Heerden, J. A., McIlrath, D. C., Ilstrup, D. M. *et al* (1988) Total pancreatectomy for ductal adenocarcinoma of the pancreas: an update. *World J. Surg.*, **12**, 658–662

van Sonnenberg, E., Wittich, G. R., Casola, G. *et al.* (1989) Percutaneous drainage of infected and non-infected pancreatic pseudocysts: experience in 101 cases. *Radiology*, **170**, 757–761

Warshaw, A. L. (1989) Pancreatic cysts and pseudocysts: new rules for a new game. *Br. J. Surg.*, **76**, 533–534

Warshaw, A. L., Richter, J. M., Schapiro, R. H. (1983) The cause and treatment of pancreatitis associated with pancreas divisum. *Ann. Surg.*, **198**, 443–452

Williamson, R. C. N. (1984) Early assessment of severity in acute pancreatitis. *Gut*, **66**, 179–183

Williamson, R. C. N. (1988) Pancreatic cancer: the greatest oncological challenge. *Br. Med. J.*, **296**, 445–446

Williamson, R. C. N. (1988) Pancreatic sphincteroplasty: indications and outcome. *Ann. Roy. Coll. Surg. Engl.*, **70**, 205–211

Williamson, R. C. N. and Cooper, M. J. (1987) Resection in chronic pancreatitis. *Br. J. Surg.*, **74**, 807–812

14

The spleen

M. J. Cooper

Anatomy and physiology

Structure

The spleen is a friable and highly vascular organ. In a normal adult it weighs about 150 g and is 12 cm long; splenic size diminishes with age. Lying within the left hypochondrium, the spleen is protected from direct injury by the 9th, 10th and 11th ribs, its long axis lying parallel to the 10th rib. The diaphragmatic surface is smooth and convex. Its visceral surface is indented by gastric, renal, pancreatic and colic impressions.

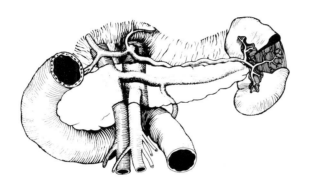

Figure 14.1 Vascular anatomy of the spleen. The splenic artery arises as a branch of the coeliac axis and runs along the upper border of the pancreas to the splenic hilum. The artery branches before entering the splenic substance and forms segmental end arteries. The splenic vein runs deep to the pancreas to form the portal vein

Blood is supplied by the splenic artery, a sinuous vessel which runs along the upper border of the pancreas (Figure 14.1). In the hilum of the spleen the artery gives off about five short gastric vessels, together with the left gastro-epiploic artery, before dividing to enter the spleen. These terminal divisions, which number between 3 and 7 with a mean of 4, are segmentally distributed; there is little blood flow between the various segments. Blood leaving the spleen drains into the splenic vein, which runs deep to the pancreas towards the origin of the portal vein. The splenic vein accounts for some 40% of portal blood flow.

Accessory spleens (splenunculi) are commonly situated near the splenic hilum within the gastrosplenic ligaments. They are found in 20% of the population.

Function

Although the spleen is not essential for life, it does have several important haematological and immunological functions. Atrophy or removal of the spleen produces long-standing sequelae.

Haematological

In health, splenic haemopoiesis is only important during intra-uterine life. Subsequently it may recur when the marrow capacity is exceeded, but in these circumstances red cell production is abnormal. Normal maturation and destruction of red blood corpuscles occurs within the splenic cords. Surface craters and pits are effaced from new cells, and old cells are removed as they become effete. In humans, the spleen acts as a storage site for iron and platelets, but not for blood.

Immunological

The spleen accounts for 25% of the body's lymphoid tissue. Most lymphocytes are produced in the bone marrow, yet the spleen has an important though not indispensable role in both humoral and cell-mediated immunity. Circulating antigens are trapped and trigger IgM production in the germinal centres. The spleen is the major site of production of the opsonins, tuftsin and properdin, which are important in the phagocytosis of encapsulated bacteria.

Effects of splenectomy

Haematological

There is an increase in the number of abnormal red cells in the circulation. Almost invariably there is leucocytosis and thrombocytosis, which peak at 7–10 days. Thrombocytosis results from increased platelet production and may persist for many years.

Immunological

The effect is aged dependent, being maximal under 1 year. IgM levels fall and take 4 years to return to normal. IgA levels rise; IgG levels are usually unaffected. There is an immediate and prolonged reduction in the ability to opsonize encapsulated bacteria, with consequently impaired phagocytosis of these organisms. Splenosis or splenuncular hyperplasia may partially restore these functions.

Indications for splenectomy

Table 14.1 lists the indications for splenectomy which are discussed below.

Trauma

A ruptured spleen is the commonest serious injury to result from blunt abdominal trauma. Rupture follows a crush injury, a blow to the abdomen or left lower thorax, or a fall onto a protruding object. Penetrating injuries are relatively uncommon in the UK; they frequently cause mixed thoracic and abdominal injuries. A force sufficient to rupture the normal spleen will often produce associated injuries to the ribs and other internal organs. A pathologically enlarged spleen is more liable to traumatic rupture.

Table 14.1 Indications for splenectomy

Traumatic rupture	Immediate
	Iatrogenic
	Delayed (spontaneous)
Hypersplenism	Primary splenomegaly
	Secondary splenomegaly
Neoplasia	Hodgkin's disease
	Non-Hodgkin's lymphoma
	Leukaemia
	Massive haemangioma
With other viscera	Total gastrectomy
	Distal gastrectomy
	Conventional splenorenal shunt
Other	Splenic cysts
	Splenic abscess

Iatrogenic injury has been a major cause of splenectomy, and although the incidence continues to fall with improving surgical technique, as many as 20–25% of all splenectomies are for this reason. Most of these injuries are capsular tears caused by the surgeon pulling on peritoneal attachments or adhesions, or sometimes by an assistant's overenthusiastic use of a retractor. They can be avoided if care is taken to divide these attachments at an early stage in any laparotomy. Iatrogenic rupture has also been reported as a complication of various endoscopic procedures.

Delayed rupture of the spleen is often actually a delay in diagnosis. However, the development of a subcapsular haematoma or post-traumatic cyst may lead to rupture hours or weeks after the injury. The true incidence of the problem is unknown; its reported incidence varies from 2% to 35% of all ruptures.

Spontaneous rupture is rare except as a complication of splenomegaly. The high mortality rate reflects late recognition of this condition.

Hypersplenism

Hypersplenism has been defined as a state characterized by splenomegaly plus a depression of one or more of the cell counts in the circulating blood that is wholly attributable to the splenic enlargement. Reduced numbers of cells result from both pooling and excess destruction. The reduction may be generalized (a pancytopenia) or specific to one element, e.g. platelets. Primary splenomegaly is uncommon and most cases represent secondary splenic enlargement in response to an as yet unknown disease. Before splenectomy is undertaken for hypersplenism, it must be established that the excess cell destruction is taking place in the spleen and that the bone marrow can provide adequate haemopoiesis once the spleen has been removed. Splenectomy may be curative in hereditary spherocytosis and idiopathic thrombocytopenic purpura.

In many parts of the world splenomegaly and hence hypersplenism result from parasitic infestations such as malaria, schistosomiasis and leishmaniasis. Splenectomy may be required, but the effect on the host immune mechanism must be carefully monitored and controlled.

Neoplasia

Lymphomas and leukaemias frequently infiltrate the spleen and can lead to gross splenomegaly. The underlying diagnosis is usually made by marrow or lymph node biopsy and should lead to treatment of the primary disease. Splenectomy is reserved for hypersplenism or pain or for purposes of staging the disease. The need for staging laparotomy in Hodgkin's disease continues to decrease as the role of chemotherapy expands. Other primary and secondary tumours to the spleen are extremely uncommon.

With other viscera

Splenectomy is an integral part of a total gastrectomy or distal pancreatectomy for neoplasia. It facilitates the operation and permits a better clearance of the regional lymph nodes. However, the spleen can be preserved by careful technique when these organs are removed for benign disease, except in severe chronic pancreatitis. Splenectomy may also be avoided during the construction of a splenorenal shunt by the use of an H-graft. Splenic artery aneurysms can usually be treated by ligation without the need to remove the spleen.

Other indications

Splenic cysts are rare. They may be congenital, degenerative, parasitic or traumatic. Although splenectomy, is the recommended treatment at present, marsupialization may prove to be as effective without the immune consequences. Splenic abscess is best treated by early splenectomy and high-dose chemotherapy, but the results are poor.

Management of the ruptured spleen

Diagnosis

This should be suspected when abdominal trauma is followed by the symptoms and signs of peritonism and shock. Difficulties arise in the unconscious or multiply injured patient, or when the bleeding is slight and contained within the splenic capsule.

The classic symptom is that of left hypochondrial pain, which is worse on moving and radiates to the left shoulder tip (Kehr's sign). The physical signs are those of hypovolaemia and evidence of local injury. There is often grazing or bruising over the left side of the abdomen; abdominal and costal movement is reduced. Peritonism is initially confined to the left upper quadrant but will spread if the bleeding continues; there may be evidence of rib fractures. If the diagnosis is in doubt, abdominal paracentesis may confirm the presence of intraperitoneal blood. Increasingly if the patient is stable many centres are employing ultrasound or CT scanning to assess the extent of the intra-abdominal injury.

The first priority is prompt resuscitation, with the establishment of adequate venous access and the cross-matching of blood. A chest radiograph will help diagnose rib fractures and associated pneumothorax or haemothorax.

Table 14.2   Splenic injury scale

Grade	Type	Injury description
1	Haematoma	Subcapsular, non-expanding <10%
	Laceration	Capsular tear, non-bleeding <1 cm depth
2	Haematoma	Subcapsular, non-expanding 10–15% Intraparenchymal, non-expanding <2 cm diameter
	Laceration	Capsular tear, active bleeding
3	Haematoma	Subcapsular >50% or expanding Ruptured bleeding haematoma Intraparenchymal haematoma >2 cm
	Laceration	>3 cm parenchymal depth
4	Haematoma	Ruptured intraparenchymal haematoma with active bleeding
	Laceration	Laceration involving segmental or hilar vessels producing major devascularization (>25% of spleen)
5	Laceration	Completely shattered spleen Hilar vascular injury that devascularizes spleen

Conservative management

Initial management is aimed at restoring a normal circulating blood volume with blood and other intravenous fluids. Many, particularly younger, patients respond well with normalization of pulse and blood pressure. In these circumstances it is reasonable to treat them conservatively without operation by careful observation and transfusion as required, with the aim of conserving the spleen. These patients require scanning to delineate the extent of the injury and in an attempt to rule out other intraoperative problems. The use of a splenic injury scale (Table 14.2) will help to determine the likelihood of success with a non-operative approach. Table 14.3 delineates the criteria which are necessary for a conservative policy of management. Cross-matched blood should always be available when pursuing such a policy, as deterioration can be sudden and unexpected. Urgent laparotomy is then indicated and may reveal other unsuspected internal injuries. A period of 10–14 days' inpatient observation is advisable in this group. Recent experience suggests that it is applicable to approximately 90% of splenic injuries in children, but only about 15–20% of adults.

Table 14.3   Criteria for non-operative management

Blunt trauma
Haemodynamically stable
Isolated splenic injury
Alert (no head injury or intoxication)

Emergency splenectomy

Access should be gained through an upper midline abdominal incision (Figure 14.2, a–a) since this can be rapidly extended (a–c) if other abdominal injuries are discovered. If the patient is bleeding heavily and access is difficult, a T-shaped extension (b) will quickly improve visibility. Initial assessment should be aimed at confirming that the spleen is the source of haemorrhage. This fact can be achieved by direct inspection or careful palpation; over-zealous handling at this stage can convert a reparable and minor injury into an irrecoverable pulp. Splenic conservation should be the aim, especially in the young, but if the spleen is shattered or bleeding profusely it should be removed at once to prevent exsanguination. The spleen is drawn medially, and the left leaf of the lienorenal ligament is divided either with scissors (Figure 14.3a) or with the fingers. Further careful traction will mobilize the spleen into the wound. The vascular pedicle can then be compressed between finger and thumb to control the bleeding, while the extent of the injury is assessed. If repair is feasible it should now be undertaken (see below).

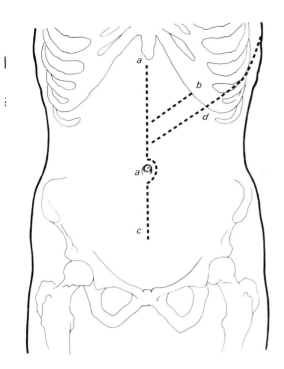

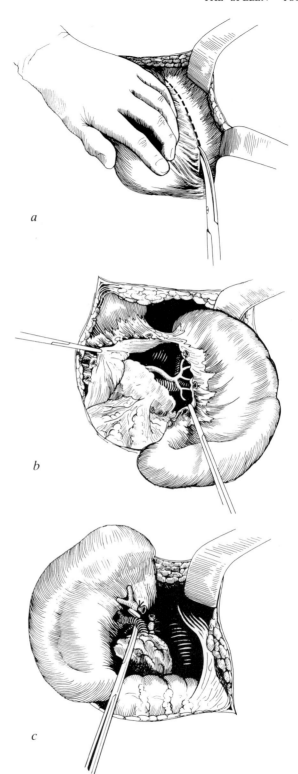

Figure 14.2 Incisions used for splenectomy. The standard incision *a–a* can be extended as a T-piece (*b*) if access is difficult or be lengthened to *c* if other pathology is discovered. For large spleens a thoraco-abdominal incision (*d*) may be helpful

If total splenectomy is unavoidable the short gastric vessel should be tied and divided, care being taken not to damage the gastric wall (Figure 14.3b). The splenic artery and vein are then identified between the pancreas and the spleen. These vessels should be doubly clamped and ligated without injuring the tail of the pancreas (Figure 14.3c). Ideally the splenic artery and vein should be ligated individually in that order. If necessary it is permissible to clamp and tie the vascular pedicle *en masse*. The spleen can then be removed by dividing any remaining peritoneal attachments. A thorough laparotomy should now be performed to exclude other associated injuries, before the abdomen is closed in the routine fashion. A drain is only required if there is associated injury to the tail of the pancreas.

Alternatives to emergency splenectomy

The role of a conservative (non-operative) approach has already been dicussed, But even if a laparotomy is performed it is not always necessary to render the patient asplenic. If at laparotomy the peritoneal blood is completely removed, it is often found that the haemorrhage has ceased. Particularly in young children it is important to conserve splenic function. Current figures suggest that with a combination of non-operative and the following operative approach, splenic salvage should be achievable in approaching 90% of children and 50% of adults. The following

Figure 14.3 Splenectomy. *a*, The spleen is displaced medially, and the lienorenal ligament is divided with scissors, allowing the spleen to be mobilized. *b*, The vasa brevia are divided between clamps. *c*. With the spleen pulled forward, the splenic artery and vein are identified and doubly ligated before division. The spleen can then be removed

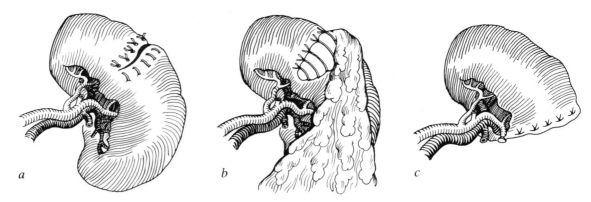

Figure 14.4 Techniques of splenic conservation. *a*, Simple mattress suture of the splenic capsule. *b*, Incorporation of omentum beneath the interrupted mattress sutures. *c*, Partial splenectomy following ligation of the lower polar artery. The capsule is approximated with sutures

techniques are of proven value; many of them require splenic mobilization.

Topical applications

Digital pressure combined with gelatin sponge, thrombin or microfibular collagen will usually suffice for simple lacerations. This approach is particularly applicable to iatrogenic injury during surgery. Packing off the spleen until the operation is completed will usually ensure that haemostasis has been secured.

Splenorraphy

Although the spleen has only a thin capsule, it is possible to suture it after all devitalized tissue has been removed (Figure 14.4a). Teflon buttresses may help to prevent the sutures cutting through. Incorporation of omentum (Figure 14.4b), cyanoacrylate adhesive or microfibrillar collagen into the mattress sutures will increase the haemostatic effect.

Arterial ligation

Ligation of the main splenic artery does not lead to splenic infarction, since there is adequate inflow from the short gastric vessels. Arterial flow can be greatly reduced by ligating the splenic artery at the upper border of the pancreas. Topical applications or splenorrhaphy may then prevent residual haemorrhage. Although arterial ligation preserves the spleen, it does impair its function. Nevertheless, the response to pneumococcal vaccination is much greater than in asplenic individuals.

Partial splenectomy

If one pole of the spleen is largely pulped and the other preserved, partial splenectomy (Figure 14.4c) may be appropriate. Most individuals have two primary lobar (intrasplenic) branches; the relevant vessel

can thus be ligated before that portion of the spleen is removed by a finger fracture technique. The cut surface of the organ is then secured with through-and-through sutures.

Auto-transplantation

If splenectomy is inevitable, some functional activity may be preserved by implanting a portion of splenic tissue. Experimental work suggests that about 40% of a spleen should be inserted into a subperitoneal or greater omentum pouch. This explant will develop a blood supply and the ability to respond to vaccination, but its capacity for pneumococcal clearance is very limited.

Elective splenectomy

Technique

The operation is usually performed through an upper midline incision. In patients with a very large and adherent spleen, a left thoraco-abdominal approach can sometimes be safer. On entering the abdomen the surgeon should perform a thorough laparotomy and make a careful search for splenunculi; these must also be removed if splenectomy is being undertaken for a blood dyscrasia.

If the spleen is very large or has many diaphragmatic adhesions, it is prudent to ligate the splenic artery at an early stage in the operation. After entry into the lesser sac and division of any adhesions, the artery is identified at the upper border of the pancreas and ligated (Figure 14.5).

The spleen is drawn away from the diaphragm and any adhesions diathermied. Strong retraction of the wound edge will assist exposure. The left leaf of the lienorenal ligament is divided, and the spleen can now be gently mobilized with the fingers. The lienocolic attachment should also be divided at this stage. The splenic bed is then packed off, and the vasa brevia are divided to free the spleen from the stomach.

The main vascular pedicle is explored to identify the individual vessels, which should be doubly ligated and tied. The spleen can now be removed. Good haemostasis is important to prevent subphrenic haematoma and abscess formation.

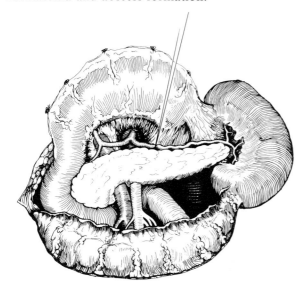

Figure 14.5 If access is difficult or the spleen is very large, the splenic artery can be tied at the upper border of the pancreas to reduce haemorrhage

Alternatives to elective splenectomy

Staging laparotomy

This is an invasive procedure with an appreciable complication rate: 30% minor, 4% major. It should be reserved for patients in whom local radiotherapy is likely to be the sole treatment as long as there is no abdominal dissemination. If a staging laparotomy is required, partial splenectomy will avoid the risk of post-splenectomy sepsis; this risk approaches 10% in children. Alternatively, patients (especially the young) should receive prophylactic penicillin or preferably be vaccinated prior to total splenectomy.

Tropical splenomegaly

Splenectomy is performed to improve the cytopenia and reduce the risk of rupture, but it will also diminish the body's immune response to the parasite. In patients with malaria, long-term chemotherapy may lead to a reduction in splenic size without the need for surgery. Alternatively, segmental splenectomy (leaving 20–30%) has been described, but whether regrowth will occur with time is unknown.

Hypersplenism

The prime indication for operation lies with prolifera-

tive disorders such as leukaemia, and here chemotherapy is the treatment of choice in the first instance. If splenectomy becomes unavoidable, however, the risk of postoperative sepsis is increased by the drug-induced immune deficiency. Partial splenectomy has been achieved by arterial embolization under antibiotic cover, thus avoiding laparotomy. The treatment can be successful provided that the operator aims for no more than a 35% infarction at each attempt. The mortality rate is high, but similar to that of laparotomy. Segmental splenectomy is clearly feasible, but the critical mass to retain is unknown. Portal decompression can be achieved by several techniques and should not involve splenectomy.

Splenic cysts

If these are echinococcal (hydatid), splenectomy remains the treatment of choice. For other cysts an attempt should be made to preserve the spleen. Simple external drainage appears to be effective, but marsupialization into the peritoneal cavity may prove superior in the long term.

Postoperative complications

Haemorrhage

Severe bleeding from the splenic vessels should be prevented by doubly ligating them during the splenectomy. Minor oozing from the splenic bed or diaphragmatic adhesions can be a problem, but this should be dealt with before the abdomen is closed. Otherwise development of the haematoma will predispose to subphrenic abscess.

Atelectasis

Minor degrees of collapse of the left lower lobe of the lung may be accompanied by a small effusion and chest infection. If fractured ribs exacerbate the problem, physiotherapy with or without intercostal nerve block should be considered to improve respiratory excursion.

Venous thrombo-embolism

The risk of generalized venous thrombo-embolism secondary to thrombocytosis is unknown, but there is reported to be a long-term increase in the risk of pulmonary embolism. In the short term, although anticoagulation is usually unnecessary, the administration of anti-platelet agents (e.g. aspirin or dipyridamole) is probably a sensible precaution if the platelet count exceeds 800×10^9/litre.

Ischaemic heart disease

The increase in whole blood viscosity and decrease in

red cell deformability following splenectomy is said to result in a two-fold increase in late death from ischaemic heart disease.

Other risks

Damage to the gastric wall or pancreatic tail may lead to fistula formation; spontaneous closure will often ensue with conservative treatment. Postoperative nasogastric suction for 24 h is a sensible precaution, but the risk of acute gastric dilatation is small.

Post-splenectomy sepsis

This syndrome results from loss of the spleen's ability to promote phagocytosis of encapsulated bacteria; about 50% of cases are due to infection with *Streptococcus pneumoniae*. Onset is insidious. The features are those of overwhelming infection, including rigors, abdominal pain, shock and disseminated intravascular coagulation. Overall only about 4% of patients develop this complication after splenectomy, but the mortality rate is between 50% and 75%. The risk of developing post-splenectomy sepsis is greatest in young children and is maximal within 2–3 years of the operation. Fortunately the risk is small following splenectomy for trauma (1–2%), but it is substantial following resection for thalassaemia or acquired haemolytic anaemias (25%).

Prophylaxis against post-splenectomy sepsis should be routinely considered. Antibiotics are effective, but they should probably be taken routinely for at least 3 years; patient compliance is a major problem. Immunization is likely to be better, although the response to vaccines is reduced after splenectomy and they do not cover all possible organisms. However, vaccines are available against 23 types of pneumococci as well as against *Haemophilus influenzae* and *Neisseria meningitidis*. They are ineffective in children under 2 years of age and of reduced value in those under 7 years. If splenectomy is a planned procedure, vaccination should be performed 1–2 months before operation.

Further reading

Cahill, C. J. and Wastell, C. (1990) Splenic conservation. *Surg. Annual*, **22**, 379–404

Pimpl, W., Dapunt, O., Kaindle, H. *et al.* (1989) Incidence of septic and thromboembolic-related deaths after splenectomy in adults. *Br. J. Surg.*, **76**, 517–521

Redmond, H.P., Redmond, J.M., Rooney, B.P. *et al.* (1989) Surgical anatomy of the human spleen. *Br. J. Surg.*, **76**, 198–201

Shackford, S.R. and Molin, M. (1990) Management of splenic injuries. *Surg. Clin. N. Am.*, **70**, 595–620

Singer, D. B. (1973) Post splenectomy sepsis. In *Perspectives in Paediatric Pathology*, Vol. 1 (ed. H. S. Rosenberg), Year Book Medical, Chicago, pp. 285–311

Vevon, P. A., Ellison, E. C. and Carey, L. C. (1989) Splenectomy for haematologic disease. *Adv. Surg.*, **22**, 205–240

15
The liver

B. R. Davidson and N. A. Habib

Anatomy

The liver occupies the right hypochondrium of the abdomen and is adherent to the undersurface of the diaphragm at its 'bare area' surrounded by the peritoneal reflections forming the coronary and triangular ligaments. It is also supported by the falciform ligament which contains the obliterated umbilical vein. The surface landmarks of the normal liver are the right 5th rib, the right costal margin and the left mid-clavicular line.

The liver derives blood from the hepatic artery (25%) and the portal vein (75%). The hepatic artery usually arises from the aorta at the coeliac axis, runs in the upper aspect of the free edge of the lesser omentum and divides into right and left branches at the hilus. Branches may arise from the superior mesenteric artery or the left gastric artery and these must be identified at the time of resection or transplantation. The portal vein is formed behind the pancreas from the superior mesenteric and splenic veins and runs at the back of the free edge of the lesser omentum, and at the hilus of the liver divides into right and left branches. Most superficially placed on the free edge of the lesser omentum is the common bile duct which drains bile from the liver via the right and left hepatic ducts.

The main venous drainage of the liver is by three large hepatic veins which have a short course between the posterior aspect of the liver and the inferior vena cava, just below the diaphragm. Three or more pairs of small veins also pass directly from the posterior aspect of the liver to the inferior vena cava.

The liver can be divided into two functioning units along a line drawn between the gallbladder fossa anteriorly and the inferior vena cava posteriorly (Figure 15.1). The surgical removal of these units is described as a right or left hepatectomy. The right and left sides of the liver can be further divided into medial and lateral sectors. The falciform ligament provides the surface landmark to the left medial and lateral sectors, whereas on the right the two sectors (right medial and lateral) are divided by an imaginary line passing from a point equidistant from the gallbladder fossa to the antero-inferior angle of the liver anteriorly to the inferior vena cava posteriorly. Within the liver the middle hepatic vein runs between the right and left sides of the liver, the right vein between the right medial and lateral sectors and the left vein between the left medial and lateral sectors.

The liver can be divided into smaller functional segments each with its own vascular supply and bile drainage. Two of these segments form each sector and are numbered as shown in Figure 15.2 in the classification of Couinaud which is widely employed to describe the regional anatomy of the liver.

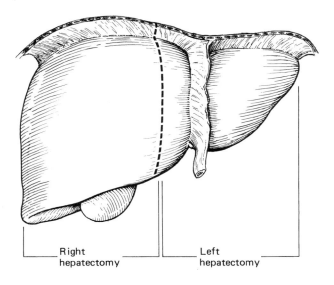

Figure 15.1 Anatomical segments of the liver in relation to partial hepatectomy

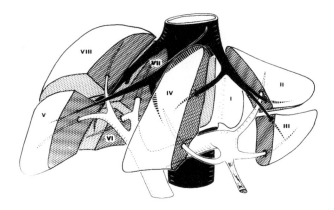

Figure 15.2 The segmental anatomy of the liver

Physiology

The functions of the liver are many and complex. Sixty-five per cent of the body's reticulo-endothelial system is contained within the liver. This is responsible for filtering and destroying bacteria absorbed from the gut and removing debris resulting from cellular breakdown. The liver detoxifies a variety of endogenous and exogenous substances, including most drugs. Hepatocytes play the dominant role in metabolism and storage of basic foodstuffs. Carbohydrates are stored as glycogen and released when necessary. Fats are metabolized, cholesterol is synthesized and the liver is the only source of albumin and alpha-globulin. It is a major storage site for vitamins, especially fat-soluble ones (A, D, K). It synthesizes many of the clotting factors. A fundamental function of the liver is the formation and excretion of bile. About half the bile flow is dependent on the secretion of bile acids, which are manufactured in the liver and are reabsorbed (all but 3%) in the terminal ileum; the remaining half derives from ductal secretion. Bile is the major excretory pathway for bilirubin, cholesterol, drugs and lipid-soluble metabolites. The formation of micelles in the gut aids the absorption of dietary lipids and solubilizes water-insoluble compounds. The most obvious sign of liver failure is jaundice which reflects the accumulation of bilirubin in the tissues. Resection of major portions of the liver is possible by the ability of the organ to regenerate. Following resection, hypertrophy and hyperplasia occur until the liver is restored to near-normal size.

Investigation of the liver and biliary tract

Biochemical

Serial measurements of bilirubin, alkaline phosphatase and transaminase levels in the serum should indicate the extent and nature of jaundice, including the presence of extrahepatic obstruction and concomitant damage to hepatocytes. Serum albumin is a guide to the synthetic capacity of the liver and the nutritional state of the patient. Since the liver produces many of the clotting factors, the prothrombin time should be assessed; hypoprothrombinaemia often responds to administration of parenteral vitamin K. Alpha-fetoprotein (AFP) is a tumour marker which is secreted by over 70% of hepatocellular carcinomas. Its level should return to normal following resection, and elevation may indicate recurrence.

Ultrasound

This is undoubtedly the most useful screening test, being non-invasive, inexpensive and repeatable. Sensitivity is reduced by obesity, excess bowel gas or a high subcostal situation of the liver. Ultrasonography is most commonly employed to confirm a dilated ductal system, but may detect cysts, abscesses and tumours. Differentiation between primary and secondary neoplasms may not be possible. Scans permit guided biopsies for histology and cytology.

Computed tomography

This has the advantage over ultrasound of defining smaller lesions, providing greater anatomical information and being unaffected by the presence of bowel gas. The scans are enhanced with oral contrast to delineate the bowel and intravenous contrast to show vascular structures.

Cholangiography

Intravenous cholangiography is only feasible in the absence of jaundice. Introduction of the Chiba ('skinny') needle has made percutaneous transhepatic cholangiography (PTC) a safe procedure, although success is limited in the absence of dilated intrahepatic ducts. PTC is of particular value in determining the level and the nature of an obstructing lesion. Endoscopic retrograde cholangiopancreatography (ERCP) similarly delineates biliary obstruction. At ERCP and PTC, bile may be aspirated for microbiology and brushing of structures performed for cytology.

Arteriography

Selective coeliac and superior mesenteric angiograms are a prerequisite for safe elective hepatic surgery. The examination has a high resolution and provides a 'road map' for the surgeon by delineating the vascular supply, including anomalies. Late-phase angiography demonstrates the portal vein, and neoplastic involvement of arterial and venous structures can be determined.

Laparoscopy

This permits direct visualization of the liver and allows accurate staging and biopsy of diseased or normal liver tissue.

Percutaneous liver biopsy

This is an invasive procedure with a risk of haemorrhage, sepsis and bile peritonitis. With care, it is safe and is valuable in the diagnosis of diffuse liver disease. Accuracy is enhanced when insertion of the needle is guided by ultrasound, CT scan or laparoscopy for localized lesions.

Preoperative precautions

Certain measures are essential for any patient with obstructive jaundice undergoing major surgery. Assessment of nutritional and clotting status should be made and corrected if abnormal. Vitamin K may reverse a clotting abnormality, but the serum albumin is unlikely to respond to parenteral nutrition if the liver is obstructed or diseased. Prophylactic antibiotics are required, as sepsis is a major cause of death. They are required to cover invasive diagnostic procedures such as PTC and ERCP. Percutaneous decompression of obstructive jaundice may improve liver function and aid postoperative recovery. Patients undergoing surgery for obstructive jaundice are prone to develop acute renal failure (the hepato-renal syndrome). This complication can be avoided by adequate preoperative hydration, the avoidance of hypotension and the use of mannitol to promote an osmotic diuresis or a renal dose of dopamine. All patients should be catheterized before operation to enable urine output to be accurately monitored.

Congenital conditions of the liver

Biliary atresia

The commonest cause of prolonged neonatal jaundice is extrahepatic biliary atresia. Uncorrected, this condition will lead to liver failure and death, with only a few infants surviving beyond 6 months. Between 10% and 20% of patients have a short length of extra-hepatic bile duct, permitting a conventional mucosa-to-mucosa anastomosis. For the majority, however, a hepatic porto-enterostomy (Kasai operation) should be attempted. The operation should be undertaken within 60 days of birth, otherwise intrahepatic fibrosis will rapidly ensue and reduce the chance of cure. Even when undertaken early the operation may be complicated by the development of cholangitis, cirrhosis and portal hypertension, resulting in a poor long-term prognosis. When evidence of deteriorating liver function is apparent, liver transplantation should be considered.

Congenital cystic disease

Cysts may be solitary or multiple. Multiple cysts are frequently associated with polycystic disease of the kidney. The cysts are often small and asymptomatic, being found incidentally at laparotomy or autopsy. If large, they may cause pressure symptoms and require surgical treatment. Small cysts usually require no treatment, but they can be aspirated and often do not recur. Larger cysts may become infected or present as a result of bleeding or rupture. They can be aspirated and treated according to the contents. Cysts filled with clear serous fluid may be marsupialized into the peritoneal cavity. Bile would indicate the need for enteric drainage into a Roux loop. Rarely a cyst may destroy the whole lobe and a partial hepatecomy may be indicated.

Caroli's disease is congenital cystic dilatation of the intrahepatic ducts (Figure 15.3). It usually presents with recurrent upper abdominal pain and cholangitis. The disease is often diffuse, in which case there is no specific therapy apart from antibiotics. Occasionally it is confined to one segment or liver lobe and in this case resection may be curative. Adequate surgical drainage of the cyst cavity may give good results.

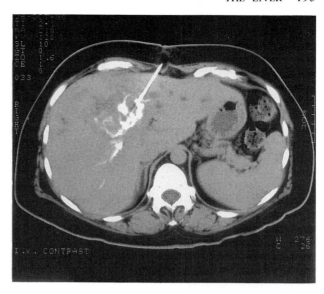

Figure 15.3 Congenital cystic dilatation of the liver (Caroli's disease) demonstrated on CT scanning

Inborn errors of metabolism

Several inborn errors of hepatic metabolism are at present untreated and lead to death at an early age. It has become apparent, with increasing experience of liver transplantation in children, that some of these problems are curable. Liver transplantations have been performed for Wilson's disease, alpha-1-antitrypsin deficiency, oxaluria, tyrosinaemia and Niemann–Pick disease.

Hepatic trauma

In the UK, liver injury is usually the result of a road traffic accident and is frequently accompanied by other serious skeletal, thoracic or abdominal injuries.

Penetrating trauma due to knives or bullets is uncommon. Stab wounds leave an obvious track and usually stop bleeding spontaneously. Low-velocity bullet wounds need only removal of the foreign body and adjacent devitalized tissue, but parenchymal shattering after a high-velocity injury is often best treated by formal hepatic resection (Figure 15.4).

The primary treatment must be to resuscitate the patient and fully assess the injuries. Penetrating wounds should be explored, with debridement and control of the haemorrhage; tetanus toxoid should be administered, together with prophylactic antibiotics. The diagnosis of hepatic injury after blunt trauma is largely made on clinical grounds. The commonest sign is abdominal tenderness often progressing to guarding and rigidity. Some patients have no specific abdominal signs or symptoms. Radiographs will show any associated chest or abdominal injuries. Abdominal paracentesis and lavage are reliable techniques for detecting intra-abdominal haemorrhage and are of particular value if the clinical signs are equivocal or the patient is unconscious. If operation is not performed soon after admission, then ultrasound scanning may show hepatic injury and the presence of a subcapsular haematoma. Laparotomy is indicated for continuing or major blood loss manifest by serial measurement of vital signs.

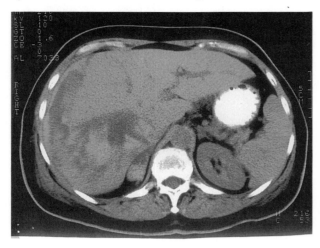

Figure 15.4 CT scan demonstrating destruction of the right liver following a road traffic accident

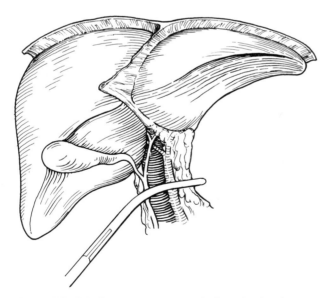

Figure 15.5 Pringle's manoeuvre. A soft clamp is placed across the free edge of the lesser omentum to occlude vascular inflow to the liver

Surgery for liver haemorrhage may be performed through a transverse upper abdominal incision which may be extended in the midline up to the xiphisternum and round the right costal margin. Clamping of the hepatic artery and portal vein at the foramen of Winslow (the Pringle manoeuvre) will provide

haemostasis if their branches have been divided (Figure 15.5). This allows the site of blood loss to be accurately determined, any non-viable liver to be removed and the damaged vessel ligated or oversewn. Bleeding from the IVC requires dissection and control of the IVC above and below the liver as well as a Pringle manoeuvre prior to full mobilization of the right lobe and suturing of the caval defect.

A satisfactory alternative to resection and repair for major liver haemorrhage is gauze packing and if carried out meticulously, may provide good initial haemostasis. After 48–72 h the packing is removed and the injury reassessed. Angiography and CT scanning may be valuable in the interim period.

Surgical treatment of liver infections

Pyogenic liver abscess

This is a rare condition which affects the elderly or debilitated. In 25–50% of cases the primary site of the infection is never established and they are termed cryptogenic. Biliary infection, usually in the form of ascending cholangitis, is the commonest source, followed by portal pyaemia from an intra-abdominal abscess related to appendicitis, pancreatitis, diverticular disease of the colon or perforations of the biliary tree or gastrointestinal tract. Other causes are direct liver trauma and haematogenous spread.

About half of all liver abscesses are multiple. Solitary abscesses are usually found in the right lobe of the liver directly under the diaphragm. Common organisms are *Escherichia coli*, Gram-positive *Streptococcus*, *Staphylococcus aureus* and anaerobes.

Presenting symptoms are variable but there is often fever, malaise, anorexia and upper abdominal pain. Laboratory investigations may show a neutrophil leucocytosis, secondary anaemia and hypoalbuminaemia. Less than half show a typical swinging pyrexia and only 10% have positive blood cultures. Abdominal X-rays may help the diagnosis by showing a raised right hemidiaphragm, right basal pleural effusion or an air-fluid level in the liver. To establish the diagnosis an ultrasound or CT scan is required, with guided aspiration for microbiology under cover of systemic antibiotics.

All patients with liver abscesses are treated with systemic antibiotics, chosen if possible by sensitivity reports. If the abscesses are multiple this may be the only form of treatment possible. Those large enough to be readily detected on imaging rarely respond to antibiotics alone and require drainage. Under ultrasound or CT guidance the abscess may be aspirated and if necessary a drain inserted percutaneously. Follow-up scans are required to assess the response to treatment.

The treatment of liver abscesses by aspiration under imaging control has the disadvantage of not dealing with the primary site and may not be successful if there is marked loculation within a chronic abscess cavity. Open surgical drainage may, therefore, be required and is performed extraperitoneally through a posterior approach through the bed of the 12th rib, if the abscess is lying at the upper posterior aspect of the right lobe (segments VII and VIII). More commonly, an anterior transperitoneal approach is employed which allows the entire liver to be inspected and the primary site to be found and dealt with. The liver abscess is aspirated with a trocar, being careful to avoid contamination of the peritoneal cavity. Any loculation is broken down and soft drains inserted which are brought out through the abdominal wall. These are left *in situ* to allow irrigation of the cavity and sinograms to be performed and are not removed until the abscess cavity is completely obliterated.

The morbidity and mortality associated with liver abscesses is high if they are multiple or inadequately drained. Early diagnosis, appropriate and prolonged antibiotic therapy, effective drainage and intensive supportive therapy are the key to a successful outcome.

Amoebic liver abscesses

About 10% of the world's population, mainly within the tropics and subtropics, are asymptomatic carriers of *Entamoeba histolytica*, but only a small percentage develop invasive amoebiasis resulting in colitis or a liver abscess. Although patients with liver abscesses are thought to develop infection by the portal spread of trophozoites, they rarely give a history suggestive of amoebic colitis. In contrast, about one-third of patients with colitis will have evidence of liver abscess.

Amoebic liver abscesses develop a liquefied centre containing necrotic liver and blood, with amoebae being identified at the spreading edge. Extension and rupture of the abscess results in invasion of the pleura, lung, pericardium and other surrounding structures. As the lesions age, they may form a fibrous capsule.

The presentation of an uncomplicated amoebic liver abscess is commonly with right upper quadrant pain accompanied by a tender hepatomegaly. Ultrasound and aspiration for culture will confirm the diagnosis and reliable serological tests such as the precipitin test are available. The treatment of uncomplicated cysts is with metronidazole and the response may be monitored clinically and ultrasonically. If an amoebic liver abscess adheres to and ruptures into a surrounding structure it is defined 'complicated'. Diaphragm, pleura, lung, bowel and the chest and abdominal wall are frequently involved. Only rarely do amoebic abscesses rupture into the peritoneal cavity, where they may present with generalized abdominal pain, ascites and abdominal distension. The commonest presentation is with localized pain in the right upper quadrant associated with hepato-

megaly and an abdominal mass. If presentation is with localized signs and the diagnosis can be confirmed, then the treatment is conservative with intravenous metronidazole. Patients presenting with generalized signs are commonly submitted to laparotomy with drainage of abscesses, although a conservative policy may be effective in this situation. Thoracic involvement may take the form of pleural or pericardial effusions developing in response to the adherence of an abscess in the right or left lobe of the liver. Abscess rupture into the right thorax produces an amoebic empyema and may result in a hepato-bronchial fistula. Rupture into the pericardium is usually fatal. Treatment is by aspiration of effusions under ultrasound or CT guidance if they produce symptoms along with metronidazole therapy.

Surgical drainage in complicated amoebic abscesses results in a shorter hospital stay. It is also indicated in the following:

1. Patients with generalized peritonitis.
2. Where the diagnosis is in doubt.
3. No clinical response to 48 h of metronidazole.
4. No improvement following aspiration of effusions.
5. Rupture into the pleura or pericardium.

Surgery is performed as described for pyogenic abscesses.

Hydatid disease

This is a common condition, particularly in the Mediterranean, Middle East and Australia. The most common form of hydatid disease is caused by the parasite *Echinococcus granulosus* whose main host is the dog and which is transferred to man by the faecal–oral route. The liver is the most commonly involved organ with the production of cysts which consist of an outer fibrous adventitia, a gelatinous laminated membrane and an inner germinal epithelium from which the infective brood capsules are derived. The cysts usually occupy the upper pole of the right lobe (segments VII and VIII) and present with right upper quadrant pain (Figure 15.6a,b). Atypical presentations may occur if the cysts become secondarily infected, rupture into the biliary tree (producing obstructive jaundice ± cholangitis) or pleural cavity. Diagnosis of hydatid cysts may be achieved by ultrasound or CT scanning and can be confirmed by serological testing using an enzyme-linked immunosorbent assay (ELISA) or radioallergosorbent test (RAST)

Calcified cysts are usually dead and therefore require no treatment. Small and deeply situated cysts may be treated conservatively with monitoring by serial ultrasound examinations. Drug therapy for hydatid disease has been more effective since the introduction of mebendazole and subsequently albendazole, but is not yet proven as a sole treatment for liver cysts. Patients presenting with obstructive jaundice or cholangitis due to daughter cysts obstructing the common bile duct may be managed initially with

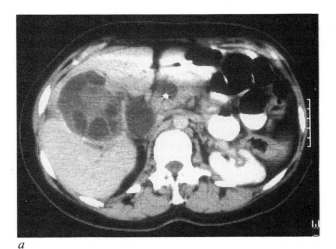

a

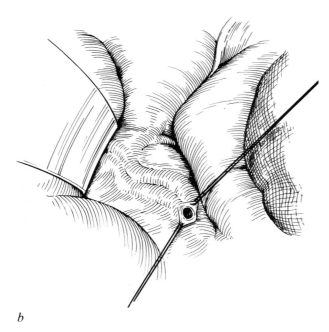

b

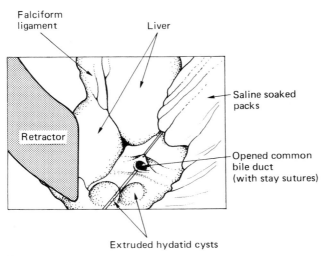

c

endoscopic sphincterotomy or nasobiliary drainage. Large and superficially placed liver hydatid cysts require surgery.

A transverse or extended right subcostal incision is usually satisfactory. A thorough laparotomy is performed prior to full mobilization of the liver. The liver is then surrounded by packs soaked in hypertonic saline which will catch and destroy any spilled brood capsules or daughter cysts. Careful aspiration of the cyst is performed and bile staining signifies a communication with the biliary tree. The cyst's wall is removed in the plane between the laminated membrane and the adventitia, with oversewing of any areas of bile leakage. The resulting cavity is filled with omentum which may be mobilized on the right gastro-epiploic vessels. Unless preoperative endoscopic sphincterotomy (ES) has been performed the gallbladder is removed, operative cholangiography performed and, if necessary, the common bile duct explored (Figure 15.6c).

Omentoplasty, as described above, is appropriate for the treatment of most hydatid liver cysts and is safe and effective. Removal of the cyst from outside the adventitia (pericystectomy) has the advantage of detecting any daughter cysts lying outside the wall of the main cyst, but the procedure may result in excessive bleeding from adherent vessels. Liver resection may be suitable in some cases, but marked distortion of normal liver architecture may produce operative difficulties, and preoperative angiography is advisable.

Neoplasms of the liver

Benign

These are uncommon and often present incidentally or by mimicking biliary disease. The usual types are haemangioma or adenoma. The latter is associated with oral contraceptive use and may regress when the drug is withdrawn. Up to 20% of all these lesions present with intraperitoneal rupture and haemorrhage, which have an appreciable mortality rate. The treatment is surgical excision which can be performed by wedge resection in most instances.

Hepatocellular carcinoma

Hepatocellular carcinoma (HCC) is uncommon in the UK, with fewer than 2 cases per 100 000 of the population per annum. Chronic liver disease, hepatitis B virus infection and alcohol abuse are important

---

Figure 15.6 *a*, Hydatid daughter cysts in the liver demonstrated on CT scanning. *b*, *c*, Exploration of the common bile duct in a patient with filling defects on operative cholangiography showing the presence of multiple hydatid daughter cysts

predisposing factors. In parts of the world where these are common, hepatoma may be the commonest intra-abdominal malignancy. In the black population in Southern Africa there are up to 30 cases per 100 000 per annum. The presenting features are often vague, especially if they are superimposed on ill health from chronic liver disease. Most patients complain of malaise, weight loss, abdominal discomfort, unexplained fever or jaundice. The liver may be enlarged and tender, often containing a palpable mass.

Liver function tests may be disordered but are nonspecific. Over 70% of patients will have increased levels of alpha-fetoprotein (AFP). The tumour may be revealed and staged by CT scanning. Angiography is important to assess the vascular anatomy of the liver (Figure 15.7). Surgery offers the only hope of cure in patients with HCC and should be carried out for all resectable lesions. Unfortunately many patients have either extensive cancers, multifocal disease or severe underlying liver disease, making a cure impossible. In cases selected as 'potentially curative' and undergoing radical surgery, a 45% 5-year survival may be obtained.

not within the bounds of this chapter, but about 30% of these tumours arise at the hepatic duct bifurcation (Klatskin tumour) and are often intrahepatic. Presentation is almost invariably with obstructive jaundice. The combination of ultrasonography, PTC or ERCP should demonstrate the lesion in most patients (Figure 15.8). Differentiation between cholangiocarcinoma and sclerosing cholangitis may be difficult and CT-guided percutaneous fine-needle aspiration cytology (FNAC) or exfoliative cytology at PTC and ERCP are often helpful. Arteriography, including venous phase studies, is important to determine vascular invasion and assess resectability.

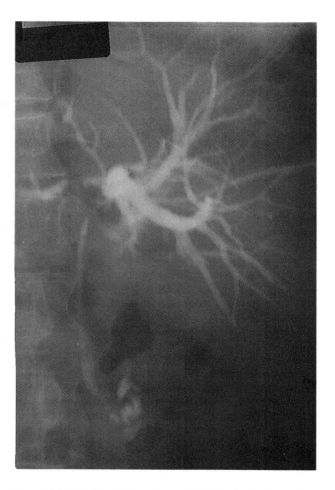

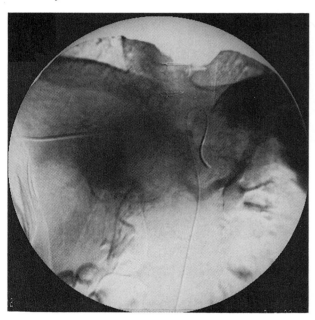

Figure 15.7 Selective coeliac axis angiography demonstrating the vascular anatomy of the liver and a 'blush' due to the tumour vascularity

Figure 15.8 A hilar stricture demonstrated by cholangiography

Patients with extensive cancers have undergone liver transplantation, but the results are generally poor, the vast majority dying from recurrent disease within the first year. Whether patients with a small primary cancer in a cirrhotic liver are best treated by resection or transplantation has yet to be resolved.

Cholangiocarcinoma

The treatment of extrahepatic cholangiocarcinoma is

Tumour resection should be the treatment of choice, but this is a major procedure which often involves a hepatic split or partial hepatic resection. It is feasible to 20–50% of patients and has an operative mortality of 15–20%. Figures up to 40% 5-year survival can be obtained with appropriate patient selection, and resection provides a good form of palliation. Other palliative options include insertion of an endoprosthesis and biliary-enteric bypass.

Metastatic cancer

This is by far the commonest liver tumour in the Western world. It is usually asymptomatic, but when advanced it results in hepatic pain, ascites, jaundice and palpable mass; other features are those of generalized malignancy such as anorexia and weight loss. Serial assays of carcino-embryonic antigen (CEA) after colonic resection may enable detection of small asymptomatic metastases. The poor prognosis of untreated metastatic disease is evident from mean survival rates of less than 3 months and a 1-year survival rate of less than 7%.

Perhaps 10% of the patients with hepatic metastases may be suitable for potentially curative resection, there being either a solitary metastasis or multiple deposits in a single segment. Published data include an operative mortality rate of about 5% and a 5-year survival rate of 20%.

Indications and contraindications to liver resection for tumours

Surgery for liver tumours may be considered for curative or palliative treatments and primary and secondary tumours may be considered for resection whether they are single or multiple, provided that they are contained within resectable area(s) of the liver.

Is the lesion technically resectable?

Liver tumours are generally considered to be resectable if there is no metastatic spread, either distant or to another area within the liver. Involvement of the inferior vena cava, the portal vein or the main biliary tree are usually considered to be contraindications to surgery. Some surgeons consider resecting the diaphragm, synchronous metastases and segments of the portal vein or inferior vena cava.

Will the patient survive the procedure?

An assessment of whether the patient will survive the procedure depends on an accurate history and examination of the patient preoperatively, with particular emphasis on the patient's age, previous abdominal surgery and history of ischaemic heart or chronic respiratory disease. The extent of liver resection which can be carried out is dependent on the function of the remaining segment or lobe of liver. This may be difficult to judge preoperatively, but patients with hepatitis or cirrhosis are in danger of postoperative liver failure. It is therefore advisable to biopsy the 'normal' liver preoperatively, where an extensive resection is planned to exclude the presence of liver cirrhosis.

Will the patient's quality or length of life be improved?

A judgement as to whether the patient's quality or length of life may be improved is perhaps the most difficult factor to assess. Palliative surgery to relieve symptoms rather than cure may be justified in centres where the morbidity and mortality of the procedure is minimal. The long-term results which have been reported for the treatment of different types of tumour should always be borne in mind prior to recommending resection.

Operative techniques in liver surgery

Positioning of patient

The patient is positioned supine on the table, but with rotation to the left by placing a wedge under the lower right chest. Elevation of the head of the table encourages the gut to remain in the lower compartment of the abdomen.

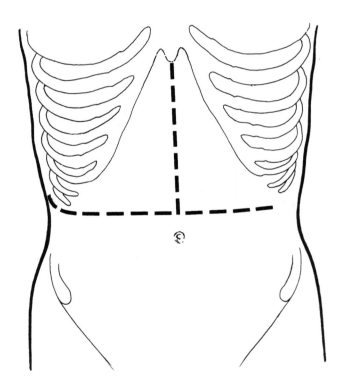

Figure 15.9 The incision for liver surgery

Skin incision

A transverse incision is made at the level of the lower rib cage with extension towards the right renal angle and upwards in the midline to the xiphisternum. This incision is sometimes called the modified Mercedes Benz incision (Figure 15.9). It gives two flaps of anterior abdominal wall which can be retracted by stitching to the skin over the chest wall. Care must be taken at the right extremity of the incision not to open the right pleural space. The incision on the right side goes around the angle of the rib cage and continues upwards parallel to the ribs in the direction of the renal angle. The last part of the incision facilitates traction of the costal margin upwards and allows direct access to the vena cava and the hepatic veins.

Retraction

For liver resection it is important to have good retraction of both right and left costal margins during the entire procedure. Fixed retractors are suitable for this purpose. Following retraction of the rib cage, one can proceed to exploratory laparotomy and exclude the presence of findings that would contraindicate the operative procedure.

Mobilization of the liver

The falciform ligament is divided in the antero-posterior direction using the cutting diathermy needle. Posteriorly the falciform ligament divides into two leaves, to the right and to the left. This point is at least 5 cm proximal to the hepatic veins or the supra-hepatic vena cava. At this stage the incision proceeds towards the left lobe of the liver by dividing the left triangular ligament, watching for a low insertion of a left subphrenic vein. To facilitate the incision of the left triangular ligament, the stomach is protected by positioning an abdominal pack between the left lobe of the liver and the stomach. Haemostasis is normally secured with the diathermy needle. After division of the left triangular ligament, mobilization of the left lobe is completed by incising the lesser omentum, being careful to avoid an aberrant left hepatic artery originating from the left gastric artery. Following mobilization of the left liver, the right leaf of the falciform ligament is divided with the right triangular ligament. This may be facilitated by the assistant's left hand rotating the liver towards the left and downwards.

Mobilization of the inferior surface of the liver starts by dividing any adhesions between the liver or the gallbladder and the large bowel, small bowel or duodenum. The peritoneum between the inferior surface of the liver and the anterior surface of the right kidney is divided and the incision proceeds towards the right to join the upper leaf of the right triangular ligament. At this stage of the dissection the assistant should retract with his right hand the inferior pole of the right liver upwards in the direction of the patient's left shoulder. It is this rotation of the liver that facilitates the posterior dissection, particularly in the bare area. To ensure full liver rotation, no swabs should be left underneath the left lobe or at the hilus. The peritoneum overlying the inferior vena cava should then be divided and the right side of the liver mobilized further. This is facilitated by the assistant retracting the right side of the liver upwards using the left hand. Any tissue remaining between the posterior surface of the liver and the posterior abdominal wall should be divided, great care being taken not to damage the right adrenal vein as it enters the IVC. At this point attention is turned to the hilar dissection.

Hilar dissection

One should identify the foramen ovale and place a sling around the structures at the free edge of the lesser omentum to gain control of the hepatic pedicle in case of sudden bleeding (see Figure 15.5). Hilar dissection starts with mobilization of the gallbladder and cholecystectomy, leaving a long remnant of the cystic duct. The common bile duct should be dissected and retracted with a sling. Dissection of the left aspect of the hepatic pedicle exposes the common hepatic artery. The right and left branches of the hepatic artery should be dissected and retracted with slings. Retraction of the common bile duct to the right and the common hepatic artery to the left, allows the portal vein to be located in the space between the two structures.

Dissection of the portal vein should be done cautiously with a blunt instrument, care being taken not to injure its small branches. Haemostasis should be secured with a 5/0 Prolene stitch. Once the portal vein is dissected, a sling is passed around to allow easy control of this structure if needed. Dissection of the portal vein towards the hilus exposes the right and left branches of the portal vein. Dissection of the right branch of the portal vein is easier when approached from the right aspect of the hepatic pedicle. To gain access the assistant rotates the hepatic pedicle (in such a way that its posterior aspect faces the right side of the patient) and the operator incises the peritoneum over the portal vein which is retracted with a sling. Upwards dissection posteriorly will expose the right branch of the portal vein. Great care is needed to avoid the caudate branches arising from the right branch of the portal vein or the upper aspect of the portal vein bifurcation feeding the caudate lobe. Likewise, the left branch of the portal vein is sometimes dissected more easily from a left, rather than an anterior approach to the hepatic pedicle.

Choice of hepatic resection

Following full mobilization of the liver, an intra-operative ultrasound should be performed to help assess tumour spread and allow the main structures in the liver to be visualized. It is at this stage that the final decision is made whether it is justifiable to proceed with a liver resection and which type of resection is appropriate.

Right hepatectomy

This procedure involves the removal of that portion of the liver to the right side of the imaginary line extending from the gallbladder fossa to the inferior vena cava (see Figure 15.1). Prior to performing the resection it is necessary to fully mobilize the liver and to gain control of the major vessels (Figure 15.10).

Inferior vena caval control

The infrahepatic portion of the inferior vena cava is dissected by extending the incision of the posterior parietal peritoneum over the lateral aspect of the inferior vena cava which may then be encircled by a sling. The suprahepatic vena cava is dissected by incising the overlying peritoneum. The entrance of the right and left inferior phrenic veins into the IVC should be avoided. Once the suprahepatic IVC has been slung, caval control has been achieved. If the cava has to be clamped during the operative procedure, a significant drop in blood pressure will result, but this may be minimized by the anaesthetist overfilling the vascular bed prior to clamping.

Prior to dissection of the right hepatic vein, the small veins to the caudate lobe are secured and this is facilitated by the left hand of the assistant rotating the liver towards the patient's left side. The veins, of which there may be 2–6 pairs, should be tied on the liver and transfixed on the side of the inferior vena cava. Bleeding from a missed caudate vein is a common cause of postoperative blood loss. After dissection and ligation of these small veins an accessory right inferior hepatic vein (approximately 30% of cases) may be encountered. It is important to recognize, dissect and transfix this vein. Further cephalad dissection will reveal the right hepatic vein which lies within a sheet of fibrous tissue. Division of this tissue allows dissection of the space between the right and left hepatic veins which should be performed cautiously with a blunt instrument. It is important to dissect clearly the plane between the liver and IVC. If this plane cannot be readily dissected no further mobilization of the right hepatic vein should be attempted, the vein being ligated following division of the liver parenchyma. If major haemorrhage occurs during dissection of the right hepatic vein, a Pringle manoeuvre along with clamping of the suprahepatic and infrahepatic vena cava should be performed until the bleeding can be arrested. The source of the haemorrhage may be isolated most readily by dividing and transfixing the right hepatic vein. Clamping of the vena cava is important in this situation as the patient may die instantaneously from a massive air embolus rather than from the haemorrhage.

Vascular control prior to parenchymal resection

The right branch of the hepatic artery and the right

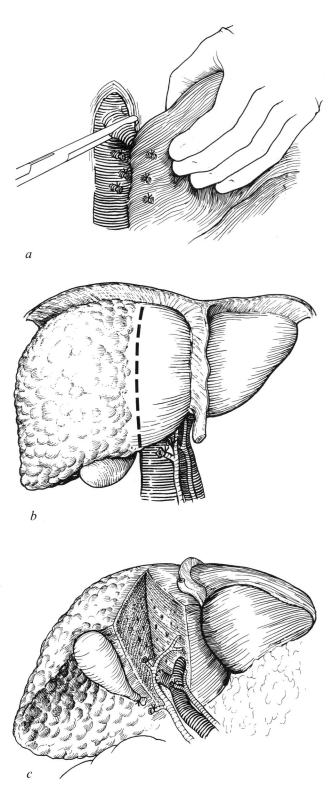

Figure 15.10 Right hemihepatectomy. *a*, After mobilizing and displacing the liver to the right, three small hepatic veins have been divided between clips and a clamp placed on the right hepatic vein. *b*, The line of parenchymal transection. *c*, After controlling the vascular inflow and outflow to the right lobe, the liver structure is divided between the right and left lobes

branch of the portal vein are ligated with silk or linen. If division of these branches is postponed until a later stage, then the decision to perform hepatectomy remains reversible. Having emptied the right liver of blood, the right hepatic vein is tied in continuity with silk or linen but is not divided outside the liver. Following ligation of the vessels to the right liver, division of the hepatic parenchyma is commenced.

Hepatic parenchymal resection

Following ligation of the right branches of the hepatic artery and the portal vein, a line of devascularization forms between the right and left lobes. The resection line should follow 1 cm to the right of this demarcation line (right side of the patient). If possible the middle hepatic vein, which lies in the plane, should be preserved. It may be located using intraoperative ultrasound. Resection commences by incising Glisson's capsule and proceeds by gently crushing the liver parenchyma with a haemostat. This technique allows separation of the parenchyma while the blood vessels and bile ducts remain intact. Alternatively, an ultrasonic dissector may be used. Remaining branches are either ligated or diathermied. If significant bleeding occurs from the liver parenchyma, the Pringle manoeuvre should be performed but released every 15 min for 2 min. The direction of liver division is important, it being towards the right side of the inferior vena cava. The dissection should keep some distance from the hilus to prevent injury to the biliary confluence. The segmental blood supply to the right liver is secured within the liver parenchyma by transfixion. Once the level of the hilus is reached, the operator's left hand should be placed behind the right side of the liver at the site of insertion of the right caudate veins in the vena cava. By placing the fingers of the left hand in the groove formed by the IVC the operator will help the direction of the dissection. Branches from the middle hepatic vein should be transfixed, as bleeding at this stage may be difficult to control. When the posterior part of the liver is reached, the right hepatic vein is clamped and transfixed from within the liver parenchyma and the right liver is removed.

Haemostasis

Time and effort should be spent in securing all the bleeding points, usually by transfixion, following the hepatic resection. Sites which require special attention to haemostasis include the cut surface of the liver, the inferior phrenic veins as they enter the IVC and the right triangular ligament. Recognized methods of securing haemostasis from the cut surface of the liver include temporary gauze packing, approximating the liver capsule by suturing or using an infrared coagulator, argon gas laser or a haemostatic glue. A bile leak may be demonstrated by injecting methylene blue into the cystic duct following a Pringle manoeuvre

and areas where the blue dye emerges are transfixed. If haemostasis is secured, there is no need for drainage. Omentum and the hepatic flexure of the colon should be 'encouraged' to occupy the place of the right liver. Rotation of the liver should be avoided by stitching back the falciform ligament.

Postoperative care

This type of procedure in experienced hands should be possible with blood loss of less than 1 litre and occasionally without intraoperative blood transfusion. In uncomplicated cases the patient can be reversed and extubated on the table and sent to the ward for postoperative care. If the procedure was prolonged or there were intraoperative difficulties, then an initial period of intensive care monitoring is preferable.

Intravenous fluid

It is important to keep the central venous pressure between 5 and 10 cmH$_2$O postoperatively by giving a combination of crystalloid and colloid. Patients with cirrhosis should initially be treated mainly with colloid in the form of plasma protein fraction or salt-poor albumin. Sufficient fluid should be administered to keep the urine output above 40 ml per hour.

Ventilation

In most cases it is not necessary to ventilate these patients artificially postoperatively and it is enough to administer 40% oxygen by mask. Physiotherapy in the immediate postoperative period is important to ensure lung expansion. A postoperative chest X-ray should be carried out to exclude a right pneumothorax which may have occurred during mobilization of the right liver. Thoracic epidural analgesia is a very effective method to keep patient pain free and to minimize the risks of right lung lower lobe collapse.

Renal function

It is important to maintain a urine output of approximately 40 ml per hour. Patients with obstructive jaundice or cirrhosis are routinely given dopamine 2–5 µg/kg per minute (renal dose). Postoperative oliguria in a patient who is normotensive, well hydrated and with a normal central venous filling pressure should be treated with an initial fluid challenge and if this does not produce a response a bolus injection of 20 mg frusemide is given.

Liver function

Patients in whom more than 50% of the liver has been removed will develop a degree of liver failure, declared by an elevated prothrombin time, INR, bilirubin, alkaline phosphatase and aspartate aminotransferase (AST). These parameters usually return to normal after 4 or 5 days. Patients with obstructive jaundice or cirrhosis are particularly susceptible to abnormalities of liver function. The patient should be actively supported with fluids, nutrition and clotting factors until liver regeneration takes place.

Complications

These can be divided into early (first 48 h) and intermediate (first postoperative week).

Early complications

The main early postoperative complications are haemorrhage and respiratory problems. The presence of a coagulopathy should always be suspected and any clotting abnormality corrected with fresh frozen plasma. Bleeding is usually encountered from the transection line, the hepatic veins or the caudate lobe veins. Respiratory problems usually arise from postoperative pulmonary atelectasis, although a pneumothorax should always be excluded. Physiotherapy or bronchial aspiration may be necessary for pulmonary collapse.

Intermediate complications

The commonest is postoperative liver failure, due to the extent of resection of liver parenchyma especially in a compromised liver (cirrhosis or obstruction). Active supportive therapy is given until liver regeneration occurs. Renal failure may occur as part of the hepatorenal syndrome associated with liver failure. Careful fluid replacement monitored by central venous pressure measurements and the administration of a renal dose of dopamine may help, and potassium canrenoate should be given routinely in patients with cirrhosis.

Sepsis

Infective complications following a liver resection are similar to those following any major intra-abdominal surgery. The collection of haematoma in the subphrenic cavity occasionally results in the development of a subphrenic abscess. Patients with ascites may develop infection within the ascitic fluid postoperatively. A bile leak should be considered if there is sepsis, and a tubogram or ERCP should be performed to confirm the suspected leak.

Chyle leak

This occurs due to damage to the lymphatics at the liver hilus and usually presents after the patient starts eating. The leak may reach enormous proportions, but lasts for 3 or 4 days before resolving. The patient should be given fluid replacement in the form of colloid.

Long-term results
Survival following surgery for hepatocellular carcinoma

The reported operative mortality varies from less than 5% to almost 50%. Many have highlighted the increased morbidity and mortality associated with surgery when cirrhosis is present and the risks may be stratified by the preoperative liver function and the size of resection required. Survival following successful resection varies from 28% to 68% of patients at 2 years, but the 5-year survival rate may be as low as 4% or as high as 45%.

Survival following surgery for liver metastases

Surgery is indicated in only a small percentage of patients with liver metastases and of these it is patients with colorectal cancer who would appear to benefit most. The natural history of untreated colorectal cancer metastases has been investigated and 8–20% of patients with untreated solitary metastases will be alive after 3 years. Surgery for solitary metastases, however, may be associated with a 30% survival at 10 years and may be performed with a minimal morbidity and mortality. Only 5% of patients with colorectal cancer develop a solitary metastasis, however, and one in four of all those presenting with liver metastases. When several metastases are present in one lobe of the liver, however, a 20–40% 5-year survival may be obtained by surgical resection. These results suggest that an active policy should be employed for the detection and surgical resection of liver metastases following surgery for colon cancer.

Survival following surgery for cholangiocarcinoma

The survival of patients with cholangiocarcinomas is generally poor, independent of their form of treatment. Surgical resection is associated with an operative mortality of 5–20%, but with good palliation in survivors. Radical surgical resection of these tumours has been employed and has shown encouraging early results, with 40% survival for 5 years. In patients who are not suitable for resection, palliative procedures may be considered including a segment III biliary enteric anastomosis, endoscopic intubation and operative insertion of a U-tube. An alternative approach for tumours unsuitable for resection is liver transplantation, with a median survival of 7.5 months in transplanted patients with regional node involvement and 35 months if nodes are not involved. There are few survivors for more than 2 years.

Intrahepatic biliary-enteric anastomosis
Liver split

Access to the hilar structures of the liver may be accomplished by extrahepatic dissection, but to enable resection of many cholangiocarcinomas it is necessary to split the liver along the median plane to open the two halves and display the confluence of the duct (Figure 15.11). This liver split or hepatotomy is particularly valuable for approaching the right hepatic duct which is completely intrahepatic.

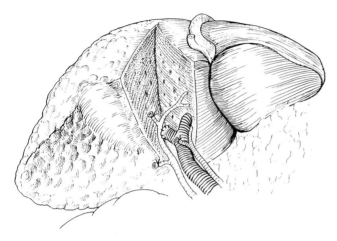

Figure 15.11 Hepatotomy (liver split). After removal of the gallbladder the liver substance is divided to provide access to the porta hepatis, particularly the origin of the common hepatic duct

The gallbladder is removed and Glisson's capsule is incised with the diathermy, heading back from the medial edge of the gallbladder bed towards the vena cava. Careful dissection at the bottom of the liver split should now display the hilar structure completely. The origin of the common hepatic duct lies anterior to the hepatic artery and portal vein. Following resection of a hilar cholangiocarcinoma, reconstruction is achieved by anastomosis of the transected bile ducts to a Roux loop of jejunum with mucosa-to-mucosa approximation (Figure 15.12). If the tumour has extended out into the liver tissue, then a central hepatic resection can be performed prior to the anastomosis.

Resection of the caudate lobe should be contemplated in cholangiocarcinoma, as most hilar tumours spread via lymphatics to this segment.

Alternatives to hilar dissection

For some patients with obstructive jaundice from a primary or secondary carcinoma at the hilus of the liver, resection is clearly not feasible. These tumours may, however, be slow growing, and biliary decompression provides good palliation. The following are some of the accepted techniques; the choice depends on the site and the extent of the tumour:

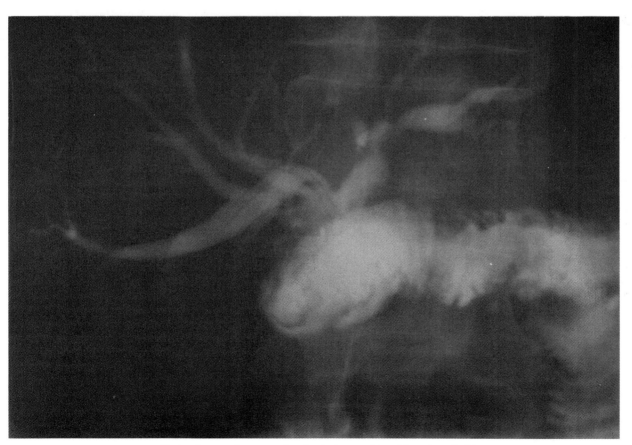

Figure 15.12 Cholangiogram demonstrating the drainage achieved by a hepaticojejunostomy

A large right-sided duct can sometimes be identified in the gallbladder bed with the use of the intraoperative ultrasound probe. Cholecystectomy is performed, and a syringe and needle with intermittent aspiration are used to explore the gallbladder bed. When bile is aspirated, the liver tissue is incised to reveal a large tributary of the right hepatic duct. Mucosa-to-mucosa suture is then possible.

A major duct on the left side can be found by opening the umbilical fissure (segment III bypass) (Figure 15.13). The round ligament is identified and followed down to the liver capsule. The thin bridge of liver tissue at its entry to the umbilical fissure is broken down. The left margin of the round ligament should then identify the duct, which at this point lies just beneath Glisson's capsule. Difficulty in identification can be resolved by needle aspiration or the use of intraoperative ultrasound. The left hepatic duct (or a major branch) can then be opened over a distance of at least 1 cm before anastomosis to a Roux loop; the liver capsule helps to strengthen this anastomosis.

This procedure is contraindicated in cases of atrophy and widespread metastases of the left lobe, as these conditions reduce the amounts of functioning parenchyma. Normally, drainage of left liver alone will resolve the jaundice and relieve itching.

Palliation of hepatic neoplasms

The overall prognosis of patients with either primary or metastatic liver cancers is poor. There have, however, been recent developments which may be of value to patients with unresectable lesions and may be considered for adjuvant therapy.

Endoscopic or percutaneous stenting of tumours

Patients with cholangiocarcinomas or liver tumours producing extrinsic compression of the bile duct present with obstructive jaundice and associated anorexia, weight loss and pruritus. This may be relieved preoperatively by endoscopic or percutaneous insertion of a biliary tract stent. In those patients in whom staging shows an unresectable lesion, it may be a definitive form of management. Prior to either endoscopic or percutaneous stenting the patient's clotting function should be checked and vitamin K and fresh frozen plasma administered as required. Antibiotic cover should be given. Initially an endoscopic approach is favoured, as this is less invasive. The papilla is cannulated and a sphincterotomy performed. Cholangiography is performed prior to passing a guide wire through the stricture under X-ray screening. An endoprosthesis is then inserted over the guide wire until the correct position is obtained, the guide wire is removed and a completion cholangiogram performed. Although biliary tract stenting may be performed as a day-case procedure in healthy patients,

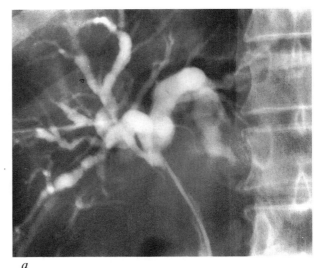

a

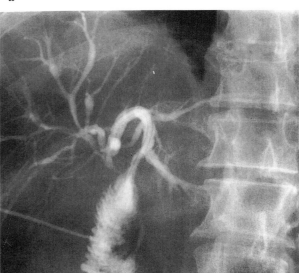

b

Figure 15.13 A hilar stricture (*a*) and a cholangiogram showing its management by a segment III bypass (*b*)

the dangers of sepsis and renal failure usually necessitate hospital admission for observation.

Endoscopic insertion will not be possible in 30% of patients, who should be referred for percutaneous drainage and stenting. The general condition of the patients improve rapidly after external biliary drainage and this may be continued, if necessary, for several days before insertion of an endoprosthesis.

Although endoscopic and percutaneous stenting provide good relief of obstructive jaundice, 25–30% of patients get stent occlusion with recurrence of jaundice or cholangitis and require the endoprosthesis to be changed. Several studies have compared the palliation obtained with stents to that of a surgical bypass procedure, and although surgery has a higher morbidity and mortality it is associated with better long-term palliation. The optimum treatment of patients with hilar cholangiocarcinomas has not been established.

Recently expandable metal stents have been introduced which can be inserted endoscopically or percutaneously. No controlled studies are available but these stents are reported to have greatly improved long-term patency rates and may, therefore, produce better long-term palliation than surgical bypass.

Hepatic de-arterialization

Hepatic neoplasms obtain most of their blood supply from the hepatic artery. Ligation of this vessel or embolization at selective hepatic angiography can be performed, resulting in shrinkage of the tumour mass with an associated symptomatic improvement. Collateral vessels rapidly form and the effect is therefore temporary and may result in acute liver failure in patients with severe underlying liver disease. The main value of de-arterialization is in patients presenting with a ruptured hepatocellular carcinoma in whom it is an effective method of producing haemostasis.

Cytotoxic therapy for hepatocellular carcinomas

The mean life expectancy of patients with untreated hepatocellular carcinoma is 2–4 months. Systemic chemotherapy may prolong survival by a short interval, but at the expense of unpleasant side effects. Regional chemotherapy administered via the hepatic artery has become the preferred form of management for unresectable primary liver cancers. This treatment may be delivered via an infusion pump placed in the hepatic artery at the time of open surgery or via a hepatic artery angiography catheter. The latter is ideal when the treatment intervals are prolonged, as with the use of ^{131}I-lipiodol. Lipiodol is a fatty acid ester which was originally used as a contrast medium because it is retained by tumour tissue following hepatic arterial injection. By this route it allows a high concentration of drug or radioisotope to be delivered directly to the tumour, with few if any systemic side effects and minimal damage to the normal liver tissue. It has been used combined with ^{131}I and a variety of chemotherapeutic drugs and may produce good disease remission in patients with hepatocellular carcinomas. In those with metastases, however, the results are generally poor. Other agents have been used for regional chemotherapy including adriamycin, mitomycin C, 5-fluorouracil and cisplatinum.

Intrahepatic alcohol injection

Alcohol may be injected directly into primary or secondary liver tumours under ultrasound guidance, producing tumour necrosis with a marked reduction in tumour size and symptoms.

Cryotherapy

Recently, cryotherapy probes have been developed which can safely destroy deeply situated lesions, even if they are in the proximity of major vessels. The area of tissue destruction during cryosurgery can be readily assessed by the use of intraoperative ultrasonography.

Laser therapy

Laser fibres are inserted into the tumour percutaneously under ultrasound guidance and the area of tumour which is destroyed by heat from the tip of the laser fibres may be accurately monitored by the use of the ultrasound probe. One advantage of this method over cryosurgery is that the latter requires a laparotomy; laser fibres may be introduced under local anaesthesia percutaneously.

Liver transplantation

Liver transplantation is now an established treatment of end-stage parenchymal liver diseases including congenital metabolic disorders (Table 15.1). Survival figures have improved due to better patient selection, anaesthesia and intensive care, organ preservation and immunosuppressives. In major transplant centres a 70–90% 1-year survival is obtained, and in those transplanted for benign disease, those surviving the first year are likely to be alive at 5 years. The results of liver transplantation in the management of primary liver tumours are universally poor and its role in this situation remains controversial.

Table 15.1 Possible indications for liver transplantation

Malignancy	Hepatocellular carcinoma
	Cholangiocarcinoma
	Sarcoma
	Liver metastases
Cirrhosis	Primary biliary
	Chronic active hepatitis
	Cryptogenic
	Alcohol
	Sclerosing cholangitis
	Secondary biliary
Metabolic	Galactosaemia
	Alpha-1-antitrypsin deficiency
	Wilson's disease
	Oxalosis
Fulminant hepatic failure, e.g. paracetamol overdose	
Budd–Chiari syndrome	
Biliary atresia	

Liver transplantation may be described as orthotopic or auxiliary. In the former the patient's diseased liver is removed and is replaced with that of the donor, whereas in the latter, part or all of the donor liver is grafted leaving the patient's diseased liver *in situ*. Most liver transplants are orthotopic in location.

Technique of liver transplantation

Harvesting the donor organ

Brain-death criteria must be fulfilled and consent received prior to organ harvesting. The general health of the donor must be investigated and liver disease, infections including viral hepatitis and AIDS and malignancy excluded. Tissue typing is carried out to find a suitable donor. The ABO blood groups should be respected during matching, but incompatibility of the HLA antigens does not preclude good results. The donor liver is exposed by forming a midline abdominal incision extending into a median sternotomy. A transverse abdominal incision with stitching back of skin flaps completes the exposure. The common bile duct, hepatic artery (all branches) and portal vein are then exposed as far distally as possible and the liver

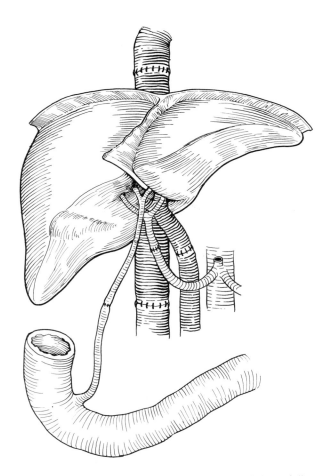

Figure 15.14 The anatomical position at completion of liver transplantation. End-to-end anastomosis of hepatic artery and portal vein restores vascular inflow. Venous return is via a segment of donor vena cava which is anastomosed above and below the liver. An end-to-end anastomosis is carried out between donor and recipient bile ducts

completely mobilized by division of the peritoneal reflections. After clamping the aorta below the diaphragm, the liver is perfused *in situ* with cold Ringer's lactate solution via a portal vein tributary and the hepatic artery via an aortic cannula. The liver is then removed with a liberal cuff of inferior vena cava above and below the liver. The hepatic artery is traced to the aorta proximally prior to its removal on an aortic patch. The portal vein and bile duct are removed with as much length as possible. On removal from the donor the liver is perfused with University of Wisconsin solution and packed in ice where it may be stored for up to 24 h.

The recipient operation

The diseased liver is removed in a similar manner to removal of the donor organ, but in this situation leaving the vessels and bile duct in the recipient as long as possible. The donor liver is flushed with human albumin solution and then the vena cava and portal vein anastomoses are performed. Following this, the donor liver may be perfused and the remaining arterial and biliary anastomoses carried out (Figure 15.14).

Postoperative care

Intensive medical management is essential in the early postoperative period following transplantation. Major complications are not infrequent and include bleeding, graft rejection and intercurrent infections.

Further reading

Adson, M. A. and Van Heerden, J. A. (1980) Major hepatic resections for metastatic colorectal cancer. *Ann. Surg.*, **191**, 576–583

Bismuth, H. (1982) Surgical anatomy and anatomical surgery of the liver. *World J. Surg.*, **6**, 3–9

Charnley, R. M., Doran, J., and Morris, D. L. (1989) Cryotherapy for liver metastases: a new approach. *Br. J. Surg.*, **76**, 1040–1041

Choi, T. K., Fan, S. T., Lai, E. C., and Wong, J. (1988) Malignant hilar biliary obstruction treated by segmental bilioenteric anastomosis. *Surgery*, **104**, 525–529

Deviere, J., Baize, M., De Toeuf, J. and Cremer, M. (1988) Long term follow up of patients with hilar malignant stricture treated by endoscopic internal biliary drainage. *Gastrointest. Endosc.*, **34**, 95–101.

Iwatsuki, S. and Starzl, T. E. (1988) Personal experience with 411 hepatic resections. *Ann. Surg.*, **208**, 421–434

Keegan-Rogers, V. and Wu, G. Y. (1989) Immunotargeting in the diagnosis and treatment of liver cancer. *Hepatology*, **9**(4), 646–648

Liver Cancer Study Group of Japan (1988) Surgery and follow-up study of primary liver cancer in Japan. Report 8. *Acta Hepatol. Jpn*, **29**, 1619–1626

Livraghi, T., Festi, D., Monti, F., Salmi, A. and Vettori, C. (1986) U.S. guided percutaneous alcohol injection of small hepatic and abdominal tumours. *Radiology*, **161**, 309–312

Lygidakis, N. J., Van der Heyde, M. N., Van Dongen, R. J., Kromhout, J. G. *et al.* (1988) Surgical approaches for unresectable primary carcinoma of the hepatic hilus. *Surg. Gynecol. Obstet.*, **166**, 107–114

Northover, J. M. A., Jones, B. J. M., Dawson, J. L., and Williams, R. (1982) Difficulties in the diagnosis and management of pyogenic liver abscess. *Br. J. Surg.*, **69**, 48–51

Ringe, B., Wittekind, C., Bechstein, W. O., Bunzendahl, H. and Pichlmayr, R. (1989) The role of liver transplantation in hepatobiliary malignancy: a retrospective analysis of 95 patients with particular regard to tumour stage and recurrence. *Ann. Surg.*, **1**, 88–89

Steger, A. C., Lees, W. R., Walmsley, K. and Bown, S. G. (1989) Interstitial laser hyperthermia: a new approach to local destruction of tumours. *Br. Med. J.*, **299**, 362–365

16
The small intestine

P. Durdey

Surgical anatomy

The small intestine, comprising jejunum and ileum, is of variable length. Measurements at post mortem suggest a range of 300–1000 cm, with jejunum comprising the proximal 40%. There is no clear demarcation of the junction between jejunum and ileum, but jejunum is easily identified by its thicker wall and prominent valvulae coniventes. The jejunal loops tend to lie in a horizontal fashion in the upper left quadrant of the abdomen, with ileum in the right lower quadrant. This is due to the attachment of the small bowel mesentery to the posterior abdominal wall running from the region of the ligament of Treitz to the right iliac fossa. Knowledge of this attachment proves useful in orientation of small bowel loops withdrawn through a small abdominal incision.

The blood supply of the small intestine arises from branches of the superior mesenteric, the artery to the foregut. The jejunal arteries arise from the left of the main trunk to form arcades. These arcades are single in the upper jejunum and double distally. The ileum is supplied by four or five arcades, often obscured by fat. Identification of the vascular arcades is necessary prior to resection and anastomosis.

The nerve supply of the small intestine is autonomic. Fibres from the autonomic plexuses travel with the blood supply.

Physiology

The function of the small intestine is digestion and absorption of nutrients. The brush border enzymes produced from the epithelium allow final digestion of carbohydrates and proteins. The majority of fats are separated from bile salts at the epithelial cell surface, absorbed and incorporated into chylomicrons which are transferred into lacteals and thence to the venous system. Medium-chain triglycerides are absorbed directly into the portal circulation.

The majority of nutrients are absorbed in the jejunum, bile salts and vitamin B_{12} in the terminal ileum. Excision of the ileum leads to loss of bile salts, with subsequent malabsorption of fat, and vitamin B_{12}.

The small intestine contains cells of the APUD series which produce a variety of gut hormones. These hormones control secretion, blood flow and motility.

Investigation of the small intestine

Investigation of the small bowel is undertaken in patients with symptoms of organic disease, malabsorption or disordered motility.

Radiology

Plain abdominal X-rays are often useful in the evaluation of acute small intestinal disorders, for example obstruction. Chronic symptoms are best investigated via barium studies.

Selective mesenteric arteriography and technetium-labelled red cell scans can help identify suspected sites of bleeding in the small bowel.

Investigation of malabsorption

A variety of investigations may help elucidate the cause of malabsorption. These are listed in Table 16.1. The most helpful are faecal fat estimation and small bowel contrast studies.

Table 16.1   Investigations of malabsorption

Faecal fat estimation
Small bowel enema
Jejunal/duodenal mucosal biopsy
D-xylose test
^{14}C conjugated bile salt breath test
Lactose tolerance test
Schilling test

Investigation of small intestine motility

A simple investigation of small bowel transit is the hydrogen (H_2) breath test. A standard dose of lactulose is administered orally. This is fermented by colonic bacteria to form H_2 gas, which is excreted by the lungs. The time from ingestion to the secondary rise in breath H_2 gives the orocaecal transit time.

More accurate techniques for quantification of small intestinal transit and motility are scintigraphic quantification and manometry via a long intestinal tube.

Surgical principles in resection and anastomosis of the small intestine

The commonest surgical procedure performed on the small intestine is resection and primary anastomosis. The indications for small bowel resection are discussed later in the chapter.

Techniques of resection and reconstruction

As with any intra-abdominal procedure the exposure must be adequate.

Division of small bowel mesentery

The first step in resection of small bowel is to divide the mesentery. For resection of short segments, or when resecting for benign conditions, the mesentery is divided close to the bowel wall. For larger resections and for malignant conditions, a V-shaped excision of the mesentery is necessary.

Once the line of excision has been decided, a superficial incision in the peritoneum will allow exposure of the mesenteric vessels (Figure 16.1). Transillumination of the mesentery from behind identifies the vascular arcades. Care must be taken in selecting the site of division to ensure an adequate blood supply to both limbs of the bowel to be anastomosed. The arteries and veins are identified, and underrun with an artery or tissue forceps and ligated individually with an absorbable ligature prior to division. Once the vessels are ligated, the viable edges of the bowel become demarcated.

Division of bowel

Once the mesentery is divided, the small bowel segment should be isolated from the peritoneal cavity by towels. The line of demarcation usually corresponds to the mesenteric edge. Crushing clamps are applied to the bowel to be resected, and are placed obliquely so as to remove more of the antimesenteric border. Non-crushing clamps are applied to the ends of the bowel to be anastomosed 3–4 cm from the line of division. The bowel is divided flush with the crushing clamps using scalpel or cutting diathermy and removed from the operating field.

Anastomotic technique

As with any anastomosis, careful technique is essential (Figure 16.2). The ends of the bowel should have a good blood supply and there should be no tension on either end. At the end of the procedure, the anastomosis should be water-tight and the lumen must not be stenosed.

End-to-end anastomosis

This is the simplest and most usual form of small intestinal anastomosis (Figure 16.2a). Division of the bowel obliquely, as above, helps prevent narrowing of the lumen. In cases of intestinal obstruction there is often disparity in diameter of proximal and distal loops. This can be dealt with by dividing the narrower diameter loop longitudinally along the antimesenteric

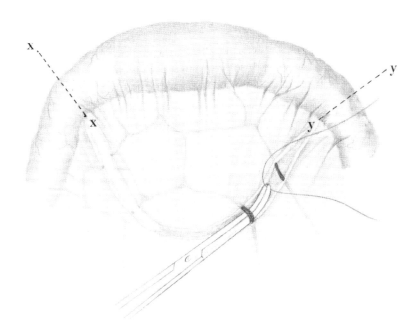

Figure 16.1 Resection of small intestine

border (Figure 16.2b) or by performing an end-to-side or side-to-side anastomosis (Figure 16.2c,d).

The precise anastomosis technique and the choice of suture is open to personal preference. The most important factor is the care with which the anastomosis is constructed.

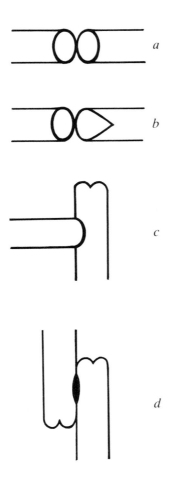

Figure 16.2 Small intestinal anastomosis. *a*, End-to-end anastomosis. *b*, Tailoring of bowel for end-to-end anastomosis when disparity in size exists. *c*, End-to-side anastomosis. *d*, Side-to-side anastomosis

Two-layer technique

The two-layer technique involves four components: (a) a posterior seromuscular layer; (b) a posterior all-coats layer; (c) an anterior all-coats layer; (d) an anterior seromuscular layer.

In practice, it is easier to perform the all-coats layer initially. Continuous or interrupted sutures may be employed.

Continuous all-coats suture

A 2/0 absorbable suture on a round-bodied atraumatic needle is ideal. This suture is haemostatic. The suture is commenced at the mesenteric border of the intestine and tied on the luminal surface. The posterior layer is constructed taking bites at 2 mm intervals through the whole thickness of the bowel wall. To avoid narrowing the anastomosis, each loop can be locked (Figure 16.3).

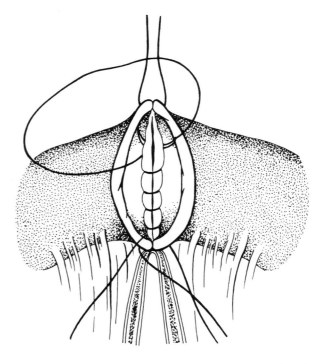

Figure 16.3 Suture of small intestine with continuous locking all-layers suture

On approaching the antimesenteric border, the technique is changed to employ the Connell (loop on the mucosa) stitch. This technique inverts the mucosa and opposes the serosal surfaces (Figure 16.4). The stitch commences on the serosal side of one limb of the anastomosis. The needle is passed into the lumen through the mucosa, and then back out through the mucosa of the same side. This creates the mucosal loop. The needle is then passed through the wall of the opposite limb from the serosal surface and a loop created on the mucosa of that side. The process is then repeated. The Connell stitch can be used for the anterior all-coats layer as it inverts the mucosa. The all-coats layer is completed by tying the suture to itself at the mesenteric border.

The seromuscular layer

The standard seromuscular layer of intestinal anastomoses is the Lembert stitch (Figure 16.5). Traditionally a 2/0 non-absorbable suture was used for this layer, usually silk or linen. A slowly absorbed suture, such as polydioxanone or polyglyconate on a 2/0 atraumatic needle, is preferable.

Due to free mobility of the small bowel, it is usually not necessary to insert the posterior seromuscular layer first, as in a colorectal anastomosis. The motility of small bowel allows rotation of the anastomosis to enable accurate placement of the posterior Lembert stitches. The seromuscular suture is commenced at the antimesenteric border. Interrupted sutures are used. The bite commences 3–4 mm away from the anastomosis and picks up serosa and muscle only. The needle is brought out immediately adjacent to the all-coats layer. The opposite limb of the bowel is picked up in a similar manner. On pulling the stitch together, the serosal surfaces are opposed. It is important to ensure that there is no 'furrow' between the two layers of the anastomosis. The sutures are placed at 2 mm intervals around the anastomosis. Care must be taken when inserting the final sutures on the posterior mesenteric border. This stitch takes the tension off the all-coats layer. By providing apposition of serosal surfaces, the anastomosis is rendered waterproof. A cross-section of the completed two-layer anastomosis is depicted in Figure 16.6. Should, for any reason, the seromuscular stitch start to cut out, the technique should be changed and horizontal mattress sutures used.

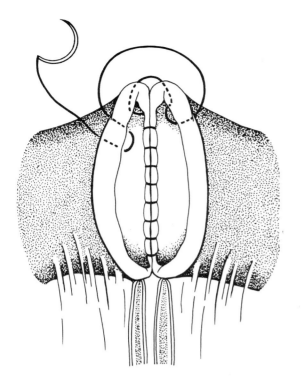

Figure 16.4 Small intestinal anastomosis. Connell inverting suture

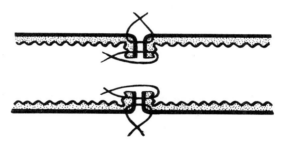

Figure 16.6 Small intestinal anastomosis using full-thickness interrupted sutures reinforced with inverting Lembert suture

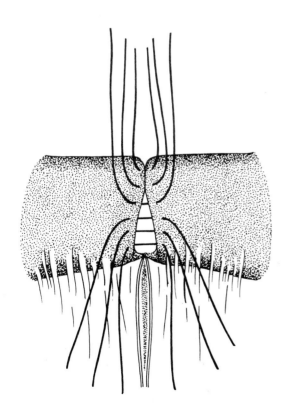

Figure 16.5 Small intestinal anastomosis. Interrupted Lembert suture

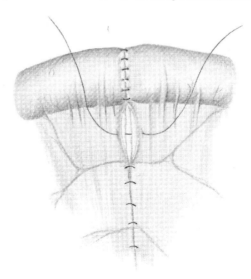

Figure 16.7 The mesentery must be closed following bowel anastomosis

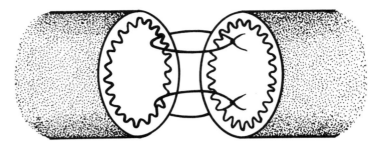

Figure 16.8 Suture of small intestine. Through-and-through all-coats with knots on the luminal side

The anastomosis is carefully inspected to ensure accurate placement of sutures, and to check for luminal narrowing. The small bowel anastomosis is completed by carefully suturing the edges of the mesenteric defect together with absorbable material, avoiding the vessels (Figure 16.7). This prevents the development of internal herniation of a loop of bowel through the mesenteric defect.

Single-layer small bowel anastomosis

An alternative method of small bowel anastomosis is the single-layer technique (Figure 16.8). A 2/0 slowly absorbed suture on an atraumatic needle is the material of choice.

The single layer can be either all-coats or, preferably, extramucosal. For either method the sutures start at the mesenteric border. For the posterior layer each stitch is inserted from the luminal surface. The bite commences 2–3 mm from the cut edge. For the extramucosal technique only the submucosa, muscle coat and serosa are picked up by the needle. The suture is passed through to the serosa and across in the opposite direction through the other limb of the anastomosis. The sutures are tied individually on the luminal surface. For the anterior half of the anastomosis, the extramucosal technique is preferred as this inverts the mucosa. The knots are tied on the serosal surface.

Either the two-layer or single-layer technique can be adapted to form side-to-side or end-to-side anastomoses.

The purse-string suture

The purse-string suture is used to close small defects in the intestine, for example after enterotomy and decompression of an obstruction, or for insertion of a jejunostomy tube (see later). The stitch is a circular series of seromuscular bites taken around the defect. On drawing the ends of the stitch together, the mucosa is buried and the defect closed. This stitch must only be used for small defects, and if the stitch narrows the lumen significantly it should be removed and a transverse closure with interrupted sutures substituted.

The three-bite stitch (Figure 16.9) is useful when closing awkward corners.

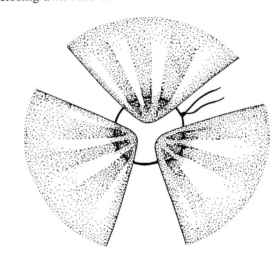

Figure 16.9 The three-bite stitch is useful for reinforcing closure at awkward corners

Stapling techniques

The advent of mechanical devices has enabled many anastomoses involving small intestine to be stapled. The principles of anastomosis by this technique are exactly similar to those for the hand-sewn method.

Enterotomy

Enterotomy is incision of the small bowel to gain access to the lumen. The main indications are for decompression of distal obstruction, insertion of a jejunostomy (see later) or rarely for removal of a foreign body (e.g. gallstone). A specialized form of enterotomy is strictureplasty in Crohn's disease (see later).

Decompression

Laparotomy for small bowel obstruction is invariably

accompanied by the problem of distended, fluid-filled proximal intestine. Decompression of the bowel is often necessary. Occasionally this can be achieved by milking contents back into the stomach which are then aspirated via a nasogastric tube. This is often not feasible and decompression via an enterotomy is required. This has the disadvantage of potential contamination of the peritoneal cavity and creates a possible site for leakage postoperatively. Small bowel decompression via an enterotomy should be undertaken only when absolutely necessary.

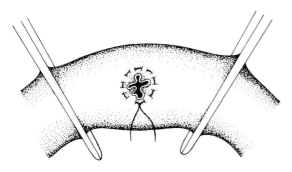

Figure 16.10 Decompression enterotomy

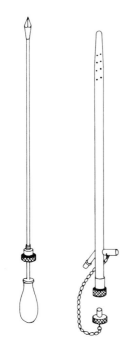

Figure 16.11 Trocar and cannula used for intestinal decompression

The chosen site should be isolated from the peritoneal cavity with abdominal packs, and a 2/0 seromuscular purse-string inserted (Figure 16.10). A small bowel decompression cannula (Figure 16.11) is a useful instrument, but a Silastic tube may be preferable. The serosa and muscle are incised carefully at

the centre of the purse-string. The decompressor is inserted and the suture tightened to prevent spillage. By intermittent suction and by telescoping the small bowel onto the cannula, decompression is achieved. On withdrawal of the cannula, the purse-string is tightened and tied. The site is oversewn with an interrupted seromuscular stitch.

Extraction of a foreign body

Obstruction of normal small bowel by a foreign body is rare. Examples include gallstone ileus and obstruction by ingested vegetable matter. If, at laparotomy, there is no evidence of perforation and the small bowel is viable, the preferred strategy is to milk the obstructing mass distally through into the caecum, obviating the necessity for enterotomy. Once in the caecum, the obstructing mass will pass spontaneously. Should this approach prove unsuccessful, the involved loop is isolated and soft clamps applied proximally and distally. The intestine is opened longitudinally along the antimesenteric border, preferably proximal to the obstruction in an area of normal bowel (Figure 16.12). This is best achieved by cutting diathermy. The foreign body is withdrawn and the enterotomy closed transversely.

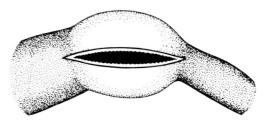

Figure 16.12 Extraction enterotomy. The longitudinal incision is closed transversely to avoid stricture formation

Jejunostomy

Feeding jejunostomy (Figure 16.13) is an attractive alternative to prolonged nasogastric feeding or intravenous nutrition in patients with a functioning small intestine. Indications include proximal obstruction, e.g. oesophageal tumour or stricture, prior to surgery, or postoperative nutrition in patients with a proximal anastomosis. In the latter case a feeding jejunostomy is easily placed at the time of surgery.

A feeding jejunostomy can be inserted under local anaesthetic or via the laparoscope. For open insertion, a transverse incision 6–7 cm long is made through the abdominal wall. A loop of jejunum, as close as possible to the duodenojejunal flexure, is selected. A small 0.5–1.0 cm incision is made in the antimesenteric border and a soft rubber Foley catheter, size 16 or 17 Fr., is inserted distally. The defect in the bowel wall is closed with an absorbable purse-string suture around the catheter which is laid along the bowel to form a gutter. The catheter and purse-string are buried over a distance of 5–6 cm by an absorbable Lembert suture. The loop of jejunum is sutured to the medial end of the incision. The catheter is brought out laterally and sutured to the skin. The abdominal wound is closed in layers. The jejunostomy can be used after 24 h.

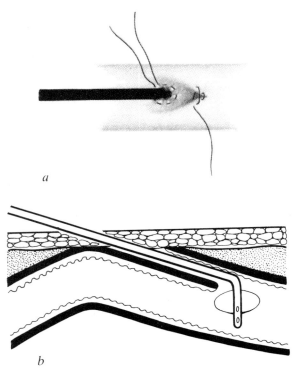

Figure 16.13 Witzel jejunostomy

Ileostomy

An ileostomy can be permanent or temporary. A temporary ileostomy is useful to defunction distal bowel or after emergency subtotal colectomy for inflammatory bowel disease.

A permanent stoma is usually fashioned as an end ileostomy. A defunctioning ileostomy is best constructed as a loop. Loop ileostomy has many advantages over loop colostomy. For either, it is essential to select the site of the stoma carefully, preferably in conjunction with a stoma therapist. In elective situations the patient should wear an ileostomy bag filled with water for 24 h to assess ease of management. In emergencies, it is still preferable to mark the site prior to surgery. The stoma site should be placed over the rectus sheath, away from the proposed scar, anterior superior iliac spine and umbilicus. If possible, the patient should be stood up to ensure that the site does not lie in a skin crease, or below a fold of obese abdominal wall.

End ileostomy

For an end ileostomy (Figure 16.14) the mesentery and vessels are divided up to the chosen point of division of the ileum. The ileum is divided between twin crushing clamps.

A 3 cm diameter of skin and subcutaneous tissue is excised at the chosen stoma site. The anterior rectus sheath is divided in a cruciate fashion. The fibres of the rectus muscle are carefully separated by blunt dissection avoiding the epigastric vessels. A cruciate incision is made in the peritoneum and approximately 5–6 cm of the ileum exteriorized. The bowel should not be under tension and must have an adequate blood supply. The mesentery is sutured to the anterior abdominal wall, obliterating the lateral space. At this stage the main abdominal wound is closed and an occlusive dressing applied.

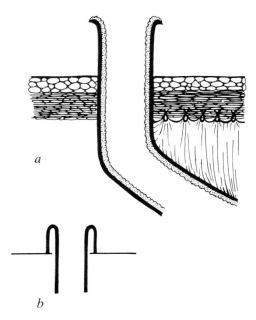

Figure 16.14 Terminal ileostomy

Several absorbable stitches are inserted between the bowel and the external oblique aponeurosis. The clamp on the ileum is removed and the crushed tissue excised. The spout is formed by inserting interrupted 3/0 absorbable sutures. Each stitch picks up the end of the bowel, takes a bite of the seromuscular layer at the level of the skin, and is then passed through the skin. The sutures are not tied until all are *in situ*. Approximately 8–10 sutures are placed around the stoma. By everting the bowel and tightening the stitches, a 3–4 cm spout will form. Careful apposition of skin and mucosa will prevent subsequent stenosis. The sutures are tied and an appliance fitted.

Loop ileostomy

A loop ileostomy is used to defunction a distal anastomosis, for example after low anterior resection, colo-anal anastomosis or creation of a pelvic ileal reservoir.

The defect in the abdominal wall is created as described above. An appropriate loop of ileum is selected. This is brought through the abdominal wall, ensuring that the mesentery is rotated in a clockwise direction until the proximal loop lies inferiorly. A short plastic rod is placed through the mesentery, immediately adjacent to the bowel wall to support the loop. A transverse incision is made in the distal limb, close to the skin level, across the anterior half of the bowel. The proximal limb is everted as previously described. The distal limb is sutured flush with the skin.

pancreatic juices into the oesophagus. One method to overcome this is to create an entero-enterostomy between proximal and distal limbs (Figure 16.15b). By stapling across the afferent limb, reflux is prevented.

The Roux-en-Y technique enables an anastomosis to be performed beyond the reach of an intact loop. The other major advantage of the technique is that afferent loop contents are diverted distally away from the anastomosis.

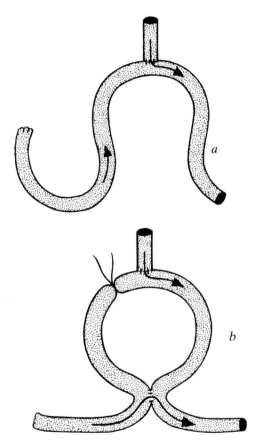

Figure 16.15   *a*, End-to-side oesophagojejunostomy. This simple loop is useful following total gastrectomy but allows bowel and pancreatic juices to reflux into the oesophagus. *b*, The creation of an entero-enterostomy with stapling or division close to the oesophageal anastomosis will minimize such reflux

Roux loops

A simple example of a Roux loop is the end-to-side oesophagojejunal anastomosis (Figure 16.15a). One disadvantage of this technique is reflux of bile and

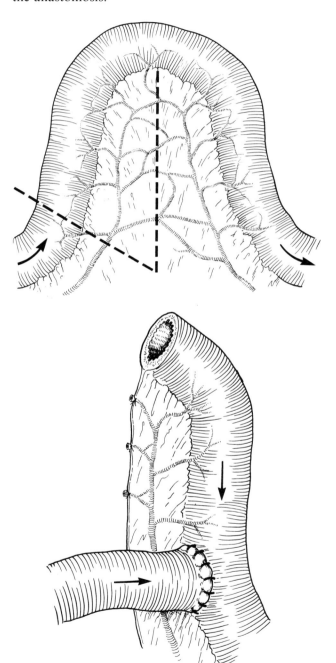

Figure 16.16   Construction of a Roux loop

To construct a Roux loop, a suitable length of jejunum is selected. The vascular arcades are carefully inspected using illumination from behind. The vessels and mesentery should be divided as shown in Figure 16.16, leaving a long efferent and short afferent limb.

The efferent limb can be anastomosed to the oesophagus after total gastrectomy, to the stomach after Polya gastrectomy (Figure 16.17) or to the bile duct after resection of the head of pancreas for biliary bypass. The afferent limb is anastomosed end-to-side 30 cm distal to the anastomosis.

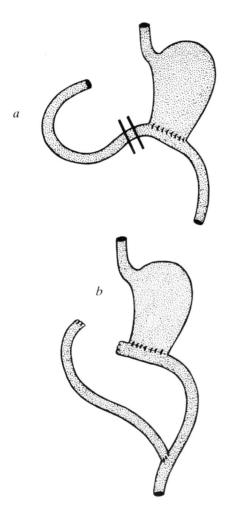

Figure 16.17 *a, b*, This variation of the Roux-en-Y is used to correct biliary reflux after Polya gastrectomy

Small bowel fistulas

Fistulas from the small intestine may be simple, involving a single track from the bowel, or complex, involving multiple loops. The fistula may communicate with an intra-abdominal abscess cavity or the skin. Causes of small bowel fistulas are listed in Table 16.2. An internal small bowel fistula, between adjac-

ent loops, may be asymptomatic. This type of fistula is often an incidental finding at laparotomy for resection of a segment of Crohn's disease.

Table 16.2 Aetiology of small bowel fistulas

Crohn's disease
Malignancy
Radiotherapy
Trauma
Anastomotic leakage:
   inadequate technique
   poor blood supply
   tension
   obstruction
   sepsis
   malnutrition

Enterocutaneous fistulas are a difficult problem. The aims of management are to obtain closure of the fistula, while maintaining adequate fluid and electrolyte balance and nutrition. Skin care around the fistula is of paramount importance and involvement of an experienced stoma therapist is helpful.

High-output fistulas may lead to severe depletion of fluid and electrolytes. Fistular output should be carefully documented and regular checks made of serum electrolytes. Small bowel fistulas, particularly if arising from proximal intestine, will lead rapidly to nutritional problems. The catabolic state is exacerbated by associated sepsis.

Management

Oral intake must be stopped to reduce intestinal secretions. Adequate and appropriate fluid replacement is essential. The majority of patients will require parenteral nutrition via a dedicated feeding line.

The anatomy and aetiology of the fistula must be carefully delineated. Contrast studies of the small bowel and fistular track are most useful. Ultrasound and computer tomography help identify abscess cavities.

Conservative management of small intestinal fistulas is employed if there is continuity of the bowel, no distal obstruction and no mucocutaneous continuity. Conservative measures will fail when there is underlying sepsis or diseased bowel, for example Crohn's disease, malignancy or radiation enteritis.

Operative intervention is required in two situations: to drain an associated intra-abdominal abscess and to secure definitive closure of a persistent fistula.

The principles involved in surgical closure of a fistula depend on careful assessment of the anatomy of the fistula and knowledge of the underlying disease process.

The area of bowel involved in the fistula should be excised. A primary anastomosis is advised only where conditions are favourable. If there is any doubt, the ends of the bowel should be exteriorized as a formal enterostomy and distal mucous fistula. Bypass should not be performed unless there is inoperable malignancy.

Traumatic injury to the small intestine

The small intestine can be injured by penetrating and blunt trauma. Incised wounds of the bowel are closed primarily. The edges of the defect are trimmed and closed transversely. Multiple lacerations over a short segment or areas of intestine of doubtful viability should be excised and primary end-to-end anastomosis performed. The peritoneal cavity is lavaged with saline.

Blunt trauma commonly occurs in road traffic accidents. Contused bowel should be inspected for viability. Doubtful segments require excision.

Mesenteric haematomas should be explored and bleeding vessels ligated. Occasionally a haematoma will mask a perforated area. Extensive tears of the mesentery may devascularize a length of small bowel which is best resected.

Inflammatory conditions

Crohn's disease

Crohn's disease is a chronic inflammatory condition which can affect any part of the gastrointestinal tract. It is typified by transmural inflammation and deep fissuring ulcers. The terminal ileum is the most common site of small bowel disease.

The mainstay of treatment for Crohn's disease is medical therapy. Surgical intervention is reserved for complications (Table 16.3).

Table 16.3   Complications of Crohn's disease of the small bowel

Obstruction
Fistulation
Abscess formation
Free perforation (rare)
Haemorrhage
Increased risk of malignancy
Growth retardation in children

The standard operation for small bowel Crohn's disease is resection with end-to-end anastomosis. Technically this may be difficult due to thickening of the mesentery. The bowel is usually resected back to an area of macroscopically normal intestine. The presence of microscopic disease at the resection margin does not influence the incidence of local recurrence.

Reoperation for recurrent Crohn's disease may require multiple resections of small bowel. This may result in the short bowel syndrome (see later). An alternative approach for narrowed areas causing obstruction is to use a technique originally designed for management of tubercular ileal strictures – strictureplasty.

Strictureplasty can be used for quite lengthy strictures. The stricture is isolated with soft bowel clamps, and the antimesenteric border incised with diathermy. The enterotomy is closed transversely in the manner of a Heineke–Mikulicz pyloroplasty with a single layer of absorbable interrupted sutures (Figure 16.18). Very long strictureplasties may require closure by a technique similar to a Finney pyloroplasty.

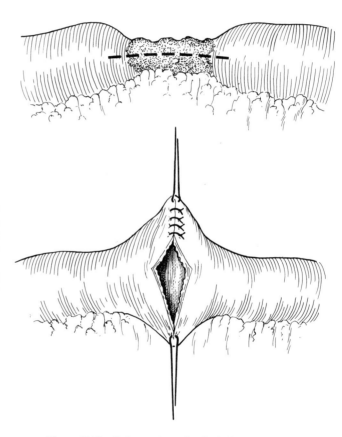

Figure 16.18   Strictureplasty for Crohn's structure

Short but clinically significant strictures in the small bowel may not be apparent macroscopically, but they may be identified by passing a small Foley catheter with a 5 ml balloon proximally and distally from an enterotomy. Fibrous strictures are easily identified, marked with a clip, and strictureplasty performed.

An extension of this technique is balloon dilatation, which can be performed via the endoscope, but the results are disappointing with a high incidence of perforation and re-stenosis.

Bypass operations for Crohn's disease should be performed only in critically ill patients. The overall results of small bowel Crohn's disease are disappointing. Recurrent disease occurs in up to 70%.

Abdominal tuberculosis

Gastrointestinal tuberculosis is no longer rare in certain parts of the UK. The majority of cases occur in immigrants, mainly of Asian origin, but the disease may occur in the indigenous population. The signs and symptoms of abdominal tuberculosis may mimic those of Crohn's disease. The presence of active disease on a chest X-ray points to the diagnosis. The mainstay of treatment is medical; surgery is occasionally required for the management of complications.

Actinomycosis

Ileocaecal actinomycosis is rare and usually follows perforation of an inflamed appendix and subsequent colonization by *Actinomyces israelii*. The infection can spread locally to surrounding structures and through the abdominal wall. This gives the typical appearance of multiple discharging sinuses with so-called sulphur granules, in the right iliac fossa. Spread to the liver via the portal venous system may occur. Treatment is a prolonged course of penicillin.

Intestinal obstruction

Obstruction of the small bowel is a surgical emergency. Acute small bowel obstruction can be classified into mechanical and adynamic paralytic ileus. Mechanical obstruction can be simple or associated with strangulation. The obstruction may be situated high in the small bowel, or low. The common causes of small bowel obstruction are listed in Table 16.4.

Table 16.4   Aetiology of small bowel obstruction

Adhesions
External hernia
Internal hernia
Volvulus
Intussusception

Pathophysiology

Obstruction to the flow of small bowel contents leads to proximal distension with fluid and gas. The loss of extracellular fluid into the obstructed loop compounds the distension. Normally, 8–10 litres of secretion are poured into the small intestine over a 24 h period. Loss of large volumes of intestinal contents by vomiting leads to rapid depletion of water and electrolytes.

A high obstruction is associated with less abdominal distension but with earlier onset of vomiting. Low small bowel obstruction is accompanied by greater distension. Vomiting occurs late.

Strangulation of intestine leads to initial venous obstruction. Futher swelling of the bowel loop leads to increasing pressure which eventually leads to occlusion of arterial flow. This is rapidly followed by gangrene, perforation and sepsis.

Diagnosis

The cardinal symptoms and signs of intestinal obstruction are pain, vomiting, absolute constipation and abdominal distension.

Pain

Small bowel colic is a characteristic, intermittent pain with acute exacerbations every 3–4 min in a high obstruction and every 10–12 min in a low obstruction. The pain is associated with increased bowel sounds which may be audible to patient and doctor. In a thin patient, episodes of colic may be accompanied by visible peristalsis evident on abdominal inspection.

Vomiting

Retrograde peristalsis of large volumes of fluid sequestered in the bowel leads to vomiting. Faeculent vomiting is a very late sign of a low obstruction.

Constipation

Complete obstruction to the small bowel results in absolute constipation. Intestinal contents distal to the site of obstruction may be evacuated after the onset of symptoms. In cases of partial obstruction, e.g. Richter's hernia, the patient may continue to pass flatus.

Abdominal distension

Abdominal distension is minimal in a high obstruction. The lower site of the obstruction, the greater the degree of distension.

The most important differentiation to be made in patients with acute obstruction of the small bowel is whether the obstruction is simple or whether strangulation is occurring. Patients with strangulation are systemically more ill than patients with simple obstruction. The diagnosis of a strangulated external hernia is relatively straightforward. The possibility of an internal strangulation must always be borne in mind in any patient with signs and symptoms of small bowel obstruction. If strangulation occurs within the peritoneal cavity, local peritoneal inflammation gives rise to continuous pain, upon which is superimposed the intermittent colicky pain resulting from obstruction. Examination of patients with intra-abdominal strangulation reveals the classic sign of localized tenderness and guarding.

Investigations

The most useful diagnostic test in a patient with suspected obstruction is a supine plain abdominal film which reveals distended loops of small bowel, the gas patterns indicating the site of obstruction. Absence of gas in the large bowel is a further indication of the site of obstruction.

Management of obstruction

The majority of cases of simple, non-strangulating obstruction can be treated by conservative measures initially. If strangulation is suspected, early laparotomy is mandatory after initial resuscitation.

Conservative management

The basic management of small bowel obstruction is replacement of fluid and decompression by nasogastric tube. Adequate fluid replacement is essential. Patients may present with hypovolaemic shock in extreme circumstances. Urinary volume must be measured accurately, if necessary by an indwelling catheter. In the elderly or in patients with cardiovascular problems, a central venous pressure line is useful in managing fluid balance.

It is essential that patients with small bowel obstruction, undergoing initial conservative management, should be carefully reassessed at regular intervals. Any deterioration in the patient's condition or the appearance of signs compatible with strangulation should lead to the abandonment of conservative therapy and immediate laparotomy. Unless there has been a significant improvement in the patient's condition after 24 h of conservative management, surgical intervention is indicated.

Operative management

The aim of surgery is to decompress the obstructed bowel and to remove the cause of obstruction. The abdomen should be opened via a midline incision and the cause of the obstruction may become apparent immediately. If not, the site of obstruction can be traced by inspecting the caecum. If this is collapsed, the obstruction must be proximal and collapsed bowel is traced proximally until the site of obstruction is reached.

If the operation is impeded by gross gaseous distension of the small bowel, this can be relieved by needle aspiration. A green needle attached to mechanical suction is effective. If there is a large amount of inspissated material in the lumen, decompression may be required via an enterotomy. Breaching the intestinal wall should be avoided whenever possible.

Once revealed, the cause of the obstruction is dealt with appropriately. Bands and adhesions can occur as a result of previous surgery or may be congenital. These are divided under direct vision. It is essential to inspect the area of bowel involved to ensure viability. If this is doubtful, the area should be resected and a primary anastomosis performed. Volvulus around an adhesion should be reduced and the offending adhesion divided. Foreign bodies can be removed via an enterotomy, whereas tumours and a Meckel's diverticulum can be resected. Idiopathic intussusception is relatively common in children, but in adults is usually associated with an intraluminal lesion, e.g. a benign tumour, and this should be removed. Where a loop of bowel is strangulated, viability should be carefully assessed on releasing the obstruction. Blood flow may be increased if the loop of bowel is wrapped in hot towels before reassessment. If viability remains in doubt, resection should be performed. Gross disparity in size of proximal and distal loops can be overcome by use of an end-to-side anastomosis.

Mesenteric vascular occlusion

Occlusion of the mesenteric vascular supply is an intra-abdominal catastrophe and carries a very high mortality. The superior mesenteric artery may be occluded by embolus or thrombosis. A less common cause is mesenteric venous thrombosis.

Success in treatment depends largely on early diagnosis and laparotomy.

Mesenteric arterial occlusion

Occlusion of the superior mesenteric artery is due to atherosclerotic narrowing of the vessel, often with superimposed thrombosis, or obstruction due to embolus. Atherosclerotic occlusion of the superior mesenteric artery occurs near its origin, the more distal trunk, and branches are often spared. Atheromatous occlusion usually occurs in elderly males. Embolus can occur in a younger age group and there is often coexisting cardiac disease. Occlusion of the main arterial trunk leads to infarction, as the collateral circulation is inadequate. Rarely, mesenteric infarction occurs in association with a dramatic fall in cardiac output, e.g. in cardiogenic shock or where there has been damage to the microcirculation of the small bowel.

Clinical presentation

Clinical presentation of mesenteric arterial insufficiency can be acute or chronic. Acute occlusion may occur without previous symptoms. The main symptom is abdominal pain. This usually occurs suddenly and can be severe. Often the presentation is more insidious. The diagnosis may not become apparent until the patient develops circulatory collapse due to intra-abdominal fluid collection and absorption of toxins following necrosis of the small bowel. A diagnosis of mesenteric vascular occlusion should always be considered in elderly patients with non-specific symptoms, in whom a picture of subacute obstruction is apparent on clinical examination and investigation. A raised leucocyte count is one of the more useful investigations. Occasionally a bruit may be heard in the right iliac fossa. Plain abdominal X-rays are often non-specific, with a few distended small bowel loops and fluid levels. The most useful aid to diagnosis remains awareness of the condition, particularly in patients with evidence of atherosclerosis, or those with cardiac arrhythmias.

Chronic ischaemia

Chronic ischaemia occurs in patients with atheromatous stenosis of the superior mesenteric artery. The symptoms are non-specific, the commonest being abdominal pain after meals. Patients often reduce oral intake in an effort to reduce this pain and there may be associated diarrhoea and weight loss. Abdominal examination is usually unhelpful unless an abdominal bruit is present. Angiography is the investigation of choice, with lateral views of the coeliac and superior mesenteric trunks.

Treatment

Acute occlusion

Once the diagnosis has been made, laparotomy should be undertaken immediately after initial resuscitation. The diagnosis is usually confirmed on opening the abdomen, particularly if the patient has presented late. Unfortunately, in the majority of cases, the operator is faced with loops of gangrenous bowel. Although the presence of a cardiac arrhythmia may suggest embolus, it is often difficult to establish the precise cause of the occlusion.

If the bowel appears viable and the patient is fit for a prolonged procedure, exploration of the superior mesenteric artery is indicated. Exposure of the root of this artery can thus be difficult, particularly in obese subjects. If embolus is suspected, the ileocolic artery should be isolated distally and a small Fogarty embolectomy catheter passed proximally. The clot or embolus can then be withdrawn. If this is unsuccessful, it is possible to attempt retrograde revascularization. The simplest method is side-to-side anastomosis between ileocolic artery and right common iliac artery or aorta. Alternative methods include a jump graft using autologous vein or a synthetic material.

Unfortunately, in the majority of cases the bowel is not viable. Complete occlusion of the main trunk of the superior mesenteric may result in gangrene of the whole small bowel and ascending colon. In elderly patients, resection of this amount of intestine is incompatible with survival. Shorter lengths of non-viable bowel can be excised and end-to-end anastomosis performed.

If initial surgical management has been successful the patient should undergo a re-exploration 24 h later to ensure that further infarction has not occurred.

Chronic ischaemia

The indications for surgical intervention in patients with chronic arterial insufficiency of the small bowel are not clearly defined. The patient is usually elderly and has systemic atheromatous disease. The mesentery can be revascularized either by a direct approach to the origin of the superior mesenteric artery or performing an endarterectomy. The arteriotomy is closed with a vein patch. If the coeliac axis is not involved by a similar process, the splenic artery can be anastomosed to the superior mesenteric, distal to the obstruction. An alternative is to insert a jump graft from the aorta or right common iliac to the superior mesenteric.

Mesenteric venous occlusion

Mesenteric venous occlusion is difficult to diagnose preoperatively. The clinical symptoms and signs are non-specific, but usually there is vague abdominal discomfort and occasional colicky pain. Abdominal distension and vomiting is a late feature. The surgical management of venous occlusion is wide resection of the affected segment of bowel. There is a significant mortality (30–40%) associated with this condition and an alternative management strategy is to perform a laparotomy to confirm the diagnosis and, if the bowel appears viable, to treat the patient by systemic anticoagulation.

Short gut syndrome

Massive resection of small bowel can result in the short gut syndrome. Conditions leading to short gut syndrome are listed in Table 16.5. The clinical outcome following massive intestinal resection depends on the site of resection, the age of the patient and the general physical state. Children are able to tolerate extensive small bowel resection better than adults. The precise length of small intestine necessary for adequate absorption is not known, but a minimum of 30 cm of jejunum is required.

In cases where there is insufficient small bowel to maintain adequate nutrition, patients are faced with lifelong home parenteral alimentation. A less extensive resection can be managed by careful dietary manipulation and supplementation. Surgical treatment of the short gut syndrome by reversed loops, forming an antiperistaltic barrier, have largely been abandoned. Small bowel transplantation provides some hope for the future.

Table 16.5 Lesions which require massive resection of small intestine

Crohn's disease
Mesenteric infarction
Volvulus
Small bowel tumours
Tumours involving the small bowel mesentery
Surgical misadventure

Radiation enteritis

The increasing use of radiotherapy for malignant conditions of the pelvic organs has led to increase in radiation damage to the small bowel. The long-term effects of radiation enteritis are due to transmural fibrosis and ischaemia from proliferative endarteritis and vasculitis. The clinical symptoms of radiation damage to the small bowel are usually encountered in the first few weeks after radiotherapy. The commonest symptoms are vague abdominal pain, diarrhoea, rectal bleeding and passage of mucus. Radiation damage may become apparent up to 20 years after the initial treatment. The most useful investigation in a patient with suspected radiation enteritis is a small bowel meal which demonstrates strictures and the presence of radiation-induced enteric fistulas.

The management of radiation enteropathy is very difficult, but a basic principle is to adopt conservative measures whenever possible. Surgical intervention is reserved for recurrent obstruction or fistulation. Prior to operation, the patient requires careful evaluation to determine the extent of the problem and to exclude recurrent malignant disease. Preoperative parenteral nutrition may be required.

The general principles in surgical management of irradiated small bowel are to perform minimal dissection to achieve objectives. Excessive division of adhesions will lead to the formation of further fistulas. Following resection, the anastomosis should be performed in healthy non-irradiated bowel. Anastomotic technique must be meticulous and consideration should be given to performing a proximal, defunctioning stoma. Occasionally, very severely damaged areas are best managed by bypass rather than resection.

Tumours of the small intestine

Small intestinal tumours are very rare. Crohn's disease, coeliac disease, dermatitis herpetiformis and Peutz–Jeghers syndrome are associated with an increased risk of development of small bowel tumours.

Benign small intestinal tumours

The majority of small bowel tumours are discovered as an incidental finding at laparotomy. Benign tumours include adenoma, angioma, lipoma and neurofibroma. Occasionally, benign tumours may form the apex of an intussusception.

Malignant small intestinal tumours

Malignant tumours of the small bowel are extremely rare. Adenocarcinomas are mucus-secreting tumours which are commoner in the more proximal part of the small intestine. The prognosis is unfavourable. The commonest tumour of the small bowel is lymphoma. This may be a primary small bowel lymphoma or may be associated with systemic disease. Other tumours of the small intestine include leiomyosarcoma and carcinoid. Carcinoid tumours may be found coincidently to have been the cause of acute appendicitis by causing luminal obstruction. Carcinoid tumours of the small intestine are usually found in the ileum. The majority of these are malignant and may be associated with the carcinoid syndrome when hepatic metastases occur.

Management

Benign small intestinal tumours can be resected locally. For malignant tumours, resection, leaving a margin of healthy bowel with removal of the draining lymph nodes, is the treatment of choice. Small bowel lymphoma requires treatment with combination chemotherapy and occasionally radiotherapy. Treatment of the primary lesion in carcinoid tumours is by resection of involved small bowel with adjacent lymph nodes.

Meckel's diverticulum

Meckel's diverticulum is the remnant of the vitellointestinal tract. It occurs in up to 4% of individuals. Meckel's diverticulum varies in length and arises from the antimesenteric border of the ileum, approximately 100 cm from the ileocaecal valve. It may contain ectopic gastric mucosa. Meckel's diverticulum can give rise to profuse gastrointestinal haemorrhage, particularly in children. An uninflamed Meckel's diverticulum is often found incidentally during laparotomy. If the diverticulum has a wide base and it feels normal to palpation, it is not necessary to remove it. If thought necessary, the diverticulum is removed using a wedge resection of the ileum and closure of the defect transversely.

Small intestinal diverticula

Rarely diverticulosis of the small bowel occurs. Diverticula are commonest in the jejunum. Bacterial overgrowth can lead to the blind loop syndrome. A small bowel diverticulum may be the site of blood loss in patients with repeated episodes of melaena. Short areas of diverticulosis can be resected. Blind loop syndrome, associated with extensive small bowel diverticula, is managed by long-term antibiotics, e.g. tetracylines.

Vascular malformations of the gut

Small intestine can be affected by vascular malformations. Hereditary haemorrhagic telangiectasia (Rendu–Osler–Weber syndrome) is an inherited disorder associated with multiple angiomatous lesions of the gastrointestinal tract. The condition leads to frequent episodes of gastrointestinal bleeding, but these are usually self-limiting and rarely require surgical intervention.

Arteriovenous malformations may be found in the small bowel. These give rise to recurrent episodes of gastrointestinal bleeding with melaena and occasionally hypotension. Patients with vascular malformations present a difficult diagnostic problem. Upper gastrointestinal endoscopy and colonoscopy are usually normal. In patients actively bleeding, selective mesenteric angiography may reveal the source of haemorrhage. An alternative is the isotope-labelled red cell scan. Often preoperative investigations do not reveal the site of the lesion. Persistent and recurrent haemorrhage are indications for laparotomy. Even with the abdomen open, vascular malformations are not easily identified. A useful technique is to inspect the lumen of the bowel with an endoscope introduced via an enterotomy. This may reveal the site of bleeding which can then be resected.

17
The appendix and colon

D. C. C. Bartolo

The appendix

Surgical anatomy (Figure 17.1)

The appendix originates from the posteromedial aspect of the caecum about 2.5 cm below the ileocaecal valve and varies in length enormously from 1 to 25 cm. Its position is extremely variable and indeed it is said to be the only organ without any consistent anatomy. Most frequently, the appendix lies behind the caecum (75% of cases). It is usually quite free, although occasionally it may lie beneath the peritoneal covering of the caecum and, if very long, may actually extend behind the ascending colon with its distal portion lying extraperitoneally against the right kidney. In some 20% of cases the appendix lies just below the caecum or hangs into the pelvis. Less commonly it passes in front or behind the terminal ileum and occasionally lies in front of the caecum or in the right paracolic gutter.

Retrocolic and retrocaecal 75%

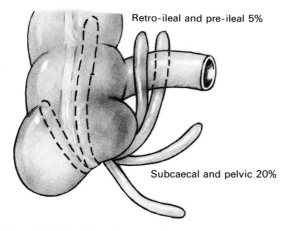

Retro-ileal and pre-ileal 5%

Subcaecal and pelvic 20%

Figure 17.1 Variations in the position of the appendix

The mesentery of the appendix carries the appendicular branch of the ileocolic artery and descends behind the ileum as a triangular fold (Figure 17.2). The appendicular artery represents the entire vascular supply of the appendix and runs first in the edge of the appendix mesentery and then, more distally, along the wall of the appendix. Thrombosis of branches of this artery in the course of acute infection must inevitably result in gangrene and subsequent perforation. This is in contrast to acute cholecystitis, where the rich collateral vascular supply from the liver beds accounts for the comparative rarity of gangrene of the gallbladder in acute cholecystitis.

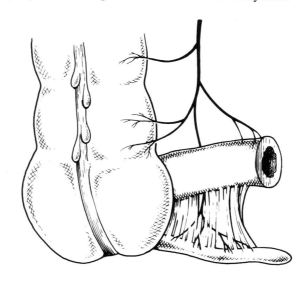

Figure 17.2 Blood supply of the appendix

Acute appendicitis

Acute appendicitis was traditionally the most important cause of the acute surgical abdomen, but its incidence is declining and the reason for this is unknown. It is a Western disease which has been attributed to a high-fat, low-fibre diet. Appendicitis is very common in Northern Europe, North America and Australia and among the white population of Southern Africa. It is rare in most of Asia, Central Africa and among Eskimos.

The diagnosis of acute appendicitis is normally made clinically. A leucocytosis provides support for the diagnosis, but a normal white cell count does not necessarily exclude it. If the appendix lies adjacent to the ureter or bladder wall, then red blood cells or pus cells may be found in the urine and indeed the patient may report pain during micturition. On careful questioning it can be ascertained that this is not dysuria but lower abdominal pain due to bladder movement that accompanies voiding. Plain X-rays of the abdomen are rarely helpful but may show blurring of the fat line in the right iliac fossa. In addition, there may be increase in the soft-tissue density.

With the rise of minimally invasive surgery there is increasing enthusiasm for preliminary laparoscopy as an adjunct to the diagnosis of appendicitis. In males the clinical diagnosis is usually easy but in females, particularly those of child-bearing age, the differential diagnosis is broader and preliminary laparoscopy where facilities are available is to be commended since in experienced hands it will reduce the incidence of unnecessary appendicectomy.

Indications for operation

Once the diagnosis of acute appendicitis has been reached, plans should be made for appendicectomy. The exceptions to this rule are as follows:

1. When the patient is desperately ill, time should be taken to resuscitate them with intravenous fluids and antibiotics. There is no doubt that this is of enormous benefit to the patient and attempts to rush into urgent surgery without careful resuscitation should be resisted.
2. In the unusual event of a patient being at sea or without reasonable access to an operating theatre, a conservative policy can be pursued since many patients can be expected to resolve on antibiotic therapy and intravenous fluids. Clearly this demands careful observation and if signs deteriorate efforts should be made to remove the appendix.
3. If it is clear that the acute attack has resolved, then appendicectomy can be deferred. In the past, most patients went on to elective appendicectomy 3 months after the acute attack. A conservative course is pursued far more frequently now. In patients considered to be at risk of caecal carcinoma, an elective barium enema should be carried out and if this is normal, most surgeons would now not advise interval appendicectomy.

Operative technique

The patient is routinely given a preoperative dose of intravenous metronidazole and a second-generation cephalosporin, such as cefuroxime. There is debate whether a suppository of metronidazole is adequate. The anxiety with this is whether adequate tissue levels can be achieved. Furthermore, not all the organisms are anaerobes and broad-spectrum cover is to be advised.

The abdomen is palpated under anaesthesia and if a mass is felt the incision can be placed directly over it. If there is no localization the author favours the transverse-pararectal incision (Figure 17.3). This starts just lateral to the lateral border of the rectus muscle approximately halfway between the umbilicus and the anterior superior iliac spine. Since the incision is placed in the skin crease, the cosmetic results are excellent and there is little temptation to make tiny incisions which afford poor access to the abdomen. The rectus sheath is then incised transversely and the

access can be increased by retracting the skin incision laterally and medially. The incision is taken beyond the lateral border of the rectus muscle. The rectus abdominus is then retracted medially and the posterior sheath incised together with the most medial fibres of the external oblique muscle. This provides immediate access to the posterior sheath and peritoneum. The traditional more laterally placed incision involved splitting the oblique muscles where bleeding may occur. The popular low-lying transverse Lanz incision starting just above and medial to the anterior superior iliac spine may provide very poor access to the high retrocaecal appendix. When extension is required, this produces an unsightly hockey-stick incision with poor cosmetic results. The importance of adequate exposure cannot be over-stressed and difficulties are normally encountered only when the inexperienced surgeon is reluctant to make an adequate incision to make the operation easy. The skin edges should be protected with swabs soaked in antiseptics and suction should immediately be available so that if pus wells up into the wound once the peritoneum has been opened, contamination can be minimized.

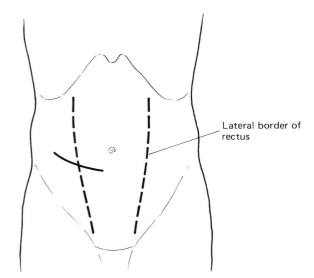

Figure 17.3 Transverse-pararectal incision

If any difficulties are encountered, the incision can be extended either laterally or medially. Once again the higher transverse incision can be extended with relative ease and if necessary the muscles can be divided if, for example, the diagnosis is incorrect and following inspection a different procedure has to be carried out. Once again this overcomes the dilemma of whether to make a midline incision where there is doubt regarding the actual diagnosis. Occasionally, when a perforated duodenal ulcer or perforated diverticulum is found, if the operator is not used to transverse incisions, the surgeon may elect to close the appendicectomy incision and embark on a formal vertical incision to deal appropriately with the pathology. The appendix can normally be delivered by drawing the caecum through the abdominal incision. If the caecum is extraperitoneal it should be mobilized by dividing its lateral peritoneal attachments. If this is the case it is important to have adequate access and, if appropriate, extend the incision. The appendicular vessels should be identified and ligated and divided, having secured haemostasis with absorbable sutures. The appendix should be crushed near its base and the artery forceps advanced a few millimetres distally. An absorbable tie is then placed around the appendix stump, ensuring that there is sufficient appendix beyond the tie to prevent slippage. The appendix is then amputated and removed. Traditionally surgeons inserted a purse-string suture to cover the stump. This is quite unnecessary and simply complicates the procedure

If the appendix is gangrenous or perforated, care should be taken not to disseminate the purulent fluid from the primary site firstly over the wound and secondly around the peritoneal cavity. Care should also be taken during mobilization of the gangrenous appendix to prevent rupture of the organ. When the caecum is oedematous it is important not to attempt inversion of the stump, which as pointed out above is unnecessary. Occasionally when the inflamed appendix is in the retrocolic position and firmly bound down along the length of the ascending colon, a retrograde appendicectomy should be performed. The base of the appendix is freed and its base ligated and divided. Traction is placed on the appendix and the vessels secured sequentially until it is removed.

Closure

The peritoneal and posterior sheath can be closed or simply left and peritonealization will rapidly occur. The anterior sheath should be closed with a strong absorbable suture using 0 or 1 Vicryl or PDS.

Where there has been excessive contamination it may be wise to dress the wound with gauze and apply Steristrips at 48 h when it has been ascertained that the wound is clean. In most instances, skin clips or a subcuticular suture of non-absorbable prolene or absorbable Vicryl can be used.

The appendix mass

The management of the appendix mass depends on the clinical setting. If the patient has a high fever and there is local tenderness, the diagnosis is of an appendix abscess and the pus must be drained. Here the incision can be centred over the centre of the abscess and no attempt should be made to carry out a laparotomy within the confines of the limited incision. The pus should simply be drained. If the appendix is accessible then it should be removed, but if not, no attempt should be made to complicate the procedure in order to remove the appendix.

If the patient's general condition is good, there is no pyrexia; with a mass in the right iliac fossa but no signs of generalized peritonitis the patient can be watched. There is no requirement for antibiotics since nature has sealed off the inflammatory process. So long as the patient's general condition continues to improve, no operative intervention is required. Clearly if the patient deteriorates, surgical intervention may be necessary.

Postoperative complications

The use of perioperative antibiotics, particularly metronidazole, has reduced the incidence of postoperative complications significantly. Complications are more likely when the appendix is gangrenous or has perforated.

PARALYTIC ILEUS

The management consists of supporting the patient with nasogastric aspiration and intravenous fluids. Antibiotics are given where appropriate. Careful clinical assessment is required to ascertain whether the ileus is the response to the initial pathology or the result of further complications which require operative intervention.

If the ileus persists and there is increasing abdominal pain, mechanical obstruction should be considered, particularly if there are active bowel sounds. Paralytic ileus is normally relatively painless with reduced or absent bowel sounds. If the symptoms begin after the patient has already passed flatus or has a bowel action, it is very likely that mechanical obstruction has supervened.

A plain radiograph can be extremely helpful. If there is a diffuse distribution of gas throughout the small bowel, large bowel and rectum, paralytic ileus is the most likely diagnosis, whereas a localized loop of distended small intestine with fluid levels, with absence of gas in the large bowel, is in favour of mechanical obstruction.

SEPTIC COMPLICATIONS

If a wound abscess develops, the sutures should be removed and pus released. Drainage should be adequate and antibiotics are not normally required unless there is evidence of cellulitis.

Pelvic abscess. A pelvic abscess may follow generalized peritonitis or the removal of a perforated appendix. The most telling sign is the onset of diarrhoea with a mucous rectal discharge. The temperature is normally elevated and may swing between peaks and troughs with the typical signs of 'pus' chart. Rectal examination reveals a tender mass which, if large enough, may be palpated abdominally.

In the majority of cases, drainage occurs into the rectum or vagina and may be assisted by digital examination. Occasionally drainage needs to be performed through the rectum or the posterior fornix of the vagina. For this purpose a pair of sinus forceps are gently passed into the softest part of the mass under general anaesthesia. Before doing this it is imperative to be certain one is dealing with pus, and ultrasonography will confirm the clinical suspicion.

Subphrenic abscess. Subphrenic abscess is much less common as a result of the routine use of antibiotics. Pus may collect in either the right or left subphrenic spaces or in the right subhepatic space forming a Morrison's pouch.

Under such circumstances the patient will have a high fever, often with little in the way of physical signs. Springing the lower ribs may produce discomfort or pain and suggests the diagnosis. The white cell count is usually raised and may be in excess of 20 000 with a polymorph leucocytosis. Radiographs of the chest may reveal elevation of the diaphragm, with pleural effusion with accompanied collapse of the lung base. In severe cases a gas and fluid level may be seen below the diaphragm. Ultrasonography is extremely helpful in localizing subphrenic infection.

In early cases, broad-spectrum antibiotics may lead to clinical improvement. If the patient's condition fails to improve, drainage is required. In the first instance this can be attempted using percutaneous drains placed under ultrasonic guidance. It is useful to place two drains so that irrigation of the cavity can be carried out. If clinical resolution still does not occur, formal drainage is required. Depending on the localization, this is performed either using a posterior approach through a small incision immediately below the 12th rib or via an anterior subcostal incision.

Carcinoid tumour of the appendix

By far the most common neoplasm of the appendix is the carcinoid tumour. This is found in about 0.1% of all appendices subjected to careful histological examination. Macroscopically the tumour consists of a yellowish plaque with intact overlying mucosa which later ulcerates. About three-quarters of the tumours occur at the tip of the appendix and only unusually are they found at the appendix base. Macroscopically the carcinoid is made up of enterochromaffin Kulchitsky cells which take up silver stains and arise in the crypts of the intestinal mucosa. Metastatic spread from carcinoid of the appendix is very rare and is practically confined to lesions which are larger than 2 cm in diameter. Such tumours occur in only about 1% of carcinoids of the appendix. The majority of carcinoids are found incidentally on routine histological study of appendices removed either at emergency appendicectomy or because they are noted to be abnormal during the course of a laparotomy for other procedures. The tumour is frequently at the tip of the organ and in this site is not expected to cause appendicitis. However, the lumen may be occluded by tumours at the base or in the body of the appendix so that carcinoid may present as a case of acute appendicitis or even an appendix abscess.

If the tumour is discovered at operation it should be removed and a careful laparotomy carried out to exclude other carcinoid tumours. In the vast majority of cases there will be no further spread beyond the appendix. In those rare cases where the tumour is large and there appear to be regional lymph nodes involved, a right hemicolectomy should be carried out.

If the diagnosis is not established until the histological examination has taken place, no further action needs to be contemplated if the tumour has been completely removed. If the base of the appendix is involved and resection is incomplete, then further surgery should be considered.

The carcinoid syndrome, which results usually from extensive hepatic metastases, is almost never seen following carcinoid of the appendix.

Colon

Anatomy

The large intestine is subdivided, for descriptive purposes, into the caecum with the appendix, the ascending colon, hepatic flexure, transverse colon, splenic flexure, descending colon and sigmoid (Figure 17.4). The large bowel may vary quite considerably in length in different individuals, with an average of about 90 cm. At operation the colon is readily identified because of its three flattened bands, the taeniae coli, which begin at the base of the appendix and run the length of the large intestine to end at the rectosigmoid junction. These represent the great bulk of the longitudinal muscle of the large bowel and because they are shorter than the gut to which they are attached, the colon becomes condensed into its typical sacculated shape. The colon, but not the appendix, caecum or rectum, also bears the characteristic flat-filled peritoneal tags, the appendices epiploicae, which are scattered over its surface and which are especially numerous in the sigmoid loop. The transverse colon is specifically identified by its attachment to the omentum.

The transverse and sigmoid colon are completely peritonealized. The ascending and descending colon have no mesocolon but adhere directly to the posterior abdominal wall; exceptionally the ascending colon may be wholly or partly peritonealized. The caecum may or may not be completely surrounded by peritoneum (the latter more likely in the female subject), and the appendix, although usually free within its own mesentery, occasionally lies extraperitoneally behind the caecum and ascending colon or adheres to the posterior wall of these structures.

The arterial supply of the colon is derived from branches of the superior and inferior mesenteric arteries. The first branch to the colon from the superior mesenteric artery is the middle colic branch, which originates from the right side of the vessel, enters the transverse mesocolon and divides into its right and left branches; the latter supplies the transverse colon to the region of the splenic flexure and represents the most distal extent of the superior mesenteric blood supply. The right colic artery is relatively small, originates some 5 cm more distally to the middle colic and supplies the ascending colon. The ileocolic artery originates another 5 cm below this and is the only constant branch of these three right-sided colonic vessels. It supplies the terminal ileum, caecum and start of the ascending colon and gives off the appendicular branch to the appendix, the most commonly ligated intra-abdominal artery. The right colic and middle colic arteries are variable and may arise from a common trunk. The right colic artery may originate from the ileocolic artery in about 10% of subjects.

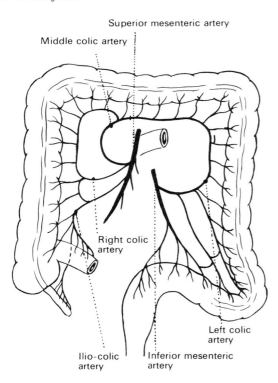

Figure 17.4 Anatomy of the large bowel and its blood supply

The inferior mesenteric artery arises from the aorta at the level of the third lumbar vertebra and gives off the left colic artery to supply the descending colon, the sigmoid branches, which supply the sigmoid colon and then descends as the superior haemorrhoidal artery to supply the rectum.

Each branch of the superior and inferior mesenteric artery to the colon anastomoses with its neighbour above and below, so that there is a continuous vascular arcade along the whole length of the large bowel.

The anastomosis of this marginal artery (of Drummond) may be small or incomplete between the left branch of the middle colic and the uppermost extent of the left colic in the region of the splenic flexure, and this is the region where ischaemic lesions of the colon are most likely to occur.

The venous drainage of the colon takes place along corresponding named veins; the inferior mesenteric vein ascends above the point of origin of its artery to enter the splenic vein behind the pancreas. The superior mesenteric vein joins the splenic vein behind the neck of the pancreas to form the portal vein.

Lymph drainage

The arrangement of the lymph nodes of the intestine is relatively uniform in both small and large bowel (Figure 17.5). Numerous small nodes lie near, or on, the wall of the intestine and these drain into intermedially placed and rather larger nodes along the vessels of the mesentery and mesocolon. These in turn drain to clumps of lymph nodes situated near the origins of the superior and inferior mesenteric vessels. From these nodes, efferent lymphatics drain into the cisterna chyli.

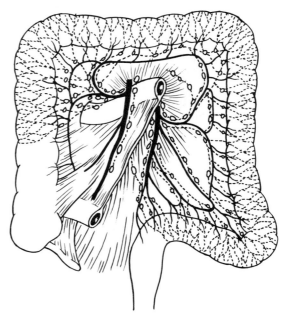

Figure 17.5 Lymph drainage of the large intestine

The lymphatic drainage field of each segment of intestine corresponds fairly accurately to its arterial supply. Thus high ligation of the vessels to the involved segment of gut with removal of a wide surrounding segment of mesocolon will remove the lymph nodes which drain the area; thus division of the middle colic vessels and resection of the wedge of transverse mesocolon would, for example, clear the lymphatic drainage in resection of a growth of the transverse colon.

Diverticula of the colon

A 'diverticulum' is an abnormal pouch which opens from a hollow organ. In Roman times the word was applied to a wayside house of ill repute and well the diverticula of the colon deserve this name.

The term diverticular disease has been applied to the condition in which there are multiple false diverticula of the colon. These arise on the mesenteric border of the bowel where the mesenteric blood vessels perforate the muscular coat.

Diverticular disease of the colon is extremely common in Western society. The vast majority of patients are asymptomatic. Clinical presentation is due to complications. Asymptomatic diagnosis of diverticular disease is made on routine barium enemas carried out for rectal bleeding or discovered at laparotomy or post-mortem examination (Figure 17.6). There are two characteristic ways in which diverticular disease can present: first, as a major complication in the previously asymptomatic patient as either perforation, with faecal peritonitis, or with haemorrhage; secondly, and more commonly, in patients with pre-existing symptoms. The presentation is characteristically with lower abdominal discomfort or pain centred in the left iliac fossa or generalized across the lower abdomen. Episodes of colic may be associated with a change in bowel habit characterized by alternating diarrhoea and constipation. These symptoms are due to the thickening and narrowing that occurs in the sigmoid colon and to the functional obstruction that occurs at the rectosigmoid junction. This is due, first, to gross muscular hypertrophy and secondly to angulation which commonly occurs at this site. The thickened pelvic colon hangs down in the pouch of Douglas causing obstruction at this site.

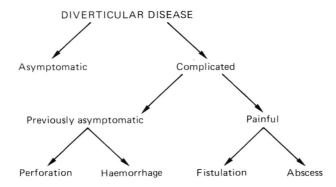

Figure 17.6 Diverticulosis and its complications

Acute diverticulitis may present with the features that have been termed left-sided appendicitis which may settle down with conservative management or progress to abscess formation with the development of a pericolic abscess in the left iliac fossa. Free perforation is more common in patients who have previously been asymptomatic; these patients present with generalized peritonitis usually associated with a massive pneumoperitoneum. This is the most serious and acute complication of diverticular disease and is usually associated with a large stercoral perforation. Where a localized abscess develops, this may progress to generalized peritonitis, but more commonly the abscess is localized and the perforation may drain into an adjacent organ, particularly the bladder (more common in men than in women). The abscess may also drain into an adjacent loop of colon, small intestine or the vagina. If an abscess points to the skin, drainage will lead to a faecal fistula onto the abdominal wall (Figure 17.7).

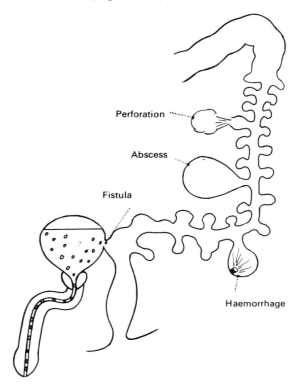

Figure 17.7 Complications of acute diverticulitis in diagrammatic form

Haemorrhage normally occurs as a major sudden rectal bleed. It is most unusual for minor blood loss to be attributable to diverticular disease. With increasing use of colonoscopy and angiography these cases are frequently due to either ischaemic colitis or angiodysplasia, and there is great debate as to how frequently diverticular disease actually causes bleeding. In the majority of cases there may be no pathological evidence of acute inflammation. Haemorrhage is particularly likely to occur in elderly patients with hypertension and arteriosclerosis and in those with diffuse diverticular disease that has previously been asymptomatic. It is considered that haemorrhage occurs because of erosion of blood vessels in the neck of the diverticulum.

Acute obstruction may result from diverticular disease, but may also be caused by adherence of a loop of small intestine to the inflamed diverticular segment.

Surgery for diverticular disease

The large majority of cases of uncomplicated diverticular disease respond to a high-roughage diet. Surgery is rarely contemplated for painful diverticular disease. Indeed the majority of these cases may be due to the irritable bowel syndrome and great caution should be exercised when contemplating surgery simply for abdominal pain.

Elective anterior resection

The indications include painful diverticular disease where conservative treatment has failed, a diverticular stricture causing obstructive symptoms, fistula into the bladder and vagina and the presence of abdominal mass where carcinoma cannot be excluded. It is important to resect the rectosigmoid junction where obstruction occurs in this condition. Failure to do this may leave part of the sigmoid loop behind and will risk recurrent symptoms and postoperative anastomotic breakdown because of distal obstruction. The patient is prepared for large bowel surgery with laxatives to empty the colon. Broad-spectrum antibiotics, including metronidazole, are given at induction of anaesthesia. The patient is placed in the Lloyd-Davis position. The author's preference is to use a transverse lower abdominal incision (Figure 17.8). This runs from above the anterior superior iliac spines and curves downward to well above the symphysis. If access proves difficult to the flexures, then it can be extended laterally. The alternative is to use a long midline incision. The advantage of the transverse incision is that access is excellent and if a stoma is required it can be brought out through the rectus sheath, leaving a large area that is separate from the actual incision. Having incised the skin, the remainder of the incision is carried out using the spray facility provided by modern diathermy. In this way, haemostasis is excellent. The inferior epigastric vessels require ligation and division and occasional large veins in the subcutaneous fat require ligation. Once the abdomen is entered the wound is covered with surgical towels and these are held in place with a Vi-drape wound protector which prevents contamination of the wound. A full laparotomy is carried out.

Attention is then directed to the pathology. The splenic flexure should always be mobilized. The reason for this is that it allows anastomosis without tension and the blood supply to the descending colon is normally excellent, based on the middle colic artery. Access to the transverse colon and splenic flexure is facilitated if the surgeon stands between the legs and an assistant retracts the wound upwards and to the left to expose the flexure. Inadvertent damage to the spleen can be prevented by placing a pack above the spleen to bring it down towards the incision prior to any mobilization. The transverse mesocolon is separated from the colon using diathermy to divide its peritoneal attachment along the colonic surface. This is normally straightforward and is facilitated by entering the correct plane. Small vessels are coagulated during the dissection. When the splenic flexure is high, it is helpful to commence the dissection along the left colon and continue towards the splenic flexure. If the operator grasps the colon with a swab and exerts gentle traction, the lateral attachments are sequentially divided. Once the lateral peritoneal attachments have been divided, the ureter is carefully separated from the mesentery of the colon. As the dissection progresses proximally, the flexure is reached and the lateral attachments between the colon are divided. Care should be taken to avoid damage to the pancreatic vessels lying along the lower border of the tail of the pancreas. The inferior mesenteric vein is then identified and ligated and divided. This is the key to adequate mobilization, since the left colon then becomes a midline structure following ligation of the inferior mesenteric artery. Although it is not strictly necessary to ligate it at its origin, the collateral blood supply is preserved between the ascending branch of the left colic artery and the branches of the middle colic artery if division occurs close to the aorta. If the inferior mesenteric artery is approached on its mesenteric aspect, it should be possible to divide it without damage to the pre-aortic sympathetics.

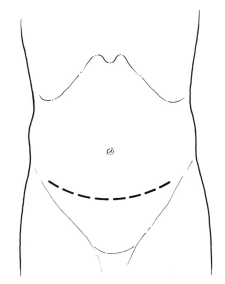

Figure 17.8 Transverse lower abdominal incision

Having fully mobilized the colon, attention is turned to the distal sigmoid and rectal dissection. This can be quite difficult in complicated diverticular disease. The sigmoid is frequently thickened and often densely attached in the pelvic pouch. Knowledge of this greatly facilitates the dissection and avoids difficulties. Having mobilized the left colon, the ureter is normally out of harm's way and there is no need to place tapes round it. The surgeon returns to the left side of the patient and continues the dissection in front of the pre-aortic sympathetic nerves in a bloodless plane which is extended lateral to the rectum. The presacral sympathetic nerves are carefully identified and preserved. The sigmoid colon which as alluded to above is frequently adherent to the back of the bladder or uterus is carefully freed by a combination of blunt and sharp dissection. If there is a fistula between the sigmoid and bladder or vagina it is gently pinched off. Often the fistulous opening is so small that the bladder and vagina do not require repair, but where the opening is larger, one or two absorbable sutures close the organ. The site of distal transection is normally at the pelvic brim and it is important to construct the anastomosis between colon and rectum rather than distal sigmoid. This is normally easily identified. The rectum does not require full mobilization, but should be freed sufficiently to allow identification of the blood supply and safe ligation of the vessels. Having decided the site of the anastomosis, the colon is clamped with a right angled clamp.

Attention is then turned to the left colon. A point with excellent vascularization is selected to construct an anastomosis without tension. The author's preference is to use one of the circular stapling devices which greatly facilitate anastomosis. With a high rectal anastomosis, the purse-string device is simple to use. A 2/0 prolene suture bearing two straight needles is inserted into the device and this will normally insert a perfect purse-string suture. The same procedure is carried out with the proximal colon, and sigmoid can then be resected. The largest stapler head that can be accommodated by the descending colon is selected, either 31 mm or 33 mm. This is normally accepted by the descending colon, but if it is narrower a smaller head is used. The stapling gun is then inserted through the anus and carefully advanced up into the bowel. The stapling head is detached and the distal purse-string suture tied. If it is clear that there are gaps, further sutures can be inserted to snug distal bowel down onto the anvil. The detached head is then inserted into the proximal bowel and having ascertained that the purse-string suture is satisfactory, the anastomosis is completed. Before the stapler is fired, care should be taken to ensure that the bowel is not twisted and that no surrounding tissues have been included. The use of air testing is controversial. If there are two good 'doughnuts' of tissue, then air testing should not be necessary.

Two fine suction drains are placed in the pelvis to remove serosanguineous collections and these can usually be removed the next day. It is our preference to lavage the abdomen with a solution of tetracycline containing 1 g per litre to try to minimize septic complications. The abdomen is then closed. The transverse incision is closed in layers using a continuous suture of loop number 1 polydioxanone. A midline incision is closed in a single layer with either prolene or polydioxanone. Recent evidence has suggested that polydioxanone is perfectly safe and has the advantage of minimizing suture sinuses without an increased risk of herniation or wound dehiscence.

Sutured anastomosis

A two-layer anastomosis is quite unnecessary for colorectal anastomosis. Despite this, many surgeons feel more secure with a continuous inner layer supported by an outer seromuscular support. The author has never used this for large bowel anastomosis. It should be stated that the most important factors for prevention of anastomotic leakage are an excellent blood supply and the absence of tension. Suture technique is largely a matter of personal preference and controlled trials fail to demonstrate any significant difference between anastomotic methods. The end result is largely a matter of careful surgical technique. Clamps are rarely necessary with adequately prepared bowel. A soft clamp may be required, to prevent spillage, if there is liquid retained in the proximal colon. Stay sutures are then placed in the four corners of the bowel. These facilitate access, and help to stabilize the colon and rectum. The author's preference is for an extramucosal appositional technique. The suture used is again a matter of personal preference but the author uses 4/0 polydioxanone. This slides well through the tissue and is of adequate strength for its purpose. It is easier first to place the posterior layer of the anastomosis and use a new suture for each of these placings. Some surgeons prefer a continuous technique, but where there is discrepancy between the bowel lumina an interrupted method is easier. A large bite of serosa colonic muscle and submucosa is taken and the needle emerges beneath the mucosa. The process is repeated in the rectum and the suture is held. Once all the posterior sutures have been placed, the bowel ends are approximated and the sutures tied. The remaining lengths of suture can be used to complete the anterior layer of the anastomosis.

Normally anastomoses between colon and the intraperitoneal rectum do not require defunctioning, but if any doubt exists a right transverse colostomy, or alternatively a loop ileostomy, can be raised. In many respects the latter is easier to manage since it can be placed in the right iliac fossa and is easier for the patient to manage. Again this is a matter of surgical preference.

Surgical management of the complications of diverticulitis

1. Perforation

A confident diagnosis of perforated diverticular disease cannot always be made. Often it is part of the differential diagnosis in the emergency management of the acute abdomen in patients with generalized peritonitis. In such cases the importance of adequate resuscitation cannot be overemphasized. It is well worth spending up to 12 h optimizing the patient's condition with broad-spectrum intravenous antibiotics, intravenous fluids, oxygen and nasogastric suction. The mortality of this dangerous condition may be significantly reduced by aggressive resuscitation, and the inexperienced surgeon should be counselled against rushing into operation despite the alarming physical and radiological signs. It is normal to use a long midline incision and once again the Lloyd-Davis position is to be preferred to allow access to the anal canal and for bowel mobilization should that be necessary. A laparotomy is carried out and the pathology in the colon ascertained. Careful peritoneal toilet should be carried out and pus, faeces and a mixture of the two carefully lavaged and aspirated. Pus should be taken for bacteriological examination.

The management of these cases demands careful judgement and clinical skill; senior help should be sought where difficulty has been encountered. The safest procedure in the presence of major peritonitis is to carry out a Hartmann's operation. The diseased segment is resected and a convenient part of left colon is exteriorized as an end colostomy. The distal rectum is oversewn. It is unwise to attempt to exteriorize the rectal stump since this involves mobilization of the rectum. Furthermore, if the rectosigmoid junction has been removed, great difficulty will be encountered if the surgeon attempts to bring the rectum out through the lower abdominal incision.

In the past such cases were frequently treated by transverse defunctioning colostomy and drainage. The advantage of this conservative procedure is simplicity, particularly for the inexperienced surgeon. The disadvantage is that the inflamed and infected segment of colon, loaded with faeces and a poorly closed perforation, persists distal to the colostomy and this may produce continued sepsis and fistula formation. The advantage of the radical resection is the removal of the septic colonic segment with the obvious benefits to the patient. It should be emphasized that this is a procedure that is safe only in the hands of experienced surgeons. Unfortunately, many patients, particularly the elderly and infirm, never have their colostomies closed following Hartmann's resection.

2. Pericolic abscess

This is considerably more common than free perforation. The initial treatment should be conservative with intravenous fluids and antibiotics. Some of these cases may be amenable to drainage under computerized tomographic guidance, particularly if the sepsis is localized. Once again, modern antibiotics with their broad spectrum and anaerobic sensitivity have encouraged surgeons to pursue a more conservative approach in septic diverticular complications.

If the condition progressively subsides, a subsequent elective resection should be advised after thorough investigation of the patient, which will include sigmoidoscopy and a barium enema.

If the mass increases in size, together with continued pyrexia, a rising pulse rate and deterioration of the patient's general condition, then surgical intervention is necessary. The diverticular segment is resected as described above and a Hartmann's resection is normally carried out. Occasionally if conditions are optimal, the surgeon may elect to carry out a primary anastomosis with a transverse defunctioning colostomy or loop ileostomy. Indeed some surgeons are happy to perform a one-stage resection and primary anastomoses. Once again, clinical judgement should be exercised.

3. Vesicocolic and colovaginal fistula

In the past the management of enterocolic fistula entailed a three-stage procedure with preliminary defunctioning colostomy followed by resection and later colostomy closure. This protracted course is rarely necessary now and in elective fistula surgery most surgeons are happy to carry out a primary resection and anastomosis. It is wise to try to place the anastomosis away from the fistula site into the bladder or vagina and if possible interpose loops of small bowel, caecum or the omentum between the fistula site and the anastomosis. In intestinal obstruction, in most instances it is possible to carry out immediate resection and, depending on the condition of the patient, primary anastomosis. Clearly the proximal colon will need to be adequately decompressed and this can be achieved either by on-table lavage using a Foley catheter inserted into the appendix stump or terminal ileum and colonic irrigation using large quantities of warm saline. The procedure is facilitated by insertion of a tube into the proximal colon which can be drained into a suitable receptacle. In order to cope with this elongated procedure, the patient's condition should be excellent and before proceeding to such measures careful discussion with the anaesthetist should take place. Where doubt concerns regarding the safety of an anastomosis, a Hartmann's resection should be carried out. If, following anastomosis, the situation is considered to be less than optimal, it is safer to bring out a proximal loop stoma. This can usually be closed 4–6 weeks after the patient has been discharged, having first ascertained on contrast studies that the anastomosis has healed.

5. Massive haemorrhage

Fortunately the majority of patients with severe haemorrhage associated with diverticular disease settle conservatively with bed rest and blood transfusion. Once the initial acute bleed has settled, colonoscopy is useful. Complete bowel preparation is usually unnecessary. A series of enemas is given and these will normally evacuate retained blood. A colonoscope is inserted until either an abnormality is seen to account for the haemorrhage or faeces are encountered. Since blood is a very effective aperient, the bleeding point is normally distal to the point where faeces are encountered. If the patient fails to stop bleeding, resection of the bowel should then be contemplated.

In most instances, angiography is to be recommended since bleeding may have occurred as a result of angiodysplasia, and right colon resection, rather than left resection, may be required. On occasion where severe haemorrhage has occurred and it is deemed inadvisable to investigate the patient further, where localization of the site of bleeding cannot accurately be made, a subtotal colectomy with ileorectal anastomosis should be performed. Lesser procedures such as multiple colotomies to determine the source of bleeding are usually unhelpful. If only a partial colectomy is performed, it may be found that further haemorrhage takes place from the residual colon forcing the surgeon to carry out a more major resection in the much more dangerous situation of a second surgical procedure on a seriously ill patient.

An alternative approach is to carry out on-table lavage as described above, followed by intraoperative colonoscopy. This may be difficult if preparation is poor, but if the bleeding point can be localized a more limited resection can be carried out.

Cancer of the colon

Carcinoma of the colon can have a very good prognosis if diagnosed early. The principle of the operation is wide resection of the tumour together with the draining lymph nodes, followed by restoration of intestinal continuity. In the emergency situation in the obstructed patient, careful judgement is required before deciding whether to restore intestinal continuity. Overall if there is an adequate blood supply and the patient's condition is good, in the absence of gross faecal loading intestinal continuity can be restored quite frequently. It is rare to have to exteriorize the bowel ends for an obstructing right colon tumour, but with left-sided lesions where there can be extensive faecal loading a number of alternatives are available and it is here that experience in judgement is so important.

Special investigations

The majority of patients will present with bleeding or a change in bowel habit. Clinical examination should include rectal examination, testing for occult blood positivity, and rigid sigmoidoscopy. Following this, if a tumour has not been seen the examination of choice is probably colonoscopy. A good-quality contrast barium enema is the alternative. The advantage of colonoscopy is that the lesion can be visualized and biopsies obtained. In addition, brush cytology increases the accuracy of a positive diagnosis. Having made the diagnosis of a colonic carcinoma, the patient should be staged ideally with computerized tomography to screen the liver for metastatic deposits and failing that with ultrasonography. Haemoglobin and liver function tests together with urea and electrolyte levels are measured. Carcinoembryonic antigen (CEA) provides a baseline measurement and if it is elevated a return to the normal range in the postoperative period suggests that a radical excision has been carried out. There is no data to show that this predicts a cure and studies continue to determine whether measurement of a postoperative CEA will provide lead time to allow better treatment of recurrent disease.

The patient is prepared for bowel surgery with laxatives in the usual manner, as described above.

When metastatic liver disease is diagnosed on ultrasonography, there is debate as to the advisability of performing a colonic resection. It should be remembered that often metastatic disease is slow to progress and a palliative resection may prevent intestinal obstruction developing in the untreated patient.

Surgical resection

It is the author's practice to place all patients in the Lloyd-Davis position. With the increased use of stapling devices, access to the anal canal is always available. Furthermore, the operator can stand between the legs to mobilize the flexures, a position that is comfortable for the surgeon and allows the assistant to retract costal margins. Again as described above, the author's preference is to use a transverse muscle-cutting incision centred below the umbilicus for left colon lesions and just skirting the umbilicus in right colon lesions. Clearly if the patient has previously had a midline incision there is no point inflicting new scars. A careful laparotomy should be carried out. There is great debate concerning the no-touch technique, but clearly excessive tumour manipulation can cause tumour emboli and should be kept to a minimum. Attention should be turned to the liver. Clinical palpation is notoriously inaccurate and misses large numbers of metastatic deposits. Currently the procedure of choice is intraoperative ultrasonography. With an experienced operator this is accurate and has a high positive predictive value when compared with follow-up computerized tomography.

When the primary tumour is operable, even if there is evidence of distant spread or metastatic disease, in most instances a palliative resection is indicated in order to save the patient the miseries of uncontrolled local disease. Occasionally with fixed tumours it is unwise to proceed to heroic surgery and the procedure should either be abandoned or, where obstruction is expected, a simple bypass can be carried out.

In the presence of wholly localized hepatic disease, hepatic resection may be considered. In the main it is wise to stage the patient properly, as the extent of disease may be underestimated. In patients with stable hepatic disease with between one and four tumours confined to one lobe, hepatic resection as a metachronous procedure can be considered 3 months after the initial colonic resection.

Contiguous invasion to adjacent structures does not necessarily confer an adverse prognosis, particularly if lymph nodes are not involved by tumour. Thus *en bloc* resection, which may include the anterior or posterior abdominal wall, the omentum, stomach, duodenum, small intestine, kidney and pelvic organs, should be offered to the patient. If there is doubt, a trial of dissection is always justified, for the results of radical surgery can be surprisingly good.

During resection, care must be taken to prevent dissemination. The tumour should not be opened and ideally should have its vascular pedicle isolated before handling. In addition, surgical tapes can be tied above and below the tumour.

Right hemicolectomy

Right hemicolectomy is indicated for operable carcinoma of the caecum, ascending colon, hepatic flexure and in some instances extended to involve tumours of the transverse colon and splenic flexures. Limited resections of the transverse colon are rarely indicated and, since they remove the middle colic artery, are more at risk of anastomotic dehiscence. Thus the author's preference, for a lesion between the caecum and the proximal descending colon, is to use right hemicolectomy or extended right hemicolectomy. Adequate access to the abdomen is imperative and facilitates safe surgery.

In tumours of the right colon the first stage is to free the peritoneal attachments; if the dissection commences at the caecum it can be extended up the right paracolic gutter and should free the terminal ileum. Frequently this portion is also retroperitoneal and lies below the caecum. In this manner the caecum and ileum can be elevated and freed sequentially from the gonadal vessels, where care is required to avoid trauma and unnecessary bleeding. The ureter is next met and the bowel separated from it. Moving proximally, the duodenum is encountered and separated from the colon. The author's preference is to use diathermy for dissection since this produces a completely bloodless field. Care is required near the origin of the hepatic flexure mesentery because frequently relatively small veins which drain into the superior mesenteric vein can be damaged if excessive traction is used. If the omentum is close to the tumour, it should be sacrificed, otherwise it can be separated from the transverse colon by elevation and dissection between the colon and the leaves of the omentum. A few small vessels proximal to the hepatic flexure require ligation and division and this should free the

whole of the right colon. As soon as possible during mobilization, tapes should be passed above and below the tumour and ligated to reduce intraluminal dissemination of cancer cells. The mesentery should then be assessed to determine the precise site of division of the bowel.

With tumours of the caecum it may be possible to preserve most of the ileocolic artery and most of the ileum, but clearly this should be judged carefully in order to allow maximum clearance of involved nodes. Feeding arteries and veins are ligated close, but at a safe distance from the superior mesenteric artery and vein to allow excision of the tumour. For tumours of the caecum and ascending colon, the transverse colon is normally removed to beyond the hepatic flexure to allow anastomosis at a well-vascularized area of transverse colon. If the middle colic artery has to be divided, because the tumour encroaches on its distribution, then the resection should be taken beyond the splenic flexure to the descending colon. This will avoid the risk of ischaemic anastomotic breakdown.

A side-to-side anastomosis is rarely necessary since any discrepancy between the ileal and colonic lumens can be overcome by carefully placing interrupted sutures with appropriate matching or, if necessary, an antimesenteric split of the ileum. With the increasing use of staples for restoring intestinal continuity, many surgeons close the two bowel ends with linear staplers using a GIA type of linear cutting stapler to form a side-to-side anastomosis and oversew the small openings required to insert this instrument. This seems an unnecessary use of hardware and saves little time for such a simple, straightforward anastomosis. The author's practice is to use interrupted 4/0 polydioxanone sutures in the four corners, picking up serosa and submucosa as stay sutures. This then minimizes the amount of handling of the tissues required with forceps. A series of appositional extramucosal sutures is then placed with the knots on the outside. This avoids having punctures through the full thickness of the bowel wall and allows the mucosa simply to flop against the two opposed ends. This allows an early seal and avoids any theoretical risk of ischaemia. Compare the mucosal surface using this technique with sutures placed every 6–8 mm, to its appearance when a continuous over-and-over all-coats suture is used. With the appositional technique, the mucosa will be of normal colour and will lie nicely. With the over-and-over technique it is often blue and bunched, a situation less conducive to normal healing. In addition, the appositional extramucosal technique avoids the theoretical risk of having a point of exit for luminal contents through the suture line tract to the exterior of the bowel. Clamps are avoided unless there is a major risk of contamination.

There is still great debate as to the advisability of using one-and two-layer anastomoses. Indeed many surgeons use a single layer of continuous prolene with excellent results. Ultimately it is a matter of personal preference and familiarization with a technique that works for the individual surgeon. Before constructing the anastomosis, it is a wise precaution to cleanse the bowel with a solution of povidone-iodine as a tumoricidal agent to remove any spilled cancer cells which could theoretically cause implantation at a future date. Overall suture line recurrence is rare. The majority of recurrent carcinomas are hepatic or spread from outside the bowel wall towards the lumen. In spite of such rarity, complacency is not called for and every effort should be made to reduce the risk of implantation.

If there is a large defect in the mesocolon this can be closed, but great care should be taken to avoid damage to the mesenteric blood vessels. In many instances, part of the omentum can be placed over the defect and loosely tacked to the bowel to prevent loops of small bowel entering the window in the small intestine.

There is normally no need to use a drain for intraperitoneal anastomoses. Haemostasis should be secured at completion of the procedure and fluid is readily absorbed by the peritoneal cavity.

At completion of the anastomosis the abdomen can be lavaged with a dilute solution of tetracycline with 1 g in a litre of normal saline.

Where extended resection is required, because the middle colic artery has been divided, the splenic flexure should be mobilized. To the inexperienced surgeon this is often a difficult technique and great care is required, first to secure adequate haemostasis and secondly to avoid injury to the spleen. A manoeuvre that can prevent capsular tears is to place a pack above the spleen prior to mobilization. This reduces the amount of retraction required, and brings the spleen down towards the operator. The omentum is lifted and the plane between the colon and the omentum entered. If it is not easily entered, simply move along the colon until a point of access can be gained and, once identified, the plane can be developed until the stomach is reached and lifted forward.

Attention can then be turned to the descending colon. The bowel wall is grasped and gently pulled towards the midline. The paracolic peritoneal attachments are divided using electrocautery and the retroperitoneal structures should gradually slip away. The gonadal vessels are freed first, followed by the ureter and, proximally, the perinephric fascia. In this way the attachments near the spleen can be freed. Occasionally the colon is almost adherent, but despite this, safe mobilization can be carried out by accurate dissection. The flexure is gradually mobilized following the plane until the inferior mesenteric vein is reached. One or two small vessels may require ligation at the inferior border of the pancreas, otherwise bleeding can be troublesome. The inferior mesenteric vein is next secured and a point for anastomosis with an adequate blood supply is selected.

Left colon resection

Tumours in the descending colon can normally be treated by anterior resection with anastomosis between the transverse colon and rectosigmoid junction. In this way the mesentery and lymph nodes can be radically removed. Attempts at less extensive resection may compromise the adequacy of the cancer procedure.

When the whole of the sigmoid has been sacrificed, anastomosis can be effected with the circular stapler passed up into the rectum or as above, with interrupted appositional sutures.

Postoperative complications

Resection of the colon may be followed by any of the local and general complications which can occur after major abdominal surgery. The most important disaster which needs a special note is leakage of the anastomosis. This is most likely to occur when the blood supply to the anastomosed ends of bowel was inadequate to allow healing. If there is tension, leakage is more likely. Faecal loading may cause pressure necrosis in certain situations.

Unfortunately the diagnosis is often delayed. Leakage should be suspected where there is an unexplained pyrexia associated with a tachycardia. Increasing abdominal tenderness should alert the surgeon to the complication. Unfortunately it is often only when the patient's condition has deteriorated to the stage of frank peritonitis that the diagnosis is made.

If anastomotic leakage has occurred or is suspected, preparation should be made to reoperate. Great care should be taken to optimize the patient's general condition by adequate resuscitation with fluids and antibiotics. Following laparotomy, careful peritoneal toilet and lavage is carried out, after which no attempt should be made to repair the leak. The natural tendency is for the surgeon to try to restore intestinal continuity. Failure of healing has occurred and in the compromised situation of faecal peritonitis in a now depleted patient, healing is even less likely to occur following a revisional anastomosis. The bowel ends should be exteriorized and the situation accepted.

Intestinal obstruction due to carcinoma of the colon

Patients presenting with intestinal obstruction due to colonic carcinoma have a significantly greater inpatient mortality compared to the elective case, and even following discharge from hospital have a significantly poorer long-term prognosis.

The haemodynamic effects of intestinal obstruction can put an added burden on the heart, particularly in patients with ischaemic heart disease; this in part explains the increased morbidity and mortality. In addition, surgical complication with intraperitoneal abscess and anastomotic dehiscence are more likely to occur in the emergency situation.

In order to minimize complications, the patient should be carefully resuscitated, with adequate replacement of intravenous fluid and blood if necessary.

Oxygen can be given to reverse hypoxia. Intravenous antibiotics may be commenced once the diagnosis has been made. The plain X-ray will point to the diagnosis of small bowel obstruction due to a caecal carcinoma or large bowel obstruction due to a tumour beyond the ileocaecal valve. The diagnosis should always be confirmed, whenever possible, with a gastrograffin enema. This will avoid the embarrassment of an operation on a patient with intestinal pseudobstruction where conservative treatment may have been appropriate. Since left colon tumours are more prone to obstruct, flexible sigmoidoscopy after a phosphate enema may reveal the site of obstruction. The majority of patients will require a nasogastric tube in order to empty a distended stomach and reduce the risk of aspiration pneumonitis, particularly during anaesthetic induction.

The patient should be placed in the Lloyd-Davis position which allows access to the abdomen and anal canal.

In general, a midline incision is used. With tumours involving the caecum, transverse colon and indeed the left colon, there is a trend towards increasing use of extended right hemicolectomy and ileal colic anastomosis. It should be emphasized that this is an operation for the experienced surgeon in a fit patient. Where doubt exists regarding the advisability of excision of the primary, a defunctioning ileostomy or proximal colostomy is to be advised.

At times it is possible to excise the tumour and mobilize the bowel to allow construction of an ileostomy with an adjacent colostomy. This allows fairly simple closure as an elective procedure once the patient has recovered.

In the majority of cases the obstruction will be found to be situated in the left side of the colon or rectosigmoid region. In the past it was common simply to perform a transverse defunctioning colostomy. Increasingly now, surgeons are prepared to carry out primary resection, often with anastomosis following on-table lavage, to obtain a clean colon.

In a very unfit patient, where the diagnosis has been made using a gastrograffin enema or flexible sigmoidoscopy, a useful option is to carry out a small upper quadrant incision and perform a colostomy which, in cases of difficulty in exteriorizing a loop of transverse colon, can be a 'blowhole' stoma with interrupted mucocutaneous sutures holding the colon to the abdominal skin. This allows the patient to decompress and, following adequate resuscitation, an elective procedure can be carried out on the next convenient list. The disadvantage of a blind transverse colostomy is the risk of leaving behind a necrotic caecum in cases of very severe obstruction, or performing a stoma at an incorrect site.

Colostomy

A colostomy is an opening made into the large bowel with a view to diversion of its contents to the exterior. The common sites are transverse colon and sigmoid colon which will be described.

1. Loop colostomy

This is usually performed as a temporary vent, for example, as a first-stage decompression before proceeding to resection of an obstructing tumour or to provide a temporary 'safety valve' above an anastomosis. It has the advantages of being simple to fashion and easy to close.

2. Double-barrelled colostomy

Here the bowel is divided and each end brought out as a separate stoma through the abdominal wall. This may be part of a Paul–Mikulicz procedure or may be performed when it is essential that no faecal material passes into the distal segment of the bowel; for example, where the colostomy is performed above a perforation or a faecal fistula.

3. End colostomy

This is a permanent colostomy in which the divided end of the sigmoid is brought out as a colostomy after abdominoperineal excision of the rectum or after a Hartmann operation, in which the rectum is excised but the anal stump is left *in situ*.

Transverse colostomy

One of the problems with a transverse colostomy is the siting of the stoma underneath the ribs. This is often difficult for the patient and is awkward for the attachment of appliances. An alternative is to mobilize the hepatic flexure and bring it down to the right iliac fossa, a much more suitable site for the stoma. Mobilization is often necessary to allow the colon to be brought through the abdominal wall. A trephine incision through the rectus abdominus is less likely to be associated with an incisional hernia than one brought out through the external oblique. The rectus sheath is incised transversely and the rectus muscle split longitudinally. It is quite unnecessary to divide the muscle and indeed this may predispose to incisional herniation. If the transverse colon is grossly distended and difficult to handle, it may require decompression by means of trocar attached to a suction pump. An alternative is to use a large hypodermic needle attached to the sucker and this will frequently allow adequate decompression. A small opening is made through the mesocolon through which a length of rubber tubing is passed. An artery forceps is passed through the wound and grasps the loop of rubber tubing. Gentle traction on the loop will withdraw the colon.

Delayed colostomy opening is never indicated and the mucocutaneous junction should be matured immediately with carefully placed interrupted sutures. This has the advantage of immediately decompressing the bowel and producing a neat colostomy which is easily managed with modern appliances. Moreover, subsequent closure is easier because there is less fibrosis.

Sigmoid colostomy

Occasionally a sigmoid loop colostomy is fashioned because of perianal sepsis or to cover an operation of the anal canal. A trephine incision is made in the left iliac fossa through the rectus abdominus; often it is possible with retraction to identify the sigmoid colon and divide its lateral attachments. An alternative is to carry out a preliminary laparoscopy, to mobilize the colon to allow sufficient mobilization to facilitate exteriorization. The sigmoid can then be gently delivered through the wound. Under such circumstances it is wise to construct a functional end colostomy. A linear stapler is used to obstruct the distal lumen, but the bowel is not divided. Just proximal to the staple line the bowel is opened and sutured to the skin in standard fashion.

Closure of colostomy

Formal closure of a colostomy is carried out once the distal anastomosis is soundly healed, and this should be confirmed with a gastrograffin enema. Although there are some advocates of early closure, it is wise to wait 4–6 weeks following major surgery as this makes closure much easier.

An incision is made around the colostomy and carried down to the wall of the colon. A relatively avascular plane is entered and the colon is freed from its attachments to the anterior abdominal wall. It is important to free completely the colon into the peritoneal cavity so that following closure it can be returned to the abdomen without fear of kinking with subsequent obstruction. The cutaneous edges are excised and trimmed away with scissors and the stoma wound sutured transversely using interrupted appositional extramucosal fine sutures. The author's preference is to use 4/0 polydioxanone. The closed loop of colon is returned to the abdominal cavity and the wound closed. The wound is often small with little tension, and an absorbable suture such as number 1 Vicryl can be used. Drainage is unnecessary, but the skin wound should be closed loosely with two or three interrupted sutures. An alternative is to use a subcuticular purse-string suture which leaves a small central aperture for drainage of serous exudate. This often looks unsightly at completion but heals with remarkably little scarring.

Total colectomy

The most common indications for total colectomy are ulcerative colitis, usually in the emergency situation, elective resection for Crohn's disease, where it is usually combined with an ileorectal anastomosis, and in selected cases for familial adenomatous polyposis with relative rectal sparing by rectal polyps. In ulcerative colitis, operation is required for two main indications. The first is in the emergency situation, in the patient with fulminating colitis complicated by toxic dilatation or haemorrhage. Under these circumstances the colon is removed and an end ileostomy is constructed. Care should be taken to preserve the ileocolic artery in its entirety and the ileum should be transected at the ileocaecal junction. This preserves adequate vascularity for subsequent reconstruction and restorative proctocolectomy with an ileal reservoir. In most instances, the procedure of choice is to bring out the distal colon through a small stab incision in the left iliac fossa or through the lower end of the midline wound. Occasionally in severe haemorrhage it may be necessary to resect most of the rectum as well, but the anal canal and a small amount of distal rectum should always be preserved for subsequent reconstruction. In the second group of indications, the operation is normally elective in ulcerative colitis that has failed to be controlled medically or the patient requests surgery because of unacceptable chronic symptoms. Nowadays, ileorectal anastomosis is rarely advised with the new advances in restorative procedures.

Volvulus

Volvulus of the colon most commonly affects the sigmoid followed by the caecum. Volvulus of the transverse colon and of the splenic flexure rarely occur. Overall this is a relatively uncommon emergency in the developed world, being more common in rural parts of Africa where large amounts of fibre are ingested.

The twisting of the bowel occurs around a very long mesentery with a somewhat narrower base. This results in a closed loop obstruction which may present acutely or as a recurring phenomenon. In many cases of sigmoid volvulus it is possible to decompress the bowel with a rigid sigmoidoscope. Volvulus not infrequently occurs in patients treated with chronic psychotropic therapy and in the first instance a conservative course may be pursued. If decompression is not possible, then laparotomy and sigmoid resection is to be advised. It is normally possible to restore intestinal continuity with a colorectal anastomosis following resection.

Volvulus of the caecum

Here the caecum and terminal ileum are involved in the twisted sigmoid and the patient presents with features of large bowel obstruction. The abdomen, as in sigmoid volvulus, is grossly distended. Plain radiographs show distension of the caecum which is located in the left upper quadrant of the abdomen and may be mistaken for a dilated stomach.

Treatment comprises urgent operative intervention after resuscitation. Resection with a right hemicolec-tomy is the treatment of choice in a patient whose condition is good, but in an ill patient exteriorization or simple fixation of the bowel is to be advised.

18

The rectum and anal canal

D. C. C. Bartolo

Surgical anatomy and physiology

Relations and structure

The rectosigmoid junction lies approximately at the level of the third sacral vertebra and is a bend of variable acuteness. The rectum, usually 12 cm in length, first follows the curve of the sacrum downwards and backwards and then downwards and forwards to become the anal canal as it passes through the puborectalis part of the levator ani muscle. At this point the bowel turns through a right angle so that the anal canal, approximately 3.5 cm in length, passes downwards and backwards to the anal orifice.

Each end of the rectum is in the midline, but the ampulla between deviates to either side. This results in folds formed by the circular muscle layer and the mucosa which are best seen at sigmoidoscopy, usually two on the left with one on the right between – the rectal valves of Houston.

The upper part of the rectum has a covering of peritoneum that is complete except for a narrow strip posteriorly. As the rectum descends, the peritoneal covering becomes reduced so that the middle part has only an anterior covering and the lower third no peritoneal covering. At the junction of the middle and lower thirds the peritoneum sweeps forwards onto the bladder in the male and onto the upper end of the vagina and uterus in the female.

On each side of the rectum below the peritoneal reflection there is a collection of fibro-fatty tissue containing the middle rectal blood vessels, the so-called lateral ligaments which tether the rectum to the side walls of the pelvis. Anteriorly, the extraperitoneal part of the rectum in the male is related from above downwards to the bladder and ureters, the seminal vesicles and prostate, and in the female to the posterior vaginal wall. This is covered with a fascial layer, the fascia of Denonvilliers, which runs from the peritoneal reflection above to the urogenital muscular diaphragm below. Posteriorly the rectum is very loosely attached to the front of the sacrum and coccyx which are covered by a thick fascial layer, the fascia of Waldeyer. Between the fascia of Waldeyer and the sacrum lie the middle sacral blood vessels. Inferiorly this fascia sweeps forwards to join the fascia of the rectum at the anorectal junction. The longitudinal and circular muscle layers of the rectum are complete. The mucosal lining is a glandular columnar epithelium.

The anal canal is related to the coccyx posteriorly, to the ischiorectal fossa on each side and, anteriorly, in the male to the membranous urethra within the urogenital diaphragm and to the bulb of the urethra, and in the female to the lower part of the vagina.

The anal canal musculature (Figure 18.1) is extremely important, for inappropriate surgery in this area may lead to incontinence. The external sphincter

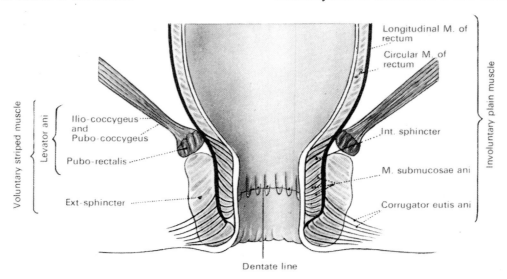

Figure 18.1 Coronal section through lower rectum and anal canal to show the anatomical features of surgical importance

consists of a cylinder of voluntary striped muscle which is continuous above with the puborectalis part of the levator ani muscle, the whole levator ani muscle and external sphincter forming an inverted cone in which the lower rectum and anal canal lie. The internal sphincter is a downward extension of the involuntary smooth circular muscle of the rectum. The longitudinal muscle layer of the rectum descends as a cylinder, but splits to send fibres through the internal and external sphincters to the skin of the lower anal canal (musculus submucosae ani) and to the peri-anal skin (currugator cutis ani). Some believe that the puborectalis is the most important part of the levator ani muscle complex, which forms a sling around the anorectal junction. Some consider that division of the muscle would inevitably lead to incontinence, whereas the remainder of the external sphincter and internal sphincter can be divided with relative impunity with only minor impairment and incontinence. If the external sphincter is preserved, that part of the puborectalis may be divided, but if the whole of the external sphincter is divided there is likely to be significant impairment of continence, although crude control may be preserved. The puborectalis muscle together with the internal sphincter at this level is known as the anorectal ring.

The upper half of the anal canal is lined to a varied extent with modified columnar epithelium, while the lower half is lined by non-hair-bearing squamous epithelium. Where the two linings meet there is the ring of anal valves, the pectinate or dentate line (Figure 19.1). Above each valve is a pocket known as an anal sinus or anal crypt of Morgagni, into which the duct of an anal gland opens. These glands, up to eight in number, lie in the submucosal layer or in the intersphincteric plane. If they become infected an abscess may result which may ultimately form a fistula-in-ano. They may rarely undergo malignant change, the resulting tumour being an adenocarcinoma.

Blood supply

The rectum is supplied by the inferior mesenteric artery which, having supplied the sigmoid colon, becomes the superior rectal or superior haemorrhoidal artery as it crosses the left common iliac artery to enter the true pelvis. At this point it is closely related to the left ureter and to the left testicular or ovarian vessels. It divides at a variable level into right and left branches which may subdivide further as they descend towards the anorectal junction. There is a good marginal communication between the last sigmoid artery and the superior haemorrhoidal artery (Griffiths, 1956). The middle rectal artery, which is variable in size and which may be absent or double, is a branch of the internal iliac artery and reaches the rectum through the lateral ligament on each side. The inferior rectal artery is a branch of the internal pudendal branch of the internal iliac artery and reaches the anal canal by traversing the ischiorectal fossa on each side. All three arteries and their branches supply all layers of the rectum and anal canal, the contribution to each being very variable (Thomson, 1975). The inferior rectal arteries are always capable of *adequately* supplying a rectal stump to a point well above the peritoneal reflection, even after division of the middle rectal arteries. The median sacral artery arises from the back of bifurcation of the aorta. It runs down between Waldeyer's fascia and the sacrum and coccyx and is encountered in mobilization of the very distal rectum. It supplies a few tiny branches to the back of the rectum.

The venous drainage closely follows the arterial supply. The superior or internal haemorrhoidal venous plexus lying in the submucosal layer of the upper anal canal contributes to three vascular pads or cushions usually found in the left lateral, right posterior and right anterior positions. From it veins drain upwards, piercing the layers of the rectal wall to form two main trunks and then a single superior haemorrhoidal or superior rectal vein (part of the portal venous system) which becomes the inferior mesenteric vein as it lies to the left side of the inferior mesenteric artery and which continues upwards to join the splenic vein. The middle rectal vein (part of the systemic venous system) is insignificant. The inferior or external haemorrhoidal venous plexus lying in the subcutaneous layers of the lower anal canal and perianal skin drains to inferior haemorrhoidal or inferior rectal veins (also part of the systemic venous system) on each side and thence to the internal iliac veins. The superior and inferior haemorrhoidal plexuses communicate to a variable degree in the subcutaneous and submucosal layers of the anal canal as well through the sphincter muscles (Thomson, 1975).

Lymph drainage

Lymph plexuses in the submucosa drain lymph to extramural vessels and nodes and accompanying the haemorrhoidal blood vessels, upwards to the pre-aortic nodes. The lymphatics accompany the superior haemorrhoidal and inferior mesenteric arteries and laterally along vessels accompanying the middle and inferior haemorrhoidal blood vessels to internal iliac lymph nodes on the side walls of the pelvis and thence to para-aortic nodes. In practice, the downward spread of rectal carcinoma is very rare beyond the mesorectum, and metastases to superficial inguinal lymph nodes via the external pudendal lymph vessels only occur if anal or perianal skin is involved. Malignant conditions of the anal canal may, of course, metastasize along any of the routes described, depending on the exact position of the neoplasm in the canal.

Nerve supply

The left side of the colon, the rectum and the anal

canal receive a sympathetic nerve supply from the sympathetic chain via the lumbar splanchnic nerves and via the thoracic splanchnic nerves by way of the plexus around the coeliac axis. These fibres converge on the pre-aortic plexus around the origin of the inferior mesenteric artery. They accompany the inferior mesenteric artery and its branches and form the presacral or hypogastric nerve which descends into the pelvis and divides to send a plexus of nerves to each side wall of the pelvis. From here, fibres pass to all the pelvic organs including the rectum and anal canal. A parasympathetic nerve supply comes from the sacral nerves via the pelvic splanchnic nerves (nervi erigentes). The fibres join the sympathetic pelvic plexus to supply the pelvic organs including the rectum and anal canal and passing up the presacral nerve are distributed to the left colon with the sympathetic fibres. Large bowel peristalsis can continue normally in the absence of an extrinsic autonomic nerve supply, but the presence of normal intramural plexuses is essential. In Hirschsprung's disease, where ganglion cells are absent from a segment of distal large bowel, peristaltic waves fail to pass and functional obstruction ensues.

It should be possible to preserve the presacral sympathetic nerves in the majority of patients with cancer of the rectum and rectosigmoid region. Careful anatomical dissection should identify this nerve which lies behind a loose areolar plane. If the presacral sympathetic nerves are divided, urinary dysfunction may develop in some situations. In the male, normal erection and orgasm will persist but ejaculation fails. The sympathetic fibres in this region were long held to be stimulatory to the internal sphincter. Recently, Loubowski et al. (1987) stimulated the presacral nerve intraoperatively and found that resting anal canal pressures fell. These observations question the previous mechanisms of the neural control of the internal sphincter. Experiments on isolated human internal sphincter muscle strips have shown that noradrenaline causes contraction, adrenaline has a variable effect and isoprenaline induces relaxation (Burleigh et al., 1979). Relaxation of the internal anal sphincter induced by sympathetic nervous activity is probably due to stimulation of beta-adrenoreceptors, since alpha-adrenoreceptor antagonists convert contraction of muscle strips into relaxation. In human volunteers, beta-adrenergic relaxation of the internal sphincter was confirmed by infusion experiments with isoprenaline, an effect which could be blocked by propananol (Gutierrez and Shah, 1975). At rest the internal anal sphincter is in a state of tonic partial contraction. Inhibition is mediated by rectal distension. This reflex is lost following rectal excision and colo-anal or ileo-anal anastomoses, and is believed to be an intramural reflex dependent on the enteric rather than the autonomic nerves. In support of this thesis, Loubowsky et al. (1987) found that when the presacral sympathetics were blocked with 0.5% bupivacaine, the recto-anal inhibitor reflex persisted. It

was maintained following complete rectal dissection down to the anal canal, but was abolished by circumferential myotomy prior to rectal excision.

The parasympathetic nerves (nervi erigentes) emerge from the sacral foraminae S2, S3 and S4. From here they travel around the side walls of the pelvis and may be seen in the extreme lateral aspects below the lateral ligaments. They then pass forward below and lateral to the seminal vesicles and are distributed to the bladder, urethra and anorectal region. It is in the anterolateral region that they are most at risk during rectal dissection. Division of these nerves inevitably results in impotence and is likely to be associated with considerable bladder dysfunction. If rectal dissection is maintained beneath Denonvilliers' fascia on the rectal aspect, as appropriate in inflammatory bowel disease, then these nerves should not be at risk.

The voluntary muscle of the external sphincter and the caudal aspects of the levator ani muscles are supplied by the inferior haemorrhoidal branch of the internal pudendal nerve and by the perineal branch of the fourth sacral nerve on each side. The levators are supplied from above by a direct branch from S3 and S4.

Sensation in the lower anal canal and perianal skin is conveyed by afferent fibres in the inferior haemorrhoidal nerve and this can be abolished by a nerve block in the ischiorectal fossa or in the caudal canal. The much less acute sensation which accompanies injection of internal haemorrhoids, in the upper anal canal for example, is probably conveyed by autonomic fibres.

Continence and defaecation

The reflexes controlling continence and defaecation are complex. From the practical point of view, patients who undergo sphincter-saving resections of the lower large bowel retain anal continence. This may be due to the fact that the autonomic pelvic plexus remains largely undisturbed, as do the somatic nerves mediating sensation from the lower anal canal and supplying the voluntary levator ani and external sphincter muscles. Following low rectal excision, resting anal canal pressure falls, but voluntary contraction is maintained. It is likely that this fall in resting pressure is due to division of the enteric nerves which exert a stimulatory influence on the internal sphincter. Voluntary contraction should not be altered following even total rectal excision with sphincter preservation. Anal sensation contributes to the maintenance of continence. The extent to which this remains intact, depends on how much anal mucosa is stripped during anastomosis to the anal canal. Rectal sensation and compliance are important in maintaining continence. Sensation in a neorectum is different, and undoubtedly diminished, although most patients retain a degree of rectal sensation. Patients in whom an ileal reservoir is attached to the upper anal canal retain a degree of rectal sensation which suggests that this is generated to some degree by pressure on surrounding pelvic structures rather than by rectal distension alone (Lane and Parks, 1977). Stretch receptors in the neorectum almost certainly contribute to the awareness of filling by gas and stool.

Defaecation is initiated by a sensation of rectal distension. Rectal emptying is of course under strong cortical control. When rectal peristalsis occurs, relaxation of voluntary anal control allows defaecation to occur. Even in the absence of all rectal sensation, however, the reflex can be initiated by voluntary straining of abdominal musculature, and patients who have had low rectal excisions can usually achieve satisfactory evacuation.

A major problem following rectal excision is the loss of the reservoir capacity. The rectum itself is normally compliant and allows defaecation to be deferred without urgency unless the continence mechanism is severely stressed by overwhelming diarrhoea. If the rectum is replaced by a narrow tube of sigmoid or ileum, high-pressure waves will be generated in the neorectum which will be associated with urgency and may indeed provoke urge incontinence.

Investigations

Investigation of the lower large bowel and anal canal starts with clinical examination of the patient. General examination with reference to the alimentary tract is carried out, abdominal examination being particularly important. The patient is then turned onto the left side with the knees drawn up and the pelvis may be elevated on a pillow. After inspection of the perineum, digital rectal examination is performed. It is important to assess whether there is any mechanical contraindication to the instrumentation which is to follow, for example spasm of the anal sphincters due to a fissure. The perineum should be examined at rest and with the subject straining down as during defaecation. Abnormal perineal descent can be noted and indeed rectal prolapse may be observed in some patients with incontinence. During digital examination, an assessment of tone and contractility of the sphincters can be made. Similarly the subject should be asked to strain, which will give an assessment of rectal mobility which may be associated with varying degrees of prolapse.

Sigmoidoscopy

The apparatus shown in Figure 18.2 may be used. Increasingly, with the worries with human immunodeficiency virus, there are calls to use disposable sigmoidoscopes which are easy and convenient to use. This investigation should form part of any examination of the alimentary tract, but it is mandatory in the presence of colorectal and anal symptoms. Bowel preparation is usually not required, but faecal loading of the lower bowel calls for an enema. Anaesthesia is not usually required, but application of a local anaesthetic preparation such as 2% xylocaine (lignocaine) gel to a tender fissure may be necessary to allow passage of the instrument. General anaesthesia may be required in children or where spasm or acute angulation in the upper reaches of the rectum cannot be negotiated. Fibreoptic endoscopy normally overcomes these problems and obviates the need for general anaesthesia.

The left lateral position is satisfactory, but the prone jack-knife position with the patient on a proctoscopy couch permits a more satisfactory examination. After digital examination the 25 cm sigmoidoscope, with its obturator in place, is lubricated and passed. Once through the anorectal junction (5 cm) the obturator is removed and a light fitting attached. The window with its bellows is attached and the instrument passed under vision with as little air insufflation as possible. Patients should be warned that lower abdominal wind pain may occur, that they may feel a desire to defaecate, and that they may pass wind. The instrument is passed upwards and backwards to the rectosigmoid junction and then downwards and forwards into the sigmoid colon. Swabbing with flat damp cottonwool swabs is carried out when necessary.

If required, a mucosal biopsy is taken with biopsy forceps as shown in Figure 18.2(b), but a heavier pair of forceps as shown in Figure 18.2(c) can be used for biopsy for a neoplasm. A biopsy is taken under direct vision, having removed the window only. Bleeding is usually not severe and can be controlled by pressure with a swab. As the instrument is withdrawn, the patient should be reassured that defaecation is not occurring.

A mucosal biopsy should be gently spread onto a piece of blotting paper prior to placing in fixative (10% buffered formaldehyde solution is suitable), while a biopsy specimen from a neoplasm can be dropped directly onto the fixative.

Proctoscopy

The apparatus required is shown in Figure 18.3. Proctoscopy is conveniently carried out after sigmoidoscopy with the patient in the same position. Many different shapes and sizes of proctoscope have been designed and a narrower instrument than the one illustrated may be needed in the presence of anal pathology or for a child.

The proctoscope with obturator and light fitting in place is lubricated and passed, initially upwards and forward and then upwards and backwards into the lower rectum. The obturator is removed. If desired, an external light source can be used beside the surgeon's right shoulder. Usually little of the rectum can be seen, except for an area of the lower anterior wall.

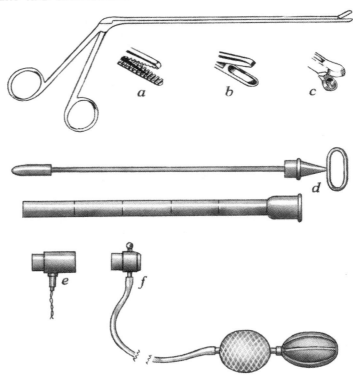

Figure 18.2 Apparatus for sigmoidoscopy. *a*, Chevalier Jackson grasping forceps with alligator jaws for swabbing. *b*, Paterson's forceps for mucosal biopsy. *c*, Officer's forceps for tumour biopsy. *d*, A 25 cm Lloyd-Davies sigmoidoscope with obturator (1.5 cm diameter); 15 cm, 20 cm and 30 cm versions of wider diameter are available but are usually reserved for use under general anaesthesia. *e*, Light fitting. *f*, Window with bellows. The second bulb is designed to maintain a constant flow of air during insufflation

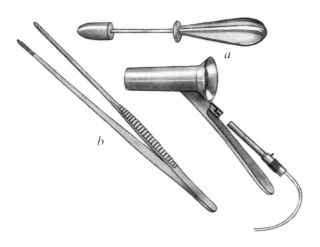

Figure 18.3 Apparatus for proctoscopy. *a*, St. Mark's pattern proctoscope with obturator and light fitting (2.0 cm diameter). *b*, Forceps for swabbing

As the instrument is withdrawn the anorectal ring closes behind the end of the proctoscope and the presence or absence of internal haemorrhoids in the upper anal canal can be assessed. This is aided by asking the patient to strain down, while providing assurance that defaecation is not occurring. The lower anal canal is then examined as the instrument is withdrawn completely.

Barium enema

A barium enema complements sigmoidoscopy. Small lesions may have been missed on sigmoidoscopy if the preparation was not optimal. It is important to use both techniques. The width of the rectorectal space can be measured in inflammatory bowel disease, where it may be abnormally large. Gross dilatation of the bowel such as occurs in Hirschsprung's disease may be seen. It cannot be overemphasized, however, that any single examination of the rectum may miss a lesion and the rectal films of a barium enema study should always be examined with great care. Even when a rectal tumour has been found, it is important either to proceed to barium enema or colonoscopy, as the patient may harbour a second cancer or additional polyps in the proximal colon.

Colonoscopy

The great advantage of colonoscopy or flexible sigmoidoscopy is that the patient will normally have been fully prepared, allowing a thorough inspection of the rectum and proximal colon to the caecum.

Lesions are not always single and metachronous tumours can be identified in the proximal bowel. Modern instruments allow excellent assessment of the rectum since they can be rectoflexed to examine the posterior rectum just beyond the anal canal. With a rigid viewing scope and with the patient in the left lateral position, it is possible to miss a small lesion in the lower posterior rectum.

Computed tomography (CT) and magnetic resonance (MR)

Scanning by CT and MR can delineate rectal tumours and clearly show direct extension of tumour into adjacent structures such as the sacrum or prostate. Such scanning adds little over and above clinical assessment, but may be useful in accurately staging the patient with advanced disease when preoperative radiotherapy is being considered. It may, however, be extremely helpful in detecting pelvic recurrence of tumour in a patient who has, for example, undergone excision of the rectum.

Rectal ultrasound

Intraluminal ultrasound probes can be inserted into the rectum. These provide excellent imaging of tumours and may accurately delineate involved pararectal lymph nodes in patients with rectal carcinoma. In experienced hands this investigation is considered to be superior to CT and MR.

Sphincter studies

The anal sphincters and their reflexes can be studied in several ways. Taken together these tests are particularly useful in evaluating cases of incontinence due either to a neurological lesion or as a result of neuromuscular injury, particularly following surgery or obstetric trauma.

The normal resting tone of the internal sphincter is measured by withdrawing a pressure-sensitive probe through the anal canal. The pressure exerted on the probe is measured together with the additional pressure which the voluntary external sphincter can exert during contraction. Rectal sensation and distensibility may be measured by means of a balloon, which is infused with air or water at a constant rate. The level of first awareness, the volume to initiate urgency, and maximum tolerance, are measured. With a balloon in the rectum and a recording probe in the anal canal, relaxation of anal tone occurs as rectal pressure rises, the recto-anal inhibitory reflex. This reflex is absent in Hirschsprung's disease. Electromyographic measurements of resting, contracting and straining action potentials in the puborectalis muscle and in the external sphincter muscles can be made with a needle electrode. These are less frequently used than manometry. The pudendal nerve terminal motor latency, an index of nerve function, can be measured using a specialized electrode. This bears a stimulating electrode which is placed on the gloved index finger and a recording electrode which lies over the proximal phalanx. The pudendal nerve at the ischial spines is then stimulated, and recordings of the electrical responses are made. The latency of this reflex is prolonged following damage to the pudendal nerve such as may occur following parturition. Electromyographic mapping of the sphincter muscles following direct damage can indicate the size and position of the gap between the divided ends of muscle, thus aiding their direct suture. In practice this is an extremely painful unpleasant investigation and has largely been superseded by endoluminal ultrasound scanning which provides excellent imaging of the sphincter complex.

In many cases, however, a good history and a careful digital examination will usually provide as much information as is necessary about the state of the sphincters to decide what local surgery may or may not be required. When doubt exists about function, or following obstetric or surgical injury, it is important to investigate patients fully, since this provides an objective assessment. This is particularly important when contemplating surgery on women of child-bearing age where operations which may weaken the sphincter may compromise continence where there has been a history of obstetric trauma.

Surgery of the rectum

Carcinoma of the rectum

The two procedures most commonly adopted for treatment of carcinoma of the rectum are excision of the rectum and anterior resection (Naunton Morgan, 1965), and several factors influence the decision as to which is used.

The most important factor is the distance of the lower edge of the tumour from the anal margin. Only a rough assessment of this can be made preoperatively by sigmoidoscopic measurement. Until relatively recently, it was considered that 5 cm of distal rectum beyond the tumour was required (Grinnell, 1954). In many cases, however, a shorter cuff will obviously suffice and it has become common practice to accept less than a 5 cm clearance. Restorative rectal surgery for very low tumours can be associated with very low recurrence rates following radical curative resections with margins of less than 2.5 cm if appropriate. The incidence of abdominoperineal resection has been steadily declining during the past 10 years.

Restorative rectal surgery can be extremely testing, especially in thickset males where the proximal dissection of the bowel is difficult because of the patient's size and the pelvis is often small. The dissection must avoid injury to the autonomic nerves and yet offer a prospect of cure with a minimal incidence of local recurrence.

The introduction of the circular stapler and peranal technique of colo-anal anastomosis (anastomosis of the colon to the anal canal just above the dentate line) has helped reduce the proportion of cases where restorative surgery cannot be undertaken. Frequently a decision cannot be made until the abdomen is opened and the bowel has been fully mobilized. Often the distal rectum can be mobilized, rendering what may appear to be a low tumour easily amenable to restorative resection. Surgery in the male is invariably considerably more difficult than in the female whose wide pelvis normally facilitates dissection.

A preoperative biopsy should always be obtained before removing a rectal tumour, since benign conditions can mimic malignancy; for example the solitary rectal ulcer syndrome. If the biopsy reveals a poorly or undifferentiated tumour, consideration may be given to offering preoperative radiotherapy to minimize the risk of local recurrence. The biopsy provides poor information for staging in terms of differentiation and grading, since the characteristics may vary within the tumour.

Other procedures such as abdominoperineal pull-through resection, transphincteric resection and per-anal resection are occasionally appropriate and will be described below.

However remote the possibility of a colostomy, the patient should be forewarned preoperatively and should be visited by a stomatherapist and by a patient with a colostomy. The site of the colostomy must be assessed and marked with the patient standing and sitting so that it is sited away from skin creases, the umbilicus, the anterior superior iliac spine and the incision. It must be at a level where it can be seen to allow the patient to change the appliance.

Mechanical bowel preparation is important, and several methods have been used. Currently the most popular use Picolax (Nordic) or ethylene glycol. The advantage of ethylene glycol is that preparation can be given rapidly. Between 4.5 and 5 litres of ethylene glycol solution are swallowed over a period of 1–4 h. This induces rapid effective bowel cleansing which can minimize the time in hospital preoperatively and reduces electrolyte disturbance. Frail, elderly patients should not go to surgery dehydrated and depleted of electrolytes from over-enthusiastic purgation. Rectal washouts and enemas are rarely required.

Antibiotic cover is normally started with the premedication or at induction and is continued for 48 to 72 h postoperatively. A broad-spectrum antibiotic such as a cephalosporin is suitable to cover the majority of large bowel operations, together with metronidazole to cover anaerobic bacteria including *Bacteroides* species specifically (Keighley, 1983).

Heparin prophylaxis and compression stockings are strongly recommended to reduce the incidence of thromboembolism.

1. Excision of the rectum

Abdominoperineal excision of the rectum can be

performed by one surgeon, the patient being turned between the two stages (Miles, 1908), but is usually done by surgeons at the abdominal incision and at the perineum working together (Lloyd-Davies, 1939) : synchronous combined abdominoperineal excision of the rectum.

Under general anaesthetic and with an intravenous infusion running, the patient is catheterized and placed in the lithotomy–Trendelenburg or St. Mark's position on the operating table (Figure 18.4). The scrotum is strapped to the right thigh and the anus closed with a purse-string suture.

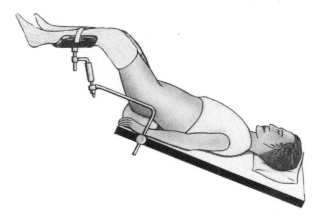

Figure 18.4 The lithotomy–Trendelenburg or St. Mark's position on the operating table for excision of the rectum and anterior resection

Through a midline or transverse incision a careful laparotomy is carried out to assess the degree of spread of the neoplasm locally and distally, the liver being the most important organ to examine. In the presence of disseminated disease, unless very extensive, it is generally agreed that removal of the primary neoplasm is desirable even if excision of the rectum is required. This will avoid the problem of obstruction at a later date and obviate the pain which local spread or a pelvic neoplasm can cause. A final decision as to whether anterior resection may be possible may have to wait until the rectum is fully mobilized.

A self-retaining retractor is inserted. The small bowel loops are placed in a bag outside the abdomen or held back by packs and retractors. The sigmoid colon is held to the right and the white line marking the junction of the visceral and parietal peritoneum incised. With sharp dissection using either electrocautery or scissors the spermatic or ovarian vessels and the left ureter are identified and separated from the vascular pedicle of the bowel. The peritoneum on the right side of the sigmoid mesentery is then incised and the vascular pedicle isolated. The inferior mesenteric artery is divided close to the aorta – the 'high tie' as shown in Figure 18.5(a). The inferior mesenteric vein lying to the left of the artery is divided at the same level. The left colic and sigmoid vessels are divided as shown in Figure 18.5. In the very old and the very fat it is prudent to divide the inferior mesenteric artery distal to the origin of the left colic artery, as shown in Figure 18.5(b). A good blood supply to the colostomy is ensured and the dissection is less difficult. The distance between a and b is approximately 2 cm, so that little in the way of lymphatic drainage is sacrificed.

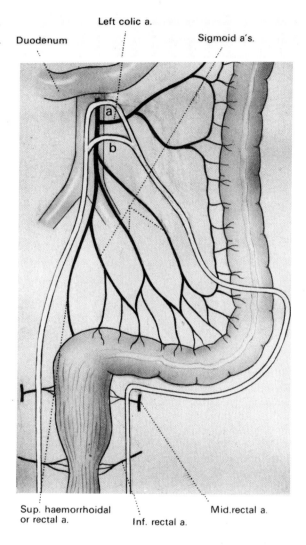

Figure 18.5 The blood supply of the lower large bowel. The white line shows the area to be resected. *a*, Ligation of the inferior mesenteric artery flush with the aorta, the 'high tie'. *b*, Ligation of the inferior mesenteric artery sparing its left colic branch

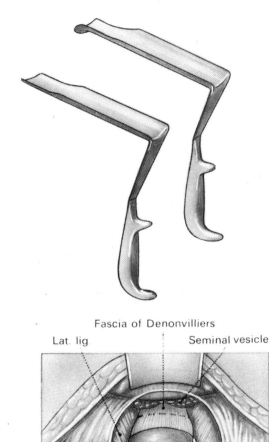

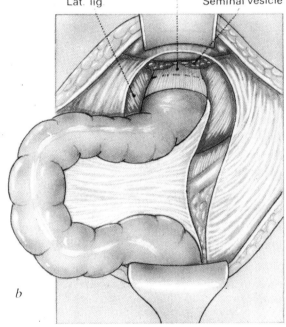

Figure 18.6 *a*, St. Mark's pattern deep pelvic retractors. *b*, Exposure of the fascia of Denonvilliers

With the pedicle divided, mobilization of the rectum can safely be undertaken. The peritoneum is incised on each side and anteriorly in front of the deepest part of the peritoneal pouch. The rectum is then lifted forwards and the almost completely avascular presacral plane opened up. The presacral nerve can usually be spared by careful dissection. Rectal dissection is facilitated by the use of electrocautery with the spray facility. This allows bloodless dissection through the loose areolar tissue that sur-

rounds the rectum, and the nerves can be carefully identified and preserved. As the posterior dissection proceeds distally, the rectum angulates anteriorly along the hollow of the sacrum. This forward dissection greatly elongates the rectum and allows it to be delivered into the abdomen. During lateral dissection of the rectum it is important to avoid 'coning' where a lateral dissection becomes progressively more medial, thus risking local recurrence. There is a clear anatom-

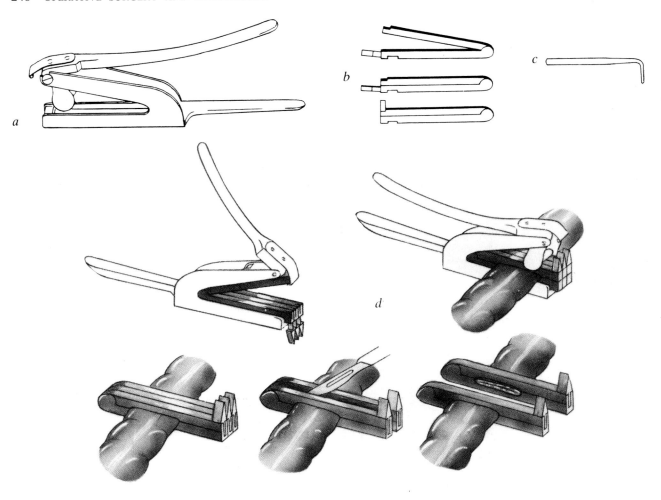

Figure 18.7 The Zachary Cope intestinal clamp. *a*, The clamp. *b*, Three hinged segments. *c*, Tommy bar for closing and opening segments. *d*, Clamp in use

ical plane which follows the side walls of the pelvis which should be followed. If the rectum is progressively displaced forwards it is relatively easy to identify the side walls of the pelvis and cut along these. The lateral ligaments are a condensation of fascia along the side walls and these do not bleed. The middle rectal vessels are below and can frequently be coagulated using electrocautery, but occasionally require ligation. Placing clamps across the lateral ligaments, particularly if sufficient tissue is maintained for a tie, will tend to make the dissection too medial and risk recurrence. The abdominal and perineal surgeons meet behind the rectum following complete mobilization. Returning to the front of the rectum, the bladder base and seminal vesicles or vaginal walls are exposed beneath the transverse peritoneal incision using a straight-lipped St. Mark's pattern retractor (Figure 18.6a). The fascia of Denonvilliers is exposed and incised, opening up the plane which passes down behind the prostate to its apex. The abdominal and perineal surgeons meet at this point.

The sigmoid mesentery is now divided, taking care to preserve the blood supply from the left colic branches and the marginal artery. The bowel is divided between crushing clamps at a point that will allow the colostomy to be formed without tension – the point at which the gently stretched sigmoid colon reaches the symphysis pubis is usually correct. A Zachary Cope clamp with three hinged segments is ideal for this step (Figure 18.7). In due course the rectum is withdrawn by the perineal surgeon.

The colostomy site is prepared. When excision of the rectum is inevitable, this step can be undertaken prior to opening the abdomen, as this ensures that the incisions in the layers of the abdominal wall are in line when the abdomen is closed. At the previously marked site a circle of skin 2 cm in diameter is removed and a trephine through the whole abdominal wall is made. It is important that the colostomy passes through the rectus muscle, as this minimizes the likelihood of paracolostomy hernia.

The perineal operator applies towels, as shown in

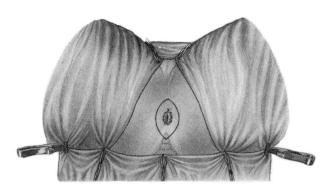

Figure 18.8 The perineal incision after closure of the anus with a purse-string suture

Figure 18.8, and a purse-string suture of stout silk is inserted around the anal canal to prevent liquid contained in the rectum contaminating the operative field. The rectum can be irrigated prior to insertion of the purse-string with a dilute solution of povidone-iodine. If the rectum is inadvertently opened, the risk of local recurrence may be reduced. An elliptical incision is made from a point midway between the bulb of the urethra and the anus anteriorly to the point of the coccyx posteriorly. Two pairs of Lane's forceps are applied to the perianal ellipse of skin. The fat in the ischiorectal fossa on each side is divided. These incisions are united posteriorly over the tip of the coccyx. A St. Mark's perineal retractor is inserted (Figure 18.9a). The fibrous attachments of the coccygeus muscles to the tip of the coccyx are divided to expose Waldeyer's fascia. The iliococcygeus muscle is now divided in a forward and lateral direction on each side, the inferior haemorrhoidal vessels being divided with diathermy or ligation. Waldeyer's fascia is incised with a scalpel, exposing the presacral space behind the mesorectum. If desired, the same plane can

be reached by excising the distal part of the coccyx, dividing the coccygeus muscles as already described and incising Waldeyer's fascia. This step may give better clearance of low rectal growths, but predisposes to coccygeal pain in the postoperative period. The abdominal and perineal surgeons meet. Anteriorly the subcutaneous fat is divided to expose the superficial transverse perineal muscles and then the deep transverse perineal muscles. The decussating fibres of the external sphincter are divided behind these pairs of muscles and the plane deepened. At each side the pubococcygeus muscle is now divided, followed by the continuation of Waldeyer's and Denonvilliers' fascia. A finger is passed behind the puborectalis muscle on each side to define the plane between the prostate and the rectum. At this point the midline anterior attachment of the rectum to the apex of the prostate and to the membranous urethra by the recto-urethralis muscle can be gently divided. The abdominal and perineal surgeons meet again in the midline and the puborectalis muscle is divided on each side (Figure 18.9b). The lower part of each lateral ligament is now divided and the rectum removed. In the female a strip of vaginal wall may be removed with the rectum, contact with the abdominal surgeon being made at the posterior fornix.

Abdominal and perineal operators collaborate to achieve complete haemostasis. The table should be levelled and a check made that the patient's blood pressure is near normal, so that troublesome reactionary haemorrhage can be avoided. The perineal wound is temporarily closed with tissue-holding forceps and the pelvic cavity filled with a cancericidal agent such as dilute povidone-iodine or distilled water for 4 min.

If haemostasis is complete, the abdominal surgeon can commence closure. It is usually unnecessary to close either the lateral space or the pelvic peritoneum. The abdominal wall is closed. A midline incision is

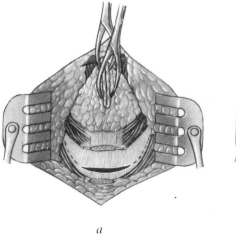

a

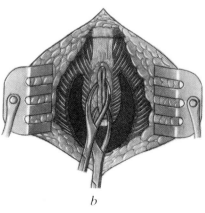

b

Figure 18.9 *a*, Incision of Waldeyer's fascia. In this case the tip of the coccyx has been divided. *b*, Division of the levator ani muscle. The iliococcygeus on each side has been divided leaving the recto-urethralis muscle and then the puborectalis fibres on each side still to be divided

usually approximated with stout continuous prolene or absorbable polydioxanone in a single layer. With a transverse incision, a two-layer technique is easier as the rectus muscle separates the anterior and posterior layers.

The colostomy is fashioned by removing the clamp from the colon, excising the crushed bowel and suturing all layers of the bowel wall to the subcuticular skin with a series of fine absorbable sutures on a tapercut needle. An adhesive colostomy bag is applied.

If pelvic haemostasis is complete, the perineal wound can be closed completely in the male with a suction drain through a separate stab incision. Suction is started immediately and continues for approximately 48 h. The levators are not sutured, but the ischiorectal fat can often be approximated with interrupted Vicryl sutures, diminishing the size of the cavity. In the female, the edges of the vaginal muscle are oversewn to control troublesome oozing and attempts to reconstitute the vagina are not required. If haemorrhage in the pelvis cannot be controlled the cavity is packed with dry gauze which is removed under anaesthetic after 72 h. If the pelvic peritoneal floor cannot be closed a plastic bag filled with gauze is placed in the pelvic cavity and this can safely be removed after 4 days without risk of bowel prolapse.

Postoperative retention of urine may require re-insertion of the catheter on one or more occasions and sometimes prostatic resection is required. Breakdown of the perineal wound requires twice-daily irrigation and dressing with an antiseptic solution until healing by secondary intention occurs. The viability of the colostomy must be checked and if the colostomy does not act spontaneously after 5 days a suppository or small enema may be required.

The specimen should be taken dry to the histopathology department where it is opened from end to end and pinned out on a board prior to fixation, photography and histological examination.

2. Anterior resection

The preparation for anterior resection should be the same as for excision of the rectum. The patient should be placed in the Lloyd-Davies or lithotomy–Trendelenburg position on the operating table to provide access to the anal canal in the event that an abdominoperineal resection is required. Mobilization of the splenic flexure is made considerably easier if the operator stands between the patient's legs looking toward the head of the table.

Following careful laparotomy and intraoperative hepatic ultrasonography the transverse colon and splenic flexure are mobilized. Morbidity following anterior resection is primarily related to sepsis. Any anastomosis between colon and rectum requires an excellent blood supply and absence of tension. The sigmoid is frequently narrow and hypertrophied due to diverticular disease in the elderly population in whom rectal cancer presents. The blood supply to the left colon, based on the middle colic artery, is excellent once full mobilization has been carried out. Low ligation of the inferior mesenteric artery preserving the ascending branch of the left colic division does not leave the same scope for mobilization and length required for low anastomosis as that achieved by complete splenic flexure mobilization.

The operator stands between the legs and the assistants elevate the omentum. Using sharp dissection with electrocautery or scissors, the plane between the omentum and the colon followed by the omentum and the transverse mesocolon is entered to enter the lesser sac. This may be difficult owing to adhesions, but dissection is complete when the stomach can be retracted forwards and the mesocolon is completely free. A useful maneuvre is to place a pack above the spleen to prevent any traction on the small vessels attached to the inferior pole where trauma can lead to troublesome bleeding from the splenic capsule. The spleen is then well within the operative field; a useful manoeuvre when the splenic flexure of the colon is intimately related to splenic hilum. Dissection allows the apex of the splenic flexure to be released, then becomes a midline structure. Attention is turned to the fourth part of the duodenum and proximal jejunum which is tethered to the base of the transverse mesocolon. The lateral peritoneal folds are freed to release the duodenum. Within the left lateral paraduodenal fossa lies the inferior mesenteric vein formed by the confluence of the left colic and middle colic veins which drains into the splenic vein. Using a combination of infracolic and supracolic dissection, the vein is freed. There are one or two smaller vessels at the inferior border of the pancreas which may require ligation. The inferior mesenteric vein is then ligated and divided. Having done this the flexure and left colon can be gently retracted anteriorly and the dissection proceeds distally to the origin of the inferior mesenteric artery.

There are few definite advantages for flush ligation, but the technique is straightforward and allows a safe ligation of a single small vessel which is a better surgical technique than mass ligation of large clumps of tissue where the ligature is more prone to slippage. Those who advise against flush ligation argue that the pre-aortic autonomic nerves are damaged. It is possible to approach this vessel via the mesenteric aspect, thus avoiding the pre-aortic plexus.

Prior to ligation it is important to free completely the left colon and sigmoid from the lateral peritoneum. This avoids any possibility that the ureter may have been inadvertently incorporated in the tie. Mobilization starts by dividing the peritoneal attachment shown by the dotted line in Figure 18.5. Once this has been separated the gonadal vein must be freed from the mesentery. The ureter lies below this and must be gently dissected free. Electrocautery facilitates this manoeuvre, since there are small veins which lead to annoying bleeding. Having divided the inferior mesentery artery, the sigmoid and proximal colon can be lifted forward. The initial dissection is carried out with the patient level or in a slightly head-up position. Once the main blood vessels have been divided the lithotomy–Trendelenburg or head-down position can be adopted. If the upper rectum and sigmoid are gently retracted forwards, the retroperitoneal dissection can continue as in Figures 18.5 and 18.6. The most important stage at this point is the presacral dissection which, as indicated above, should preserve the presacral sympathetic nerves. Rectal mobilization is then continued as before. It is important to mobilize well beyond the tumour. Heald advocates near total rectal excision including the whole of the mesorectum for the majority of rectal cancers (Heald and Ryall, 1986), because in some patients lymph nodes are found in the mesorectum lying distal to the primary tumour. A reasonable rectal stump should be retained, since function is worse when the dissection and excision encompass the whole rectum. When the anastomosis lay 6 cm from the external anal verge, function was considerably better than when it lay 3 cm away (Karanjia *et al.*, 1992).

A crushing clamp of the right angled variety is placed beyond the tumour. If the fingers of the left hand are placed over the tumour the clamp should be positioned just beyond and an adequate distal resection will be carried out. When there is a villous component to the tumour the clamp site should be checked by endoscopic examination, since soft parts of the tumour may not be palpable. Where the tumour is bulky this technique will afford increased clearance because of the added amount of bowel contained between the fingers and the clamp. Having done this, the rectum is irrigated for a second time with povidone-iodine solution.

With the stapled anastomosis there are several methods for dealing with the rectal stump:

1. After rectal irrigation the rectal stump can be stapled closed using a linear stapler. In the narrow male pelvis this may be extremely difficult.
2. With the right-angled clamp in place, a cut and stitch technique can be used. Using a 0 prolene suture the anterior wall of the rectum is incised and an over-and-over purse-string suture taking 2 mm deep bites 4 mm apart is inserted. The importance of small bites cannot be overemphasized since larger ones lead to bunching which risk an incomplete 'doughnut'. The posterior layer is continued by a series of cuts and suture placements. It is important when dealing with the posterior rectum to be aware of the tendency for the muscular part of the rectum to retract well beyond the mucosa, leading to the mucosa only being inserted in the stapling device.
3. When the rectum is bulky in a small pelvis it is often easier to remove the rectum and ask the assistant standing between the legs to apply perineal pressure with the fist directed towards the anus. Once again, attention should be directed towards ensuring that the rectal muscular layers are included in the stitch.

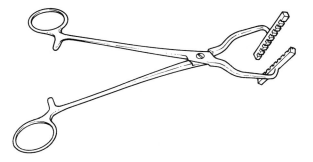

Figure 18.10 Purse-string clamp. This facilitates the insertion of a purse-string suture

4. Purse-string clamp (Figure 18.10). The clamp is placed beyond the right angle occluding clamp and a 2/0 prolene suture bearing two long cutting needles is passed through the eyes of the clamp. In the narrow male pelvis these do not pass all through the instrument and it is necessary to bend the needles as they emerge and withdraw them from the device. An automatic purse-string device is available (Autosuture, US Surgical Corporation) and this is placed beyond the occluding clamp and using a series of staples a purse-string is inserted. Great care is required using this technique since inadvertent proximal traction will lead to the staples pulling out of the rectal stump. The new detachable stapling heads have made anastomosis considerably easier than it was in former times (Figure 18.11). Using the stapled technique described in 1, the head can be removed and the spike withdrawn into the device. The stapling head is advanced through the anal canal, and once into the small rectal stump the spike can be advanced through the stapled rectum as close as possible to the staple line. If this technique is not used the complete device is gently inserted into the anal canal and opened. It is advisable to irrigate the pelvis with dilute povidone-iodine since there is a theoretical risk that malignant cells will be pushed into the pelvis if the rectum has not been adequately cleansed. With the head of the stapler detached, the purse-string can be tied and its adequacy checked. If appropriate, reinforcing sutures can be inserted.

The important part of the anastomosis is dependent on the viability of the left colon. The advantage of mobilizing the colon at the beginning of the procedure is that the demarcation will be obvious by the time of anastomosis and a section of bowel which bleeds freely can be selected. If there is no tension and the cut vessel ends bleed freely, it is most unlikely that problems will ensue. The purse-string clamp is extremely useful for the proximal purse-string suture

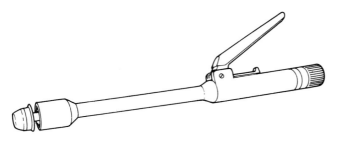

Figure 18.11 A circular stapler for intestinal anastomosis

and saves time. Once again a povidone-iodine wash is carried out and the stapler head is inserted. The two ends are reattached and the anastomosis completed. If there are two good 'doughnuts', no air or water testing should be necessary.

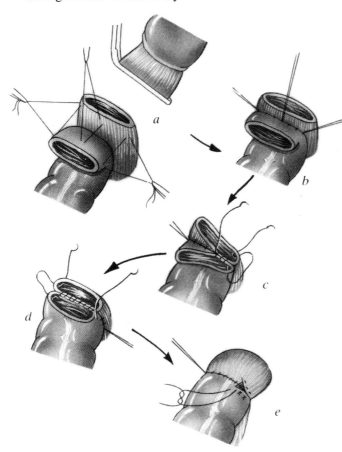

Figure 18.12 Two-layer anastomosis. *a*, Posterior layer of five, or ideally seven, non-absorbable 3/0 silk Lembert sutures placed as shown and left untied. Stay sutures on each side of rectal stump not shown. *b*, Proximal colon railroaded down to the rectum and sutures tied. The central and lateral sutures are held. Stay sutures removed. *c*, All-layers continuous suture started in midline posteriorly using double-ended 2/0 chromic catgut suture. Over-and-over stitch used except at the corners where a Connell or loop on the mucosa stitch negotiates the turn onto the anterior surface. *d*, Connell or over-and-over suture along the front. If used, the cottonwool ball must be removed from the lumen of the proximal colon. *e*, Anterior layer completed with interrupted non-absorbable 3/0 silk seromuscular horizontal mattress Lembert sutures

Alternatively, a one- or two-layer anastomosis can be performed (Figures 18.12 and 18.13). Some use an inner layer of catgut with outer silk as shown in Figure 18.12. The two-layer technique is difficult deep down in the pelvis, but is relatively straightforward in the wide access afforded by the female pelvis.

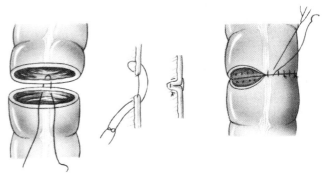

Figure 18.13 One-layer anastomosis. The posterior sutures are tied on the mucosal surface. The anastomosis is completed anteriorly with horizontal mattress sutures

A single-layer technique is shown in Figure 18.13. An alternative approach uses appositional extramucosal sutures which do not pass through the mucosa, allowing the mucosa to form a flap over the suture line leading to early mucosal continuity.

Following completion of the anastomosis there is no need to close the pelvic space which is filled by loops of bowel which fall into the pelvis. If omentum is available it is a wise manoeuvre to detach the right side and create a pedicle which can be placed in the pelvis behind the anastomosis and, if there is sufficient, this can be brought round to the front. This should minimize complications should leakage occur. Two fine suction drains are placed in the pelvis behind the anastomosis and these can usually be removed the next day. Drains remove blood which may become an infected haematoma or abscess. Once formed, pelvic abscesses tend to discharge through the anastomosis leading to leakage and the consequent risk of a fistula. Others argue that a drain should be placed adjacent to the anastomosis to allow a fistula to develop if leakage occurs. The complication of anastomotic breakdown and subsequent pelvic infection is best avoided by meticulous attention to haemostasis and avoidance of tension at the anastomosis. If there is any doubt about the safety or adequacy of the procedure, then a defunctioning stoma should be constructed as a transverse colostomy or loop ileostomy. The advantages of the latter are that it is easily placed in the right iliac fossa and is considerably easier to manage compared with a stoma placed under the ribs in the right hypochondrium.

Anal dilatation at the end of the procedure does not make passage of flatus easier and does not reduce the risk of leakage. Anal function may be compromised with subsequent leakage. Sphincter pressures fall following anterior resection confirming that this is an unnecessary manoeuvre (Horgan *et al.*, 1989).

3. Colo-anal J-pouch anal anastomosis

A factor which adversely affects the result after total rectal excision and colo-anal anastomosis is the relative non-compliance of the neorectal reservoir. Descending colon and particularly sigmoid tend to generate rather higher pressures in the early period following reconstructive surgery and patients are unable to defer defaecation. Following surgery, many patients have intense stool frequency, albeit during the first few months postoperatively. These problems may be overcome by the construction of a 6–8 cm J-shaped reservoir by side-to-side anastomosis of the terminal portion of the proximal colon to be used for reconstruction.

This technique is particularly applicable to reconstruction of radiation-induced rectovaginal fistulae following treatment of cervical cancer.

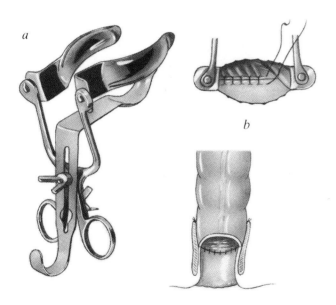

Figure 18.14 Peranal anastomosis. *a*, Parks anal retractor with detachable third blade. *b*, The colon anastomosed to the anal canal just above the dental line

4. Peranal anastomosis (Parks, 1977)

On occasion the tumour lies so close to the dentate line that dissection beyond it will mean that the 'doughnuts' excise a substantial portion of the internal anal sphincter. It is then preferable to construct the anastomosis endo-anally. The technique is as described at 2 above, except that the rectum is transected beyond the tumour without insertion of a purse-string suture. The surgeon then moves to the perineum and inserts an anal retractor. The options are the Parks retractor shown in Figure 18.14 or two Gelpi retractors (Figure 18.15). The principle of safe colo-anal anastomosis requires the absence of tension and a good blood supply. From the functional aspect excessive anal dilatation must be avoided. The Parks retractor is bulky and adequate exposure is only afforded with excessive anal dilatation. If dilatation can be minimized, better function can be expected. The Gelpi retractor can be inserted and opened to allow the equivalent of two fingers to be inserted into the anal canal which is adequate to perform a mucosectomy and does not dilate the sphincter excessively. The mucosa is injected with adrenaline diluted at 1:200 000 with normal saline. The mucosa is elevated from the level of the dentate line and excised, taking great care to avoid damage to the underlying internal sphincter. Following adequate haemostasis the colon is brought through and the whole thickness of the bowel sutured to the dentate line or just above it with a series of interrupted sutures such as 4/0 PDS which has a sharp needle that easily passes through the tougher tissues of the internal sphincter. Previously used long rectal cuffs have largely been abandoned because they are unnecessary for continence and sepsis was more common.

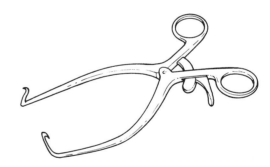

Figure 18.15 Gelpi retractors, used to display the anal canal for ileo-anal anastomosis while minimizing dilatation

5. Fulguration

There is limited place for fulguration of lower rectal neoplasms which are very early tumours, or in patients who are medically unfit to undergo routine resection. Full-thickness excision of neoplasms 4 cm or less may be removed with a clear margin of the normal tissue using a diathermy needle. Regular re-examination is required to look for and to treat any residual tumour.

6. Trans-sphincteric resection (see page 254)

7. Peranal or endo-anal approach to the rectum (see page 255)

The trans-sphincteric approach to the rectum
(York Mason, 1974)

With a suitable proximal defunctioning colostomy the rectum can be exposed by an incision starting at the anal margin in the midline posteriorly and lying to one side of the coccyx and sacrum. The external anal sphincter is then divided, followed by the lower part of the levator ani muscle and a few fibres of the gluteus maximus muscle. This exposes the rectum. A complete tube of rectum can be removed with subsequent anastomosis (Figure 18.16a). If necessary the muscle coat of the rectum and anal canal (internal sphincter) can be divided and the mucosal lining of the rectum and anal canal exposed. Submucosal resection of extensive benign lesions such as rectal adenoma can then be carried out. If necessary a complete tube of mucosa can be removed with subsequent mucosal anastomosis (Figure 18.16b). Alternatively the rectum can be opened and a transrectal full-thickness resection carried out (Figure 18.16c). This approach can be used to repair rectoprostatic or rectovaginal fistulae.

For small tumours an endo-anal approach remains acceptable and for bulkier lesions it is usually preferable to carry out a restorative low anterior resection using staples or colo-anal anastomosis. Troublesome complications of the York Mason procedure are local recurrence and fistula through the perineal wound.

The Kraski approach to the rectum

The rectum can be approached through a midline incision over the sacrum, coccyx and anococcygeal raphe. The muscular and ligamentous attachments to the coccyx are divided. The anococcygeal raphe is divided in the midline from coccyx to external sphincter and the coccyx removed. The fifth and, if necessary, the fourth sacral vertebrae can also be removed. Waldeyer's fascia is now exposed and when divided in the midline access to the whole rectum is achieved. Procedures as described in the previous section can be carried out. The technique offers little advantage over the trans-sphincteric approach, except perhaps in the removal of an extensive retrorectal lesion such as a teratoma or dermoid cyst. The

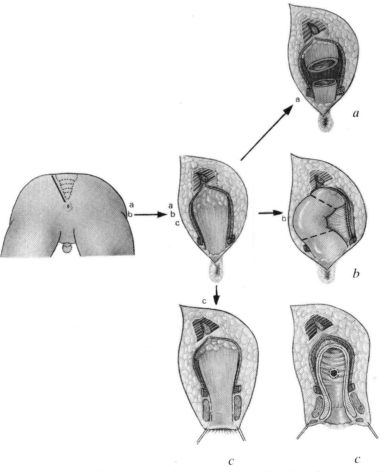

Figure 18.16   The trans-sphincteric approach to the rectum. *a*, Resection of a segment of rectum after division of the external sphincter and levator ani. *b*, Resection of rectal mucosa after division of the rectal muscle layers. *c*, Transrectal procedure after opening the rectal mucosa and if necessary the whole anal canal

divided sacrum can cause discomfort postoperatively when the patient is sitting.

The peranal or recto-anal approach to the rectum

1. Rectal polyp

Rectal polyps should all be removed for histological examination. Barium enema or colonoscopy and sigmoidoscopy are essential to exclude other pathology and to detect other polyps. The bowel is prepared with a disposable phosphate enema. General anaesthesia is usually employed, but caudal anaesthesia which allows adequate relaxation of the external anal sphincters can be used. The patient is placed in the left lateral or prone jack-knife position.

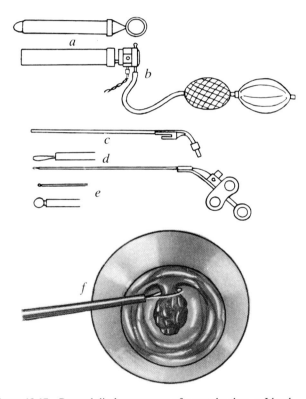

Figure 18.17 Peranal diathermy snare of a rectal polyp. *a*, Lloyd-Davies operating sigmoidoscope with obturator – 15 cm or 20 cm in length. *b*, Light fitting with windows and bellows. *c*, Sucker. *d*, Diathermy snare. *e*, Diathermy buttons. *f*, Stalk of polyp encircled by snare

Through an operating sigmoidoscope (Figure 18.17a–e) the stalk of the polyp is encircled with a diathermy snare and with a low-intensity coagulating current the whole lesion is removed for histological examination (Figure 18.17f). Any bleeding can easily be arrested with a diathermy coagulation button. In the lower rectum some polyps can be delivered to the outside so that the stalk can be ligated and the polyp excised.

2. Sessile rectal adenoma (Parks, 1966)

Preparation is as described for the removal of a rectal polyp. The lithotomy, left lateral or prone position is used according to the site of the lesion. With a Parks or Eisenhammer anal retractor in place the submucosal layer may be infiltrated with normal saline containing adrenaline (1 in 300 000). Alternatively, using a modern diathermy hand-held instrument in the coagulation mode the tumour can be dissected under direct vision and if appropriate the full thickness of the bowel wall can be taken, with a cuff of adjacent normal mucosa. The underlying muscle can be left bare to allow epithelialization to occur. If the full thickness of the bowel is taken, then the defect should be repaired. In the case of circumferential lesions, many feel that it is necessary to cover the rectum by advancing the proximal bowel. Clearly this is mandatory if the full thickness of the bowel has been entered, but with large villous adenomas it is possible to elevate carefully the whole of the tumour and preserve the underlying muscle layer. Epithelialization occurs, and healing takes place without scarring and stricturing. If there are anxieties it is often relatively easy to advance the proximal bowel over the denuded layer and suture it to the distal rectum or anal canal.

3. Rectal carcinoma

Very small rectal carcinomas may be removed per anum. Full-thickness resection of the anal wall is required and the defect closed using a single layer of absorbable sutures. The indications for such a procedure are rare as there must be no extrarectal extension of the tumour (difficult to assess clinically and impossible to assess histologically as no lymph nodes are removed), and lesions of high-grade malignancy must be excluded. In very old patients, those who are medically unfit or in someone who refuses to have major surgery, the procedure may be justified. With lesions of 3 cm or less, which have not invaded deeply into the muscle, the prognosis is excellent irrespective of whether this is treated by radical resection or local excision. Approximately 10% of apparently superficial rectal carcinomas will have involved local lymph nodes. The tumour then becomes a Duke's C lesion and the prospect of cure is dramatically reduced. The advantages of radical surgery in the elderly patient must be balanced by the operative mortality. Endoluminal ultrasound may improve the staging of tumours, but the accuracy of predicting lymph node status is only about 80%.

Conservative excision of the rectum for inflammatory bowel disease

Conservative excision of the rectum is carried out in patients undergoing proctocolectomy for ulcerative colitis without malignant change or for Crohn's proctocolitis or in patients who have initially undergone subtotal colectomy, usually for ulcerative colitis in a toxic phase, in whom the rectum is not suitable for ileorectal anastomosis. A much less extensive procedure can be carried out than is required for malignant disease of the rectum.

The patient is prepared in the usual way and under general anaesthetic is placed in the lithotomy–Trendelenburg position on the operating table. Two methods of dissection are used in patients with inflammatory bowel disease. The first is the so-called close rectal dissection. This is in a very vascular plane because the rectal mesentery is divided between it and the rectal wall. This is a somewhat tedious procedure since each vessel has to be individually ligated. It preserves most of the mesorectal fat and leaves a very small cavity in the pelvis. The lateral ligaments are divided close to the rectum and anteriorly the dissection involves high division of Denonvilliers' fascia to enter the plane behind the prostate or vagina. An alternative approach uses the anatomical plane favoured, and using electrocautery blood loss can be kept to a minimum and the presacral nerves can be carefully identified. The lateral and anterior dissection is kept close to the rectum, and using a careful technique it should be possible to avoid compromising the patient's sexual and bladder function.

The perineal surgeon closes the anus with a stout suture. The intersphincter plane between the internal and external anal sphincters needs to be identified. Once entered, the plane, which is relatively avascular, can be followed into the pelvis. The dissection allows the muscles to be closed with interrupted absorbable sutures and this leads to rapid healing of the perineal wound in the majority of patients. In perineal Crohn's disease there may be fistulae which require to be laid open and these can be excised or simply curetted. Healing is much more rapid if the wound can be closed, but clearly if there is extensive sepsis this is unwise. Antibiotic cover is essential and the skin can be conveniently closed with absorbable sutures.

Restorative proctocolectomy (ileo-anal pouch procedure)

In 1947 Ravitch and Sabiston described a restorative procedure for ulcerative colitis using a straight ileo-anal anastomosis following total rectal and colonic excision. Functional results were poor because there was no neorectal reservoir and patients had urgency, stool frequency and mucous or faecal leakage, particularly at night time. Parks and Nicholls (1978) created a reservoir which was anastomosed to the anus. They used an S-shaped pouch, constructed from three limbs of small intestine (Figure 18.18) with an efferent limb which was anastomosed to the anal canal. During straining for evacuation, the efferent limb would occlude, leading to inefficient emptying of the pouch. A number of patients had to resort to

pouch catheterization. Utsunomiya et al. (1980) advocated a J-shaped reservoir and a number of other designs have been used including the W reservoir described by Nicholls and Parks. The W and S reservoirs need to be sutured and the technique is time consuming. The J reservoir can be stapled and this reduces operating time. Approximately 40 cm of terminal ileum is used to construct a reservoir and this gives a pouch capacity of 300 ml. This is adequate to give the patient acceptable stool frequency without urgency.

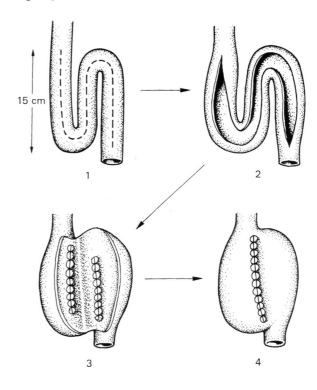

Figure 18.18 Three-limbed S-pouch

Technique for colectomy

Unless the patient has a cancer complicating ulcerative colitis, a relatively conservative colonic excision can be carried out with vessel ligation close to the colon. It is advantageous to preserve the ileocolic artery in its entirety and caecal dissection takes place close to the colonic wall to keep the arcade between the terminal branches of the inferior mesenteric and ileocolic arteries. If there is a problem with inferior reach of the ileum, selective vessel ligation can be carried out. The terminal ileum is transected close to the ileocaecal valve to maximize ileal preservation. If a J reservoir is to be constructed, a point 20 cm from the ileocaecal junction is taken and if it easily reaches beyond the inferior border of the symphysis pubis a safe ileo-anal anastomosis can be constructed. If not, then mesenteric lengthening manoeuvres must be carried out. These are as follows:

The small bowel mesentery should be carefully separated near its origin from the transverse mesocolon and its remnants. At this site, if the peritoneum overlying the small bowel mesentery is divided, 2–3 cm of added length can be achieved. Mobilizing the duodenum and the pancreas in the plane between it and the vena cava and aorta can provide added length by freeing the whole of the small bowel. Complete mobilization of the duodenum will add length. In addition, if problems are encountered in an obese or tall patient, extensive excision of the small bowel mesenteric peritoneum can be carried out without adverse effects, provided that the vasculature is preserved. If there is still inadequate length, the mesentery should be transilluminated and appropriate vessels selected for division. Vascular occlusive clamps are placed over the vessel to ensure that the collateral supply is adequate. If it is, the vessel can be divided. It is usually possible to obtain adequate length.

1. RECTAL EXCISION AND MUCOSECTOMY

Using this technique, rectal mobilization is carried out as described above. At a suitable level, which is normally 4–5 cm from the external anal verge, the rectum is transected. The surgeon having constructed the ileal reservoir then moves to the perineum and carries out a mucosectomy as described in colo-anal anastomosis. The ileal reservoir with an opening at its apex is then placed in the pelvis and the distal aperture is delivered through the anal canal and sutured using a series of interrupted 4/0 PDS or Vicryl sutures. The strength of the suture is less important than that of the needle which has to be passed through the rather fibrous internal sphincter. If there is a problem with reach, the perineum can be pushed inward by the assistant to facilitate anastomosis.

2. STAPLED ILEO-ANAL ANASTOMOSIS

This technique is considerably easier and two methods are available: the double stapled anastomosis and the end-to-end conventional stapled approach. In the former the rectum is transected approximately 5 cm from the external anal verge and, as described above in anterior resection, the stapler head is detached and the spike inserted close to the transverse staple line. Using the conventional approach, a purse-string is inserted by one of the manoeuvres described above.

The protagonists of mucosectomy argue that the whole of the colitic mucosa should be removed to minimize the risk of subsequent carcinoma in the distal inflamed rectal mucosa. Those who advocate the stapled anastomosis claim the results are superior and accept the small risk of malignant transformation. The relative ease with which restorative proctocolectomy can be carried out using the stapler has led to an increase in the popularity of this technique.

3. LOOP ILEOSTOMY

Because of the complexity of the ileal pouch and ileo-anal anastomosis, it is advisable to protect the anastomosis with a loop ileostomy. Some surgeons carry out the operation without a defunctioning stoma, but clearly this requires careful judgment and patient selection.

Complete rectal prolapse

This is a distressing condition which is commonly accompanied by faecal incontinence. Abdominal rectopexy corrects the prolapse but incontinence may persist. Abdominal procedures are superior to the perineal techniques in that impaired incontinence is more prone to persist after operations like the Altmeier procedure which entails perineal rectosigmoidectomy sometimes accompanied by plication of the pelvic floor muscles (Watts et al., 1985; Solla et al., 1989). About 75% of patients can expect continence to be improved following abdominal rectopexy. A large number of patients become constipated and this has been suggested as the mechanism of improved postoperative continence. Other reports have ascribed restoration of continence to recovery of internal sphincter pressures.

Four techniques of abdominal rectopexy are commonly used:

1. NON-RESECTIONAL RECTOPEXY (Figure 18.19a)

The rectum and distal sigmoid colon are fully mobilized down to the top of the anal canal. The lateral ligaments are divided and the rectum is then sutured low down, as shown in the illustration, and further sutures may be inserted below the level of sacral promontory to prevent intussusception occurring.

2. IVALON RECTOPEXY (Figure 18.20b)

Rectal mobilization is carried out in the same way and a square of Ivalon (Downs Surgical, UK) is placed in the pelvis. It is sutured to the pre-caecal fascia and sufficient width is retained to cover half the posterior circumference of the rectum. This is sutured using a series of non-absorbable sutures to the side of the rectal wall.

3. MARLEX RECTOPEXY (Figure 18.20c)

This is a modification of the Ivalon procedure. As shown in the illustration, Marlex (C. R. Bard Inc., USA) is inserted and this excites less reaction and is less prone to troublesome infection. To avoid problems with anterior rectal wall prolapse, a strip of Marlex may be placed in the rectovaginal septum. This technique was popularized by Nicholls and Simson (1986). In the original description by Ripstein, Marlex was placed to surround the full circumference

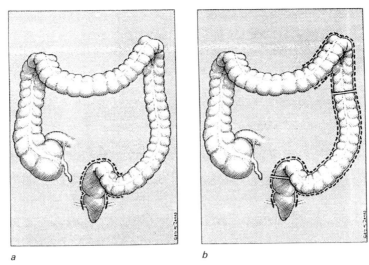

a

b

Figure 18.19 Colorectal mobilization for rectopexy. *a*, For non-resectional procedures (lateral ligaments divided), *b*, For resection and rectopexy (lateral ligaments divided)

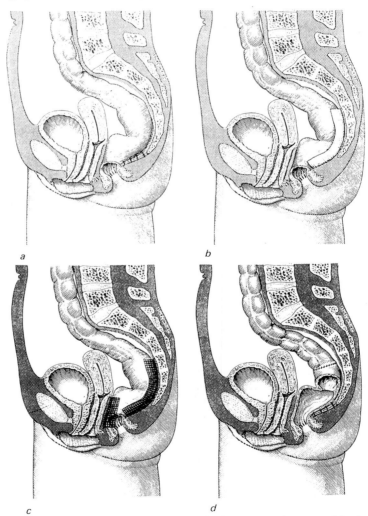

a

b

c

d

Figure 18.20 *a*, Simple suture rectopexy – four sutures fix the rectum to the presacral fascia. *b*, Posterior Ivalon sponge rectopexy. *c*, Anterior and posterior Marlex rectopexy. *d*, Resection and rectopexy – the rectum is sutured as in *a* but the sigmoid colon and upper rectum have been excised with colorectal anastomosis

of the rectal wall (Figure 18.21). This may lead to intestinal obstruction due to the elongated, redundant sigmoid colon flopping down in the pouch of Douglas.

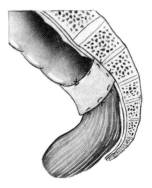

Figure 18.21   Ripstein operation for complete rectal prolapse

4. RESECTION AND RECTOPEXY (Figure 18.20d)

This technique was described by Frykman and Goldberg (1969). Here the redundant sigmoid is excised and an anastomosis constructed approximately 12 cm from the external anal verge. In patients who have severe constipation preoperatively, more extensive resection can be carried out as shown in Figure 18.19b).

Duthie and Bartolo (1992) compared the outcome following the four operations and found that continence was more likely to be improved significantly following resection rectopexy or suture fixation. The functional results and continence restoration were less satisfactory following implant surgery with Marlex or Ivalon. The worst functional results were following Ivalon rectopexy. Non-implant surgery was associated with a rise in sphincter pressures, which was not seen when Ivalon or Marlex were used.

There is continued debate surrounding which is the most appropriate procedure.

Perineal operations for rectal prolapse

The Tiersch wire or suture technique has largely been abandoned because the wire may ulcerate and may leave the patient with difficulty with defaecation often compounded by faecal impaction above the perineal wire. The most popular perineal operations are the Delorme procedure and the Altmeier or perineal rectosigmoidectomy. These should be reserved for the frail elderly patients who would be unfit for abdominal surgery because reported functional results are inferior to those of the abdominal procedures.

The Delorme procedure (Figure 18.22)

Here the mucosa is excised from the everted rectum. Dissection commences just distal to the dentate line. The diathermy technique facilitates haemostasis and

the operation is more convenient in the prone jack-knife position. Anaesthesia can be induced using a caudal or spinal anaesthesic in the unfit patient. The mucosal tube is excised and the dissection extends as far proximal as possible. A series of 0 or 1 Vicryl sutures are inserted around the circumference to plicate the underlying rectal muscle. A series of bites are taken in the proximal bowel. Approximately eight of these are placed around the circumference and following insertion they are tied. This normally leads to inversion of the everted prolapse which lies snugly within the pelvis. The postoperative course is normally uneventful and the patient is usually able to eat from the first day postoperatively. It is remarkably well tolerated by the frail and elderly patient.

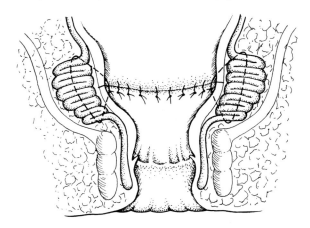

Figure 18.22   The Delorme procedure at completion. The mucosa has been stripped, and the underlying muscle has been plicated with interrupted sutures

The Altmeier procedure

The difference between this and the Delorme procedure is that the whole thickness of the prolapse is excised. The mucosal dissection, commencing at the dentate line, is deepened through the full thickness of the bowel wall. The peritoneal cavity is usually entered anteriorly, since there is a deep pelvic pouch in the majority of patients with prolapse. It is then a matter of sequentially dividing the mesorectal vessels until the redundancy in the sigmoid has been excised. A colo-anal anastomosis is constructed at a point where there is no undue tension. Interrupted full-thickness sutures are used. It may be possible to staple such an anastomosis, but direct suture is usually straightforward.

A modification of this procedure is to plicate the levator ani and sphincter muscles with interrupted prolene sutures prior to anastomosis. This is similar to the post-anal repair described below.

Rectovaginal fistula

Preliminary preparation for surgery should include

examination under anaesthetic, sigmoidoscopy (and if necessary colonoscopy), radiography and biopsy of the rectum and of the fistula track to determine the part of the bowel to which the fistula connects and whether there is any underlying pathology such as Crohn's disease or malignancy.

A traumatic fistula of obstetric origin can usually be dealt with in a conservative repair in which the anatomical layers (rectal mucosa, sphincter muscle layers and vaginal mucosa) are identified and closed separately using either a vaginal or an anal approach. Alternatively the fistula can be converted into a third-degree perineal laceration with repair of the resulting defect in layers and reconstitution of the perineal body. A covering colostomy is not normally needed. In some patients the fistula can be approached through the anus using a Parks retractor and occasionally a York Mason trans-sphincteric approach is appropriate.

A very high rectovaginal fistula due to obstetric trauma or a fistula associated with inflammatory bowel disease usually requires a bowel resection with restoration of continuity and possibly a hysterectomy. This approach is occasionally suitable for a fistula associated with malignant disease or an irradiation fistula if normal bowel is present on each side of the affected area. Occasionally, restoration of continuity may not be possible and excision of the rectum with colostomy is the only alternative.

Adult megacolon: full-thickness rectal biopsy

Adult megacolon may be due to adult Hirschsprung's disease or to intractable constipation which has required long-standing use of laxatives to which the bowel has become unresponsive. It is important to distinguish between these two conditions and although X-rays and sphincter studies may be helpful, a full-thickness rectal biopsy is conclusive.

The bowel must be mechanically cleansed, and this may take many days in the face of long-standing constipation. With the patient under general anaesthesia and in the lithotomy position an anal retractor is inserted. A stay suture is placed through the full thickness of the rectal wall just above the anorectal ring in the left lateral quadrant and is tied, leaving the needle attached. A second suture is placed 3 cm proximal to the first and this also tied. The bowel wall is then incised just proximal to the first stitch and a strip of bowel wall 3 mm wide is removed between the two sutures. The edges of the defect are then oversewn using the first stay suture, which is tied to the second at the upper end of the wound.

Patients with adult Hirschsprung's disease require a Duhamel procedure or colo-anal anastomosis. For the rest, a total colectomy with ileorectal anastomosis may be indicated in those with a thin dilated large bowel.

Hirchsprung's disease

Patients presenting in the first few months of life should be given a defunctioning colostomy, using a right transverse colostomy, as the primary treatment. For those in later life, a period of rectal irrigation may prepare the bowel sufficiently prior to the definitive procedure at which it is usual to add a covering colostomy. Three principal procedures are used and frozen section examination of a piece of bowel wall must confirm that the colon to be brought down for anastomosis is normal.

1. Colo-anal anastomosis

In this procedure the aganglionic segment is resected and a colo-anal anastomosis constructed.

2. Duhamel's operation

In this procedure (Figure 18.23) the rectum is preserved and a retrorectal peranal pull-through performed. The rectum is transected in the adult at approximately 8 cm from the external anal verge. Dissection is continued in the midline posteriorly and an opening made just above the anorectal ring. Using an anal retractor, the proximal normal diameter colon is then anastomosed just above the anal canal. This anastomosis can be stapled. A septum is left between the rectum and the transposed loop of colon. This can either be crushed by placing a clamp on it, which is left to fall off, or alternatively it can be stapled using a linear stapler to transect it. It is important to avoid the proximal bowel mesentery which should lie posteriorly otherwise clamping may induce ischaemia. Faecal stasis may occur in the rectal stump and many advocate the colo-anal procedure to overcome this disadvantage. The overall advantage of the Duhamel procedure is that it does not involve anterior rectal dissection with the risks of damage to the nervi errigentes (see above).

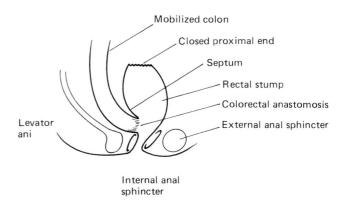

Figure 18.23 The Duhamel procedure

Surgery of the anal canal

Internal haemorrhoids

1. Conservative treatment

The single most important prophylactic treatment is the avoidance of straining at stool, best achieved by the addition of bulk to the diet in the form of fibre to achieve a satisfactory stool consistency.

Application of ointments and creams and insertion of suppositories rarely produce anything but temporary relief of anal discomfort or irritation and do nothing for bleeding.

A. INJECTION

The symptom of bleeding resulting from first-degree internal haemorrhoids can usually be controlled by injection treatment (Gabriel and Milligan, 1939). Some patients with second-degree internal haemorrhoids achieve similar relief and injection therapy is worth trying in combination with banding (see below). Third-degree haemorrhoids require other forms of treatment. Pregnancy is no contraindication to injection treatment.

After general examination and sigmoidoscopy to exclude other pathology such as colitis or neoplasm, proctoscopy is performed to establish the diagnosis. Bowel preparation and anaesthesia are unnecessary. No assistant is required. The proctoscope is passed and it is convenient to insert a cottonwool swab into the lower rectum to hold back any faecal material and to put the rectal wall slightly on the stretch. A 10 ml Gabriel syringe with a bayonet-locking guarded needle is used. The solution for injection is 5% phenol in almond oil, with 0.5% menthol added. The menthol helps to dissolve the phenol crystals during preparation and is said to reduce the discomfort of the injection. The needle is inserted into the submuco-sal layer just above each haemorrhoid and approximately 5 ml injected into each of three sites (Figure 18.24). Ideally the mucosa should balloon up as the injection proceeds. If it is too superficial the mucosa goes quite white and the injection must be discontinued or an ulcer will result which may lead to secondary haemorrhage. The needle can be inserted too deeply, in which case no ballooning will be seen. It is possible to inject into the prostate, in which case haematuria, haematospermia or epididymitis may result. In this event broad-spectrum antibiotics should be administered immediately. Occasionally following an otherwise satisfactory injection, a submucous abscess occurs or rarely an oleogranuloma.

During the injection the patient will feel nothing or a sensation of distension. The rectal swab is removed and a clean swab inserted at the level of the injection site before withdrawing the proctoscope. If the injection site bleeds, a swab should be placed at the anorectal junction and the proctoscope removed. After a few minutes bleeding will have stopped in the majority of cases. If bleeding persists, local application of a swab soaked in adrenaline (1:1000) will be effective. Very rarely, packing as for secondary haemorrhage after haemorrhoidectomy is required. Patients should be warned that they may see the cottonwool swab, that they may notice more bleeding than usual at defaecation for a day or two, and that they may be aware of leakage of mucus for a few days.

A second injection can be given if the haemorrhoids are sizeable, but this should not be done for 6 weeks to allow the first injection to have a full effect and to avoid mucosal ulceration.

B. BARRON BAND LIGATION (Barron, 1963)

This can be used as primary treatment of second-degree internal haemorrhoids, or for residual secondary haemorrhoids after haemorrhoidectomy or for

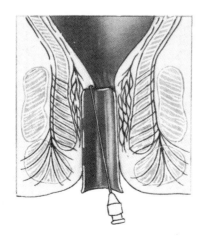
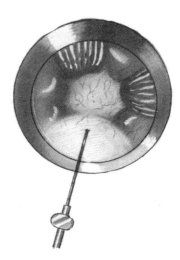

Figure 18.24 Injection of internal haemorrhoids

recurrent haemorrhoids which are suitable for banding. The procedure can be carried out following the routine examination described above, without bowel preparation or anaesthetic.

A proctoscope is passed and held by an assistant. The instrument for banding is shown in Figure 18.25(a). It consists of a double metal cylinder (i) onto which a rubber band is mounted using a detachable cone (ii). Once loaded, the haemorrhoid to be banded is grasped near its base with forceps (iii) through the double cylinders. The instrument is then fired and this places the bands in position as shown in Figure 18.25(b).

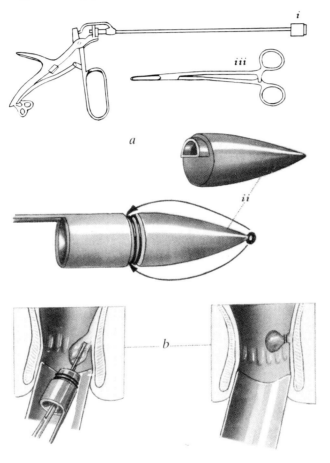

Figure 18.25 Barron band ligation of internal haemorrhoids. *a*, The instrument – i, double cylinder; ii, cone for mounting the rubber bands; iii, grasping forceps. *b*, The firing of the instrument and the end result

Oral analgesia may be required. Sloughing occurs between 4 and 10 days and may be accompanied by bleeding. Rarely this is severe and requires hospitalization and packing as for secondary haemorrhage after haemorrhoidectomy. It is wise only to band one or two haemorrhoids at any one session and to wait at least 3 weeks before contemplating further banding.

2. Surgical treatment

A. HAEMORRHOIDECTOMY – LIGATION AND EXCISION (ST. MARK'S OR MILLIGAN–MORGAN TECHNIQUE)

This operation (Milligan *et al.*, 1937) is indicated for internal haemorrhoids that are large and prolapse and fail to respond to conservative measures. The presence of a skin tag, fissure or superficial fistula is an additional indication. Pregnancy is not a contraindication, but palliative treatment is best until the pregnancy is over as the situation will then improve and surgery may be avoided. With modern anaesthetic techniques, old age is not a contraindication. Great caution should be exercised in carrying out haemorrhoidectomy in elderly in whom the sphincter may be weakened and the haemorrhoids are really a manifestation of mucosal prolapse as a result of anal laxity. Likewise, caution should be exercised in multiparous women where obstetric trauma may have weakened the sphincters. Prolapsed thrombosed internal haemorrhoids can be removed by the technique to be described, within 48 h of the event, but thereafter there is a small risk of portal pyaemia, and a conservative regimen of bed rest and local applications of lead lotion, or other astringents, can be advised. Other causes of symptoms must be excluded prior to surgery. This entails general examination and sigmoidoscopy and, if indicated, a barium enema. It is particularly important to exclude a colonic or rectal neoplasm. Haemorrhoidectomy should not be carried out in the presence of dysenteric infection or any form of colitis, as the wounds will prove difficult to heal and a flare-up of the colitis may ensue. Reassurance is required that this need not be the painful procedure that it is sometimes made out to be.

The patient may be admitted on the day of operation or the night before. No preparation is required. Indeed it has been claimed by some that bulking agents given prior to surgery reduce postoperative pain. They may work by encouraging early defaecation which dilates the sphincter, thereby relaxing it. Shaving is quite unnecessary. Clearly it is unhelpful if the rectum is faecally loaded and if this is the case, a phosphate enema should be given. General, caudal or spinal anaesthesia are all eminently satisfactory.

The patient may be placed either in the lithotomy or preferably in the prone jack-knife position. The latter is considerably more comfortable for the surgeon and his assistant. Moreover if local or regional anaesthesia is used it is much more dignified for the patient who does not have to lie awake with his or her legs in the air supported on potentially uncomfortable lithotomy poles. The perineum should be cleansed with either cetrimide or povidone-iodine.

If the patient is under general anaesthesia the operation can be commenced with an inferior haemorrhoidal nerve block. This allows a much lighter general anaesthetic to be given and reduces postoperative discomfort. Lignocaine 1% with adrenaline

(1:200 000) is used, provided that there is no cardiac contraindication to the use of adrenaline. The skin behind the anus is swabbed with antiseptic. With a finger in the anal canal, a no. 19 Fr. gauge 50 mm needle on a 20 ml syringe is inserted in the midline and passed in turn into each ischiorectal fossa where 7 ml of solution are injected. Three artery forceps are now placed on the perianal skin in the left lateral, right posterior and right anterior positions, corresponding to the usual sites of the primary internal haemorrhoids. Traction on these brings the internal haemorrhoids into view and three more artery forceps are placed near the apex of each haemorrhoidal mass. Secondary haemorrhoids can be clipped with a

further pair of forceps and included with the nearest primary mass for dissection. Traction on all six forceps reveals the 'triangle of exposure' between the three haemorrhoidal pedicles (Figure 18.26a). By holding each pair of Dunhill forceps apart in turn, the mucocutaneous junction is put on the stretch and 2 ml of the above local anaesthetic solution are injected subcutaneously using a no. 25 Fr. gauge 16 mm needle. This reduces troublesome minor haemorrhage significantly and it is worth waiting a few minutes for this effect.

The dissection starts using scissors, surgeon's straight scissors being suitable. It is very important throughout to make sure that mucocutaneous

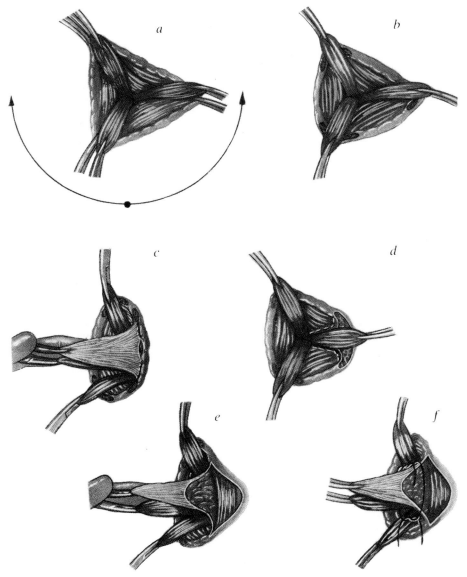

Figure 18.26 Ligation and excision of internal haemorrhoids (St. Mark's or Milligan–Morgan technique). *a*, Site of inferior haemorrhoidal nerve block and the 'triangle of exposure'. *b*, A cut on each side of the haemorrhoidal mass at the anal margin. *c*, Cut outside the haemorrhoidal mass. *d*, Mucosal incision on each side of each haemorrhoidal mass. *e*, Dissection of the haemorrhoidal mass off the internal sphincter. *f* Ligation of the pedicle

'bridges' are maintained between each area of dissection. A cut on each side of the haemorrhoidal/skin tag mass at the anal margin marks the limit of the sideways dissection of each haemorrhoid. When learning the technique this can be done to all three haemorrhoid/skin tag masses at this stage, thus marking the base of each 'bridge' at the start (Figure 18.26b). The two forceps on the left lateral haemorrhoidal/skin tag mass are now held in the left hand with the index finger of the left hand in the anal canal and a cut is made outside the mass midway between the two cuts already made (Figure 18.26c). These three cuts are then joined along the dotted line in the illustration. To be certain that the 'bridges' are maintained, with narrow-bladed scissors (McIndoe scissors) the mucosa on each side of the mass in the anal canal is divided as far as its apex (Figure 18.26d). The index finger of the left hand is then reinserted into the anal canal and with blunt scissors the dissection of the haemorrhoid/skin tag mass from the whitish circumferential fibres of the internal sphincter continues to the apex of the haemorrhoid (Figure 18.26e). The pedicle of the haemorrhoid/skin tag is then transfixed and ligated (Figure 18.26f). This process is repeated for each haemorrhoid mass. Any residual veins beneath the bridge edges are removed by filleting, residual tags of skin trimmed and bleeding points treated with diathermy.

A bulk-forming laxative is prescribed and continued in diminishing dosage until the anal canal is healed and an easy bowel action with a formed motion is achieved. Adequate analgesia should be given.

Complications include retention of urine which may require catheterization, reactionary haemorrhage from an external wound, which is usually slight and responds to local application of a swab soaked in adrenaline (1:1000), haemorrhage from a slipped ligature on a pedicle which requires religation under general anaesthesia, and the formation of a fistula due to the edges of the wound falling together. The most serious complication is secondary haemorrhage which usually occurs at about the 8th postoperative day. This normally responds to evacuating the rectal haematoma under general anaesthesia. Often no bleeding point is found. If one is seen it can be oversewn. It is rare for there to be recurrence of secondary haemorrhage.

B. CLOSED HAEMORRHOIDECTOMY

This technique, not widely practised in the UK, aims to preserve as much of the lining of the anal canal as possible. Healing by first intention is usually achieved and postoperative pain is reduced.

Dissection of each haemorrhoid/skin tag mass starts at the anal margin (Figure 18.27a) and as narrow a strip as possible of the skin and mucosa is removed together with the underlying haemorrhoidal tissue until the internal sphincter is exposed (Figure 18.27b). Further haemorrhoidal tissue is removed from beneath the edges of the wound (Figure 18.27b) and the wound is closed with a continuous absorbable suture (Figure 18.27c).

C. HAEMORRHOIDECTOMY – LIGATION AND EXCISION (PARKS' TECHNIQUE)

This technique (Parks, 1956) aims to remove haemorrhoidal tissue, restore sensitive prolapsed anal skin to the lower anal canal and remove an equivalent amount of mucus-secreting columnar epithelium from the upper anal canal and lower rectum.

A Parks retractor is used (Figure 18.28). Normal saline containing adrenaline (1:300 000) is injected subcutaneously and submucosally at the site of each haemorrhoidal complex in turn. The dissection starts at the anal margin and as little anal skin as possible is removed (Figure 18.28a). As the dissection proceeds, flaps of anal skin and mucosa are raised (Figure 18.28b). The small piece of anal skin and underlying haemorrhoidal tissue is dissected from the internal sphincter, ligated and excised (Figure 18.28c). The two flaps of anal skin and mucosa are then advanced up the canal and sutured as shown in Figure 18.28(d) using 0 strength chromic catgut. The stitches should include internal sphincter muscle fibres to fix the flaps more securely. Postoperative pain is said to be less than in the standard ligation and excision operation and anal stenosis is rare.

Parks speculated that this operation was less painful than the conventional ligation excision technique. Parks' original objective of preserving anal sensation was achieved using this operation, but it was no less painful than the ligation excision procedure (Roe et al., 1987).

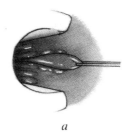
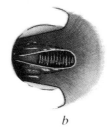
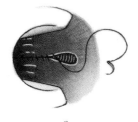

a   *b*   *c*

Figure 18.27 Closed haemorrhoidectomy

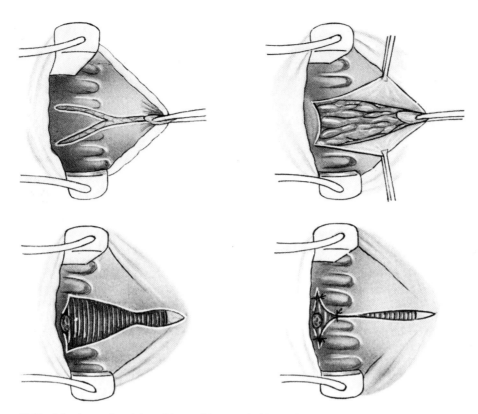

Figure 18.28 Ligation and excision of internal haemorrhoids (Parks' technique). *a*, Small amount of tissue at skin edge raised. *b*, Dissection of haemorrhoidal mass. *c*, Dissection completed. *d*, Anal mucosa advanced up the canal and sutured

D. DIATHERMY HAEMORRHOIDECTOMY

There are two aspects to postoperative pain following haemorrhoidectomy. The first results from sphincter spasm which may be avoided by carrying out anal dilatation. This is unwise, however, since haemorrhoidectomy is followed by a fall in sphincter pressures and further reductions may result in incontinence (Roe *et al.*, 1987). Pain may originate from the sutures inserted to transfix the haemorrhoidal pedicle. If these pick up internal sphincter, they may cause pain. An alternative approach uses diathermy for the whole dissection. With care no bleeding ensues and the proximal excision which is taken well above the anorectal ring leads to secure haemostasis. In practice there is little risk of anorectal stenosis so long as adequate bridges are left between the haemorrhoidal excision.

Anal skin tags

Skin tags alone rarely give symptoms but if hygiene is difficult, pruritus may be troublesome. They often occur in association with other conditions, such as internal haemorrhoids, and may be removed in the treatment of these conditions. Small tags can be removed as an outpatient procedure under local anaesthetic. No sutures are required and a simple dry dressing is needed for a few days. Larger tags require caudal or general anaesthesia for their removal.

Fibrous anal polyp (hypertrophied anal papilla)

Rarely one or more fibrous polyps may develop at the dentate line and if prolapse occurs they are noticed by the patient. They may occur with other conditions such as fissure-in-ano and may be treated with that condition. If they occur alone they should be ligated and excised under anaesthesia using an artery forceps and 0 strength Vicryl.

Perianal haematoma (thrombosed external haemorrhoid)

Thrombosis in an external haemorrhoidal vein is usually an acutely painful condition associated with the appearance of a tender bluish swelling of variable size.

If very painful and comparatively small the whole area can be excised under local anaesthetic. A Hibitane-soaked dressing is applied for 24 h and thereafter frequent hot baths and dry dressings are all that are necessary. A gentle aperient is advisable. Relief of pain by incision of the lesion and evacuation of the clot can be dramatic, but a troublesome oedematous tag may be left.

If a large area is involved the haematoma can be evacuated under local anaesthesia. This is one of three anal conditions in which emergency surgery can afford considerable relief and reduce immense suffering. The other two are anal fissure and intersphincteric abscess. If left untreated, resolution is usually complete in 2–3 weeks. A complete proctological examination is then essential to exclude other pathology.

Fissure-in-ano

Simple anal fissure occurs in the lower half of the anal canal, in the midline posteriorly in 75% of patients, in the midline anteriorly in 15% and at the sides in 10%. It is associated with spasm of the anal sphincters. In women, anterior fissures are more common and occur in approximately 30%.

Inspection of the anus will usually reveal the lower end of the fissure, even in the presence of marked spasm. Digital examination is usually possible if 2% lignocaine lubricant is used and if great care is taken. Sigmoidoscopy or proctoscopy may not be possible initially. A fissure that is not in the midline, is extensive and irregular or which is multiple is suspicious of other pathology such as inflammatory bowel disease. This must be investigated appropriately; syphilis must be diagnosed by dark-ground illumination of a smear and a neoplasm must be biopsied.

As a fissure passes from the acute to the chronic stage several changes occur (Figure 18.29a–f). Initially the vertical muscle fibres of the musculus submucosa ani are seen (a), but as the fissure deepens the horizontal fibres of the internal sphincter are seen

(b). A sentinel tag of skin may then develop at the lower end of the fissure (c), together with a hypertrophied anal papilla on the dentate line at the upper end (d). Undermining of the edges may lead to abscess formation (e) and finally a subcutaneous fistula may develop at the lower end (f).

Stages (a) and (b) can be treated conservatively with a high-fibre diet and supplementary bulking agents like Fybogel or Lactulose to soften the stool. If conservative treatment fails, then lateral subcutaneous internal sphincterotomy is indicated (Hawley, 1969).

This procedure can be performed under local anaesthetic as a day case. No bowel preparation is necessary. A caudal anaesthetic is ideal, but if this is too extensive it may delay the patient's discharge if there is associated limb weakness or urinary retention. This usually resolves rapidly, but if the operation is carried out late in the day it may be unwise to discharge the patient in the evening.

With the patient in the prone jack-knife position the fissure should be confirmed. A tiny incision is made at the three o'clock position with a no. 15 blade. A pair of small scissors is then inserted into the intersphincteric plane and gradually withdrawn, following which the submucosal plane is elevated. Each arm of the scissors blade is then inserted, one in the superficial plane created and one in the intersphincteric plane. The internal sphincter is then divided to the top of the fissure (I. P. Todd, personal communication).

Identification of the internal sphincter and the groove between it and the external sphincter may be facilitated by inserting an Eisenhammer bivalve speculum. Using this technique it is usually not necessary to suture the wound. This is thought to minimize postoperative pain. An alternative technique is to use

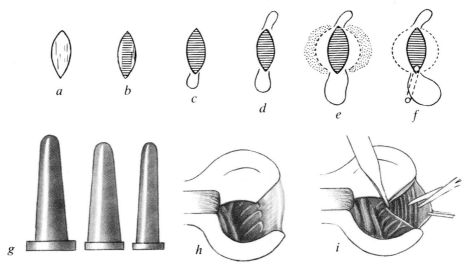

Figure 18.29 Fissure-in-ano. *a*, Vertical fibres of musculus submucosae ani exposed. *b*, Horizontal fibres of internal sphincter exposed. *c*, Sentinel tag of skin develops. *d*, Anal papilla develops. *e*, Undermining and abscess formation. *f*, Subcutaneous fistula develops. *g*, St. Mark's pattern and dilator – three sizes. *h*, Bivalve speculum inserted into anal canal. *i*, The internal sphincter exposed

an iridectomy knife which is placed through a similar tiny incision. The knife can either be advanced along the submucosal plane and the cut made laterally towards the external sphincter or, alternatively, it can be placed in the intersphincteric plane and cut medially towards the lumen of the anal canal stopping short of dividing the mucosa and submucosa.

The open technique is shown in Figure 18.29. Here a longer incision is made and the internal sphincter is identified under direct vision. It can then be cut for the appropriate length. The wound is then closed with absorbable sutures. A sentinel skin tag or anal papilla is removed. Undermined edges are trimmed and a fistula if present is laid open. The temptation to carry out the sphincterotomy in the base of the fissure should be resisted as a dorsal wound may not heal well and may lead to troublesome incontinence due to the keyhole deformity thus created. At completion of the procedure a dry gauze dressing is applied. Postoperatively, bulking agents and analgesics are given.

Perianal sepsis

There have been many theories to explain perianal sepsis. The simplest one is based on that shown in Figure 18.30 in which an intersphincteric abscess is the primary cause of the problem. The hypothesis is that one of the anal glands which lies deep to internal anal sphincter becomes infected, leading to an intersphincteric abscess which can spread laterally into the ischiorectal fossa, inferiorly to the perianal space and superiorly into the intermuscular space to form a high intermuscular abscess.

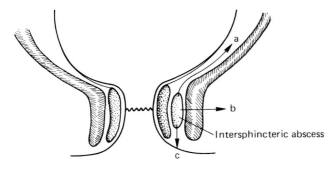

Figure 18.30 Perianal sepsis. *a*, High intermuscular abscess. *b*, Ischiorectal abscess. *c*, Perianal abscess

Whereas the ischiorectal and perianal abscess is often quite obvious clinically, this is not often the case with the intersphincteric and high intermuscular abscess. The patient will have a painful fluctuant indurated swelling just lateral to the anal canal, in the case of a perianal abscess, and further out when the sepsis is in the ischiorectal fossa. An intermuscular abscess is one of the differential diagnoses of severe acute anal pain. With intersphincter sepsis, little may be obvious and rectal examination may be impossibly painful. If there is an obvious perianal or ischiorectal

abscess, then an incision can be made over the most fluctuant part. A swab of the pus is sent for bacteriological culture and the cavity is explored digitally to assess its extent and to break down loculi. Instruments should never be used for fear of penetrating the levator ani muscle and causing a supralevator extension of the sepsis. The wound edges are trimmed to allow free drainage and the corner of a piece of gauze soaked in Betadine or Hibitane is inserted to keep the wound open. It should not be packed. The dressing is changed at 24 h and thereafter the patient has a twice daily bath with reapplication of the dressing. In appropriate situations the patient can be discharged with the dressings carried out by a district nurse or relative.

Perianal sepsis may be the result of a sebaceous cyst or folliculitis. In these instances the pathology is helpful in that culture will usually reveal a skin pathogen such as *Staphylococcus aureus*. If the culture yields an enteric pathogen it is highly probable that the patient has an enteric communication with the anal canal and will be at risk of subsequently developing a fistula.

Fistula-in-ano

A fistula-in-ano will not heal spontaneously and apart from causing recurrent abscess may in very rare cases become malignant. Inflammatory bowel disease and large bowel neoplasia must be excluded by sigmoidoscopy and proctoscopy and if necessary by barium studies prior to surgery. The nomenclature associated with this condition is difficult and several classifications of fistula-in-ano exist (Hawley, 1975; Parks *et al.*, 1976). To describe a fistula as 'simple', if it consists of a radial track running from an external opening to an internal opening in the anal canal, and all others as 'complex', is insufficient. To describe a fistula as 'low' when it arises from an anal gland regardless of whether it tracks above the levator muscle, and 'high' only if it has an opening in the bowel above the levator muscle, is helpful. Many would regard any extension above the levator muscle as being a 'high' extension, but this again is insufficient. What is required from the practical point of view is an accurate understanding of the anatomy of the anal canal musculature together with a clear appreciation of the relationship of the fistula track and its opening to these muscles. Several complicated situations can arise which are very difficult to deal with but which are fortunately very rare. Only the more common situations are dealt with in this chapter and only nomenclature about which there is no debate is used.

A fistula nearly always arises from an infected anal gland (Figure 18.31a) and in 80% of cases the gland involved is in the midline posteriorly. The duct of each gland opens into a crypt at the dentate line (Figure 18.31b) and this becomes the internal opening of the fistula. The glands themselves are in the inter-

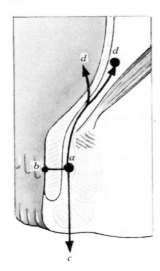
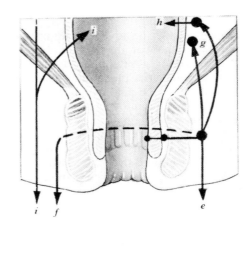

Figure 18.31 Fistula-in-ano. *a*, Anal gland. *b*, Opening of gland into a crypt. *c*, Low intersphincteric fistula. *d*, High intersphincteric fistula. *e*, Trans-sphincteric fistula with opening directly to the outside. *f*, Trans-sphincteric fistula with circumferential extension. *g*, Trans-sphincteric fistula with supralevator extension. *h*, Trans-sphincteric fistula opening into the rectum. *i*, Extrasphincteric fistula

sphincteric plane and a resulting abscess can extend in one of several directions. If it extends downwards to the perianal skin, the most common situation, it is a low intersphincteric fistula (Figure 18.31c). If it extends upwards and opens into the rectum it is a high intersphincteric fistula (Figure 18.31d). Extension upwards and downwards and circumferentially in this plane can all occur in the same fistula. Very rarely the track of such a fistula may pass up in the intersphincteric plane to the supralevator space and down through the levator muscle to the ischiorectal fossa to the outside. This is a suprasphincteric fistula (not shown) and calls for very careful management (Parks *et al.*, 1976). If infection spreads through the external sphincter the fistula becomes trans-sphincteric and the track may then pass directly to the outside (Figure 18.31e), or spread circumferentially outside the external sphincter beneath the levator muscle and then to the outside (Figure 18.31f) occasionally by several openings, or rarely upwards through the levator muscle where again it may track circumferentially (Figure 18.31g). Very rarely such a track may enter the rectum (Figure 18.31h).

In cases of inflammatory bowel disease a fistula may pass from the rectum or more proximal diseased bowel to the outside directly (Figure 18.31i), there being no connection with the anal canal. This is an extrasphincteric fistula, cured by dealing with the proximal disease. Very rarely such a track may pass down in the intersphincteric plane (not shown).

The patient is admitted the day before surgery and given a phosphate enema. The patient can be placed in the lithotomy or prone jack-knife position.

Instruments

A set of Lockhart-Mummery directors is required (Figure 18.32a). There are four instruments in the set and they are characterized by a groove running the whole length of the instrument down which a scalpel blade can be passed. A malleable silver probe-ended director, together with a set of fine malleable silver probes, may be helpful.

Intersphincteric fistula

A low intersphincteric fistula is the type most commonly encountered. With one finger in the anal canal, a director is gently passed from the external opening. Under light anaesthesia the anorectal ring can be clearly felt above the track containing the director (Figure 18.32b). The point of the director is then brought to the outside (Figure 18.32c). The track is laid open by cutting along the groove on the director with a scalpel. The track is curetted and the tissue sent for histological examination. A careful search is made for communicating tracks which are laid open if found. The main track is extended outwards for a short distance and the whole wound trimmed to make a triangular wound which is as shallow as possible (Figure 18.32d). If there is an upward extension in the intersphincteric plane without an opening into the rectum, it will usually drain satisfactorily when the lower part is laid open as described.

A flat gauze dressing soaked in Betadine or Hibitane (1:2000) is tucked into the wound in the anal canal to reach the apex of the triangular wound. A wool pad is applied to absorb secretions. The inner dressing is kept moist with Betadine or Hibitane and is soaked off in a hot bath after 48 h and thereafter reapplied twice daily after a hot bath. Two people are required to do the dressing in order to ensure that it reaches the apex of the wound in the canal each time. A gentle laxative is given.

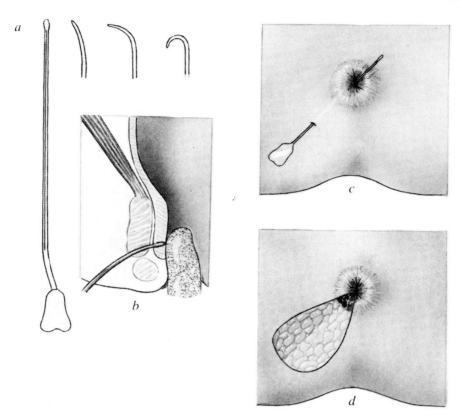

Figure 18.32 Fistula-in-ano. *a*, Set of Lockhart-Mummery directors. Low intersphincteric fistula-in ano. *b*, Probing of fistula. *c*, Director passed to the outside. *d*, Track laid open

If the abscess in the intersphincteric plane tracks upwards only, then it calls for different management. With an anal retractor in place, a director is passed up the track in a cranial direction from the opening in the anal canal to the rectal opening if there is one. If there is no rectal opening, one is made artificially with the director and the track is laid open with a cutting diathermy needle. No dressing is required.

Trans-sphincteric fistula

Sometimes such a fistula can be laid open as already described for a low intersphincteric fistula. Often, however, when the director is passed into the external opening of this fistula it passes parallel to the anal canal to the apex of the ischiorectal fossa of one side rather than to the internal opening in the anal canal (Figure 18.33a) and great care must then be taken not to push it through the levator muscle or, worse still, on into the rectum. The ischiorectal part of the fistula is laid open first by passing the director forwards and then backwards (Figure 18.33b–d). If the track passes to the other ischiorectal fossa this too must be laid open (Figure 18.33e). A search is then made for the internal opening, which is often in the midline posteriorly, and this too is laid open provided that it is below the anorectal ring.

Dressings are applied and changed as for low fistulae, but initially a general anaesthetic may be required for the dressing if the wound is extensive. Weekly revision, under general anaesthetic if necessary, is needed throughout the healing process and if any missed tracks become apparent (a bead of pus in otherwise healthy granulations) they must be laid open. Active sphincter exercises are encouraged and a gentle laxative given.

Extension of such a fistula through the levator muscle to the supralevator space will close satisfactorily provided that adequate drainage is established, and if there is an opening into the rectum this should be closed with absorbable sutures. Of prime importance in the management of these more difficult and fortunately rare fistulae is the integrity of the puborectalis muscle. In such difficult cases a covering sigmoid colostomy may be necessary.

Many of these patients do not require prolonged inpatient care, and modification of the surgical technique by minimizing the amount of skin cut can reduce the postoperative discomfort and allow early ambulation. In this respect, with a simple track, it is possible to marsupialize it by suturing the cut edges of the skin to the edges of the granulation lined track. Once all the granulation tissue has been curetted, a clean track is left. If the skin edges are loosely

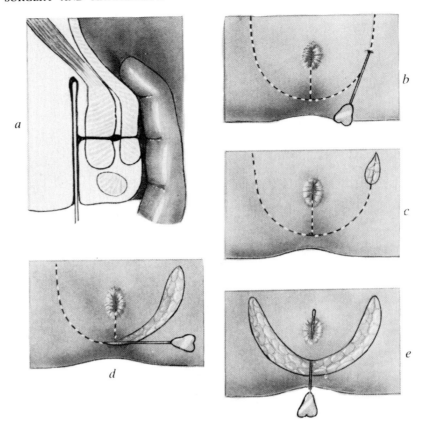

Figure 18.33 Trans-sphincteric fistula-in-ano. *a*, Probing of fistula. *b–d*, Ischiorectal part of fistula laid open. *e*, Track to internal opening probed and laid open

apposed with interrupted fine Vicryl or PDS the skin tends to keep the track open and allows the patient to be discharged on the day of operation or the following day. They are carefully managed as outpatients.

The major problem in this area is the high trans-sphincteric or suprasphincteric fistula. There are several ways in which these can be dealt with. One option is to deal with all the extrasphincteric sepsis and insert a seton through the primary fistula track. This can be a loop of silk, nylon or a vascular vessel loop. Setons can be loosely tied to act as drains, or tightly to divide muscle. The theory behind the tight seton is that because it cuts through the muscle slowly there is time for the cut edges above to reunite. This is more theory than reality and in truth patients treated in this manner often end up with a rather deficient sphincter with poor control of liquid and flatus, albeit preserving reasonable continence to solid stool.

A variety of procedures have been adopted to avoid dividing extensive amounts of muscle. The most popular of these is the advancement flap in which the primary fistula track is either excised or thoroughly curetted. The full thickness of the rectal wall is then elevated, the internal opening is closed with an absorbable suture and the resulting defect is then repaired with interrupted sutures. This technique

is effective in simple fistulae and in some due to Crohn's disease. Clearly in the more complicated fistula there is a risk of recurrence, but if muscle can be preserved this is obviously to the patient's benefit.

The procedure for advancement flaps is as follows. The patient is given full mechanical bowel preparation, antibiotic prophylaxis and, under general anaesthesia, is placed in either the lithotomy or prone jack-knife position. The tract(s) is identified with a fistula probe and marked with a nylon loop. The internal opening is exposed using two Gelpi's retractors (Seward, Middlesex, UK) or an Eisenhammer speculum, and is excised with an elliptical incision (Figure 18.34). Approximately half the circumference of the rectal wall is dissected proximally using cutting diathermy to minimize bleeding (Figure 18.35). The mucosa distal to the internal opening is elevated for a short distance. The internal opening of the fistula track is closed with Vicryl. The mobilized rectal wall is then advanced over the closed end of the track and anastomosed to the anal canal with interrupted absorbable sutures. The external component of the fistula's track is managed by drainage rather than excision. Skin around the external opening is excised and the granulation tissue surrounding the track curetted. The resulting cavity is drained externally using a no. 8 Foley catheter or mushroom drain which may be left *in situ* for periods of up to 1 month postoperatively (Lewis and Bartolo, 1990).

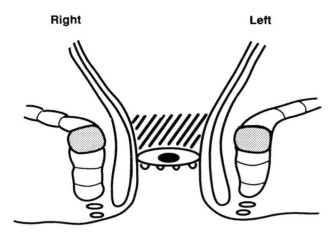

Figure 18.34 Coronal section of the anorectal region showing excision of the internal opening

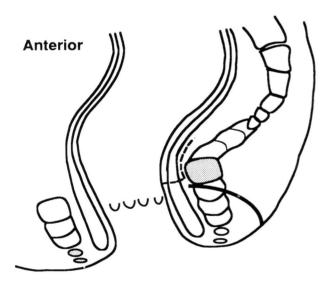

Figure 18.35 Sagittal section of the anorectal region showing the full thickness rectal flap, dissected proximally using cutting diathermy

Malignant neoplasms of the anal canal

Anal neoplasms are relatively rare. The three most common malignant conditions of the anal canal are adenocarcinoma arising in the lower rectum or anal glands, squamous cell carcinoma of the anoderm and malignant melanoma.

Adenocarcinoma should be treated by abdomino-perineal excision of the rectum, with wide clearance of the perineal and ischiorectal tissues. Because of the lymphatic drainage of the perianal skin, close attention must be paid to the inguinal glands. Excision

biopsy and frozen section examination of a superficial inguinal lymph node may be called for, if necessary, followed by a block dissection of groin nodes.

Squamous cell carcinoma may require excision of the rectum, but wide local excision may be feasible if the upper part of the sphincter mechanism is uninvolved when dealing with a comparatively less aggressive tumour. Interstitial radiotherapy with or without external beam irradiation may also give adequate control of such tumours, the treatment being covered by a defunctioning colostomy where appropriate. External beam irradiation may also be used to treat metastatic inguinal lymph nodes.

Malignant melanoma may require excision of the rectum, but because of the very poor prognosis, local excision if possible is perhaps a more sensible and humane procedure.

Anorectal incontinence

This distressing symptom can occur as a result of sphincter damage, for example after fistula operation, or after difficult childbirth or other trauma. It is best treated by direct repair of the sphincters. It can also occur in association with complete rectal prolapse and in a group of patients who have minimal prolapse but who have weakness of the pelvic floor muscles, including the sphincters, for other reasons, for example, due to nerve damage during a difficult labour. In the latter two groups postanal repair of the sphincters may be appropriate. Sphincter studies which may be helpful in the evaluation of these difficult patients have been described.

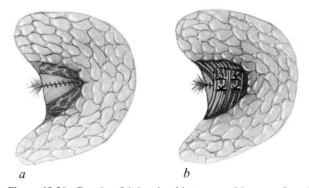

a   *b*

Figure 18.36 Repair of injured sphincters. *a*, Mucosa of anal canal repaired. *b*, Sphincter ends overlapped and sutured

1. Repair of injured sphincters

When divided, the ends of the sphincter muscles spring apart and the gap between them becomes filled with fibrous scar tissue. A large circumferential incision around the anus is made, centred on the site of maximal damage as determined by electromyographic or ultrasound studies. The scar tissue is carefully dissected and the muscle ends identified. The mucosal

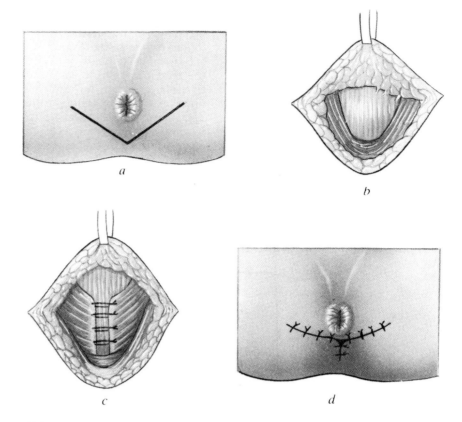

Figure 18.37 Postanal repair of sphincters. *a*, Incision. *b*, Plane between internal and external sphincters opened up. *c*, Loose repair of levator ani and external sphincter. *d*, Closure of incision

lining of the anal canal is separated from the muscle layers and repaired with continuous chromic catgut (Figure 18.36a). The muscle ends are then overlapped and loosely sutured with prolene (Figure 18.36b). The free edge of the anal mucosa is sutured to the muscle and the wound left open to granulate. A covering colostomy may be used.

2. *Post-anal repair* (Parks, 1975)

The aim of this repair is to plicate the sphincter muscle cylinder from within (in order to preserve its nerve and blood supply) and so reform the right-angled anorectal angle which is invariably lost in these patients, the puborectalis part of the levator ani being the most important factor in this respect.

The patient is placed in the lithotomy or prone jack-knife position and a solution of normal saline with adrenaline (1:300 000) infiltrated into the post-anal tissues. A V-shaped incision is made 6 cm behind the anus and the anterior flap of skin elevated as far as the anal margin (Figure 18.37a). The plane between the white internal sphincter muscle and the reddish external sphincter is then opened up round half the circumference of the anal canal and lower rectum. Waldeyer's fascia is divided to enter the

pelvirectal space (Figure 18.37b). Two or three sutures of prolene are then inserted loosely to approximate the two sides of the iliococcygeus part of the levator ani (Figure 18.37c). Below this, similar sutures are placed in the pubococcygeus part of the levator ani, with a third layer in the puborectalis and a final layer in the lower part of the external sphincter muscle.

The anterior flap of skin is taken up into the anal canal by this procedure and the wound is therefore closed as a V–Y with suction drainage (Figure 18.37d). Magnesium sulphate is given for 10 days to achieve diarrhoea and avoid straining. Thereafter a hydrophilic laxative is used regularly and glycerin suppositories inserted every morning to achieve an easy bowel action.

Anal and perianal warts (condylomata acuminata)

These must be distinguished from condylomata lata of syphilis. A full proctological examination is essential as they may occur in the anal canal and more rarely in the lower rectum. The external genitalia must be examined, for if all warts are not treated recurrence is inevitable.

If confined to the perianal skin, small numbers of warts can be treated with 25% podophyllum in tincture of benzoin compound. This is applied to the warts twice weekly until all have gone. Care must be taken not to touch the normal skin as it tends to burn and it is advisable for the patient to have a bath 4 h after each application.

More extensive perianal warts or warts in the anal canal call for excision under general anaesthesia. A phospate enema is given. The affected area is infiltrated with normal saline containing adrenaline (1:300 000). This elevates the warts on a balloon of skin or mucosa and they can then be cut off with fine-pointed scissors preserving as much normal skin as possible. Diathermy excision tends to destroy slender skin bridges and thus healing takes longer.

If very extensive, the operation may have to be done in stages to avoid anal stenosis. Close follow-up is essential as recurrence is common, but any such recurrences can usually be treated successfully with podophyllum.

References

Barron, J. (1963) Office ligation of internal haemorrhoids. *Am. J. Surg.*, **105**, 563–570

Burleigh, D. E., D'Mello, A. and Parks, A. G. (1979) Responses of isolated human internal anal sphincter to drugs and electrical field stimulation. *Gastro*, **77**, 484–490

Duthie, G. S. and Bartolo, D. C. C. (1992) Abdominal rectopexy for rectal prolapse: a comparison of techniques. *Br. J. Surg.*, **79**, 107–113

Frykman, H. M. and Goldberg, S. M. (1969) The surgical treatment of rectal procidentia. *Surg. Gynecol. Obstet.*, **129**, 1225–1230

Gabriel, W. B. and Milligan, E. T. C. (1939) Haemorrhoids. *Br. Med. J.*, **2**, 412

Goligher, J. C. (1976) Cryosurgery for haemorrhoids. *Dis. Colon Rectum*, **19**, 213–218

Griffiths, J. D. (1956) Surgical anatomy of the blood supply of the distal colon. *Ann. R. Coll. Surg. Engl.*, **19**, 241–256

Grinnell, R. S. (1954) Distal intramural spread of carcinoma of the rectum and rectosigmoid. *Surg. Gynec. Obstet.*, **99**, 421–430

Gutierrez, J. G. and Shah, A. M. (1975) Autonomic control of the internal anal sphincter in man. In *Fifth International Symposium of Gastrointestinal Motility* (ed. G. van Trappen), Typoff Press, Belgium, pp. 363–373

Hawley, P. R. (1969). The treatment of chronic fissure-in-ano: a trial of methods. *Br. J. Surg.*, **56**, 915–918

Hawley, P. R. (1975) Anorectal fistula. *Clin. Gastroenterol.*, **4**, 635–649

Heald, R. J. and Ryal, R. D. H. (1986) Recurrence and survival after total mesorectal excision for rectal cancer. *Lancet*, **i**, 1479–1482

Horgan, P. G., O'Connoll, P. R., Shinkwyn, C. A. and Karwan, W. O. (1989) Effect of anterior resection on anal sphincter function. *Br. J. Surg.*, **76**, 783–786

Jones, I. T., Fazio, V. W. and Jagelman, D. G. (1987) The use of trans-anal rectal advancement flaps in the management of fistulas involving the ano-rectum. *Dis. Colon Rectum*, **30**, 919–923

Karanjia, N. D. Schache, D. J. and Heald, R. J. (1992), Function of the distal rectum after low anterior resection for carcinoma. *Br. J. Surg.*, **7**, 114–116

Keighley, M. R. B (1983) Perioperative antibiotics. *Br. Med. J.*, **286**, 1844–1846

Lane, R. H. S. and Parks, A. G. (1977) Function of the anal sphincters following colo-anal anastomosis. *Br. J. Surg.*, **64**, 596–599

Lewis, P. and Bartolo, D. C. C. (1990) Treatment of trans-sphincteric fistulae by full thickness ano-rectal advancement flaps. *Br. J. Surg.*, **77**, 1187–1189

Lloyd-Davies, O. V. (1939) Lithotomy–Trendelenburg position for resection of rectum and lower pelvic colon. *Lancet*, **ii**, 74–76

Lord, P. H. (1972) A new approach to haemorrhoids. *Prog. Surg.*, **10**, 109–124

Loubowski, D. Z., Nicholls, R. J., Swash, M., Jordan, M. J., Nuer, A. L. (1987) Control of the internal anal sphincter. *Br. J. Surg.*, **74**, 668–670

Miles, W. E. (1908) A method of performing abdomino-perineal excision for carcinoma of the rectum and of the terminal portion of the pelvic colon. *Lancet*, **ii**, 1812–1813

Milligan, E. T. C., Naunton Morgan, C., Jones, L. E. *et al.* (1937) Surgical anatomy of the anal canal, and the operative treatment of haemorrhoids. *Lancet*, **ii**, 1119–1124

Naunton Morgan, C. (1965). Carcinoma of the rectum. *Ann. R. Coll. Surg.*, **36**, 73–99

Nicholls, R. J. and Simson, J. N. L. (1986) Anteroposterior rectopexy in the treatment of solitary rectal ulcer syndrome without overt rectal prolapse. *Br. J. Surg.*, **73**, 222–224

Parks. A. G. (1956) The surgical treatment of haemorrhoids. *Br. J. Surg.* **43**, 337–351

Parks, A. G. (1966) Benign tumours of the rectum. In *Clinical Surgery*, Vol. 10, *Abdomen and Rectum and Anus* (eds C. Rob, R. Smith and C. Naunton Morgan), Butterworths, London, pp. 541–548

Parks, A. G. (1975) Anorectal incontinence. *Proc. R. Soc. Med.*, **68**, 681–690

Parks, A. G. (1977) A technique of colo-anal anastomosis. In *Operative Surgery: Colon, Rectum and Anus* (eds C. Rob and R. Smith), Butterworths, London, pp. 164–167

Parks, A. G., Gordon, P. H. and Hardcastle, J. D. (1976) A classification of fistula-in-ano. *Br. J. Surg.*, **63**, 1–12

Parks, A. G. and Nicholls, R. J. (1978) Proctocolectomy without ileostomy for ulcerative colitis. *Br. Med. J.*, **2**, 85–88

Ravitch, M. M. and Sabiston, D. C. (1947) Anal ileostomy with preservation of the sphincter. *Surg. Gynecol. Obstet.*, **84**, 1095–1097

Roe, A. M., Bartolo, D. C. C., Vellacott, K. D., Locke-Edmunds, J. C., Mortensen, N. J. McC. (1987) Submucosal versus ligation excision haemorrhoidectomy: a comparison of anal sensation, anal sphincter manometry and postoperative pain and function. *Br. J. Surg.*, **74**, 948–951

Solla, J. A., Rothenberger, D. A. and Goldberg, S. M. (1989) Colinic resection in the treatment of complete rectal prolapse. *Neth. J. Surg.*, **41**, 132–135

Thomson, W. H. F (1975) The nature of haemorrhoids. *Br J. Surg.*, **62**, 542–552

Utsunomiya, J., Iwama, T., Imajo, M. *et al.* (1980) Total colectomy, mucosal proctectomy, and ileo-anal anastomosis. *Dis. Colon Rectum*, **23**, 459–466

Watts, J. D., Rothenberger, D. A., Buls, J. G., Goldberg S. M. and Nivatvongs, S. (1985) The management of procidentia: 30 years experience. *Dis. Colon Rectum*, **28**, 96–102

Wells, C. and Naunton Morgan, C. (1962) Polyvinyl alcohol sponge prosthesis: the use of Ivalon sponge. *Proc. R. Soc. Med.*, **55**, 1083–1085

York Mason, A. (1974) Trans-sphincteric surgery of the rectum. *Prog. Surg.*, **13**, 66–97

19

The biliary system

J. P. Neoptolemos

Cholecystitis

Most cases of cholecystitis are due to gallstones, although 5–10% are due to unusual but nevertheless important causes, for example acalculous cholecystitis.

Gallstone disease

About 45 000 cholecystectomies are performed in the UK each year and at least 600 000 in the USA. Gallstones are commoner in women. Ten per cent of men aged 60–70 years have gallstones compared with 30% of women. The prevalence in older men approaches that of older women. Approximately 20% of individuals with gallstones eventually develop symptoms, a plateau being reached at 15 years, and 20% of patients with symptoms present with acute cholecystitis. Between 25% and 50% of symptomatic patients undergo cholecystectomy.

Types of gallstone and their formation

Racial and environmental factors are involved in gallstone formation. The prevalence of gallstones is high in Europe, Australia and the USA and low in Greece and Africa; it is very high in North American Indians, in Chile, Sweden and Czechoslovakia.

The types of gallstone are shown in Table 19.1. There are three important varieties: cholesterol, black-pigment and brown-pigment stones. Only cholesterol stones are amenable to dissolution therapy, unless they are radio-opaque (15%).

Table 19.1   Types of gallstone

Cholesterol stones	Pigment stones	Rare stones
Mixed cholesterol	Black pigment	Calcium carbonate
Pure cholesterol	Brown pigment	Calcium phosphate
Composite	Salt and pepper	Fatty acid calcium

Gallstones form when bile is supersaturated by one or more components and when the conditions exist for nucleation. Bile is the only vehicle by which cholesterol can be excreted from the body. It is held in solution by mixed micelles composed of phospholipid (lecithin) and bile salts. Supersaturation of cholesterol will, therefore, occur if the balance of this system is changed, for example interruption of the entero-hepatic circulation of bile salts (e. g. ileal disease or resection and cystic fibrosis). Impaired gallbladder motility predisposes to stone formation: pregnancy, menstruation, truncal vagotomy, starvation and prolonged parenteral nutrition. Cholesterol stones are found in 70% of gallbladders from Westernized people.

Black-pigment stones which are small (<0.5 cm) and multiple are found in 30% of gallbladders. They are composed of tightly packed polymerized chains of (deconjugated) bilirubinate; 60% are calcified. They are commonly found in patients with cirrhosis and haemolytic disorders.

Brown-pigment stones are formed in the bile ducts from calcium bilirubinate secondary to increased bacterial β-glucuronidase activity. They are large, soft and commonly occur in patients from the East. They are found in the bile ducts of 30% of Western patients at the time of cholecystectomy, but in 70% of those with 'recurrent' bile duct stones. Retained suture material is the cause in at least 30% of cases. They are rarely radio-opaque. Both cholesterol and brown-pigment stones may be amenable to treatment by extracorporeal shock wave lithotripsy (ESWL).

Chronic cholecystitis

The cardinal feature is the formation of intramural mucosal diverticula between the gallbladder wall muscle bundles (Rokitansky–Aschoff sinuses). Some of the complications which may develop are shown in Table 19.2.

Pain is constant rather than intermittent. Important differential diagnoses include myocardial infarction, peptic ulcer disease and in young women the Curtis–FitzHugh syndrome. 'Biliary dyspepsia' (flatulence and fullness) is not specific to gallstones. The diagnosis needs to be established by ultrasonography (US) which is 95% accurate. Oral cholecystography (OCG) and endoscopic retrograde cholangiopancreatography (ERCP) are occasionally required.

Acute cholecystitis

Obstruction to the cystic duct may lead to a chemical cholecystitis in the first 12–24 h, usually followed by secondary bacterial infection (60–80%). The gallbladder wall becomes oedematous and hypervascular. There is often patchy gangrene of the gallbladder wall

Table 19.2 Possible complications of chronic and acute cholecystitis

Mucocele	Septicaemia
Empyema of the gallbladder	Mirizzi's syndrome
Acute or chronic cholecystitis	Cholecystoduodenal fistula
Gangrenous cholecystitis	Gallstone ileus
Perforation with biliary peritonitis	Cholecystocolic fistula
Emphysematous acute cholecystitis	Cholecystocutaneous fistula
Sub-hepatic abscess	Porcelain gallbladder
Liver abscess	Gallbladder carcinoma

with thrombosis of the cystic artery and its branches. The incidence of bacterial infection increases with age, especially with anaerobic organisms. Spontaneous resolution occurs in about 85% of cases.

There is a fever, a leucocystosis and a rapid pulse. Murphy's sign is usually positive. An impression of a mass in the right upper quadrant is found in 25%. Mild jaundice is present in 10–25%, but this is usually due to Mirizzi's syndrome (see below). Hyperaesthesia (Boas's sign) and cutaneous oedema (Leake's sign) are rare.

Plain radiography is essential to exclude a perforated viscus; it may reveal acute emphysematous cholecystitis (especially in patients with diabetes mellitus) or calcified stones. The diagnosis is established by US. Radionuclide biliary scanning (RBS) using ^{99m}Tc-HIDA may be of value.

Treatment of gallbladder stone disease

The mortality from elective cholecystectomy is 0.5%, with a morbidity of 5%. The mortality is 1% or more in older patients with medical problems. In patients with cirrhosis the overall mortality is higher (5%) and depends on the degree of cirrhosis: the mortality is 1% in those with normal clotting, increasing to 80% if the prothrombin time is >2.5 normal.

Empyema of the gallbladder carries a mortality of 15–25% and is usually caused by a delay in diagnosis, particularly in the elderly.

There is no indication for undertaking cholecystectomy in patients with asymptomatic gallstones unless they have diabetes mellitus or mild cirrhosis.

Patients presenting with biliary colic require analgesia and intravenous fluids and these need to be continued if there is acute cholecystitis. Intravenous antibiotics are required. Surgery should be undertaken during the same admission and indications for urgent intervention are: (a) general clinical deterioration: (b) spreading or generalized peritonitis; (c) empyema of the gallbladder or abscess formation; (d) acute emphysematous cholecystitis

CHOLECYSTODUODENAL FISTULA AND GALLSTONE ILEUS

About 1% of patients develop an internal fistula, 70% of which are cholecystoduodenal which may lead to gallstone ileus. The mortality is high (10–30%) and is related to delay in diagnosis. Stones impact in the terminal ileum (70%); jejunum (15%); duodenal bulb (Bouveret's syndrome) (10%); and rarely the sigmoid colon (usually in association with diverticular stricture). The diagnosis is suggested by (a) pneumobilia (30–50%), (b) 'tumbling obstruction' due to the stone moving, and (c) air in the gallbladder and duodenal bulb, or Balthazar's sign (25%). The simplest operation should be performed (enterotomy). The gallbladder and the gastrointestinal tract need to be palpated to ensure there are no other stones. If there are large stones in the gallbladder, cholecystectomy is carried out. Bile duct stones (20–30%) are managed surgically or endoscopically, depending on the patient's general condition.

MIRIZZI'S SYNDROME AND CHOLECYSTOCHOLEDOCHAL FISTULA

A distended gallbladder may compress the bile duct to cause jaundice. Contraction of the gallbladder due to fibrosis leads to erosion into the main bile duct. Cholecystectomy is indicated for Mirizzi's syndrome. For cholecystocholedochal fistula, a cholecystoduodenostomy is a safer operation. In more complex situations a choledochoplasty (using part of the gallbladder wall) or a choledochojejunostomy Roux-en-Y may be required. The mortality is 1% for the simplest type of fistula, rising to 12% for situations in which the whole circumference of the bile duct has been eroded by the gallbladder stone. Preoperative ERCP is helpful in deciding the best type of operative approach.

Acalculous disease

Chronic acalculous cholecystitis may occur in 5–10% of all chronically symptomatic patients. Acalculous cholecystitis may be primary (50% of cases) or be associated with a predisposing cause (Table 19.3). Gallbladder dysfunction can be diagnosed by serial US or computerized RBS, etc.

Acute acalculous cholecystitis

Ischaemia of the gallbladder (from various causes) is probably the single most important aetiological fac-

Table 19.3   Associated conditions in acalculous cholecystitis

Cholesterolosis	Major sepsis
Adenomyomatosis	Metabolic conditions
Xanthogranulomatous cholecystitis	Torsion of gallbladder
Specific infections:	Porcelain gallbladder
Typhoid	Malignancy
Leptospirosis	Atherosclerosis
Staphylococcus spp.	'Colloid' disorders
Brucellosis	Crohn's disease
Actinomycosis	Kawasaki syndrome
Clonorchiasis	Intraportal chemotherapy
Ascariasis	Sclerosing cholangitis
Trauma:	Haemobilia
Blunt trauma	
Burns	
Surgery (abdominal and extra-abdominal)	

tor. Secondary bacterial infection is similar to that of calculous acute cholecystitis (60–80%). There is, however, a much higher incidence of gangrenous cholecystitis, empyema of the gallbladder and free biliary perforation. Patients with specific underlying infections need appropriate chemotherapy. Urgent cholecystectomy is advised, but this depends on the aetiology and general state of the patient.

Diseases of the bile ducts

Choledocholithiasis

The true prevalence is not known – in one large autopsy series the incidence was 4%. Some 8% of patients with gallstones present with jaundice, but the incidence of bile duct stones at routine cholecystectomy is 15–20% and 45% may remain asymptomatic. Ten per cent of patients with biliary colic pass stones from the gallbladder into the bile duct and then into the duodenum (compared with 100% in patients with acute pancreatitis).

About 10% of patients with symptomatic bile duct stones present with acute cholangitis and 6–8% present with acute pancreatitis.

Acute cholangitis

This is characterized by Charcot's triad: obstructive jaundice, a swinging pyrexia (38°C or more) with rigors, and pain and tenderness over the liver. Jaundice may be occasionally absent (2%). Acute cholangitis may be mild or severe, with complete bile duct obstruction and frank pus in the bile ducts (mortality up to 100%). In severe cholangitis, shock and mental confusion coexist (Reynold and Dargan's 'pentad'). If there is a rise in bile duct pressure to $25\,cmH_2O$ due to obstruction, bile and bacteria are forced across the sinusoids into the hepatic veins and into the systemic circulation. In Western patients, acute cho-

langitis is associated with bacterial infection (80–100%) and is usually secondary to bile duct stones. Strictures of the bile ducts from benign and malignant causes are responsible for acute cholangitis in 5–15%.

Recurrent pyogenic cholangitis (RPC)

This is a common disease of the East and is known as Oriental cholangitis. In contrast, the primary cause is infective (usually due to *Escherichia coli* and sometimes *Clonorchis sinensis*), with secondary bile duct stone formation. Stones are almost always of the brown-pigment variety and less than 30% of patients have stones in the gallbladder. Recurrent pyogenic cholangitis is characterized by biliary strictures of the extrahepatic and/or intrahepatic systems. Liver abscesses and destruction of the liver parenchyma from chronic sepsis occur.

Treatment of choledocholithiasis

Jaundice is not an indication for emergency treatment, but for prompt correction of metabolic disturbances and investigation. Ultrasonography will only detect bile duct stones in 20–50% of cases and direct cholangiography (ERCP) and sometimes percutaneous transhepatic cholangiography (PTHC) is frequently required.

Treatment for acute cholangitis includes hydration with crystalloids and colloids if there is septicaemia, parenteral vitamin K and intravenous antibiotics. Most patients will respond (85%) and semi-elective bile duct decompression can be undertaken with cholecystectomy if the patient is otherwise fit. If the patient does not respond within 24–48 h, this is an indication for urgent decompression. Endoscopic sphincterotomy (ES) is the treatment of choice: surgery carries a mortality (20–30%) several times that of ES (4–5%). If ERCP is not available, percutaneous drainage (at PTHC) will help reduce the operative mortality.

Biliary fistulae

Internal biliary fistulae are usually caused by gallstones (90%); other causes are peptic ulcer (6%), cancer, trauma, parasitic infestation and congenital anomalies. In Western gallstone disease the incidence is about 1%, compared with 15% in Oriental gallstone disease.

Periampullary fistulae are due to iatrogenic trauma from bile duct exploration (Bâkes dilators, etc.) or from stones eroding into the duodenum.

Bronchobiliary and pleurobiliary fistulae presenting in the neonate or young child is a congenital anomaly and needs surgical treatment. In adults this is secondary to gallstones, trauma or parasitic infestation. Endoscopic stenting and/or surgery is required, depending on the exact nature of the fistula.

External biliary fistulae are usually due to iatrogenic injury. Most will spontaneously resolve, provided that there is no distal obstruction. Continued major bile loss (>1 litre/24 h) results in the choledochostomy acidotic syndrome with hypokalaemia, hyponatraemia and acidosis. Fluid replacement is essential and if conservative treatment fails, surgical identification and repair of the site of leakage, clearance of any obstruction, or the establishment of an alternative internal drainage route is required.

Biliary stricture

Iatrogenic trauma is the commonest cause and occurs in 0.3% of cases following cholecystectomy due to failure to demonstrate the biliary anatomy properly, usually owing to inexperience.

If the injury is recognized at the time of surgery, a primary repair should be undertaken. An end-to-end anastomosis is made using interrupted sutures and a T-tube is placed at the site of the anastomosis. If a separate hole is made for the T-tube below the anastomosis, this can compromise the blood supply.

If the stricture is recognized postoperatively, the preferred approach is a Roux-en-Y left hepaticojejunostomy. If the hilum has been destroyed, a direct hilar approach will be required, anastomosing two or more of the main ducts to the Roux-en-Y limb. Good long-term results are obtained in up to 85% of cases, but repeat operations are often required and the long-term mortality is at least 10%.

Sclerosing cholangitis

This is a chronic inflammatory disease producing fibrosis and stricturing of the bile ducts. The aetiology is unknown but may be associated with inflammatory bowel disease (50%) and occasionally with AIDS, recurrent biliary infections, cystic fibrosis and chronic pancreatitis. There is no predisposing factor in 30–40%. It may be predominantly intrahepatic (30%),

extrahepatic (30%) or diffuse (40%). The diagnosis is largely based on cholangiography (ERCP or PTHC). It may be difficult to distinguish sclerosing cholangitis from cholangiocarcinoma with which it is associated.

Treatment is generally unsatisfactory, but useful palliation may be obtained in patients with predominantly extrahepatic involvement by a Roux-en-Y hilar anastomosis. Intrahepatic biliary strictures may be dilated. The additional insertion of two stents through the right and left hepatic ducts may be used to keep the biliary tree and the anastomosis free of obstruction. Progressive liver failure and portal hypertension are important indications for liver transplantation.

Choledochal cysts

These may be classified according to Todani: type I, a solitary fusiform extrahepatic cyst into which the cystic duct drains (80%); type II, a supraduodenal saccular cyst draining into the extrahepatic bile duct (5%); type III, an intraduodenal diverticulum (choledochocele) (5%); type IV, multiple extrahepatic cysts with or without intrahepatic cysts (10%); type V, multiple small intrahepatic cysts (Caroli's disease) (<1%).

They commonly present in neonates or childhood, but 20% present in adults. The clinical features often suggest bile duct stone disease, but a mass may be felt or the patient may present with acute pancreatitis.

The cyst must be excised and this is all that is necessary for type II; a transduodenal sphincteroplasty is required for type III, and a Roux-en-Y hepaticojejunostomy for type I. Extensive intrahepatic involvement will necessitate partial hepatectomy with excision of the extrahepatic biliary tree and a Roux-en-Y cholangiojejunostomy.

Post-cholecystectomy syndrome

Up to 50% of patients develop significant symptoms after cholecystectomy. The syndrome defines a clinical situation in which the patient complains of a return of the original symptoms without jaundice. A third of patients have extrabiliary disease such as peptic ulcer, irritable bowel syndrome and diverticular disease. A proportion have psychiatric problems.

Important biliary causes are retained bile duct stones, strictures, chronic pancreatitis and tumours of the pancreas and biliary tree. Thorough investigation, including ERCP, is necessary. Approximately 10% of patients have genuine sphincter of Oddi dysfunction (either stenosis or dysmotility). This may be diagnosed by manometry of the sphincter at ERCP. The treatment of sphincter of Oddi dysfunction is endoscopic sphincterotomy or transduodenal sphincteroplasty. Good long-term results are obtained in about 70% of patients.

Tumours of the gallbladder and extrahepatic biliary tree

Gallbladder cancer is the commonest form of biliary tract cancer, with an incidence of 10–20% relative to that of pancreatic cancer. It occurs predominantly in females (3:1) and is nearly always associated with gallstones. The peak age incidence is 70–75 years. Most patients present with an abdominal mass due to advanced malignancy. Long-term survival is poor unless the diagnosis is made preoperatively or is found as a histological surprise following cholecystectomy for gallstones (3%). The 5-year survival for the latter group is 15%.

Carcinomas of the ampulla of Vater and lower bile duct are much less common but the resectability rate is higher (60%). The 5-year survival rates for ampullary cancer vary from 30% to 60% and for low bile duct cancers 10–25%. A number of bypass procedures are available for obstructive jaundice, operative and non-operative (endoscopic or percutaneous). In younger patients, the surgical option is preferred. It is important to ensure that a suitable bypass is feasible prior to laparotomy. Laparoscopy may prove useful in avoiding laparotomy altogether.

Anatomical variations

It is important to understand common variations to undertake safe biliary surgery. The usual arrangement of the cystic duct (Figure 19.1a) occurs in only 70% of cases. Low entry of the cystic duct (Figure 19.1b,c) occurs in 25%. Unusual arrangements of the main hepatic ducts are uncommon, but failure to appreciate these anomalies (Figure 19.2) can cause major postoperative problems. The blood supply of the extrahepatic main bile duct comes from a vascular arcade between the gastroduodenal artery and the right hepatic artery (Figure 19.3). Excessive destruction of this arcade during dissection can lead to postoperative stricture.

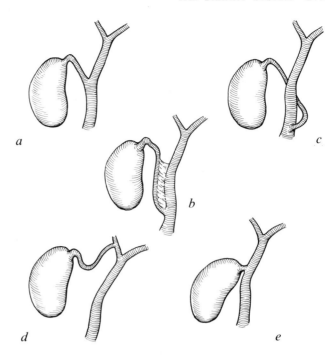

Figure 19.1 Variations in the site of the cystic to the biliary tree. *a*, Most common site of insertion into the main bile duct (MBD). *b*, A low insertion into the right side of the MBD with a long parallel course. *c*, A low insertion into the MBD following a posterior course. *d*, Insertion into the right hepatic duct. *e*, Direct insertion of the gallbladder neck into the MBD

Calot originally described an important anatomical triangle between the common hepatic duct, cystic duct and cystic artery. Currently, the superior border is taken as the inferior surface of the liver between the right hepatic duct and Hartmann's pouch, since this contains all the important structures. The hepatic portal vein, right hepatic portal vein and left hepatic portal vein lie posterior to the respective bile ducts and hepatic arteries. Important variations of the cystic artery are shown in Figure 19.4. Note that the right hepatic artery or proper hepatic artery can lie in

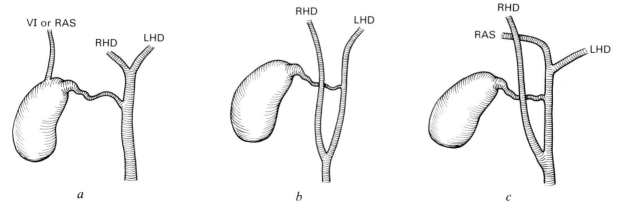

Figure 19.2 Abnormal variations of the extrahepatic biliary system. *a*, The segment IV or right posterior sectorial (RPS) duct drains directly into the gallbladder. *b*, The right and left hepatic ducts combine distally from the hepatic hilum; *c*, The right anterior sectorial (RAS) duct joins the main bile duct distal to the hilum (RHD, right hepatic duct; LHD, left hepatic duct)

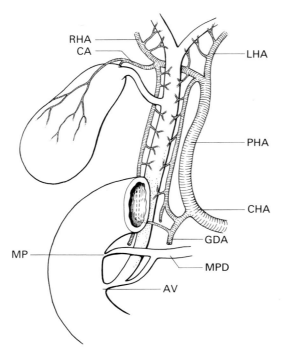

Figure 19.3 Arterial blood supply to the extrahepatic biliary tree. The main supply comes in from the 3 o'clock and 9 o'clock arteries laterally positioned (RHA, right hepatic artery; LHA, left hepatic artery; CA, cysticartery; PHA, proper hepatic artery, CHA, common hepatic artery. GDA, gastroduodenal artery, MP, minor papilla; MPD, main pancreatic duct; AV, ampulla of Vater)

Calot's triangle at sites where they can easily be damaged (Figure 19.4e,f). The right hepatic vein can also be quite superficial and be prone to injury in the triangle.

The liver is divided into eight anatomical segments, each with its own bile duct, hepatic venous drainage and hepatic portal venous and hepatic arterial supply. The right liver consists of segments V–VIII and the left liver segments I–IV (Figure 19. 5). In about 30% of individuals the right hepatic artery is either entirely replaced (10%) or there is an additional (accessory) branch (10%) arising from the superior mesenteric artery (SMA). Similar anomalies (20%) occur for the left hepatic artery arising from the left gastric artery. In 3% the entire hepatic artery arises from the SMA and rarely (0.2%) from the left gastric artery. Anomalies of the portal vein are rare, but may involve the hepatic portal vein lying completely anterior to the duodenum.

It is essential that patients with complex biliary disease have preoperative cholangiography by ERCP, PTHC or both, and those undergoing surgery involving hilar structures or liver resections must have preoperative selective hepatic arteriography. The venous phase of this procedure may provide useful information regarding the hepatic portal venous system. Computed tomography (CT) scanning is essential in patients with cancer, for staging and planning resection.

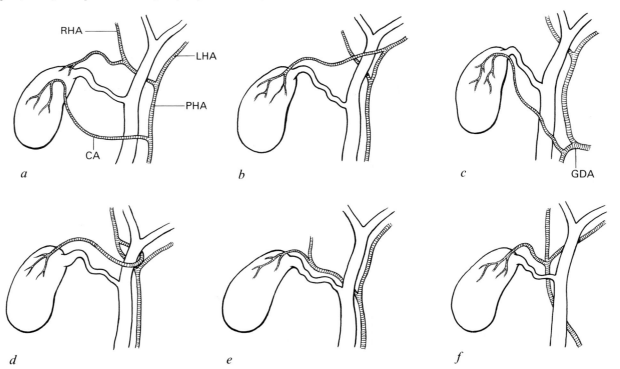

Figure 19.4 Common variations of the cystic artery (CA). *a*, The main (anterior) CA leaves the proper hepatic artery (PHA) and crosses the main bile duct (MPD) distally while the posterior branch of the CA arises from the right hepatic artery (RHA). *b*, The CA arises from the left hepatic artery (LHA). *c*, The CA artery arises from the gastroduodenal artery (GDA). *d*, the CA artery arises from the LHA but first travels posteriorly around the MBD. *e*, The RHA travels parallel to the cystic duct. *f*, The bifurcation of the RHA and LHA occurs within Calot's triangle

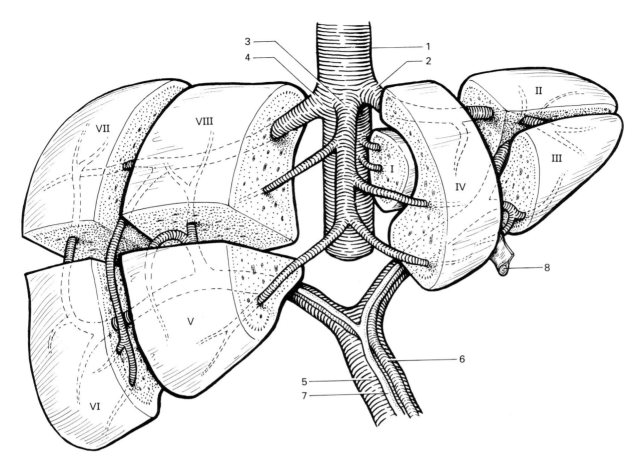

Figure 19.5 The eight segments (I–VIII) of the liver exploded to show the ductal and blood supply (1, inferior vena cava; 2, left hepatic vein; 3, middle hepatic vein; 4, right hepatic vein; 5, hepatic portal vein; 6, proper hepatic artery; 7, common bile duct; 8, round ligament)

Biliary surgery – general considerations

The operation should be explained to the patient beforehand and consent obtained. It is important to discuss likely problems with the patient and relatives if a major procedure is planned. With rare exceptions, a general anaesthetic with endotracheal intubation is used. Patients undergoing relatively straightforward biliary procedures require:

1. Prophylactic heparin.
2. Prophylactic antibiotics.
3. Blood grouping and serum saved.

Patients with obstructive jaundice require:

1. Adequate preoperative hydration: intravenous crystalloids for at least 24 h prior to surgery.
2. Bladder catheter for preoperative, operative and postoperative urine measurement.
3. Preoperative correction of anaemia (< 10 g/dl).
4. Preoperative correction of low albumin (< 30 g/dl) with human albumin.

5. Correction of clotting disorders with parenteral vitamin K and fresh frozen plasma.
6. Prophylactic antibiotics.
7. Blood cross-matched (2–6 units depending on the situation) and fresh frozen plasma freely available.
8. Mannitol (100 ml of 20%) given at the start of surgery and subsequently to maintain a urine output of > 60 ml/h.

Lactulose 20 ml orally b.d. preoperatively is recommended to reduce the endotoxin load to liver. Intravenous H_2 blockade is recommended perioperatively to reduce the risk of postoperative haemorrhage (which is increased in jaundiced patients).

The patient lies supine. The skin is prepared with antiseptic solution from the mid-chest to below the groin and draped to expose the right upper quadrant for benign procedures. If peroperative cholangiography using X-ray plates is contemplated, the patient's position is checked on the table before starting the operation. Appropriate venous access and monitoring (blood pressure, pulse, ECG and respiratory gases) are mandatory.

In patients undergoing major resections for gall-bladder or bile duct cancer, additional venous access, CVP measurements and an arterial pressure line are required.

For routine gallbladder and bile duct operations, the following incisions may be used: (a) Kocher's right subcostal (good access); (b) right upper quadrant transverse (good cosmesis); (c) midline; (d) right paramedian. Patients undergoing major resections for cancer or difficult bypass procedures usually require a bigger incision, (e) bilateral subcostal ('rooftop' or 'chevron' incision) – if there is a narrow costal angle an upwards midline extension is helpful ('Mercedes Benz' incision).

Drainage is collected using a small soft tube drain or vacuum drain. Many surgeons do not place drains.

Catgut should not be used in biliary surgery except to obtain minor haemostasis. Non-absorbable sutures such as silk should also be avoided. Fine prolene should be used for vascular repair or vascular anastomosis. Slowly absorbed sutures such as Vicryl (braided) for ties and PDS (monofilament) for biliary anastomosis are recommended.

The subcostal incisions may be closed in two layers using slowly absorbable and/or non-absorbable monofilament (such as prolene); some surgeons use mass closure, but this can be difficult in the obese. The skin is closed with a subcuticular suture.

Biliary operations for benign disease

Cholecystectomy

The surgeon stands on the patient's right, the first assistant on the left and the second assistant on the surgeon's right side. The gallbladder, liver and hepatoduodenal ligament are inspected and palpated to confirm the diagnosis and exclude other pathology. Any congenital or inflammatory adhesions between the gallbladder, duodenum and/or hepatic flexure are divided with scissors following counter-traction.

A pack is inserted into the right paracolic gutter to hold bowel out of the operating field. A folded pack is placed over the hepatoduodenal ligament and the first assistant's left hand is used to provide left oblique-downwards traction. A retractor (Deaver or short Lloyd-Davies) is used by the first assistant's right hand to provide right oblique-upwards traction from the liver hilum. A small swab is placed between the retractor and the liver to prevent displacement and liver injury. The neck of the gallbladder is grasped with forceps (Moynihan's) and right oblique-down-wards traction is applied by the second assistant. This three-way traction fully exposes Calot's triangle. With an adequate incision, a self-retaining wound retractor is not usually required (and can make the operation more difficult).

A small swab is placed in the pouch of Rutherford Morison to collect any blood or spilt bile. The peritoneal edge at the junction of the gallbladder and cystic duct is divided with scissors. Using the closed tips of the scissors, the peritoneum over Calot's triangle is lifted anteriorly. This is now divided towards the liver hilum: the deeper blade of the scissors should be seen through the transparent peritoneum clearly with no intervening structures (Figure 19.6). Using a small pledget ('peanut' swab), the peritoneum is pushed away from the gallbladder towards the main bile duct. If there is a lot of fatty tissue in the triangle, squeezing and rubbing this between the right index finger and thumb will help to reveal the anatomy.

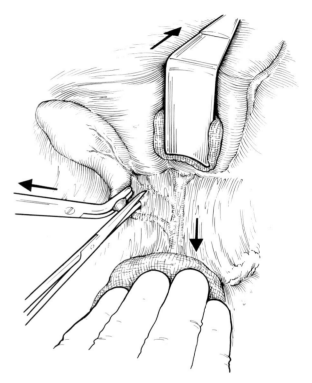

Figure 19.6 Cholecystectomy 1. Three-way traction being applied to Calot's triangle by the liver retractor, the assistant's left hand over the hepatoduodenal ligament and Moynihan's forceps grasping the lower edge of the gallbladder (arrows). The taut anterior peritoneum over Calot's triangle can now be safely divided by scissors

The cystic duct is cleared of surrounding tissue from its origin to the border of the main bile duct. This can be done with curved forceps (Lahey's) being inserted into Calot's triangle adjacent to the duct and gently opened. It is not necessary to identify the entry of the cystic into the main bile duct in all cases. This can be dangerous in the 25% or so cases in which there is a low entry. The cystic duct should be palpated to feel for any small stones which can be milked back into the gallbladder with finger and thumb or partly closed curved forceps.

The arrival of the cystic artery onto the gallbladder must clearly be seen. It is nearly always associated with a sizeable cystic duct lymph node. With traction on the gallbladder, the artery feels like a taut string and relaxation will allow a pulse to be felt. A ligature is passed around this using an aneurysm needle and tied away from the gallbladder. A second ligature is applied, tying towards the gallbladder; if the artery is long, the distal end can be diathermied on the gallbladder. The cystic artery is divided. The proximal part of the cystic duct is similarly ligated and an artery forceps applied to the ligature is used to retract the cystic duct to the right (Figure 19.7). A loose ligature is applied around the distal part of the cystic duct and a peroperative cholangiogram (POC) is performed. Once the cholangiogram has been performed, the cystic duct stump is ligated. Excessive force in tying the knot should be avoided as this can cause necrosis of the cystic duct stump at the site of the ligature. The cystic duct is divided.

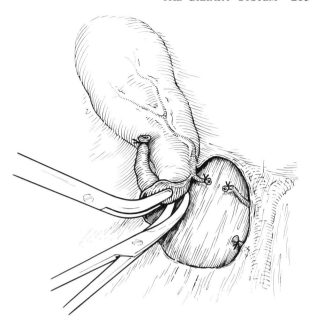

Figure 19.8 Cholecystectomy 3. The cystic duct has been divided and ligated. Traction on the gallbladder neck reveals the plane of dissection. The scissors are used to divide the fascial attachments keeping close to the gallbladder wall

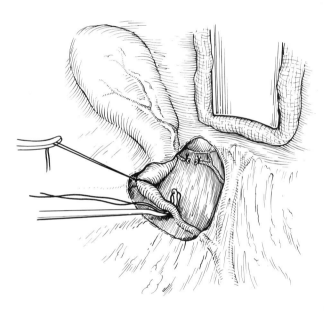

Figure 19.7 Cholecystectomy 2. The peritoneum has been divided and swept away from Calot's triangle. The cystic artery has been ligated and divided. The proximal cystic duct has been ligated and made taut by traction on the undivided ligature, enabling the aneurysm and the second cystic duct ligature to be introduced

The gallbladder can be removed in a neck or fundus-first manner. The neck of the gallbladder is grasped with tissue forceps and pulled towards the surgeon. The gallbladder is dissected from the liver bed using scissors. It is important that the tips of the scissors should always face the gallbladder and the scissor cuts must be made on the gallbladder wall to avoid trauma to the liver (Figure 19.8). Bleeding from the cut edge of the peritoneum or liver bed is dealt with by diathermy as the dissection proceeds. After cholecystectomy, residual bleeding in the gallbladder fossa is dealt with by diathermy. The peritoneum over the gallbladder fossa need not be closed.

In the fundus-first approach, 10–20 ml of N/saline are injected into the potential space between the liver and the gallbladder. The fundus of the gallbladder is grasped with tissue forceps (Duval's) and pulled towards the first assistant. A cutting diathermy point may be used instead of scissors to remove the gallbladder from the liver bed (Figure 19.9). It is important to stay close to the gallbladder as the neck of the gallbladder is approached. The natural plane of the gallbladder plate of fascia is towards the hilum. If dissection has veered towards the liver side of this plate, inadvertent injury can occur.

The gallbladder should be opened to confirm the pathology and an additional opening may indicate an 'accessory' cystic duct which should then be looked for at the operation site. Rarely, a part of the common bile duct and/or common hepatic duct may be attached to the cystic duct, indicating a major iatrogenic injury. These types of injuries can be entirely avoided by careful dissection and appreciation of anatomical variations (see Figures 19.1, 19.2 and 19.4) and distortions that can occur during surgery (Figure 19.10).

Peroperative cholangiography

The origin of the cystic duct is secured and a small artery forceps is used to hold the loose ends of the suture. Light traction is placed on this suture towards the right. A second suture is loosely placed around the distal end of the cystic duct but not tied. Using scissors, a small cut is made in the cystic duct close to the gallbladder. A probe may be required to break down the valves of Heister and identify the direction

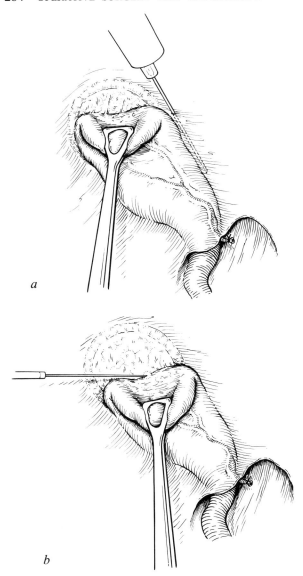

a

b

Figure 19.9 Fundus-first dissection of the gallbladder. *a*, A Duval's tissue forceps is used to retract the fundus of the gallbladder to the left and 10–20 ml of saline injected into the space between the gallbladder and the liver. *b*, Diathermy is now used to dissect the gallbladder free

of the duct. A variety of cannulas can be used including the Stoke-on-Trent cannula and a ureteric cannula. The Gourevitch metal cannula combines the best features of the Stoke-on-Trent instrument, but being metal cannot be occluded by the fixing ligature and can be used as a probe.

The cannula, with a long transparent extension tube, is filled with saline, excluding air bubbles. With an attached syringe it is inserted into the cystic duct with the syringe plunger continuously pressed by an assistant. Once in the duct, the loose ligature is tied and the cannula withdrawn so the tip lies in the cystic

duct (Figure 19.11). If there is any doubt about the anatomy, a snugging ligature is used (Figure 19.12). The proximal end of the extension tube is held outside of the abdomen below the level of the cystic duct and the syringe removed. Retrograde bile flow should then appear in the extension tubing. The 20 ml syringe containing contrast (40% Hypaque diluted 1:1 with *N*/saline) is then connected.

All packs and clamps are removed from the abdomen. A drape is placed over the operation site and its centre marked with a drop of saline. The patient is rotated slightly towards the right. The portable X-ray machine is centred over the biliary system and three films are taken. The amount of contrast used depends on the size of the ducts, but for the average individual, successive volumes of 3 ml, 5 ml and 12 ml give excellent results (total = 20 ml). The anaesthetist is asked to stop ventilation of the patient just before each of the three radiographs is taken.

The POC is considered normal if (a) both the extrahepatic and intrahepatic systems are clearly visualized; (b) contrast has entered the duodenum; (c) there are no filling defects; and (d) there is no leakage of contrast.

If no contrast has entered the duodenum, delayed films are taken with the use of a spasmolytic.

Screening cholangiography allows the observation of contrast in the biliary tree during contrast injection. It may occasionally detect anomalies missed by other techniques.

If difficulties are encountered during POC, the need for continuing with the procedure should be reviewed as injury or damage may occur. Many surgeons pursue an effective selective policy of performing POC (Table 19.4). Following completion, the ligature around the cystic duct is cut using a small blade on a long handle. The end of the cyst duct is grasped with curved forceps and ligated. If the cystic duct cannot be cannulated and a POC is strongly indicated, this can be undertaken by inserting a butterfly needle with long extension tubing directly into the main bile duct and the procedure repeated. Occasionally, postoperative leakage follows this technique.

Table 19.4 Criteria associated with an increased chance of finding bile duct stones and used as the basis for selective cholangiography during cholecystectomy

History of jaundice
History of acute biliary pancreatitis
Multiple small gallbladder stones
A wide cystic duct
Main bile duct > 10 mm
Elevated serum bilirubin or liver enzymes

Difficulties encountered during cholecystectomy

Good assistance, adequate exposure and good lighting are essential. In some patients the fundus-first

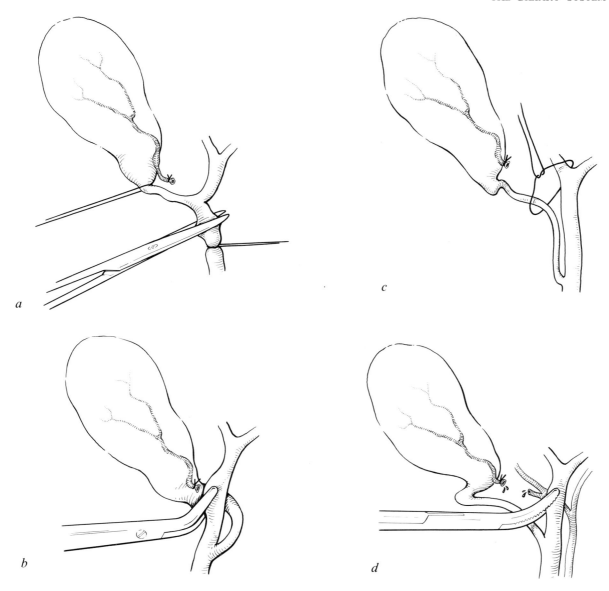

Figure 19.10 Ways in which extrahepatic anatomy can be damaged iatrogenically. *a*, A narrow common bile duct has been misinterpreted as a continuation of the cystic duct. *b*, The common hepatic duct has been grasped at the same time as the gallbladder neck. *c*, The ligature around the cystic duct also includes the right hepatic duct. *d*, In an attempt to place an arterial forceps around the base of a torn cystic artery, the right hepatic artery and common hepatic duct are included

approach may be the only practicable approach to removing the gallbladder. There is often no tissue plane and it is important to stay close to the gallbladder. A useful manoeuvre in this situation is to open the fundus of the gallbladder, aspirate the bile and remove the stones. The left index finger is then inserted into the gallbladder to help delineate the gallbladder among the mass of fibrotic tissue. A probe may be inserted into the cystic duct to identify this structure. Detection of the cystic artery may be difficult or impossible and is only recognized once it is divided!

If the main cystic artery, or an accessory artery, is divided before it is ligated, no attempt should be made to grasp this with forceps. A swab is pressed into Calot's triangle and any pooled blood aspirated. The swab is removed and the bleeding vessel secured with a transfixion suture picking up tissue which is immediately adjacent to the artery. If a main hepatic artery or the right hepatic portal vein is injured, this should be repaired with a 5/0 prolene arterial suture avoiding application of artery forceps. In the case of an artery, the bleeding point may be pinched with dissecting forceps while the prolene is inserted. Dissecting forceps applied to a bleeding, partly embedded, right hepatic portal vein can be dangerous by

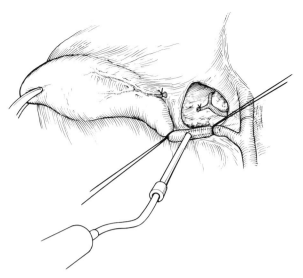

Figure 19.11 Insertion of a Gourevitch metal cannula for performing a peroperative cholangiogram

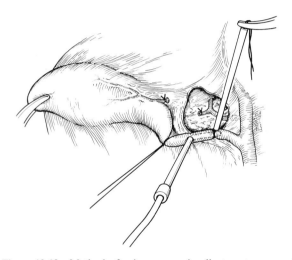

Figure 19.12 Method of using a snugging ligature to secure the Gourevitch metal cannula

producing tearing. Pringle's manoeuvre (pinching the hepatoduodenal ligament) may help in reducing bleeding while the bleeding site is sutured.

The blood supply to the gallbladder in acute cholecystitis or acute or chronic cholecystitis may largely derive from the liver bed, since the cystic artery is often thrombosed. Bleeding from the liver bed can be troublesome. A gauze swab should be pressed into the gallbladder fossa for 5–10 min. Bleeding is then arrested with diathermy forceps or ball-end diathermy. If the liver parenchyma is torn, this is secured with a figure-of-eight transfixion suture. Large needles should be avoided as there are major structures deep to the gallbladder fossa which can be damaged. Small bile leaks, either from a small superficial bile duct in the gallbladder fossa or an

'accessory' cystic duct, are secured with a transfixion suture.

Occasionally it will be found that the cystic duct is congenitally absent (rare) or more likely it has been destroyed by fibrosis and has been replaced by a small cholecystocholedochal fistula. If there is any doubt an on-table cholecystogram should be performed by needle puncture of the gallbladder or the gallbladder opened and the opening into the bile duct shown by a probe. In this case, a 95% cholecystectomy is performed. The remaining gallbladder wall attached to the bile duct is closed (choledochoplasty).

Partial cholecystectomy

Rarely the gallbladder is so involved with fibrosis that safe cholecystectomy cannot be performed. In this case, the gallbladder wall as it attaches to the liver can be removed with cutting diathermy. Any remaining gallbladder mucosa should be fulgurated. It may have been destroyed by the inflammation. A POC can be performed from inside the gallbladder through the opening of the cystic duct. It is not often patent. No attempt should be made to identify the cystic artery. If patent, the cystic duct can be occluded by transfixion sutures as it opens into the gallbladder (Figure 19.13).

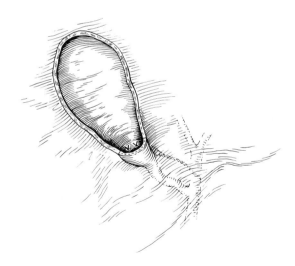

Figure 19.13 Partial cholecystectomy for severe chronic cholecystitis. Note that Calot's triangle has not been dissected. Interrupted sutures have been used to ensure obliteration of the cystic duct as it opens into the remaining part of the gallbladder

Cholecystostomy

Occasionally cholecystostomy under local anaesthesia is indicated. It is important to locate the gallbladder accurately using ultrasonography. Following infiltration of the skin, muscle and peritoneum with 1% lignocaine, a 3 cm incision is made through the skin

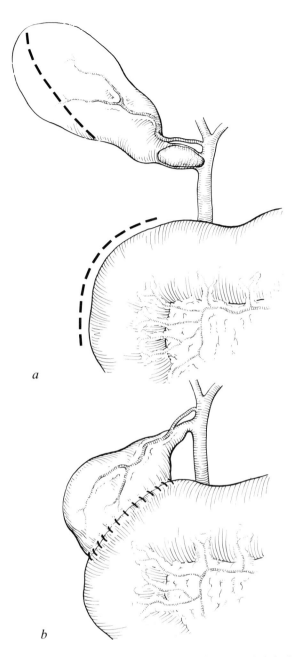

a

b

Figure 19.14 Partial cholecystectomy for a cholecystocholedochal fistula. *a*, The duodenum is Kocherized and the fundus of the gallbladder is excised, enabling removal of the gallstone. *b*, A side-to-side cholecystoduodenostomy has been fashioned

and aponeurosis and then splitting the muscle. Intravenous analgesia (pethidine) and sedation (short-acting benzodiazepine) may be required. A purse-string suture is placed in the fundus and an incision is made in the centre of this and bile aspirated. The stones are removed, paying particular attention to removing stones lodged in Hartmann's pouch. Clearance should be confirmed by inserting a flexible choledochoscope into the gallbladder.

A large Foley or Malecot catheter is placed into the gallbladder and secured with the purse-string suture. The incision is closed with interrupted sutures. The catheter may be used for subsequent cholecystography. If there are retained stones, the tract is used for clearance using a choledochoscope. The catheter should be removed at 4–6 weeks.

A similar technique may be employed at laparotomy, but cholecystectomy is to be preferred.

Cholecystoduodenostomy

A cholecystocholedochal fistula is often involved with intense fibrosis of the gallbladder. In this situation, a partial cholecystectomy is performed and a cholecystoduodenostomy is fashioned using a single layer of interrupted sutures (Figure 19.14) following Kocherization of the duodenum. Any stones in the bile duct should be removed and this may be possible through the fistula itself (see below).

Supraduodenal choledocholithotomy

The anterior part of the extrahepatic main bile duct lying just above the duodenum is cleared of peritoneum for 3 cm. Two fine stay sutures are placed in the centre of this area, one on each side of the midline of the duct. The bile duct is lifted up with the stay sutures and an incision of 0.5 cm is made with a small scalpel. Confirmation of the anatomy is obtained by proof puncture before incising. The incision is enlarged using angled Pott's scissors and bile aspirated by a suction tube.

The number of stones and their location should have been determined by POC and any lying near the choledochotomy are milked out using finger and thumb. Unless the second part of the duodenum is very mobile, it should be Kocherized. The attachment of the hepatic flexure and transverse mesocolon to the mid-portion of the second part of the duodenum is retracted downwards and divided. The upper and lower parts of the second part of the duodenum are grasped with two pairs of Duval's forceps and retracted towards the left. The posterior peritoneum 1 cm to the right of the duodenum is picked up with tissue forceps and divided with scissors parallel with the second part of the duodenum. Small vessels running in the peritoneum are diathermied, avoiding injury to the veins supplying the duodenum, the inferior vena cava and the right renal vein. Further retraction of the duodenum will allow the left-hand fingers to be inserted behind the duodenum and the head of the pancreas. Any stones in the lower end of the bile duct can be felt between the fingers and thumb.

Various techniques are used to remove stones:

1. Simple flushing of the bile ducts with a Nelaton's catheter and saline.
2. Désjardins forceps: the acutely angled forceps

should be used for exploring the lower bile duct; slightly angled forceps for entering the right and left hepatic ducts (Figure 19.15).

3. Fogarty balloon catheter retrieval.
4. Dormia basket or balloon via the flexible choledochoscope.

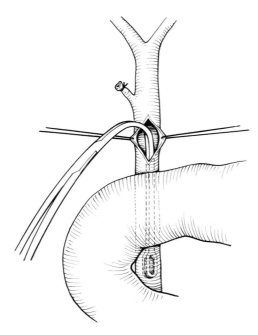

Figure 19.15 Exploration of the main bile duct. The choledochotomy is held open by stay sutures and an acutely curved Désjardin's forceps is being used to retrieve a stone from the lower common bile duct

At the end of the procedure, duct clearance is checked by flexible choledochoscopy. One disadvantage of this technique is that it tends to push small stones into the small intrahepatic biliary radicles. If this is suspected, at least three passes into the intrahepatic ducts are needed as the turbulence of the flushing saline often forces the stones out.

The use of choledochoscopy has significantly reduced the incidence of retained stones, but insertion of a soft T-tube (latex) is prudent. The T-limbs should be shortened to avoid blocking the junction of the hepatic ducts proximally and occluding the pancreatic duct distally. It should also be guttered and a central 'V' cut out to minimize trauma on its removal. The bile duct is closed around the T-tube by a single layer of interrupted sutures and is brought out laterally through the skin by the straightest route. It may be secured to the skin indirectly by pulling the T-tube through a small cylinder of the same tubing which is sutured to the skin (Figure 19.16).

A T-tube cholangiogram is performed at 5–6 days. If there are no retained stones, the T-tube is cut close to the skin and clamped. If there are no symptoms,

the patient is discharged home to return 4–6 weeks later for removal of the T-tube as a day case. Some remove the tube at 10 days. The length of hospital stay can be reduced and the risk of bile leakage, which may occur if the tube is pulled out earlier, is lessened.

Retained stones can be dealt with by saline flushing and spasmolytics such as sublingual GTN may help. Endoscopic sphincterotomy can be used to remove the stones during the same admission. Alternatively, the T-tube tract can be dilated at 4–6 weeks and the stones removed using a choledoscope or steerable Dormia basket.

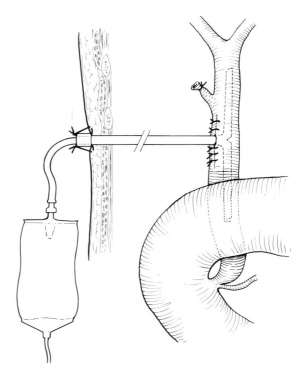

Figure 19.16 A secured T-tube following insertion into the main bile duct. Note that the T-tube has been guttered and has a central 'V' cut out. Interrupted sutures have been used to close the bile duct. The T-tube has been secured using a small cuff of the T-tube itself, the latter only being sutured to the skin

Transduodenal sphincteroplasty

This approach should not be used to explore the bile duct routinely as there is a small but significant risk of severe acute pancreatitis. The main indications are:

1. An impacted stone in the ampulla of Vater which cannot be removed from above.
2. Re-exploration for retained stones when the main extrahepatic bile duct is < 1.5 cm in diameter or is involved in dense fibrosis.
3. Dysfunction of the ampulla of Vater.
4. Choledochocele.

The transverse mesocolon is dissected off the second part of the duodenum which is then Kocher-

divided for 0.5 cm with Pott's scissors and both edges on each side are sutured with interrupted 4/0 sutures. One end of the sutures is kept long for traction with fine artery forceps. The procedure is repeated until 2–3 cm of the sphincter is divided (Figure 19.17b). The diameter of the sphincteroplasty will be 6–10 mm depending on the size of the duct. The apical suture is very important in order to avoid retroperitoneal bile leakage. The duodenum is closed using a single layer of interrupted sutures.

Choledochoduodenostomy

This is an excellent procedure, especially in elderly patients. The indications are:

1. Main extrahepatic bile duct >15 mm.
2. Multiple stones (<5).
3. Acute cholangitis.
4. Reoperation for retained stones.
5. Benign stricture of the lower bile duct.

The duodenum is Kocherized. A 3 cm longitudinal incision is made in the supraduodenal bile duct. A 3 cm incision is made at right angles to this in the duodenum centred over the bile duct (Figure 19.18a). A single-layer anastomosis using interrupted sutures is fashioned. The posterior layer is first made, with the knots on the inside of the anastomosis (Figure 19.18b). The anterior layer has the knots on the outside of the anastomosis.

A minority develop 'sump' syndrome with bacterial overgrowth in the lower end of the bile duct, due to food debris or narrowing of the stoma. Treatment is endoscopic by removal of the food debris, performing an endoscopic sphincterotomy or enlarging the stoma.

Hepaticojejunostomy and choledochojejunostomy

Roux-en-Y

If the hilum is not involved, the operation of choice for a bile duct stricture is a Roux-en-Y left hepaticojejunostomy. The course of the left hepatic duct is largely extrahepatic. It is approached by lowering the liver plate at the hilum. A retractor at the hilum is used to retract the liver cranially. The fascia over the hilum is divided using dissection forceps and scissors. The bifurcation of the bile duct should be clearly seen, with the left hepatic artery running along its inferior margin. The fascia over the left hepatic duct is divided for 4–6 cm (Figure 19.19). Care should be taken as it courses into the liver parenchyma because it is often crossed by a vessel at this point.

A longitudinal incision of 4–5 cm is made in the left hepatic duct. About a dozen sutures are passed through the upper border and held individually with small artery forceps without cutting the needles off. These are used to retract the upper border of the bile

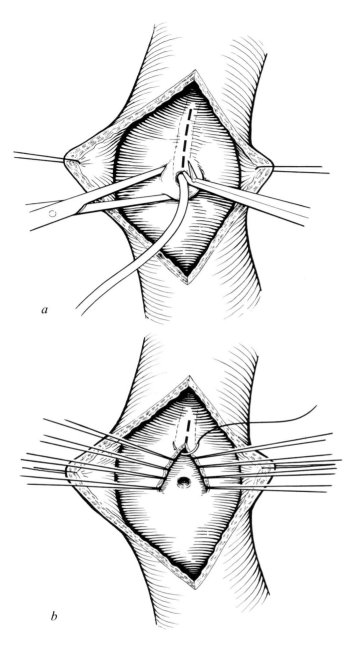

Figure 19.17 Transduodenal sphincteroplasty. *a*, A longitudinal duodenotomy has been made after Kocherization and the duodenum is held open by two stay sutures. Tissue forceps lift the side of the ampulla upwards. The ampulla is being divided by Pott's scissors along the line of a catheter passing from (or into) the bile duct. *b*, The bile duct mucosa is sutured to the duodenal mucosa as the division of the ampulla proceeds. The pancreatic duct is visible

ized. A longitudinal 4 cm incision is made opposite the ampulla of Vater, which is two-thirds of the way down the second part of the duodenum. A tissue forceps is placed on the right side of the ampulla which helps to bring it comfortably into the operating field on retracting anteriorly (Figure 19.17). A fine catheter is passed into the ampulla which should then be felt in the supraduodenal bile duct. The ampulla is

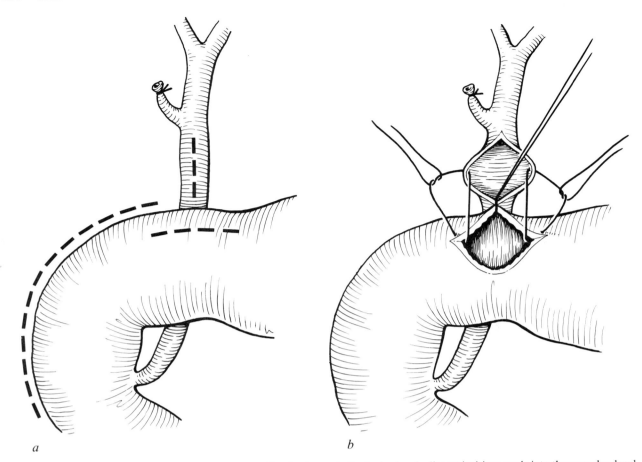

a   *b*

Figure 19.18   Side-to-side choledochoduodenostomy. *a*, The duodenum is Kocherized and adjacent incisions made into the supraduodenal bile duct and proximal duodenum. *b*, A central posterior suture has secured the lower end of the bile duct incision to the mid-point of the upper (right) side of the duodenal incision. Lateral sutures have also been placed but not tied. The posterior layer will be completed using interrupted sutures (knots inside). The anterior layer will be fashioned, first starting centrally (knots outside)

duct upwards. The lower (posterior) anastomosis to the Roux-en-Y is then fashioned using interrupted sutures, knots on the inside. The upper (anterior) anastomosis is then made using the sutures already inserted into the bile duct, knots on the outside (Figure 19.20). There should be no tension on the Roux-en-Y limb. Additional sutures between the ligamentum teres and the Roux limb can be used to relieve any angular tension.

If the junction of the right and left hepatic ducts is involved in the stricture, it will be necessary to trace the right and left bile ducts until they are of normal calibre. In order to do this, a hilar liver split may be necessary. The ducts are anastomosed in an end-to-side manner using interrupted sutures.

In patients with sclerosing cholangitis or RPC with intrahepatic strictures, it may be desirable to dilate these and leave stents *in situ*. When the dilatation is complete, a dilator is pushed through the liver parenchyma to the surface. A silastic tube of appropriate size with drainage holes is forced over the nipple of the dilator and pulled through into the site of the anastomosis, before the anterior layer has been com-

pleted. This is passed through the anastomosis and out through an enterotomy lower down. The anterior anastomosis is now completed. Both ends are brought out through the skin and an O-tube established with a connecting piece. The tube may be flushed or changed when necessary because of clogging.

By leaving the proximal limb of the Roux-en-Y long, it can be brought out of the abdomen and secured just below the skin. This access hepaticojejunostomy can be used to insert a choledochoscope into the hepatic ducts for treatment of recurrent strictures by balloon dilatation or removal of stones by Dormia extraction in RPC (Figure 19.21).

A side-to-side Roux-en-Y hepatic or choledochojejunostomy may be used for major bile duct defects following trauma. An end-to-side hepaticojejunostomy is required following excision of a choledochal cyst.

It is important to observe three important principles with these types of anastomoses.

1. A side-to-side anastomosis is performed if it is possible, rather than an end-to-side anastomosis.

2. A single-layered anastomosis using interrupted sutures is used (as in all biliary anastomoses).
3. The most difficult anastomosis is performed first (the posterior layer).

Stents are not usually required unless the bile duct anastomosed is small or is likely to restricture.

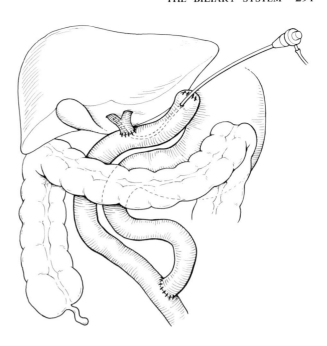

Figure 19.21 Access Roux-en-Y hepaticojejunostomy for recurrent hepaticolithiasis

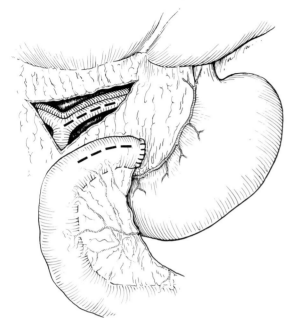

Figure 19.19 Left hepaticojejunostomy. A Roux-en-Y jejunal loop has been advanced up to the exposed left hepatic duct which lies in the left hilar area extrahepatically. The sites of incision for the side-to-side anastomosis are shown

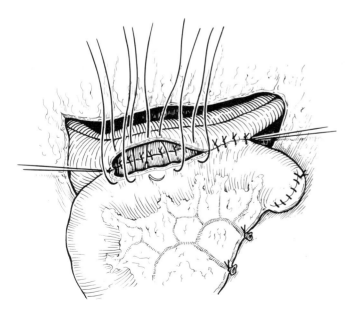

Figure 19.20 The posterior anastomosis is fashioned first using interrupted sutures (knots inside). The figure shows the outer anastomosis (knots outside) being completed.

Biliary operations for malignant disease

Radical resection of the gallbladder

Appropriate planning can be undertaken with US and CT if the diagnosis is made preoperatively. If an apparently resectable gallbladder cancer is found unexpectedly at laparotomy, it may be more appropriate to take a biopsy and close the abdomen. Further investigation with a view to early definitive surgery should be undertaken. If the diagnosis is made from histological examination, the need for further surgery will depend upon the stage.

The usual extent of a radical gallbladder resection is shown in Figure 19.22 which includes resection of liver segments IVa and V. In principle, the lymphatic resection begins at the common hepatic artery. It is identified at its origin from the coeliac axis following division of the lesser omentum. The right gastric artery and pyloric vein are divided in order to achieve complete lymphatic clearance. The duodenum is Kocherized. The hepatoduodenal ligament is opened longitudinally and slings are placed around the main bile duct and hepatic artery. The bile duct is ligated and divided as it enters the pancreatic parenchyma. Retraction of the bile duct reveals the hepatic portal vein, which is dissected up to the hilum.

Full mobilization of the liver is required and is achieved by dividing the falciform, right triangular and coronary ligaments. The hilar structures are exposed following division of Glisson's capsule. The left and right portal tracts are dissected for 3–4 cm on

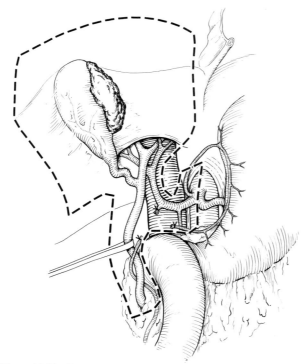

Figure 19.22 Extent of dissection for a radical gallbladder resection for gallbladder cancer. Segments IVa and V are resected *en bloc* with the gallbladder, extrahepatic biliary tree and the lymph node chain up to the coeliac axis

each side; if a middle hepatic artery is present (supplying segment IVa) this is divided. The parenchymal dissection is deepened just to the right of the umbilical fissure. It is continued arteriorly across the surface of the liver, then around and inferiorly below the gallbladder. By keeping to the anatomical segments, there is relatively little blood loss. The use of intraoperative US for mapping the anatomy is helpful. An ultrasonic dissector makes identification of tubular structures easier. The common hepatic duct is divided below the bifurcation if possible and internal drainage is established with an end-to-side Roux-en-Y reconstruction. Occasionally, more extended resections are justified (such as an extended right hepatectomy involving segments IV–VIII with an end-to-side left hepaticojejunostomy), provided that complete clearance can be achieved.

Radical resection of lower bile duct and ampullary carcinomas

Ampullary carcinomas

The operation of choice is a Whipple's operation.

Palliative bypass operations for obstructive jaundice

The commonest indication is for advanced cancer of the head of pancreas. Less commonly, bypass is required for non-resectable cancers of the ampulla of

Vater, extrahepatic bile duct and gallbladder and occasionally for metastatic disease. Histology should be obtained if resection is not planned. Sometimes 'pseudotumours' may be apparent at the liver hilum or ampulla of Vater. A lymphoma in the region of the head of pancreas may be clinically indistinguishable from adenocarcinoma but be amenable to non-operative treatment.

Following biliary bypass for jaundice, 15% of patients with pancreatic cancer require surgery for duodenal obstruction. Since there is no evidence that a gastrojejunostomy alters operative morbidity, this is routinely added by some surgeons.

Surgical bypass is to be preferred for younger patients with no significant co-morbidity; even so, there is a 10–15% mortality. Older patients are best treated by non-surgical stenting. The long-term survival of patients is similar irrespective of the type of biliary bypass (mean 4–10 months). There are a number of surgical options; the level of bypass is partly dictated by the level of obstruction.

Choledochoduodenostomy (see above)

This is a relatively simple, quick and reliable method for low-lying cancers. It is particularly suitable for elderly patients in whom non-operative means of stenting have failed.

Roux-en-Y hepaticojejunostomy (see above)

This should be done as a side-to-side hepaticojejunostomy. It is liable to remain patent for longer than a choledochoduodenostomy.

Left hepaticojejunostomy (see above)

This is an excellent bypass procedure for obstruction of the common bile duct or lower common hepatic duct.

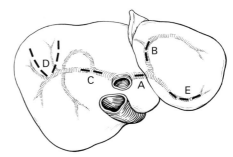

Figure 19.23 Possible sites of access to the biliary tree for bypass of high strictures. *a*, Extrahepatic left hepatic duct. *b*, Round ligament or segment III approach, *c*, Right hepatic duct through the gallbladder fossa. *d*, Segment V duct following excision of a V-shaped segment of liver. *e*, A superficial segment II duct

Round ligament approach

A Roux-en-Y may be taken up to a dilated segment III duct (Figure 19.23). The pons hepatis is divided by inserting a groove retractor into the umbilical fissure and using a cutting diathermy point. The pons hepatis is a bridge of liver tissue which joins segments III and IV anterior to the umbilical fissure and does not contain vital structures. Prominent fibres on the left of the ligament are divided between ligatures, care being taken not to injure the left hepatic portal vein. The dilated segment III duct lies just below this and to the left.

Other procedures

Occasionally none of the above is suitable. A dilated segment II duct may be found near the liver surface (Figure 19.23). A needle and syringe may be used to detect the right hepatic duct through the gallbladder fossa following cholecystectomy.

A limited hepatotomy (liver split) or V-shaped hepatectomy may be used to identify a dilated segment V-duct which is to the right of the gallbladder.

A silastic stent can be used for tumours proximal to the common bile duct (Figure 19.24). The procedure is similar to that described for benign strictures (see above). The lower end of the silastic tube is pulled out through the common bile duct. The choledochotomy is closed snugly around the tube with interrupted sutures and the tube converted to an O tube. Patients may do very well with this for several years.

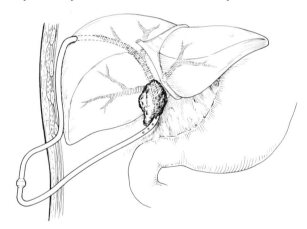

Figure 19.24 An O-tube in position for decompressing the biliary tree because of malignant hilar obstruction

A cholecystojejunostomy can sometimes be used successfully for tumours of the head of the pancreas, but there are disadvantages. Drainage may be incomplete because of gallbladder stones, a narrow cystic duct and because the cystocholedochochal junction becomes involved with cancer.

Further reading

Adson, M. A. and Farnell, M. B. (1981) Hepatobiliary cancer – surgical considerations. *Mayo. Clin. Proc.*, **56**, 686–699

Andren-Sandberg, A., Alinder, G. and Bengmark, S. (1985) Accidental lesions of the common bile duct at cholecystectomy. Pre- and perioperative factors of importance. *Ann. Surg.*, **201**, 328–332

Aranha, G. V., Sontag, S. J. and Greenlee, H. B. (1982) Cholecystectomy in cirrhotic patients: a formidable operation. *Am. J. Surg.*, **143**, 55–59

Baker A. R., Neoptolemos, J. P., Leese, T., James, D. C. and Fossard, D. P. (1987) Longterm follow-up of patients with side-to-side choledochoduodenostomy and transduodenal sphincteroplasty. *Ann. Roy. Coll. Surg. Engl.*, **68**, 253–257

Bismuth, H., Houssin, D. and Castaing, D. (1982) Major and minor segmentectomies. 'Reglees' in liver surgery. *Wld J. Surg.*, **6**, 10–24

Blumgart, L. H. and Kelly, C. J. (1984) Hepatico-jejunostomy in benign and malignant high bile duct stricture: approaches to the left hepatic ducts. *Br. J. Surg.*, **71**, 257–261

Cameron, J. L., Pitt, H. A., Zinner, M. J., Herlong, H. F. *et al.* (1988) Resection of hepatic duct bifurcation and transhepatic stenting for sclerosing cholangitis. *Ann. Surg.*, **207**, 614–622

Clavien, P. A., Richon, J., Burgan, S. and Rohner, A. (1990) Gallstone ileus. *Br. J. Surg.*, **77**, 737–742

Csendes, A., Diaz, J. C., Burdiles, P., Maluenda, F. and Nava, O. (1989) Mirizzi syndrome and cholecystobiliary fistula: a unifying classification. *Br. J. Surg.*, **76**, 1139–1143

De Aretabala, Y., Roa, I., Araya, J. C., Burgos, L. *et al.* (1990) Operative findings in patients with early forms of gallbladder cancer. *Br. J. Surg.*, **77**, 291–293

Hickman, M. S., Schwedinger, W. H. and Page C. P. (1988) Acute cholecystitis in the diabetic: a case control study of outcome. *Arch. Surg.*, **123**, 409–411

Leese, T., Neoptolemos, J. P., Baker, A. R. and Carr-Locke, D. L. (1986) Management of acute cholangitis and the impact of endoscopic sphincterotomy. *Br. J. Surg.*, **73**, 988–992

McSherry, C. K. (1989) Cholecystectomy: the Gold standard. *Am. J. Surg.*, **158**, 174–178

Neoptolemos, J. P., Davidson, B. R., Shaw, D. E., Lloyd, D. *et al.* (1987) Study of common bile duct exploration and endoscopic sphincterotomy in a consecutive series of 438 patients. *Br. J. Surg.*, **74**, 916–921

Neoptolemos, J. P., Hofmann, A. F. and Moossa, A. R. (1986) Chemical treatment of stones in the biliary tree. *Br. J. Surg.*, **73**, 515–524

Nevin, J. E., Moran, T. J., Kay, S. and King, R. (1976) Carcinoma of the gallbladder. Staging, treatment and prognosis. *Cancer*, **37**, 141–148

Sarfeh, I. J., Rypins, E. B., Jakowatz, J. G. and Juler G. L. (1988) A prospective, randomised clinical investigation of cholecystenterostomy and choledochoenterostomy. *Am. J. Surg.*, **155**, 411–414

Taylor, T. V., Armstrong, C. P., Rimmer, S., Lucas, S. B. *et al.* (1988) Prediction of choledocholithiasis using a pocket computer. *Br. J. Surg.*, **75**, 138–140

Terblanche, J., Kahn, D., Bornman, P. C. and Werner, D. (1988) The role of U tube palliative treatment in high bile duct carcinoma. *Ann. Surg.*, **103**, 624–632

Williamson, R. C. N (1988) Acalculous disease of the gallbladder. *Gut*, **29**, 860–872

Winslet, M. C. and Neoptolemos, J. P. (1991) The place of endoscopy in the management of gallstones. *Clinical Gastroenterology*, **5**, 99–129

20

Endoscopic procedures for the general surgeon

D. Alderson

Gastrointestinal endoscopy, using flexible telescopes and fibreoptic illumination, was first introduced by Hirschowitz in the mid-1950s. By the mid-1970s endoscopic assessment of the upper gastrointestinal tract, biliary and pancreatic ductal systems and colon had become widespread throughout the Western world. The addition of invasive therapeutic techniques, to the diagnostic capabilities of endoscopy, occurred almost simultaneously. These therapeutic modalities offer genuine alternatives to conventional surgery for a wide variety of conditions and have rendered certain operations virtually obsolete. The further introduction of new technologies, such as video endoscope systems, which have revolutionized teaching, and endoscopic laser treatments, which have added a new dimension to endoscopic therapy, have continued to widen the scope of endoscopic surgery.

This chapter focuses on these therapeutic endoscopic manoeuvres, rather than on the diagnostic capabilities of endoscopy. All surgeons with an interest in gastrointestinal surgery should be capable of carrying out the appropriate endoscopic procedures relevant to their area of interest, so that proficiency in colonoscopy, for instance, should be considered a mandatory element in the training of a colorectal surgeon.

Oesophagogastroduodenoscopy

This is the most widely practised endoscopic procedure and is considered the gold standard examination for a wide variety of conditions lying between the cricopharyngeus muscle and the second part of the duodenum.

The treatment of benign oesophageal strictures

The most common cause of stricture formation in the oesophagus is gastro-oesophageal reflux disease. All oesophageal strictures should be brushed for cytology and biopsied. Strictures secondary to reflux disease are characteristically short and occur immediately above the gastro-oesophageal junction. The majority present in elderly patients and can be satisfactorily managed by intermittent endoscopic dilatations, supplemented with appropriate general measures and medical therapy.

Satisfactory dilatation should result in patients requiring the procedure not more than three times annually. Failure to achieve this merits consideration of alternative strategies. This is particularly important in young patients where surgery should be carefully considered before embarking upon a prolonged programme of dilatation. Dilatation can be accomplished using graduated dilators (Savary Gilliard or Celestin types), olivary dilators (Eder–Puestow), or rigid cylindrical balloon catheters (Figure 20.1). Conventionally, the stricture is negotiated with a flexible tipped guide wire under direct vision, which usually passes easily into the stomach. The endoscope is removed and the stricture gradually dilated by passing dilators over the guide wire. It is not usually necessary to perform this procedure with X-ray control, as the risk of instrumental perforation in the dilatation of benign strictures is extremely low. It is important, however, that the guide wire should pass easily through the stricture, and the procedure should not be carried out if the endoscopist is in any doubt that this has occurred. Under such circumstances the procedure should be repeated with X-ray facilities. This problem is more commonly encountered with malignant strictures and is discussed in more detail later. An alternative form of dilatation is to use a pneumatic through-the-scope balloon system. The adult human oesophagus can be safely dilated up to 51 Fr. (17 mm) diameter.

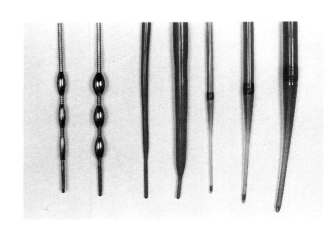

Figure 20.1 Oesophageal dilators. Left to right, Eder–Puestow × 2; Celestin × 2; Savary Gilliard × 3

Dilatation for achalasia

Pneumatic dilatation of the lower oesophageal high-pressure zone for achalasia should be considered the first treatment of choice for this condition. Surgery is indicated only in that group of patients where pneumatic dilatation has failed to provide adequate symptom relief over a prolonged period. The procedure can be repeated and is particularly appropriate in elderly patients. Both through-the-scope and guide-wire mounted balloon systems can be used. Wide-diameter (35 mm) balloons produce a satisfactory result in over 90% of patients. It is vital that the balloon is correctly located in the high-pressure segment and X-ray control is therefore required. The balloon is inflated to about 200–300 mmHg and kept at this pressure for 30–60 s. There is little risk (1–5%) of oesophageal rupture, but chest X-ray should be obtained afterwards to ensure that this has not occurred. Such perforations can be managed conservatively, but the presence of shock, sepsis, haemorrhage or communication with the pleural and/or peritoneal cavities should all be considered indications for exploration.

Treatment of malignant oesophageal strictures

Endoscopic treatment of malignant oesophageal strictures is widely practised. Carcinomas of the oesophagus, cardia and invasion of the oesophagus by bronchogenic carcinomas represent the most common pathologies encountered. The majority of patients selected for endoscopic therapy are those who are unfit for surgery or who are known to have widespread metastatic disease. Endoscopic treatment, nevertheless, can become part of a radical treatment programme, either as a preliminary to surgical therapy to maintain adequate swallowing while the patient is undergoing further evaluation, or as a method of maintaining patency during a course of radiotherapy.

There are essentially two approaches to endoscopic treatment of malignant oesophageal strictures. These involve either splinting the lesion using a prosthetic tube, or recanalization of the oesophagus using a laser. The two techniques are complementary and should not be viewed as mutually exclusive. Laser therapy is preferred in patients with high oesophageal obstruction, i.e. within a few centimetres of the distal edge of the cricopharyngeus muscle, and for those tumours which represent anastomotic recurrences following previous surgery. In the case of the former, this is because the collar on an oesophageal prosthesis produces a sensation of gagging and the constant desire to swallow if it abuts against the upper oesophageal sphincter, and in the case of the latter, anastomotic recurrences regularly produce a degree of angulation which can make them technically more difficult to deal with by guide-wire dilatation and prosthesis insertion. Conversely, intubation is preferred for extrinsic neoplasms involving the oesophagus, since this avoids the risk of fistula formation. In addition, most patients with long, i.e. >4 cm strictures, usually fare no better in terms of their quality of swallowing after laser therapy versus intubation. For this reason, intubation is the preferred first treatment of choice for such long strictures as it avoids the need for the repeated therapies.

A recently introduced alternative to laser recanalization is the use of intralesional alcohol injection which results in sloughing of intraluminal tumour within a few days. This may be a realistically cheap alternative to laser therapy.

Intubation of malignant oesophageal strictures

The upper end of the neoplasm is visualized and a guide wire passed through the narrowed area. The same constraints which apply to the dilatation of benign strictures apply here, although the risk of the guide wire not proceeding smoothly is more common with malignant obstruction. Again, in such cases, the procedure should be stopped until X-ray control can be obtained. Some strictures are extremely tortuous and a useful method for negotiating these is to use an angiography catheter with its steerable guide wire. This has the added advantage that contrast material can be injected and seen to enter the gastrointestinal tract, distal to the stricture. Once the guide wire has been passed successfully through the stricture into the stomach, the narrowed area is dilated to a size equal to the external diameter of the body of the prosthesis chosen. A variety of tube designs is available, in a variety of materials, over all lengths and diameters (Figure 20.2). Expandable metallic mesh stents have recently been introduced. These may be easier to insert since there is no need for preliminary wide dilatation. The theoretical problem of tumour regrowth through the mesh interstices will probably be easy to manage with the laser.

There are two basic systems for the insertion of conventional tubes. The Nottingham Introducer System consists of two metal rods and a distal expandable olive, which can be opened to grip the inside of the prosthesis, as shown (Figure 20.2). The alternative is to mount the tube over a cylindrical balloon, which is inflated to grip the internal surface of the prosthesis (Figure 20.2). It is important to measure the distance from the patient's incisor teeth to the upper end of the stricture carefully, using the endoscope, and to mark an identical distance from the collar of the prosthesis to a point on the introducing system. When this marker is at the patient's teeth, the prosthesis will then be appropriately located in the oesophagus. When the expanded olive of the Nottingham Introducer System is let down, or the balloon deflated, the introducing system can be withdrawn and the position of the prosthesis checked by endoscopy. A chest X-ray should be obtained to confirm that the position is correct and, again, to exclude oesophageal perforation. With either technique, the risk of perforating the oesophagus is less than 5% in experienced hands. If a tear has occurred, then provided that the prosthesis is in the correct place, it can usually be satisfactorily managed conservatively with broad-spectrum antibiotics and restriction of oral intake.

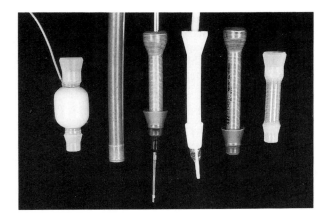

Figure 20.2 Oesophageal endoprostheses and insertion devices. Left to right, endoprosthesis for tracheo-oesophageal fistula with inflatable balloon to occlude the fistulous opening; pusher tube; Nottingham Introducer System; Celestin balloon introducer system; flanged rubber and metal wire prosthesis; unflanged silastic and wire prosthesis

Endoscopic laser recanalization

Endoscopic recanalization of the oesophagus can be achieved using a Nd YAG laser via the biopsy channel of the endoscope. There are certain precautions which must be observed in the use of laser therapy, which essentially involve protection against accidental firing of the laser into the eyes. The Nd YAG laser emits light at wavelengths of 1064 and 1318 nm and thus lies in the near infrared part of the spectrum. Such lasers therefore incorporate a low-powered red helium–neon laser aiming beam for appropriate targeting. The laser can be used both in a non-contact or contact mode, the former requiring higher energy levels because of back-scattering of some laser light. Until recently, contact therapy required a special artificial sapphire tip to conduct the laser energy, but recent developments in bare-fibre technology have made this unnecessary. Because there is little or no selective absorption of laser energy by tumour tissue, attempts have been made to develop tumour photosensitizers which selectively absorb laser light to maximize effects to the tumour and minimize those to surrounding tissue. The principal aim of laser recanalization is destruction of the endoluminal tumour, which is accomplished by photocoagulation of the tissue followed by carbonization and vaporization, as further laser energy is applied.

In the non-contact mode, laser energies of up to 100 W, applied to a 2–3 mm area of tumour from a distance of about 1 cm, over 1–2 s, will produce vaporization of that area. As the tissue carbonizes, the characteristics of light absorption alter and intravascular coagulation means that further laser energy cannot be dissipated by blood flow. It is important, therefore, that the laser light should not be applied perpendicularly to the oesophageal wall, but instead, virtually parallel to it, in order to prevent perforation. Recanalization of a typical oesophageal tumour might therefore require the application of 5000–10 000 J of energy, using a non-contact Nd YAG laser. When used alone, significant regrowth usually occurs within 4–6 weeks, necessitating further treatments at about these time intervals.

Injection sclerotherapy of oesophageal varices

Injection sclerotherapy is the most frequently used therapy for control of the acute haemorrhage from oesophageal varices and will successfully control bleeding in 85–90% of patients. The techniques used for sclerotherapy are far from standardized; a variety of sclerosing agents can be used (5% ethanolamine oleate, 3% sodium tetradecyl sulphate, absolute alcohol), with direct or para-variceal injection techniques, with or without manoeuvres to produce compression of a varix after it has been injected. Although the precise value of each of these is in some doubt, the most important point is to ensure that bleeding varices are injected close to the oesophagogastric junction, since the majority of varices which bleed do so within 2 cm of this region. It may be necessary to make up to ten 2 ml injections in order to achieve haemostasis. Because it is frequently difficult to be sure that this has occurred, balloon tamponade may be necessary following injection sclerotherapy, using a 4-lumen tube. The tube is removed at 24 h, when repeated sclerotherapy may be necessary. The goal of sclerotherapy is the complete obliteration of varices, which is usually accomplished by a series of injections every few days initially, and then monthly until the varices have disappeared. About 30% of patients will develop an oesophageal ulcer at the injection site and these ulcers themselves are difficult to treat and can be associated with a considerable risk of mortality in their own right, if they bleed. Only about 5–10% of patients who have undergone successful sclerotherapy develop strictures which require dilatation, and the risk of perforation is only about 1%.

A recently developed alternative to sclerotherapy is band-ligation, similar to that used for haemorrhoids. In one study, this method produced initial control in 95% of subjects. Gastric varices are difficult to treat by endoscopic sclerotherapy.

Endoscopic treatment for upper gastrointestinal bleeding

Upper gastrointestinal bleeding is a common clinical

problem. The causes identified in a recent series of over 2000 cases, collected by the American Society for Gastrointestinal Endoscopy, are shown in Table 20.1. There are many arguments concerning the role of endoscopy in the management of such bleeds, centred on the failure of some studies to demonstrate survival benefit as a result of endoscopy. Against these, it should be remembered that endoscopic examination of the upper gastrointestinal tract is the most useful method for arriving at a definitive diagnosis, which is possible in over 80% of patients, provided that endoscopy is carried out within 24 h of the onset of bleeding. Certain endoscopic findings are known to be associated with a high risk of re-bleeding, an occurrence recognized for the past 30 years as the single most important factor which contributes to surgical mortality. Nowadays endoscopy, in addition to its diagnostic capability, also provides therapy, of which three methods are popular.

Table 20.1 Causes of gastrointestinal bleeding

Cause	Percentage
Duodenal ulcer	24.3
Gastric erosions	23.4
Gastric ulcer	21.3
Varices	10.3
Mallory–Weiss tear	7.2
Oesophagitis	6.3
Erosive duodenitis	5.8
Neoplasm	2.9
Stomal ulcer	1.8
Oesophageal ulcer	1.7
Vascular anomalies	0.5
Other causes	6.3

Therapeutic techniques

1. *Laser photocoagulation.* Photocoagulation of a bleeding lesion, using the Nd YAG laser, is effective with a perforation rate less than 2%. The application of laser energy through a continuous jet of water may be superior to the conventional non-contact therapy, both in terms of initial success and less treatment-induced bleeding. The principal disadvantage of laser therapy is its cost.
2. *Electrocoagulation and heater probes.* These work by producing thermal coagulation from direct contact between the device and the bleeding lesion. Both methods require some form of tip irrigation in order to prevent adhesion between the coagulated tissue and the probe tip, in order to reduce the problem of re-bleeding when the probe is removed from the coagulated tissue. A number of commercial devices are available and can be shown to be effective in reducing the further risk of bleeding.
3. *Sclerotherapy.* This has already been outlined for oesophageal varices, but has become increasingly popular within the past 5 years as a method of

dealing with bleeding ulcers. A combination of sclerosant and vasoconstrictor is used, injected in a ring around the ulcer base.

Technical aspects

Upper gastrointestinal endoscopy for bleeding should be carried out only by experienced endoscopists and requires experienced assistance. Endoscopy should never be attempted prior to appropriate resuscitation and should form part of the overall plan of management for each individual patient. In a small percentage of patients, the risk of aspiration during endoscopy is significant, particularly for variceal bleeds in encephalopathic individuals, and in these circumstances it may be wise to perform the procedure under general anaesthesia.

At all other times, endoscopy is started with the patient lying in the left lateral position, with the head lower than the feet. Once the endoscope is passed to the stomach, an assessment needs to be made whether or not an adequate examination can be performed based on the contents of the stomach. If too much blood is present, the endoscope should be removed, replaced by a large orogastric tube and the stomach contents siphoned out. One should avoid attempting to suck out the stomach contents with a syringe under force, as this can produce marked mucosal artefact. The installation of water or saline down the orogastric tube can make lavage proceed more easily. The endoscope is then re-passed, to enable an appropriate examination to be performed. It is nearly always best to get the endoscope into the duodenum before attempting to look for pathology in the oesophagus or stomach. After inspection of the duodenum, it may be necessary to roll the patient in order to carry out an adequate examination of the stomach, and this requires good assistance.

The endoscopist should strive to answer four questions:

1. Can the site of bleeding be localized?
2. What is the nature of the bleeding lesion?
3. Is there active haemorrhage?
4. Is there a visible protruding vessel present in the base of a peptic ulcer?

The last two points critically affect a decision to offer therapy. Both active bleeding and the presence of a visible protruding vessel are indications for intervention. There is some debate about the value of other endoscopic findings, and the one which causes most debate is the presence of a large clot in the ulcer base. Some of these lesions will contain a vessel which is obscured by the clot, so that there are only two sensible strategies to deal with this endoscopic appearance. One is to wash the clot away to see if there is a visible vessel and then institute treatment as appropriate; the alternative is to inject the ulcer base of all of these lesions, accepting that this may be unnecessarily aggressive for some patients. Thermal methods cannot be applied when the clot is in the way.

Endoscopic treatments can substantially lower the risk of re-bleeding. Surgeons should nevertheless remember that not all lesions are endoscopically accessible. Endoscopic therapy, like surgery, needs to be carried out correctly and should be viewed as part of the overall management plan and not as a technique which replaces an operation.

Percutaneous endoscopic gastrostomy (jejunostomy)

The endoscopic insertion of feeding tubes into the stomach or upper small bowel has become increasingly popular in recent years. The technique is suitable for all patients with severe problems affecting deglutition, provided that endoscopic access can be obtained and there is no distal gastrointestinal obstruction. The most common groups of patients are those with neuromuscular incoordination in the pharynx such as a brain-stem stroke where inhalation can be a major problem. Endoscopic jejunostomy insertion is a viable alternative to a long per-nasal feeding tube in surgical patients with impaired gastric emptying.

A number of commercial kits are available which are of two basic designs. With any system, the first manoeuvre is to transilluminate the abdominal wall by shining the gastroscope through the anterior wall of the distended stomach. The gastric wall is then punctured from the skin with a sheathed needle so that a guide wire can be passed into the stomach to be visualized by the endoscopist. With the small size gastrostomy tubes (Figure 20.3) placement is made by serial dilatation of the track over the guide wire, followed by insertion of the feeding tube which will incorporate some form of retention system.

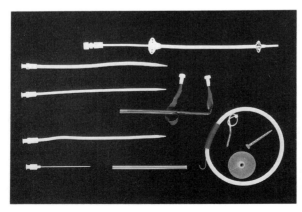

Figure 20.3 Endoscopic gastrostomy kit (Malecot type) for percutaneous trans-gastric insertion

Wider tubes (Figure 20.4) are difficult to insert in this way, so the guide wire is grasped in the stomach with a snare and the endoscope/guide wire assembly

brought out through the patient's mouth. The guide wire in this system has a looped end which can be attached to the feeding tube. This is then pulled into the stomach by traction on the guide wire at the abdominal wall until the tube is in place. The gastrostomy tube is cut at an appropriate level. With either technique it is important that the retaining device is snugly against the gastric mucosa, but should not blanch it in order to prevent necrosis and possible displacement.

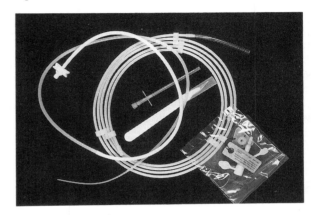

Figure 20.4 Endoscopic gastrostomy kit for trans-oral insertion

Jejunostomy insertion is most easily done with a side-viewing endoscope. The guide wire through the abdominal wall in the stomach is grasped with a snare and taken down at least to the third part of the duodenum. The feeding tube is then passed over the guide wire after releasing the snare. Provided that some redundant feeding tube can be left in the gastrointestinal tract, the tube will tend to move distally. Wound infection at the insertion site can be minimized using antimicrobial prophylaxis.

Therapeutic techniques during endoscopic retrograde cholangiopancreatography (ERCP)

Successful cannulation of the papilla of Vater was first described by McCune and colleagues in 1968. The technique involves using a side-viewing endoscope to visualize the papilla and cannulation of either the bile duct or pancreatic duct as appropriate. The technique therefore has diagnostic capabilities under the following circumstances:

1. Investigation of jaundice.
2. Assessment of the bile duct before or after cholecystectomy.
3. The assessment of abdominal pain, thought to be of pancreatic origin.

The widespread popularity of ERCP, however, is largely based upon the therapeutic offshoots of diagnostic ERCP: the treatment of common duct stones and the palliation of biliary and pancreatic strictures using stents.

Management of choledocholithiasis

Endoscopic sphincterotomy has become the established treatment of choice for most patients with stones in the biliary tree. These can present either before or after surgery for gallstones.

Management of choledocholithiasis with the gallbladder *in situ*

Two factors are of prime importance in determining the management of this problem: the age of the patient and the mode of presentation.

Age is important because, at the young end of the spectrum, some surgeons feel apprehensive about the potential long-term effects of duodenal reflux into the biliary tree, after endoscopic sphincterotomy. At the other end of the age scale, it has become accepted that in some patients the gallbladder itself is asymptomatic and may not need to be subsequently removed after dealing with the common duct problem.

ERCP should be performed urgently on all patients, irrespective of age, with acute cholangitis who fail to show signs of clinical improvement after 12 h of intensive medical therapy. This is one of the few indications for emergency ERCP and sphincterotomy. It is imperative that the endoscopist should ensure that biliary drainage has beeen achieved by sphincterotomy, ± stone extraction, ± the insertion of a drainage tube. If biliary drainage cannot be obtained endoscopically, then such patients must go on to urgent surgery.

Urgent ERCP (within 24 h) is desirable for all patients with acute pancreatitis thought to be of biliary origin, but particularly for that subgroup designated to have a severe biochemical attack as predicted by Imrie or Ranson criteria. There is good evidence that ERCP and attempted stone extraction can reduce the mortality in this group of patients.

The decision to carry out ERCP on all other patients, with the gallbladder *in situ*, is based largely on the perception of risk of a stone being present in the bile duct, the patient's age and the range of treatments available within an institution. The advent of laparoscopic cholecystectomy has had a pronounced effect in this group. A history of jaundice, abnormal liver function tests, multiple small stones in the gallbadder and a dilated common bile duct on ultrasound are the most useful features which imply an increased risk of a stone in the bile ducts, and an acceptable philosophy is to subject such individuals, irrespective of age, to diagnostic ERCP, and convert this to a therapeutic procedure if stones are present in elderly patients or any who are unfit for surgery. Within this group who have undergone sphincterotomy, some are known to have gallbladder symptoms

as well, and therefore come to a laparoscopic cholecystectomy, but many elderly patients have no symptoms from the gallbladder itself and there is little justification in subjecting them to cholecystectomy at a later date, since the risk of developing complications is known to be small ($< 10\%$).

No firm view can be expressed at this time regarding the wisdom of offering younger patients endoscopic treatment of their common duct stones, followed by laparoscopic cholecystectomy, intraoperative cholangiography and exploration of the common bile duct as appropriate. There are no published prospective trials to indicate which will be the most beneficial and cost-effective method.

Choledocholithiasis following cholecystectomy

There are two possible clinical scenarios here: patients who have a T-tube *in situ* and those who do not. For the former group, stones may be extracted via the T-tube which has to be left in place for about 4 weeks to produce a mature track, or endoscopic sphincterotomy can be performed, followed by stone extraction. The two techniques should be viewed as complementary. For all other patients, endoscopic therapy is the treatment of choice, with a lower morbidity than a second operation.

Technique of endoscopic sphincterotomy and stone extraction

A variety of sphincterotome designs is available (Figure 20.5). Some endoscopists use the sphincterotome for both the diagnostic and therapeutic parts of the procedure, if it is felt that a common duct stone is likely to be encountered. Because contrast material can escape from some designs of catheter at the site of the sphincterotomy wire, rather than solely at the tip, it is important to achieve deep cannulation in order to produce a good-quality cholangiogram without a large amount of dye in the duodenum. Conversely, some endoscopists begin with a diagnostic catheter and exchange this over a guide wire for a sphincterotome. Since insulated guide wires are now available, it is not necessary to remove the wire prior to using the sphincterotome. With most designs of sphincterotome it is necessary to insert about two-thirds of the wire into the papilla and check that the tip is in the bile duct by injecting a small amount of contrast. As the wire is tightened, this creates a bow-string effect, and it is important that this wire tightening should occur between about 11 o'clock and 1 o'clock on the papilla. By using a diathermy current, the roof of the papilla and the biliary sphincter complex is incised vertically upwards. Throughout this procedure, it is important to maintain this deep cannulation using the endoscope up-down tip control and/or the bridge mechanism to keep the catheter firmly against the roof of the papilla. The adequacy of the sphincterotomy is usually easily apparent but can be subsequently tested by withdrawing an inflated balloon catheter through the sphincterotomy to check its size. Cholangiograms obtained before sphincterotomy, must be of high quality and the likely number of stones thought to be present clearly identified, since it is less easy to obtain good cholangiography after sphincterotomy, owing to the presence of air in the biliary tree and rapid emptying of dye. Occlusion cholangiography, by inflating a balloon catheter just inside the bile duct and injecting dye above it, is a useful way of visualizing the biliary tree after sphincterotomy.

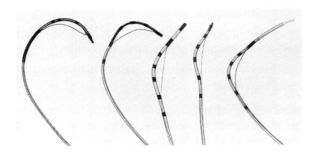

Figure 20.5 Differing designs of endoscopic sphincterotomy wires

Stones can be removed using balloon catheters or baskets as shown in Figure 20.6. Special problems occur in patients with stones impacted at the ampulla, multiple stones, large stones greater than 2 cm in diameter and stones in the presence of a biliary stricture. Stones impacted at the ampulla can make biliary cannulation difficult. Special needle-knife sphincterotomes which project from the catheter like a bee-sting can be used to incise the papilla above the biliary opening, directly onto the stone, to facilitate stone extraction and sphincterotomy performance. Some endoscopists feel this manoeuvre is sufficiently hazardous to recommend its performance only by very experienced operators! The bile duct filled with multiple calculi may be difficult to clear and is frequently found in patients with severe acute suppurative cholangitis. A technical failure can occur here, when after clearing the lower bile duct, a mass of biliary debris still causes obstruction. Insertion of a nasobiliary drain or a biliary stent, of the type used as an internal prosthesis for malignant obstructive jaundice, can provide effective biliary drainage leading to a repeat ERCP under more favourable circumstances.

Large stones pose a particular problem. Although the problem can usually be overcome by widening the sphincterotomy, truly giant calculi require special consideration. In some elderly patients it may be permissible to place a stent alongside such a large calculus, simply to prevent stone impaction in the sphincterotomy The alternative is to attempt some form of lithotripsy and this can be either mechanical, electrohydraulic or via a laser. The first method uses a

rigid basket, the latter two a mother and baby system, in which a small end-viewing endoscope is passed down the biopsy channel of the duodenoscope into the common bile duct. An alternative approach is to use extracorporeal shock-wave lithotripsy, using a catheter placed into the bile duct for precise stone visualization under X-ray control.

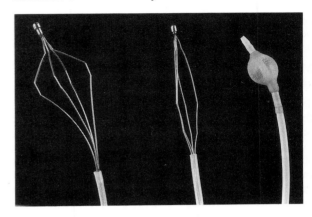

Figure 20.6 Basket and balloon catheter designs for gallstone extraction

Stones occurring in the presence of strictures are common in the Orient (Oriental cholangiohepatitis). In Western societies they usually occur after previous biliary surgery. Preliminary balloon dilatation may allow stone removal, but the long-term results of endoscopic balloon treatment of benign biliary strictures seem inferior to surgery.

Endoscopic sphincterotomy and stone extraction have a low morbidity and mortality. Bleeding, pancreatitis and perforation are the three most commonly recognized and collectively lead to significant morbidity in about 5% of subjects. Numerous authors have published large series with a mortality of around 1%.

The insertion of biliary and pancreatic endoprostheses

The insertion of a biliary stent has become a popular method of dealing with malignant obstructive jaundice. The stent can be considered a permanent device with an anticipated lifespan of between 3 and 6 months, or viewed as temporary in those patients who are to undergo further assessment with a view to surgical resection of the tumour. Stent placement in the biliary tree requires a wide-channel duodenoscope capable of carrying a minimum diameter stent of 10 Fr. Although some endoscopists routinely create a sphincterotomy before attempting stent insertion, this is not essential unless it improves access to the distal bile duct. A Teflon catheter containing a guide wire is passed up the bile duct to the site of obstruction. If the catheter itself will not go through the obstruction, the spring-tipped guide wire is advanced from the catheter to see if it will pass. Steerable wires are available for difficult strictures. Once the wire passes through the strictured area, the catheter is then advanced over the wire and the position checked fluoroscopically. Stent insertion is facilitated by using a relatively stiff Teflon tube over the wire. The stent is inserted over this guide wire/catheter assembly and pushed down through the endoscope with a pusher tube, which is the same diameter as the stent. It is important to select the stent of the appropriate length and stents are manufactured with varying distances between the retaining flanges at either end. The stent is pushed through the stricture, so that the upper end lies above the obstruction, with the lower end in the duodenum. It may be necessary for hilar strictures to have a stent in each side of the biliary tree, although many groups believe this is best accomplished using a combined radiological/endoscopic technique. This combined technique is particularly useful for hilar strictures and for those strictures which cannot be negotiated with a guide wire from below. A standard percutaneous transhepatic cholangiogram is performed and external biliary drainage established for 48 h. During this time, there is some biliary decompression which makes negotiation of the stricture from above easier. A guide wire inserted from above is used to traverse the stricture and the distal end of the wire left in the duodenum. This can be subsequently retrieved via the endoscope and the prosthesis manoeuvred into place from below, in the usual fashion.

Pancreatic stents can be inserted using the same principles as for the insertion of biliary prostheses. There are encouraging early results from Europe regarding their role in pancreatic ductal decompression for chronic pancreatitis and subsequent pain relief, although as yet they are not popular in the UK.

The principal complications associated with stent insertion are blockage and sepsis. The extent to which stents encourage low-grade infection within the biliary tree is not clear, nor is the exact nature of the biofilm which seems to occur on the insides of plastic stents and which leads to their occlusion. While stents can be changed by simply pulling out the previous stent and inserting a new one in its place, an alternative approach recently has been to use expanding stents made of metallic mesh. These are considerably more expensive than plastic stents but do have a longer life expectancy. There may be some risk of blockage due to tumour regrowth into the interstices of the mesh and back into the lumen, but the true extent of this problem still requires evaluation.

Therapeutic colonoscopy

This centres on the methods necessary to deal with colonic polyps, strictures, tumour recanalization and the management of colonic bleeding.

Colonoscopic polypectomy

The removal of polyps via the colonoscope is both safe and effective. Significant haemorrhage is a risk in only about 1% of patients and perforation occurs in less than 0.5% of patients. The mortality of the procedure is consequently minuscule.

There are, in essence, two techniques to deal with polyps which largely relate to their shape and size. Pedunculated polyps are most appropriately dealt with using a snare which is closed around the stalk of the polyp. By applying diathermy current to the stalk, this is gradually cut through, allowing the polyp to be removed. There are certain hazards to be avoided, the most important of which relates to large polyps measuring greater than 4 cm in diameter, which may virtually fill the colonic lumen. The rule for such polyps is never to snare more polyp than can be adequately seen and remove them in a piecemeal fashion. Bleeding from a polyp stalk is uncommon, but if it occurs, the most effective way of dealing with it is to attempt to re-snare the stalk and occlude the vessel by tightening the snare around the stalk. It is usually not necessary to reapply further diathermy, but simply to hold the snare in place for 10 min. Sessile polyps without a stalk can be difficult to snare, but it is surprising how many of these lesions can be satisfactorily snared and a pseudo-stalk created of mucosa. There is a danger of producing a tenting injury in the colon wall, but by moving the snared polyp to and fro under direct vision and confirming that the mucosa moves but not the entire bowel, this usually means that snare polypectomy can be effected safely. An alternative for sessile polyps, and also for very small polyps, is either to use a mini-snare or so-called hot biopsy forceps which allows electrical current to be passed to the tips of an insulated forceps after the specimen has been trapped within the jaws of the instrument.

A variety of tricks is available for the recovery of multiple polyps, which can be a tedious job. The most thorough and accurate way of dealing with multiple polyps is obviously to remove each one separately by withdrawing the colonoscope and reinserting the instrument each time. This is laborious and can be difficult if, for instance, the sigmoid colon is tortuous. The use of a split over-tube can speed this up considerably. The most useful alternative to this approach is to incorporate a sputum trap in the suction line and to deliberately aspirate small polyps into such a trap from where they can be recovered. Sometimes polyps are dropped and apparently seem to disappear. The injection of water down the biopsy channel and watching the direction of flow is a good indicator of the likely route the polyp will have taken, as a result of gravity. If all of these measures prove unsuccessful, the instillation of 500 ml of warm water above the most proximal biopsy site, immediately prior to removal of the colonoscope, will allow most polyps to be evacuated easily by the patient after the procedure.

Colonoscopic dilatation and recanalization

The majority of colonic strictures are obviously due to cancer or diverticular disease. They frequently preclude total colonoscopy, as they can be impossible to negotiate. There are, however, two conditions which respond well to dilatation; these are post-radiotherapy strictures and anastomotic strictures. The former usually lie in the pelvis and are amenable to either graduated dilatation (Savary Gilliard type) or the use of a rigid cylindrical balloon. Through the scope, balloon systems are adequate and will produce a functional diameter with an acceptable clinical outcome. Although anastomotic strictures are also more common in the pelvis, those in the abdominal cavity proper are amenable only to balloon dilatation.

A minority of patients with colonic cancer are not suitable even for palliative resections and, again, this particularly pertains to bulky neoplasms in the rectum. These can be successfully recanalized using the Nd YAG laser, in exactly the same way as for the oesophagus. This is, however, a relatively slow technique and the use of a transanal resectoscope as an alternative should be strongly considered, provided that the lesion lies within reach.

Colonoscopy for lower gastrointestinal bleeding

Despite many favourable reports from enthusiasts, acute colonoscopy for lower gastrointestinal bleeding has never been widely popular. Its value, however, should not be underestimated, particularly in that small subgroup of patients who have major haemorrhages with haemodynamic instability, which are proven not to arise in the oesophagus, stomach or duodenum. Under these circumstances, it should be remembered that blood is an excellent cathartic and formal preparation of the colon is not necessary. If adequate colonoscopic views cannot be obtained, however, it is better to cleanse the colon from above using a per-nasal tube, than to administer enemas from below, which tend to wash the blood proximally and increase interpretive difficulties. The nature of the bleeding lesion obviously dictates the treatment required, but arteriovenous malformations and colonic angiodysplasia are the two conditions in which colonoscopic treatment is most appropriate. To date, there seems to be no clear advantage for sophisticated laser systems, in dealing with either of these problems, over standard electrocoagulation.

Conclusion

The surgical endoscopist should remember that he or she has the unique opportunity to use the advantages of endoscopy intraoperatively. No part of the gastrointestinal tract is out of reach and the technique can certainly be used profitably in the diagnosis of obscure causes of gastrointestinal bleeding, particularly when it arises in the small bowel. The indications for endoscopic techniques seem to widen annually, and with the current enthusiasm for minimal access surgical techniques, the likelihood of combining these with endoscopic approaches is high. This is already clear in the relationship between laparoscopic cholecystectomy, ERCP and trans-cystic exploration of the common bile duct, using ultra-thin choledochoscopes. It is imperative that the surgeon remains at the forefront of this new technology, fully prepared to evaluate new treatment strategies for the next century.

Further reading

Berry, A. R., Souter, R. G., Campbell, W. B. and Mortensen, N. J. McC. (1990) Endoscopic transanal resection of rectal tumours – preliminary report of its use. *Br. J. Surg.*, **77**, 134–137

Breunetaud, J. M., Maunoury, V., Cochelard, D., Adenis, A. *et al.* (1990) Lasers in rectosigmoid cancers: factors affecting immediate and long-term results. In *Baillière's Gastroenterology*, Baillière, London, pp. 615–629

Cotton, B. P. (1990) Management of malignant bile duct obstruction. *J. Gastroenterol. Hepatol.*, Suppl. 1, 63–77

Gelfand, M. D. and Kozarek, R. A. (1989) An experience with polyethylene balloons for pneumatic dilatation in achalasia. *Am. J. Gastroenterol.*, **84**, 924–927

Huibregtse, K., Cheung, J., Coene, P. P. L. O., Fockens, P. *et al.* (1989) Endoscopic placement of expandable metal stents for biliary stricture – a preliminary report on experience with thirty-three patients. *Endoscopy*, **21**, 280–282

Huibregtse, K., Schneider, B., Vrij, A. A. and Tytgat, G. N. A. (1988) Endoscopic pancreatic drainage in chronic pancreatitis. *Gastrointest. Endosc.*, **34**, 9–15

Ingoldby, C. J. H., El-Saadi, J., Hall, R. I. and Denyer, M. E. (1989) Late results of endoscopic sphincterotomy for bile duct stones in elderly patients with gallbladders in situ. *Gut*, **30**, 1129–1131

Payne-James, J. J., Spiller, R. C., Misiewicz, J. J. and Silk, D. B. A. (1990) Use of ethanol induced tumour necrosis to palliate dysphagia in patients with oesophago-gastric cancer. *Gastrointest. Endosc.*, **36**, 43–46

Paynes, J., Forne, M., Bagena, F. and Viver, J. (1990) Endoscopic sclerosis in the treatment of bleeding peptic ulcers with a visible vessel. *Am. J. Gastroenterol.*, **85**, 252–254

Pitt, H. A., Kaufman, S. L., Coleman, J., White, R. I. *et al.* (1989) Benign post-operative biliary strictures: operate or dilate? *Ann. Surg.*, **210**, 417–427

Sander, R., Poesl, H., Zuern, W., Spuhler, A. *et al.* (1989) The water jet-guided Nd-YAG laser in the treatment of gastroduodenal ulcer with a visible vessel. *Endoscopy*, **21**, 217–220

Siegel, J. H., Ben-Zvi, J. S. and Pullano, W. E. (1990) Mechanical lithotripsy of common duct stones. *Gastrointest. Endosc.*, **36**, 351–356

Stiegmann, G., Goff, J., Michaletz, P., Korula, J. *et al.* (1990) Endoscopic variceal ligation versus sclerotherapy for rebleeding oesophageal varices: early results of a prospective randomised trial. *Gastrointest. Endosc.* **36**, 189

Terblanche, J., Burroughs, A. K. and Hobbs, K. E. F. (1989) Controversies in the management of bleeding esophageal varices. *N. Engl. J. Med.*, **320**, 1393–1398 and 1469–1475

Tytgat, G. N. J. (1990) Endoscopic therapy of oesophageal cancer: possibilities and limitations. *Endoscopy*, **22**, 263–267

Williams, C. B. and Bedenne, L. (1990) Quadrennial review: management of colonic polyps – is all the effort worthwhile. *Gastroenterol. Hepatol.*, **5**, 144–165.

21

Laparoscopic cholecystectomy

H. J. Espiner

The first laparoscopic cholecystectomy was completed by Philippe Mouret of Lyon in March 1987. Dubois *et al.* (1990) presented the first detailed account of the operation and the Americans Reddick and Olsen (1990) followed with their technique which has largely been the one adopted by an expanding number of surgical centres.

The operation has become possible with the development of the new chip camera which, when mounted on a 10 mm telescope, gives a sufficiently clear image to allow the surgeon and his team to conduct the procedure on television monitors. High-powered light sources provide sufficient illumination for fine dissection and high-flow insufflators maintain the essential pneumoperitoneum when additional punctures are made for retraction and dissection. The hand instruments used are simple graspers, dissectors, scissors and diathermy hooks; these were already available from gynaecological laparoscopic surgery, but clips and their applicators have been specially designed for cholecystectomy.

Indications

All patients with symptomatic gallstones should be considered, but most would agree with Cuschieri *et al.* (1991) that the following are contraindications: (a) pregnancy; (b) portal hypertension; (c) jaundice; (d) severe acute cholecystitis or empyema.

Extensive previous upper abdominal surgery, morbid obesity, acute pancreatitis, ductal calculi (persistent after failed endoscopic removal) and coagulation disorders are relative contraindications. With experience the more severe inflammatory complications of gallstones are being treated successfully. It must be stressed, however, that a proper training in all the techniques of open biliary surgery is essential before a surgeon embarks on this new approach; conversion to open operation might be required in up to 5–10% of elective cases because of technical difficulty or anatomical uncertainty.

The operation

The operation consists of raising a pneumoperitoneum, inserting the laparoscope, establishing ports for retraction and dissection and retrieving the gallbladder. The whole procedure is carried out with the surgeon standing on the left side of the patient. A trolley with the insufflator and monitor comfortably in view is parked on the patient's right side, close to the table at the point of the shoulder; a similar trolley with a second monitor is placed on the left for the scrub nurse and first assistant.

Pneumoperitoneum

If the Veress needle is to be placed through the lower abdomen or umbilicus, the bladder must be emptied. The needle is tested for free release of the cannula and correct alignment of the side hole with the bevel of the needle. With the insufflator switched to 1 litre flow, the pressures generated into free air and against a closed tap are noted; the insufflator is set to deliver gas up to 12–15 mmHg pressure. The safest site for insertion is just suprapubically with the patient horizontal: the needle is held on the shaft like a dart and vertical to the skin. It is passed directly through the rectus sheath and peritoneum with a decisive thrust into the free space of the pelvis – a distinct click indicates peritoneal puncture and the needle should then move freely from side to side. With the gas flow at 1 litre/min, the pressure will read 5 mmHg, fluctuating, but always below 8 mmHg. Liver dullness is quickly lost as insufflation proceeds to 3–5 litres and the abdominal wall is seen to be uniformly distended; slow insufflation may reduce the costal and shoulder pain sometimes noticed after any laparoscopy.

Laparoscopy

A 10 mm trocar and cannula is used for access with the telescope. By pressing firmly on the abdominal wall above the umbilicus the lower abdomen is rendered tense and prominent: an incision is made in the umbilicus and with the trocar and cannula held in the right hand with the index finger extending along the shaft to prevent too deep an entry, the instrument is introduced with a steady pressure and a twisting movement aiming at the anus – clear of the sacral promontory. It is helpful to palpate this landmark before insufflation to be sure of avoiding injury to the aorta and vena cava. As with the Veress needle, a distinct 'pop' is felt as the peritoneum is breached.

The trocar can be withdrawn and inspection begun. The telescope with attached camera and light cable is passed and the pelvis is inspected for any injury caused by the needle or the cannula. It is then rotated to inspect the abdominal cavity generally and the right upper quadrant in particular. The presence of adhesions is carefully noted, especially those in relation to the liver. It may be helpful to pass a nasogastric tube to decompress the stomach, and the colon and omentum will usually fall away if the patient is placed in the reverse Trendelenburg position with the right side uppermost.

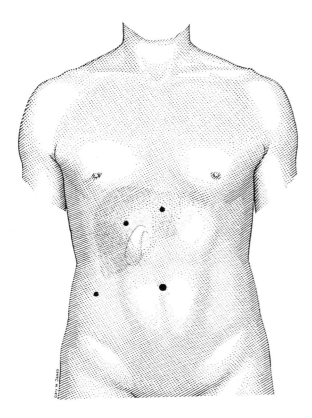

Figure 21.1 Port placement for exposure and dissection

Exposure

Three secondary ports are used (Figure 21.1). In the first, a 5 mm trocar and cannula is placed under direct vision on screen in the right mid-clavicular line just below the costal margin. Finger pressure on the abdominal wall will show the projected site which should be just over the gallbladder and if possible in line with the liver edge. If the course of the superior epigastric artery is marked beforehand using a hand held doppler, a potential source of haemorrhage is avoided. Closed grasping forceps are passed to sweep omentum and colon aside and expose the fundus of the gallbladder which is then grasped. A second 5 mm cannula is inserted in the anterior axillary line normally level with the umbilicus, but higher or lower depending on obesity and where the liver edge lies – if the patient is thin with a narrow costal margin

the insertion point may be just above the anterior superior iliac spine. Lockable grasping forceps are then used to take the fundus and rotate the liver to show its inferior surface. The surgeon must be sure there are no adhesions to the capsule which will tear into the liver with displacement. The success of the operation depends on good fundus elevation; if grasping is difficult, needle decompression of bile or mucus may help; if inflammatory thickening is a problem, changing to a 10 mm cannula and using large-toothed grasping forceps will help.

The third and main operating port is a 10 mm trocar and cannula passed in the midline just below the xiphoid at a level judged by the position of the liver edge; it must not be too low. The trocar tip is angled to pass through the peritoneum just to the right of the falciform ligament to avoid bleeding. The mid-clavicular line forceps are applied to the neck of the gallbladder which is then drawn anteriorly and inferiorly and to the right, pivoting on the firmly held fundus. This opens out Calot's triangle and presents the left side of Hartmann's pouch for dissection from the upper midline port using 5 mm instruments through an appropriate reducing sleeve (Figure 21.2).

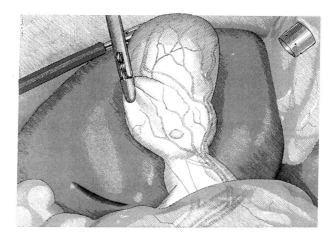

Figure 21.2 Balanced traction is used to expose Calot's triangle

Excision

The principles are the same as for open operation. Blunt dissection is used to display the cystic duct first, starting as close to the neck as possible working from the outer 'free' edge; the artery is then sought and may be clipped but not divided if a cholangiogram is to follow. Phillips *et al.* (1990) stress that confirmation of the anatomy before any structure is divided is important in the prevention of ductal injury. Special cholangiography forceps have been devised (Olsen, 1991), but a simple method is to pre-bend a plastic catheter to give it a smooth curve and pass it through an angiocath cannula inserted over the exposed cystic duct (J. B. Petelin, personal communication). Rotation will bring the catheter in line with the incised duct for grasping forceps to complete the insertion. A lightly closed clip secures the catheter and prevents leakage of contrast on injection.

The alternative 'close dissection' technique is based on the 'fundus down' method developed for open cholecystectomy (Espiner, 1982). Because fundus traction hinders the view, dissection is begun on the lower third and is carried across Hartmann's pouch to the neck and thence down the cystic duct (Figure 21.3a–c). By dividing the vascular and peritoneal connections to the gallbladder in the plane immediately adjacent to its wall and always on its surface, formal identification and division of the cystic artery becomes unnecessary. If inflammation or fibrosis has tethered a nearby right hepatic duct or artery close to the gallbladder wall, this method will ensure that such structures are pushed aside as the dissection line continues always well up on the gallbladder wall. Because all the small branches of the artery are sealed by diathermy forceps before division, the field is kept bloodless throughout. Once the neck is freed and the cystic duct identified and doubly clipped, there is then no need for cholangiography or display of the junction of the cystic and common ducts. In the author's opinion this technique offers the best guarantee of safety, especially in difficult dissections.

Removal of the gallbladder from below upwards is straightforward, provided that dissection is conducted in the plane close to its wall. Veins and Luschka ducts in the liver bed are easily entered if lasers or diathermy hooks transgress the areolar tissue of the bed, and bleeding from the liver edge can be tiresome if the division of the peritoneal attachments strays into the liver capsule. Proper tension is the secret of easy removal and a firmly held fundus is essential. Much of the dissection can be completed from the left side with the neck held over to the right, but later rotation of the neck to the right combined with downward traction on the fundus to the left displays the peritoneal attachment of the right side for easy division. As the fundus is reached, the neck forceps are pushed up and over the liver edge to expose the last attachments which may be quite vascular. Before the gallbladder is finally removed, the liver bed is inspected for haemostasis. It is an important principle of laparoscopic surgery that bleeding points are secured immediately and a reliable suction irrigation system is essential.

Retrieval

Removal of the gallbladder is usually straightforward through the umbilicus. If the telescope is slowly withdrawn into its cannula as the neck-holding forceps are kept in view and moved towards the cannula, the neck of the gallbladder can be delivered into the mouth of the cannula and then grasped with a 10 mm forceps as the telescope is taken and placed in the midline port. Under direct vision the neck is drawn carefully into the cannula and the cannula and

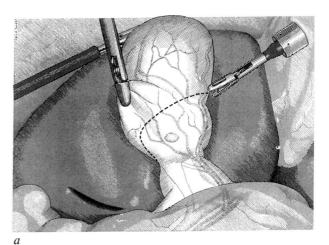

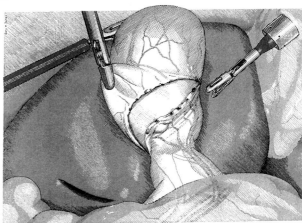

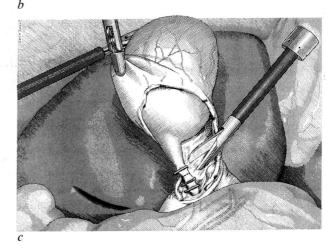

Figure 21.3 *a*, The line of dissection across the lower third and above the cystic node. *b*, The peritoneal and vascular connections are separated always on the surface of the gallbladder. *c*, Provided direct mural continuity between neck and cystic duct is confirmed, dissection is complete

forceps together gently withdrawn through the abdominal wall. Holding the neck outside with artery forceps, the gallbladder is opened, bile is aspirated, stones removed or crushed and the collapsed viscus removed. Because the site of entry at the umbilicus is the first and blind puncture, it is fully inspected from above before withdrawal of the cannula, so that any bowel injury which would otherwise go unnoticed can be excluded. If the gallbladder wall is thick or the stones larger than 1.5 cm diameter, the puncture site is incised and closure by suture will then be necessary.

An alternative technique is to employ a retrieval system (Maple Medi-Tech, UK), consisting of a large, wide-mouthed pouch, which can be deployed over the anterior surface of the liver while the fundus forceps easily place the gallbladder inside; an elongated tail draws up the mouth of the pouch like a drawstring into the end of the midline cannula which is then withdrawn over the tail. The mouth of the pouch is then opened externally and the contents, securely contained, are easily removed without enlarging the puncture site. This retrieval system is very useful in difficult cases where deliberate opening of the gallbladder and piecemeal removal is the only way to proceed; early deployment into the subhepatic space allows progressive collection of stones and debris as they appear. Large stones which cannot be crushed can be shattered easily by electrohydraulic lithotripsy, an instrument present in most urology theatres.

Closure

A tube drain is placed in the gallbladder bed via the anterior axillary line port and retained for 6–8 h, helping to remove residual carbon dioxide from the peritoneum. In the absence of any bile drainage it is removed. Bupivacaine hydrochloride (0.5%) is infiltrated into each portal site down to the peritoneum and the wounds are gently irrigated with Savlon (1%) before subcuticular Vicryl and Steristrip closure of the skin.

Postoperative course

There are no restrictions; patients can leave hospital as soon as they are fully recovered from anaesthetic. Simple analgesics are prescribed and opiates are avoided. Older patients and those with acute cholecystitis or empyema usually stay a day or two longer.

Complications

As with any laparoscopy there is a risk of gas embolism, mediastinal emphysema and pneumothorax, laceration of the aorta or vena cava leading to immediate or delayed haemorrhage, and bowel injury – all may follow blind insertion of the first trocar. Intraabdominal haemorrhage from torn adhesions and large haematomata in the abdominal wall may follow insertion and instrument manipulation through secondary ports. The surgeon must be fully aware of the pitfalls of laparoscopy and their avoidance and should receive formal training in the technique.

Bile duct injury is the most serious complication and mistaken judgement of the anatomy is the usual cause. Cholangiography may help to minimize this. Excessive traction in the presence of inflammation has led to tearing of the junction of the cystic and common bile ducts, and inappropriate laser or cautery dissection in the vicinity of the right hepatic duct may cause significant bile leakage. If there is any doubt about a particular structure, resort to open operation is essential. Haemorrhage is usually the result of faulty technique and dissection in the wrong plane. Instant tamponade with forceps pressure might control the immediate problem, while extra ports for clip application or endoloop placement are established. Adequate suction irrigation apparatus must be in readiness at all times. Bile leakage postoperatively may indicate a duct injury, slipped clip or breach of a Luschka duct in the liver bed and should be suspected if pain persists or recurs in the right upper quadrant after a few days; increasing tenderness, fever and elevated white count may be noted. Computerized scanning with needle drainage should solve a sealed leak, and endoscopic nasobiliary drainage or stenting may have a part to play in a more persistent fistula and laparotomy should always be considered.

There are no long-term complications of this operation as yet, but where umbilical access has been by initial incision or the puncture site enlarged to remove a thickened gallbladder with large stones, there is a risk of herniation, and strangulation requiring operation has been reported.

Many teachers stress the importance of learning basic techniques on trainers and simulators, but nothing can replace the direct experience gained in the operating theatre. Acting first as camera person and then as first assistant gives the trainee an invaluable feel for the instruments, while basic dexterity can be quickly acquired with a simple home video camera and television.

References

Cuschieri, A., Dubois, F., Mouiel, J. et al. (1991) The European experience with laparoscopic cholecystectomy. *Am. J. Surg.*, **161**, 385–387

Dubois, F., Icard, P., Berthelot, G. and Leavrd, H. (1990) Coelioscopic cholecystectomy. *Ann. Surg.*, **211**, 60–63

Espiner, H. J. (1982) Emergency cholecystectomy: towards guaranteed safety. In *Care of the Acutely Ill and Injured* (eds D. H. Wilson and A. K. Marsden), Wiley, New York, pp. 385–387

Olsen, D. (1991) Laparoscopic cholecystectomy. *Am. J. Surg.*, **161**, 339–344

Phillips, E. H., Berci, G., Carroll, B. et al. (1990) The importance of intraoperative cholangiography during laparoscopic cholecystectomy. *Am. Surgeon*, **56**, 792–795

Reddick, E. J. and Olsen, D. O. (1990) Laparoscopic laser cholecystectomy. *Surg. Endoscopy*, **3**, 131–133

22

Hiatal hernia

D. B. Skinner

Proper surgical management of hiatal hernia and gastro-oesophageal reflux is based on principles and understanding learned only recently. Hiatal hernia was not diagnosed in a living human being prior to the introduction of oesophageal radiography early in this century. Until the mid-century, hiatal hernia was thought to be an anatomical problem similar to hernias elsewhere in the body, and the usual surgical treatment emphasized obliteration of the hernial sac and suturing of the diaphragmatic crura to narrow the oesophageal hiatus. In 1951, Allison's description of gastro-oesophageal reflux and reflux oesophagitis established this as the disease causing the symptoms of heartburn and regurgitation and the complications of stricture and bleeding. Subsequently, Hiebert and Belsey (1961) convincingly demonstrated that patients could have abnormal ooesphageal reflux causing complications in the absence of a hiatal hernia, and it became gradually appreciated that most patients with hiatal hernia did not require treatment.

Now it is generally accepted that hiatal hernia and gastro-oesphageal reflux are different conditions which commonly occur together, but may occur independently. A large number, estimated at 10% of the adult population of North Americans and Europeans are known to have a hiatal hernia, but very few of these people are troubled by the symptoms or complications of reflux. On the other hand, approximately 80% of those with pathological degrees of reflux causing symptoms and complications have an associated hiatal hernia, but 20% do not. It is the frequent entry and prolonged presence in the oesophagus of acid peptic secretions, and occasionally pancreaticobiliary secretions, which cause the symptoms of heartburn and regurgitation and the complications of reflux.

Types of hiatal hernia

The very common type I, axial or sliding hiatal hernia by itself generally causes no symptoms or complications unless associated with abnormal reflux. Accordingly, the type I hiatal hernia should not be considered to be a disease, and does not require any type of medical or surgical treatment. The rarer type II, para-oesophageal or rolling hiatal hernia presents a different problem (Figure 22.1). In this instance the herniation of stomach is into a free peritoneal sac extending into the thorax. Since abdominal pressure is consistently higher than thoracic pressure, this sac will naturally tend to enlarge until the entire stomach is in an intrathoracic location. Even though such hernias may be asymptomatic, they are potentially lethal because of the high incidence of gastric obstruction, volvulus, infarction, bleeding and intrathoracic

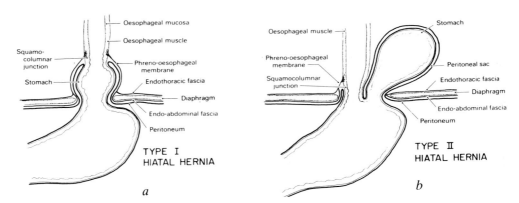

Figure 22.1 The anatomical abnormalities for a type I sliding or axial hernia (*a*) and a type II rolling para-oesophageal hiatal hernia (*b*). In the type I defect the phreno-oesophageal membrane remains intact but is displaced in a cephalad direction. This membrane is formed by the fusion of the endo-abdominal and endothoracic fascia coming off the diaphragm. Normally it inserts 3–4 cm above the junction of tubular oesophagus with gastric pouch. The insertion of the membrane is into the submucosa of the oesophagus. If insertion of the membrane occurs at a normal level, the hiatal hernia pouch remains intra-abdominal, as does the lower oesophagus, so no reflux may occur.

In the type II hiatal hernia there is a defect in the phreno-oesophageal membrane permitting a true peritoneal sac to enter the thoracic cavity. The junction of oesophagus and stomach remains at the normal location and is fixed by the insertion of the remainder of the intact phreno-oesophageal membrane

gastric dilatation. For this reason, the large type II para-oesophageal hernias should be repaired surgically when they are encountered, even if they are asymptomatic. This type is the only variety for which surgical repair of hiatal hernia is always indicated.

The diagnosis of hiatal hernia is generally made by radiography. Since the common type I hiatal hernia is not always a disease and may not require therapy the diagnostic problem is documentation of gastro-oesophageal reflux. For this purpose, radiography is much less effective than in diagnosing hiatal hernia. Only about 40% of those patients who eventually are proved to have abnormal degrees of reflux are shown to have reflux demonstrated spontaneously during radiographic studies including cine barium swallow techniques.

Oesophageal function tests

To make the diagnosis of abnormal gastro-oesophageal reflux, oesophageal function tests are frequently required. Several of these tests are widely employed and are generally done at the same sitting.

Manometry

The first of these tests to be introduced was oesophageal manometry. Observations of oesophageal peristalsis dated back many years, but modern oesophageal manometry was developed in a systematic fashion by Code and associates at the Mayo Clinic in the mid-1950s (Fyke *et al.*, 1956). The technique was refined (Winans and Harris, 1967) to provide more quantitative data by using infused catheters.

To perform oesophageal manometry a triple lumen fluid-filled catheter with orifices spaced 5 cm apart is introduced like a nasogastric tube into the stomach. The catheter channels are connected through pressure transducers to a recorder. Alternatively, miniaturized electronic transducers may be used in place of the open-tipped water-perfused catheters. The train of catheters or transducers is slowly withdrawn from the stomach into the oesophagus. Normally each pressure detector passes from the stomach characterized by baseline pressure slightly higher than atmospheric, through a zone of high pressure between the stomach and oesophagus, and finally into the less than atmospheric pressure environment of the oesophagus (Figure 22.2). The high-pressure zone usually measures between 3 and 4 cm in length. One-half to three-quarters of this high-pressure zone is located within the abdominal environment as indicated by positive-pressure deflections with respiration. The functional level of the diaphragm is determined as the place where respiratory pressure deflections reverse as the thorax is entered. The high-pressure zone is believed to represent the distal oesophageal segment which extends several centimetres within the abdominal cavity before the gastric pouch is entered (see Figure 22.1). There is a statistical correlation between the magnitude, length and abdominal segment of the high-pressure zone and the presence or absence of gastro-oesophageal reflux in a population of patients and normal subjects. However, the overlap in pressures recorded in patients with or without abnormal reflux is too great to employ manometry as a diagnostic measurement of reflux in an individual patient.

Besides assessing and locating the distal oesophageal high-pressure zone, manometry provides other valuable information. Findings diagnostic for achalasia, scleroderma or oesophageal spasm may be observed in patients with symptoms of oesophageal disease which might otherwise be confused with some manifestations of reflux. The principal function of manometry is the exclusion or diagnosis of other motor disorders which may accompany or be confused with an incompetent cardia and gastro-oesophageal reflux.

pH reflux tests

Oesophageal pH studies are another commonly used test of oesophageal function, and are routinely employed in conjunction with oesophageal manometry. A long gastrointestinal pH electrode is passed like a nasogastric tube into the stomach. As this electrode is slowly withdrawn, a sharp rise in pH is noted over a 1 cm distance corresponding to the level of the distal oesophageal high-pressure zone. Such a sharp rise in pH is seen in approximately 80% of normal people. Patients with an incompetent cardia frequently have gradual and prolonged rise in pH. Unfortunately this may occur in normal individuals if acid and mucous material from the stomach are coated on the pH electrode. Although this pH electrode withdrawal technique is the first pH test for reflux described (Tuttle and Grossman, 1958), it is not widely used because of the high rate of false-positive examinations.

A *standard acid reflux test* developed in the mid-1960s places the pH electrode 5 cm above the top of the high-pressure zone and after an acid load is placed in the stomach (Kantrowitz *et al.*, 1969). Patients are asked to perform a series of respiratory and postural manoeuvres to challenge the cardia while pH is being recorded in the oesophagus. During a standard acid reflux test, patients perform coughing, deep breathing, Valsalva manoeuvre and Müller manoeuvre, in the supine, right side down, left side down and head down positions. After each bout of reflux, time is allowed for pH to return to above 4 before the test is resumed. More than two drops in pH during the performance of these manoeuvres is determined to be abnormal when compared with healthy controls (Skinner and Booth, 1970). This test is performed in conjunction with oesophageal manometry and provides a rapid and effective screening test for patients with abnormal reflux. It is more accurate than manometry alone or the Tuttle test for the diagnosis of

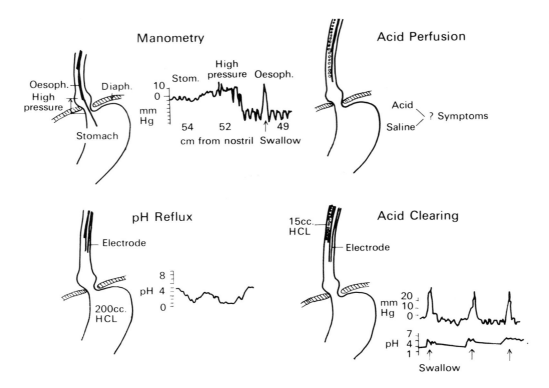

Figure 22.2 Diagram of commonly used oesophageal function tests. Manometry is performed with triple-lumen catheter to record pressures across the gastro-oesophageal junction. The pH reflux test detects drops in pH 5 cm above the gastro-oesophageal junction after placement of an acid load in the stomach. The acid clearing test determines the ability of the oesophagus to empty 15 ml of 0.1 N HCl from the mid-oesophagus. Normally this occurs with swallowing. The acid perfusion test correlates the presence of the patient's own symptoms with the perfusion of acid or saline into the mid-oesophagus (From Skinner and Booth, 1970, by permission)

abnormal reflux. Because the test is of limited duration and imposes severe stress on the cardia, it still carries an incidence of false-positive and false-negative results.

Acid clearing

It requires two abnormalities for reflux oesophagitis to develop. A patient must have frequent episodes of gastro-oesophageal reflux and, in addition, must have some disorder of normal oesophageal clearing which permits the regurgitated gastric contents to have prolonged contact with the squamous epithelium. It is normal for everyone to have reflux on occasion, particularly after meals. Regurgitated gastric contents are cleared from the oesophagus only by coordinated peristalsis. The small amount of residual acid is then neutralized by swallowing saliva (Helm *et al.*, 1984). A disorder in oesophageal clearing permits refluxed contents to remain in the oesophagus.

A test of acid clearing is used routinely in conjunction with the standard acid reflux test. After the reflux test is completed, a 15 ml bolus of 0.1 N hydrochloric acid is placed in the mid-oesophagus. Distal oesophageal pH is monitored while the patient is asked to swallow at 30 s intervals. Normal individuals without

reflux oesophagitis clear this acid from the oesophagus in 10 swallows or less. Those with oesophagitis are likely to have a marked prolongation of clearing, or to have repeated drops in pH during the test as further reflux occurs. This test is useful as a screening method to identify those at greatest risk for having oesophagitis.

Acid perfusion

The symptoms of epigastric pain and heartburn are non-specific, and may be caused by a variety of other conditions including coronary heart disease, other oesophageal diseases, gastritis, gastric ulcer or duodenal ulcer, pancreatitis or biliary tract disease. For this reason the acid perfusion test is often performed when symptoms are atypical to determine if the patient's symptoms may be provoked by infusion of acid into the oesophagus. The test is generally conducted at the end of the battery of oesophageal function tests. The infusion catheters are left in the mid-oesophagus and 0.1 N HCl or normal saline are alternately perfused for 10 min intervals into the oesophagus without the patient being informed as to which substance is being infused. If the patient's spontaneous symptoms are elicited by acid and relieved by saline, it can be stated that the symptoms are acid induced and of oesophageal origin. When coupled with the documentation of abnormal reflux, the presumption of reflux causing symptoms may be made. With the use of oesophageal manometry, standard acid reflux test, acid clearing test and the acid perfusion test, the functional disorders of the oesophagus, including gastro-oesophageal reflux, may be diagnosed in a high proportion of patients with studies which are simple to perform on an outpatient basis. These tests provide the most commonly and effectively employed methods for diagnosing abnormal gastro-oesophageal reflux.

Prolonged oesophageal pH monitoring

Continuous oesophageal pH monitoring over 24 h or longer provides additional insight into the disordered pathophysiology of reflux, and is of great value in the diagnosis of the atypical or difficult patient. The technique employed is that described by Johnson and DeMeester (1974) in which the long gastrointestinal pH electrode is left in position 5 cm above the high-pressure zone. Commercially available systems have the earth electrode incorporated in the catheter assembly. The long electrode is connected to a portable pH meter and recorder so that the patient may be at home during the time of observation. The subject is instructed to note changes in position, symptoms or other activities so that correlations may be made between activities and intra-oesophageal pH. The patient is maintained on a diet adjusted to eliminate low pH foods. A portion of the test is performed while the patient is in the sitting or upright position, and the other half of the test is performed while the patient is lying flat in bed overnight. From the tracing obtained over a 24-hour period it is possible to calculate the proportion of time in the upright position or supine position in which oesophageal pH is less than 4, the total number of reflux episodes in each position, the number of episodes longer than 5 min, the longest episode of low pH and the total time during which pH is abnormally low. A scoring system is devised to take each of these factors into account.

Studies in normal healthy individuals demonstrate that everyone has some reflux, usually after meals. This generally occurs in the upright position, and the bouts of reflux are limited in number and of short duration. Individuals with pathological reflux demonstrate three patterns (DeMeester et al., 1976). Most commonly seen is the patient who has multiple and prolonged bouts of reflux in both the upright and supine positions. These individuals tend to be both symptomatic and subject to oesophagitis. Another smaller group of patients has reflux only in the supine position. Since this reflux generally occurs while the patient is asleep at night, the individual may be unaware of the reflux. Swallowing occurs rarely at night, so the duration of contact of the regurgitated substances and the oesophageal mucosa may be pro-

longed. These prolonged bouts of reflux are correlated with an increased incidence of oesophagitis. If this occurs only while the patient is asleep, he or she may not be aware of reflux until the onset of dysphagia occurs. This may explain an earlier observation that 20% of patients seen with oesophageal strictures do not request medical help for their symptoms prior to the onset of dysphagia.

The third subset of abnormal reflux is that which occurs only in the upright position. These patients reflux frequently with any change of activity or body position during the daytime while they are up and around. They are often highly symptomatic, but protect themselves against complications of reflux by swallowing air, antacids or food. They complain frequently of belching as well as heartburn, and are often overweight. If these patients have no supine reflux, the chance of oesophagitis is small since the acid is cleared by the swallowing manoeuvres which the patient employs. Most of these individuals acquire the habit of oesophagia which may be difficult to correct after a successful anti-reflux repair. These patients may be more subject to abdominal distension and the gas bloat syndrome after successful anti-reflux surgery, but have a small risk of oesophagitis. Accordingly, it seems inadvisable to operate on such patients, and great efforts are made to treat them medically unless frank oesophagitis develops.

The 24-hour continuous pH monitoring studies are especially useful in diagnosing those patients in whom reflux causes pulmonary symptoms, and those individuals in whom an alkaline component to reflux is present. Respiratory symptoms are common in North America and Europe. It is well known that chronic or acute aspiration of gastric contents into the lung may lead to respiratory disease. The frequency of respiratory symptoms in patients with reflux is as high as 60%. However, it is often difficult to demonstrate a direct cause-and-effect relationship between reflux and respiratory complaints. By continuous pH monitoring it is possible to identify those patients in whom bouts of reflux regularly precede the onset of coughing and respiratory symptoms. This occurs in less than 10% of patients with abnormal reflux. In others the coughing itself is a cause of abnormal reflux. When respiratory symptoms are prominent and are considered as a possible indication for anti-reflux surgery, the use of continuous pH monitoring will determine whether this is a justifiable indication for surgery in an effort to relieve the respiratory disease (Pellegrini et al., 1979).

It has been known for some time that acid-reducing gastric operations such as pyloroplasty and vagotomy or antrectomy with or without vagotomy do not relieve, and may aggravate, symptomatic reflux and oesophagitis. Careful analysis of 24-hour pH recordings demonstrates a small group of patients in whom the pH intermittently rises above 7 to the range of 7.6 which is equivalent to the alkalinity of pancreatic and biliary secretions. This may occur with or without acid reflux, depending on the amount of acid production by the stomach. Based on such studies, patients are identified with oesophageal strictures in spite of achlorhydria, and in whom the alkaline regurgitation is frequent and the probable cause of the oesophagitis and stricture.

When the symptoms are atypical and radiographic studies do not convincingly demonstrate spontaneous reflux, the oesophageal function tests serve as the standard for diagnosis of functional disorders including an incompetent cardia and gastro-oesophageal reflux. In difficult or unusual cases, continuous pH monitoring in the oesophagus provides additional valuable information. Once the diagnosis of abnormal gastro-oesophageal reflux is established by one of these methods, further investigation for the presence of complications is indicated.

Diagnosis of oesophagitis

Oesophagitis is the most common complication of reflux and the precursor to stricture and bleeding. Since oesophagitis is a pathological diagnosis it requires direct observation of the condition of the lower oesophagus, most frequently by flexible fibre-optic endoscopy. Based on the appearance of the distal oesophagus, oesophagitis may be graded from 0 to IV. Grade I oesophagitis is recorded when erythema of the oesophagus near the gastro-oesophageal junction is seen but there are no frank ulcerations. A biopsy of the mucosa may show hyperplasia of the basal epithelial layers of the squamous epithelium and close proximity of the rete pegs and vascular bundles to the surface giving the red appearance. However, no inflammatory cells are seen and this should not be considered as true oesophagitis. Grade II oesophagitis is noted when there is a break in the mucosa with frank ulceration. Oesophagitis progresses to grade III when the ulcerations are confluent and accompanied by fibrosis and rigidity of the wall. When a frank stricture develops so that the oesophagoscope cannot be passed, grade IV oesophagitis is recorded. The degree of oesophagitis is an important determinant when considering indications for surgery.

Anti-reflux surgery

Indications

After completion of the work-up, including barium swallow, oesophageal function studies and endoscopy, and a general evaluation of the patient's health, consideration of treatment is undertaken. Surgery is reserved for those patients with the complications of reflux including ulcerative oesophagitis, stricture, bleeding documented to come from oesophagitis, complicated Barrett's oesophagus and documented repeated bouts of aspiration causing lung disease. All other patients with uncomplicated reflux should be treated medically in an effort to relieve their symptoms. Only if symptoms are clearly known to be caused by reflux, and cannot be relieved by rigorous medical treatment over approximately 6 months, should a patient with uncomplicated reflux be considered for surgical treatment. Even in these circumstances the pure upright refluxer who has the habit of aerophagia is probably not a surgical candidate because of the high incidence of symptomatic gas bloat syndrome after operation. As indicated above, only the large type II para-oesophageal hiatal hernia is an indication for surgery based on the diagnosis of hiatal hernia. The rationale for recommending surgery when ulcerative oesophagitis is present is that recurring bouts of ulcerative oesophagitis may lead to fibrosis and stricture which are much more difficult to treat, and have less chance of being cured. Ulcerative oesophagitis may progress to frank stricture formation in a remarkably short time, so that surgical treatment is generally advisable when oesophagitis reaches this degree of mucosal damage and cannot be reversed promptly by intensive medical therapy.

Principles

Once a decision to operate is reached, the operation to be performed should be an anti-reflux repair rather than simply an obliteration of the hiatal hernia sac and narrowing of the oesophageal hiatus. A number of anti-reflux repairs have been advocated in recent years. Allison (1951) initially described a repair which he hoped would prevent reflux by reattaching the phreno-oesophageal membrane to the margins of the hiatus. This did not succeed in correcting reflux in many patients, and Allison eventually acknowledged this after long-term follow-up of his cases (Allison, 1973). The Allison repair is not now recommended for anti-reflux surgery.

There are a number of effective anti-reflux operations under evaluation. Each of these recognizes similar principles. For an anti-reflux operation to be successful, it should restore the normal or somewhat exaggerated length of intra-abdominal oesophagus. Evidence compiled in recent years indicates that it is the intra-abdominal segment of narrow-diameter swallowing tube entering the large-diameter gastric pouch within a common pressure chamber of abdomen which accounts for the normal control of reflux. When described in this way, it is obvious that the law of Laplace governing wall tension of tubes applies. This causes the smaller-diameter swallowing tube to remain closed and requires a greater force to distend its lumen than is the case for the larger diameter stomach.

If the intra-abdominal segment of oesophagus is lost so that the swallowing tube is in the less than atmospheric pressure environment of the thorax as it enters into the gastric pouch, then it will tend to have a larger diameter and be a less effective barrier to reflux when challenged by increased gastric pressure. The evidence for this mechanism is documented by a number of experimental and clinical observations (DeMeester *et al.*, 1979; Skinner, 1985). A true anatomical sphincter in the distal oesophagus of human beings has never been convincingly demonstrated, and current evidence indicates that a sphincter muscle *per se* is not present or necessary in the distal oesophagus to prevent reflux. Rather, the anatomical location of the intra-abdominal oesophagus and its geometric relation with the gastric pouch is critical in preventing reflux. Each of the successful anti-reflux repairs emphasizes the restoration of the intra-abdominal segment of the oesophagus and restricts the diameter of the lumen by a partial or full plication of stomach around the intra-abdominal oesophageal segment.

Selection of approach

In Europe and North America, the anti-reflux repairs developed independently by Nissen (1961) and by Belsey (Skinner and Belsey, 1967) both in 1955, are most widely used. The repair described by Hill (1967) of Seattle has many advocates in North and South America, and a repair described by Guarner of Mexico City recognizes similar principles (Guarner *et al.*, 1975). The Belsey Mark IV operation can only be performed through a thoracotomy incision. The Nissen fundoplication may be performed transthoracically or transabdominally. The Hill posterior gastropexy and calibration of the cardia are performed through an abdominal approach, and the Guarner operation is similarly done transabdominally. Unfortunately the choice of operation is often governed more by the experience and credentials of the surgeon rather than by the needs of the patient. When a surgeon is familiar and comfortable with anti-reflux operations being done either transthoracically or transabdominally, indications for one approach or the other are recognized. A common cause of failure of anti-reflux surgery is insufficient reduction of enough length of intra-abdominal oesophagus or reduction of it under too much tension. The transthoracic approach allows more oesophagus to be completely mobilized which facilitates establishment of the intra-abdominal segment of swallowing tube. For this reason the transthoracic approach is preferred in patients with severe oesophagitis or in patients who have recurrence following previous efforts at anti-reflux surgery. The transthoracic approach offers advantages in the obese patient in whom exposure of the cardia through an abdominal incision may be unduly difficult. The abdominal approach is highly satisfactory for the first-time anti-reflux operations in thin patients, and is clearly the procedure of choice when other intra-abdominal disease requires correction at the same time.

Because the Belsey Mark IV operation and Nissen fundoplication are probably most widely used, and because of space constraints in this chapter, only these two repairs will be described in detail. The interested reader is encouraged to investigate the techniques and attributes of the Hill and Guarner repairs by using the cited references. The placement of a prosthetic device around the cardia as described by Angelchik and Cohen (1979) is not advocated because of the seriousness of complications when they occur.

Mark IV anti-reflux repair

The Belsey Mark IV operation was so named because it represented the fourth modification or variation employed by its developer, Ronald Belsey of Bristol, England. Finding that the original Allison repair did not succeed in preventing reflux, Belsey instituted a series of modifications until the Mark IV operation proved to be a successful anti-reflux procedure. These modifications proceeded between approximately 1949 and 1955.

The operation is performed through a left 6th interspace thoracotomy. The 6th interspace is chosen both because a higher thoracotomy seems to cause less postoperative pain and discomfort due to less rib motion, and because this repair is used when extensive mobilization of the oesophagus up to the aortic arch is desired. It is essential to avoid undue stretching, breaking of ribs, or damage to the chest wall during the performance of this operation, so as to minimize post-thoracotomy discomfort. Often the serratus muscle need not be divided.

After the thorax is opened, the pulmonary ligament is divided, ligating a small vessel at its free margin. An incision in the pleura is made just anterior to the aorta. The oesophagus is dissected from its bed, ligating two or three direct branches from the aorta to the oesophagus. Because of the extensive submucosal collateral circulation of the oesophagus, these vessels may be ligated without fear of causing ischaemia. As the oesophagus is elevated from its bed the adherent right pleural surface is dissected free bluntly to prevent opening of the right thorax with accumulation of blood in the downside chest during the remainder of the procedure. Anteriorly the oesophagus is dissected free from the pericardium from which some of the oesophageal muscle fibres arise. Eventually the entire oesophagus with its adjacent vagus nerve branches is completely freed from the rest of the mediastinum up to the level of the aortic arch (Figure 22.3).

The reflection of the greater peritoneal sac onto the anterior surface of the oesophagus is incised by pulling up on the oesophagus and cutting directly into the tissues at the anterior margin of the oesophageal hiatus. After the pleura is divided, the next layer is the phreno-oesophageal membrane which represents a fusion of the endo-abdominal and endothoracic fascia. This membrane inserts into the submucosa of the oesophagus several centimetres above the oesophagogastric junction. After incising the phreno-

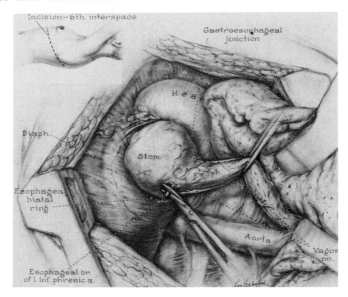

Figure 22.3 A transthoracic anti-reflux repair is generally performed through the left 6th intercostal interspace. The oesophagus is mobilized up to the arch of the aorta to enable reduction of the intra-abdominal segment of oesophagus. All attachments to the hiatus are divided. In this figure the ascending branch of the left inferior phrenic artery is being divided (From Belsey and Skinner, 1972, by permission)

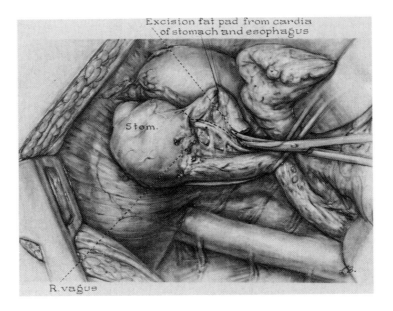

Figure 22.4 After full mobilization of the oesophagus the hiatal hernia sac and redundant fibro-fatty tissue on the cardia are excised to permit close apposition of the fundus of the stomach to the oesophagus when the fundoplication is performed. The vagus nerves are preserved (From Belsey and Skinner, 1972, by permission)

oesophageal membrane, retroperitoneal fat is encountered. Deep to this lies the peritoneal reflection which is opened. The cardia is completely freed from its attachments to the diaphragm by incising the phreno-oesophageal membrane circumferentially. An ascending branch of the left inferior phrenic artery is encountered laterally close to the left vagus nerve.

This artery is ligated and divided but the nerve is carefully preserved. Medially the hepatic branch of the vagus nerve should be preserved. Just posterior to this lies the ascending, communicating branch of the left gastric artery (Belsey's artery) which is ligated and divided. Once this is done the lesser peritoneal sac reflection off the intra-abdominal oesophagus is easily identified and entered. The dissection is completed preserving the two main vagus nerve trunks and their branches. At the end of this dissection it should be possible to pass a right-angle clamp or the operator's fingertip completely around the free edge of the hiatal muscle.

The fibro-fatty tissue remaining on the anterior and lateral oesophageal wall is excised so that the fundo-plication of the stomach serosa will be against bare oesophageal muscle to encourage adhesion (Figure 22.4). Several vessels are usually encountered in this fat pad. It is important to dissect this tissue from a cephalad direction distally. Otherwise the dissection is likely to follow the phreno-oesophageal membrane into the submucosal layer of the oesophagus.

The pleura overlying the junction of diaphragm and pericardium is incised medially. The pericardium is bluntly elevated off the right portion of the diaphragm so that the tendinous origin of the diaphragm may be identified. By pulling the diaphragm forward with a tenaculum, the tendinous right pillar of the diaphragm is identified. A spoon bowl may be introduced posteriorly into the hiatus to protect the liver while large needles bearing silk sutures are passed through the right and left margins of the oesophageal hiatus to narrow it posteriorly (Figure 22.5). The number of sutures required to obliterate the posterior hiatus from its vertebral origin anteriorly varies with the size of the hiatal hernia, but three such sutures is an average number. These sutures are laid in place but not tied until the fundoplication is completed. Up to this point, the dissection is the same whether a Belsey or Nissen type of fundoplication is subsequently employed.

If the Mark IV operation is chosen, a first row of three 2/0 silk sutures is placed. Laterally the first stitch passes from fundus of stomach to the oesophageal muscle 2 cm above the gastro-oesophageal junction just adjacent to the left vagus nerve. The suture is reversed and passed back through the oesophagus catching both transverse and longitudinal muscle fibres by a slightly oblique direction of the stitch. The stitch then passes through the fundus of the stomach. The mattress suture is tied to begin the approximation of the gastric fundus to the distal oesophagus. A similar stitch is placed anteriorly, and the third suture in this row is placed medially adjacent to the right vagus nerve. This brings approximately 2 cm of distal oesophagus within the gastric wrap.

A second row of sutures is placed passing initially through the diaphragm, then fundus of stomach and oesophagus and reversing back through the three structures in reverse order (Figure 22.6). The suture passing through the diaphragm is placed into the bowl of a spoon inserted beneath the diaphragm to protect the intra-abdominal organs. The diaphragm suture should catch the edge of the central tendon of the diaphragm rather than the muscular layers of the margins of the hiatus since the muscles do not hold sutures well. The first stitch is again placed laterally

through the diaphragm, fundus of stomach and oesophagus 4 cm above the gastro-oesophageal junction. The stitch is then reversed and passed back obliquely through the oesophagus, stomach and diaphragm. The two additional sutures are placed anteriorly and medially. These sutures are held until all three are inserted.

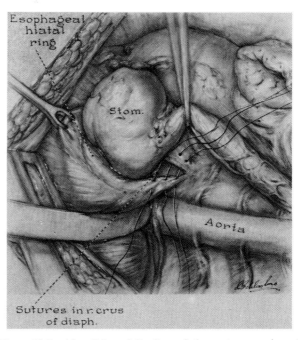

Figure 22.5 After full mobilization of the gastro-oesophageal junction the repair is started by narrowing the hiatus posteriorly. Up to this point the steps in the transthoracic anti-reflux operation are the same for either a Belsey Mark IV or Nissen fundoplication procedure (From Belsey and Skinner, 1972, by permission)

The gastro-oesophageal junction is placed manually beneath the diaphragm where it should remain without tension prior to the sutures being tied (Figure 22.7). When it is seen that the repair is satisfactory, the sutures are pulled up individually to avoid sawing through the oesophageal muscle. Sutures are tied without tension so that they do not cut through the fragile muscle of the oesophagus. When the fundoplication is completed in this fashion, the posterior sutures in the diaphragmatic crura are ligated also avoiding strangulation of the muscle. A chest tube is inserted, and the chest is closed in layers avoiding overtight suturing which increases post-thoracotomy discomfort.

A nasogastric tube is not routinely used but may need to be inserted postoperatively if the patient develops abdominal distension. Preoperative and intraoperative antibiotics are given because of the possibility of a needle entering the oesophagus and contaminating the mediastinum with mouth organisms. The chest tube is removed when drainage has decreased to less than 200 ml in 24 h. Liquids are given by mouth as soon as bowel sounds return which

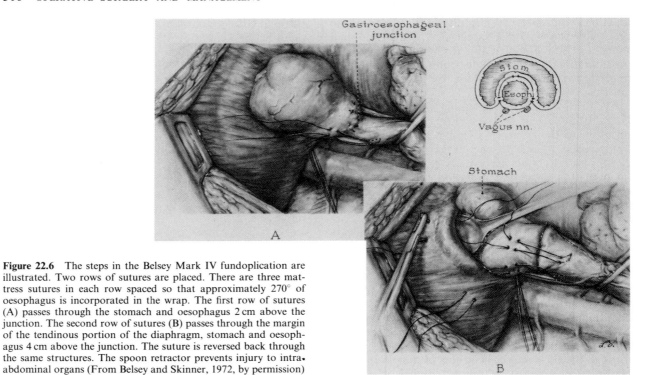

Figure 22.6 The steps in the Belsey Mark IV fundoplication are illustrated. Two rows of sutures are placed. There are three mattress sutures in each row spaced so that approximately 270° of oesophagus is incorporated in the wrap. The first row of sutures (A) passes through the stomach and oesophagus 2 cm above the junction. The second row of sutures (B) passes through the margin of the tendinous portion of the diaphragm, stomach and oesophagus 4 cm above the junction. The suture is reversed back through the same structures. The spoon retractor prevents injury to intra-abdominal organs (From Belsey and Skinner, 1972, by permission)

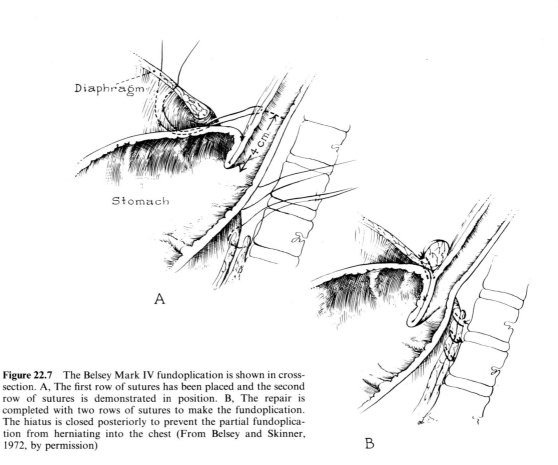

Figure 22.7 The Belsey Mark IV fundoplication is shown in cross-section. A, The first row of sutures has been placed and the second row of sutures is demonstrated in position. B, The repair is completed with two rows of sutures to make the fundoplication. The hiatus is closed posteriorly to prevent the partial fundoplication from herniating into the chest (From Belsey and Skinner, 1972, by permission)

is generally on the 2nd postoperative day. The patient receives a barium swallow study prior to discharge to document the effectiveness of the repair. On discharge, patients are cautioned to chew their food well, eat slowly, and to avoid a large bolus or sticky foods for several weeks after surgery.

Nissen fundoplication anti-reflux repair

The Nissen fundoplication may be performed either transthoracically or abdominally. When done through the thorax, the incision and dissection are identical to those used for the Mark IV repair and described above. After complete mobilization of the intrathoracic oesophagus and cardia from the diaphragm and removal of the para-oesophageal fibro-fatty tissues, the posterior sutures are placed to narrow the hiatus and again left untied until the fundoplication is finished.

amount of gastric fundus is folded into the wrap to ensure that it will not be too tight. Normally, three additional such sutures are placed progressing in a cephalad direction until 3–4 cm of distal oesophagus has been included in the fundoplication (Figure 22.9). At this point it is important to ascertain that the wrap is not too tight. The operator's finger should slide easily through the tunnel caused by the full fundoplication, or a no. 60 Fr. gauge bougie may be passed by mouth by the anaesthesiologist and be shown to enter easily into the stomach without tearing the sutures of the fundoplication. Once this is done the fundoplication is placed beneath the diaphragm where it should remain without tension. The posterior sutures are tied to complete the repair (Figure 22.10). Chest closure is similar to that described for the Mark IV operation.

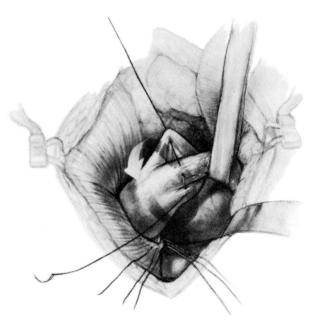

Figure 22.9 After the posterior sutures are placed in the hiatus, the fundoplication is performed. The lateral fundus is wrapped posteriorly behind the oesophagus. A series of sutures is placed through anterior and posterior stomach and oesophagus on the medial aspect of the oesophagus (From Skinner, 1976, by permission)

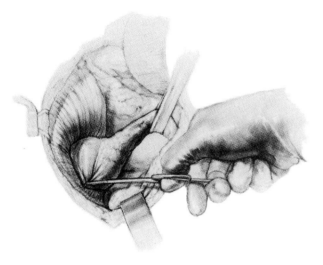

Figure 22.8 If a transthoracic Nissen fundoplication is selected, the highest short gastric vessels are divided as they are drawn up into the hiatus. The dissection of the oesophagus and cardia is the same as for the Mark IV repair (From Skinner, 1976, by permission)

To facilitate a loose and easy complete wrap of stomach around the oesophagus, the two or three highest short gastric arteries from the spleen to stomach are divided by drawing them up into the hiatus and individually ligating and dividing them (Figure 22.8). The posterior fundus is passed behind the oesophagus and the anterior fundus is passed medially so that the suture line is placed on the medial or right aspect of the oesophagus. This causes the least distortion of the stomach. The first suture is passed between the posterior fundus of the stomach, muscle of the gastro-oesophageal junction, and anterior aspect of the fundus just at the cardia. The vagus nerves are left adjacent to the oesophageal wall. These sutures should be placed far out on the fundus of the stomach on each side so that a substantial

When performed transabdominally, the Nissen operation may be done through several incisions. Some surgeons prefer a midline incision, others choose a left paramedian incision. Some employ a bilateral subcostal incision. The author generally prefers a right subcostal incision extended across the midline to the left costal margin just missing the tip of the xiphoid cartilage. After thorough abdominal exploration, the left lobe of the liver is taken down by dividing the triangular ligament. The triangular ligament is divided past the midline avoiding the junction of phrenic and hepatic veins. The stomach is pulled down and to the left to avoid tension on the short

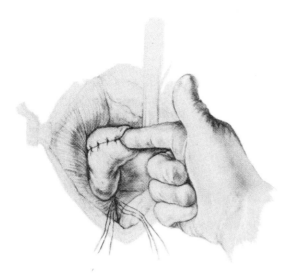

Figure 22.10 After completion of the fundoplication, which should be 4 cm in length, the operator's finger is passed through the tunnel along the oesophagus to be certain that it is not tight. The repair is then reduced into the abdomen and the posterior sutures in the hiatus are tied (From Skinner, 1976, by permission)

gastric arteries. This reduces the hiatal hernia sac and exposes the intra-abdominal segment of oesophagus. A transverse incision is made through the peritoneum overlying the oesophagus. This incision should be carried the full width of the hiatus, taking care not to divide the hepatic branch of the vagus nerve which passes in the top of the gastrohepatic ligament. To the left this incision is carried out onto the crus of the diaphragm. The operator's finger is inserted in the groove between the exposed oesophagus and left crus of the diaphragm. By dissecting bluntly in a straight posterior direction, the aortic pulse is palpated. The operator's finger should use the aorta as a guide and slide off the aorta onto the vertebral column and then back up medially to encompass both the oesophagus and adjacent vagus nerves. When the blunt dissection is carried out in this manner there is little danger of injury to the oesophagus itself which may occur if the dissection is carried too close to the oesophageal wall. After the oesophagus and adjacent nerves are encircled, a tape is placed around them to provide subsequent traction.

The reflection of the peritoneum from the gastro-oesophageal junction over the spleen is incised and the highest short gastric vessels are exposed. Two or three of these are dissected, ligated and divided to provide mobility to the fundus. When this is completed the posterior fundus should easily pass behind the oesophagus without putting undue tension on the remaining short gastric vessels. The lower oesophagus is dissected bluntly from the mediastinum to be certain that at least 4 cm of distal oesophagus can be delivered into the abdomen. When this is accomplished the oesophagus is drawn down and retracted to the left to expose the decussation of the diaphrag-

matic crura. With the operator's finger protecting the coeliac axis, a large needle bearing a 1/0 silk suture is passed through both crura, being certain to include endo-abdominal fascia in each bite (Figure 22.11). Usually three or four such sutures are placed in a cephalad direction to narrow the oesophageal hiatus so that it will accept only one of the operator's fingers without being too tight. The diaphragmatic sutures are tied at this time.

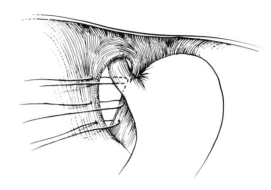

Figure 22.11 Following full mobilization of the gastro-oesophageal junction, sutures are placed through the hiatus posteriorly to narrow the orifice (From Skinner *et al.*, 1972, by permission)

The mobilized fundus is passed posteriorly behind the oesophagus and grasped with a non-crushing clamp such as the Lockwood clamp. A portion of the anterior fundus near the greater curvature is rolled over the anterior aspect of the oesophagus. The first suture of the fundoplication is inserted from the anterior fundus through the muscle of the oesophagus at the gastro-oesophageal junction and through the posterior fundus. These sutures are placed widely out onto the fundus to roll a good amount of gastric wall into the tunnel around the oesophagus to prevent the repair from being too tight. As with the thoracic approach, four or five such sutures are placed until a measured 3–4 cm length of intra-abdominal oesophagus is completely wrapped by gastric fundus (Figure 22.12). The vagus nerves are left within the wrap. When this is achieved, a no. 60 Fr. gauge bougie or operator's finger is passed through the tunnel to be sure that it is loose and will not obstruct the lower oesophagus. After careful inspection for haemostasis, the wound is closed with great care, as ventral hernia is one of the known complications of this approach.

When done transabdominally, great care must be taken to be certain that enough lower oesophagus is mobilized to prevent the repair from being performed on the upper stomach. If the repair is done too low or if the oesophageal sutures do not hold and the repair slides down onto the stomach, a portion of the stomach above the wrap is partially obstructed and leads to severe reflux as a complication of the operation. This is the so-called 'slipped Nissen' effect. The most certain way to avoid this is to leave intact

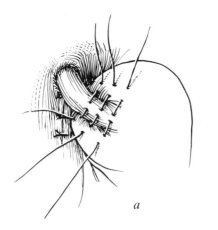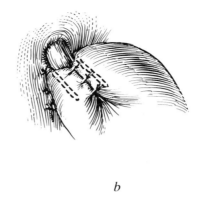

a   *b*

Figure 22.12 To complete the transabdominal Nissen fundoplication a series of sutures is placed through the anterior and posterior stomach and oesophagus. The fundus is brought posteriorly behind the oesophagus. Approximately 4 cm of intra-abdominal oesophagus should be included in the fundoplication. It should be loose enough to accept the operator's finger (From Skinner *et al.*, 1972, by permission)

the high gastrohepatic ligament including the hepatic branch of the vagus nerve, and perform the wrap cephalad to this.

As with the Mark IV operation, preoperative and intraoperative antibodies are used in case one of the sutures has been placed too deeply in the oesophageal wall. With the full fundoplication postoperative intubation of the stomach may be more difficult, so a nasogastric tube is routinely left in the stomach until bowel sounds have returned and feeding can be started. A barium swallow is routinely obtained before the patient's discharge from the hospital to ascertain that a proper repair has been achieved without complication.

Postoperative results

A properly performed Mark IV operation or fundoplication should demonstrate the intra-abdominal segment of oesophagus on the postoperative barium swallow. If this is not seen, the patient is unlikely to have a successful anti-reflux repair. When a 4 cm segment of intra-abdominal oesophagus is restored, early postoperative standard acid reflux tests or 24-hour pH monitoring demonstrate that both of these repairs are highly effective in restoring competency to the cardia. Both repairs generally cause a rise in magnitude of the distal oesophageal high-pressure zone (Skinner and DeMeester, 1976). The Nissen fundoplication causes a higher and more consistent rise which is probably caused by the fact that a full fundoplication rather than partial fundoplication around the oesophagus is done. Both repairs as well as the Hill and Guarner repairs are highly effective in relieving the patient's symptoms and complications of reflux. Which of the repairs will prove to be most effective in the long run remains to be determined as long-term randomized follow-up studies of the several repairs by the same team of surgeons are not yet completed and reported.

In a 10-year follow-up study, the success rate in patients followed for more than 10 years after the Belsey Mark IV operation is 85% with all symptomatic patients undergoing oesophagoscopy, and all patients being followed with barium swallow examinations during the follow-up period (Orringer *et al.*, 1972). Similar results are reported for the other repairs (Vansant and Baker, 1976; Rossetti and Hell, 1977; Guarner *et al.*, 1980; Negre, 1983).

Recurrences may develop at any time following operation even up to 10 years after the repair, so short-term reports of success with anti-reflux surgery are not very meaningful. Which repair is best depends not only on long-term success in eliminating recurrences of hiatal hernia and reflux, but also on which repair has the least incidence of side-effects such as persisting dysphagia and the gas bloat syndrome. When a satisfactory anti-reflux repair can be achieved at the initial operation, it can be expected that at least 85% of patients will have successful long-term control of their symptoms and complications of reflux.

Reflux stricture

Management of the patient with a stricture of the oesophagus caused by reflux is much more difficult. This may require oesophageal resection and replacement, as described in Chapter 9. A variety of methods short of resection are described. When a stricture is formed, the overall experience is that any repair short of resection and reconstruction has approximately a 70% success rate at best in eliminating postoperative dysphagia and recurrence of reflux and the hiatal hernia. Our policy is to invest substantial time in the preoperative preparation of patients with strictures prior to their first anti-reflux operation. The preoperative preparation includes intensive medical therapy and daily dilatation until a no. 40 Fr. gauge dilator can be passed easily for several consecutive days prior

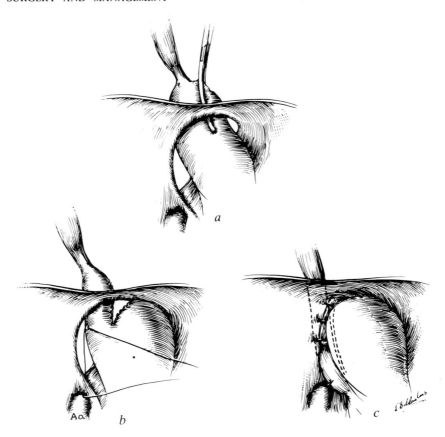

Figure 22.13 The gastroplasty originally described by Collis is illustrated. A tube is cut from the lesser curvature of the stomach to lengthen the distal swallowing tube. Collis initially described anchoring this to the arcuate ligament. However, a standard Belsey or Nissen fundoplication may be added to complete the anti-reflux repair (From Skinner *et al.*, 1972, by permission)

to surgery. When this is achieved it is usually possible to continue dilating the stricture to a no. 60 Fr. at the time of operation. Repairs for stricture should be performed transthoracically to allow extensive mobilization of the oesophagus in an effort to restore the intra-abdominal segment of oesophagus. In nearly all cases this can be accomplished. However, some patients continue to require dilatations after a Mark IV or fundoplication procedure for stricture, and the recurrence rate is higher in these patients.

Reflux-induced strictures consist of elements of inflammation, oedema and muscle spasm, as well as fibrosis of the oesophageal wall. The spasm and oedema may be eliminated by intensive preoperative preparation, but the fibrosis may not be reversible. When the latter is severe, it may be difficult or impossible to reduce the swallowing tube to an intra-abdominal location. Several alternatives other than resection are available, and are employed at the first anti-reflux operation. When reoperation is necessary for recurrence after treatment of a stricture, resection and reconstruction as described elsewhere are preferable.

The three most commonly used operations short of

resection include a Nissen fundoplication left in the thorax, an extension of the swallowing tube by a gastroplasty (Collis, 1957) coupled with a Nissen or Belsey reconstruction, or the Thal gastric patch procedure (Thal *et al.*, 1965) coupled with a fundoplication left in the thorax. Because the Nissen fundoplication is a 360° wrap, it is effective mechanically even if left in the chest (Safaie-Shiraze *et al.*, 1974). However, this operation has several disadvantages in that the incidence of progressive enlargement of the iatrogenic hiatal hernia is high. The intrathoracic gastric pouch seems to be subject to gastric ulceration, bleeding and perforation as has been observed in several series. For this reason, treating the strictured shortened oesophagus by intrathoracic fundoplication alone is not widely practised. When this is done, the stomach must be carefully sutured to the margins of the hiatus in an effort to prevent further herniation, and the hiatus must be left widely open to prevent congestion and obstruction of the gastric pouch.

A more widely favoured alternative is the Collis gastroplasty manoeuvre (Figure 22.13). In this procedure the swallowing tube is lengthened by fashioning a tube of lesser curvature of the stomach as an extension of the oesophagus. This is done by passing a bougie through the stricture into the stomach and fashioning a tube around a no. 40 or larger dilator. The tube may be formed by the use of a stapler or by clamping and oversewing the stomach on both sides of the incision between the fundus and the lesser curvature tube. The remaining exaggerated gastric fundus is used as a plication around the intra-abdominal segment of swallowing tube (Pearson et al., 1978). Either the Mark IV or the Nissen fundoplication may be employed for this manoeuvre. In this fashion a narrow-diameter swallowing tube consisting of stomach is placed beneath the diaphragm to achieve control of reflux. It is important that the diameter of this tube be similar to that of the oesophagus, and that the tube does not flare out as it enters the stomach to avoid an inverted funnel effect which encourages subsequent reflux.

Some surgeons employ the Thal procedure coupled with a fundoplication (Hollenbeck and Woodward, 1975). This is particularly useful when the stricture is very difficult to dilate or when it is split in the course of operation. An incision is made across the stricture which is allowed to gape open. A skin graft is applied to the defect with the adjacent gastric fundus sutured to the margins of the open oesophagus incorporating the skin graft in the suture line. If simply left as a gastric patch across the stricture, free reflux will occur and recurrent oesophagitis and stricture will be the outcome. Accordingly, a full fundoplication of stomach around the lower oesophagus must be employed when this operation is chosen. Both the Collis gastroplasty and Thal procedure with fundoplication have been reported in several series to give approximately 70% relief of dysphagia and long-term control of reflux. Since similar results are achievable with fundoplication alone after intensive preoperative preparation of the patient, we continue to prefer the anti-reflux repair without the Collis or Thal manoeuvre whenever possible.

Until long-term results are reported which clearly establish one repair or another as the best anti-reflux operation, individual surgeons should be encouraged to learn one or more of these procedures, to employ them in carefully selected and fully evaluated patients, and to observe their own postoperative results both by barium swallow studies and postoperative oesophageal function testing to ascertain that they are indeed achieving control of reflux.

References

Allison, P. R. (1951) Reflux oesophagitis, sliding hiatal hernia, and the anatomy of repair. Surg. Gynecol, Obstet., 92, 149

Allison, P. (1973) Hiatal hernia. Ann. Surg., 178, 273–276

Angelchick, J. and Cohen, R. (1979) A new surgical procedure for the treatment of gastroesophageal reflux and hiatal hernia. Surg. Gynecol. Obstet., 148, 246–248

Belsey, R. H. R. and Skinner, D. B. (1972) Surgical treatment: thoracic approach. In Gastroesophageal Reflux and Hiatal Hernia (eds D. B. Skinner, R. H. R. Belsey, T. R. Hendrix et al.), Little, Brown, Boston

Collis, J. L. (1957) An operation for hiatus hernia with short oesophagus. J. Thorac. Cardiovasc. Surg., 34, 768

DeMeester, T. R. et al. (1976) Patterns of gastro-oesophageal reflux in health and disease. Ann. Surg., 184, 459–470

DeMeester, T. R. et al. (1979) Clinical and in vitro analysis of determinants of gastroesophageal competence. Am. J. Surg., 137, 39–46

Fyke, F. E., Code, C. F. and Schlegel, J. F. (1956) The gastro-oesophageal sphincter in healthy human beings. Gastroenterologia, 86, 135

Guarner, V., Degollade, J. R. and Tore, N. M. (1975) A new antireflux procedure at the oesophagogastric junction. Arch. Surg., 110, 101–106

Guarner, V., Gavino, J. and Martinez, T. N. (1980) Ten-year evaluation of posterior fundoplasty in the treatment of gastroesophageal reflux. Am. J. Surg., 139, 200

Helm, J. F., Dodds, W. J., Hogan, W. J., Soergel, K. H. et al. (1984) Effect of esophageal emptying and saliva on clearance of acid from the esophagus. N. Engl. J. Med., 320, 284–288

Hiebert, C. A. and Belsey, R. (1961) Incompetency of the gastric cardia without radiologic evidence of hiatus hernia. J. Thorac. Cardiovasc. Surg., 42, 352

Hill, L. D. (1967) An effective operation for hiatal hernia: an eight-year appraisal. Ann. Surg., 166, 681

Hollenbeck, J. I. and Woodward, E. R. (1975) Treatment of peptic oesophageal stricture with combined fundic patch-fundoplication. Ann. Surg., 182, 472

Johnson, L. F. and DeMeester, T. R. (1974) Twenty-four hour pH monitoring of the distal oesophagus: a quantitative measure of gastro-oesophageal reflux. Am. J. Gastroenterol., 62, 325

Kantrowitz, P. A., Corson, J. G., Fleischli, D. L. et al. (1969) Measurement of gastro-oesophageal reflux. Gastroenterol., 56, 666

Negre, J. (1983) Post-fundoplication symptoms. Ann. Surg., 198, 698

Nissen, R. (1961) Gastropexy and fundoplication in surgical treatment of hiatal hernia. Am. J. Dig. Dis., 6, 954

Orringer, M. B., Skinner, D. B. and Belsey, R. H. R. (1972) Long-term results of the Mark IV operation for hiatal hernia and analyses of recurrences and their treatment. J. Thorac. Cardiovasc. Surg., 63, 25

Pearson, F. G. et al. (1978) Gastroplasty and fundoplication in the management of complex reflux problems. J. Thorac. Cardiovasc. Surg., 76, 665

Pellegrini, C. A. et al. (1979) Gastro-oesophageal reflux and pulmonary aspiration: incidence, functional abnormalities and results of surgical therapy. Surgery, 36, 110–119

Rossetti, M. and Hell, K. (1977) Fundoplication for the treatment of gastroesophageal reflux in hiatal hernia. Wld J. Surg., 1, 439

Safaie-Shiraze, S. et al. (1974) Nissen fundoplication without crural repair. Arch. Surg., 108, 4

Skinner, D. B. (1976) Surgical Techniques Illustrated, Vol. 1, No. 2, Little, Brown, Boston

Skinner, D. B. (1985) Pathophysiology of gastroesophageal reflux. Ann. Surg., 202, 546

Skinner, D. B. and Belsey, R. H. R. (1967) Surgical management of oesophageal reflux and hiatus hernia. J. Thorac. Cardiovasc. Surg., 53, 33

Skinner, D. B., Belsey, R. H. R., Hendrix, T. R. *et al.* (eds) (1972) *Gastro-oesophageal Reflux and Hiatal Hernia*, Little, Brown, Boston

Skinner, D. B. and Booth, D. J. (1970) Assessment of distal oesophageal function in patients with hiatal hernia and/or gastro-oesophageal reflux. *Ann. Surg.*, **172**, 627

Skinner, D. B. and DeMeester, T. R. (1976) Gastro-oesophageal reflux. *Curr. Probl. Surg.* **13**, January

Thal, A. P., Hatafuku, T. and Kurtzman, R. (1965) New operation for distal oesophageal stricture. *Arch. Surg.*, **90**, 464

Tuttle, S. G. and Grossman, M. I. (1958) Detection of gastro-oesophageal reflux by simultaneous measurement of intraluminal pressures and pH. *Proc. Soc. Exp. Biol. Med.*, **98**, 225

Vansant, J. and Baker, J. (1976) Complications of vagotomy in the treatment of hiatal hernia. *Ann. Surg.*, **183**, 629

Winans, C. S. and Harris, L. D. (1967) Quantitation of lower oesophageal sphincter competence. *Gastroenterology*, **52**, 779

23
Subphrenic abscess

D. J. Leaper

Introduction

A subphrenic abscess can be defined as a collection of infected fluid within the subhepatic or subphrenic spaces. Their causes are mainly the localization of generalized peritonitis, or iatrogenic. Less common causes are related to blood-borne infections caused by pneumoccocus or mycobacterium (particularly after splenectomy) or to urological disease leading to perinephric abscesses which present in the extraperitoneal subphrenic space.

Perforated organs which may lead to a subphrenic abscess include the stomach, duodenum, biliary tree and intestine (related to the supracolic compartment), but when the patient lies supine, infected fluid may gravitate upwards from the pelvis (from a perforated appendix for example). Peptic ulceration, cholecystitis and inflammatory or neoplastic bowel diseases are the principal specific causes. Subphrenic abscesses may be sequels to penetrating or blunt injury.

Iatrogenic causes include postoperative complications involving similar abdominal organs, when a collection of fluid (haematoma, seroma or bile leak) becomes contaminated by infected visceral contents. Anastomotic leakage is another, often masked, cause. Endoscopy in the gastrointestinal tract may rarely lead to a subphrenic collection, if there is bleeding or perforation; and similarly laparoscopy, particularly when procedures are undertaken. Pancreatitis following ERCP or splenectomy may also lead to a lesser sac abscess.

Microbiology

When an intestinal viscus is the source of infection there is usually a combination of organisms found in the pus – an aerobe (Gram-negative bacillus) and an anaerobe (*Bacteroides* or *Streptococcus faecalis*) – which act in synergy. Abscesses unrelated to open viscus pathology or surgery are more likely to contain staphylococci. The progression of contamination and localization to subphrenic abscess depends on inoculum size, the pathogenicity of organisms present and the patient's host defence.

The use of antibiotics should be based, if possible, on microbiological sensitivities, but their use is controversial. Empirical use of a broad-spectrum combination (e.g. a penicillin, aminoglycoside and metronidazole) or monotherapy (e.g. imipenem) should be reserved for patients who have clear evidence of septicaemia, toxicity or multiple organ systems failure. The harvesting of some pathogens such as clostridial gas-gangrene spp. or β-haemolytic streptococci, indicates the use of specific antibiotic therapy.

Anatomy (Figures 23.1–23.3)

Only 10% of subphrenic abscesses are extraperitoneal and relate mainly to the bare area of the liver (relating to liver abscesses) or the perinephric areas (relating to genitourinary disease). The remainder are intraperitoneal and there are five potential spaces: right suprahepatic and infrahepatic and left suprahepatic, anterior infrahepatic and posterior infrahepatic.

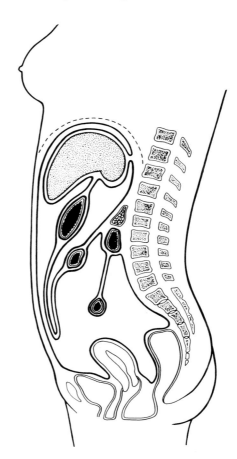

Figure 23.1 The intraperitoneal and subphrenic spaces

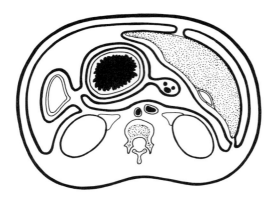

Figure 23.2 The intraperitoneal and subphrenic spaces

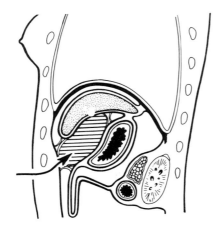

Figure 23.3 Left anterior infrahepatic abscess. The left posterior infrahepatic space (the lesser sac) lies posteriorly to the stomach

The right suprahepatic space lies between the diaphragm and right lobe of the liver, limited posteriorly by the superior layers of the coronary and right triangular ligaments and medially by the falciform ligament. The right infrahepatic space is bounded above and in front by the right lobe of the liver and gallbladder, below and behind by the diaphragm, the upper pole of the right kidney, the right suprarenal gland, the second part of the duodenum, a part of the head of the pancreas, the right colic flexure and the right extremity of the transverse colon and mesocolon.

The left suprahepatic space is large and complicated. It separates the diaphragm from the left lobe of the liver, fundus of stomach and spleen. It is limited medially by the falciform ligament. Posteriorly it is limited medially by the left triangular ligament lateral to which it extends backwards between the diaphragm and spleen and then inwards between the kidney and spleen and the lienorenal ligament.

The left anterior infrahepatic space lies between the left lobe of the liver above and in front and the stomach and lesser omentum below and behind. The left posterior infrahepatic space or lesser sac lies behind the caudate lobe of the liver, the stomach and the lesser omentum and extends downwards to a variable distance into the greater omentum. Behind it are the transverse colon and mesocolon, the neck and body of the pancreas, the upper pole of the left kidney, the left suprarenal gland and a considerable part of the diaphragm.

History, examination and laboratory findings

There is usually an antecedent history of peritonitis or inflamed viscus, penetrating injury or surgery. In addition to signs of toxicity the patient may complain of localized abdominal pain and there is localized tenderness in 30%. Only 10% of patients have a palpable upper abdominal or loin swelling and there may be oedema of the overlying skin. The patient has a tachycardia and church spire temperature (Figure 23.4), but the latter may be hidden by the use of antibiotics. There is usually a markedly raised white blood cell count, mainly neutrophils, but neutropenia is a poor prognostic sign, and there may be a fall in haemoglobin.

Multiple systems organ failure, reflected in laboratory investigations, may be the only sign of a subphrenic abscess. Hepatic failure presents with falling albumin and jaundice, a prolonged ileus is associated with hypovolaemia, and eventually intrinsic renal failure with rising blood urea and creatinine, stress gastritis and bleeding (disseminated intravascular coagulation) is reflected in haematological parameters and fibrinogen degradation products, and there may be respiratory failure with adult respiratory distress syndrome.

Investigations

Plain X-ray and contrast studies

A chest X-ray may show a pleural effusion or basal collapse and a raised diaphragm above a subphrenic abscess. Immobility of the diaphragm is shown on screening, but this may be a non-specific sign. Plain abdominal X-rays may show a localized mottled appearance with a gas fluid level (Figure 23.5). In addition there may be signs of a localized ileus, displacement of organs or loss of normal radiological anatomy (such as the line of a psoas muscle or renal shadow). Contrast studies show displacement (such as anterior displacement of stomach by a pancreatic lesser sac abscess) or extravasation (Figure 23.5).

Ultrasound scanning

Ultrasound scanning (USS) is accurate in diagnosis, showing echo-free areas and localization in 60–80%

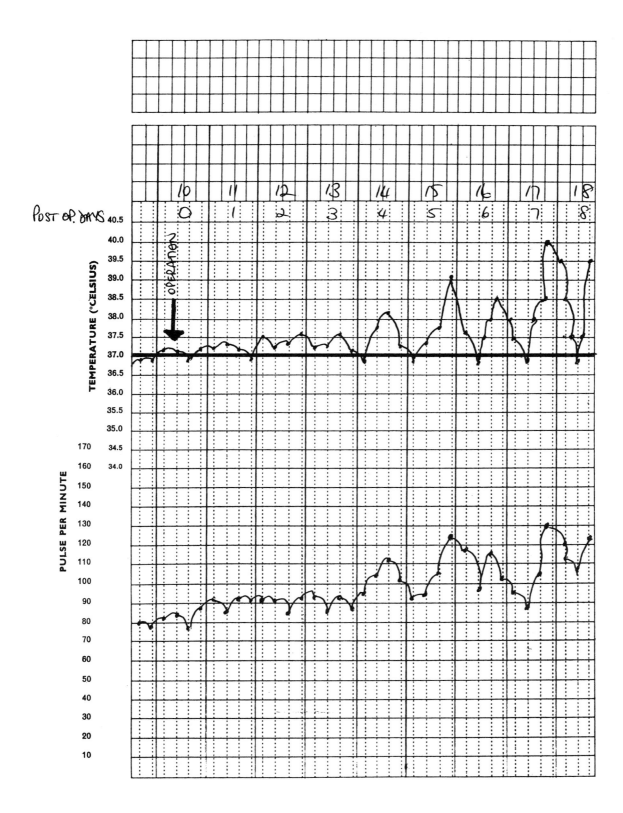

Figure 23.4 Typical pulse and temperature relating to development of a subphrenic abscess after total radical gastrectomy and a leak from the oesophagojejunal anastomosis

of subphrenic abscesses (Figure 23.6) and like computed tomography (CT) scans allows guided aspiration. Loops of bowel affected by ileus make diagnosis difficult.

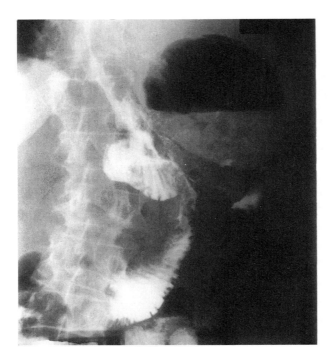

Figure 23.5 Gastrograffin swallow from the same patient as in Figure 23.4. The leak from the anastomosis is shown with a mottled abscess and a gas fluid level

Computed tomography

Investigation by CT is accurate in up to 95% of patients, particularly after oral or intravenous contrast which enhances the low-density attenuation typical of an abscess.

Radionuclide scanning

Radionuclide scans using ^{67}Ga or ^{111}In isotope-labelled white cells image areas of inflammation, but may give false positives when there is not a localized area of suppuration. Their accuracy is not likely to exceed 80%.

Nuclear magnetic resonance

This is a promising technique, but there is not sufficient data to establish its use, nor is it widely available.

Treatment

Like all abscesses, those in the subphrenic spaces need prompt drainage and the method of choice and first line of treatment is by USS- or CT-guided percutaneous techniques. Abscesses tend to point to the skin surface through planes of least resistance and are amenable to percutaneous drainage. An extraserous route is preferable. When the subphrenic abscess is unilocular and contains thin material, this technique is successful in over 80% of patients. When there are

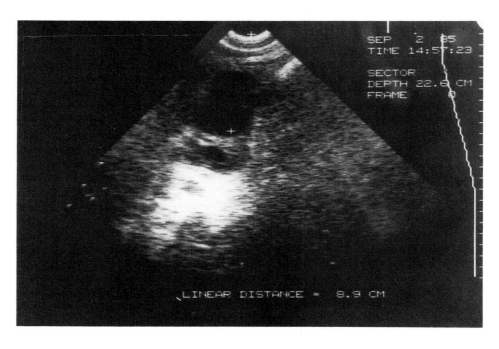

Figure 23.6 Abdominal ultrasound scan showing an echo-free area typical of a subphrenic abscess

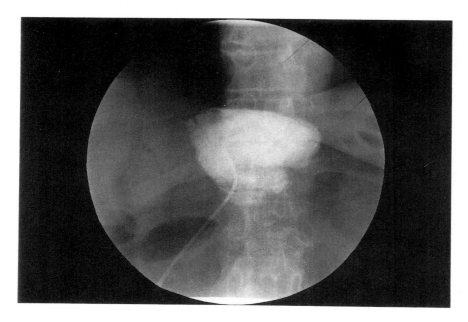

Figure 23.7   Sinogram using a pigtail drainage catheter to assess sequential resolution of an abscess cavity

loculations or thick pus, success may only be achieved in 20%. The technique involves a preliminary tapping with a needle under guidance, then the insertion of a self-retaining pigtail catheter through a trocar or by a Seldinger technique. The catheter allows irrigation or instillation of antibiotics when the abscess contains thick pus or highly infective material. Drainage is effected with a sterile non-return valved system (as in T-tube bile drainage). Sequential sinograms to show effective resolution may be taken using the catheter before its removal (Figure 23.7).

Open drainage

Operative intervention needs to be undertaken when USS- or CT-guided percutaneous drainage cannot be safely undertaken, or when it has failed, particularly with multilocular collections not well identified by imaging techniques, and when there is a fistula. The transpleural route, through a lower rib posterior approach, should be abandoned, even if effective obliteration of the pleural cavity is undertaken. This risks pulmonary complications such as pneumonia, empyema or bronchial fistula, damages the diaphragm and does not allow any peritoneal exploration.

Anterior extraserous approach (Figures 23.8–23.10)

An oblique incision is made 2.5 cm below and parallel with the costal margin on the side of the abscess, starting over the middle of the rectus muscle and extending well lateral to it. This is deepened through the three anterolateral abdominal muscles and trans-

versalis fascia, lateral to the unopened rectus sheath. The extraperitoneal alveolar tissue and peritoneum are exposed.

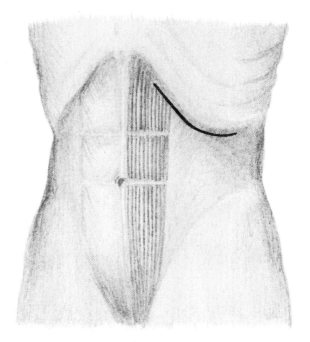

Figure 23.8   Anterior extraperitoneal approach for drainage of subphrenic abscess

To reach the suprahepatic space on either side, the fingers peel the peritoneum off the undersurface of the diaphragm. This is easily accomplished, especially

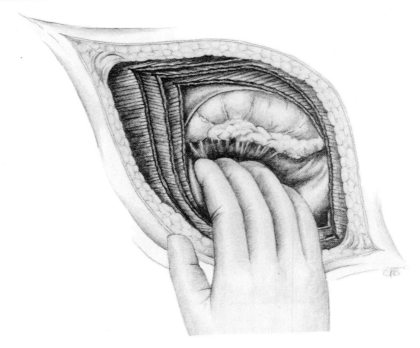

Figure 23.9 Anterior extraperitoneal approach to subphrenic abscess. The oedematous abscess wall is exposed by blunt dissection

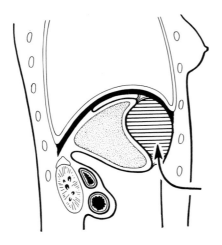

Figure 23.10 Right anterior subphrenic abscess. Anterior extraperitoneal approach

when inflammatory oedema is present. When the abscess is reached, as indicated by induration, a finger is inserted through its wall. Pus is evacuated with a sucker, some being kept for bacteriology. The opening into the abscess is then enlarged and any loculi within it are broken down. Thorough exploration of the entire suprahepatic region on either side is possible if the whole hand is inserted through the incision. Suprahepatic abscesses on the right side are located between the diaphragm and the right lobe of the liver

those on the left may be between the diaphragm and the left lobe of the liver, the fundus of the stomach or the spleen.

The right infrahepatic space is explored by passing the fingers upwards and backwards below the right lobe of the liver and above the hepatic flexure and right extremity of the transverse colon. The left anterior infrahepatic space is easily reached by pushing the fingers backwards and upwards below the left lobe of the liver and above the stomach and lesser omentum.

Extraperitoneal abscesses on either side can also be reached by the anterior extraserous route if the incision allows entry of the whole hand.

Posterior extraperitoneal approach
(Figures 23.11–23.13)

The patient is placed as for nephrectomy. The incision starts 2.5 cm from the midline and runs downwards and forwards over or just below the 12th rib, extending beyond its tip far enough to allow insertion of the whole hand. Division of latissimus dorsi and serratus posterior inferior exposes the rib. Its periosteum is divided with diathermy and stripped from the whole length of its upper and lower borders and deep surface. Erector spinae must be retracted backwards to gain access to the posterior end of the rib, and care is required to avoid injuring the pleura. After excising the whole rib subperiosteally, its bed is incised transversely at the level of the spinous process of the first lumbar vertebra to avoid injuring the pleura. The incision extends inwards from the periosteum to divide fibres of the serratus posterior and quadratus lumborum muscles, and outwards to sever the muscles of the 11th intercostal space. The exposed attachments of the diaphragm, which may be well or poorly developed, are divided. At the inner end of the incision the subcostal and iliohypogastric nerves must be preserved. Blunt dissection in the perinephric fat reveals the smooth, shiny, thin, fibrous posterior layer of the renal fascia through which the perirenal fat is visible. Blunt dissection outside the renal fascia exposes the upper pole of the kidney and the suprarenal gland.

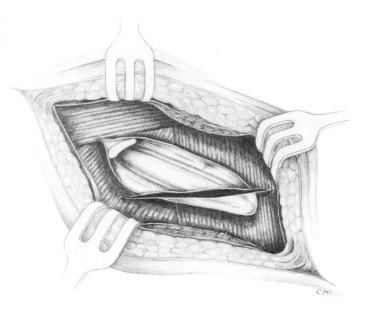

Figure 23.12 Posterior extraperitoneal approach to subphrenic abscess. The 12th rib has been resected subperiosteally and its bed incised transversely

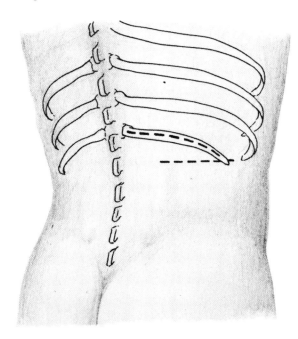

Figure 23.11 Incision for extraperitoneal approach to posterior subphrenic abscess. The line of the pleura is shown well below the 12th rib

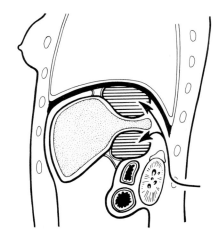

Figure 23.13 Posterosuperior and posteroinferior subphrenic abscesses. These are readily approached via the posterior extraperitoneal route

The suprahepatic and extraperitoneal spaces on either side are easily explored by passing the fingers upwards under the diaphragm. To explore the right infrahepatic space, the fingers are pushed forwards and downwards through the junction of the renal and diaphragmatic fascias, about and in front of the kidney and suprarenal gland and below and behind the right lobe of the liver.

Transperitoneal (laparotomy) approach

This approach should be considered to exclude complications, such as a leaking anastomosis, or to drain multiple loculated abscesses. A laparotomy is necessary as a 'second-look' procedure when a subphrenic abscess is suspected, and particularly when recurring sepsis is anticipated. Acute necrotizing pancreatitis leading to recurrent abscesses is an example. Incor-

poration of a Marlex mesh or a 'zipper' into the abdominal wall allows easy peritoneal access, even on ventilated patients in the intensive care unit.

Open drainage allows the placement of large-bore drains (14 mm or more) which can easily be used for irrigation. One or several drains should be brought out through separate stab incisions and secured with a monofilament non-absorbable suture. Siphon drains work as well as suction drains, but sump suction drainage avoids the blocking of drainage holes. Closed systems with non-return valves are preferable to avoid secondary exogenous infection and secondary skin irritation, which is difficult to achieve with sump drainage.

Prognosis

Spread of a localized infection, leading to peritonitis, intestinal or faecal fistula or liver abscess, is a complication of treatment, although liver abscess is rare now with appropriate antibiotic prophylaxis. Mortality, even after uncomplicated abscesses, can reach 30% but can exceed 50% in older patients (>65 years) who are obese or have an intercurrent disease such as diabetes, cancer or immunosuppression. A serum albumin falling <30 g/litre is a poor prognostic sign and if shock or multiple organ failure is present, mortality may be 100%.

Further reading

Deveney, C. N., Lurie, K. and Deveney, K. E. (1988). Improved treatment of intra-abdominal abscess. *Arch. Surg.*, **123**, 1126–1129

Gerzof, S. F. and Johnson, W. C. (1984) Radiologic aspects of diagnosis and treatment of abdominal abscesses. *Surg. Clin. N. Am.*, **64**, 53–65

Goldman, M., Ambrose, N. S., Drolc, Z., Hawker, R. J. and McCollum, C. (1987) Indium-111-labelled leucocytes in the diagnosis of abdominal abscess. *Br. J. Surg.*, **74**, 184–186

Harley, H. R. S. (1987) Subphrenic abscess. In *Operative Surgery and Management*, 2nd edn (ed. G. Keen), John Wright, Bristol, pp. 314–319

Hau, T., Haaga, J. R. and Aeder, M. I. (1984) Pathophysiology, diagnosis and treatment of abdominal abscesses. In *Current Problems in Surgery* (ed. M. M. Ravitch), Year Book Medical Publishers, Chicago, pp. 8–82

Joseph, A. E. A. (1985) Imaging of abdominal abscesses. *Br. Med. J.*, **291**, 1445–1446

Lurie, K., Plzak, L. and Deveney, C. N. (1987) Intraabdominal abscess in the 1980's. *Surg. Clin. N. Am.*, **67**, 621–632

Murray, H. W. (1990) Secondary peritonitis and intraabdominal abscess. *Hosp. Pract.*, **25**, 101–120

Nichols, R. L. (1986) Management of intra-abdominal sepsis. *Am. J. Med.*, **80**: 204–209

Ochsner, A. and Debakey, M. (1938) Subphrenic abscess: collective review and analysis of 3,608 collected and personal cases. *Int. Abstr. Surg.*, **66**, 426–438

Polk, H. C. and Lamont, P. M. (1983) The search for pus. *Br. J. Hosp. Med.*, **30**, 199–202

Rhys-Davies, E. and Thomas, W. E. G. (1988) *Nuclear Medicine: Applications to Surgery*, Castle House Publications, Tunbridge Wells, UK

Stone, H. H, Mullins, R. J., Dunlop, W. E. and Strom, P. R. (1984) Extraperitoneal versus transperitoneal drainage of the intra-abdominal abscess. *Surg. Gynecol. Obstet.*, **159**, 549–552

Neck, face and jaws

24

The thyroid gland

N. E. Dudley

Surgical anatomy

General orientations

The thyroid gland is situated in the anterior triangle of the neck, weighs approximately 20 g and consists of two lateral lobes (right and left) which are joined by a midline isthmus. A small pyramidal lobe (of Lalouette), of varying size, commonly joins the isthmus at its junction with the left lateral lobe by a fibrous band or strand of muscle fibres known as the levator glandulae thyroideae. The lobes measure approximately $5 \times 3 \times 1.5$ cm (slightly larger in women) and extend from the middle of the thyroid cartilage above to the sixth tracheal ring below. Each lobe fills the space between the trachea and oesophagus medially and the carotid sheath laterally. A strong condensation of vascular connective tissues, known as the suspensory ligament of Berry, binds the gland firmly to each side of the cricoid cartilage and this ligament, together with the pretracheal fascia splitting to invest the gland, makes the thyroid move up and down on swallowing. The fascia (false or surgical capsule) sends fibrous septa into the gland substance, dividing it into numerous lobules. These consist of 30–40 follicles which contain colloid and are the main secretory and storage elements.

Development of the thyroid

The thyroid develops from two distinct embryological structures – the primitive pharynx and the neural crest. A median pharyngeal downgrowth migrates between the first and the second arch components of the tongue and descends caudally along a line from the foramen caecum at the back of the tongue to the pyramidal lobe of the thyroid, in a track which passes ventral to the hyoid bone and then loops behind it. The track becomes obliterated but parts may persist giving rise to a thyroglossal cyst or fistula which will rise on protrusion of the tongue. Rarely the thyroid bud fails to descend and develops *in situ* at the back of the tongue (lingual thyroid). It may descend too far and result in a primary mediastinal or retrosternal goitre. Rarely the thyroid bud may fail to divide, resulting in one lateral lobe, usually the left being absent. The parafollicular or C cells, scattered between the cuboidal epithelial cells which line the thyroid follicles, are derived from the neural crest. They first migrate to the ultimobranchial bodies of the fourth and fifth branchial pouches and then to the thyroid. These cells in later life have the potential to undergo hyperplastic and malignant change and result in the calcitonin-producing medullary carcinoma of the thyroid.

Blood supply

The vascular supply of the gland is significant and becomes greater in hyperactive thyroid states. The main supply is via two paired arteries and an occasional third vessel to the lower pole of one or other lobe. The superior thyroid artery, the first branch of the external carotid, runs downward on the inferior constrictor to reach the apex of the lateral lobe where it divides into a large anterior branch and a usually smaller, but important posterior branch. Occasionally a tributary comes off high on the left to reach and supply the pyramidal lobe fairly near the midline. The inferior thyroid artery is generally much larger than the superior thyroid artery but is less constant, being absent or duplicated on one or other side in 10% of individuals. It arises from the thyrocervical trunk and, passing upwards for a variable distance, then loops down running medially behind the carotid sheath to reach the posterolateral aspect of the gland at the junction of the middle and lower thirds. Numerous unnamed accessory arteries arise from the oesophagus and trachea, but the most frequently encountered is the thyroidea ima (Neubauer's artery), which courses up anteriorly on the trachea to reach the isthmus or one of the lower poles and takes origin from the aorta or brachiocephalic artery. In the absence of the inferior thyroid artery on one side, the thyroidea ima may be the principal source of blood supply to the lobe and therefore substantial.

The named thyroid veins are subject to greater variation. The superior thyroid vein, formed by a confluence of vessels from the upper pole, crosses the common carotid artery high in the neck to drain into the internal jugular. The middle thyroid vein, which overlies the inferior thyroid artery, also ends in the internal jugular vein after crossing the common carotid artery. The inferior thyroid veins pass down from the isthmus and inferior poles of the lateral lobes to join the internal jugular or brachiocephalic veins in the anterior mediastinum and are intimately associated with the thyrothymic ligaments which expand inferiorly as the lobes of the thymus.

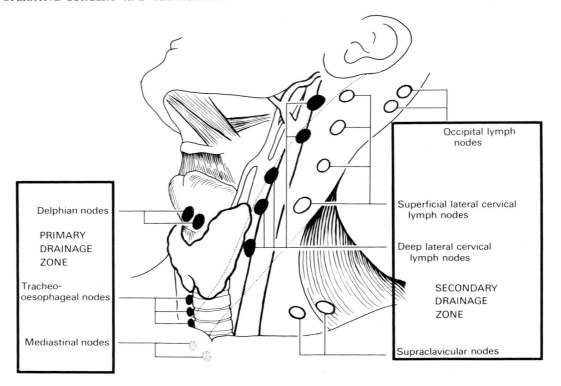

Figure 24.1 Lymphatic drainage of the thyroid gland

Lymphatic drainage

A rich network of lymphatics ramify throughout the gland. They drain primarily into mediastinal nodes inferiorly, tracheo-oesophageal nodes laterally and the midline Delphian nodes superiorly. Dye studies suggest that the majority of lymph from the thyroid returns to the thoracic duct without passing through the deep cervical lymph node chain or the nodes of the posterior triangle, although these pathways may open up secondarily (Figure 24.1). This factor has implications in the assessment of a patient with carcinoma of the thyroid who may develop lymph node deposits outside the primary drainage areas even on the contralateral side (Crile, 1957).

Important anatomical relations

Recurrent laryngeal nerves (Figure 24.2)

There are several structures in relation to the gland with which a surgeon must be familiar. The most important of these is the recurrent laryngeal nerve, which is a branch of the vagus. The latter, having entered the mediastinum, gives off the recurrent nerve which returns to the neck having circled around the arch of the aorta on the left and the right subclavian artery on the right. It ascends in the tracheo-oesophageal groove and has a variable relationship with the inferior thyroid artery on each side (Figure 24.2).

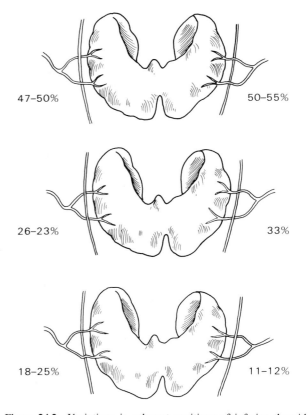

Figure 24.2 Variations in relevant positions of inferior thyroid artery and recurrent laryngeal nerve

Table 24.1 Disadvantages of anti-thyroid drugs, radioactive iodine and surgery in the management of hyperthyroidism

Anti-thyroid drugs	Conservative ^{131}I	Surgery
1. Requires compliant and highly motivated patient to cope with variable drug regimen	1. Prospect of radiation therapy may be unacceptable to the patient	1. Prospect of neck surgery may be unacceptable to the patient
2. Needs close clinical and laboratory supervision over 18–24 months	2. Uncertainty about long-term carcinogenic effects of low radiation doses – known to be more oncogenic than high doses	2. Unsuited to patients of advanced age or poor medical status
3. Danger of over-treatment leading to hypothyroidism and thyroid enlargement	3. Uncertainty about teratogenic effects which restrict reproduction post-therapy	3. Scar inevitable with possibility of keloid formation
4. Risk of side-effects from drugs – rashes and nausea plus potentially dangerous marrow depression	4. Slow response to therapy (3–6 months), especially large multinodular goitres	4. Results are highly operator dependent
5. Poor response with large multinodular goitres	5. Not appropriate for cosmetically unacceptable toxic goitres	5. Small but definite risk of serious complications in skilled hands: Recurrent laryngeal nerve damage <1% Permanent hypoparathyroidism <0.5%
6. Not appropriate for cosmetically unacceptable toxic goitres	6. Cumulative (high) hypothyroidism rate requiring long-term follow-up	6. Modest rate of hypothyroidism
7. High relapse rate		

In general the nerve runs deep to the artery, but may actually pass through or anterior to the branches of the artery as it breaks up close to the gland (Hollingshead, 1952). Occasionally the nerve itself divides early and branches around the artery (10%). In less than 1% of individuals the recurrent laryngeal nerve on the right is non-recurrent and passes directly from the vagus to the cricothyroid muscles. As it takes the same course as the inferior thyroid artery, it is particularly vulnerable if unrecognized when this vessel is ligated laterally. Whichever course the nerve takes, it ultimately enters the larynx with the inferior laryngeal artery posterior to the cricothyroid articulation and supplies all the intrinsic muscles of the larynx together with some sensory supply to the mucosa below the vocal cords. The principal effect of division of this nerve is paralysis of the vocal cord on that side.

The superior laryngeal nerve

This also arises from the vagus (inferior ganglion) and divides at the level of the hyoid bone into a large internal laryngeal nerve and a smaller external laryngeal nerve. The latter runs close to the superior thyroid artery but at a deeper plane, immediately above the superior pole of the thyroid. It terminates as the nerve supply to the cricothyroid muscle which acts as a tensor of the vocal cords on the same side.

The cervical sympathetic chain

This underlies the carotid sheath just medial to the vagus on the prevertebral fascia and is in close proximity to the inferior thyroid artery as it arches around medially.

Indications for surgery

Thyrotoxicosis

There are three methods of treatment for this condition: anti-thyroid drugs, radio-iodine and surgery. Fashions have waxed and waned, but a marked preference for the use of radio-iodine persists in the USA compared with the UK where its use is more selective. The merits of each individual treatment have been argued and frequently overstated, but each has its advantages and disadvantages. The latter are summarized in Table 24.1. Ultimately it is for the patients to decide which treatment is most acceptable to them. In the author's opinion, surgery is clearly most appropriate in the following five situations:

1. Large toxic multinodular goitre/Plummer's disease

The thyroid function of patients with this condition is often very labile while being treated with anti-thyroid drugs and relapse rates are high when medication is withdrawn (greater than 50%). This is true even after prolonged therapy. There is no reliable test to identify those patients who will relapse off therapy, although attempts have been made on the basis of HLA status and thyroid-stimulating antibody levels. Radioactive iodine treatment is least suited for Plummer's disease as uptake is variable, has minimal impact on the size of the gland and response is slow. Surgery is best carried out early before the airway and the cardiovascular system are compromised. The specific surgical procedure is a subtotal thyroidectomy reducing the gland to an acceptable size and especially removing those parts of the gland shown to be active on radio-iodine scanning.

2. Large diffuse toxic goitre (Graves' disease)

Patients affected with this condition are likely to be the most florid cases, with the additional problem of cosmetic embarrassment. The policy of prompt elective surgery after preoperative preparation with anti-thyroid drugs and beta blockers has much to commend it. It is debatable whether surgery should be offered when patients have a small gland, since the risks of hypothyroidism are greater than when a bulkier gland is the target. In women, especially in their reproductive years, who have relapsed after 12–18 months of a well-monitored course of anti-thyroid drugs or in whom medication has proved impractical (poor compliance, unacceptable side effects, etc.), then surgery is the first choice provided that it is acceptable to the patient and the necessary surgical skills are available. The operative procedure undertaken is a subtotal thyroidectomy.

3. Toxic solitary nodular goitre/toxic adenoma/autonomous 'hot' nodule

Resecting the physiologically hyperactive part of the gland (demonstrable on radio-iodine uptake scan) by surgery is so straightforward that other methods of treatment need be considered only when the medical state of the patient identifies him or her as an unacceptable risk. The disadvantage of anti-thyroid drugs is that they need to be given lifelong; radio-iodine therapy irradiates surrounding normal tissue with the possibility of inducing malignant change and with these methods the nodule usually persists. The operative procedure is subtotal lobectomy or isthmusectomy, depending on which part of the gland contains the active nodule.

4. Childhood Graves' disease

Children with hyperthyroidism are more prone to relapse after withdrawal of medical therapy and radio-iodine is contraindicated due to the high incidence of benign and malignant nodules after exposure to radiation (Duffy and Fitzgerald, 1950). Unless medical therapy is quickly effective, surgery is the treatment of choice. Since hypertrophy of the remnants and recurrent thyrotoxicosis rates are higher in children, surgery needs to be more radical. An experienced thyroid surgeon used to operating on children is essential if unacceptably high myxoedema rates and complications are to be avoided. Long-term follow-up is essential.

5. Thyrotoxicosis in pregnancy

This is a rare combination (0.2% of pregnancies), but can present a difficult management problem. Anti-thyroid drugs given to the mother cross the placental barrier and may result in hypothyroidism and a goitre in the fetus – iatrogenic cretinism. After delivery, anti-thyroid drugs are excreted in the milk but not in sufficient quantities to cause comparable effects. Radio-iodine is never given in view of the possible teratogenic effects on the developing fetus, especially in the first trimester or later when the fetal thyroid is trapping iodine. If maternal thyrotoxicosis is moderate or severe and if cardiac symptoms are prominent, heralding possible cardiac failure late in pregnancy, then subtotal thyroidectomy should be undertaken electively in the middle trimester when it is safe and effective.

Non-toxic goitre

Benign enlargements of this type occur for several reasons – lack of iodine in the diet causing an *endemic goitre*, inherited enzyme defects preventing iodine trapping and normal metabolism of thyroxine causing a *dyshormonogenetic goitre* or an acquired enzyme defect due to other factors such as ageing in a *sporadic goitre*. In each instance the gland initially is typically diffuse and soft – a *simple goitre* – but over several years becomes larger and nodular.

1. Diffuse non-toxic goitre

Goitres of this type occurring as a result of iodine deficiency rarely present until well established, but if modest in size may become less evident in response to iodine or eradication of the offending goitrogen in the diet. The process may be arrested by giving thyroxine which depresses the thyroid stimulating hormone (TSH) drive to the gland. If there is no response, partial thyroidectomy may be indicated on cosmetic grounds.

2. Multinodular non-toxic goitre

Large goitres of this type may well cause the patient concern due to cosmetic disfigurement, incipient or established pressure symptoms and discomfort. All of these are good indications for surgery, the extent of which is dependent on the size and number of nodules present. Following operation, a small dose of thyroxine (0.1 mg daily) reduces the risk of recurrence.

3. Solitary nodular non-toxic goitre

Due to the high prevalence of solitary nodules (over 50% thought to be solitary are in fact part of a multinodular process), a policy of removing all of them surgically, although sound, is simply not practicable. Fine-needle biopsy (aspiration biopsy cytology), popularized in Sweden, has reduced surgical exploration rates for thyroid nodules by 24% and has the merit of being quick, painless and convenient, being performed as an outpatient procedure (Hamberger *et al.*, 1985). It suffers from the limitations of all biopsy techniques – the skill and ability of the operator to obtain a representative sample and the experience and accuracy of the cytopathologist reporting the specimen. The only serious limitation of this technique is the failure to differentiate between follicular adenomas and follicular carcinomas which can be made only by studying the overall histological pattern and, in particular, the presence of capsular and vascular invasion. Unless the surgeon can depend on a cytology service which has a very low false-negative rate, total lobectomy is advocated, and especially in children and in males under 40. Fine-needle biopsy quickly identifies a cystic nodule or simple cyst for which, if less than 2 cm in diameter, drainage may be curative. Ideally the cyst wall should also be biopsied to ensure that a papillary carcinoma is not being missed.

Carcinoma of the thyroid

This is a rare cancer, but the incidence appears to be increasing. The indications for and extent of surgery in carcinoma of the thyroid depends primarily on the histological type, but age of onset and mode of presentation influence management. These aspects will be considered in relationship to the five main types.

1. Papillary carcinoma

This is by far the commonest carcinoma (60% incidence overall, rising to 80% if only children and those under the age of 40 are considered). Women are affected twice as often as men. Occasionally in older patients it occurs in association with follicular lesions when the papillary pattern of behaviour predominates. The typically unencapsulated pale homogeneous primary tumour spreads via the lymphatics and there is a 90% incidence of microscopic tumour foci when the whole gland is meticulously examined (Russell *et al.*, 1963).

Multiple macroscopic deposits will be evident at operation in 20% of patients and extrathyroid spread to the regional nodes in 50%. These are usually on the same side as the lesion and within the area of primary lymphatic drainage, namely the central group of paratracheal nodes.

There is controversy about the extent of surgery required. The conservative approach is to perform a total lobectomy on the side of the solitary macroscopic primary without evident lymph node involvement, secure in the knowledge that for the majority of patients the prognosis is excellent if kept on TSH suppressive doses of thyroxine (usually 0.1 mg/day). Total thyroidectomy is reserved for patients with macroscopic multifocal disease and/or demonstrable lymph node involvement (Wade, 1983). Those who advocate a more aggressive strategy perform total/near total thyroidectomy for all cases, accepting a greater morbidity especially with regard to hypoparathyroidism. The advantage of this approach is that multifocal tumour throughout the gland is always removed, the risk of anaplastic change in residual foci is excluded and postoperative surveillance may be possible through serial thyroglobulin estimation. Deciding between the two strategies is resolved by a scoring system which has been devised (Hay *et al.*, 1987) to identify low- and high-risk patients based on four variables, easily remembered by the initials AGES (Age, Grade, Extent and Size) and for each, higher indices reflect a poorer prognosis and the need for more radical surgery. When DNA flow cytometry becomes more readily available (possible on fine-needle aspirate samples), this may provide additional or more precise guidance on treatment.

Surgery for papillary carcinoma should always include clearance of nodes in the primary lymphatic drainage zone. The thymus need not be disturbed unless obviously involved, as ectopic parathyroids are frequently located in the thyrothymic ligament. Nodal involvement in the secondary drainage areas may be suspected by their blue/black discoloration which often appear fleshy or cystic. Clearance of all such involved nodes should be carried out by a modified neck dissection, only sacrificing the internal jugular vein and sternomastoid muscle if directly involved. There is no justification for the classical radical block dissection which has been shown to confer no improvement on tumour recurrence rates or survival and leaves the patient with disfigurement and the risk of lymphoedema of the face. When lymph node recurrences do occur, often years later (less than 10% of cases treated by total lobectomy), they can easily be excised being well encapsulated, aptly termed 'berry picking'. Patients with successive recurrences treated in this way do not appear to have compromised survival. When local invasion or distant spread not amenable to surgery occurs, radio-iodine uptake occurs in approximately 20% of papillary metastases and therapeutic radio-iodine can be considered for eradication.

2. Follicular carcinoma

This differentiated tumour accounts for 20% of all thyroid cancers and, since the incidence world wide is higher in endemic goitre areas, would appear to be related to iodine lack and TSH drive. Three times as many women as men are affected and the peak age at diagnosis is 45, a decade later than for papillary carcinoma. On microscopic examination the tumour is typically solitary and encapsulated, but may occasionally be multiple and occupy the entire lobe. The degree of malignancy of a follicular carcinoma depends on the extent to which its capsule has been breached and the blood vessels invaded, which can accurately be assessed only by examination of the whole nodule. The tumour characteristically metastasizes by the blood stream and rarely via the lymphatics. Presentation, therefore, is typically as a non-toxic solitary nodule with or without evidence of distant spread. Metastases occur in the lungs, bones and occasionally the brain. It is rare for distant metastases to arise without a clinically impressive primary tumour and subsequent management is guided by mode of presentation. Most tumours will be suspected on fine-needle biopsy and confirmed on frozen section after total lobectomy, as for papillary carcinoma.

If the pathologist can state unequivocally that the malignant features of capsular and vascular invasion are present, the surgeon should proceed to total thyroidectomy as the treatment of choice (Reeve et al., 1988). If the appearances are not clear-cut, it is better to wait until the definitive paraffin sections are available. These may reveal micro-angio invasion without capsular involvement, in which case suppression of the TSH drive to the gland with T4 (0.1–0.2 mg/day for life) is likely to be all that is required. If, however, overt vascular or capsular invasion is seen, reoperation is strongly advised, converting to total thyroidectomy. This should be carried out within 7–10 days because thereafter surgery becomes difficult due to new vessel growth and fibrosis. Total thyroidectomy is advocated not because multifocal disease is common but because removal of the main 'iodine trap' enables distant metastases to be identified and ablated using radio-iodine. The usual routine is to withhold thyroxine after thyroidectomy until the patient becomes hypothyroid, usually within 3–6 weeks, so that the increased TSH drive makes the secondaries avid for iodine and therefore more likely to be identified.

3. Anaplastic carcinoma

This tumour typically occurs in elderly women and accounts for 10–15% of thyroid cancers. It is notable for its speed of growth and extreme malignancy, invasion occurring locally with distant spread via the blood stream and lymphatics. In the rare stituation of its occurrence in middle age, total thyroidectomy followed by external radiotherapy may extend survival for a time. It may do the patient a disservice if implantation of tumour occurs in the surgical incision. The surgeon's role is mainly to establish the diagnosis beyond doubt, and in view of the bulky nature of most anaplastic tumours a good representative sample can be obtained with a Tru-cut needle. Occasionally relief of pressure on the trachea can be achieved by removal of the isthmus, but generally local radiotherapy offers the only prospect of worthwhile palliation. The 12-month survival rate is zero and chemotherapy marginally improves the prognosis.

4. Lymphoma

Some of these tumours, which may mimic anaplastic carcinoma in presentation and histological appearances, arise in patients with long-standing Hashimoto's thyroiditis or widespread lymphoma. Some are very sensitive to radiotherapy and remarkable regression can be obtained. Worthwhile 5-year survival is recorded. Chemotherapy is reserved for patients with disseminated disease. The role of surgery therefore is diagnostic and attempts to remove a thyroid lymphoma are rarely appropriate.

5. Medullary thyroid carcinoma (MTC)

This rare tumour has attracted great interest since it was first described in 1959 (Hazard et al., 1959) and, clinical awareness having been aroused, now accounts for 5–10% of tumours in reported larger series of thyroid malignancies. It arises from the parafollicular C cells which are distributed throughout the gland but are in highest concentration in the upper poles (Roediger, 1976), where these tumours are most likely to be to be located. If the tumour is solitary the disease is more usually sporadic (80%) (Sizemore et al., 1977), but if multiple the familial form (20%) must be strongly suspected. The latter shows an autosomal dominant pattern of inheritance, men and women being equally affected. Successive generations tend to be diagnosed at a progressively younger age, but this may reflect the improved efficiency of screening. Familial MTC is associated with a tumour of one or both adrenals (medulla) – phaeochromocytomas – and with parathyroid hyperplasia. This endocrine triad is recognized as multiple endocrine neoplasia (MEN type IIA or Sipple's syndrome). A phenotypically distinct group of patients with medullary thyroid carcinoma and phaeochromocytoma but without parathryoid disease is described (MEN IIB). These patients have characteristic facies, marfanoid habitus and submucosal neurofibromas of the tongue and lips. In sporadic and familial MTC, the C cells produce a near-specific tumour marker – calcitonin – which provides guidance in detection and management. Hypercalcitonaemia is not always present and affected individuals may have a normal basal immunoreactive calcitonin level (ICT). The diagnosis of MTC may be assumed if grossly elevated basal calcitonin levels, in the absence of any other malignancy, are recorded. Normal basal calcitonin levels can be provoked to abnormal and diagnostic levels by giving an intravenous injection of pentagastrin (0.5 μg/kg) and a calcium infusion sufficient to raise the serum 0.6 mmol/litre. The degree of elevation may reflect the presence of a small occult tumour or C-cell hyperplasia and the latter is recognized and treated as a premalignant condition.

Surgical management should initially identify familial patients and, having done so, exclude a phaeochromocytoma and hyperparathyroidism. This is because the dangers of thyroid surgery in the presence of an undiagnosed phaeochromocytoma are considerable. Opinions are divided as to whether affected patients should be subjected to bilateral adrenalectomy when disease is demonstrable on one side only. Although medullary hyperplasia, or a frank tumour, occurs on both sides in 50% of patients, the morbidity of total adrenalectomy for the other 50% is hard to justify. No such reservations apply to the extent of surgery on the thyroid, which should be total thyroidectomy (Russell *et al.*, 1983) in view of the high incidence of multicentric lesions in the familial (80%) and sporadic (20%) disease. Particular attention is paid to the completeness of resection of the upper poles and of the primary lymphatic drainage areas. Dissection of the lymph nodes in the central compartment of the neck extends from the hyoid bone to the innominate vessels, since up to 75% of nodes will be found to contain metastatic disease (Gordon *et al.*, 1973). Lymph nodes in the lateral compartment should be sampled and, if positive, removed as a modified block dissection (described later). A patient with medullary thyroid carcinoma which is revealed unexpectedly after total lobectomy for a non-toxic solitary nodule need only be submitted to total thyroidectomy if familial disease is subsequently discovered or elevated basal or provoked calcitonin levels are demonstrated. A serial rise in serum calcitonin is a strong indicator of recurrent disease which may be detected by pentavalent DMSA scanning (Udelsman *et al.*, 1989). Metastases may be suitable for surgical removal, radiotherapy, radioiodine or chemotherapy. Results, however, are often disappointing.

6. Secondary tumours of the thyroid

Although rare, these most commonly arise from breast, kidney, ovary or colon. Thyroidectomy may be indicated if the secondary deposits are confined to the thyroid and the primary tumour is under control.

Other thyroid conditions

1. Acute suppurative thyroiditis

When antibiotics fail to eradicate a rare pyogenic infection of the thyroid, an abscess may develop requiring drainage by aspiration or open operation.

2. Hashimoto's disease/lymphadenoid goitre

This is a common cause of enlargement of the thyroid, women being affected 15 times more frequently than men. It is most often seen between the ages of 35 and 55 and onset is rapid over several months. The patient is euthyroid initially, but progresses to a hypothyroid state as the lymphocytic infiltration advances throughout the gland. Occasionally there is a toxic phase of variable duration. The goitre is characteristically diffuse and rubbery, but may become multinodular and asymmetrical, then shrinking to become fibrotic. Symptoms of pressure on the trachea and oesophagus are common. These may be relieved by exogenous thyroxine (0.1–0.2 mg/day) and a course of prednisolone 20 mg daily. If there is still no response, removal of the affected lobe or isthmus is indicated. Hashimoto's goitres are relatively avascular and easily separable from the false capsule. The development of malignant lymphoma and differentiated thyroid cancer in a Hashimoto's gland is now considered to be a minimal risk. Antibody levels help discriminate between Hashimoto's disease and cancer, although high microsomal and thyroglobulin titres occur in 12% of cases of thyroid carcinoma. Surgery is indicated in any patient with Hashimoto's disease where malignancy is suspected on clinical or cytological grounds – total lobectomy or total thyroidectomy depending on the extent of the disease process.

3. Riedel's thyroiditis/woody thyroid/ligneous thyroiditis

This is extremely rare. Some even doubt its existence as an entity distinct from Hashimoto's and de Quervain's thyroiditis which can both produce a very hard and fibrotic gland. If the fibrosis is particularly dense and extends beyond the thyroid tethering it to the trachea, strap muscles, etc., then the diagnosis must be considered with a differential diagnosis of thyroid carcinoma. The cause is unknown, but is probably one of a group of conditions characterized by multifocal midline fibrosis, including fibrosing mediastinitis, retroperitoneal fibrosis, sclerosing cholangitis and orbital pseudotumour. Relief of symptoms may follow division of the thyroid isthmus which is hard and brittle and which can be literally snapped off the trachea with the fingers.

4. Thyroid cyst

The prevalence of cysts of the thyroid increases with age and often reflects a degenerative process in a multinodular goitre. Benign cysts are frequently tense and, due to their location, render the sign of fluctuation unreliable and hard to elicit. Thyroid ultrasound should reliably identify them as a well-circumscribed echolucent area, but intracystic debris should raise the suspicion of cystic degeneration in a tumour which occurs, notably in papillary carcinoma. Cysts which are smaller than 2 cm in diameter are treated by aspiration, submitting the fluid for cytological examination and the patient to re-examination. Larger cysts are likely to recur when tapped, and may well be cosmetically unacceptable. These carry a risk of sudden airways obstruction due to intracystic haemorrhage and are, therefore, best dealt with electively by partial thyroidectomy.

Preoperative preparation

All patients require haemoglobin estimation, chest radiograph and an ECG, but an intraoperative blood transfusion is rarely required for any of the procedures to be described. Much laboratory time and effort may be saved by blood grouping and storage of serum only. Patients with disturbance of thyroid function will have had appropriate investigations, but the serum thyroxine is the single most appropriate baseline test for the remainder.

When the airway is compromised cervical views, anteroposterior and lateral, may help to delineate the trachea above the sternal notch. The anatomical relationship at the thoracic inlet, preferably using a body scanner, is particularly helpful when a substantial retrosternal goitre is suspected, so that the full extent of the problem can be assessed and appropriate precautions taken by the surgeon and anaesthetist. Vocal cords are examined routinely by indirect laryngoscopy, as a small number of patients have an unsuspected idiopathic unilateral palsy (Neil et al., 1972). The recognition of this is important to ensure integrity of the nerve on the other side. Likewise, laryngoscopy is essential if the patient has had previous surgery or developed hoarseness of the voice which might indicate thyroid malignancy or independent laryngeal pathology.

Thyrotoxic patients require special preparation and it is essential to establish a euthyroid state or control the peripheral effects of the circulating high levels of thyroid hormone. The majority of patients referred for surgery will be receiving anti-thyroid drugs but are likely to be unstable; hence the need for operation. Where toxicity is modest and surgery can be undertaken quickly, the beta blocker propranolol in a dose of 20–40 mg 8-hourly is given for 10 days preoperatively. When toxicity is severe the anti-thyroid drugs are continued up to the time of surgery, ensuring that the white blood count and clotting mechanisms are not compromised. Ideally the patient should be hospitalized for 48 h so that the dose of propranolol can be adjusted to a level which controls the sleeping pulse rate to below 70 beats/min. It is essential to give propranolol with the anaesthetic premedication to ensure control intraoperatively. After surgery, the dose of propranolol is reduced over the next 7 days, in line with the half-life of serum thyroxine. Some authors (Peden et al., 1982) favour the newer, longer-acting beta blockers which can be given daily but require the same precautions. Beta blockers are contraindicated in patients with bronchial asthma, sinus bradycardia, second- and third-degree heart block and heart failure due to pulmonary hypertension. Lugol's iodine 10 drops orally t.d.s. for 10 days (given in milk to make it more palatable)

is now rarely used. It inhibits organic binding of iodine and thyroid hormone release and reduces the vascularity of the gland but it increases the bulk of the goitre due to colloid deposition, rendering surgery more difficult.

Patients with significant thyrotoxicosis traditionally receive a 6–8-week course of carbimazole 10–15 mg 8-hourly, reducing to a 5 mg 8-hourly maintenance dose for the next 12–18 months once a euthyroid state is achieved. If the patient has an adverse reaction to the drug, propylthiouracil may be given as an alternative, 100 mg 8-hourly. Extended use of any of the thiourea group of drugs may cause prothrombin deficiency (Naeye and Terrien, 1960), leucopenia and rarely bone marrow depression.

Standard surgical approach to the thyroid

The first requirement is to ensure that the patient is comfortably placed and the diathermy-indifferent electrode is in firm contact with the buttocks. Good access to the anterior compartment of the neck is best achieved by placing a pillow beneath the shoulders to gently extend the cervical spine. Support and stabilization of the head on a padded ring or U-shaped neurosurgical rest is important, especially in the elderly, to prevent severe pain and headaches postoperatively. In patients with short, stocky necks or large goitres it is helpful to pull the shoulders down by gentle traction on the arms in their long axis, securing them to the sides of the body with foam wedges (Figure 24.3). The table is then tilted 15° head up to reduce engorgement in the neck veins and minimize subsequent bleeding. This manoeuvre relieves pressure on the superior vena cava in patients with a retrosternal goitre which is compressing the thoracic inlet. A flat board, supported by a pillow, placed horizontally on the upper abdomen and lower chest or a magnetic pad provides a convenient instrument tray (Figure 24.3).

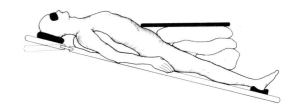

Figure 24.3 Position of patient for operation on the thyroid gland

The skin is prepared with aqueous chlorhexidine and the operative area draped. There are several ways of doing this. The author favours a four-towel technique with large cottonwool or gauze packs, one on either side of the neck being pushed well down with long-handled forceps into the recess between the head support and the shoulder pillow – these absorb any blood loss from the lateral extent of the neck incision. The head towel is reflected forward, rather than using a conventional head towel, which permits ready access to the airway for the anaesthetist in the event of any dislodgement of the endotracheal tube. Although the skin of the head and neck is rich in small vessels, infiltration with 1 in 1000 adrenaline in saline is now rarely practised. Much of the bleeding at the skin edge stops spontaneously and more persistent bleeding vessels are best recognized and coagulated at the time, rather than relying on the vasoconstrictive properties of adrenaline.

Routine operations on the thyroid are carried out using a Kocher collar incision which is placed in one of the natural skin creases (Langer's lines) approximately two finger-breadths above the sternoclavicular joint (Figure 24.4). This may conveniently be marked on the skin using a length of silk held taut against the convexity of the neck. Symmetry is important, for maturation of collagen in the scar may contract unevenly if the lines of stress are unequal which will result in a poor cosmetic appearance. It is therefore helpful to check the symmetry by standing at the head end of the table, looking down on the proposed incision directly from above. In view of the risk of keloid formation, the practice of cross-hatching, using a stylus and ink, or scarifying the skin with a needle is to be avoided. Matching the skin flaps at the end of the operation is rarely a problem for an experienced surgeon. The incision is deepened through the sub-cutaneous fat and platysma muscle, below which the deep cervical fascia is encountered, investing the strap muscles centrally and the sterno-mastoid muscles laterally. The anterior jugular veins course beneath this fascial layer and, provided that the surgeon keeps to the plane between the platysma and the fascia, blood loss is minimal.

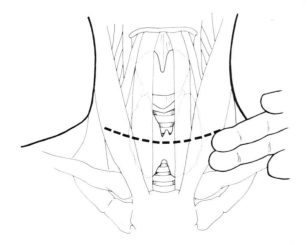

Figure 24.4 Standard incision for operation on the thyroid gland

Once the layer has been established, Babcock or Allis tissue forceps applied to the subdermal layer of each skin flap enable initial, deft scalpel dissection

of these using a technique of traction and counter-traction and blunt dissection with a swab on the index finger. Mobilization is extended superiorly to the thyroid notch and inferiorly to the suprasternal notch. The diamond-shaped surgical field is held exposed with a Joll's self-retaining retractor, the wound edges being protected with tetra towels. The deep cervical fascia is then incised vertically in the midline raphe from the prominence of the thyroid cartilage to the suprasternal notch and isthmus of the thyroid. Dissecting in this plane as it extends laterally over the lateral lobes beneath the sternothyroid muscle requires considerable care. Difficulties may arise when the strap muscles are thinned by compression or adherence to the thyroid secondary to the inflammation of auto-immune thyroiditis or direct invasion by thyroid malignancy. Exposing the thyroid further requires delivery of each lobe in turn into the wound. In young patients the strap muscles usually present no impediment and the lobe can be freed by sweeping the areolar connections between it and the overlying sternothyroid muscle with the index finger. Alternatively the tissue plane can be gently spread open by widening the jaws of a pair of artery forceps held vertically. In the rare event where the strap muscles limit exposure and prevent forward dislocation of the lobe, there should be no hesitation in dividing them. These muscles derive their nerve supply segmentally from the ansa hypoglossi as it loops down from the carotid sheath and it is desirable to preserve this innervation. The patient suffers no detectable functional deficit if these muscles have to be resected as part of a cancer clearance. In practice the jaws of a pair of long forceps inserted under the strap muscles at the junction of the upper one-third and lower two-thirds can be brought out at the medial border of the sternomastoid muscle, allowing identification and preservation of the nerve before dividing the muscle with diathermy. Stay stitches to the divided upper and lower muscle flaps are then placed and hitched over the Joll's retractor ratchets (Figure 24.5).

Specific thyroid procedures

Subtotal thyroidectomy

The aim is to remove sufficient thyroid tissue to abolish toxicity yet preserve a posterior remnant of the gland on each side sufficient to maintain the patient in a euthyroid state. Each lobe is dislocated forward in turn and most surgeons find it preferable to stand on the opposite side of the table to the lobe being delivered. Retraction of the strap muscles is conveniently carried out with a Vaughan–Hudson angled retractor which reduces the risk of damage to the sympathetic chain. The middle thyroid vein is usually the first structure seen crossing to the gland at its midpoint, and this must be ligated and divided

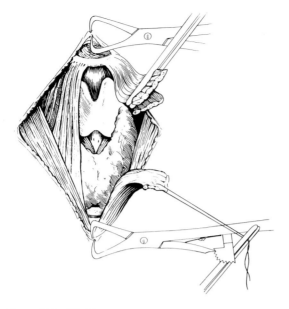

Figure 24.5 Division and mobilization of strap muscles

before the lobe can be further delivered. This is done with a ligature passed on a small aneurysm needle and then, keeping the gland retracted medially and downwards with a gauze swab, the superior pedicle is defined. It is only after this has been done that the lobe can be fully mobilized. The adherent sternothyroid muscle is conveniently pushed off the surface of the upper pole with a Lahey swab mounted on forceps (beware of a fairly constant high unnamed vein running from the pole to the internal jugular). A thyroid director is then passed between the larynx and the thyroid pedicle. This is a subtle and useful manoeuvre and if damage to the recurrent laryngeal nerve is to be avoided, the point of the director should be aimed upwards and laterally, ensuring by fingertip pressure that the point of the director has passed behind all the upper lobe thyroid tissue (Figure 24.6). Keeping the director in place, the pedicle is doubly ligated with a transfixion suture of 2/0 linen passed behind and then anteriorly to secure both branches of the superior thyroid artery. Formal division of the pedicle can often be deferred until the final resection of the lobe is undertaken. The lobe is now secured with Lahey grasping forceps and rotated medially. The inferior thyroid artery is identified by opening up the space between the trachea and common carotid artery with blunt forcep dissection and then is under-run cleanly and precisely with a ligature on an aneurysm needle. If this is placed as far laterally as practicable, it is ready for typing in continuity once the recurrent laryngeal nerve and parathyroids have been identified. Gentle traction on this ligature often throws the recurrent laryngeal nerve into prominence, as it runs up at an acute angle from the mediastinum to reach the tracheo-oesophageal groove before assuming its intimate relationships with the branches of

this artery. When it is not evident, an aberrant course should be suspected, notably lateral or anterior to the trachea or even non-recurrent. The nerve can be confidently identified by its white colour, fine longitudinal surface artery, lack of pulsation and lack of elasticity. Proceeding with the operation at this stage without having identified the nerve is hazardous. The inferior thyroid artery ligature is now tied and the thyroid lobe is freed inferiorly by isolating and dividing between ligatures the inferior thyroid veins and thyroidea ima artery where present. During this manoeuvre the recurrent laryngeal nerve should be kept in view and avoided at all times. The inferior parathyroid gland may be seen at this point, especially if ectopic, lying in the thyrothymic ligament. This and its blood supply will be preserved if the veins are swept medially and secured close to the gland. In this form of thyroidectomy the parathyroids do not need to be identified formally and, indeed, attempting to do so may hazard their blood supply. If one is inadvertently excised or devascularized it should be diced into 1 mm cubes and auto-transplanted into the adjacent sternomastoid muscle.

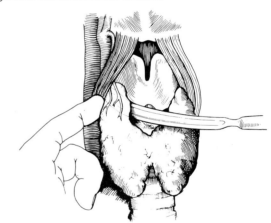

Figure 24.6 Mobilization of superior lobe of the thyroid gland

At this stage the surgeon must make the important decision about how much thyroid tissue to leave behind. The empirical formula of resecting seven-eighths and leaving one-eighth of the gland is a useful guideline and results in a majority of euthyroid patients. The merit of this approach is that it requires no modification for varying sizes of gland, but it has the disadvantage that it does not take into account the age of the patient (generally the younger the patient, the more radical the resection needs to be) or high thyroid auto-antibody titres (which call for less radical excision). Attempts to standardize the size of the thyroid remnant by linear measurement, dental wax stents (Murley and Rigg, 1968) or clinical judgement (Hedley *et al.*, 1972) have been shown to be highly inaccurate, so that the recommendation to leave 3 or 4 g of tissue on each side is meaningless.

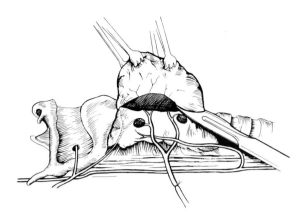

Figure 24.7 Removal of thyroid lobe by sharp dissection, preserving parathyroid glands

which produce a better result than routine suturing which tends to tattoo the skin at the needle entry points. After securing the drains with a fine non-slip silk suture, a loose thyroid dressing may be applied.

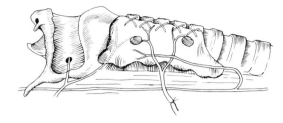

Figure 24.8 Haemostatic suture of residual thyroid

Having decided on the size of the residual thyroid, small artery forceps are placed on the posterolateral aspect of the surgical capsule, and injury to the recurrent laryngeal nerve and parathyroids should be avoided if resection is started above the level defined by the anterior surface of the trachea. The gland is then incised with a scalpel blade directed medially and obliquely towards the trachea (Figure 24.7). The identical sequence of events is then performed on the opposite side of the neck when some fine adjustment of remnant size will be possible to give an overall one-eighth residue. Both lobes and the isthmus having been freed, the gland now remains attached only by the pyramidal lobe or fibrous remnant of the thyro-glossal tract. This requires careful dissection upwards so that no additional thyroid tissue or blood supply is overlooked. The thyroid remnants are then sutured to the pretracheal fascia with continuous chromic catgut in a herringbone fashion, picking up the surgical capsule and rolling the thyroid towards the midline and away from the recurrent laryngeal nerve (Figure 24.8). This is not only haemostatic but if, for any reason, the neck requires further exploration the fibrotic reaction around the thyroid remnants is well away from important structures. The thyroid bed may be drained and if the dead space is modest a Redivac drain is ideal, but if large or haemostasis has been difficult, a wider bore drain of the Drayvac type is preferred. It is exteriorized by a separate small stab incision on each side of the neck. The drains cross in the midline and run for some distance beneath the platysma layer so that superficial as well as deep drainage is provided, avoiding the risk of a subcutaneous seroma. After flexing the head by adjustment of the headrest, the strap muscles are reconstituted using interrupted 2/0 chromic catgut and then approximated with their overlying fascia in the midline with a continuous catgut suture. Finally, the platysma is closed with a running 3/0 plain catgut, picking up the edge of the muscle with evenly matched, very small bites so that the overlying skin is accurately realigned. The author favours skin closure with (Avlox) clips

Partial thyroidectomy

The standard exposure of the thyroid and the sub-total excision techniques as already described are performed, leaving as much normal tissue as possible consistent with a modest lateral remnant on each side which will not be evident when the patient swallows. It is inadvisable to leave the isthmus or pyramidal lobe even when apparently normal, for if compensatory hypertrophy occurs it will be cosmetically unacceptable at that site.

Removal of a retrosternal goitre

The surgeon will know of the ectopic site of the gland by preoperative symptoms, examination and investigation, and operating theatre staff will have been alerted to the possible need to split the sternum. In practice, almost all retrosternal goitres can be delivered and removed through the neck, but the incision should be placed lower. The anterior chest wall is shaved, skin prepared and draped accordingly and if the airway is severely compromised the services of an experienced anaesthetist are imperative. It is usually safer in these cases to withhold sedative agents for premedication and rely on speedy intubation with the patient awake, having sprayed the vocal cords with local anaesthetic. The combination of a paralysed patient and one with a difficult airway such as this may result in failure to intubate and fatal anoxia. Wholly or partially intrathoracic goitres derive their arterial supply from the superior and inferior arteries in the neck and these should be secured in the usual way, likewise the superior and middle thyroid venous drainage. Once the upper pole has been freed, an attempt should be made to dissect the retrosternal portion of the lobe with the index finger and gently ease it upwards. Minimal force should be used, otherwise the recurrent laryngeal nerves, which cannot always be visualized, due to the limited space, may be avulsed or severely stretched. If this manoeuvre fails, the surgeon has one of two choices – intracapsular enucleation or formal splitting of the sternum.

The latter is probably only necessary or justified if thyroid malignancy is suspected or when operating for a recurrent goitre. Intracapsular enucleation involves incision of the thyroid just above the sternal notch, after which the fibrous septa and colloid nodules within the lobe are broken down with a finger. The contents can then be scooped out with a large Volkmann spoon or a Yanker's sucker. It may then be possible to deliver the capsule to secure the inferior thyroid veins, but if there is still concern about the location of the recurrent laryngeal nerve and haemostasis is good, it is best left *in situ*. Two large suction drains are recommended. When the sternum needs to be split, an incision is made in the midline down to the periosteum with cutting diathermy from the suprasternal notch downwards for an appropriate distance (Figure 24.9). The space between the manubrium and the great vessels is gently opened up by finger dissection as far as the digit can reach. Introducing a vertical mechanical saw, the manubrium, or sometimes the whole sternum, is divided longitudinally, keeping the saw handle forced upwards at all times. A self-retaining sternal retractor is racked open to spread the divided manubrium or sternum (Figure 24.10). Bleeding from the periosteum is controlled with electrocautery and from the marrow with bone wax. The parietal pleura is freed in the midline and pushed laterally. Removal of a retrosternal goitre proceeds along routine lines and the chest is then closed by accurately reapproximating the sternum using wire sutures. These are passed through the bone with an awl, the underlying structures being protected by a malleable copper spatula. The wires are held taut with strong forceps, twisted, clipped and the tips of the wire then buried into the periosteum. A retrosternal drain is brought out superiorly and attached to an underwater seal to control a small pneumothorax which may have been produced. The subcutaneous fat is closed with interrupted catgut and the skin with a running subcuticular prolene or absorbable suture.

Total thyroid lobectomy or total thyroidectomy

Thyroid lobectomy is undertaken when the surgeon knows or suspects that the patient has thyroid carcinoma in one half of the gland, and if confirmed on frozen section a total lobectomy may in addition be carried out on the other side, completing a total thyroidectomy. The approach to the thyroid is standard, but the subtotal excision technique described earlier is modified in several important ways. At no stage is the gland grasped with tissue forceps for traction, otherwise a malignant focus may be ruptured inadvertently with spillage of tumour cells. It must also be assumed that multicentric tumour deposits may exist or capsular invasion be present, hence the need to give a solitary nodule a wide berth by removing the entire lobe, isthmus and a midline portion of the contralateral lobe. This ideal should

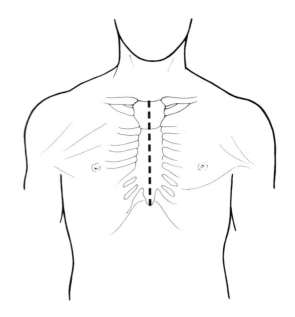

Figure 24.9   Incision for partial or complete splitting of the sternum to gain access to large retrosternal goitre

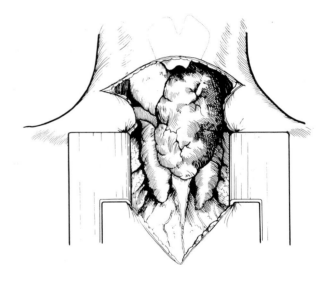

Figure 24.10   Exposure of retrosternal goitre following splitting of the upper sternum

not be pursued in a way that may endanger the recurrent laryngeal nerve or parathyroids, and where these could be compromised it may be better to leave a little residual thyroid tissue and ablate this later with radio-iodine. The main blood supply of each parathyroid is from the inferior thyroid artery, but before the end artery to each parathyroid is reached collaterals are picked up from the oesophageal and tracheal vessels. In this procedure it is best, therefore, not to ligate the inferior thyroid artery in continuity but to trace out each of its terminal branches, preserving the one to the parathyroids and individually clipping and dividing the rest between mosquito forceps as they enter the false capsule. Concurrently, the recurrent laryngeal nerve is traced along its course and it often helps to have this gently retracted laterally on a soft, silastic sling. The relationship of the nerve to Berry's ligament is variable, passing medial to its attachment in 65% of instances, through the ligament in 25% and through the thyroid gland itself in 10%. Damage will be avoided by dissecting the gland free from the nerve under direct vision, especially when the ligament is divided to release the upper pole. Occasionally, local invasion by tumour prevents complete removal, notably at the side of the larynx and oesophagus. In these circumstances the extent of the residual tumour should be marked with small liga-clips to assist the radiotherapist in planning treatment fields.

The safe performance of a standard, total lobectomy should be within the capabilities of most general surgeons, but an effective total thyroidectomy with acceptably low morbidity is more demanding and not for the inexperienced.

Modified block dissection for thyroid carcinoma

The standard Kocher incision is extended on one or both sides (Figure 24.11) and routine exposure of the thyroid gland undertaken. Having raised the skin flaps to their full extent, a clearer field may be obtained by suturing the apex of each skin flap to the drapes rather than using two Joll's retractors which tend to get in the way. Operability is assessed and where there is clear involvement of the strap muscles or sternomastoid on one side, these are resected *en bloc* with the total thyroidectomy specimen, as described above. The plane between the sternomastoid and strap muscles is opened up and the carotid sheath exposed. Where there is heavy nodal involvement along the internal jugular chain extending to the posterior cervical and supraclavicular groups, the author finds it easiest to detach the sternal and clavicular heads of the sternomastoid and rotate this muscle upwards. This provides excellent exposure yet allows preservation of the blood supply (occipital artery) and nerve supply (accessory) so that it may be reattached on completion of the node dissection. Great care is needed when removing the upper and lower deep cervical nodes and their surrounding fat from the surface of the internal jugular vein. Silastic slings placed around the vessel, above and below, provide counter-traction and control the vein wall which, if breached, could cause an air embolus as well as serious bleeding. The internal jugular vein may have to be sacrificed (see Chapter 27). Involved supraclavicular and posterior triangle nodes are dissected in continuity with the deep cervical chain and occasionally the posterior belly of the omohyoid muscle may require excision with division of the transverse cervical and supraclavicular vessels. The vagus and phrenic nerves are substantial and easily identified and preserved, but the thoracic duct on the

left and the main lymphatic duct on the right are easily damaged. If this occurs, the affected duct should be tied off rather than an attempt made to effect a repair.

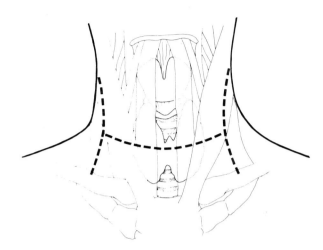

Figure 24.11 Modification of thyroid incision to include bilateral lymph node dissection

Postoperative care

It is important to recognize promptly any of the possible complications, the management of which will be individually discussed in the next section. The patient is extubated on the operating table. If there has been any concern about the integrity of the recurrent laryngeal nerves, the anaesthetist is requested to examine the vocal cords. Ideally, the patient is observed in a recovery area close to the theatre until fully conscious and should haemorrhage occur or airway obstruction develop, surgical and anaesthetic help will readily be available. The vital signs, and the appearance of the neck, should be checked regularly in the first 12 h and thereafter 4-hourly until the patient is stable. Thyrotoxic patients whose operations have been covered with beta blockers require monitoring of the pulse over several days while the dose is progressively decreased. The suction drains remain for 48 h by which time the wound is usually dry. Alternate clips are removed at 48 h and the remainder at 72 h. On discharge from hospital, generally on the third or fourth postoperative day, the patient is instructed to massage the skin gently in the region of the incision with lanolin which keeps the scar supple and helps to prevent adhesion of the platysma to the underlying strap muscles. The latter causes unsightly puckering of the skin on swallowing.

Postoperative complications

In competent hands all surgical procedures on the

thyroid carry low rates of morbidity and no mortality. There are, however, potentially dangerous local and specific complications which can severely compromise the outcome and be life threatening. The majority are avoidable with sound surgical technique and good preparation (notably of thyrotoxic patients).

Haemorrhage

This is typically reactionary and a potential problem in the first 24 h after surgery. Failure to secure the superior thyroid vessels efficiently, preferably with a transfixion suture, runs the risk of serious blood loss. Inadequate control of the inferior and middle thyroid vein may also have serious consequences. Major haemorrhage deep to the strap muscles must be recognized quickly, as there is a problem of pressure within a confined space on the airway and the rapid development of laryngeal and subglottic oedema. Medical and nursing staff need to be aware of the significance of pallor, respiratory difficulty, stridor and swelling of the wound. No reliance should be placed on the absence of blood loss from drains because these can block easily. Immediate action to evacuate any haematoma and secure an airway by intubation or tracheostomy may be necessary to avert a potentially life-threatening situation. At the bedside of all patients following thyroidectomy, clip removers and a pair of artery forceps should be readily available. These will allow the incision and the strap muscles to be opened up. If stridor persists, then skilled anaesthetic help is needed for intubation which may be very difficult due to oedema. In the absence of such help, a mini-tracheostomy or large medicut needle and cannula (no. 12 blue) inserted percutaneously through the cricothyroid membrane or between the tracheal rings should stabilize the situation until the patient can be returned to theatre for the arrest of haemorrhage.

Recurrent laryngeal nerve damage

This complication is the most publicized and feared by patient and surgeon, alike, yet the incidence of permanent damage and transient damage is extremely low (less than 0.1% and 2–4%, respectively). It is largely avoidable if the surgeon routinely seeks to identify the nerve on each side during all operations on the gland. Loss of power and huskiness of the voice which is often evident for two or three days after surgery is most likely to be due to oedema and is relieved by local anaesthetic lozenges and/or humidified air. Persistence of symptoms may indicate neuropraxia which is caused by stretching or crushing of the nerve. The damage is reversible and recovers over several weeks or months. If the nerve is divided or ligated, then permanent damage will result. The injury is more likely when the anatomy is distorted, for example with recurrent or malignant goitres.

Unilateral injury may be asymptomatic and pass undetected due to compensatory adduction of the uninvolved cord. It will only be detected if routine postoperative laryngoscopy is performed. Symptomatic patients with unilateral cord paralysis can anticipate improvement of their voice if the affected cord is stabilized in adduction by submucous injection of Teflon under direct laryngoscopy. The effects of bilateral nerve injury are likely to be temporary, but pose an immediate problem when the patient is extubated at the end of surgery. The unopposed adductor action of the cricothyroid muscles close the glottis to such an extent that the least exertion results in airway obstruction. The patient must be promptly reintubated, paralysed and ventilated while hydrocortisone is given 100 mg t.d.s. to combat the oedema and inflammatory response. Usually the patient can be successfully extubated within 48 h. If a trial of extubation again fails, tracheostomy is performed. It is wise to wait for 9 months before accepting the fact of permanent damage, at which stage several surgical approaches are possible. Exploration and resuture of the nerve with grafting when necessary is now feasible using microsurgical techniques, as is the anastomosis of the hypoglossal and recurrent nerves.

Superior laryngeal nerve paresis

The true incidence of this injury is unknown due to lack of any objective test of function until recently. If the patient experiences a change in the voice – loss of pitch and inability to make explosive sounds – damage is likely. Voice analysis using a Visipitch oscilloscope will help to confirm this damage, which may occur in up to 25% of patients (Kark et al., 1984). The majority will usually recover if the nerve has only been stretched. If no improvement is evident after 3 months, it is unlikely to occur. Bilateral damage is said to produce a very flat, hoarse voice which tires easily.

Hypoparathyroidism

The serum calcium level should be checked routinely postoperatively because patients who are not overtly hypoparathyroid may suffer vague lethargy and depression or insidiously develop cataracts, mental deterioration and psychosis (Rose, 1963). Hypocalcaemia due to parathyroid deficiency will usually be evident within 1 week of operation and should be suspected if the patient appears unduly agitated, depressed or hyperventilates. Circumoral tingling is generally the first and most sensitive indicator of a low serum calcium and paraesthesia in the fingers and its preceding frank tetany is seen when hypocalcaemia is profound. Tapping over the facial nerve will cause contraction of the facial muscles (Chvostek–Weiss sign), but this phenomenon may be observed in 10–15% of normal individuals (Barnes and Gann, 1974). Carpopedal spasm, provoked by occlusion of the circulation to the arm (Trousseau's sign), indicates severe hypocalcaemia and requires intravenous calcium infusion (10 ml of 10% calcium gluconate, given slowly to avoid cardiac arrest in systole). This infusion may need to be repeated 4–6 hourly. Oral effervescent calcium is commenced at the same time, 4–16 g daily, dose depending on response. If hypocalcaemia persists, vitamin D (calciferol 25 000–100–000 u as well as 2–3 g oral calcium per day are given until return to normocalcaemia. Patients lacking parathyroid reserve will produce these signs and symptoms in the future if challenged, e.g. during pregnancy or at the menopause, etc.

Hypothyroidism and recurrent hyperthyroidism

The ability of the thyroid to produce sufficient thyroxine after thyroidectomy reflects not only the size of the remnant but also the pre-existing pathological processes within the gland. Hypothyroidism is inevitable after total thyroidectomy or malignancy, but less predictable, for example, after a thyroid lobectomy for a benign solitary nodule. Avoiding hypothyroidism is one of the main challenges when operating for thyrotoxicosis. In this instance, postoperative function is dictated by several factors:

1. The severity of disease prior to surgery.
2. The age of the patient.
3. The presence of high levels of preoperative thyroid auto-antibodies.
4. The size of the gland and evidence of lymphoid infiltration on histology.
5. The surgical judgement which evaluates the foregoing and dictates how much of the gland to remove.

In experienced hands, consistent hypothyroidism rates of 10–15% can be achieved while avoiding levels of persistent hyperthyroidism greater than 5%, which would be unacceptable. Hypothyroidism should be allowed to develop with rising TSH levels over 6 weeks after total thyroidectomy for malignancy (notably follicular lesions). A radio-iodine scan is then performed to identify possible distant metastases which are then ablated. Thereafter, tri-iodo-L-thyronine (T3) 50–100 µg/day is given in preference to L-thyroxine (T4) by virtue of its shorter biological half-life of 1 week which enables repeated scans to be performed with minimal delay. Once isotope ablation of residual disease has been achieved, conversion to T4 is appropriate. The replacement dose for individual patients varies considerably, the majority only requiring 0.2–0.3 mg/day. Nearly all patients operated on for thyrotoxicosis become biochemically hypothyroid for 2–3 months after surgery and no correction is necessary as the majority will then stabilize in a euthyroid state. However, follow-up for at least 2 years is important for clinical assessment and to check serum thyroxine and TSH levels, as a small percentage of patients will become clinically hypo-

thyroid and require a modest dose of T4 in the order of 0.1–0.2 mg daily. Routine T4 (0.1 mg daily) is recommended for all patients operated on for non-toxic, diffuse or multinodular goitres, since failure to suppress TSH drive can result in recurrent goitre, even if hypothyroidism is subclinical.

Tracheal collapse

In this condition the wall of the trachea has become softened by 'chondromalacia', so that collapse occurs when the goitre is removed. It is seen occasionally following removal of a long-standing goitre, especially if retrosternal. In such cases there is likely to be a degree of laryngeal oedema and reduced movement of the vocal cords following difficult intubation and delivery of the lobes. Whenever the trachea is noted to be markedly soft and narrow, an elective tracheostomy should be performed.

Thyroid crisis

Now a very rare event with the improved methods of control of thyrotoxicosis, this state, when fully expressed, is characterized by high fever, tachycardia (atrial fibrillation), extreme restlessness and delirium. Treatment should be given promptly and is based on high doses of anti-thyroid drugs (Neo Mercazole (carbimazole) 30 mg stat and then 15 mg 8-hourly) plus 1 g of sodium iodide intravenously. The beta blocker propranolol 2 mg is given slowly intravenously with electrocardiographic control. Fluid replacement, ice-pack cooling and sedation may help to abort the crisis.

Cervical sympathetic damage

This is a rare complication resulting from deep, forceful retraction on the carotid sheath producing Horner's syndrome, notable by the absence of the vascular dilatation component (Smith and Murley, 1965). The myosis and ptosis are frequently permanent.

Wound complications

Keloid – the deposition of excessive collagen in the scar – is the most unpredictable complication but is said to be more prevalent in Negroes, redheads and during pregnancy. Unless the scar can be excised and adapted to conform more readily to Langer's lines, reoperation is unlikely to confer any improvement but topical steroids and low-dose irradiation may prevent recurrence. Infection is an uncommon complication and when it occurs a foreign body should be suspected, the most common offender being non-absorbable suture material. Rarely, nickel sensitivity from the clips used for the skin closure results in blistering and breakdown.

References

Barnes, H. V. and Gann, D. S. (1974) Choosing thyroidectomy in hyperthyroidism. *Surg. Clin. N. Am.*, **54**, 289

Crile, G., Jr. (1957) The fallacy of the conventional neck dissection for papillary carcinoma of the thyroid. *Ann. Surg.*, **145**. 317

Duffy, B. J., Jr. and Fitzgerald, P. J. (1950) Cancer of the thyroid in children. *J. Clin. Endocrinol. Metab.*, **10**, 1296–1308

Gordon, P. R., Huves, A. G. and Strong, E. W. (1973) Medullary carcinoma of the thyroid gland. *Cancer*, **31**, 915

Hamberger, B., Gharib, H., Melton, , L. J. *et al.* (1985) Fine needle aspiration biopsy of the thyroid nodules. Impact on thyroid practice and cost of care. *Ann. J. Med.* (in press)

Hay, I. D., Grant, C. S., Taylor, W. F. and McConahey, W. M. (1987) Ipsilateral lobectomy versus bilateral lobar resection in papillary carcinoma. A retrospective analysis of surgical outcome using a novel prognostic scoring system. *Surgery (St Thomas's)*, **102**, 1088–1095

Hazard, J. B., Hawk, W. A. and Crile, G., Jr. (1959) Medullary (solid) carcinoma of the thyroid: a clinicopathological entity. *J. Clin. Endocrinol.*, **19**, 153–161

Hedley, A. J., Michie, W., Duncan, T. *et al.* (1972) The effect of remnant size on the outcome of subtotal thyroidectomy for thyrotoxicosis. *Br. J. Surg.*, **59**, 559–563

Hollingshead, W. H. (1952) Anatomy of the endocrine glands. *Surg. Clin. N. Am.*, **32**, 1115–1140

Kark, A. E., Kissim, M. W., Auerbach, R. *et al.* (1984) Voice changes after thyroidectomy: the role of the external laryngeal nerve. *Br. Med. J.*, **289**, 1412–1415

Murley, R. S. and Rigg, B. M. (1968) Post-operative thyroid function and complications in relation to a measured thyroid remnant. *Br. J. Surg.*, **55**, 757–760

Naeye, R. L. and Terrien, C. M. (1960) Haemorrhagic state after therapy with propylthiouracil. *Am. J. Clin. Pathol.*, **34**, 254–257

Neil, H. B., III, Townsend, G. L. and Devine, K. D. (1972) Bilateral vocal cord paralysis of undetermined aetiology: clinical course and outcome. *Ann. Otol. Rhinol. Laryngol.*, **81**, 514–519

Peden, N. R., Gunn, A. and Browning, M. C. K. (1982) Nadolol and potassium iodine in combination in the surgical treatment of thyrotoxicosis. *Br. J. Surg.*, **69**, 638–641

Reeve, T. S., Delbridge, L. *et al.* (1988) Thyroid cancers of follicular cell origin. *Prog. Surg.*, **19**, 78–88

Roediger, W. E. W. (1976) Thyroidectomy for non-familial medullary carcinoma. *Br. J. Surg.*, **63**, 343–345

Rose, N. (1963) Investigation of post-thyroidectomy patients for hypoparathyroidism. *Lancet*, **i.**, 124–127

Russell, C. F., van Heerdeen, J. A., Sizemore, G. W. *et al.* (1983) The surgical management of medullary thyroid carcinoma. *Ann. Surg.*, **197**, 42–48

Russell, W. O., Ibanez, M. L., Clark, R. L. *et al.* (1963) Thyroid carcinoma classification. Intraglandular dissection and clinicopathological study based upon whole organ section of 80 glands. *Cancer*, **16**, 1425–1460

Sizemore, G. W., Carney, J. A. and Heath, H., III (1977) Epidemiology of medullary carcinoma of the thyroid gland: a 5-year experience (1971–76). *Surg. Clin. N. Am.*, **57**, 633–645

Smith, I. and Murley, R. S. (1965) Damage to the cervical sympathetic system during operation on the thyroid gland. *Br. J. Surg.*, **52**, 673

Udelsman, R., Dudley, N. E. *et al.* (1989) Medullary carcinoma of the thyroid: management of persistent hypercalcitonaemia utilizing [^{99m}Tc] (v) dimercaptosuccinic acid scintography. *Br. J. Surg.* **76**, 1276–1281

Wade J. S. H. (1983) The management of malignant thyroid tumours. *Br. J. Surg.*, **70**, 253–255

25

The parathyroid glands

J. R. Farndon

Surgical anatomy

There are normally four parathyroid glands, but there can be a larger or smaller number. Gilmour's study of 428 cadavers (Gilmour, 1938) found two glands in 0.2%, three in 6.1%, five in 6% and six in 0.5%. Only 87% of patients will have a normal complement of four glands. The normal gland weighs 30 mg and measures 3–6 × 2–4 × 0.5–2 mm, is characteristically tan in colour and difficult to palpate even when enlarged. The glands move freely within an envelope of surrounding fat and are usually discrete from the thyroid.

The upper parathyroids develop from the dorsal endoderm of the fourth pharyngeal pouch, the ventral part of which is fused laterally to the developing thyroid gland on the floor of the primitive pharynx. Ninety-two per cent of upper parathyroid glands remain in close contact with the dorsal aspect of the thyroid above the level where the recurrent laryngeal nerve crosses the inferior thyroid artery. In 1.6% they are found between the thyroid and the oesophagus, in 1.5% they lie between the pharynx and oesophagus and in 0.5% within the carotid sheath (Figure 25.1). Pathological enlargement favours dorsal displacement either by forces of deglutition or negative intrathoracic pressure and an upper parathyroid tumour may reach the posterior mediastinum. The upper glands, however, will usually be found on the posterolateral aspect of the thyroid lobe at or just below the level of the cricoid cartilage. They are frequently near the branches of the inferior thyroid artery as they enter the false capsule of the thyroid.

The lower parathyroid gland develops from the dorsal endoderm of the third pharyngeal pouch which also gives rise to the thymus. In contrast to the fourth pouch, which remains fairly static in position during embryological development, the third descends to the anterior mediastinum leaving a discrete mass of parathyroid in the neck and a thymus retrosternally. Excessive disruption produces an accessory parathyroid and thymic tissue, while failure to disrupt at all results in an intrathymic mediastinal parathyroid. In 20% of patients the parathyroids will actually be within the thymus and this is usually bilateral in 50% (Proye, 1978). The lower parathyroid on each side will normally be found on the posterior aspect of the lateral lobe of the thyroid just below and ventral to the level where the recurrent nerve crosses the inferior

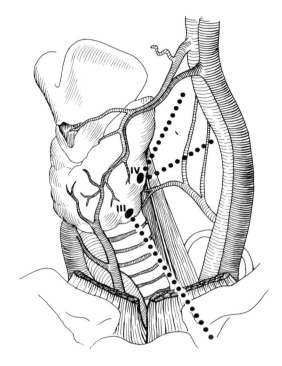

Figure 25.1 Normal and abnormal position of the parathyroid glands

thyroid artery. The glands may lie within the thyro-thymic ligament.

A frequency distribution diagram of the possible locations of the superior and inferior parathyroid glands has been produced by Åkerström et al. (1984).

The blood supply to the parathyroids is almost exclusively via the inferior thyroid artery. Tracing the terminal branches of this vessel may aid recognition of the glands. In 5% of cases the upper parathyroids derive their blood supply from the superior thyroid artery and then the gland is likely to be situated above the upper pole of the thyroid gland itself. Although the ultimate arterial branch of supply to each gland is an end artery, collateral circulation can be observed at a point proximal to the hilum of the parathyroid and is derived from oesophageal, tracheal or superior thyroid arteries.

Preoperative preparation

If patients present with bone disease (osteitis fibrosa

cystica) as a result of primary hyperparathyroidism or secondary hyperparathyroidism, then after removal of the abnormal overactive glands, a calcium debt remains and, in combination with atrophy of the residual normal glands, symptomatic hypocalcaemia may occur. Preoperative preparation using 1-alpha-hydroxycholecalciferol, at a dose of 2–4 µg/day, for a few days preoperatively, may help reduce the profound hypocalcaemia seen in the postoperative period. This hypocalcaemia is often described as the 'hungry bones syndrome'. The degree of preoperative hypercalcaemia may preclude treatment with vitamin D analogues.

Patients may rarely present with hypercalcaemic crisis. This is characterized by severe dehydration, mental confusion or coma, weakness and nausea and vomiting. Preoperative preparation requires intensive resuscitation including rehydration and treatment with diphosphanates and/or calcitonin.

No preoperative localization studies are advocated unless a previous neck exploration has been undertaken. Surgery for hyperparathyroidism should be undertaken by those with a special interest and there is no place for the occasional surgeon. In the hands of competent surgeons, successful localization of the abnormal parathyroid gland will occur in over 95% of patients without preoperative localization.

Preoperative counselling is an important element of preparation. Patients should be told that, rarely, the abnormal gland may not be found at cervical exploration. An explanation should be given to the patient that this usually means that the abnormal gland is within the anterior or posterior mediastinum. Patients should be told that a mediastinotomy is not usually carried out at the first exploration upon failure to locate abnormal glands in the neck.

Patients should be warned about the possible complications of surgical intervention. They should be told about the possibility of hypocalcaemia requiring treatment with calcium – sometimes a confusing concept for patients, especially when they have been told that they have an excess of calcium in the system!

The recurrent nerve will be seen and protected during exploration, but patients should be warned about the possibility of neuropraxia and of the very rare possibility of permanent damage to one or other of the recurrent laryngeal nerves. The forewarned and counselled patient is less aggrieved than the ill-informed, distressed patient. Medicolegal wranglings occur more commonly when communication between surgeon and patient has been poor.

The risk of primary or secondary haemorrhage is small and might be mentioned, but in a way not to disturb or frighten the patient.

Some surgeons use methylene blue, given as a preoperative infusion to aid localization of the glands. There is no clear evidence that this brings any particular advantage or more successful exploration and it may be associated with cardiotoxicity and thrombophlebitis in the infused vein. The coloration of the patient's skin by methylene blue can be frightening to nurses and anaesthetists!

Indications for surgery

Symptomatic primary hyperparathyroidism

The surgeon should be sure of the biochemical diagnosis. Indicators are hypercalcaemia, detectable or abnormal levels of parathyroid hormone, hypophosphataemia, hyperchloraemia, hypercalciuria and possibly a raised alkaline phosphatase. Nephrogenous cyclic AMP may be raised and some laboratories measure hydroxyprolene excretion as a marker of bone breakdown. The importance of measuring the urinary calcium excretion must be emphasized. The finding of a low normal or excretion level below normal must raise the suspicion of familial hypercalcaemic hypocalciuria. In this condition there is an abnormality of the renal tubule and no abnormality in the parathyroid glands. The patient does not normally benefit from neck exploration! The surgeon must play a part in being sure of the preoperative biochemical diagnosis.

There is good evidence that symptomatic disease will regress after parathyroidectomy whether this is the incidence of renal stones and renal tract infection (McGeown, 1961) or improvement in osteitis fibrosa cystica, resolution of subperiosteal bone resorption and diminution in bone and joint pain (Kaplan et al., 1976). Peptic ulceration may regress (Wilder et al., 1961) and psychological disturbance may resolve (Aurbach et al., 1973). Hypertension will be seen in association with primary hyperparathyroidism in perhaps 40–50% of patients. Its aetiology may be tenuously linked, but there is no evidence that blood pressure will be improved following restoration of normocalcaemia (Salahudeen et al., 1989).

Asymptomatic primary hyperparathyroidism

With the advent of the routine use of biochemical screening, asymptomatic hypercalcaemia has been a frequently detected biochemical abnormality. It is seen in patients who are relatively asymptomatic or truly devoid of symptoms. The distinction between symptoms and normal ageing changes can be very difficult. Most people feel tired if asked! As patients increase in age, then so the number of musculoskeletal symptoms usually increases and these need not be due to primary hyperparathyroidism. Mental changes and depression occur frequently in old age.

The incidence of primary hyperparathyroidism in women over the age of 60 is as high as 200 per 100 000 per year (Heath et al., 1980). Only limited information is available about the natural history of mild hyperparathyroidism. Recent evidence suggests that mild neuromuscular symptoms and mental changes may be ameliorated following parathyroidectomy. In patients under the age of 50 and in whom follow-up is difficult or impractical, surgery may be indicated. It is presumed that early mild disease would eventually progress to the more classic presentation with bones, stones and abdominal groans. Early tissue damage may be seen by examining the eyes and observing metastatic corneal or conjunctival calcification. In truly asymptomatic patients with no evidence of tissue damage and mild hypercalcaemia (less than 3 mmol/litre), then observation and regular review is acceptable.

Secondary hyperparathyroidism

This is seen in patients with chronic renal failure and in those being treated by peritoneal or haemodialysis. This occurs secondarily to the hyperphosphataemia and other metabolic disturbances associated with chronic renal failure. Occasionally it is seen in patients with long-standing, severe intestinal malabsorption. Prolonged hypocalcaemia stimulates the parathyroids with abnormal release of parathyroid hormone. Similar pathological bone changes, as seen in primary hyperparathyroidism, occur with soft-tissue calcification (periarticular and arterial), pruritus and myopathy. When medical therapy (vitamin D analogues) fails, subtotal parathyroidectomy or total parathyroidectomy and autotransplantation may be required.

Tertiary hyperparathyroidism

This is a rare condition which is thought to occur in patients with long-standing secondary hyperparathyroidism. Diffuse parathyroid hyperplasia evolves into nodular hyperplasia and it is thought that one of the nodules within a gland becomes autonomous. In this situation, correction of the underlying primary cause does not allow resolution of the primary hyperparathyroidism. After successful renal transplantation and restoration of normal renal function, for example, if tertiary hyperparathyroidism exists this often becomes more obvious and clinically manifest. Urgent parathyroidectomy may be required in the days or weeks following successful renal transplantation.

Operative procedures

1. Routine approach

The initial approach to the parathyroid glands is identical to that described for the thyroid. Meticulous haemostasis is crucial, especially at the stage of freeing the thyroid from the strap muscles laterally and opening up the space between the gland and the carotid sheath. If blood extravasates, it stains the surrounding connective tissues, including the para-

thyroids, and identification is made more difficult. When present, the middle thyroid vein is divided between silver clips to allow full mobilization of the thyroid lobe medially and forwards. It is preferable to keep the lobe retracted with a gauze swab on the finger rather than using transfixion sutures or grasping forceps, both of which can lead to bleeding. The inferior thyroid artery and recurrent laryngeal nerve are indentified. This is to help prevent nerve damage and to localize the parathyroids which largely derive their blood supply from the inferior thyroid artery. The parathyroids have an intimate anatomical relationship with nerve and artery, but several other factors help the surgeon identify normal and abnormal parathyroid glands:

(a) The gentlest compression or contact of the parathyroid gland will cause a 'blush' or bruise due to the richness of its blood supply. The 'blush' is due to subcapsular haemorrhage.
(b) Compared with lymph nodes, thyroid nodules and fat globules, parathyroids are soft and almost impalpable. They are very mobile within a fatty envelope.
(c) The cut surface of a parathyroid is homogeneous, shiny and vascular and contrasts with the cut surface of a lymph node which has a visible cortex, is duller, relatively avascular and granular in appearance.
(d) The parathyroid gland has a characteristic red/brown or tan colour. Large glands may be cystic.
(e) There is usually a definite sharp edge to the parathyroid adjacent to its vascular pedicle once it has been freed from the surrounding fat.

Nodules of thyroid tissue may be quite separate and distinct and away from the thyroid gland, and may mimic a parathyroid adenoma in appearance. Even frozen section may be incorrectly positive and the situation is complicated by the fact that some parathyroid adenomas sometimes have a follicular appearance on microscopy.

Surgery for hyperparathyroidism is not for the occasional operator. Patients should be referred to surgeons with recognized training and experience in surgery for primary hyperparathyroidism. The incidence of nerve damage is lower and the success of surgical exploration is higher in these circumstances.

2. Surgery for primary hyperparathyroidism

Various operative strategies are described. Some surgeons (a minority) advocate unilateral neck compartment exploration. The side chosen is determined by the use of preoperative localization scans (including thallium subtraction scanning, ultrasonography and/or magnetic resonance imaging). The sensitivity and specificity of the procedure are not sufficiently great to allow this strategy to be uniformly successful. The finding of an adenoma and an accompanying normal gland on one side is also no guarantee that there could not be a second or third adenoma in the unexplored compartment. This might occur in up to 5% or 10% of patients, depending upon the series. If a localization procedure were found to be close to 100% sensitive and specific, then unilateral exploration, perhaps under local anaesthetic, might be advocated.

The more radical approach describes exposure and biopsy of all four glands. This, however, has been shown to be associated with a higher incidence of hypocalcaemia. A 'middle ground' strategy would seem sensible and in most people's hands is associated with high rates of successful exploration. This involves exploration of right and left compartments and the identification of all four (or more) parathyroid glands. The exploration might be scan-directed in that, if positive localization has been obtained preoperatively, then this side of the neck could be explored first and the adenoma and half the normal gland be sent for frozen section biopsy. While awaiting the frozen section results, the opposite compartment could be explored and the hoped-for two normal glands seen but not necessarily biopsied unless one or other appeared macroscopically abnormal. A frozen section return of an adenoma (perhaps with a compressed rim of normal gland and low adipocyte content) along with a fragment of a normal gland (atrophic with high numbers of fat cells) is almost certain to mean that the patient does not have four-gland diffuse hyperplasia. The chance of there being a second or third adenoma is probably of the order of 1% or 2%.

If at exploration four normal appearing glands are found within the neck and there is certainty of the diagnosis, then sliver biopsies of all four glands should be obtained to exclude the possibility of hyperplasia. If the glands are reported as normal, then the patient's disease is almost certainly due to a fifth or sixth ectopic gland.

Sliver biopsies from normal glands are best taken using silver clips. The clip is applied away from the feeding vessels into the parathyroid. The clip marks the site of the normal gland and provides haemostasis. The sliver biopsy is removed with a scalpel blade from the surface of the silver clip.

It is imperative that operative notes include an accurate drawing of the surgical findings, indicating the precise location of the glands removed and of those remaining. An indication should also be made of which glands were biopsied and what the frozen section and definitive histopathology showed.

Difficulties in exploration

When routine exploration of the normal anatomical sites for the parathyroid fails to reveal an adenoma, then a methodological dissection of both sides of the neck must be undertaken.

Abnormal localities for a missing upper parathyroid are examined initially. The upper pole vessels and the area around the upper pole and the tracheal/oesophageal groove from just below the cricoid cartilage to the posterior mediastinum must be examined by careful, bloodless dissection. The recurrent laryngeal nerve must be carefully protected, especially low in the neck as it crosses the thyrothymic ligament. The retro-oesophageal prevertebral space must be examined and lateral exploration must be carried out. Care must be taken to protect the cervical sympathetic chain in this area.

The carotid sheath must be opened throughout its length, since ectopic additional glands can be found in this site.

When the lower parathyroid gland cannot be found or when all four parathyroids have been identified and shown to be normal on frozen section, then it is likely that the missing gland or a fifth gland will lie within the thymus. Two superior extensions are to be found from each thymic lobe. These extend to the lower pole of the thyroid as the thyrothymic ligament. Enlarged parathyroid glands can often be seen as mobile red/brown structures within the capsule of the thymus or the thyrothymic ligament. Even if the adenoma is not visible, the capsule of the thyrothymic ligament and the upper pole of the thymus must be incised to allow careful exploration of these areas. Cervical thymectomy should be carried out when only three or four normal glands have been found in the exploration so far and especially if a lower parathyroid is still not identified.

Intrathyroidal parathyroid adenomas occur in 10–15% of patients. Intraoperative ultrasound may help the identification of such lesions and avoid the need for 'blind' incisions into the thyroid in an attempt to locate an adenoma.

The amount of parathyroid tissue to excise is sometimes not easily determined. Patients come to surgery with earlier disease and the degree of enlargement of a single parathyroid adenoma may not be more than four times the upper limit of normal. The identification of a 150–200 mg adenoma is not easy!

If an adenoma cannot be found, then normal glands should not be removed 'willy-nilly', since this may lead to hypoparathyroidism during this or subsequent explorations.

A marginally enlarged gland, although called normal on frozen section, may prove to be an adenoma on paraffin section histology. Such a gland should be removed. The normal size and weight of a parathyroid gland has been previously defined.

When all four glands are enlarged, then this is almost certainly due to primary hyperplasia and either a three-and-a-half gland resection is performed, leaving no more than 30 mg of one gland, or all four glands are removed and slivers taken from the most normal gland on frozen section can be autotransplanted in a forearm muscle bed (see below). If a fragment of one gland is left *in situ*, then its position should be marked with a silver clip or a non-absorbable suture such as silk so that, should reoperation be required, the site of the recurrent disease should be more readily uncovered.

3. Surgery for primary or secondary parathyroid hyperplasia

In the case of secondary hyperplasia, the diagnosis will usually be obvious from the patient's underlying primary disease (chronic renal failure or malabsorption, for example). Patients with primary hyperplasia usually come from well-identified families in whom the condition is inherited as an autosomal dominant. The condition occurs either as a pure inherited form of primary hyperparathyroidism or as part of the multiple endocrine neoplasia type I syndrome.

In either situation, all four parathyroid glands are usually easily identified since they are uniformly enlarged and hyperplastic. Occasional asymmetrical hyperplasia is seen and mistakenly reported as multiple adenomas. In those patients with chronic renal failure, the tissues are generally more friable and oedematous and bleeding is more likely to be encountered.

A standard approach in patients with hyperplasia is to remove three-and-a-half glands and leave behind half or less of the most macroscopically and microscopically normal gland with an intact blood supply. The remnant is marked with a silver clip and/or a non-absorbable suture. A recording in the operation note is made of the location of the remnant.

Total parathyroidectomy and a lifelong requirement for vitamin D analogues and calcium is inadvisable.

An alternative surgical strategy, popularized by Wells in the USA, is to perform a total parathyroidectomy and autotransplantation of some parathyroid tissue into the flexor muscle mass of the forearm. As in the subtotal parathyroid option, the gland chosen for transplantation must be that which looks macroscopically and microscopically most normal. Tissues which show adenomatous hyperplasia should not be left in the neck and should not be transplanted into the forearm muscle. The forearm muscle is preferred to other intramuscular sites since it is readily accessible should persistent or recurrent disease occur, when futher parathyroid tissue can be removed under local anaesthetic. The additional advantage is that the degree of function can be monitored by measuring parathyroid hormone gradients by drawing blood between the grafted arm and non-grafted arm from similar antecubital veins. The grafted arm levels should be higher than those in the non-grafted arm (positive gradient). Prior to muscle implantation, half of each gland is separately identified and placed within tissue culture medium or saline at 4°C in an ice bath. This allows the parathyroid tissue to become firm. Frozen section confirmation will identify the most normal gland and, from this gland, slivers of parathyroid tissue measuring 1 mm × 1 mm × 3 mm are produced by scalpel cuts. Twelve to 15 such slivers

should produce about 40–50 mg of tissue (equivalent to a normal gland) and these are implanted into separate muscle pockets in the brachioradialis of the non-dominant forearm (Figure 25.2). Fine instruments should be used and haemostasis should be secure. The muscle pockets should be dry so that revascularization of the fragment occurs within 7 days. Each pocket with its enclosed fragment is closed over with a non-absorbable suture to prevent extrusion of the fragment and ready recognition if re-exploration is subsequently required.

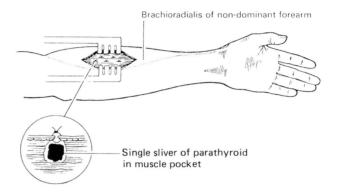

Figure 25.2 Transplantation of the diced parathyroid gland into a forearm muscle

The patient may be protected against early or late graft failure by cryopreservation of some remaining excised parathyroid tissue. Most clinics do not find this is an essential component of patient care since graft failure is exceedingly rare.

Attention must be paid to the site of implantation, taking note of any existing arteriovenous fistulae in those patients on haemodialysis or to place the graft away from arterial or venous sites where fistulae may have to be constructed in the future.

4. Surgery after failed cervical exploration for hyperparathyroidism

The first responsibility to a patient who presents in this way is to make a vigorous appraisal of previous biochemical data, pathology reports and the operative findings of the first exploration. It is essential to ensure that the patient did have primary hyperparathyroidism. If the diagnosis is confirmed, then further steps of localization and re-exploration can be considered.

If there is a history of several members within the family with unsuccessful neck explorations, then the possibility of familial hypocalciuric hypercalcaemia needs to be considered.

If there is a family history of previous failed neck exploration and the diagnosis seems certain, then the possibility of primary hyperplasia needs to be considered and that inadequate amounts of tissue were excised in the first exploration.

When the general health of the patient, balanced against the severity of the disease, calls for re-operation, then appropriate localization studies are essential, especially if the first exploration was performed by a surgeon of experience. Current localization procedures with sufficient accuracy, sensitivity and specificity include thallium/technetium subtraction scanning (Figure 25.3), CT scanning and magnetic resonance imaging. Ultrasonography may not be easy because of the previous exploration and obliteration of tissue planes.

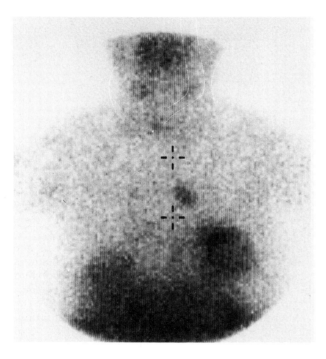

Figure 25.3 Thallium/technetium subtraction scan showing a mediastinal parathyroid tumour. The patient's body outline can be seen with the head superiorly and the tumour located between the crosses above the heart shadow

Selective venous sampling with parathyroid hormone estimations may have to be carried out if the less invasive localization techniques do not show evidence of a missed adenoma. Arteriography may complement selective venous sampling and it may be of therapeutic use, especially if a missed parathyroid adenoma is found within the mediastinum. Anterior mediastinal parathyroid adenomas are frequently fed by end arteries as branches of the internal mammary artery. Selective cannulation of the feeding vessel may then allow injection of autologous clot or gel foam which would cause infarction of the adenoma and non-surgical cure of the persistent hyperparathyroidism.

Before exploration, it is usual to have concordant localization data from at least two investigations. The re-exploration then is carried out as above, checking methodically all possible sites. The adenoma should be uncovered by following the guidance of the positive localization procedures.

Mediastinal adenomas should be removed by splitting the sternum. The sternotomy need not be full length, especially if the adenoma is found within the thymus.

5. Surgery for parathyroid carcinoma

This accounts for about 1% of all patients with hyperparathyroidism. Suspicion of the existence of this condition should occur if there is gross biochemical disturbance, for example serum calcium greater than 3.5 mmol/litre. Parathyroid carcinomas can often be felt as a mass in the anterior triangle of the neck. Operatively the situation is different in that the gland is usually firmer, grey or white in colour and adherent to surrounding structures which frequently include the recurrent nerve. If the diagnosis is suspected operatively and confirmed on frozen section, then the best treatment is block dissection of the tumour and all involved soft tissues surrounding. If there is thyroid invasion, then total thyroid lobectomy is frequently required. Care must be taken not to rupture the tumour and spill cells, as this leads to local recurrence which is almost impossible to eradicate. Lymph nodes should be excised *en bloc*.

A situation may be encountered which mimics parathyroid carcinoma. If during a previous exploration for primary disease a parathyroid cyst or tumour is ruptured, then cells may 'seed' into surrounding muscles and structures. The cells become functional and recurrent hyperparathyroidism occurs. This condition is sometimes called parathyromatosis. It is equally difficult to treat and the only hope of reducing the serum calcium to normal is by removing infiltrated, seeded muscle and structures where possible.

Wound closure and postoperative care

After completing the cervical operation, the neck wound is irrigated with warm saline. This aids identification of small bleeding points which can be diathermied before neck closure. Small clots are removed.

The neck wound can then be closed, reapproximating the strap muscles and platysma with interrupted absorbable sutures. The skin should be closed with interrupted clips which can be removed on the second day.

There is no need to leave drains within the neck. With meticulous haemostasis and despite the fact that no drains are left, bleeding should not be a problem in current surgical practice.

Cord movement can be checked by the anaesthetist on extubation, but this gives no guarantee that continued normal recurrent nerve function will be maintained. Intraneural haematoma formation or bruising may subsequently lead to neuropraxia. The nerve should have been seen and protected throughout the exploration and therefore non-continuity of the nerve should not be an option unless it had to be divided because of involvement by the tumour – sometimes seen with inflammatory benign adenomas where the nerve is intimately bound to the capsule of the adenoma. Adequate preoperative counselling and warning should be given to all patients.

Postoperative complications

Secondary haemorrhage should not occur!

Small seromas may occur within the wound and are easily dealt with by needle aspiration. Wound infections are exceedingly rare.

Persistent hypercalcaemia in the immediate postoperative period must challenge the original diagnosis and/or the accuracy of intraoperative surgical findings and frozen section reports. The possibility of a fifth or sixth abnormal ectopic gland must be entertained.

Recurrent hypercalcaemia occurring after 6 months or more is almost certainly due to inadequate excision of four-gland hyperplastic disease.

Hypocalcaemia is seen infrequently in current practice, but the serum calcium must be checked in the postoperative period. Relative hypocalcaemia (even within the normal range) may produce symptoms in a patient who has been 'used to' a higher circulating serum calcium level.

Continued hypocalcaemia which produces symptoms is likely due to suppression of residual normal parathyroid glands, associated with too vigorous a biopsy policy or due to a calcium deficit in bones which have to heal as a result of long-standing osteitis. In patients who have had removal of a large adenoma (several grams), bone disease and normal gland suppression are usually of sufficient magnitude that the patient will require intravenous calcium supplements in the first day or two after surgery and thereafter require oral calcium and vitamin D analogue supplements. The calcium should be given in a dilute infusion into a central vein to avoid peripheral thrombophlebitis.

Oral effervescent calcium tablets and 1-alpha-hydroxycholecalciferol can then be given and the patient allowed home, to return for fairly frequent serum calcium checks until the bone disease is healed and/or the atrophic parathyroid glands have recovered.

References

Åckerström, G., Malmeus, J. and Bergstrom, R. (1984) Surgical anatomy of the human parathyroid glands. *Surgery*, **95**, 14–18

Aurbach, G. D., Mallette, L. E., Patten, B. M. *et al.* (1973) Hyperparathyroidism: recent studies. *Ann. Intern. Med.*, **79**, 566–581

Gilmour, J. R. (1938) The gross anatomy of the parathyroid glands. *J. Pathol Bacteriol.*, **46**, 133–149

Heath, H., III, Hodgson, S. F. and Kennedy, M. A. (1980) Primary hyperparathyroidism incidence, morbidity and potential impact in a community. *N. Engl. J. Med.*, **302**, 189–193

Kaplan, R. A., Snyder, W. M., Stewart, A. *et al.* (1976) Metabolic effects of parathyroidectomy in asymptomatic primary hyperparathyroidism. *J. Clin. Endocrin. Metab.*, **42**, 415–426

McGeown, M. G. (1961) Effect of parathyroidectomy on the incidence of renal calculi. *Lancet*, **i**, 586–587

Proye, C. (1978) Exploration parathyroididienne pour hyperparathyroidie. *J. Chir.* (Paris), **115**, 101

Salahudeen, A. K., Thomas, T. H., Sellars, L. *et al.* (1989) Hypertension and renal dysfunction in primary hyperparathyroidism: effect of parathyroidectomy. *Clin. Sci.*, **76**, 289–296

Wilder, W. T., Frame, B. and Haubrich, W. S. (1961) Peptic ulcer in primary hyperparathyroidism: an analysis of 52 cases. *Ann. Intern. Med.*, **55**, 885–893

Further reading

Åckerström, G., Rudberg, C., Grimelius, L. *et al.* (1992) Causes of failed primary exploration and technical aspects of reoperation in primary hyperparathyroidism. *Wld J. Surg.*, **16**, 562–569

Brennan, M. F., Doppman, J. L., Krudy, A. G. *et al.* (1982) Assessment of techniques for parathyroid gland localization in patients undergoing re-operation for hyperparathyroidism. *Surgery*, **91**, 6

Carmalt, H. L., Gillet, D. J., Chu, J. *et al.* (1988) Prospective comparison of radionuclide, ultrasound, and computed tomography in the preoperative localisation of parathyroid glands. *Wld J. Surg.*, **12**, 830–834

Dunlop, D. A. B., Papapoulos, S. E., Lodge, R. W. *et al.* (1980) Parathyroid venous sampling: anatomic considerations and results in 95 patients with primary hyperparathyroidism. *Br. J. Radiol.*, **53**, 183

Hollingshead, W. H. (1952) Anatomy of the endocrine glands. *Surg. Clin. North. Am.*, **32**, 1115–1140

Marx, S. J., Stock, J. L., Attie, M. F. *et al.* (1980) Familial hypocalciuric hypercalcaemia: recognition among patients referred after unsuccessful parathyroid exploration. *Ann. Intern. Med.*, **92**, 951

Neil, H. B., III, Townsend, G. L. and Devine, K. D. (1972) Bilateral vocal cord paralysis of undetermined aetiology: clinical course and outcome. *Ann. Otol. Rhinol. Laryngol.*, **81**, 514–519

Nichols, P., Owen, J. P., Ellis, H. A. *et al.* (1990) Parathyroidectomy in chronic renal failure: a nine year follow-up study. *Q. J. Med.*, **283**, 1175–1193

Purnell, D. C., Scholtz, D. A., Smith, L. H. *et al.* (1974) Treatment of primary hyperparathyroidism. *Am. J. Med.*, **56**, 800–809

Sandelin, K., Auer, G., Bondeson, L. *et al.* (1992) Prognostic factors in parathyroid cancer: a review of 95 cases. *Wld J. Surg.*, **16**, 724–731

Shantz, A. and Castleman, B. (1973) Parathyroid carcinoma. A study of 70 cases. *Cancer*, **31**, 600–605

Smith, I. and Murley, R. S. (1965) Damage to the cervical sympathetic system during the operation on the thyroid gland. *Br. J. Surg.*, **52**, 673

Tibblin, S., Bondeson, A. G. and Ljungberg, O. (1982) Unilateral parathyroidectomy due to a single adenoma. *Ann. Surg.*, **195**, 245–252

Wells, S. A., Gunnells, J. C., Gutman, R. A. *et al.* (1975) Transplantation of the parathyroid glands in man. Clinical indication and results. *Surgery*, **78**, 34–44

Wells, S. A., Gunnells, J. C., Gutman, R. A. *et al.* (1977) The successful transplantation of frozen parathyroid tissue in man. *Surgery*, **81**, 86

Young, A. E., Grant, J. I. Croft, D. N. *et al.* (1983) Location of parathyroid adenomas by thallium-201 and technetium-99^m subtraction scanning. *Br. Med. J.*, **286**, 1384

26

The salivary glands

R. W. Hiles

The parotid gland

Surgical anatomy (Figures 26.1–26.3)

The surface markings of the boundaries of the parotid gland are the zygomatic arch *above*, the anterior margin of the auricle together with the mastoid process *behind*, and a line drawn from the tip of the mastoid process to the angle of the jaw *below*. *In front*, the gland may extend as far as the anterior border of the masseter muscle, which is readily felt when the teeth are clenched. The line of the parotid duct can be drawn from the lower border of the tragus of the ear towards a point midway between the base of the ala of the nose and the upper limit of the upper lip vermilion. It occupies the middle third of this line and opens on the buccal mucous membrane opposite the second maxillary molar tooth.

The gland is wedged deeply between the mastoid process and the external auditory meatus behind and the posterior border of the mandible in front. The base of this wedge lies outwards and extends forwards over the masseter muscle and constitutes the superficial lobe. The thin edge of the wedge is usually called the deep lobe and extends upwards to reach the glenoid fossa behind the temporomandibular joint.

Behind the gland, the mastoid process is sandwiched between the sternomastoid and the deeper digastric muscle. In front, the mandible is sandwiched between the masseter outside and the medial pterygoid muscle inside. The accessory portion of the gland lies on the masseter muscle, between the parotid duct and the bone of the zygomatic arch.

The gland is enclosed within a sheath of fascia so that tension and pain are produced when the gland swells. On the surface of the parotid beneath this fascia lymph nodes lie on and in the superficial substance of the gland. Three other structures pass through the gland; the most superficial is the facial nerve with its several divisions and terminal branches. More deeply lies the posterior facial vein and deeper still the external carotid artery. The deepest narrowed edge of the wedge-shaped gland lies against the internal jugular vein. The upper part of this deep portion of the gland is also in contact with the auriculotemporal nerve which gives the gland its secretomotor branch from the otic ganglion.

Blood is supplied to the gland by branches from the external carotid artery and returns via the posterior facial vein. Lymphatic drainage is first to the glands within the parotid and then on to the anterosuperior group of the deep cervical lymph glands.

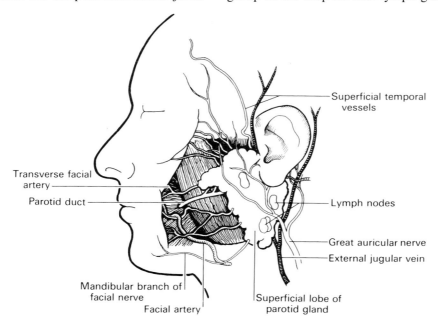

Figure 26.1 The superficial lobe of the parotid gland and its relations

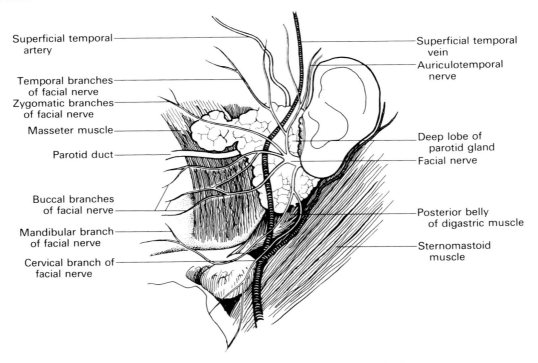

Superficial temporal
artery

Temporal branches
of facial nerve
Zygomatic branches
of facial nerve

Masseter muscle

Parotid duct

Buccal branches
of facial nerve

Mandibular branch
of facial nerve

Cervical branch of
facial nerve

Superficial temporal
vein
Auriculotemporal
nerve

Deep lobe of
parotid gland
Facial nerve

Posterior belly
of digastric muscle

Sternomastoid
muscle

Figure 26.2   The facial nerve in the parotid gland

When the gland has been removed, its bed is seen to be made up posteriorly of the posterior belly of the digastric, the styloid process of the temporal bone and the stylohyoid muscle arising from it. Deep to these is the internal jugular vein passing downwards over the lateral mass of the atlas and being crossed by the accessory nerve. Anteriorly, not quite in touch with the gland, is the internal carotid artery crossed by the tip of the styloid process above and the glossopharyngeal nerve lying on the stylopharyngeus muscle below.

The most important structure in surgery of the parotid gland is the facial nerve. It emerges from the stylomastoid foramen with the digastric muscle origin below and lateral and the root of the styloid process and the tympanomastoid sulcus above and deep. The main trunk of the nerve commonly divides, after a variable distance, into two main divisions and subsequently into branches going to five main areas: temporal, zygomatic, buccal, mandibular and cervical. The mandibular branch is notable in that it emerges from the lower border of the parotid gland passing below the angle of the mandible into the neck. Later it crosses the inferior border of the mandible lying on the facial artery, running upwards into the face again to supply the depressor muscles at the angle of the mouth. There are considerable variations in the pattern of divisions and branches of the nerve, with numerous cross-connections between them. It is best never to take the anatomy of the nerve divisions for granted and to dissect each nerve as if it was the first ever to have been followed.

Special investigations

Simple radiographs of the parotid area will often reveal calculi, but those in the deep lobe are sometimes obscured by the irregular opacities of the skeletal outlines.

Recent developments in imaging have transformed the quality of visualization of the parotid, and any pathology that might arise in it, that can be achieved.

Ultrasound is rapidly becoming the first choice of imaging technique to determine the extent and possible nature of a lesion in the parotid region.

Magnetic resonance imaging offers a high degree of differentiation and discrimination in the nature of soft-tissue tumours.

Computed tomography is of greatest assistance in determining whether or not there is any bony involvement from a tumour in the parotid and the extent of that involvement.

Sialography is particularly relevant to the diagnosis of chronic parotitis and duct stenosis, when sialectasis may be evident. It is of little practical value in the differential diagnosis of masses in the parotid area as these almost invariably warrant exploration and resection.

More sophisticated *tests of salivary function* involving the collection, measurement and analysis of salivary fluid from the duct are rarely used in busy surgical practice, although specific findings are documented.

Needle aspiration biopsy can be useful for diagnosis but can give false negatives if not directed at the exact site of suspected pathology within the gland. Ultra-

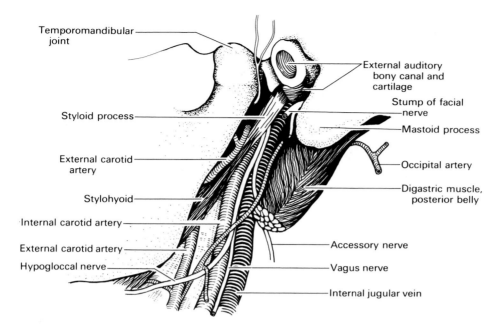

Temporomandibular joint

External auditory bony canal and cartilage

Stump of facial nerve

Styloid process

Mastoid process

External carotid artery

Occipital artery

Stylohyoid

Digastric muscle, posterior belly

Internal carotid artery

External carotid artery

Accessory nerve

Hypogloccal nerve

Vagus nerve

Internal jugular vein

Figure 26.3 The deep bed of the parotid gland

sound scanning can be used to direct the needle more accurately in order to achieve a representative biopsy. Some consider that, since the commonest parotid tumour, pleomorphic adenoma, is so prone to local recurrence, there is a risk of seeding along the needle track once this tumour's integrity is breached during such a preoperative biopsy.

Operations

Before any operation on the parotid gland the patient should be warned that the facial nerve is at risk. Also he or she should be warned that, if adequate tumour treatment demands it, all or part of the nerve may have to be sacrified.

Warning of the occasional postoperative complication of gustatory sweating in the skin normally overlying the parotid should be given.

Incision of abscess

Acute suppurative parotitis is now quite rare except when patients suffering from other conditions, such as intestinal obstruction or typhoid fever, are allowed to become dehydrated. Prevention is better than cure.

Early infection can be successfully treated with systemic antibiotics, but once suppuration is established surgical drainage becomes necessary. If the abscess is already pointing, incision is best made directly through the skin at the site of pointing. Once through the skin and the abscess entered and drained, the incision should only be enlarged in a transverse direction so as to minimize the risk of damage to the

facial nerve. If no pus is pointing but the gland remains swollen and tender, the parotid is explored through a skin incision as for superficial parotidectomy, the parotid fascia is incised transversely and the gland probed with blunt instruments to release any loculi of pus. The wound is closed loosely with drainage.

Removal of calculi

Parotid stones are not common and are usually situated deep within the gland. If in the main duct and palpable from the mouth, they can be removed by an approach from the mucosal aspect, slitting open the duct longitudinally. Calculi within the gland are often multiple and if producing symptoms will require parotidectomy. They may occur in association with chronic parotitis.

Exploration of the gland

Any firm painless mass in the parotid gland is an indication for exploration in the absence of any evidence of systemic disease. Haemangioma, cyst and lipoma all occur occasionally and can usually be diagnosed clinically by compressibility, fluctuance and non-fluctuant softness respectively. Occasionally malignant tumours are found within, or in association with, cysts having a short history. If large and troublesome any of these benign tumours may require formal excision. This can be done using an incision as for superficial parotidectomy and then dissecting out the tumour with due regard to preservation of the integrity of the facial nerve.

Enucleation of mixed salivary tumours

This is mentioned only to be dismissed, as it carries with it a high risk of 'seeding' the operative wound with tumour cells, which may subsequently produce multiple recurrences which are difficult to resect.

Superficial parotidectomy

This operation is carried out for any firm tumour involving the superficial portion of the gland in the absence of preoperative facial paralysis. Such a tumour usually proves to be pleomorphic adenoma, but less commonly adenolymphoma or early carcinoma is encountered. Rarely, in the course of developing the dissection for superficial parotidectomy, it is discovered that the tumour is a neurilemmoma affecting the facial nerve. Such a tumour is best dissected meticulously from the nerve, if necessary using microsurgical techniques, so as to preserve as much nerve function as possible consistent with total removal of the neurilemmoma. Occasionally pleomorphic adenoma is small, only occupying a small portion of the superficial parotid. In these cases localized resection of the parotid can be performed provided that great care is taken not to breach the integrity of the capsule of the tumour, which would invite recurrence. If in doubt, a formal superficial parotidectomy should be carried out.

Surgical procedure

Anaesthesia

Parotid surgery should always be performed under general anaesthesia because it is imperative that the patient should be absolutely still and the procedure can sometimes be lengthy.

The anaesthetist is asked not to use any long-acting muscle relaxant which would make it impossible to check on facial nerve function with a nerve stimulator during operation.

It is a great advantage to have a relatively bloodless field which can add to the safety and speed with which the facial nerve can be dissected. This can be achieved with the technique of hypotensive anaesthesia which is safely induced by experienced anaesthetists. Similar operative conditions can be achieved by the infiltration of a solution of adrenaline (1 in 250 000) into the operative area. This should be done by the surgeon at least 5 minutes before beginning the dissection. However, it should not be forgotten that local anaesthetic agents can prevent nerve conduction and invalidate the use of a nerve stimulator to aid in the identification of the main trunk and branches of the facial nerve.

Position

The patient is placed supine on the operating table with the head supported by a rubber ring and turned to the contralateral side. Slight head-up tilt of the whole body prevents venous congestion in the operative field. The head is towelled with the whole face exposed so that muscle activity can be observed when the facial nerve is stimulated.

Exposure

The main limb of the incision runs in the pre-auricular skin crease and is extended upwards above the ear running slightly anteriorly within the temporal scalp. Downwards, the incision is carried around the lobe of the ear to run posteriorly in the post-auricular groove for 2–3 cm. The incision is then angled acutely downwards and forwards to form a flap of skin over the mastoid process and then runs approximately two finger-breadths below the angle of the mandible, preferably in a convenient skin crease. Incision should extend at least as far as the anterior border of the sternomastoid (Figure 26.4).

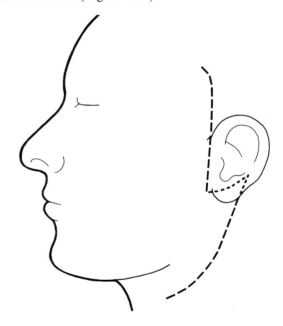

Figure 26.4 Skin incision to approach the parotid gland

The skin anterior to this irregularly curved incision is then raised at a level deep to the subcutaneous fat. With care the parotid fascia can be identified and raised and preserved with the skin and subcutaneous fat flap. This fascia forms an effective barrier to postoperative auriculotemporal innervation of cutaneous sweat glands and thus greatly reduces the incidence of Frey's syndrome. Alternatively, the parotid fascia can be raised as a separate flap once the skin has been raised at the conventional level, which is the deep extent of the subcutaneous fat, which is a slightly easier and less hazardous plane of dissection bearing in mind the proximity of the branches of the facial nerve, particularly in the anterior parts of the superficial parotid gland. The skin and parotid fascia flaps can be held at the edge by fine skin hooks and the correct level for developing dissection of these flaps can often be seen best by tenting the skin towards the operator. A thin whitish fornix of air-filled fascia will develop to guide the dissection in the appropriate plane.

Meticulous haemostasis is carried out with the tips of the diathermy forceps so as to keep the operative field unstained with blood. It is preferable to use bipolar diathermy in the interests of reducing the risk of damage to adjacent facial nerve branches. The skin is dissected as far anteriorly as just beyond the anterior border of the masseter, superiorly to just above the zygomatic arch and inferiorly to expose the upper part of the anterior triangle of the neck (Figure 26.5).

served intact with care. The deeper plane of dissection can be developed with relative safety above and below the mastoid and is then developed with caution in the angle between the cartilage of the external auditory meatus and the anterosuperior aspect of the mastoid process. The small posterior auricular artery is almost invariably encountered, divided and ligated before reaching the vicinity of the main trunk of the facial nerve as it emerges from the stylomastoid foramen (Figure 26.7). Retraction of the parotid gland should be done with great gentleness, otherwise traction forces may be transmitted to the facial nerve and can cause axonal damage.

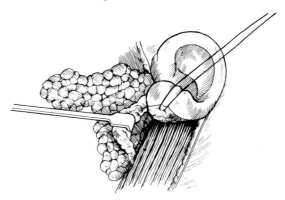

Figure 26.6 Elevation of the parotid 'corner'

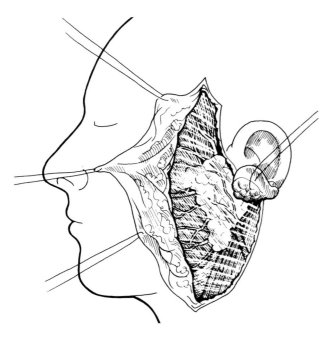

Figure 26.5 Dissection of the anterior skin flap to reveal the parotid gland

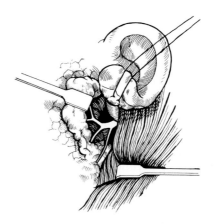

Figure 26.7 Exposure of the facial nerve

Dissection

A deeply penetrating natural fascial plane is then opened up running medially between the anterior cartilage of the external auditory meatus and the parotid, in the pre-auricular groove. This plane will readily open up with blunt dissection. Sharp dissection is then used to extend this plane deep to the ear lobe, inferior to the external auditory meatus and on to the base of the mastoid process. Thence, the deep dissection proceeds downwards along the antero-superior border of the sternomastoid, thus raising the extreme posterolateral, 'corner' of the parotid gland (Figure 26.6). It may be necessary to divide the great auricular sensory nerve but it can usually be pre-

The nerve is usually covered with a thin fascial sheath which has to be entered before the nerve can be seen clearly. When in the vicinity of where the nerve should be, it often helps to use a nerve stimulator which can detect its position accurately, even before it can be seen. It is necessary to be able to recognize in detail the several distinctive anatomical landmarks in the region of the stylomastoid foramen in order to approach the nerve with careful confidence and not too much anxiety. If the anteroinferior extremity of the conchal cartilage is sought, as it

forms the support of the inferior wall of the membranous part of the external auditory canal, it will be seen to form the shape of an arrowhead which points to the nerve. Deep to the tip of this cartilage is the rim of the bony external auditory canal. This rim sits alongside the base of the mastoid process forming a groove between the two which leads downwards in a very short distance to the stylomastoid foramen and the main trunk of the facial nerve emerging from it. If the styloid process can be identified just superior and deep, even merely by touch, this will add confirmation to the supposition that the surgeon is in the right place and looking at the right nerve. The posterior facial vein will be lying deep to the main trunk.

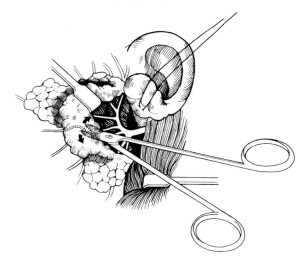

Figure 26.8 Dissection of the superficial parotid gland from the facial nerve branches without traction

Once the main trunk of the facial nerve has been identified and confirmed by stimulation, the superficial parotid can then be methodically removed as the trunk is traced forwards to its division and branches. Separation of the parotid gland from the nerve can only be achieved with safety by gentle and meticulously accurate dissection. The nerve must not be traumatized by traction or crushing, nor by disturbance of its delicate blood supply which can often be seen running along the epineurium. Small, fine, blunt, curved scissors are used superficial to the nerve by introducing them closed, pushing them gently between the nerve and the superficial parotid in an anterior direction and then gently opening the blades (Figure 26.8). With patience the whole of the nerve can be displayed in this way. Occasionally, fine filaments of nerve, usually cross-connections between the divisions or branches, will be so closely adherent to tumour that it is wiser to sacrifice them, provided they are small. The functional deficit will be barely detectable paresis, postoperatively. As the dissection proceeds anteriorly, the nerve branches become more and more superficial and they often appear to take

an abrupt turn laterally as they reach and cross the masseter. It is at this point that they are often most vulnerable to surgical injury, when confidence is running high. Once the anterior border of the masseter has been reached, the plane of the deep dissection can be cautiously joined to that of the subcutaneous dissection. The superficial parotid and its contained, intact tumour will then have been resected (Figures 26.9 and 26.10).

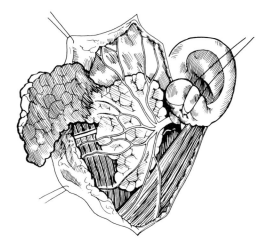

Figure 26.9 Superficial parotid gland almost resected

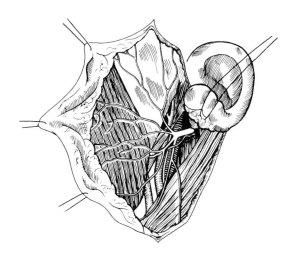

Figure 26.10 The surgical field after total parotidectomy with preservation of the facial nerve

With large tumours which become wedged between the mandible and mastoid process it is sometimes impossible to approach the main facial nerve trunk as a prelude to the safe dissection of its nerve branches from proximal to distal. In such circumstances, in experienced hands, it is best to initiate the nerve dissection first by careful identification of the mandibular branch of the nerve within the lower parotid and then to follow this branch proximally until it leads to the main trunk of the nerve. In this way the tumour and the parotid tissue surrounding it can be lifted laterally and upwards from its wedged position as the full extent of the pes anserinum of the facial nerve is revealed by careful dissection. It should not be forgotten that a tumour within the parotid can lie either superficial or deep and sometimes both and can thus distort the normal route of the nerve.

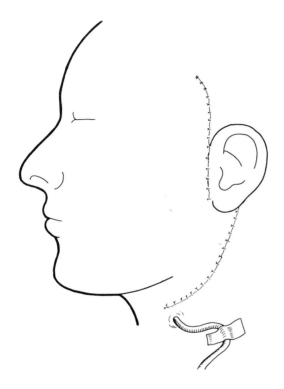

Figure 26.11 Skin closure with suction drainage of the parotid bed

Meticulous haemostasis is then secured, taking care not to include finer branches of the facial nerve in ligatures or diathermy points. The wound is drained by a fine perforated plastic tube to a closed suction drainage bottle (Figure 26.11). Skin closure is effected with interrupted 6/0 absorbable sutures. If fine, sub-cutaneous, absorbable sutures are also used, skin sutures can be removed early (after 3 or 4 days) and suture cross-hatch scars of the skin avoided. Suction is maintained until the aspirate is minimal, usually for 2–4 days. The drain is then withdrawn.

Postoperative complications

1. Facial nerve injury

2. Fistulas

Occasionally salivary fistulas will occur through the scar of the incision but the majority of these close spontaneously. A short course of Pro-Banthine (pro-pantheline) will reduce salivary flow and aid spontaneous closure if used at the first sign of trouble. It is rare for fistulas to persist, but if this happens either the residual parotid is resected or the fistula is dissected out and drained into the mouth.

3. Auriculotemporal (or gustatory sweating) syndrome (Frey's syndrome)

This is not uncommon several months after parotid-ectomy. The patient experiences sweating of the skin over the site of the parotidectomy while eating. It is generally considered to be due to inappropriate inner-vation of the cutaneous sweat glands by the secreto-motor fibres which have regenerated from the divided ends of the auriculotemporal nerve and which pre-viously supplied the resected parotid. Once the syn-drome is explained, most patients are able to tolerate it and fortunately the severity of the symptoms tends to diminish over a number of years. Surgical treat-ment aimed at more central disconnection of the secretomotor fibres is usually reserved for extremely severe cases and is not always of lasting benefit.

Topical sweating inhibitors, such as aluminium chloride hexahydrate 20% (Anhydrol forte solution) normally used for axillary hyperhidrosis, can be use-ful in suppressing troublesome sweating of the cheek skin, but must be applied with extreme caution to avoid contact with the eye. It is probably best pre-scribed under the supervision of a dermatologist.

Total parotidectomy with preservation of the facial nerve

Indications

Neoplastic indications for this operation are multiple benign tumours, large benign tumours in the deep portion of the gland and early and low-grade malig-nant tumours with no or very limited involvement of the facial nerve branches. In the latter case the preser-vation of the facial nerve is incomplete.

Perhaps the most difficult and hazardous parotid-ectomy is that required to treat chronic parotitis where the nerve is engulfed in scarred parenchyma.

Surgical technique

The skin flap is raised as for superficial parotidectomy and the main trunk of the facial nerve identified. If the tumour is large and deep, direct access to the main trunk of the facial nerve may be difficult and it can be easier to find the mandibular branch in the lower part of the operative field in the neck. (This can prove difficult and hazardous for the inexperienced oper-ator.) Once this branch is found it can be traced posteriorly, which will lead to the main inferior div-ision and eventually the main trunk. It is imperative that the nerve be handled extremely gently. Its trunk, divisions and branches all need to be separated from the parotid tissue deep as well as superficial to it and have to be gently retracted from side to side in order to deliver the deep portion of the gland. If there is any danger of reducing the adequate and clean clearance of a malignant tumour by striving to preserve the nerve intact, the nerve or offending part of it is best sacrificed. In order to resect the deep portion of the gland, the posterior facial vein and the external carotid artery have to be ligated at the points at which they leave and enter the gland. Before the gland can be separated anteriorly, the parotid duct is ligated and then divided as it dips behind the buccinator muscle.

Total parotidectomy with sacrifice of the facial nerve

Indications

Total clearance of the gland together with all its contained and some of its neighbouring structures is indicated when it holds a malignant tumour which is already involving the facial nerve and/or the structures bordering on the gland. Such a malignancy may have arisen in a pre-existing pleomorphic tumour and can be either squamous or adenocarcinoma. Another particularly aggressive tumour is the cylindroma (adenoid cystic carcinoma). More uncommonly an acinic carcinoma is encountered.

Surgical technique

The positioning, approach and initial dissection are as for superficial parotidectomy. The external carotid artery is divided and ligated above the hypoglossal nerve and digastric muscle as it enters the parotid region. The approach may be complicated by involvement of other structures by the tumour, for instance skin or mandible, which must be removed.

Involved skin must be resected but there may be sufficient skin remaining to allow direct closure. Otherwise a skin flap will be necessary, such as a transposition flap from the neck or, in the male, a scalp flap. Alternatively, pedicled axial flaps from the neck or chest can be used or a free flap, such as the latissimus dorsi flap, requiring microvascular anastomosis.

If the mandible is involved, resection of the ascending ramus and angle, together with the attached muscles, may be required. It is sometimes possible to leave the anterior part of the ascending ramus and thus preserve the inferior dental nerves intact. The Gigli saw is passed from the angle of the mandible upwards along the medial aspect of the bone and posterolateral to the inferior dental nerve to reach the sigmoid notch. After section of the bone, the maxillary artery is divided and the condyle of the mandible detached from the glenoid fossa. The mandible or sections of it can be reconstructed using bone grafts. These can be either free, non-vascularized grafts or free bone flaps requiring microvascular anastomosis.

If bone and skin has to be resected the defect can be repaired, after appropriate careful planning, with composite free flaps of skin and bone, sometimes containing muscle taken to preserve the integrity of the vascular network within the free flap which can also contribute useful bulk to the repair.

If a 5 mm length or more of the proximal stump of the main trunk of the facial nerve can be preserved, immediate nerve reconstruction can be carried out using sensory nerve, such as the great auricular, as a bridge graft. Because of the proximity of the tumour it may not be wise to take the nerve graft from the same side but one can readily be taken from the opposite neck. The graft is taken with an appropriate number of branches from any of the sensory cervical outflow nerve systems (C2 and C3). Nerve suture is carried out with 8/0 or 10/0 nylon, if necessary with the aid of an operating microscope. It is not yet established which technique of nerve suture gives the best regeneration, but it has been known for many years that a simple cuff of interrupted fine epineural sutures can give gratifying results. The principle is to effect the most accurate apposition of the nerve ends that is possible while doing the minimum amount of damage to the axons, neurilemmal sheaths and their blood supply.

If cervical lymph node involvement is present or suspected, then total parotidectomy will be performed in continuity with a radical *en bloc* dissection of the cervical lymph nodes (see Chapter 27). In this case the internal jugular vein will be resected from the deep aspect of the bed of the parotid.

Submandibular gland

Surgical anatomy

As its name suggests, this gland lies under the cover of the body of the mandible. It is cradled by the anterior belly of the digastric muscle in front, the insertion of the stylohyoid below and the stylomandibular ligament behind. Enclosed by deep fascia, it is covered by the skin and platysma and crossed superficially by the anterior facial vein and the mandibular branch of the facial nerve. Similar to the parotid, lymph nodes are found in association with it and a few embedded in it. The facial artery making its way to the face is embedded in a groove, at first in the deep and then in the lateral surface of the gland (Figure 26.12).

The superficial part of the gland lies against the mylohyoid muscle and the nerve and vessels supplying this muscle. The gland is then hooked around the posterior margin of the muscle so that its deep part rests between the medial aspect of this muscle laterally and the hypoglossus medially. On the hypoglossus its deep relations, in succession from above downwards, are the styloglossus, lingual nerve, submandibular ganglion, the hypoglossal nerve and the deep lingual vein (Figure 26.13).

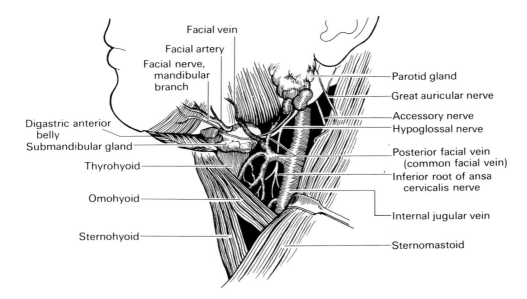

Figure 26.12 Superficial relationships of the submandibular gland

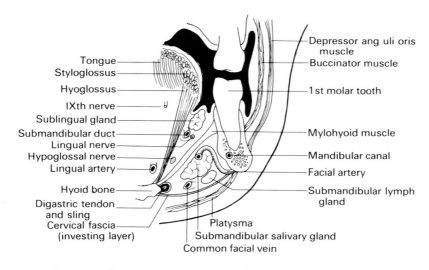

Figure 26.13 Comprehensive view of the main relationships of the submandibular gland

A 5 cm long duct, which emerges from the hilum gland at the posterior border of the mylohyoid, runs forwards in the floor of the mouth and passes to the opening on the summit of the sublingual papilla at the side of the base of the frenulum of the tongue. Posteriorly, the lingual nerve is above the duct but crosses it laterally at the anterior border of the hypoglossus to pass beneath the duct before turning forwards medially and upwards again into the tongue. The hypoglossal nerve is below the duct. Occasionally, a few small ducts from the sublingual gland, which lies alongside the anterior portion of the duct, open into it. The submandibular ganglion, from which the gland receives its secretomotor fibres, is found attached to the lingual nerve as it approaches the gland and its duct from above (Figure 26.14).

Special investigations

Simple radiography is the most useful investigation in the case of recurrent submandibular gland enlargement related to meals and will help locate any calculi that may be present. Stones in the duct can often be palpated in the floor of the mouth. Calculi within the glands sometimes have a low mineral content and they are not noticeably radio-opaque.

Sialography is of little value in submandibular disease.

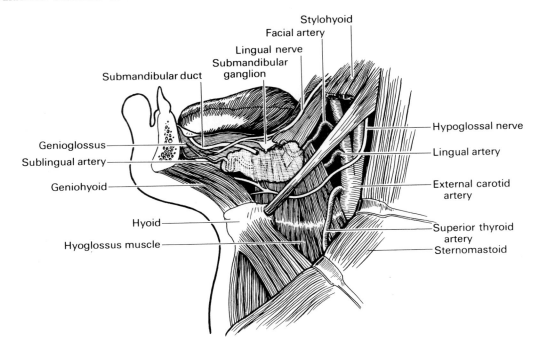

Figure 26.14 A ghost of the resected submandibular gland showing its deep bed

As in the case of the parotid gland, the newer imaging techniques of ultrasound scanning, magnetic resonance imaging and computed tomography can be extremely useful in providing a much more detailed and accurate visualization of the gland and the nature and extent of any associated pathology than was previously possible. Needle aspiration biopsy can also be useful.

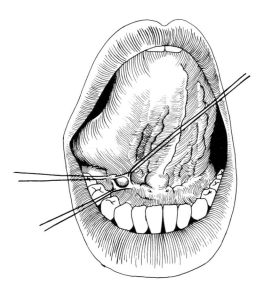

Figure 26.15 Securing the release of a submandibular duct calculus

Operations

Removal of stone from the duct (Figure 26.15)

Operative removal of a stone can be carried out under local analgesia or with general anaesthesia. A retraction suture passed below the duct behind and in front of the stone traps it and facilitates longitudinal incision of the duct over it. The stone can then be readily delivered from the floor of the mouth and the open duct is left unsutured.

Removal of calculus in the hilum of the gland

The whole gland and its duct should be resected in these cases.

Resection of submandibular salivary gland

General anaesthesia is usually employed and the patient is positioned as for parotidectomy. An incision is made almost the whole length of the body of the mandible but some two finger-breadths below it. A convenient skin crease is used for preference (Figure 26.16). Platysma is divided at a low level within the skin wound and elevated with care so as to avoid damaging the mandibular branch of the facial nerve which runs deep to the platysma in the upper part of the operative field. The facial artery and vein are divided and ligated as they reach the lower border of the mandible (at this point the mandibular branch of the facial nerve is particularly vulnerable but

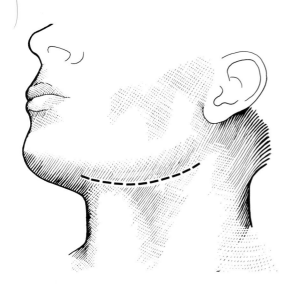

Figure 26.16 Skin incision for submandibular gland resection

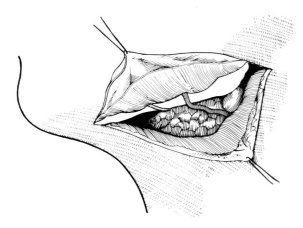

Figure 26.17 The superficial approach to the submandibular gland. The mandibular branch of the facial nerve is preserved on the back of the platysma muscle sheet

should be preserved) (Figure 26.17). The common facial vein is located and divided posterior to the gland. The anterior margin of the sternomastoid muscle is dissected free and the facial artery is ligated again, below the submandibular gland, where it arises from the external carotid artery. The superficial portion of the gland will now be clear and can be dissected from the underlying mylohyoid muscle until the posterior margin of that muscle is reached and the hypoglossal nerve is preserved below the gland. The muscle border is then retracted and the deep part of the gland delivered by careful dissection to separate it from the lingual nerve above. The submandibular ganglion is then divided from the lingual nerve. Careful, complete haemostasis is achieved on the plexus of sublingual vessels in that area. The gland now remains attached only by its duct which is divided and ligated well forward in the floor of the mouth (Figure 26.18).

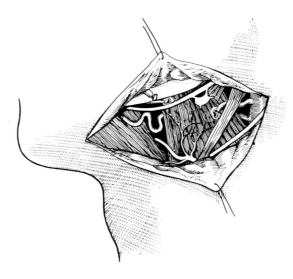

Figure 26.18 The surgical bed after the submandibular gland has been resected

The wound is closed with fine absorbable sutures to the platysma, taking care not to entrap the already carefully preserved mandibular branch of the facial nerves. A small corrugated or closed suction drain is inserted into the deep bed from which the gland has been removed. The skin is closed with 6/0 non-absorbable sutures. The drain can usually be removed in 24–48 h.

Gland resection for tumour

Neoplasm occurs in the mandibular gland only one-tenth as frequently as in the parotid. Tumours can be benign (pleomorphic adenoma) or malignant. Pleomorphic adenoma and low-grade malignancy restricted to the gland are treated by resection as described for recurrent sialoadenitis and calculi within the glands.

Radical resection for aggressive malignancy

In order to establish the diagnosis, an excision biopsy of the *total* gland may be necessary, with frozen section histology. If the aggressive nature of the tumour is evident by its short history and fixity, formal radical resection can be carried out *ab initio*, as the diagnosis is obvious. Local recurrence after the rare poorly differentiated tumours is common, distressing and difficult to treat, particularly if less than a radical operation has been performed. Full radical resection will often mean resection of the hemi-mandible on the affected side, full clearance of both submandibular triangles and an *en bloc* excision of the ipsilateral cervical lymph nodes. If involvement of the mucosa of the floor of the mouth is extensive, plastic surgical repair of the lining may be required using a forehead flap of skin based on the superficial temporal vessels. If neck skin is also involved and requires resection, fresh cover may be required. Transposition neck flap is sometimes feasible but often a deltopectoral axial pattern skin flap or a myocutaneous pectoralis major flap will be necessary. A more sophisticated repair by composite free flap of iliac crest bone and groin skin can be used in suitable cases after radical clearance of tumour. Such a free flap is raised on the deep circumflex iliac artery and vein which is then divided and anastomosed, by microvascular technique, into a convenient neck artery of compatible size.

27

Block dissection of the glands of the neck

R. T. Routledge

Surgical ablation of the lymph nodes and the lymphatic network remains the most effective method of controlling lymphatic metastases from primary tumours of the head and neck, despite recent claims of 'neck node control' by radiotherapy. The incidence of recurrent tumour after a skilfully performed radical neck dissection is extremely low and most recurrent problems in dealing with tumours of the head and neck relate to inadequate clearance of the primary.

Indications

The question is often posed, 'At what stage, when dealing with head and neck malignancies, should a neck node clearance be carried out?' We have learned, over the years, to be somewhat more selective and have concluded that bigger and better operations do not necessarily bring larger rewards. No self-respecting surgeon will embark on mutilating surgery without good justification for its use and the day of the so-called 'prophylactic neck dissection' has, hopefully, disappeared. There are always those who can produce the series of cases who have undergone neck dissection when clinically there has been no evidence of secondary involvement of nodes, and in which careful microscopical studies have shown in a small percentage of cases malignant cells in lymph glands. But we recognize that not all such malignant cell inclusions necessarily prosper and that the body is capable of dealing with many of them; and we have no evidence that removal of affected nodes at this early stage gives better results than neck dissection carried out when a node is first discovered. It is certain that if a policy of 'prophylactic neck dissection' is carried out, very many patients will be subjected to mutilating surgery who might never have needed it.

With some few exceptions it is sound policy to institute a careful follow-up of all patients treated for a primary malignant growth of the head and neck, with a particularly rigorous search for any possible involvement of neck nodes at 3-monthly intervals, and to proceed to neck dissection if nodes are palpable or if, indeed, there is any doubt that involved nodes are present in the neck. No policy, however, should be adhered to invariably and there could be occasions when it would seem politic to carry out a neck dissection at the same time as ablation of the primary growth, even though neck nodes are not clinically involved. In those cases in which reconstruction following ablative surgery of the primary involves introducing tissue employed in the reconstruction into the neck, it is safer to clear the neck first. Potentially infiltrated tissue is being opened up and tissue introduced which may mask nodes which later become enlarged so that they would have been palpated but for the bulk of material introduced beneath the neck skin. This applies particularly in cases where pectoralis major myocutaneous flaps are routed on a muscle pedicle beneath the skin of the neck or where a sternomastoid-clavicle myo-osseous repair of an ablated mandible is carried out.

On occasions the biological behaviour of the primary, usually of posterior tongue or upper pharynx, is so disturbingly aggressive that wisdom dictates that early lymphatic spread is inevitable and an *en bloc* clearance of primary and neck nodes is advisable. Similarly, patients who present late in the course of their disease with an uncontrolled primary growth probably merit neck dissection, even though nodes are not clinically palpable.

Having said all this, it remains a fact that the majority of patients with primary tumours of the head and neck will have a neck clearance only if and when nodes become clinically evident.

There is no indication for needle biopsy of suspect nodes. If there exists that much doubt concerning a node, it is better to take the decision to carry out a formal neck clearance.

The term 'block dissection of neck' covers a number of related procedures which may be summarized as follows:

1. Radical.
2. Suprahyoid.
3. Supra-omohyoid.
4. Function-preserving.
5. Bilateral.

1. Radical dissection

This is the standard full clearance of neck nodes, the most usually employed procedure and one which forms the basis of all types of neck clearance.

Preoperative considerations

It goes without saying that a full standard preoperative preparation of the patient is mandatory. Age, *per se*, is no contraindication to operation. There will be times when no amount of preoperative therapy will get a patient as fit as one would have desired, but in such cases it must be remembered that this is an emergency procedure. Without it the affected gland may become uncontrollable and risks may have to be taken in order to spare the patient a miserable death from eventual fungating neck growth.

Anaesthesia

Standard general anaesthesia via an endotracheal tube suffices for most cases. In certain ear, nose and throat procedures a preliminary tracheostomy is prepared and anaesthesia is continued via this route. Similarly, major lower jaw resections involving excision of the entire symphyseal region so disturb tongue fixation that a preliminary tracheostomy becomes essential. In those cases where it is safe to employ it, hypotensive anaesthesia controls bleeding and speeds the operation. In other cases simple head-up tilt and maintenance of an unobstructed airway produce effective control of bleeding and enable the surgeon to carry out the operation in the manner of a strict anatomical dissection which, in effect, it is.

The patient lies flat on his or her back with the neck extended and the chin turned towards the opposite side. Skin towels are conveniently fixed by suturing them, in places, to the skin and are arranged to provide access to the whole neck, the lower face and upper chest.

Incisions

Numerous patterns of incision have been employed since Crile described linked double horizontal incisions which were standard for many years. In essence, incisions must provide unobstructed access to the entire operative field and ideally should be placed, so far as is possible, within normal skin crease lines. Two forms of incision will be described which adequately provide for most eventualities.

The McFee incision is mostly commonly employed (Figure 27.1). This is an unlinked, double horizontal pattern which raises a wide strap of skin to expose the whole of one side of the neck and submandibular region. The upper component extends from just beyond the midline in the symphyseal region at the level of the lower border of the mandible, downwards and backwards in a deep curve to the posterior border of the mastoid process. Taking this incision beyond the midline medially facilitates thorough clearance of the submental glands, an important group and one that is often missed. The lower incision extends from the midline at the suprasternal notch along the line of the clavicle to beyond the anterior border of the trapezius.

This is the safest and most elegant of all the incisions described for the operation of block dissection of the neck. Being an unlinked combination of two parallel, horizontal neck incisions there are no awkward 'T' junctions, which commonly lead to delayed healing, and no vertical component to lead to postoperative webbing of the scar. In those cases who have received preoperative radiotherapy, with consequent diminution in vitality of the treated soft tissues, it is by far the safest pattern of incision to use. Breakdown is uncommon and the final cosmetic result could not be improved.

It is, however, not so suitable for function-preserving neck dissections, and an alternative pattern is recommended and is described later.

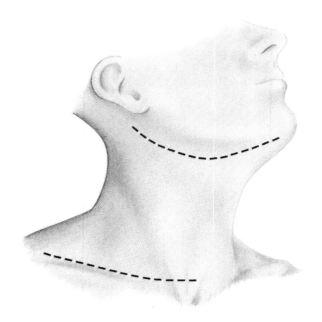

Figure 27.1 McFee unlinked double horizontal incisions for block dissection of the neck

Procedure

Lower dissection

When the horizontal incisions have been made, down to platysma, the upper skin flap is raised in full length to a level above the lower border of the mandible. This flap may then be conveniently anchored out of the way by means of a temporary suture fixed to the head towel.

The whole of the neck skin, bounded by the two horizontal incisions, is then raised by sharp dissection in the form of a wide strap extending from the midline anteriorly to beyond the anterior border of the trapezius posteriorly. It is essential that the whole of the anterior border of the trapezius is displayed, so that it can, during the course of the dissection, be stripped of its fatty-fascial investment. There is a posterior group of deep cervical nodes which it is important to remove with the main specimen.

There remains controversy as to what should be the

fate of the platysma; whether this muscle should be taken with the specimen or left on the skin flaps in the belief that the flaps will be protected from necrosis. It is difficult to see what protection to a skin flap can be provided by denervated devascularized muscle. Skin flaps, properly designed and handled, should not necrose and in order to adhere to the monobloc principle the author feels that it is essential that the platysma be removed with the contents of the neck (Figure 27.2).

safely and easily be ligatured and divided. There is, quite constantly, at the level of the clavicle, a fairly large tributary running medially and it is good practice to display this clearly, so that the lowest ligature may be placed just above the junction. This avoids accidental damage to the tributary and consequent bleeding in a particularly inaccessible area. Two ligatures are tied above and below the point of division of the vein and it is wise to secure the lower stump with a transfixation tie.

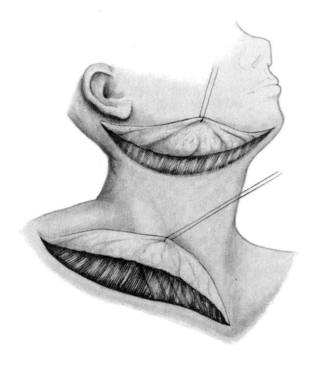

Figure 27.2 The platysma muscle is separated from the skin flaps

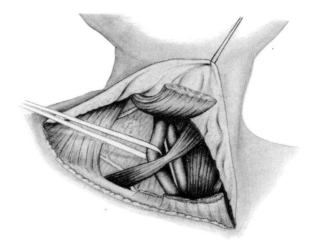

Figure 27.3 The sternomastoid muscle is divided almost at its insertion and the internal jugular vein mobilized

Elevation of the skin strap displays the platysma, a well-defined muscle sheet except for the posterior and inferior margins where it tends to tail off. This muscle sheet is divided along its entire length in the midline and inferiorly, ligating and dividing the external jugular vein low down. Retraction in an upward direction, by means of a tissue forceps gripping the lower border of the muscle, will begin to display the deeper structures at the root of the neck. The medial, intermediate and lateral supraclavicular nerves will be seen fanning out across the clavicle and these are divided.

The insertion of the sternomastoid into the clavicle and the upper border of the sternum is clearly displayed and then divided (Figure 27.3). Tissue forceps grasp the thick, divided muscle and retract upwards to expose part of the lower belly and the tendon of the omohyoid. This muscle is divided below its intermediate tendon and is lifted upwards by an artery forceps gripping the tendon. Immediately deep is the internal jugular vein. About a 2 cm length of this vein, just above the clavicle, is carefully cleaned so that it can

Careful finger dissection deep to the vein will free it for 1 or 2 cm from the carotid sheath and the vagus nerve, which must be identified and preserved.

Attention now focuses on the areolar content of the root of the neck. Working from medial to lateral, a combination of sharp and finger dissection will allow the fatty pad to be swept outwards and upwards off the scalene muscles and the brachial plexus. The phrenic nerve running obliquely across the face of the scalenus anterior will come into view and the transverse cervical vessels will be encountered in the fatty tissue. They can usually be cleared of fat but a constant branch running vertically upwards towards the levator scapulae will need to be ligated and divided. Sharp dissection continues up the anterior border of the trapezius, dividing the accessory nerve as it enters the muscle, having emerged from the sternomastoid at the junction of its middle and lower thirds, and is extended as far as access from the lower skin incision will allow, and then the medial portion of the operative site is cleared, again as far as access from the lower incision permits. The internal jugular vein together with the carotid sheath is easily stripped from the common carotid artery and vagus nerve (Figure 27.4).

At this stage in the dissection the skin strap is retracted downwards and the dissection specimen is passed under it and upwards, to appear in the upper wound and the dissection can then be completed from this access point.

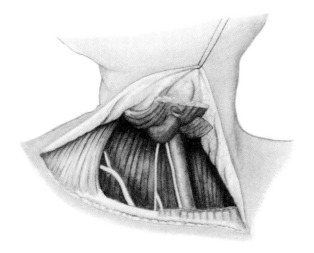

Figure 27.4 The internal jugular vein is ligated and divided at its lower end and the dissection specimen is cleaned and passed under and above the skin flap

Middle dissection

Special care must be taken at this stage to avoid damage to the phrenic nerve. This nerve arises mainly from C4 but has connections from C5 and C3 as well. As freeing of the internal jugular vein proceeds, deep to it can be seen the cervical plexus with the individual nerves emerging from between the scalenus anterior and the scalenus medius, and it is all too easy, if care is not exercised, to lift forwards the upper end of the phrenic nerve, by retraction on the overlying vein, and damage it as the cervical nerves are cut. The author makes it a rule to divide the cervical nerves well forward of the roots of the phrenic nerve and to avoid heavy retraction on the specimen at this stage, so that distortion of the underlying structures is minimized.

Broadly speaking, the internal jugular vein is the key to the operation. Dissection proceeds in its plane, separating it and the carotid sheath from the carotid artery and vagus nerve and extending posteriorly to the anterior border of the trapezius and anteriorly to denude the strap muscles up to the midline, so that the neck contents are removed in one and the same plane. Large thyroid venous tributaries are divided between ligatures.

The first major arterial branch to be encountered is the superior thyroid artery as it turns over and runs for a short distance parallel to the carotid artery. With primary tumours of the oral cavity it can be left intact, though it will need to be sacrificed with primary growths of the larynx and thyroid. The carotid bifurcation can be seen at about the level of the hyoid

and at this stage the cervical fascia may be boldly incised from the attachment of the intermediate tendon of the digastric to the greater horn of the hyoid, along the line of the anterior belly of the digastric as far as its insertion into the symphysis. Posteriorly the fascial incision is continued up to the mastoid process and these two manoeuvres then permit rapid advance of the dissection into the submandibular triangle. The internal jugular vein and carotid sheath are stripped upwards until the origin of the occipital artery is visualized (Figure 27.5). The hypoglossal nerve hooks round at this point to cross the internal and external carotid arteries, and it should always be secured at this stage so that it may be protected in the rest of its course towards the tongue. It will be necessary, now, formally to divide between ligatures the large lingual tributary of the internal jugular vein. It is often duplicated and easily damaged, to cause considerable bleeding which can be difficult to secure.

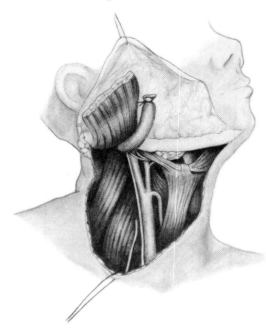

Figure 27.5 The dissection is completed into the submandibular triangle and the internal jugular vein is dissected up until the origin of the occipital artery is visualized

If, at this point, the carotid artery and vagus nerve are displaced forwards the sympathetic trunk, with the superior and middle ganglia, are clearly seen lying parallel and deep to the vessels. Aimless dissection from behind forwards, in the middle part of the neck, could damage the trunk. The capsule of the submandibular salivary gland is freed from its attachments to the digastric muscle and a tissue forceps grasping the lower pole of the gland lifts it upwards and outwards to expose the gland bed comprising the mylohyoid and hyoglossus muscles.

Upper (submandibular) dissection

Periosteum is divided along the lower border of the anterior part of the mandible and the fibro-fatty contents of the submental triangle are swept away from before backwards from the muscle bed. At the anterior border of the masseter the facial artery and anterior facial vein are divided between ligatures. Traction on this superoanterior corner of the specimen will now expose, in full, the muscle bed of the submandibular gland, crossed diagonally by the hypoglossal nerve. Upward traction shows the facial artery entering the posterior part of the gland accompanied by the common facial vein. The vessels are divided and ligated (Figure 27.6). Downward traction pulls a U-loop of lingual nerve into the operative field. The lingual nerve is attached to the deep lobe of the submandibular gland and the origin of the submandibular duct by means of its branches to the submandibular ganglion, which supplies the gland. The ganglion is usually quite obvious and, as it is divided from the deep lobe, the lingual nerve tracks back into place, deep to the ramus of the mandible. The submandibular duct is ligated as close to the oral mucosa as possible, and divided, and the whole contents of the submandibular triangle are then free.

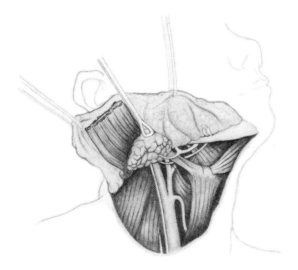

Figure 27.6   The facial artery and the facial vein are exposed and divided following dissection of the fibro-fatty contents and the submental triangle

In the posterosuperior angle of the field the lower pole of the parotid gland is transected. It contains a large venous trunk, the posterior facial vein, which is divided between ligatures. The upper attachment of the sternomastoid is cut through to expose the posterior belly of the digastric. Deep to this lies the upper end of the internal jugular vein and the accessory nerve, and from these the whole of the specimen is now suspended. The nerve is closely applied to the

vein and is separated and divided. The jugular vein is divided between ligatures and the upper end is further secured by a transfixation tie. The specimen is now free (Figure 27.7).

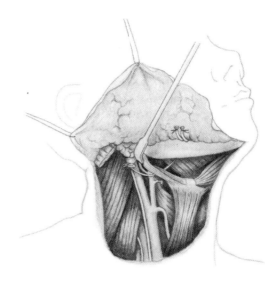

Figure 27.7   The lower pole of the parotid gland is transected, the upper attachment of the sternomastoid is divided and the jugular vein is ligated and divided as high as possible

Complete haemostasis is secured, and the wounds are then closed in layers with suction drainage.

Postoperative management

Postoperative therapy is determined by the extent of any other ablative procedure, which may be carried out together with the neck dissection, such as a jaw or laryngeal resection. No special postoperative care is required following a straightforward block dissection of neck. The operation can be fairly swiftly concluded and, in many cases, without blood transfusion. Morbidity is not marked and patients are usually ambulant by the day after operation. Suction usually continues for 48–72 h, and sutures are removed at 7 days.

Complications

The incidence of serious complications is low. Using a McFee incision even minor wound breakdown is uncommon, and frank skin necrosis is almost never seen.

Wound breakdown with carotid blowout is always quoted as a complication, yet the author has only encountered this on two occasions and in both very heavy irradiation had been followed by ill-planned incisions. If there is very real doubt that heavy irradiation may have lowered soft-tissue viability to a point where skin necrosis is inevitable after added surgical trauma, before closing the wounds the levator scapulae can be freed and turned over medially as a hinged flap in order to provide muscle cover to the denuded carotid.

If, in spite of everything, there is a major skin breakdown, so as to threaten exposure of the carotid, swift action to replace non-viable skin using a convenient deltopectoral or pectoralis major flap will save the day.

On occasions dissections at the root of the neck may damage the thoracic duct. Even if the duct is visualized during the dissection it can be difficult to secure between ligatures, as it so easily tears. Division of the thoracic duct leads to a discharge of milky fluid from the wound, which is mostly of nuisance value. Such fistulas always close spontaneously in time, though they may give trouble for several weeks. No special treatment is indicated.

Postoperative sequelae

It cannot be denied that sacrifice of the accessory nerve does pose problems for the patient in the way of a paralysed trapezius, often with complaints of continuing discomfort in the neck and shoulder. The surprising feature is that so few patients have difficulty in adjusting to this disability, which will, of course, be permanent. Very often I have been intrigued to find, 6 months after a radical neck dissection, a surprisingly powerful shoulder shrug against resistance. This can be due to only two factors. First, that the levator scapulae compensates in large measure for the lost trapezius action. Secondly, that there is an additional motor supply to the trapezius, which is not routinely damaged in a neck dissection.

Further investigation revealed that it is possible to identify a nerve trunk of not inconsiderable size, posteriorly in the lower third of the neck, which arises from the cervical plexus and joins the accessory nerve within the substance of the sternomastoid muscle at a point about 2 cm from its posterior border. Routinely, now, when performing a radical neck clearance, the author dissects out this cervical branch and divides the accessory nerve proximal to the junction. Careful postoperative assessment has demonstrated that in all cases some trapezius function is preserved and patients have made no complaint of shoulder weakness or stiffness, or of the constant dragging ache which so commonly follows trapezius paralysis. The minimal added dissection required in no way compromises the radical nature of the operation as, for most of its course, the cervical component runs in the plane of the scalene muscles deep to the block of tissue to be excised and, having carefully sectioned the accessory nerve, the sternomastoid muscle can be elevated and removed as previously described.

Excision of the mandibular branch of the facial nerve, as it loops down into the neck and then ascends to cross the facial vessels as they overlie the mandible at the anterior border of the masseter, leads to paralysis of half the lower lip with a very obviously asymmetrical appearance, particularly when the face is in animation. It has to be accepted, though, that this is a small price to pay to ensure a complete clearance. A small lymph node is constantly encountered just at the point where the nerve crosses the facial vessels, and any attempt to dissect out the nerve must jeopardize a total clearance.

2. Suprahyoid clearance

The suprahyoid clearance is a poor substitute for a radical neck dissection and I believe that it has no place in the treatment of head and neck cancer. It was said to be indicated in an unfit patient in whom lymphatic involvement was limited to mobile nodes confined to the submandibular triangle, or in cases of bilateral node involvement where a full block dissection was carried out on the more heavily involved side, and a suprahyoid clearance on the less affected side, in order to avoid the complications of a bilateral radical neck dissection.

The suprahyoid dissection, as such, is little more than a clearance of the submandibular triangle and removes the gland and its duct, the fascial investments of the triangle and only the extreme upper part of the carotid sheath, and fascial coverings of the jugular vein. It must be considered to be a pale, inadequate imitation of a radical neck node clearance and cannot be justified on any grounds.

3. Supra-omohyoid clearance

This extended operation does have rather more indication and can be considered in grossly unfit patients whose glandular involvement is limited to a single, mobile node in the submandibular triangle, or in cases with bilateral, palpable nodes in whom, on one side, there is only one mobile node in the submandibular triangle.

Only one incision is required, corresponding to the upper horizontal incision of the radical operation. The upper flap is raised and retracted as already described in the radical neck dissection, and the lower skin edge is undermined and retracted downwards so that dissection can begin at a point well below the carotid bifurcation. It is not usual to transect the sternomastoid which can be retracted posteriorly to obtain a good view of the middle of the neck. The internal jugular vein is divided between ligatures just above the superior thyroid tributary, and the carotid sheath is stripped from this level upwards. The remainder of the dissection proceeds as already described for radical dissection, save that the upper end of the sternomastoid remains attached to its origin on the mastoid process, and because of this the internal jugular vein has to be ligated at its upper end, lower down than can be attained in a radical block dissection.

It is to be noted that this procedure does not permit clearance of the nodes at the root of the neck, nor along the anterior border of the trapezius.

It does not match up to the standards required of curative surgery for malignant conditions, in that a deliberately incomplete procedure is being carried out and the field is seriously jeopardized if glands, which are left behind, become involved, so that further surgery of the neck has to be undertaken.

4. Function-preserving neck dissection

The 'function-preserving' neck dissection is an interesting concept and is a valuable procedure so long as fairly limited indications are adhered to. Described by Bocca for the treatment of lymphatic spread from primary laryngeal growths, it has been applied to other malignant head and neck conditions, notably to patients with primary growths of the oral mucosa.

As originally envisaged, the procedure was carried out as prophylactic clearance so that it can, with justification, be employed in patients with aggressive tumours or late tumours in whom no nodes are palpable but where experience dictates that an elective neck dissection is indicated. It is probably safe also to advise such a procedure in patients in whom a single, small, mobile node is noted in the submandibular triangle. Any suspicion of multiple nodes or of fixation of nodes to deeper structures, or overlying muscles, should rule out this more limited clearance.

Paradoxically, though the dissection is less radical it is a more difficult procedure to carry out, because so many structures have to be identified and preserved and because, to an extent, surgical access is more restricted. For these reasons the McFee approach tends to be too limiting and an alternative incision is recommended. It consists of a horizontal and a vertical component (Figure 27.8). The horizontal limb corresponds exactly to the usual long submandibular incision, which is the upper component of the McFee procedure. From the midpoint of this limb an incision extends in lazy S form to the midpoint of the clavicle. Three skin flaps are thus outlined and are raised to expose a wide triangle of neck. If required, greater access to the root of the neck may be achieved by incorporating an additional horizontal component to the vertical neck incision at the level of the clavicle. Bocca describes a thorough clearance of all fascial and aponeurotic investments from the line of the posterior border of the sternomastoid to the midline, preserving the sternomastoid muscle, the accessory nerve, the internal jugular vein and the submandibular salivary gland.

It is claimed that the procedure from a cancer 'cure' standpoint is as effective as other methods, yet avoids all the major disabilities associated with these methods. The concept has gained in popularity over the past few years, but it should be emphasized that its main indication is in those cases in whom no lymph nodes are palpable – that is to say as a prophylactic procedure, an attitude to treatment which is by no means accepted by the majority of head and neck surgeons. It would seem to the author that a great danger of this method is that attempts may be made to apply it to totally unsuitable cases and that a full radical neck dissection, with preservation of trapezius function, as already described, provides safer management from the cancerological viewpoint, with little increase in postoperative disability. Its chief value may lie in the management of patients with bilateral node involvement, where a radical neck dissection can be performed on one side, and a function-preserving clearance, which leaves the internal jugular vein intact, on the other.

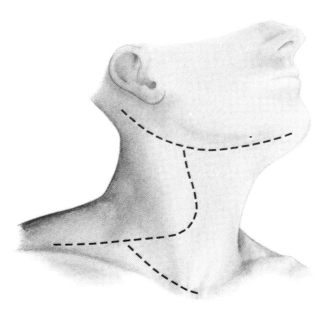

Figure 27.8 Incisions for 'function-preserving' block dissection of the neck

5. Bilateral neck dissection

The prognosis for any patient suffering from primary malignancy of the head and neck, who presents with bilateral cervical node involvement, must necessarily be grave. This does not mean that the case is lost and that energetic salvage attempts should not be instituted. Many such patients have been saved and, indeed, cured by an aggressive policy.

A bilateral, radical block dissection of the neck performed at one operation carries postoperative hazards so severe and a mortality rate so high as to preclude its justification in any case. The dangers stem from the removal on both sides of the internal jugular vein. This vein provides almost all the drainage from the head and neck and sudden simultaneous bilateral interruption causes severe congestion of all the territory drained. The risks of irreversible brain damage, due to venous stasis, are high, particularly so as we are dealing with patients in the older age groups whose cerebral reserve, in any event, is probably low. If a period of not less than 3 months can be allowed to elapse between the two block dissections, morbidity and mortality are greatly reduced, probably as a result of vertebral vein hypertrophy following ligation of the internal jugular vein on one side.

A standard radical clearance can therefore be performed on both sides of the neck, so long as the two procedures can be separated by not less than 3 months. Such a policy can be applied to those cases in whom glands appear on the other side of the neck after one side has already been cleared.

Often, however, on clinical examination glands are palpable bilaterally and the need arises for simultaneous attack on both sides of the neck. It is advised that a radical operation be carried out on the most affected side or on the side of the primary if both gland groups are equally involved, and some form of internal jugular vein-preserving clearance on the other side – either a function-preserving operation or supra-omohyoid clearance as described earlier.

28
Maxillofacial surgery

J. W. Ross

Infection

Acute alveolar abscess

This arises within the bone of either jaw and is usually due to a tooth with dead pulp or nerve. It can also arise between the gum and a tooth and often will have been preceded by chronic inflammation of the area. Other pathological conditions in the jaws may produce abscesses, such as cysts, buried teeth or fractures. If a tooth is involved, it becomes very tender to pressure. The infection may resolve, discharge into the mouth or penetrate into the soft tissues, and whether the latter produces cellulitis or an abscess depends on the infecting organism and the patient's resistance. Extension into the various potential spaces around the jaws can result in external swelling, trismus and danger to the airway when sublingual, submandibular and pharyngeal spaces are involved (Figures 28.1 and 28.2).

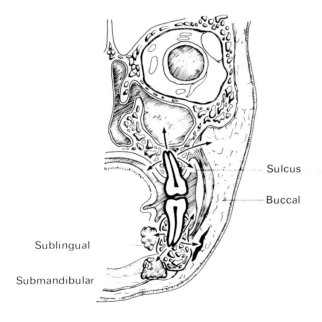

Figure 28.1 Possible pathways of infection arising from an apical abscess. The promixity of the maxillary sinus is clearly shown (coronal section)

Pus formation, which may be detected by fluctuation or pointing, should be relieved as soon as possible by incision and drainage, either intra-orally or extra-orally at dependent points. The best place for incision can often be located by asking the patient to indicate the most painful spot with one finger. Intubation of the patient is sometimes needed for operation but can be difficult and dangerous when there is poor mouth opening or potential airway obstruction. Forced opening of the mouth or manipulation with a laryngoscope may cause premature bursting of an abscess intra-orally which could result in inhalation of pus and airway restriction.

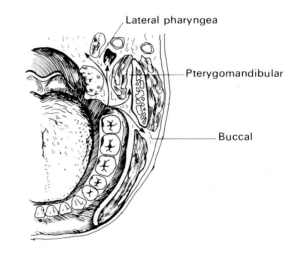

Figure 28.2 Possible pathways of infection arising from infection around wisdom tooth (transverse section)

External incision should extend to the subcutaneous level and continue with sinus forceps to avoid damage to important underlying structures, such as the facial nerve. The sinus forceps should be inserted closed until the pus is reached and then withdrawn open to ensure free drainage. A careful check should be made that all loculi have been entered and a finger is effective for this purpose.

An essential part of the operation is the drainage but removal of the cause is usually carried out under the same anaesthetic.

It is uncommon to insert drains into intra-oral wounds but this is usually necessary for external drainage. A corrugated rubber drain, trimmed at a 45° angle but with the point removed to avoid vessel erosion, is inserted to the depth of the cavity. Multiple drains are used if there is more than one loculus.

The drain is usually retained for 48 hours only but, if pus is draining freely at that time, it may be kept in place or shortened and removed later. After 4 days, retention of the drain may induce discharge by acting as a foreign body.

Complications

Actinomycosis

If there has been surgery in the mouth or fracture of the mandible some few weeks before the acute episode, or there is an unusual amount of induration associated with the swelling, the first sample of pus should be taken in a tube rather than on a swab for investigation in the laboratory for actinomycosis. This is a chronic condition but may produce an acute abscess. Colonies of the bacterium (*Actinomyces israelii*) may be seen as 'sulphur' granules in the pus which may be crushed and examined under the microscope, revealing a typical pattern of radiating filaments or 'ray fungus'. If actinomycosis is diagnosed, prolonged antibiotic treatment is indicated, usually with penicillin.

Facial sinus

Rarely, an alveolar abscess will track to the skin surface and discharge, producing a chronic discharging sinus which may be some distance from the tooth. These sinuses are commonly misdiagnosed and a dental opinion should always be obtained when there is uncertainty about the diagnosis.

Treatment is removal of the cause and excision of the sinus tract, if the sinus is not of recent origin.

Cavernous sinus thrombosis

Although rare, cavernous sinus thrombosis is a serious complication of infection in and around the jaws. Spread is presumed to take place by infected thrombi in the pterygoid plexus or anterior facial vein which connects with the cavernous sinus. The patient will develop rigors and a high swinging temperature with oedema around the eyes and exophthalmos. Involvement of the nerves in the sinus results in ophthalmoplegia on the affected side.

Treatment is by anticoagulants and antibiotics and again removal of the cause and drainage where required. The patient should be under neurosurgical care.

Sterile abscess

This condition is becoming more common and is sometimes known as 'antibioma'. It is due to treating abscesses with antibiotics but without drainage, and occurs when the antibiotic sterilizes the pus, leaving a fluctuant abscess which, when incised, does not grow an organism.

Clinically, the patient presents with a fluctuant swelling and is afebrile. Incision and drainage are indicated.

Osteomyelitis

Occasionally, infection in or around the jaws can result in extension through the medulla. When acute, the patient has a high temperature, severe pain, loosening of teeth, lymphadenitis, swelling of the face and eventually multiple discharging sinuses within the mouth and on the face. Pus may discharge around the teeth.

In the lower jaw, involvement of the mandibular nerve may produce anaesthesia of its distribution.

The condition is predisposed by systemic and local factors causing lowered resistance, including diabetes, agranulocytosis, hypogammaglobulinaemia, typhoid, marble bone disease, Paget's disease, radiotherapy and, of course, fractures.

The mandible is more commonly affected and this is thought to be because of its denser bone and poor collateral circulation. However, in infants the condition occurs more commonly in the maxilla and is believed to be haematogenously spread or due to local trauma. Metastatic osteomyelitis may spread to or from the mandible.

It is considered that an important factor in the spread of osteomyelitis may be the stripping of the periosteum from the bone by the pus, thus depriving it of its blood supply. As the infection spreads, pieces of bone become isolated from their blood supply and die. These sequestra may be seen on radiography and are related to the areas of bone destruction.

As with the treatment of acute alveolar abscess, pus is collected as soon as possible for identification of the organisms and a sensitivity test.

Although the organism is usually *Staphylococcus aureus*, a wide variety of organisms has been associated with the condition.

Surgical drainage and sequestrectomy are carried out under general anaesthesia, care being taken not to strip healthy periosteum from the bone.

Control of the disease process has to be exercised mostly on clinical evidence as the radiographic appearance lags some 10–20 days behind the clinical state.

Weakening of the mandible can advance to the stage where fracture readily occurs and care must be taken to continue antibiotic treatment until the condition is completely under control. Inadequate treatment may lead to chronic osteomyelitis which is most difficult to treat.

There is good evidence that some cases of chronic osteomyelitis of the mandible are associated with the 'incompetent leucocyte syndrome'.

Maxillofacial injuries

Most fractures of the facial skeleton are due to road

traffic injuries. Maxillofacial injuries commonly occur in association with injuries to other parts of the body and the most important of these is the head injury, which occurs in approximately one-third of the cases. Impact to the head is transmitted not only to the brain but to the cervical spine and a careful check must be made for injuries in this region. A general examination of the patient must be carried out and one should suspect other injuries if the patient is in shock as this generally does not occur with facial injuries in isolation.

As the facial skeleton consists of thin bones with certain reinforced buttresses, it collapses in a relatively easy manner when the body is projected on to a stationary object. The face therefore acts as a shock absorber and lessens trauma to the brain.

Severe injuries are common in the driver and front seat passenger, and fragmentation of the windscreen may cause permanent disfigurement and disabilities, such as blindness and facial palsy, a condition which is seen less frequently since the legislation on the wearing of seat belts was introduced.

External haemorrhage is rarely a problem with maxillofacial injuries and the correct treatment is reduction of the fractures and suturing of the lacerations as soon as possible.

The most likely cause of problems in these cases, particularly where there is unconsciousness, is the airway. Careful pharyngeal toilet with suction should be carried out wherever possible and with swabs and forceps where suction is not available. The hazards include blood, vomit, broken teeth, dentures, oedema and falling back of the tongue where the anterior part of the mandible and the attachment of the tongue are separated from the rest of the jaw.

With fractures of the maxilla, there will be swelling of the palate and spasm of the pterygoid muscles which tend to draw the maxilla downwards and backwards, thus aggravating the compromised airway. Therefore, the face-down position is most important and, where necessary, the tongue should be held forward together with the maxilla, if this is displaced, to free the airway until intubation.

It is a good working rule that patients with severe facial injuries in combination with a head injury should have a tracheostomy performed at the earliest opportunity, to protect the airway and also facilitate future treatment by removing the endotracheal tube from the areas of injury. The chest should always be radiographed for missing tooth fragments and dentures.

The fractured maxilla may be displaced by the pull of muscles, which also occurs in the mandible when the muscles of mastication cause upward rotation of a ramus fragment where the fracture is anterior to the attachments of medial pterygoid and masseter muscles.

When fractures of the mandible are bilateral, inframandibular muscles will cause downward and backward displacement of the symphysis.

Fractures of the mandible

Fractures of the mandible occur in any situation but the common sites are the subcondylar, the angle, the body, the canine and symphysis regions. Those fractures of the jaw which involve teeth are inevitably compound to the mouth and, where the teeth are grossly involved, or are themselves damaged in the root, they should be removed or they will tend to retard healing.

Fractures of the maxilla (Figure 28.3)

As the bones of the maxilla are thin, they do not tend to fracture along simple lines but tend to comminute and collapse. Le Fort carried out trauma experiments on cadavers and showed that there were three main levels of maxillary fracture.

The first and lowest is the Le Fort I, which is a horizontal fracture passing above the floors of the antra and nose, through the septum and lateral walls of the nose, zygomatic buttresses and pterygoid plates.

A Le Fort II fracture is the so-called 'middle-third' or 'pyramidal' fracture which ascends from zygomatic buttresses through the infraorbital margins and high into the nasal cavity.

A Le Fort III fracture is at a higher level and involves the roof of both orbits and, as the zygomas are below the level of the fracture, the face as a whole is separated from the skull. The latter is a rare fracture, but a possible complication of both the Le Fort II and III fractures is involvement of the base of the skull in the region of the cribriform plate, causing a dural tear and consequent leakage of cerebrospinal fluid. There is a danger of infection passing from the nose and becoming established within the cranium, causing meningitis.

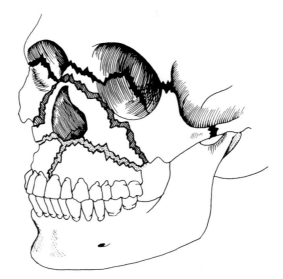

Figure 28.3 Le Fort I, II and III fractures with split palate

These patients, whether they show cerebrospinal fluid leak or not, are treated prophylactically with antibiotics in some centres.

About 20% of maxillary fractures include a split of the palate which is sometimes severe enough to cause rupture of the oral mucosa but usually results only in a widening of the maxillary arch. It is important that this fracture is recognized if correct reduction is to be achieved.

Fractures of the nose

The nasal bones may be fractured and displaced in any direction but are usually pushed backwards. If the blow is severe enough, the ethmoids are collapsed and the medial walls of the orbits and canthal ligaments shifted laterally, producing a condition known as 'telecanthus'. The lateral cartilages of the nose may be displaced and one side override the other and the cartilaginous septum may be displaced from its groove in the vomer and curved to one side or the other.

Fractures of the zygoma

One or both zygomas are commonly fractured in combination with a fractured maxilla and may be depressed, producing a flattened cheek prominence. The main fractures occur at the zygomatic buttress, infraorbital margin, involving the infraorbital canal and at the zygomaticofrontal and zygomaticotemporal sutures, or some other place on the arch.

Fracture and displacement of the zygoma can, of course, occur in isolation, and fracture of the zygomatic arch with depression is commonly seen. This depression consists of a triple fracture with the apex of the two fragments pushed medially, which is usually the direction of the trauma. However, downward displacement rarely takes place because of the strength of the investing temporal fascia.

Blowout fracture

Since this injury was first described there has been much debate about its cause. It was originally believed that a blowout fracture of the orbital floor was caused by compression all around the rim of the orbit from an injury, such as a ball striking the orbit. It is now considered that a blow to the inferior orbital rim is sufficient to cause this type of fracture in the orbital floor without the rim itself fracturing.

Characteristically, the blowout fracture of the orbit shows radiographically that some of the contents of the orbit have dropped through into the antrum and will appear as a 'teardrop'. Confirmation of this is by coronal computerized axial tomography which may show a trapdoor deformity of the thin bones of the orbital floor. It was said that trapping of the inferior rectus or inferior oblique muscles was the cause of the diplopia which often results from this injury.

However, recent work has shown that the eye is held in position in the orbit by radial fibrous bands and it is believed that it is the trapping of the fibrous bands which produces the immobility of the eye.

Whatever the cause of injury in these cases, the eye itself may have sustained trauma and careful inspection should be made by an ophthalmic surgeon.

Treatment of maxillofacial injuries

Fractures of the mandible, where most of the teeth are present, are treated by interdental or eyelet wiring (Figures 28.4 and 28.5). This consists essentially of passing a wire loop around two teeth, twisting to tighten into the concavities of the teeth at the gum margin. This leaves an eyelet protruding and the process is continued with other pairs of teeth in both jaws until sufficient eyelets have been applied to allow the eyelets themselves to be joined from upper to lower jaw, fixing the jaws together. This can be carried out under local anaesthesia but general anaesthesia is commonly used.

Consideration of the airway must be given at all times and the patient's stomach must be empty before the jaws are fixed together. The patient is returned to the ward with wire cutters so that, in an emergency, the fixation can be cut to open the jaws. Since the teeth have been brought together in their correct occlusion, the attached bone will be reduced into its correct position but problems arise where there are few or no natural teeth.

When without teeth and with dentures, fixation of the jaws is achieved by wiring the jaw fragments into the dentures using circumferential wires and then wiring the dentures together, producing reduction of the fractures.

These methods will stabilize those fractures which have teeth attached to them or which can be included in dentures. However, fractures behind this region may require separate fixation by direct bone wiring, either from the mouth or through the skin. The choice will depend on the position, extent and displacement of the fracture. One simple wire loop is usually sufficient to fix this proximal fragment because the anterior part of the jaw has already been fixed.

Where there are no teeth and dentures have been lost or broken, it is necessary to construct facsimiles of the dentures without teeth and wire these into position as one would have done with the dentures. The lower four incisors are usually removed from the dentures to facilitate feeding but, with the acrylic splint, provision is made anteriorly for a feeding gap.

With unilateral fracture in the subcondylar region, patients can often achieve their correct bite with effort and take a soft diet. When they are unable to bite correctly, as with marked displacement of the fracture, the jaws are wired together for 10–14 days. With bilateral subcondylar fractures, jaw fixation is necessary for 4 weeks at least or shortening of the ascending rami may develop.

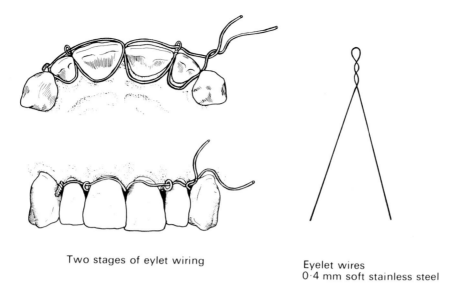

Two stages of eylet wiring

Eyelet wires
0·4 mm soft stainless steel

Figure 28.4 Eyelet wiring of teeth for immobilization of fractured jaw

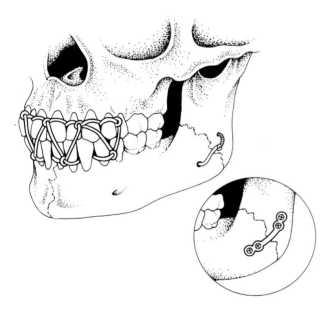

Figure 28.5 Eyelet wiring of a fractured symphysis; interosseous wiring of angle fracture

Reduction and fixation of the fractured maxilla are invariably carried out under general anaesthesia and, because the bite relationship is important in achieving correct reduction, the anaesthetic is administered via a nasal tube.

If there are fractured zygomas it may be necessary to elevate these to allow for disimpaction of the maxilla, and these movements are carried out with care to avoid penetration of sharp bone fragments into the orbits.

When the palate is split reduction is necessary, which requires compressing the posterior ends of the arch of the teeth together with either finger pressure or a special instrument. It will be clear that when reduction has been achieved the upper and lower teeth will match and bite together accurately.

When the maxilla has been set in the correct position, judged in a lateral and anteroposterior plane by the matching of the bite, it is necessary to displace it upwards into the correct position to re-establish facial height. This is a matter of judgement as over-correction can be achieved where there is comminution, and if the face is too long, healing will be delayed because of the lack of bone contact. Interdental wiring may be applied between the teeth to fix the bite when it is then necessary to hold the face height until healing takes place. There are a number of methods available for this, of which the most common is four-screw fixation, comprising a screw on each side of the mandible, anterior to and below the mental foramen. There are special self-tapping bone screws which are inserted with a hand drill through a small incision in the skin. Two screws are applied to the supraorbital region in the same way and the face height assessed. Vertical bars and joints are used to lock the upper and lower set of pins together. It is then necessary to join the screws horizontally to brace this apparatus, sometimes known as the 'box frame' (Figure 28.6).

With the combined injury of mandible and maxilla, it is essential that a platform be formed to allow reduction of the maxilla into the correct position. It may therefore be necessary to insert intraosseous wire across the fracture lines in the mandible to render it 'intact', and a suitable basis on which to build the rest of the face.

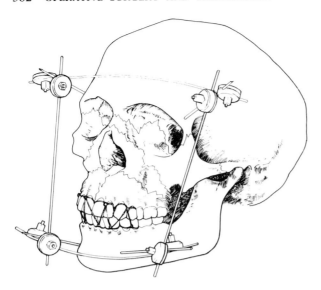

Figure 28.6 Screw fixation of fractured maxilla using 'box frame'

Before the application of external fixation, it is necessary to deal with the zygomas and naso-ethmoidal complex.

Zygomatic fractures will usually respond to the Gillies approach from the temple, when Bristow's elevator is inserted through a small incision above the hairline between the temporal fascia and the temporal muscle, passed easily down under the zygomatic arch or zygomatic body and pressure is applied outwards to elevate the fragments.

Care must be taken to avoid inward pressure on the temporal bone. This method leaves a scar which cannot be seen when the hair grows. If the zygoma proves unstable, it may be necessary to carry out open reduction of the fractures with wiring.

The advent of miniature bone plates has enabled big strides to be taken in maxillofacial surgery since we can now avoid, in many cases, a patient returning from the theatre to the intensive therapy unit to protect the airway in that the fractures can be treated without fixing the jaws together. As shown in Figure 28.5, a bone plate can be applied across a fracture through the cheek, if this is more convenient, and will hold that fracture in position against gentle stresses of function. Where there is doubt about this, two plates can be used in parallel. These mini plates can also be used for fixing fractured maxillas and zygomas and even nasal fractures in some cases. They are made of titanium and are malleable.

Fractures of the nose are treated by manipulating the lateral cartilages and nasal bones with Walsham's forceps; the outer blade is covered with rubber tubing to protect the skin. The septum is repositioned if displaced and the nasal bones brought forward using Asch forceps. A problem arises when the ethmoids have been compressed as it is necessary to apply strong pressure with thumb and forefinger far back on the medial walls of the orbits while bringing the septum and nasal bones forward with the forceps. This squeezing-in action helps to restore the medial canthi to their correct postion but, if the canthi are completely free from the skeleton, it may be necessary to make small incisions to pick up their ends and wire them together across the nose. If these are still attached to bone and if it possible to collect them with the rest of the nasal fragments, they may be controlled using thin lead plates on each side, which are wired across the nose and maintained for 10 days.

The problem of soft-tissue injury should be considered before extubation, and after fracture fixation. Even in the most severe facial injuries, there is usually no loss of tissue but, in cases where tissue has been lost, e.g. a piece of lip, initial treatment is to suture the mucosa to the skin accepting the defect temporarily and later carrying out a secondary plastic surgical repair.

The patient is carefully extubated and the pack removed before the jaw fixation is finally tightened. The pharynx is sucked out through the mouth and via the nose and, if there is no tracheostomy, it is wise to leave an endotracheal or nasopharyngeal tube in position to maintain the airway until such time as this can safely be removed.

Postoperative care

The patient should be returned to the ward with wire cutters where the jaws are wired together, and when there is external fixation of the box-frame type it will be necessary to send a spanner back to the ward with the patient. All staff dealing with the patient postoperatively should know exactly which procedures are required to open the mouth and should appreciate that the patient may still have food in the stomach and may therefore vomit.

The patient takes a purely fluid diet after the operation, but if there is any doubt about the patient's ability to do this, an intravenous line is left in place and a nasogastric tube should be inserted before the patient leaves the operating theatre.

It is important that all patients have thorough oral hygiene to keep the mouth scrupulously clean, and regular checks of the fixation should be carried out, particularly in the restless patient; loosening of wires can occur and there may be disturbance of external fixation.

The average time for union of fractures is 3 weeks for the maxilla and 4 weeks for the mandible.

Surgery of the temporomandibular joint

Indications for temporomandibular joint surgery include:

1. Ankylosis.
2. Dislocation – recurrent or long standing.

3. Arthrosis – not responding to conservative methods.
4. Osteoarthritis with pain.
5. Jaw deformities, e.g. condylar hyperplasia.
6. Fractures.

The pre-auricular incision is the most common approach to the temporomandibular joint. The upper end of the incision should be about 3 cm in length, angled forward at about 45°. Its posterior end should be at the groove where the helix joins the scalp. The incision then continues in the groove anterior to the helix and tragus and ends anterior to the lobe attachment.

The incision is therefore above the main trunk of the facial nerve but care must be taken to avoid the upper branches crossing the zygomatic arch superficial to the periosteum.

Dissection is carried out anterior to the external auditory meatus cartilage and the temporal part of the incision deepened until the temporal fascia is reached. This is incised exposing the temporal muscle and subperiosteal dissection is carried out along the zygomatic arch. This will expose the joint capsule and its thickened lateral ligament. Incision of the capsule from above and posteriorly will expose the condyle (Figure 28.7).

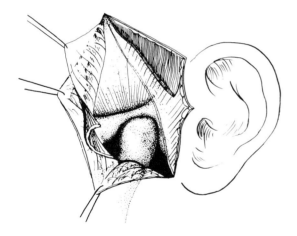

Figure 28.7 Pre-auricular approach to temporomandibular joint

1. Ankylosis

In severe cases of bony or fibrous ankylosis of the joint, dissection is extended well along the arch to expose the affected area. The aim of the operation is to produce a gap between the mandible and the skull to allow free movement. This gap may be left open or filled with a foreign material, such as silastic, to prevent reattachment.

Costochondral grafting is used when a space maintainer or functional hinge is required. This will require augmentation of the pre-auricular incision with a submandibular approach as the rib will be wired to the ramus and the cartilage inserted into the

fossa at the base of the skull, which is prepared to receive it if necessary.

2. Dislocation

Cases of long-standing dislocation of the mandibular condyle are rare and even fewer require open reduction. However, chronic recurrent dislocation is more common and occurs unilaterally or bilaterally. Reduction is usually possible without general anaesthetic, local anaesthetic or sedation and, as it becomes more frequent, reduction becomes easier and can quite often be achieved by the patient.

Its occurence is nevertheless an inconvenience and many operations have been devised in the past to prevent it. These range from plication of the capsule of the joint to removal of the articular eminence, and have met with varying degrees of success. Dautrey's operation has proved to be successful (Figure 28.8), but the prognosis can be improved by grafting a block of iliac bone to the articular eminence.

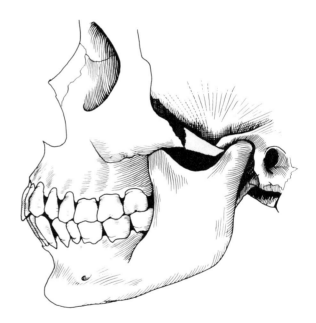

Figure 28.8 Dautrey's procedure for recurrent dislocation of the temporamandibular joint. The zygomatic arch is transected and the posterior end is depressed to prevent forward movement of the condyle.

3. Arthrosis

This is a very common affliction of the temporomandibular joint, particularly in young females. It is believed to arise from a disturbance of the complex neuromuscular control of the joint. This painful disturbance is often associated with anxiety and tension, but after conservative methods have been fully explored surgery may be necessary.

Some success is claimed with condylotomy, which can be carried out as a blind procedure using a Gigli saw, or as an open procedure via a pre-auricular incision, or through the mouth.

It has become apparent due to improved diagnostic methods, e.g. video-arthrography and MRI, that some of the problems are due to disc detachment or instability and these can be repaired surgically.

4. Osteoarthritis

Severe pain may occur in the proliferative phase of this disease and surgery is often the only way to deal satisfactorily with the problem. The aim is the removal of the irregular part of the condylar head undertaken as a high condylectomy, or so-called 'shave'.

5. Condylar hyperplasia

Unilateral growth of the condyle may occur after normal skeletal growth has ceased, and may be associated with deformity of the condyle. In these patients, removal of the condyle (condylectomy) is indicated.

6. Fracture

Gross displacement of the fractured condyle in children may have serious growth consequences and occasionally open reduction is required. The pre-auricular incision is used often with a submandibular incision to allow manipulation of the fragment or fragments into position.

Treatment of oral malignancy

The commonest form of oral malignacy is the squamous carcinoma, 50% of which involve the tongue. Leucoplakia is said to predispose to malignancy, but only 4% of these white patches become malignant. Leucoplakia, when it arises in the floor of the mouth, produces a higher incidence of malignancy, thought to be due to pooling of carcinogens or possibly to the endodermal origin of the floor of the mouth.

Tumours are usually classified on the STNM classification:

S – Site.
T – Extent of primary tumour.
N – Involvement of regional lymph nodes.
M – Presence of distant metastases.

Each category is graded and the grades are combined to ascribe a staging to the tumour. Some sites are known to have a poorer prognosis than others, e.g. those situated towards the posterior of the mouth in the oropharynx or posterior tongue.

The extent of the primary is obviously important in the prognosis as well as being an important consideration in the mutilating effect of any surgery.

Involvement of the regional lymph nodes implies serious spread of the disease and the presence of distant metastases a bad prognosis. The rate of growth of a tumour is a most important prognostic index.

Preoperative considerations

A careful examination of the mouth should be carried out, particularly down the sides of the tongue and back in the floor of the mouth, using spatulas or dental mirrors. The patient should be asked to lift the tongue into the palate so that the root of the tongue, sides of the tongue and floor of the mouth can be examined anteriorly. The examiner will then be able to assess the full extent of the tumour already seen and may possibly detect other primaries.

Fixation of the tongue is an ominous sign.

Pre-malignant lesions

Localized pre-malignant lesions are generally excised but can be treated by cryosurgey. The more extensive pre-malignant lesions which can involve much of the mucosa inside the mouth, producing the so-called 'hot mouth', may eventually result in multiple primary tumours. Serial excision with skin grafting has been carried out in these cases, although some authorities advocate the use of radio-active yttrium, which has a very low penetration.

Methods of treatment

Choice of treatment for oral cancer is as follows:

1. Surgery.
2. Radiotherapy.
3. Cytotoxic drugs.
4. Combinations of these treatments.

The choice of treatment will depend on the stage of the disease, the biological activity of the tumour, the general fitness of the patient and the question of whether any treatment has already been attempted and been unsuccessful. The commonest combination therapy is to carry out excision of the tumour and follow this by radiotherapy. Cytotoxic drugs can be administered by intra-arterial perfusion but are more usually given systemically. Lymphomas and sarcomas are rarely treated by surgery.

Surgical treatment of tumours

The tumour is excised with a margin of surrounding normal tissue to an extent which depends on the location and histology of the tumour, but is usually about 2 cm. Allowance must be made for special situations where the tumour is known to spread preferentially, such as into the mandibular canal and greater palatine canal. These excisions may mean loss of large portions of upper or lower jaw and, if there is lymph gland involvement, block dissection is performed in continuity with the tumour.

CARCINOMA OF THE LIPS

Small carcinomas involving the vermilion of the lip can be excised by wedge excision allowing 1 cm on each side of the tumour and closed directly with little deformity. If this excision of the tumour would result in the loss of more than one-third of the length of the lip, the defect can be filled by a cross-lip flap, i.e. swinging a flap from the other lip on a pedicle to help fill the defect. Larger excisions than this will need more complicated flaps to restore the sphincter to a reasonable aesthetic and functional size.

CARCINOMA OF THE MANDIBLE

In the mandible, where excision of the tumour has resulted in loss of the body or angle on one side, it is preferred to disarticulate the condyle and coronoid process in continuity if immediate reconstruction is not contemplated. Otherwise, the proximal fragment will flex and will cause extreme discomfort if the upper natural teeth are present or will rub on the upper denture.

If the excision terminates anteriorly between the canine region and the centre line of the mandible, it is possible to leave the patient without any reconstruction, apart from that necessary to restore lost soft tissue. The importation of a pedicle or flap to provide soft-tissue cover helps to prevent the swing of the mandible to the operated side and also serves partly to fill in the defect caused by the loss of bone.

Many patients can wear lower dentures on edentulous remaining fragments of lower jaws provided that they extend across the midline to the excised site, and most, when faced with the proposition of reconstruction, invariably prefer to accept the situation and wear a new reduced lower denture.

Because the tongue tends to fall backwards without anterior support, postoperative nursing and feeding can be difficult should it be necessary to excise the symphysis. The airway may be so at risk that tracheostomy is necessary, and feeding will be by nasogastric tube inserted at operation, in combination with an intravenous infusion. Fortunately, symphysis tumours are quite rare but, for the above reasons, an attempt is made to reconstruct the anterior mandible even if this is only on a temporary basis, e.g. by a titanium implant allowing the tongue to be sutured forward and stabilized.

When the tumour is confined to the floor of the mouth or alveolus and is superficial in a reasonably deep mandible, it is permissible to cut out a block of mandible with the tumour, leaving a lower border strut intact. This also enables one to stabilize the tongue, but the same rules of excision apply as far as the safety margin is concerned and it is not therefore always possible to leave a deep strut. The patient must take care postoperatively as fracture may readily occur.

CARCINOMA OF THE TONGUE

The tongue may be involved primarily in a tumour or by extension. This may necessitate excision of a small part of the tongue which may be closed directly or a large part may need removal, care being taken to give a good margin around the tumour. This may cause difficulty in swallowing and speaking, but most patients adapt quickly to the smaller tongue.

If the excision is large, the tongue tip can often be rotated and sutured to cover a raw area anteriorly and large superficial defects can be covered with quilt grafts. A split-skin graft is applied to the raw area and sutured to it around the edges and to the bed of the graft. The grafted skin is then perforated in a number of places to allow free escape of blood – this is the so-called 'quilt' graft.

CARCINOMA OF THE MAXILLA

Malignant tumours of the maxillary alveolus invariably require removal of a section of the maxilla and quite frequently this entails a hemimaxillectomy and includes the removal of varying amounts of soft tissue from the cheek. The hemimaxillectomy includes the lateral nasal wall, but it is often possible to leave the septum intact and attached to the remaining part of the maxilla, although there should be no hesitation in removing whatever structures may be involved in the tumour. Superiorly, the excision usually stops at a level which leaves the infraorbital rim intact. If, at operation, it is found that the tumour involves the roof of the antrum or the infraorbital rim, this is excised and, if the orbit is involved, enucleation of the eye may be required.

Only rarely does the tumour involve the overlying skin and this is more common with alveolar tumours than with those originating within the antrum, which may themselves present on the alveolus. When skin is involved, it is excised with the usual normal margin.

Occasionally, maxillary tumours extend from the orbit or nasal cavity into the ethmoidal air cells or into the base of the skull. On these occasions it is usual to carry out the operation in cooperation with a neurosurgeon, but spread to this extent implies a very poor prognosis. Enucleation of the eye is usually followed by excision of the edges of the eyelids which are sutured together and the defect is eventually covered by a prosthesis attached to spectacles. Defects in the skin can often be covered by locally mobilized flaps when small but larger defects will need imported skin from other sites.

Although it is possible to carry out a limited hemimaxillectomy without incision of to the skin, in those cases where the operation is likely to be more extensive a Ferguson incision is used. This passes upwards through the vermilion of the lip and philtrum and around the ala of the nose in the crease at the lateral margin towards the medial canthus and from there laterally under the eyelid as far as is necessary to achieve access. After excision is complete, the maxillary defect is filled with a gutta percha mould covered with a split-skin graft. The mould is held in place by some form of dental appliance which is made before the operation and which can be supported by a frontal bar and external screws or by bilateral circumzygomatic wiring, if the zygomatic arch on the affected side is intact. In some cases of excision of carcinoma of the maxilla, removal of the coronoid process on the affected side will facilitate the wearing of an obturator without affecting function.

Complications

These include salivary fistulas, breakdown of wounds with exposure of bone grafts and implants, and necrosis of flaps or pedicles. The early postoperative complication, once the airway has been ensured, is bleeding, the source of which is sometimes difficult to detect and can be rapidly fatal.

When the histological report is received after the operation, it may reveal that excision is incomplete. A decision is then made whether further surgery will be carried out or whether the patient will have radiotherapy or cytotoxic therapy. This will depend on the type of tumour and the surgeon's impression of the extent and spread of the tumour gained at operation and discussion with the oncologist.

Jaw reconstruction

Defects and deformities of the jaws occur in the following circumstances:

1. Excision for malignancy.
2. Excision of large benign tumours and cysts.
3. Severe accidents including missile injuries.
4. Osteomyelitis and osteoradionecrosis.
5. Congenital anomalies.

The aim of treatment is to restore mastication, deglutition without leak into the nose, speech and appearance.

1. After excision for malignancy

In the maxilla, restoration of function and appearance is usually achieved by fitting a prosthesis known as an 'obturator' (Figure 28.9). A rapidly constructed temporary obturator is inserted 7–10 days postoperatively when the plastic foam or mould is removed. This is replaced by an appliance, hollow for lightness, which can be of an elastic material to allow insertion into undercuts to improve retention.

Defects in the maxilla can be repaired by the use of rib grafts covered by nasal and oral mucosal flaps but this is rarely necessary as obturators are well tolerated.

In the mandible, reconstruction is complicated by the inevitable loss of soft tissue which may be extensive and will certainly include the periosteum. Lost soft tissue may be replaced by flaps.

When it is necessary to maintain space between the bone ends or to establish postoperative stability of the tongue, foreign material may be used until such time as bone grafting can be safety undertaken. It is not common practice to carry out primary bone grafting in malignant cases, because of the difficulty in achieving adequate soft-tissue coverage, and also on account of the possibility of recurrence of tumour. The presence of hidden metastases must also be considered.

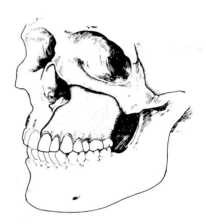

Figure 28.9 Obturator replacing resected maxilla

Many materials have been used as implants between the bone ends. These include stainless steel strip, titanium bars and Kirschner wires. The importance of symphysis replacement has been mentioned in the postoperative forward fixation of the tongue and any of these materials may be used for this. All except the Kirschner wires are attached to the fragments by screws of the same metal.

Unfortunately, many of these cases suffer perforation of mucosa or skin postoperatively in relation to the implant, or wound breakdown, in spite of prophylactic antibiotics and double suturing of the mucosa. In the mouth, this is considered to be due to the movements of the mucosa over the implant, possible impairment of blood supply and contracture of scar tissue.

However, exposure is not always a disaster as loss of the implant can be deferred until the patient is over the dangerous postoperative phase, when fibrosis will tend to hold the tongue forward as well as retaining some separation of the fragments. When it is decided eventually to replace the implant by bone, grafting can be carried out in a variety of ways.

Figure 28.10 shows grafting of the symphysis using a rib that has been notched on its inner surface to allow it to bend without breaking after skewering it with a Kirschner wire of about 2 mm diameter. The ends of the wire are inserted at least 2.5 cm into the medulla of the mandibular remnants. The ramus and gaps in the body can be replaced by iliac crest or rib grafts, which are wired into place.

Clinical experience suggests that chip and medulla grafts have a higher resistance to infection than solid pieces of bone and, to this end, grafting of these into a mesh trough has been used in the mandible. The trough can be made of titanium or Dacron and is attached by screws to the cut end of the mandible. Suitable medulla can be excavated from the iliac crest via a small incision.

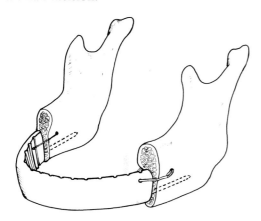

Figure 28.10 Replacement of symphysis and parts of lower jaw using rib autograft. The rib is notched on its inner surface to allow bending without fracture

Following radiotherapy, the blood supply to the soft tissues is impaired, and this will have an adverse influence on the survival of the bone graft. This difficulty may be overcome by the removal of a piece of iliac crest or rib with its arterial supply and venous drainage, followed by microvascular anastomosis of these to suitable vessels in the neck. These operations have enabled primary grafting of large sections of jaws with iliac crest and skin combined. Myocutaneous flaps with rib attached and based on pectoralis major are also used to reconstruct both jaws.

More recently, split clavicle including part of the sternal articulation and skin has been used to replace parts of the mandible, including the condyle. The microvascular anastomosis is based on the acromiothoracic axis.

2. After excision of benign lesions

Immediate reconstruction is carried out, which avoids the difficult dissection often encountered in secondary grafting.

A great advantage of benign tumour excision is that periosteum may be retained, maintaining some osteogenic potential. Iliac crest or rib grafting is used.

3. After traumatic loss

In general, immediate grafting is avoided owing to wound contamination and soft-tissue loss, and is postponed until the wound is cleanly healed and adequate soft tissue is available for cover, either by importation from other regions as pedicles or flaps or locally from advancement or rotation.

In the meantime, the space for the graft must be maintained without insertion of foreign material in the wound.

When teeth are present, the upper and lower jaws are fixed together with the wires or splints and external fixation is used to hold the bone fragments. This consists of bone screws inserted into the bone at each side of the gap and joined by external bars and joints, and is used without joining the jaws in edentulous cases.

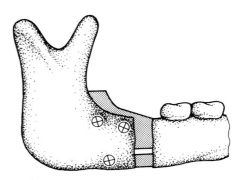

Figure 28.11 Sagittal split of the mandible may be used for correction of prognathism or retrognathism as there is a large area of bone contact between the fragments. It is now no longer necessary to fix the jaws together after this operation, as direct screwing of the fragments can take place through the cheek and gentle function is possible from the time of operation. Care, of course, must be taken not to screw through the mandibular nerve

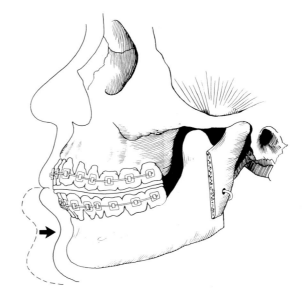

Figure 28.12 Vertical subsigmoid osteotomy for prognathism can be performed intra-orally or extra-orally. Intra-oral operation avoids potential damage to the facial nerve

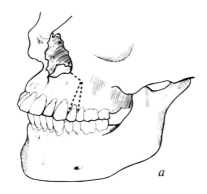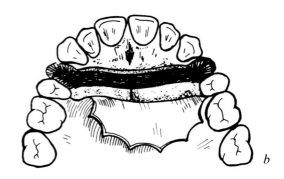

Figure 28.13 *a, b* Osteotomies can be performed on the maxilla at any level up to and including the base of skull in extreme deformity, e.g. Crouzon's disease. Minor local deformities are corrected by segmental osteotomies, e.g. anterior maxillary osteotomy

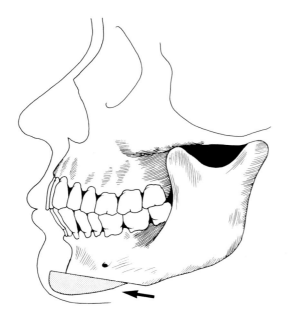

Figure 28.14 A retruded chin, with teeth in a normal bite, can be corrected by genioplasty carried out intra-orally. For protruding chins the movement is backwards

4. After osteomyelitis and osteoradionecrosis

Bone grafting may be required after oesteomyelitis once infection has been controlled and healing is complete. Periosteum is often present and the above techniques are used (see Figure 28.13a,b).

Following bone loss due to osteoradionecrosis, bone grafting is avoided, as healing is unlikely on account of poor blood supply, both in the bone and soft tissue, and the likelihood of chronic infection. The main problem is that the bone affected by radiation, and which should be excised, cannot be defined. These cases are rare but the use of bone grafts with their own blood supply must improve the prognosis.

A new technique after excision in these circumstances is to fill the defect to the angle and ramus with a rotated temporal muscle flap which has the advantage of bulk and its own blood supply.

5. Congenital anomalies (Figures 28.11–28.14)

Further reading

Cawson, R. A., McCracken, A. W. and Marcus, P. B. (1982) *Pathologic Mechanisms in Human Disease*, C. V. Mosby, St. Louis

Epker, B. N. and Wolford, L. M.(1980) *Dentofacial Deformities. Surgical-Orthodonic Correction*, C. V. Mosby, St. Louis

Jones, J. H. and Mason, D. K. (1980) *Oral Manifestations of Systemic Disease*, W. B. Saunders, Philadelphia

Rowe, N. L and Willams, J. Ll. (1985) *Maxillofacial Injuries*, Churchill Livingstone, Edinburgh

Shafer, W. G., Hine, M. K. and Levy, B. M. (1983) *Textbook of Oral Pathology*, W. B. Saunders, Philadelphia

Breast, skin grafting and lymphoedema

29

Principles of skin cover

J. Lendrum

The importance of the skin's integrity cannot be over-emphasized. Whenever breached, its function of maintaining the *milieu intérieur* is impaired. Control of body fluid and heat is lost; protection from toxic fluids, rays and solids is lost; colonization by micro-organisms is inevitable and invasion likely. The skin's sensory and expressive roles may be destroyed.

Subsequent scar contracture may destroy the function of the structures, particularly joints, which skin clothes. The patient's body image and acceptability in society may be altered, making him or her a psychiatric cripple.

The principles of skin cover are to restore form and function as rapidly as possible, leaving as inconspicuous scars as possible, without creating further avoidable damage.

The priority of skin cover must follow only maintaining the airway and control of bleeding, for without an intact skin envelope all deep structures are at risk of continuing damage, and elaborate surgery on brain, bowel or bone will have been wasted.

To heal and function skin must be live and cover live tissue. The diagnosis of dead, dying or irrevocably damaged skin and the recognition of impending or potential risks to its blood supply are therefore fundamental to its handling.

The assessment of skin viability is often difficult and can only be made from experience. The successful handling of skin can be learned, but not taught, and depends on gentleness, sympathy and imagination. The colour and feel will guide the surgeon who may persuade but never compel skin.

Basic principles of skin handling

Gentleness is the key to success. Skin should be handled as little as possible. The major enemies are tension and haematoma.

1. The patient

Patients should be as fit as possible. Diabetes, anaemia and malnutrition should be corrected. Arteriosclerosis, particularly in the legs, delays healing.

2. The operation site

This must be anaesthetic and well illuminated.

3. The surgeon

The surgeon must be comfortable and relaxed.

4. Colourless antiseptic

Skin preparation is essential. Dyes obscure colour and make vitality impossible to assess.

5. Instruments

These need be few and simple. Suction should be available. Knives should be sharp. Hooks should be used to move skin. Holding in the fingers, crushing in heavy dissecting or ratchet forceps must be avoided.

6. Retraction

This must be done cautiously. Bruising, crushing and kinking under forceful retraction will damage skin. Continuous rubbing with instruments and sutures will burn it as effectively as hot compresses or careless diathermy.

7. Skin edges and raw surfaces

These must be kept moist. Desiccated tissue dies.

8. Stop all bleeding before closure

Haematoma becomes colonized by bacteria and will form an abscess. Haemostasis must be accurate and delicate so that no damage is done to other tissue.

Where bleeding cannot be stopped completely, wounds should be drained, left open or temporarily covered by a dressing.

The commonest cause of postoperative wound sepsis is inadequate operative haemostasis and is usually an avoidable technical disaster.

9. Remove all dead and foreign material

Avascular fat, muscle and bone necrose to form abscesses.

10. Avoid all 'dead' spaces

Wounds should be closed in layers, taking care not to leave gaps which will inevitably fill with exudate or blood and form abscesses.

The minimum amount of buried suture material should be used to achieve this. Each suture acts as a potential nidus for infection. Heavy, tightly tied sutures strangulate tissue.

Where subcutaneous fat does not survive between the skin and the deep fascia or periosteum the scar will adhere to the deep layer and produce a tender, puckered, obvious, depressed scar.

11. Bony ridges and depressions

These should be smoothed down or padded over with soft tissue. Skin stretched tight over a ridge will necrose.

12. Skin edges

These must come together easily *without tension*: the ultrastructure of dermis permits a certain limited amount of stretch and no more. Attempts to force skin beyond this inbuilt limit are disastrous.

Judgement of the amount of extension possible can be learned only by experience and is critical. Hauling on skin with thicker and thicker stitches, placed further and further from the edge ending with 'deep tension sutures', shows a lack of understanding of skin physiology and a lack of judgement which ends at best in a hideous scar, but more often in wound breakdown.

If sutures cheese wire through, thicker ones will not relieve the tension. If the skin feels tight as it is closed, postoperative oedema will make it tighter still. If skin blanches as it is moved its circulation has stopped and no amount of hyperbaric oxygen will keep it alive.

There is always an alternative method of closure which should and must be used.

13. Dressings

These should protect the wound from shearing, pressure and rubbing. The old concept of the 'pressure' dressing has been shown to exert either no pressure or so much that venous return is prevented, thereby causing necrosis. The idea has been abandoned. Wound immobilization postoperatively for a few days relieves pain, reduces bleeding and reduces the risk of external forces disrupting the wound. This may be achieved by a soft, bulky gauze pad, firmly bandaged in place, which protects the patient and his or her relatives from an unsightly wound. This type of dressing may be used to absorb exudate from a wound, but it must be thick enough to remain dry on its outer surface and stable enough to remain in apposition with the wound. A wet or displaced dressing will militate against healing and must be removed.

Skin itself is the best wound dressing and often needs no additional cover. Micro-organisms will not invade a well-closed wound from outside, but will always disrupt a badly closed wound from within.

14. Sutures

These should never be tied tightly. The area enclosed in a tight suture will necrose. Postoperative oedema makes tight sutures tighter still, and the stitch will cut through the skin.

Sutures should be removed as soon as possible; no later than 48 h from the eyelids, 4 days from the rest of the face and 7 days elsewhere. If the wound then opens, it was not correctly closed in the first place.

Non-absorbable sutures should not be used on the pinna or genitalia: their removal from these sites causes agony. Absorbable materials such as catgut and Dexon should not be used as percutaneous sutures.

The methods of covering skin defects are:

1. Direct approximation.
2. Transplantation.

Direct approximation

Indications

1. Surgical incisions.
2. Clean lacerations.
3. Small areas of skin excision/loss.

Method

Plan the incision or excision to lie in or parallel to a natural skin crease where tension is least and scarring least conspicuous (Figure 29.1). There is never any indication for vertical incisions in the neck. (N.B. Abdominal striae run across the lines of minimal tension.)

Draw on the skin a plan of the proposed incision, checking the line of skin crease and the available skin that can be removed by gently pinching it up between finger and thumb.

The amount that may be excised will depend on:

1. *The site.* Beware the presternal, infraclavicular and deltoid regions, which almost invariably produce hypertrophic scars. Thick skin of the palms, sole and back are least extensible.
2. *Local anatomical landmarks.* Landmarks such as the mouth, eye or nose will limit what can be removed without distortion.
3. *The age of the patient.* The patient's age is proportional to what may be excised. Infants' skin is not extensible. Increasing age diminishes tension and produces folds of stretched skin which permit large areas to be sacrificed. Cut the skin with a sharp knife. Avoid stretching and tearing. Cut perpendicular to the surface. Bevelled edges heal with a heaped-up conspicuous scar.

Stop all bleeding.

Check tension before suturing by the feel and colour of the skin on drawing it together with hooks.

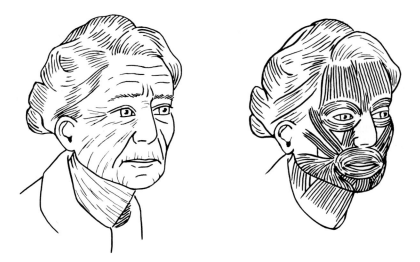

Figure 29.1   The lines of facial wrinkles which correspond to the elective site of scar direction when compared with the underlying muscles

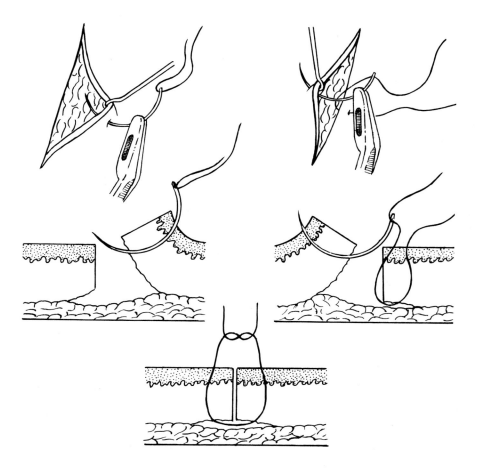

Figure 29.2   Suturing with eversion of the skin edges. Note that the skin is lifted with a hook and not crushed with dissecting forceps

If it feels tight a little more gain may be made by cautiously undermining the adjacent skin, but beware, especially in the leg, that this does not destroy the blood supply (Figure 29.2).

Check that local landmarks are not distorted, for example by pulling a lip or eyelid into ectropion.

Edge-to-edge skin apposition must be exact. Fine sutures should be used on curved cutting needles: 3/0 is the strongest needed; the maximum on the face is 5/0 and on the eyelids 6/0.

Types of direct closure

The defect must be converted into either a fusiform or wedge shape

FUSIFORM

This is usually incorrectly known as 'elliptical'. The length-to-breadth ratio should be as great as possible to avoid pleats at the apices known as 'dog ears'. A length at least four times the breadth is usually necessary. The two sides must be of equal length (Figures 29.3 and 29.4).

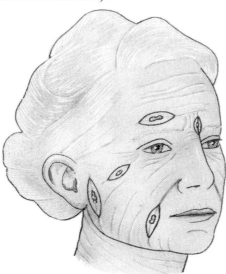

Figure 29.3 'Elliptical' facial incisions and excisions. Lines of election

WEDGE

Where skin of the margin of lip, eyelid, nostril or pinna is to be removed this may be done by excising a wedge of the full thickness of the structure.

Up to one-quarter of the length of the free margin of these may be sacrificed with a good structural and functional reconstruction by careful closure of each separate layer (Figures 29.5 and 29.6)

Contraindications

1. Where tension would result.
2. Where displacement, distortion or destruction of anatomical landmarks would result.
3. Where the resulting scar would cross a natural skin crease.

Transplantation

Definition

Movement of live tissue from one site to another where it can produce a lineage of live cells.

Types of transplantation

1. Grafts.
2. Flaps.

Indications

Wherever skin loss is too wide for the area to be closed directly.

Skin grafts

Definition

Skin removed from one site, with complete division of its vascular connections, transplanted to another site where it revascularizes by capillary anastomosis. Skin grafts are classified according to:

1. Their donor–recipient relationship.
2. Their thickness.

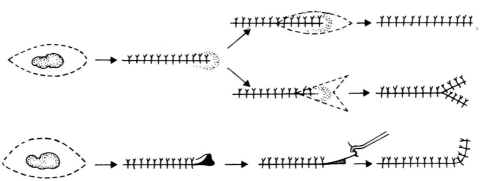

Figure 29.4 Alternative methods of excising the 'dog ear' produced by a short ellipse

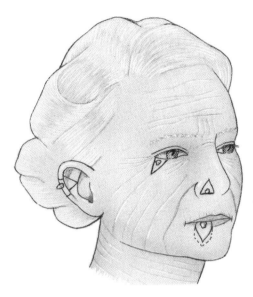

Figure 29.5 Wedge excision through the full thickness of the pinna, eyelid, nostril and lip

These two categories are the only ones which can provide permanent skin cover.

3. Homograft (American equivalent: allograft). Tissue transferred from one individual to another of the same species who is not genetically identical.

Homografts even of close genetic similarity are rejected after a very variable unpredictable time, ranging from days to months. Their use is restricted to the temporary cover of large raw areas resulting from burns, while awaiting healing of the donor site before recropping.

4. Heterograft (American equivalent: xenograft). Tissue transferred from an individual of one species to one of a different species.

Freeze-dried pigskin, often used as a skin substitute dressing in extensive burns, is incorrectly named a 'graft' as it is dead and does not 'take'.

Take. Of a graft, this means its biological reattachment to its recipient area and consequent normal physiological behaviour.

TYPES OF GRAFT CLASSIFIED BY DONOR–RECIPIENT RELATIONSHIP

1. Autograft. Tissue transferred from one part of an individual to another part of the same individual.

2. Isograft. Tissue transferred from one individual to another of identical genetic constitution (identical twins).

TYPES OF FREE SKIN GRAFT CLASSIFIED ACCORDING TO THICKNESS (Figure 29.7).

1. Split-skin grafts (partial-thickness or Thiersch grafts).

2. Full-thickness grafts (whole-thickness or Wolfe grafts).

3. Composite grafts.

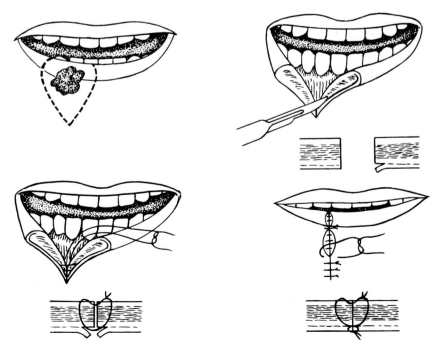

Figure 29.6 Two-layer closure of wedge excision defect of the lip

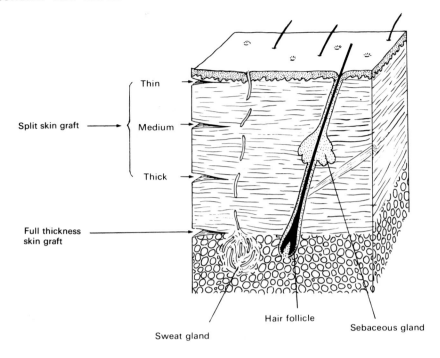

Figure 29.7 Thickness of skin grafts. Split-skin graft

1. Split-skin grafts

These consist of epidermis and the subjacent dermis, the thickness of which may be thin, intermediate or thick according to the depth of dermis included.

Indications

Split-skin grafts are used for free skin grafting where skin or mucosal defects too large to be closed directly have a base (graft bed) which has a vascular supply sufficient to support the graft.

Free grafts begin to necrose and autolyse when detached from their donor site. If they revascularize before this happens they will survive and regenerate. The recipient graft bed must therefore be capable of producing granulations.

It is, however, unnecessary and usually inadvisable to wait for granulations to form before applying a graft. Delay allows the exudate from the raw surface to be converted to fibrin through which capillaries cannot penetrate. Massive bacterial colonization of the raw surface also prevents take.

Contraindications

1. Where the raw area has an avascular bed formed by:

    (a) Bare cortical bone deprived of its periosteum (medullary bone readily accepts grafts).
    (b) Bare cartilage deprived of its perichondrium.
    (c) Bare tendon deprived of its paratenon or sheath.

    (d) Open joints or other fistulas.
    (e) Prostheses and foreign bodies.

2. On major arteries, veins and nerves which are not only unable to support grafts, but which need padding between themselves and the skin.
3. Where it is planned to do subsequent surgery. Skin grafts cannot be lifted as flaps without necrosing.
4. On irradiated tissue.
5. As a substitute for conjunctiva. Desquamating skin, especially if hairy, abrades, ulcerates, and causes vascularization and consequent corneal opacity.

Principles of split-skin grafting

1. The patient should be as fit as possible.
2. The thinner the graft the more rapidly does the critical basal cell layer revascularize so that the more certain is successful take. Thin grafts therefore take on areas where the blood supply is least good, such as fat and fibrous tissue, or where there is some bacterial contamination.

Thin graft donor sites heal more rapidly with less scarring. However, thin grafts have disadvantages when compared with thick ones:

(a) Contracture is inversely proportional to graft thickness.
(b) Thin grafts are more likely to change colour than thick ones. Mottled areas of de-, hypo- and hyperpigmentation alternate within the same

sheet of graft to a greater extent in thin than in thick grafts.

(c) Graft skin consistency is less like the normal. Thin grafts tend to remain shiny and stiff for longer.
(d) They are less robust and stand less wear and tear. They are more prone to breakdown and ulceration after trivial trauma.
(e) Hair regeneration is less common and sparser with thinner grafts.

For these reasons the thickest graft which will take on the recipient area should always be used.

Thin grafts should be used only:

(a) In the emergency cover of burns.
(b) For temporary repair, following trauma, and for covering the raw surfaces of open flaps.
(c) On chronic ulcers the beds of which cannot be excised completely.
(d) Where the defect is not over or near a joint.
(e) Where the graft is not easily seen.

Thick grafts should be used:

(a) For the release of contractures.
(b) Over or near joints.
(c) On the face, hands and feet.
(d) When the donor site can be hidden.

Wherever possible a single sheet of skin should cover the whole defect. Where there are joints in a graft, hypertrophic scars result.

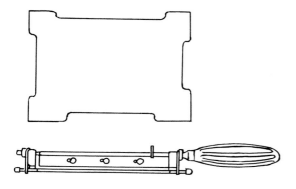

Figure 29.8 Gabarro board. Skin graft knife

Mesh grafts

Multiple parallel rows of offset slits cut in a graft permit its expansion in both planes by up to six times its original dimensions. When stretched, a latticework of holes appears, so that it resembles a string vest. The holes epithelialize within a few days by growth from the edges of the strings. These grafts are useful for:

1. Grafting areas larger than the available donor sites (i.e. burns over 30–40% of the body surface area).
2. Grafting uneven surfaces, especially small radius

convexities such as the scrotum or concavities such as the defect following maxillectomy or orbital exenteration where sheet grafts would pleat.

DISADVANTAGES

1. Until epithelialization is complete the recipient area is still open.
2. They contract more than do sheets.
3. The 'string vest' appearance remains as a permanent cosmetic deformity.

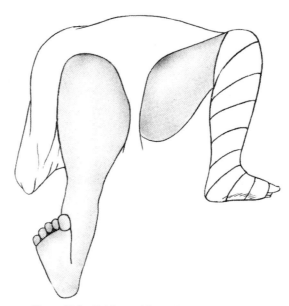

Figure 29.9 Taking a skin graft. Position of patient

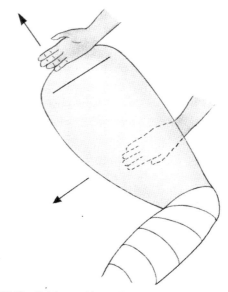

Figure 29.10 Taking a skin graft. Position of assistant. The left hand is flattening the thigh by lifting and pushing in the direction of the lower arrow. The right hand is tensing the skin by pulling in the direction of the upper arrow

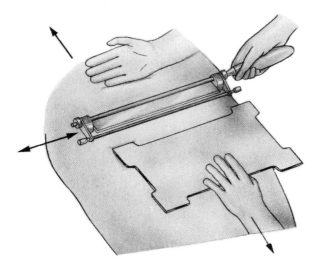

Figure 29.11 Taking a split-skin graft. Continued tension and stretching of the thigh in the direction of the arrows by the assistant is imperative, while the action of the surgeon is at right angles to this

Donor site (Figures 29.8–29.11)

Almost any area may be used as a source of donor skin. In extensive burns whatever is undamaged may be used to repair what is. Where there is a choice:

1. Like should replace like if possible. Each area of skin is unique and only identical with the same area on the opposite side of the body.
2. Broad, smooth, flat or convex surfaces are easiest to shave.
3. Take the nearest colour match. (The post-auricular sulcus and upper medial aspect of the arm are best for the face.)
4. Take the graft from an area which is normally hidden. Shaving off a layer of skin leaves permanent scarring: the thinner the graft the less conspicuous this will be.

In young girls the first choice must be the buttock. The front of the chest should be avoided.

The face, hands, feet and genitalia are always the last resort. When grafting a defect resulting from excision of a malignant neoplasm the same limb should never be used as a donor site. The donor site is a large raw wound which should be protected until healed by an occlusive dressing.

The healing time of the donor site is proportional to the thickness of graft taken from it. A thin graft donor site should heal within 7 days and a thick one within 3 weeks by coalescence of epithelium spreading from hair follicles, sebaceous and sweat glands in the base.

A thin graft donor site will leave barely detectable discoloration, whereas a thick one will always remain shiny, mottled and noticeable and is best treated by covering with a thin graft.

Skin storage

Split-skin grafts may be stored in airtight containers suitably labelled with the patient's name and date of operation:

1. For up to 3 weeks at 4°C wrapped in a gauze well wrung out of normal saline.
2. For up to 6 months at −196°C wrapped in a glycerol gauze, the container being bathed in liquid nitrogen.

The recipient area

The success of a graft is proportional to the care with which the recipient area is prepared. Ideally, this should be a clean, vascular (but not bleeding), smooth, flat, raw surface.

Fluid or solid between graft and bed will prevent take.

Haematoma and exudate are the most common causes of graft failure and must be prevented by meticulous haemostasis. Patient pressure on a raw bleeding surface is an investment which will save time, trouble and regrafting later.

Foreign bodies should be removed. Old scar tissue and exuberant, proud, oedematous, gelatinous, grey or yellow granulations must be excised, for example from chronic ulcers. This process is called 'debridement'. Irradiated tissues must be excised.

Avascular structures should be covered by vascular ones. Bare limb bone can be covered by transposing a muscle belly over it. The outer table of the skull may be sacrificed to graft the diploë. Major vessels and nerves should be covered by vascular soft tissue. Open joints or fistulas should be closed.

The base should be levelled to permit the graft to adapt accurately to its surface. Hollows fill with exudate through which capillaries cannot grow.

The wound should be free from beta-haemolytic streptococci, even small numbers of which destroy grafts. Small numbers of other pathogens do not prevent graft take, but heavy infestation by *Staphylococcus* and *Pseudomonas* may.

A single sheet of skin graft should be applied to the defect whenever possible, making sure that there are no pleats or overlaps, especially at the graft edge. When two or more sheets are needed to cover a single defect they should be butt jointed accurately. Whenever there is skin overlap both layers and the surrounding graft will die.

When a graft is put on to deep fascia the skin at the perimeter should be sewn both to the graft and the deep fascia, so that there is no shearing between them.

Check that no haematoma is present under the graft after its application. This is visible through all but the thickest grafts and must be removed before dressing.

Graft dressing

More grafts are lost because of bad dressings than are

saved by good ones. Dressings therefore should be avoided whenever possible and made simple and secure when they are used.

The objective is fixation of the graft to its bed, so that capillary anastomosis can take place without mechanical interference. This is a natural process which does not require a cover, but does need protection from shearing, sliding or rubbing forces moving the graft on its bed and protection from pressure which prevents capillary blood flow.

The 'pressure dressing' should be regarded as a means of preventing pressure necrosis of the graft rather than a means of squashing the graft home.

AIMS OF DRESSINGS

1. To immobilize the graft in relation to its bed.
2. To protect the graft from pressure.
3. To protect the patient and those around him or her from the unsightly appearance of the patch.

INDICATIONS FOR USE

1. When treating outpatients.
2. When treating an elderly or arthritic patient who must be kept mobile with a graft on the leg.
3. When grafting concavities, such as the orbit, maxilla or mouth.
4. When grafting over paratenon or tendon sheath.
5. When using mesh grafts.
6. When a double surface or a full circumferential area on trunk or limb makes it necessary partially to bear weight on the graft.

METHOD

The graft edge should be sutured accurately on the perimeter of the defect without overlap. The sutures should pass through a covering single layer of tulle gras and overlying piece of polyurethane foam sponge cut accurately to fit the defect. These sutures should be tied radially over the foam.

Where grafts are used over or near joints these should be immobilized by appropriate splints.

The dressings should be removed as soon as possible for inspection. Haematoma or seroma which have lifted small areas of graft (less than 1 cm diameter) should be expressed by nicking the graft and pressing it back to its bed. Larger areas should be removed and replaced by stored skin.

CONTRAINDICATIONS

1. On the neck.
2. On the trunk, especially the back.
3. Where a previous graft has failed.

EXPOSED GRAFTING

Grafts not covered by dressings may be watched and haematoma and seroma expressed before they cause skin necrosis.

It is not necessary to suture the graft to its bed. Immobilization of the area is mandatory. Infants need immobilization of all limbs.

The graft must be protected from accidental knocks and rubbing. Great ingenuity is required to devise protection by cages, splints or cradles.

Delayed grafting

Grafts applied to unconscious patients are often disturbed as the patient regains consciousness. Changes of blood pressure and violent movements may cause bleeding under the graft.

To obviate these risks it is preferable to store the graft and wait for 48 h before applying the graft to the defect. At operation the recipient area is prepared for grafting, but covered instead by a dressing of tulle gras and saline- or povidone-iodine-soaked gauze.

The dressing can be removed painlessly 48 h later, blood and serum washed off with a gentle saline douche and the skin graft applied as a dressing and left exposed.

Extensive burns and areas of skin loss where the debridement cannot be guaranteed should not be grafted primarily.

It is better to give a second general anaesthetic at 48 h and if necessary complete the debridement before applying the grafts.

Postoperative care

Grafts should be protected from mechanical injury and underlying fluid aspirated or expressed whenever necessary until take is assured at 8 or 10 days. By then grafts are sufficiently adherent to withstand washing and gentle handling. A graft which moves on its bed at this time has failed to take and should be replaced (remember the fault lies with the bed and not the graft).

The graft subsequently scales, crusts at the edges and becomes shiny. It does not secrete sebum. It remains insensitive and therefore liable to damage from unnoticed trauma over the next few months. It should therefore be gently but thoroughly washed and greased by massage with lanolin or ung. aquosum for at least 6 months until supple, sensitive and matt surfaced.

Grafts should be protected by clothing or barrier creams from bright sunlight for at least 12 months.

Cosmetics may be used to disguise the graft as soon as it has completely healed.

Excess scar tissue forms under grafts and their edges hypertrophy unless continuously compressed for 6 months after they have taken.

As soon as take is assured and healing complete a two-way stretch compression garment should be worn to minimize this risk. To be effective it must be worn 23 h per day.

Graft contracture continues for at least 3 months and cannot be prevented by splints. Early mobilization and compression may prevent joint stiffness, but are not always successful.

Causes of graft loss

1. Fluid between the graft and bed. Common. Usually due to bleeding.
2. External mechanical force:
   (a) Inadequate immobilization.
   (b) Poor dressing. Common. Usually due to carelessness.
3. Necrotic or avascular tissue in the graft bed. Common. Usually due to inexperienced surgery.
4. Poor general health of the patient. Usually due to diabetes or anaemia.
5. Infection. Rare. Usually due to beta-haemolytic streptococci.

Antibiotics are only indicated if beta-haemolytic streptococci are grown from the wound or an infection elsewhere merits appropriate treatment. Neither systemic nor topical antibiotics will induce graft survival if anything prevents capillary anastomosis between bed and graft.

Graft inadequacies

Failure to restore form and function may result from:

1. Graft loss.
2. Graft contracture. This flattens normal contours, bridging concavities and grooving convexities. Joint movement is limited particularly in the neck and over joint flexures.
3. Junctional scars hypertrophy and add to the contour distortion. They are inelastic. Grafts commonly wrinkle adding to the contour problem.
4. The colour seldom perfectly matches the surrounds and is often mottled.
5. Hair may be inappropriately transferred and causes problems in mucosal replacement. On the scalp, free grafts do not grow sufficient hair to match normal scalp.
6. Fragility of the grafts. Thinner than normal dermis and less subcutaneous padding make grafts less robust than normal skin. In early months they lack sensation and are therefore at greater risk of injury, especially on soles, palms and shins. Protective sensation usually returns within 2 years.

2. Full-thickness grafts

These require perfect apposition to a perfect bed for survival. Their use is therefore limited to replacement of small areas on the face and hand where the recipient area blood supply is excellent, where contracture would be disastrous, and where their excellent cosmetic and wear properties are required.

Donor sites

The post-auricular sulcus is the best match for the face. An area of skin adequate to cover an eyelid can be removed from behind one ear and the secondary defect closed by direct suture. Larger areas of less good colour match and consistency for facial reconstruction can be taken from the supraclavicular fossa, with direct closure of the donor site. This area should be avoided in girls.

Small areas can be taken from groin, elbow and wrist flexures for use on the hand with direct closure of the donor site.

On the rare occasion when large grafts are needed the secondary defect must itself be grafted by split skin.

Principles of use

Full-thickness grafts should never be used in the emergency cover of injuries. All subcutaneous fat must be removed from the grafts. They must be made to fit the defect exactly in shape and size and must be sutured under their original tension. They must be efficiently immobilized and applied under a tie-over dressing. They cannot be stored nor can their application be delayed. They will not take on granulations.

3. Composite grafts

These are unreliable and are seldom used. They consist of skin and subcutaneous fat, usually with enclosed cartilage. Their survival depends on very rapid revascularization through their cut edges and they must therefore be very small; 1 cm is a wide composite graft.

Their use is restricted to reconstruction of the nose tip, columella or alar margin by grafts from the pinna and occasionally transfer of a toe tip to a finger or thumb.

They should never be used in the emergency management of trauma. They cannot be used on granulations, stored or delayed.

No sutures should be used to hold them in place. They should be fixed by Micropore tape.

Flaps

Definition

Tissue transferred from one site in an individual to another site in the same individual while maintaining its vascular supply.

The pedicle

This is the area by which the blood supply is maintained and is a necessary part of every flap. The term 'pedicle flap' is therefore a tautology. The terms 'tube pedicle' and 'tube pedicle flap' are archaic.

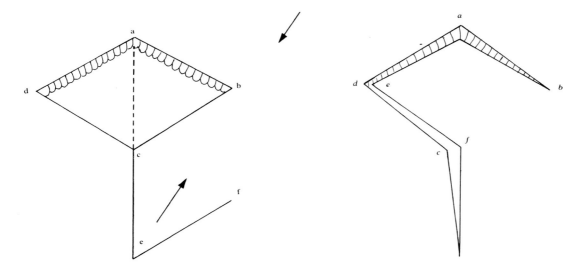

Figure 29.12 The rhomboid transposition flap. The arrows in the left-hand diagram are in the line of the skin crease

The range of flaps used in the cover of skin defects is vast and continually increasing. Even the classification is altering annually.

Indications for flap transfer

1. Where the defect has an inadequate blood supply to support a graft.
2. When a second operation in the area will be required.
3. To cover tendons which have lost their paratenon or sheath.
4. Over divided nerves.
5. For restoring contour.
6. For padding bony prominences.
7. To replace unstable scars or grafts.

Principles of raising skin flaps

The meticulous planning, lifting, transfer and postoperative care of flaps constitute the ultimate challenge to plastic surgeons and are more an art than a science.

Their use should be restricted to those aware of the full range of available methods, with the experience and intuition to choose the most appropriate, the technical skill to achieve transfer safely and who have nurses adequately trained to safeguard the flaps postoperatively. The rewards are great, but the dangers and potential disasters of flap transfer are at least as great.

Planning

The area of the defect is first accurately defined. This may be much larger than apparent, especially if pre-

vious scar or graft contracture has dragged surrounding skin into the defect.

The depth of the defect must be gauged and skin, deep tissues and mucosal lining replaced if they have been lost.

The most appropriate flap donor site is chosen, safely to fill the defect with the tissue of nearest functional and cosmetic match. Like should wherever possible replace like. In general the nearer the donor to recipient area the better will be the match.

Local flaps, which move in one stage to an immediately adjacent area, are preferred to distant flaps, of which each stage of transfer adds to their risk and may involve the patient in several weeks of immobilization in uncomfortable positions.

The safety of the flap depends on maintaining its blood supply throughout transfer.

The patient's age and ability to cooperate must be taken into account in planning the most appropriate source and method of transfer.

The flap is designed in reverse; first making a jaconet pattern of the defect and transferring this through each step of the sequence to its donor site. The flap should be designed slightly larger than the defect if more than one stage of transfer is involved, to allow for shrinkage and trimming. In transferring the pattern each stage must be checked to ensure that there is no tension or kinking, and that there is no pressure on the flap. Any of these hazards may occlude the venous return from the flap and cause its necrosis.

Types of flap

The rhomboid flap (Figure 29.12)

This is an elegant example of the local flap. It usually

has a *random* pattern blood supply (lacking an anatomically distinct arteriovenous system) and is very safe because the ratio of its length to breadth is nearly equal. If a named artery and vein run in its subcutaneous tissue it is an *axial* flap.

The main use is on the face and the trunk. *The defect* must first be converted into a parallelogram, the sides and short axis of which are equal and the acute angles of which are 60°.

The donor site is the adjacent area of skin which most readily can be spared. There are four possible areas for each rhomboid. The line of the short axis of the rhomboid (a–c) is extended on to the adjacent skin for an equal distance (c–e) and a second line (e–f) drawn from its end equal in length to, and parallel with, one side of the defect (c–b), so that the angle between the two lines enclosing the flap is 60°.

The incision is made along this line into the subcutaneous fat, which is raised with the skin and transposed through 60° to fill the defect. This involves direct approximation of points c–f, which should therefore lie in the plane of maximum skin extensibility (at right angles to the creases). The feasibility of this closure should be checked in the planning by pinching up the skin between these two points.

Latissimus dorsi flap

Originally described in 1896 to reconstruct the ablated breast, it is a historical tragedy that this flap has only recently gained the popularity that it deserves. It consists of the latissimus dorsi muscle with some, all or more than its overlying skin and is classified as a 'musculocutaneous compound flap' as it consists of more than one type of tissue.

Most areas of skin receive their blood supply from vessels that leave the muscle to traverse the deep fascia and supply the immediately overlying skin. Latissimus dorsi occupies a large area of the back, and the skin over and immediately around it can survive solely on these radiating vessels. The blood supply to the muscle comes mainly from the thoracodorsal artery, which is the terminal branch of the subscapular artery, with a corresponding venous drainage. Thus a huge area of skin, measuring up to 30 × 15 cm, may be moved on a pedicle lying in the axilla.

USE OF THE LATISSIMUS FLAP (Figure 29.13)

1. As a *local* flap to reconstruct the chest wall and breast. This is a *transposition* flap which retains a skin pedicle in addition to its thoracodorsal vessels.
2. As a *distant* flap on the:
   (a) Upper limb.
   (b) Neck (including the mucosal lining of the oesophagus and pharynx).
   (c) Face (for cheek lining or skin cover).
   (d) Head.

The required area of skin is detached entirely from its surroundings, and only its muscle attachment on its vascular pedicle is left. The flap is tunnelled under the intervening skin to reach its new destination. It is then known as an 'island flap'.

3. As a *free* flap. Skin and muscle are detached as an 'island' of which the artery and vein (which have diameters of about 2 mm) are also divided and anastomosed under the operating microscope to suitable vessels adjacent to the recipient areas, which may be anywhere on the body but are most commonly in the leg.

OPERATIVE TECHNIQUE

The defect is first outlined and a pattern transferred to the skin overlying the muscle. When used as a transposition or island flap the pattern is used to check that the proposed pedicle is long enough easily to reach the recipient area.

The skin and subcutaneous fat are incised directly down to the muscle and the cut edge of the flap sutured temporarily to the muscle to prevent shearing damage during the remaining dissection. These sutures are removed before suturing the skin to the recipient area.

The lateral border of the muscle is identified and lifted. The origins are divided from their inferior and medial attachments to the iliac crest, the lumbar fascia and the thoracic vertebrae. The muscle is turned upwards from the underlying deep muscles of the back, dividing two posterior rami of the lumbar segmental vessels in the process. Care must be taken at the inferior angle of the scapula to avoid raising serratus anterior with the latissimus muscle. The neurovascular bundle appears deep to the latissimus near the lateral border of the scapula, and its branches to serratus anterior are divided. If more mobility of the flap is needed the insertion of the latissimus to the humerus may be divided. If, as is usual, the bulk of the muscle is greater than required, its motor nerve, the thoracodorsal, may be divided to induce atrophy without prejudicing the blood supply to the overlying skin.

Both muscle and skin are sutured into their new positions. Usually the donor site can be closed by direct suture, but if a wide flap has been raised from a thin patient the secondary defect should be grafted with split skin rather than close the wound with tension. Suction drains should be inserted at the lower end of the donor site and retained until dry.

The loss of function resulting from this musculocutaneous transfer is surprisingly small. Forced adduction of the arm is probably taken over by teres major.

Management of wounds inflicted outside the operating theatre

This depends on the type and site. Such wounds

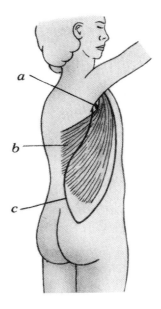

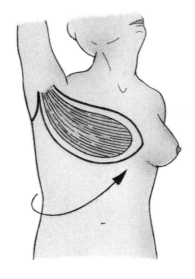

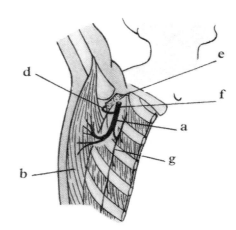

Figure 29.13 The compound myocutaneous latissimus dorsi flap. *a*, Thoracodorsal neurovascular bundle. *b*, Latissimus dorsi muscle. *c*, Outline of skin flap. *d*, Circumflex scapular vessels. *e*, Scapula. *f*, Subscapular vessels. *g*, Lateral thoracic vessels

should all be treated with suspicion and a careful eye for the unexpected. The surgeon should aim to repair the wound with full skin closure by the most rapid means, even where this means temporary loss of form or function. Reconstruction should never be attempted at the time of initial repair; it must always be planned, timed and executed under ideal conditions on a fit patient.

Avoid making the damage worse. Attend first to the airway and the blood loss. Conserve all viable tissue. Excise all dead tissue and foreign bodies.

1. Abrasions

Tattooed dirt should be scrubbed out with a wire suede brush and hydrogen peroxide. Superficial dermal damage should be covered by a non-adherent bulky dressing. If there is complete dermal destruction or friction burning a skin graft dressing should be applied.

2. Clean lacerations

Explore the full extent of the wound and repair:

1. Damaged deep structures such as tendons and nerves.
2. The wound in layers.
3. The skin after trimming dead or bevelled edges – if these can be done within the first few hours of injury. If not, await resolution of oedema before repair.

3. Crush injuries

Caused by blunt impact, these injuries produce skin and subcutaneous fat necrosis which may not be immediately obvious. Complex patterns of tissue disruption may be difficult to piece together. These wounds are usually ragged, untidy and dirty. Simplify them as much as possible. Cut back skin and subcutaneous fat to bleeding tissue. Convert a stellate to a circular or elliptical shape. Remove all haematoma and foreign bodies. Cover with a temporary graft or perform delayed primary suture (q.v.).

4. Avulsion injuries

These are injuries in which a tangential impact tears up a flap of skin. They must be treated with the utmost care. Successful healing is a tribute to surgical judgement.

Gently lift the flap, clean the whole bed and stop all bleeding. Further management depends on the site of injury:

(a) *Head, face, neck and hand.* Err on the side of conservation. Flaps of dubious viability should be laid back on their site of origin without sutures. Trim the minimum skin from the flap margins.
(b) *On the arm, trunk and genitalia.* It is preferable to excise the whole flap and replace by an immediate graft.
(c) *On the leg.* It is mandatory to excise the whole flap and replace by an immediate graft.

A major cause of morbidity is the mismanagement of the trivial avulsion flap injury of the skin of the shin in the elderly and in patients on long-term corticosteroid treatment. The anatomy of the blood supply to the skin of the shin precludes flaps surviving and they must always be replaced by grafts.

5. Projectile injuries

The management depends on the type and velocity of the missile.

(a) *Shotgun pellets.* These should be removed unless they have penetrated deeply and a search for them would inflict worse damage.
(b) *Shrapnel and low-velocity bullet wound.* The wound tracks should be laid open and drained. The missile should only be removed if it can be found without extending the damage. Skin entry and exit wounds should be excised and packed loosely open and, if extensive, grafted secondarily.
(c) *The modern high-velocity bullets.* These bullets leave tiny entry and often as tiny exit wounds, but expend their enormous kinetic energy in the deep tissues which are therefore torn up and disrupted for a wide distance round the track.

All fascial planes traversed by these bullets must be opened widely, and no attempt made to close anything except major vessels. Only in this way can oedema be prevented from occluding the circulation to the part and making damage worse. Delayed primary closure is essential.

Loss of full thickness

Lips, eyelids and noses should be closed as a wedge if possible, but loss of more than one-quarter of the free border should be closed by loose approximation of skin to mucosa. Reconstruction should only be started when healing is complete.

Burns

Nice judgement is required to determine the depth of dead tissue which should be excised and grafted. This should be done as soon as the decision is made:

1. That the depth of injury is greater than will heal under a dressing within 10 days.
2. That the patient's general condition and particularly fluid balance are stable.

Delayed primary closure

Make haste slowly is the rule for all dirty and untidy wounds. As soon as possible after injury:

1. Lay the wound open widely to allow drainage, to relieve compression, to promote blood circulation, to explore and to remove all dead, damaged and foreign material.
2. Stop as much bleeding as possible.
3. Close open joints and cover major vessels and nerves with local soft tissue. Cover exposed brain by dura or a fascial patch.
4. Loosely pack the wound with well-padded gauze, firmly bandaged.
5. Splint fractures comfortably.

After 48 h reanaesthetize the patient and remove all the packing. Check and if necessary complete the debridement. Close the skin, usually best done with a thin split-skin graft.

Correct primary or delayed primary treatment of skin loss usually obviates the need for subsequent scar revision. The majority of scars and areas of skin loss sent to plastic surgeons for revision result from inept initial management. If these simple guidelines are followed patients will be saved from delayed healing, disfigurement and demoralizing additional surgery.

Further reading

Converse, J. M. (1977) *Reconstructive Plastic Surgery*, Vol. 1, 2nd edn, W. B. Saunders, Philadelphia

Dowden, R. V. and McCraw, J. B. (1981) Myocutaneous flaps, In *Recent Advances in Plastic Surgery* (ed. I. T. Jackson), Churchill Livingstone, Edinburgh, pp. 29–44

Gillies, H. D. (1920) *Plastic Surgery of the Face*, Hodder and Stoughton, London

Grabb, W. G. and Smith, J. W. (1973) *Plastic Surgery*, 2nd edn, Little Brown, Boston

Hunt, T. K. and Dunphy, J. E. (1979) *Fundamentals of Wound Management*, Appleton-Century-Crofts, New York

McGregor, I. A. (1980) *Fundamental Techniques of Plastic Surgery*, Churchill Livingstone, Edinburgh

30

The breast

A. J. Webb

In dealing with breast disease the major consideration is for the female breast: a small section on diseases affecting the male breast is placed at the end of the chapter. Benign and malignant breast lesions are an exacting aspect of general surgical practice. They cause great anxiety for the patient and her family and it behoves the surgeon to make a precise diagnosis and deal with the problem in an efficient, compassionate and informed manner. Breast carcinoma is an unrelenting scourge; epidemiological studies would suggest that the numbers will increase. In the USA it is expected that around 10% of all women will develop breast cancer. A total of 142 900 new cases were recorded in 1987. Currently in the UK around 24 000 new patients with breast cancer will be discovered and annually some 15 000 women will require some form of treatment for recurrent disease. It is salutary to realize that 35% of women still present with inoperable disease (Roberts, 1990). There exist interesting differences in the age-adjusted incidence of breast cancer between countries. Hawaii shows a high incidence at 80/100 000 women. Oxford, England, is 54/100 000 and Osaka, Japan, 12/100 000 women. There are, in addition, inexplicable variations in incidence between social classes (Henderson *et al.*, 1984).

The possible relationship between long-term hormone replacement therapy (HRT) and the incidence of breast cancer in women beyond the age of 50 years is uncertain. It is possible that the increase which has already been documented in the USA (Grant, 1989) is related to HRT and could subsequently occur in the UK.

The past decade has witnessed an upsurge in interest and research related to the biological characteristics of breast cancer (Baildam *et al.*, 1989). There is little doubt that in the foreseeable future it will continue as a perplexing and capricious disease which requires informed and dedicated team management.

Clinical examination

Clinical errors are a frequent event in clinical practice even among experienced surgeons, and more so among general practitioners. Forrest (1974) states an accuracy rate at 80% and this level is confirmed by other studies. Carelessness in examination is seldom the reason for mistakes: the physical form of female breast tissue accounts for much of the difficulty.

Small cancers can present within a large breast and the signs are masked by breast tissue and fat. Buried cysts are often referred to outpatient clinics as an 'undoubted malignancy' because the smooth cyst outline is obscured. Areas of nodularity are often difficult to assess.

The surgeon must perform a careful clinical examination. Although there are many good descriptions and illustrations available in the literature (Handley, 1964; Widow, 1968; McKinna, 1983; Thomas and Boulter, 1984), it is worth while emphasizing certain aspects. Inspection is essential, preferably with the patient sitting up and arms braced on the hips. Contraction of the pectoral muscle will reveal any deep tethering or skin attachment and elevation of the arms above the head will confirm. Sometimes it is valuable to palpate the breasts as they lie away from the chest wall. But the best position is the patient lying on her back and the hands placed on the head or behind the neck. Careful reinspection, especially of the nipple area, should precede palpation. Feel the breast with the flat of the slightly flexed fingers

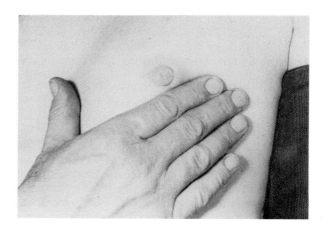

Figure 30.1 Examination of the breast using the flat of the fingers

(Figure 30.1). It is sensible to use the dominant hand but a certain degree of ambidexterity can be rewarding. A finger-and-thumb feel is sometimes needed to elucidate a deeply placed feature or to gently express discharge from the nipple. Often the patient will be successful in expressing discharge in order that smears can be made. Delicate finger-and-thumb palpation is essential to assess thickening of the lactiferous ducts.

There is much to be said for examining with a light soapy lathering of the breast skin. Alternatively 0.5% Hibitane (chlorhexidine) in spirit is equally effective. Haagensen (1971) preferred talcum powder for a similar purpose. Skin friction is diminished and the palpatory features are significantly enhanced. Cysts in particular are far easier to identify by this simple trick.

Axillary examination is even more unreliable than breast palpation. There is at least a 30% error in feeling the axillary contents (Fentiman and Mansell, 1991). Provided the axillary fascia is relaxed by the position of the arm and the examiner's fingers pass gently high into the axilla, sweeping its contents against the medial axillary wall, then there is some chance of a useful yield. It is easy to neglect the axillary tail and the pectoral nodes lying close to it. The supra- and infraclavicular regions must be carefully palpated.

Two-view mammography employed in the diagnostic breast clinic setting at the correct age (greater than 35 years) and accepting well-recognized limitations is essential for proper breast practice.

A sensitivity rate for defining breast cancer of between 80% and 90% is commonly achieved.

For national breast screening in the UK, single oblique mediolateral films are taken with true lateral, craniocaudal and magnification views being added should the patient be recalled for further assessment. A proportion of women find mammography an uncomfortable procedure.

NHS breast screening programme

From the burden of statistics which consistently record around 24 000 new cases of breast cancer, 15 000 deaths per year, 15 000 women alive with recurrent and metastatic disease and the fact that England and Wales have the highest standardized mortality rate at 28.4/100 000 (1985), it came as no surprise that breast screening was proposed.

Political, lay and some medical pressure was irresistible. The Report on Breast Cancer Screening by a working party chaired by Professor Sir Patrick Forrest was published in 1986 (HMSO) and formed the basis for the National Health Service Breast Screening Programme (NHSBSP). It is a comprehensive document and essential reading for general surgeons at all levels. In January 1991 a further report 'Breast Cancer Screening 1991: Evidence and Experience since the Forrest Report' was published from a committee study under the chairmanship of Professor Martin Vessey (Breast Cancer Screening, 1991a). A letter from the Chief Medical Officer (Breast Cancer Screening, 1991b) affirmed the conclusions of this publication.

The Forrest Report was based on previous trials of breast screening from New York, Sweden and the Netherlands which purported to demonstrate a reduction in cancer mortality of 30% at 10-year follow-up.

The programme, which began in Avon during July 1989, involved single lateral oblique mammograms for women aged between 50 and 64 years and hoped for at least a 70% take-up from invited women. It was estimated that for a target population of 41 150 women, 13 716 would be invited each year of a 3-year round which would then be repeated. If 10 800 women were screened, then 1080 (10%) would be recalled for assessment and further radiographs: 162 (1.5%) would be referred for surgical biopsy and 59 (0. 55%) breast cancers be detected. At the end of the first year of Avon Screening, 11 000 women attended, 27 palpable invasive cancers were discovered and 97 impalpable mammographically suspicious lesions were outlined of which 36 were malignant (11 non-invasive, 25 invasive). A total of 63 cancers were therefore brought to light in 1 year.

The Forrest Report has been the subject of much criticism (Skrabanek, 1988; Roberts, 1989; Rodgers, 1990) because of overstating the potential value of screening at a significant cost of resources to implement the programme (especially surgical requirements). The general conclusion of Vessey's committee was supportive and emphasized the need to consolidate the programme. Additional evidence for the benefit of screening has been published (Chamberlain et al., 1988; Collins, 1991).

It would be unrealistic to obscure the facts. Problems have arisen in administration, radiology, surgical management and organization, histopathological diagnoses and psychological disturbances in the patients. A consistent dedicated team, to include a nurse counsellor, is obligatory and regular monthly audit sessions are both essential to good practice and invaluable educationally.

A few of the surgical aspects are itemized:

1. The attendees are supposed to be fit, asymptomatic women. Due to screening they may be 'converted into patients'. They are sometimes both unfit and demonstrate obvious clinical breast cancer detectable without the aid of mammography.
2. Minimal clinical features (nodularity or slight deformity) may be highlighted by a visible mammographic change and the diagnosis of cancer becomes clear.
3. It is possible, at surgical assessment, to confirm the presence of cancer by fine-needle aspiration cytology (FNAC) of both palpable and impalpable solid lesions.
4. The potential of complementary breast ultrasound examination is affirmed by a sensitivity in malignancy of around 70–80%. The status of stereotactic FNAC is more uncertain but worthy of investigation (Masood et al., 1990).
5. Guided biopsies for impalpable mammographic abnormalities become commonplace. They de-

mand skilled radiological needle guiding; stereo-tactic sense from the surgeon; good theatre and radiological organization; and a simple but reliable scheme for specimen marking to assist and not confuse the histopathological team.

6. Adequate theatre sessional time is necessary to allow unhurried surgery coupled with the opportunity for teaching junior surgeons.

7. For mammographic calcification, adequacy of excision is a problem when ductal carcinoma in situ (DCIS) and/or lobular carcinoma in situ (LCIS) are reported and the edge biopsies are not histopathologically clear. Further excision is then necessary for at least a 5 mm measured clearance. Should the second procedure be inadequate, then total mastectomy emerges as the only sensible choice. Opinion differs regarding axillary surgery for pure DCIS (Silverstein et al., 1990) as the incidence of involvement is low. Perhaps a limited level 1 biopsy will become the vogue. If micro-invasion is discovered, then a level 1 and 2 clearance carries much sense.

8. A paradoxical situation may arise in perhaps 10% of impalpable cases. Serial histopathology results oblige the surgeon to offer total mastectomy to a woman; whereas had she presented with a small (<2 cm diameter) invasive tumour at a favourable anatomical site, then segmental mastectomy (wide local excision or quadrantectomy) with node dissection and breast irradiation could be the favoured procedure. For widespread minimal disease, more extensive surgery than that acceptable for an invasive tumour!

9. The distinction between well-defined, well-differentiated breast cancer and cryptic mature fibroadenoma is not always reliable from mammography and ultrasound. Equally, if a lump is palpable, whatever the radiological features FNAC should always be carried out. The same comments apply to the distinction between small scirrhous cancers and complex sclerosing lesions (Page and Anderson, 1987).

10. The psychological reactions from some patients and relatives can be difficult to handle, especially as the service is well organized and free! Some women and their spouses are frankly annoyed at having to be brought back to the Screening Centre for further radiographs and surgical assessment. Engendered anxiety, especially where there is unavoidable delay in securing admission for guided biopsy, leads to unreasonable criticisms of nursing and medical staff.

11. In the absence of knowledge on the natural history of DCIS and significant misgivings on the good sense of a trial proposed for surgical management (Hamilton and Buchanan, 1990), it is difficult to counsel patients as to the wisest surgical procedure.

12. Within the current controversy over breast screening, a sensible attitude for surgeons to adopt is to regard the exercise as an important experiment.

Breast abscess

Three types of breast abscess occur. First, infection of an areolar tubercle of Montgomery. This presents like a boil and is incised. Occasionally, chronic folliculitis develops and is difficult to treat. Chronic abrasion may be the cause (Levit, 1977).

Secondly and more frequent is inflammation connected with the nipple area and elsewhere in the breast related to the mammary duct ectasia/periductal mastitis (MDE/PDM) syndrome. This important pathological entity may be acute or subacute. Rarely, a four-quadrant swelling develops, accompanied by erythema and 'peau d'orange', simulating an inflammatory carcinoma. Rapid and precise diagnosis is imperative and for this purpose FNAC is invaluable and sensitive.

Ectatic inflammation can respond to a combination of antibiotics. Flucloxacillin and metronidazole are helpful and may assist in partially resolving the sepsis into localized collections of pus which are then drained. Recurrent abscesses are not unusual and each requires wide drainage. The more usual sub-areolar sepsis forms a localized abscess which is drained through a direct incision. Unfortunately a para-areolar or mammary duct fistula may follow and subsequent surgical excision will become necessary (Hadfield, 1960; Hughes et al., 1989).

Thirdly, intramammary abscess may develop during lactation. The process begins as a congested and obstructed area of the breast due to nipple oedema from a fissure or a 'creamy plug' obstructing a duct orifice.

Early local treatment with heat, expression of milk and systemic antibiotics may induce resolution. The infant feeds from the other breast. After 3–4 days, persistent induration with oedema should lead to aspiration of pus with an 18-gauge needle and incision.

Incision is made over the induration and the cavity entered to evacuate the pus. All locules are broken down by digital dissection. The cavity is lightly packed and a rubber corrugated drain left in situ. A second, dependent cannula incision is necessary if the cavity is large. A plastic stent is favoured for facilitating drainage (Hughes et al., 1989).

Occasionally, a deep chronic abscess deriving from an infected cyst, localized ectatic infection or lactational abscess overtreated with multiple antibiotics presents clinically as a hard dominant mass. The unusual lesion, breast granuloma, can similarly appear sometimes with erythema nodosum (Koelmayer and MacCormick, 1976). A perverted tissue reaction to the MDE/PDM syndrome may be the cause of this lesion. FNAC will usually reveal the true nature of such a mass, but excision is sometimes required.

Biopsy of the breast

Biopsy is the removal of tissue or cellular material from an organ during life for the purposes of pathological examination. Following clinical examination it is the essential sequel to establish a definitive diagnosis. It is the classic and widely held view that such proof must be histological. An increasing number of practitioners now accept cytological diagnosis alone (Dixon *et al.*, 1984). Controversy abounds regarding the most convenient, safe and accurate method of biopsy (Burn, 1973; Editorial, 1977; Rilke, 1984). Needle biopsy and surgical procedures are the two contenders:

1. Needle biopsy embraces three differing techniques.
   (a) Fine-needle (18–23 gauge size) aspiration cytology, incorporating some form of constant suction obtains a yield for cytological examination and enjoys scattered but increasing popularity in Europe, the USA and Great Britain (Grubb, 1981; Trott, 1983).

   Its accuracy in skilled hands is undeniable and too often its detractors have failed to employ the technique correctly (Magarey and Watson, 1976; Davies *et al.*, 1977). It possesses many advantages, being supremely convenient, atraumatic, swift to report and economical. Very small (0.5 cm diameter) breast lumps, regional lymph nodes and soft-tissue deposits are all suitable for this technique (Webb, 1982; Smallwood *et al.*, 1985).
   (b) Large-needle (Tru-cut style) biopsy employs a small trocar and cutting cannula principle to remove a core of tissue from the breast for histology (Roberts *et al.*, 1975: Davies *et al.*, 1977; Baum, 1981; Baildam *et al.*, 1989). The procedure necessitates a small skin incision under local anaesthesia and is reported to be rather inaccurate for lumps less than 2 cm in diameter.
   (c) Drill biopsy (Burn *et al.*, 1968) aims for a similar tissue yield by an ingenious high-speed pneumatic drill apparatus (Morrison and Deeley, 1955). Like large-needle biopsy, this procedure is a compromise to obain histological material while avoiding surgical incision or excision.
2. Incision biopsy for cancer has received the support of eminent surgeons in the past (Haagensen, 1971). For possible benign dysplastic lesions, incision is the rule; there seems to be no sense in wide excision of an area of fibrocystic dysplasia when the aim of the intervention is to sample the area in doubt for histological proof of its innocence or otherwise. The same principle applies to mammary ectasia and excision of the major duct system.
3. Excision biopsy is ideal for the removal of fibroadenomata, small cysts and clinically uncertain nodules less than 5 cm in diameter (Hughes, 1982).

For benign lumps, diagnosis and treatment are achieved. In some circumstances, marginal local excision prior to total mastectomy and axillary clearance is required. Wide local excision (2–3 cm margin), segmental resection or quadrantectomy is favoured by some surgeons for small cancers (up to 2 cm diameter) previously identified by needle biopsy. Medially placed cancers are very suitable for this approach (Greening, 1983). Excision biopsy coupled with frozen or urgent paraffin section is popular where needle biopsy has failed, is indeterminate or is not used. Malignancy having been confirmed, it is then possible to discuss with the patient which surgical approach she favours (Cady, 1989).

There is an increasing tendency in British surgeons to employ minimally invasive biopsy procedures. FNAC still suffers from some prejudice and there is a relative lack of trained cytologists, but it is the least traumatic procedure (Webb, 1970, 1975; Coleman, 1982; Melcher *et al.*, 1984; Dixon *et al.*, 1987). Each biopsy procedure is now described in more detail.

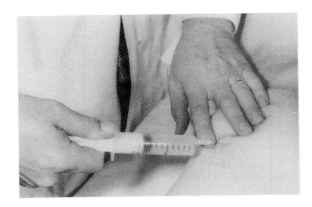

Figure 30.2 Fine-needle aspiration cytology of a lump in the breast which is steadied by the fingers of the left hand. The braced-thumb method of constant suction is shown

Fine-needle cytology (FNAC or ABC)

The lump or lumpiness is steadied with the fingers of the left hand and a disposable no. 1 (21-gauge) needle, with a 20 ml syringe attached. Draw back 2–3 ml of air into the syringe. The needle is then delicately inserted after cleaning the skin. Constant suction is produced either by a syringe pistol or more simply by the braced thumb (Figure 30.2). The needle is moved delicately through the lesion in several directions, sucking tissue juice and cells into the bore of the needle and syringe stem. Suction is reduced before withdrawing the needle. The contents are carefully blown onto slides and spread into smears. Rapid air drying is essential, followed by fixation in methanol (5 min). Giemsa staining gives uniformly reliable results, but wet fixation and Papanicolaou staining are performed by some cytologists. The procedure should be repeated at a different site if required.

The total biopsy procedure from puncture to microscopy and diagnosis can be achieved well within 30 min in perhaps 80% of breast lumps. This procedure may be applicable in a breast clinic to inform the patient of her probable diagnosis and treatment plan at the first visit. This style of practice demands considerable resources and is controversial in its concept (Nicholson *et al.*, 1988).

Fine-needle aspirates have been found suitable for refined immunocytochemistry to measure ER receptor status (Coombs *et al.*, 1987; Lundy *et al.*, 1990).

Large-needle and drill biopsies (Baum, 1981; Hughes, 1982; Baildam *et al.*, 1989)

Cutting edge cannulas and trocars, together with drill biopsies, demand a very similar procedure. Common to both styles is the insertion of local anaesthetic and a 3–5 mm skin incision to allow entry into the breast tissue. The large needle is inserted into the lesion which is steadied in the standard manner. The needle is thrust into the breast mass and rotated to obtain a core of tissue. Syringe suction is applied to withdraw the specimen. The drill biopsy needle attached to the apparatus is inserted through the skin and the drill speed adjusted to obtain a cut core. The needle is detached and syringe suction applied to withdraw as for large-needle biopsy. The biopsy specimen is gently extruded onto a slide and carefully transferred to fixative. The standard and variable laboratory processing time for paraffin sections applies, but frozen sections may be feasible if necessary. A sensitivity rate of 95% is reported (Baildam *et al.*, 1989).

Excision biopsy

For small, superficially placed lesions in selected patients, sedation and local anaesthesia is acceptable and widespread office practice in the USA. For the majority, general anaesthesia is preferred, although this can be arranged on an outpatient, day-stay basis. The patient is towelled with the arm abducted on a board. The incision depends on the site of the lesion, its probable nature and the size of the breast. Ideally para-areolar circumferential skin crease or marginal (Galliard–Thomas) incisions are made for cosmetic and aesthetic reasons, provided that there is no likelihood of malignancy (Figure 30.3). After skin incision, fat is reflected to reveal the breast tissue proper. The lesion is relocated and this may be difficult as all breast lumps become less obvious once the skin is incised. The breast tissue is held with Poirier or Allis tissue forceps. For a very mobile lump, fixation with a no.1 needle is recommended. Using sharp dissection the breast is incised and the lesion exposed. Three alternatives are then possible:

1. For fibroadenoma, the lump is totally excised with a narrow (1–2 mm thick) margin of breast tissue. Because of their extreme mobility fibroadenomas do carry the risk of eluding excision unless a precise technique is followed.
2. For fibrous dysplasia, a sample is excised, preferably in a coronal rather than a radial segmental direction. It is sometimes possible to 'shape' the residual edges of dysplastic breasts after excision to improve cosmesis.
3. If careful palpation of the cavity reveals suspicious induration, then this should be removed *in toto*.

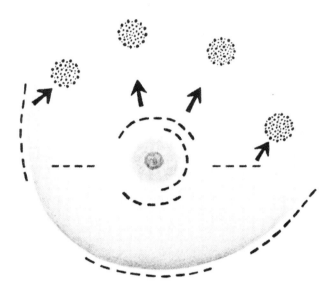

Figure 30.3 Excision biopsy. Para-areolar, circumferential skin crease or marginal (Galliard–Thomas) incisions are made for cosmetic and aesthetic reasons

If cysts are found during biopsy they can be aspirated or emptied by incision. Painstaking haemostasis is essential following biopsy. Obvious major vessels on the surface are ligated with 3/0 Vicryl or catgut; smaller bleeding points are coagulated with diathermy. To facilitate this, the edges of breast tissue are held up with tissue or artery forceps and small retractors to expose the depths of the biopsy space. Drainage is a matter of judgement. Large cavities are best drained using thin corrugated rubber. The drain is tethered with a silk suture, and a 3/0 prolene, 'pullout' suture tied after removal of the drain adds neatness. Breast tissue should never be sutured after excision. The fat may be loosely sutured before skin closure to avoid an unsightly hollow. Skin suture by fine silk or nylon gives tidy results, but if a thick corium dermis is present, then a subcuticular 4/0, polyglycolic or monofilamentous suture gives excellent results.

If doubt exists as to whether the lesion is malignant, the biopsy incision must then lie within the bounds and line of a possible subsequent mastectomy or further local excision.

Incision biopsy

This procedure should rarely be required in current practice. It may be considered for a possible malignant mass greater than 5 cm in diameter. The aim is to obtain a representative sliver of tissue for macroscopical frozen section and diagnosis. Incision biopsy is an unsatisfactory procedure. The incision should avoid obvious subcutaneous veins and be as small as is feasible, cutting directly through skin, fat and breast tissue. It is important that the depth of the incision should reach the cancer. Diathermy haemostasis is ideal and the skin should be closed with a tight inverting suture, hopefully to prevent contamination during the mastectomy. Some surgeons prefer to insert a swab soaked in a cancerocide such as cetrimide before skin closure.

Guided excision biopsy (Michell and Ebbs, 1989)

The inception of a National Breast Screening Programme has increased the number of guided breast biopsies for impalpable mammographically revealed densities or suspicious calcifications.

Following assessment by a designated breast surgeon aided by magnification views and clinical examination, the patient is fully informed. Prior to operation the patient attends the X-ray department with all relevant films. A specialist radiologist inserts a thin-needle trocar into the lesion site and confirms correct positioning by mammography. The trocar is removed, leaving the needle *in situ* and fixed beneath a dressing. Several commercial types of needle are in current use.

The patient appears in theatre with the needle in position. The dressing is carefully removed without dislodging the needle and the site prepared. It is essential for the surgeon to study the guided films in order to plan the incision. This usually lies below the needle entry. A circumferential incision is made and the skin edges reflected for 1–2 cm, allowing the needle to be drawn through into the wound, and a small tissue forcep (Allis or Poirier) applied to fix the surface site of needle entry. By scalpel or scissor dissection a block of tissue is removed to include the guiding needle and lesion. It is helpful to palpate this block during the excision process.

The specimen and mammograms are sent to the department of radiology for confirmation of excision. If the lesion has been missed, then further excision is carried out and the specimens X-rayed. For some calcified lesions it may be helpful to mark the orientation of the block by designated silk sutures. The cavity is inspected and small edge biopsies taken for supplementary breast pathology. The wound is closed with drainage. All material is submitted to the specialist breast pathology department.

Mammodochectomy

This procedure is excision of the major duct system. It is a simple and usually effective operation which was initially described by Adair and Urban and popularized in Great Britain by the reports of Hadfield (1960, 1968). The indications for it are troublesome mammary duct ectasia, para-areolar fistula, which is a complication of ectasia, and intraduct papillomata. Inverted nipples can also be corrected by this procedure. Some surgeons prefer the operation of microdochectomy for possible intraduct papilloma in young women, having localized and cannulated the offending duct. Others prefer to remove all the ducts in those over the age of 40 in the light of sound evidence that more than one duct is commonly involved (duct papillomatosis).

Mammary duct ectasia or the periductal-mastitis syndrome is a prevalent and perplexing disease; its incidence is probably underestimated and it frequently passes unrecognized. The aetiological basis of the underlying abnormality is poorly understood and some surgeons prefer the term 'periductal mastitis' (Thomas *et al.*, 1982; Dixon *et al.*, 1983; Hughes *et al.*, 1989). In its milder forms the clinical presentation may be as follows:

1. Pain in the nipple and surrounding breast.
2. Discharge from the papilla; varying in amount and character.
3. Small tender areas in the sub- and para-areolar region.
4. Progressive retraction of the papilla
5. Mild, self-resolving episodes of sub-areolar inflammation.
6. A discrete breast lump.

Confirmation of the diagnosis can usually be made on clinical grounds by palpating the breast ducts, supplemented by mammography, fine-needle aspiration cytology of any masses and microscopy of the nipple discharge. The indication for surgery depends on the severity of the symptoms and the presence of a discrete lump.

Mammary duct fistula following abscess formation demands intervention, whereas intermittent nipple discharge seldom requires it unless atypical cells are found by cytology or the discharge is persistent and a social nuisance.

In young women with abscess formation, some surgeons prefer to drain the abscess and later excise the single involved duct (Hughes *et al.*, 1989).

Technique (Figure 30.4)

The nipple is stretched to expand the area and small skin scratches are made to ensure precise suturing. Usually an inferior hemicircumferential skin incision is made at the precise junction between areola and

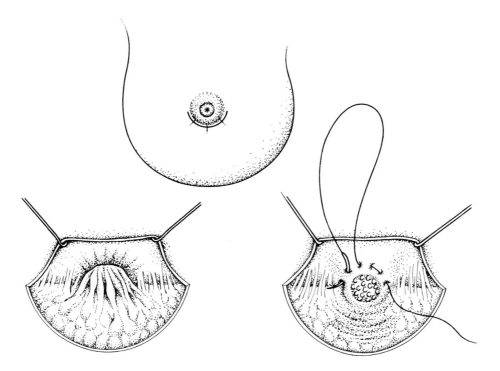

Figure 30.4 Mammodochectomy. Excision of the major duct system or lactiferous sinuses through a peri-areolar skin incision

breast skin proper. The areola is elevated by skin hooks. Very careful scalpel dissection is begun towards the papilla remaining between the ducts and smooth muscle corium of the areola. Thickened ducts are easy to see and are detached from the papilla by sharp dissection. The duct cluster is held with an artery forceps. Once the papilla has been cleared the ducts are incised at their emergence from the breast tissue. If necessary, and it often is so, thickened breast or a sub-areolar mass of uncertain nature is excised. Where possible the ducts are ligated with fine catgut or underpinned as they emerge from the breast stroma. Gentle bimanual pressure on the breast will usually reveal large abnormal ducts by the issuing discharge. This stage of the operation can be technically difficult. Fine ligature and diathermy haemostasis having been achieved, everting sutures of 4/0 plain catgut are inserted behind the papilla to lightly protrude it. In some circumstances, and particularly in recurrent para-areolar fistula formation, it is worth attempting to close over the breast surface by gently suturing the edges together with fine (2/0 or 3/0) catgut sutures.

Drainage may be necessary using a thin corrugated rubber strip. Skin closure is by 3/0 prolene sutures or by subcuticular material. The vascularity of the mammillary skin may be impaired if the dissection is excessive or carried too close to the corium of the areola.

However carefully performed, the operation sometimes fails as the fistula recurs. Further excision is required and it may be advisable to leave open the wound and pack with gauze soaked in antiseptic. The wound is sutured secondarily. Occasionally mastectomy is needed.

Microdochectomy (Hughes *et al.*, 1989; Berna *et al.*, 1990)

A bloodstained nipple discharge is uncommon and happens less frequently than patients will allege. It is often caused by an intraduct papilloma and thickened ducts may be felt. A distinct mass and a bloody discharge are far more suggestive of intraduct and invasive carcinoma. Cytology of the discharge is essential and will confirm the presence of erythrocytes together with clumps of benign and often atypical papillary epithelium. Carcinoma cells are distinctive and easy to identify (Fung *et al.*, 1990). Mammography should be arranged, but its sensitivity for demonstrating malignancy is low (Welch *et al.*, 1990).

Ductograms are sometimes diagnostic. If the

offending duct can be reliably located, then under anaesthesia a lacrimal probe is inserted into it and by a radial incision extending from papilla to areola the duct and papilloma are excised. A no. 15 scalpel blade is ideal for this dissection. Subcuticular 4/0 plain catgut or 4/0 interrupted prolene sutures will give an excellent cosmetic result.

Carcinoma of the breast

The surgical alternatives

Once the diagnosis of carcinoma has been established by some form of biopsy, then there is a choice of procedures. There are five operations currently favoured.

1. Limited excision with only enough surrounding tissue to allow a clear margin together with axillary dissection of variable extent: otherwise known as 'lumpectomy' or 'tumourectomy' (Harris *et al.*, 1981; Hermann and Esselstyn, 1982; Fisher *et al.*, 1985).
2. Segmental mastectomy or quadrantectomy involving a wide removal of the cancer to include a palpable margin of 2.5–3 cm normal breast tissue (Veronesi *et al.*, 1981). Through one incision, it may be possible to dissect the axilla also – or a separate approach is dictated depending on the site of the primary. In the Veronesi procedure, pectoralis minor is removed together with the apical and central axillary contents.
3. Simple or total mastectomy where axillary nodes remain.
4. Extended simple or total mastectomy where axillary node sampling or clearance is added (Forrest, 1982).
5. Subradical or Patey mastectomy where complete axillary dissection is attempted with removal of the breast and pectoralis minor. Pectoralis major is preserved. Alternatively, pectoralis minor is detached from its origin and left *in situ*.

Classical radical mastectomy is probably never performed in the UK at the present time.

1. Lumpectomy

2. Segmental mastectomy and axillary dissection

These procedures are followed by adjuvant radiotherapy to the breast region alone. The techniques are controversial and require a very precise surgical skill. Some 10-year surgical results in respect of sizeable series have been published (Brady and Bedwinek, 1984; Fisher *et al.*, 1985). For a variety of reasons an attempt to construct a controlled randomized trial comparing them with extended simple mastectomy and irradiation for both modalities has proved difficult.

Perhaps these procedures are acceptable practice in the following circumstances:

(a) A patient who refuses total mastectomy.
(b) An elderly unfit patient with a limited life expectancy from other causes.
(c) A small cancer within a large breast without mammographic evidence of multicentricity.
(d) Biologically favourable (low and intermediate grade) biopsy-proven cancers of size <2 cm diameter on mammographic films.
(e) A cancer placed at least 3 cm from the areolar edge.
(f) Most medially placed cancers.

Clinical judgement should be exhibited in all cases. In the proven presence of systemic disease, segmental resection might remain the ideal method of controlling local disease.

The patient is towelled as for mastectomy. It is necessary to remove a modest skin ellipse to include the biopsy site. The skin edges and fat are reflected and a segment of breast including the growth is removed, incising 2.3 cm beyond palpable limits. It may be possible to extend the incision to include the axillary biopsy. Otherwise a separate skin crease incision from the pectoralis major margin to the anterior border of latissimus dorsi is made. Despite precise haemostasis by ligature and diathermy, drainage is wise. A vacuum suction system is possibly best avoided. The hollow induced by the suction is cosmetically ugly and a corrugated drain is better. With long incisions extending to the axilla, two suction drains left for 2–3 days only may suffice and leave minimal distortion.

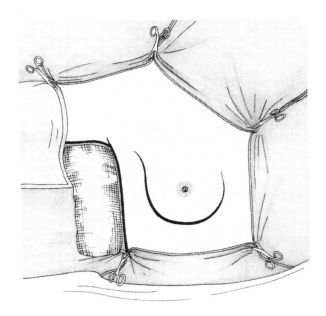

Figure 30.5 A towelling arrangement suitable for right mastectomy. For Patey or subradical mastectomy, the arm should be towelled separately

3, 4. Simple and extended simple mastectomy
(Figures 30.5 and 30.6)

These are popular operations and rightly so. The cosmetic and functional results are excellent and the long-term results match those obtained by more radical procedures. Provided the diagnosis of carcinoma has been confirmed by preliminary needle or excision biopsy the patient can be towelled with the arm abducted. The area is painted with antiseptic and towelled. It is necessary to paint the arm, axilla and posterolateral chest most carefully. The chest should lie on a sterile waterproof sheet covered by a towel; a roll of cottonwool wedged into position between chest wall and table preserves sterility there and absorbs oozing from the posterior skin flap. Raising the skin flaps requires special care.

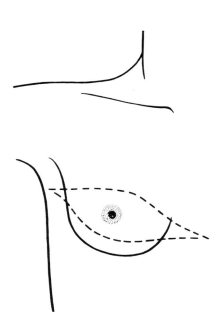

Figure 30.6 Diagram of mastectomy incision adequate for simple, extended simple and Patey operations

Mammography has confirmed the anatomical fact that two elements comprise the panniculus adiposus overlying the breast, namely the subcutaneous fat proper and the breast fat. The latter is looser and coarsely lobular. When raising the skin flaps, optimal vascularity is preserved by the dissecting between these two layers; scalpel or curved scissor dissection is equally effective, it is a matter for personal preference. Primary healing is anticipated, so a reliable guide to the amount of skin excision with the breast is helpful. The author marks the skin incisions with Bonney's blue dye, taking a clearance of around 2–3 cm from the tumour edges.

First, the upper flap is raised, lifting the skin by hooks applied to the corium dermis (Figure 30.7). Alternatively, the skin edge may be held in swabs.

Elevation of the skin and counter-pressure on the breast over a swab reveals the correct tissue plane. Clearance extends to pectoralis major beyond breast tissue to the level of the second costal cartilage, passing laterally to the border of pectoralis major. For simple or total mastectomy the suspensory ligament of the axilla (brachiopectoral fascia) is not opened but the breast tail, usually with adherent lymph nodes, is detached downwards from serratus anterior. The posterior flap is elevated, beginning laterally. Counter-traction between breast and skin edge allows dissection to reach the anterior border of latissimus dorsi and entry into the axilla posteriorly. The subscapular vessels and nerve to latissimus are sought and preserved.

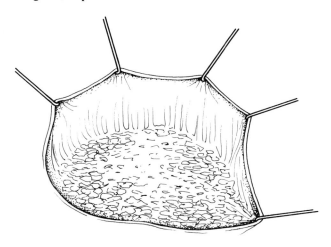

Figure 30.7 Elevation of the upper mastectomy flap, illustrating the separation between the fatty components of the skin and of the breast

For extended simple mastectomy, once the lateral half of the anterior flap is raised the axilla may be entered anteriorly. From above, the breast including the pectoral fascia is stripped away from the muscle. The anterior border of pectoralis major is elevated and the suspensory ligament opened to expose the axillary contents. The simplest manoeuvre at this stage is to dissect all the gross axillary contents from the vein downwards to the axillary tail. Alternatively a sample of nodes is taken. The axillary fat and nodes are dissected away by delicate scissor work, ligating the central or apical vein of the axilla early. By pledget and a scissor this tissue mass is detached from the axillary walls and includes any subscapular nodes, but avoiding damage to the neurovascular bundle. The lateral thoracic vessels and nerve to serratus anterior are sought and preserved: the intercosto-brachial nerve and lateral cutaneous branch of third dorsal segment are often preserved. Laterally the axillary tissue is freed from axillary skin and the tendon of latissimus dorsi. Haemostasis is by careful ligature and diathermy to small bleeding points, following which the axillary contents and breast are drawn downwards to meet the already partially detached breast lying over the pectoralis major. The raising of the lower flap is then completed and the breast is removed from above downwards, ligating perforating vessels with 2/0 and 3/0 silk. Both inferiorly and over the anterior axillary fold 'scissor pruning' of fat may be required to ensure a pleasing cosmetic result.

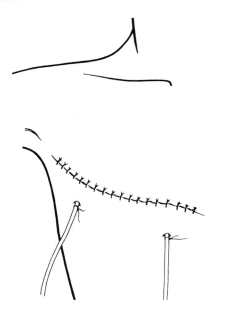

Figure 30.8 Skin suture and drainage following simple mastectomy

The skin edges are assessed for apposition and vascularity; trimming may be necessary. Marker sutures are placed along the line of the incision to ensure alignment and two vacuum suction drains are inserted through the lower flap, one to lie medially and the other in the axilla (Figure 30.8).

The suction drains are removed when drainage is minimal and the sutures at 8 days, provided healing looks adequate. Occasionally there is scabbing and superficial loss at the edge of the upper flap. Some povidone-iodine paint is applied daily. This simple and inexpensive measure prevents significant secondary infection and ensures that healing proceeds under the scar. Despite drainage, serous fluid may collect beneath the flaps; it is repeatedly aspirated with a fine needle and syringe as required. In certain circumstances, tethering the edges of skin to the underlying muscle seems to limit seroma production. Radiotherapy apart, the scar is ready to accept a prosthesis at 4 weeks from the time of operation.

5. Patey mastectomy (subradical mastectomy) (Figures 30.9–30.11)

Some surgeons insist that surgical clearance of the axilla is essential to clear all local disease and enable proper staging. Yet they wish to avoid the morbidity associated with radical mastectomy. The operation described by Patey and Dyson (1948) enables these criteria. The towelling preparation differs from that customary for simple mastectomy as the arm is prepared separately to allow abduction when the axilla is dissected. Otherwise the skin flaps are raised as for

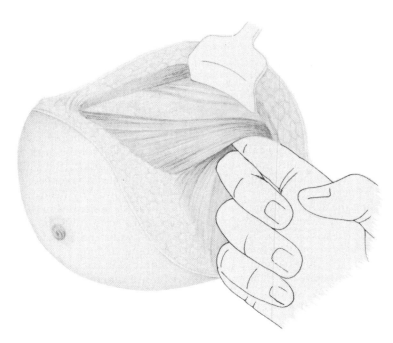

Figure 30.9 Patey mastectomy. Pectoralis major has been retracted and pectoralis minor defined prior to detachment from the coracoid process

simple mastectomy and the axilla is approached. The ipsilateral assistant then flexes the arm with the elbow held at a right angle. Pectoralis major is retracted and pectoralis minor exposed. This muscle is detached from the coracoid process and turned downwards to expose the apex of the axilla. The fatty and nodal contents are removed from above and below the axillary vein which necessitates ligating the small veins which drain from the chest wall into the main trunk. It is essential to preserve the lateral pectoral nerve and pectoral branch of the acromiothoracic artery which pass through the clavipectoral fascia to supply pectoralis major. The medial pectoral nerve component to that muscle is sacrificed when the minor is detached. The dissection proceeds downwards towards the central contents which are delicately cleared as for extended local mastectomy, apart from the medial side. Here pectoralis minor is detached from the ribs by cutting diathermy; any interpectoral nodes are included in the specimen. Alternatively, pectoralis minor is not removed but after axillary dissection is left *in situ* or reattached to its origin. Thereafter the operation proceeds as for local mastectomy.

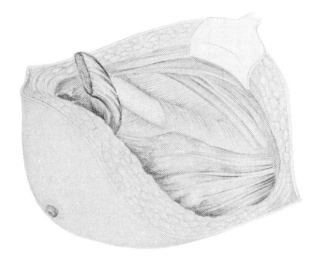

Figure 30.10 Patey mastectomy. Pectoralis minor, the axilla contents and the breast have been dissected away and drawn downwards

6. Radical mastectomy

Despite a large amount of evidence to the contrary, a few surgeons in Great Britain, the USA and Australasia still consider that radical mastectomy offers the most effective treatment for stages 1 and 2 carcinoma of the breast. The approach to T1b and T2b tumours in the absence of detectable distant metastases is problematical. Such cases are few but some opt for radical mastectomy in such a presentation. Similarly, local recurrence after simple mastectomy or local excision and irradiation might be suitable. The alleged benefit is related to diminished local and

axillary recurrence and there is well-documented evidence to support such a view (Osborne and Borgen, 1990). For an unrivalled account of the technical minutiae integral to radical mastectomy, the reader is referred to Riddell (1954).

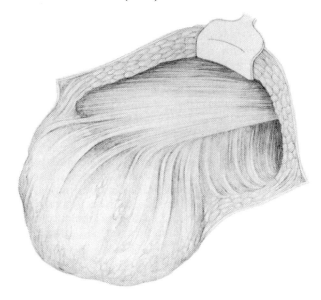

Figure 30.11 Patey mastectomy. The total specimen is almost fully detached from the pectoralis major

POSTOPERATIVE CARE FOLLOWING TOTAL MASTECTOMY

Limited arm and shoulder movements are allowed from the start, but it seems sensible to restrict abduction movements until around 14 days postoperatively, by which time most of the serum collections have been aspirated. If serum re-collects it must be regularly aspirated. Serum collections may also develop after excision biopsy and should be cleared. The patient should be warned of the possibility of lymphatic vessel thromboses in the axilla and arm. These are manifested by tight, painful wire-like strands extending as far as the cubital fossa; arm movements should continue and the process will resolve.

When the wound has healed, or after radiotherapy has been completed and the skin recovered, a light dusting powder to the chest wall is soothing and a mammary prosthesis can be inserted inside the brassière. Until that time, a light prosthesis is worn.

Regional node biopsy

To assess the spread of breast cancer and prescribe surgical and other measures accordingly, some surgeons favour biopsy of the apical, axillary and internal mammary nodes (Blamey *et al.*, 1979). The principle has not gained wide acceptance.

The argument is reasonable: if the apical axillary

nodes are involved, then cure is unlikely, even more so if the internal mammary nodes contain tumour. If both sites are invaded, then this simple biopsy evidence is as reliable a predictor of widespread micrometastases as skeletal and liver isotopic scanning.

The principle and practice of this type of biopsy does remain controversial, and many surgeons are happier assuming the presence of disseminated disease if a certain number of axillary nodes contain tumour. Deposits >2 mm in diameter are significant and over four nodes affected is a marker of poor prognosis.

Isolated axillary biopsy

This applies when the mammary incision for segmental excision or lumpectomy cannot be conveniently extended. A skin crease incision is made to extend from the palpable borders of the pectoralis major and latissimus dorsi. The axillary space is opened through the suspensory ligament and wide exposure developed by gentle blunt dissection and retraction. A generous representative sample of the central contents and palpable nodes is effected. The exposure tends to be modest; obsessive haemostasis and drainage are advisable.

Internal mammary node biopsy

It is probably wise to confine biopsy to the second and third interspaces, through a short vertical or transverse incision. Pectoralis major is detached from the sternal edge and perforating vessels are ligated. For a distance of 4 cm lateral to the sternal edge, the intercostal muscle and anterior intercostal membrane are incised to expose the internal mammary vessels. Fatty and nodal tissue is isolated by delicate pledget dissection, taking care to avoid puncturing the pleura. The nodes may be as small as 2–3 mm diameter. Haemostasis accomplished, the pectoral is reattached with interrupted 3/0 or 4/0 sutures.

Apical axillary node biopsy

A short incision of around 6–8 cm in length is made below and parallel to the middle third of the clavicle. The pectoral is detached subperiosteally from the clavicle and retracted downwards. The clavipectoral fascia is divided and the axillary vein identified. The space between the axillary vein and the upper chest wall is cleaned. One expects to find fibro-fatty tissue, including some apical nodes.

There are occasions where, following any form of total mastectomy or wide local excision for wound recurrence, skin grafting is required. The wound gap is closed as far as reasonable tension will allow and a split-skin graft taken from the thigh is cut to match the defect. A reliable skin knife (e.g. Humby–Bodenham) must be in a perfect state of function and the

operator familiar with how to set the blade.

The graft is laid on petroleum jelly gauze over a skin board and trimmed to size: spare skin is saved in a sterile jar and refrigerated. The graft is laid on the raw surface or sutured at the edges with 3/0 or 4/0 braided silk sutures which are left long and tied over a plastic foamy pressure pad. A skin-graft mesher allows coverage of larger defects using smaller areas of donor skin.

Reconstructive surgery

Subcutaneous mastectomy with insertion of prosthesis or reconstructive prosthetic mammoplasty following mastectomy

There is disagreement over the advisability of prosthetic reconstruction following total mastectomy. Aside from the potential resource implication for the NHS, the biological considerations should dominate decisions.

The American approach is more in favour of immediate reconstruction on request (Cady, 1990) and the caveats far less restrictive (Bostwick, 1990; Vinton et al., 1990).

Reasonable points for consideration might be:

1. A small primary tumour <2 cm diameter.
2. Widespread or extensive ductal carcinoma in situ (DCIS and ECIS).
3. Absence of invasive multicentricity on mammography and histopathology.
4. A low or intermediate Bloom and Richardson grade tumour without lymphatic involvement and other adverse prognostic features.
5. No previous radiotherapy.
6. Complete understanding by the patient and her partner of the risks and potential complications.

There is much to be said for delaying reconstruction for 2 years following mastectomy. This allows most of the biologically unfavourable tumours (Fox, 1979) to be declared by local or distant spread.

Cronin and Gerow (1964) reported on the reliability and suitability of Silastic gel mammary prostheses, for augmentation mammoplasty and replacement. Williams (1972) wrote that during the previous 9-year period Dow-Corning Corporation sold over 50 000 Silastic prostheses: since then interest in reconstructive breast surgery has increased (Georgiade, 1977). Adjacent editorial articles by Freeman (1972) and Weiner (1972) counselled caution and enthusiasm, respectively. Current practice in the USA is reviewed by Dowden and Dinner (1984). The issues involved are fundamental and may be itemized as follows:

1. There are no long-term studies of subcutaneous mastectomy with prosthetic inserts.
2. In North America there is an increasing tendency

to offer mastectomy and prosthetic replacement for non-malignant lesions or symptoms, e.g. mastodynia, recurrent breast cysts, multiple biopsies for dysplasia, atypical epitheliosis, a strong family history of breast cancer and familial and hereditary breast cancer (Lynch, 1990).

3. Troublesome complications may arise following prosthetic insertion, the sole aim of which is to retain a cosmetic effect. The prosthesis does not bounce naturally with movement; nipple sensation is significantly altered and may be lost. Skin healing may fail and the prosthesis becomes exposed. The cosmetic effect may be marred by a firm subcutaneous reaction producing skin wrinkling and prosthesis encapsulation. For malignancy, a total mastectomy with a well-fitting prosthesis serves superbly well for most women. It is common experience that most cope psychologically with physical loss.

Operative details

A selection of sterile Silastic prostheses should be available in the theatre, together with a scale to weigh excised breast tissue. General anaesthesia without intentional hypotension is required, but a 20–30° head-up tilt is useful. The towelling arrangement includes elevation to paint the back and lie the patient on a sterile towel. Both breasts are exposed and the towels are sutured in place; the opposite side is covered initially, to be exposed later for comparison.

A submammary incision is ideal but a reasonable alternative is an oblique approach behind the anterior axillary fold. Previous biopsy scars may dictate another incision such as sub-areolar or lateral radial. By firm retraction over swabs, the skin edges are separated and it is critical to the success of the procedure to enter the correct plane. The separation lies between the breast fat and subcutaneous fat. The latter contains a network of veins, and the fat is finely lobular; it varies in thickness according to build. Delicate elevation of the skin edges by skin hooks or Allis tissue forceps is performed, followed later by appropriate retractors. When the nipple is reached, the ducts are divided, leaving a thick corium layer to preserve vascularity and hopefully eventual sensation. It is sensible to mobilize an edge of the breast and elevate it from the pectoral fascia. Thereby the breast tissue can be turned deep side out and dissection simplified. The major arterial supply to the breast skin enters on the medial and lateral side, so it is prudent to dissect very carefully there in order to ligate the arterial branch entering the breast while preserving the skin vessel.

Careful and patient retraction will enable the breast to be removed and preferably a biopsy of low axillary (pectoral) nodes also. Total haemostasis is achieved by fine 3/0 silk ligatures or very precise fine diathermy coagulation. The incision is held open by retractors, and the gel-filled, round prosthesis is slipped into the

vacated space and checked for size; the opposite breast is exposed and comparison made. If necessary, the prosthesis is replaced to fit. The skin is then closed in two layers. A deep subcutaneous layer of 2/0 or 3/0 chromic catgut is carefully placed followed by subcuticular or fine interrupted skin sutures according to preference. The wound is sealed with mastiche or Nobecutane (resin wound dressing, Astia), followed by some form of supportive dressing. A cotton brassière is applied over the dressing.

Variations in technique

It is important to mention these; they are interesting and instructive. Watts (1977), who has assembled a wide experience of subcutaneous mastectomy, requires careful resterilization of the prosthesis, despite assurance from the manufacturer. Also a 'no touch' technique is used throughout the mastectomy, in particular for insertion of the prosthesis, when new gloves are taken. He avoids both drainage and antibiotics. Others employ a far less rigid technique, seemingly content to handle both skin and prosthesis. In one large American series (Williams, 1972) local steroid (triamcinolone acetate) and antibiotic (cephaloridine) are injected into the space. Suction drainage is widely used. Insertion of the prosthesis following subcutaneous mastectomy may be immediate or delayed for 3–6 months. Immediate insertion carries a greater risk of complications, especially where the skin is thin and biopsy scars are present. Delayed insertion allows skin vascularity to reach an optimal state, but sadly the cosmetic result tends to suffer. Some surgeons routinely excise and resuture previous biopsy scars at the time of mastectomy.

Postoperative management

Certain details are very important. A soft lateral pad of sterile cottonwool is inserted inside the brassière cup to prevent the prosthesis from sliding laterally into the axilla. Arm and shoulder movements are restricted for 2 weeks. Occasionally a collection of serous fluid requires careful aspiration.

Complications

If a significant haematoma develops, it is sensible to evacuate it at around 48 h. Skin loss of minor degree can be excised down to the prosthesis and resutured. Gross exposure of the prosthesis necessitates its removal with resuturing or grafting. Skin loss may not be immediate, but may take many weeks to develop. Later complications have already been mentioned. They include rupture of the prosthesis, its dislocation into the axilla and the formation of a firm or even hard fibrous capsule. The latter may respond to firm massage but, as with the others mentioned here, reoperation and a new prosthesis may be required.

A modification in the insertion of Silastic mammary prostheses has recently appeared. To overcome the very troublesome complication of capsule formation some surgeons insert the prosthesis deep to the pectoralis major. The route is either by splitting the muscle centrally, by incising serratus anterior laterally and tunnelling behind pectoralis; alternatively, the sternocostal origin of pectoralis is detached and the prosthesis slipped upwards. This site for the prosthesis has become the preferred choice for both immediate and delayed reconstruction following total mastectomy (Forrest, 1982; Hughes et al., 1989; Bostwick, 1990). A modest-sized (200–250 ml) prosthesis may be inserted, but the procedure is controversial and awaits further evaluation. An additional modification is to use tissue expansion incorporating a prosthesis which is progressively inflated over a period of weeks with saline injections (Radovan, 1982).

The principal use of this technique is to expand a space for insertion of a prosthesis where, due to the previous mastectomy, skin is tight and of poor quality.

Additional techniques and aspects of breast reconstruction

The present position has been well reviewed by Hughes (1984), but there is much controversy in the philosophy and practice of this branch of breast surgery. First, if less radical procedures for selected breast cancers are successful, then the need for reconstruction will be less than if mastectomy is the rule.

The overwhelming reason for reconstruction is to relieve the psychological distress consequent on mastectomy in many women. Whereas some 20–30% of women suffer a significant psychological reaction to mastectomy (Maguire, 1984), the reaction is much improved by 1 year afterwards (Dean et al., 1983). The results of reconstruction are generally rather discouraging, so there would appear to be sound reasons for delaying it beyond 2 years. The majority of women adjust very quickly to a tidy mastectomy and a neatly fitted external prosthesis.

Any further questions are perhaps best reserved for either plastic surgeons or general surgeons with a dominating interest in breast cancer and a belief in reconstruction. The procedures are the latissimus dorsi flap and the rectus abdominis flap – both rather complex techniques. Details are provided in publications by Bostwick et al. (1978), Webster and Hughes (1983) and Nash and Hurst (1983).

Subcutaneous mammary prostheses have been attended by rather modest results (Dean et al., 1983; Ward and Edwards, 1983) and have not gained great acceptance. It remains to be seen if 'flap' techniques are more successful. The indications for their use need to be very precisely defined. For more current and detailed reviews the reader is referred to Morgan (1987) and Bostwick (1990).

Plastic surgery procedures in relation to the breast

The most dramatic of these procedures is mammoplasty, but this is a difficult and unpredictable technique even in skilled and experienced hands (McKissock, 1972). A variety of procedures is currently employed, which probably means that the perfect operation is elusive. The operation should not be undertaken by a general surgeon. Nevertheless, he may feel competent to excise resistant locally recurrent breast carcinoma or an area of radionecrosis. To close a chest wall defect, a simple split-skin graft or a rotation flap with grafting of the exposed area is employed (Dudley, 1977). This is not a difficult technique; it demands clean excision even down to and through the muscle layer if necessary and the construction of an adequate rotation flap. The need for this operation arises very infrequently and it should only be performed if there is no evidence of distant metastases. Otherwise, hormonal measures or local intra-arterial chemotherapy are the logical approach.

Augmentation mammoplasty

This commonly performed operation, which employs a Silastic silicone gel prosthesis, is considered for hypoplastic breasts or where, following childbirth and lactation, the breasts undergo a degree of atrophy and ptosis. The indication is a relative one and is purely concerned with cosmesis. The stress and unhappiness which some women allege in these circumstances should be carefully evaluated by the surgeon. The technique is not difficult and in the absence of available plastic surgical expertise could reasonably be acquired and practised by a general surgeon concerned with breast disease.

Operative details

Under general anaesthesia an incision is made just above the inframammary crease in order to preserve a small fringe of breast tissue attached to the chest wall close to the lower skin edge. The incision is deepened to the pectoral fascia and the breast is lifted away from the fascia by blunt swab or digital dissection. Unlike subcutaneous mastectomy, the dissection is easy and there is little risk to blood supply. After a suitable bed is fashioned and haemostasis secured, a round, correctly sized, low-profile Silastic prosthesis is eased in and manipulated into place. According to Williams (1972) a safe size is 225 ml and a volume of 315 ml should never be exceeded. Alternatively, a subpectoral placement may be selected.

The skin is closed in two layers, the first by 2/0 plain or chromic catgut, making use of the fringe of breast and fatty subcutaneous tissue to produce a ledge which will prevent the prosthesis from slipping downwards. Skin closure is according to the preference of the operator.

An alternative approach relies on an oblique axillary incision hidden by the anterior axillary fold. The breast is dissected away from pectoralis major as with the inferior approach, and to reach the lower quadrants of the breast a thick blunt metal sound has been advocated. The prosthesis is inserted as previously described and the use of topical steroids and antibiotics is favoured by some surgeons.

The complications match those which may follow subcutaneous mastectomy. For 608 patchless Silastic prosthetic augmentations, Williams (1972) reported infection in 3, exposure due to skin loss in 6 and ptosis of the prosthesis in 14.

It is essential that during preoperative counselling another important element is understood by the patient. Following any type of prosthetic or flap reconstruction, the ease and efficacy of postoperative clinical examination and breast screening is prejudiced. The patient must be warned. A particular scenario in relation to silicone gel implant augmentation and screening is discussed in full by Silverstein *et al.* (1990). High-risk women should probably avoid augmentation entirely or opt for the subpectoral position if the operation is judged to be imperative.

Carcinoma in situ of the breast

This important clinical and pathological entity has been well recognized for decades. Breast screening programmes have heightened awareness because of the increasing frequency with which ductal carcinoma in situ (DCIS) is revealed in asymptomatic women. Lobular carcinoma in situ (LCIS) looks rather different microscopically and is usually an incidental histopathological discovery within or around a surgical excision biopsy for anticipated benign disease. This is quite separate from some invasive lobular cancers which present in the standard manner. Both variants arise from the terminal duct–lobular unit (Wellings *et al.*, 1975) and must be regarded as malignant change within confined areas at a pre-invasive stage.

The incidence and natural history of DCIS is uncertain. From autopsy studies, DCIS is present in 5–6% of assumed normal breasts. Breasts amputated for invasive cancer contain coexistent DCIS in at least 40% of cases. The uncertainty lies in forecasting which patients with DCIS will progress to invasive disease and how quickly. DCIS comprises a heterogeneous histopathological entity. Comedo (with central necrosis), solid, cribriform and micropapillary patterns are identified. Clinically three types are evident:

1. Small calcified microfocal lesions most commonly found by guided excision biopsies from screen-detected disease.

2. Symptomatic, tumour-forming palpable lumps (5% of all breast cancers).

3. Diffuse, segmental or spreading disease demonstrable on screening films and confirmed by surgical biopsy (EISC or ECIS) (Banerjee, 1990).

From screening mammography in asymptomatic women without any palpable breast nodularity, fine microcalcification(s) are a signal and important feature. The pattern favouring DCIS includes > 15 calcifications with a branching or fine, linear and irregular pattern. Differentiating benign from malignant features can be difficult and the extent of calcification underestimates the spread of DCIS in 40% of biopsies. It is apparent regarding mammographically discovered breast cancers, that 15% at least are DCIS.

Natural history and biological prediction should dictate surgical management, but information is modest and the only real certainties relate to the large-cell comedo-type with central necrosis.

This pattern is easily discerned from histopathology and cytology, but if reassurance is necessary for the surgeon, modern studies of ploidy (cellular DNA content), proto-oncogene expression and thymidine labelling (cell turnover studies) confirm its aggressive potential. Current concepts include:

1. Total mastectomy without node surgery or radiotherapy will secure a virtual 100% rate of cure (Wanebo *et al.*, 1974; Rosen *et al.*, 1979).

2. Local excision alone will be followed by a recurrence later which varies from 13–17% at 5-year follow-up to 55% at 7 years (50% invasive) (Price *et al.*, 1989). Such recurrence may not prejudice survival (Millis and Thynne, 1975; Rosner, 1980).

3. Based upon a careful study by Silverstein *et al.* (1990), small lesions of ±2 cm diameter with at least 5 mm clear margins may be treated by local excision only. Larger lesions and those with margins involved by DCIS deserve mastectomy. Unless micro-invasion is found by histopathology, axillary surgery is unnecessary as the occurrence of node invasion is less than 1% of patients.

4. Clinical trials devised for the management of DCIS, assuming optimal accrual for localized disease, will require between 10 and 15 years to provide reliable answers.

5. Conservative surgery enrols the patient in annual mammography (whether single or double views is uncertain) and 6-monthly clinical review. Radiation therapy would make such assessment more difficult. Mastectomy is a supportable option particularly for comedo DCIS: perhaps here, immediate reconstruction carries a sound biological basis in contrast to many women with invasive disease (Carpenter *et al.*, 1989; Phipps and Rayter, 1990).

The place of tamoxifen adjuvant treatment is an important consideration. Irradiation following local excision is more of a problem and a trial is under way (CRCC Trial) to assess its potential. As expected the matter is controversial and a well-reasoned caution has been published by Hamilton and Buchanan (1990).

Lobular carcinoma in situ (LCIS) is more of a mystery than DCIS and is not associated with pathological microcalcification. It functions as a risk predictor for later breast cancer, whereas DCIS is regarded as a precursor of invasive cancer (Cady, 1990). After diagnostic biopsy, long-term follow-up at 3-monthly intervals is obligatory. LCIS frequently affects both breasts. One series (Rosen et al., 1978) followed 99 patients for an average of 24 years, discovering 18% ipsilateral and 13% contralateral invasive cancers. Check mammography every 2–3 years would seem sensible in such cases.

Invasive lobular carcinoma portrays indefinite mammographic features and FNAC smears are difficult to interpret. The cells are small and false-negative reports are frequent. Excision biopsy, when in any clinical doubt, is the safest approach.

Management of the breast cancer patient

The early 1970s were associated with new concepts in relation to breast cancer and its management. Diagnosis was improved by the adoption of low-dose mammography and the recognition that the identification of a cancerous lump by some form of needle biopsy in the clinic led to more enlightened investigations. The concept of micrometastases and the faltering importance of radical local surgery were easily accepted by most surgeons. The implications and irregular availability of cellular hormone receptors were and are more difficult. Adjuvant chemotherapy and hormonal treatment for high-risk groups enforced on all the importance of an oncological team to sustain long-term treatment for all cases.

The recognition of early metastases and the near-total eclipse of radical surgery led to greater emphasis on rehabilitation and an as yet unfulfilled and unsubstantiated requirement for breast reconstruction.

The formulation and execution of controlled clinical trials for breast cancer treatment may have created more problems than provided solutions. Some are of much greater potential than others. Hopefully the maturation of important studies within the next few years will be rewarding.

It is difficult within a few pages to appraise a problem which taxes modern oncology to its limit and concerning which so much is written. Apart from understanding up-to-date and substantial scientific fact, one needs a basic philosophical approach to this killing disease. It is sensible to begin by relating certain dilemmas in basic knowledge apropos breast cancer – it is understandable that so many disagreements still exist. Over the past 45 years there has been no improvement in the survival rate from breast cancer (Bonnadonna et al., 1976), although disease-free intervals have been increased. Figures differ for survival, but they suggest that at 10 years 30–50% of all cases are alive. Forrest (1974) reported that for stages 1 and 2 only, the 15-year survival rate was around 30% and these figures were confirmed by other British workers. At 30-year follow-up, Adair's series reported around 20% of patients alive and disease free on clinical grounds (Adair et al., 1984).

Breast cancer is an extremely capricious and unpredictable disease. It has been suggested that it is several different diseases (Baker, 1977).

Fox (1979) has proposed the separation of breast cancer into slow and rapidly dying patterns. The latter group recur swiftly following surgery and are deceased by 7 years. In the slow group it is possible to detect recurrence in the 18–25 years follow-up interval and beyond.

Although statistics show trends within large groups of cases, there is significant tumour heterogeneity in breast cancer and variations in tumour – host balance. Increasingly, however, the expressed hope is to 'tailor' management to the biological state.

It is possible that the next decade will be associated with better prediction and consequently more logical therapy.

A reliable clinical stage system is necessary. The style adopted from the Union International Centre-Cancer, and the American Joint Committee on Cancer joint report (UICC/AJCC), is as follows:

T_1 Tumour <2 cm in diameter
T_2 Tumour >2 cm but <5 cm in diameter
T_3 Tumour >5 cm in diameter
T_4 Tumour with direct extension to chest wall or breast skin
T_{1-3a} Tumour not fixed to pectoral *fascia or muscle*
T_{1-3b} Tumour fixed to pectoral *fascia or muscle*
N_0 No palpable adenopathy
N_1 Abnormal movable ipsilateral axillary nodes
N_2 Abnormal fixed or matted ipsilateral axillary nodes
N_3 Ipsilateral supraclavicular or infraclavicular adenopathy or arm lymphoedema
M_0 No evidence of distant metastases
M_1 Metastases present

Stage I = $T_1 N_0 M_0$
Stage II = $T_2 N_0 M_0$ $T_{1-2} N_1 M_0$
Stage IIIA = $T_2 N_{0-1} M_0$ $T_{1-3} N_2 M_0$
Stage IIIB = $T_4 N_{0-2} M_0$ $T_{1-4} N_3 M_0$
Stage IV = $T_{1-4} N_{0-3} M_1$

The past decade, with a crescendo in the past 5 years, has witnessed an enormous amount of clinical and laboratory investigation into all aspects of breast cancer. Much of it is controversial and much uncertainty still exists.

We are entering an era of highly selective therapy based on more sophisticated analysis of the primary cancer. . . . Such individual factors will enable more selective therapy.
(Blake Cady, 1990)

To enable the reader – especially the surgical trainee – to make sense of recent advances, controversies and popular practice, it will be helpful to itemize these in sections.

1. There is considerable and increasing public interest in breast cancer. Around 1 in 12 women in the UK will develop the disease. Most patients attend with a palpable lump, but the importance of impalpable disease (DCIS and LCIS) must be accepted and recognized. There is good evidence that DCIS, as a precursor lesion, begins locally and slowly evolves into diffuse disease and finally invasion over a span of 5–10 years. Current information suggests that 50% of DCIS lesions will eventually become invasive (Lagios et al., 1982, 1989).

2. The 'new biology' of 'biological predeterminism' of breast cancer, which infers that systemic haematogenous spread into micrometastases occurs very early in the stage of tumour growth, is widely accepted. The similar survival rates despite a variety of local treatments is adduced to support the theory. There are critics, however, and one detects a current move to reject minimal local surgery in view of the high incidence of local recurrence. Extensive local surgery exemplified by radical mastectomy conferred very low locoregional recurrence rates (2–6% at 10 years) (Osborne and Borgen, 1990; Collins, 1991).

The significance of local recurrence after lumpectomy (wide local excision) and segmental mastectomy is considered to be less serious than skin or chest wall recurrence after total mastectomy (Cady, 1990). The fact that patients continue to die of metastatic disease well beyond 15 years after surgery and that the survival curve even after 30 years never becomes horizontal supports the widely accepted need for systemic therapy.

3. Breast screening is in progress and, despite all the evidence, might be more properly regarded as an 'experiment'. At least 10 years will elapse before the anticipated benefits will appear. Whether screening should be extended beyond the age of 64 remains uncertain. Why there are no survival benefits from screening below the age of 50 years is a fascinating and incompletely explained question. The whole screening problem is complex and embraces cost effectiveness, radiological technique and quality control. Cady (1990) infers that patient expectation and the legal climate in the USA will prevent objective studies. The outcome will be awaited with considerable interest. Certainly the Department of Health is impressed with the early results.

4. For impalpable lesions a standard radiological, surgical and pathological sequence is essential. A reasonable guide to surgery might be:

(a) For local DCIS, <2.5 cm diameter, wide local excision with 5–10 mm margins should be adequate; node sampling is unnecessary but, in a trial setting, tamoxifen could be of long-term benefit.
(b) Lesions between 2.5 and 5 cm in diameter, segmental mastectomy with clear margins as above

and node sampling (4 nodes) is sound.
(c) For DCIS >5 cm in diameter or positive margins after an initial resection or widespread mammographic microcalcification, total mastectomy with node sampling is a logical operation.
(d) Should micro-invasion be detected on histopathology, then an axillary level 1 and 2 clearance is sensible.
(e) Patients with proven DCIS and LCIS who have a positive family history show a higher risk of developing invasive disease. Total mastectomy and subpectoral reconstruction would seem an option for such women.

5. Limited invasive breast cancer is a term used for tumours up to 1 cm diameter. Minimal breast cancer is an unwise description for such small growths (Collins, 1991). Survival rates for limited disease are good, at around 97–98% (8 years). The incidence of lymph node metastases in palpable 1 cm tumours is 14% (Rosen et al., 1981), and only 9% for impalpable tumours of the same size. Unless the tumour is centrally placed, wide local excision is suitable for such lesions.

6. For tumours up to 4 cm in diameter, the NSABP trial B-06 advises local resection. This has been the subject of much criticism (Fisher et al., 1985). Many surgeons, however, prefer to limit wide local excision with 2 cm clearance margins – for lesions no greater than 2 cm mammographic diameter (Veronesi et al., 1990). The tumour should be at least 3 cm from the areolar edge; the breast size should be suitable, and adjuvant postoperative irradiation to the breast area is standard treatment. In Fisher's reported series (1985), the local recurrence rate (at 5 years) was at least 32% (Collins, 1991), reduced to 7% by radiotherapy. In such cases, high-risk features might sway the surgeon in favour of mastectomy, and include:

(a) high Bloom and Richardson histological grade (Bloom and Richardson, 1957)
(b) poor nuclear grade with tumour necrosis
(c) inflammatory features
(d) low-density mammographic shadowing
(e) lymphatic and vascular invasion.

Preoperative irradiation and preoperative chemotherapy may have a place in treating patients with these high-risk tumours.

Some idea of feasibility is shown as follows: 195 patients with primary breast cancer were separated into two groups by standard criteria for either breast conservation or mastectomy. Eighty-five patients were unsuitable for conservation; 110 were ostensibly considered, but 56 opted for mastectomy. Further investigations excluded 10 of the remaining 54, so 44 patients from 195 (23%) eventually achieved conservative surgery.

7. Total mastectomy might be reserved for T_{2a}–T_{3a} (5 cm maximum) tumours and for smaller lesions fitting the above criteria and where the tumour (of

whatever size) is central in position. For lobular invasive tumours, total mastectomy as opposed to wide local excision is logical. In cases where wide local excision and radiotherapy fails, mastectomy is the next step. If local conditions are adverse, myocutaneous flaps or skin grafting becomes necessary.

8. Considering axillary surgery, the ascendency of breast conservation surgery in the past 20 years secured the eclipse of radical mastectomy and the axilla became an uncertain area for the surgeon. Perhaps the axillary nodes, whatever metastatic tumours they harboured, could be safely included in radiotherapy.

Alternatively, a non-exacting dissection of around four lower nodes might suffice (Forrest, 1982) for staging, leaving adjuvant treatments to cope with residual tumour.

Seemingly, the inclination to leave the axilla alone if it was palpably negative was an irresistible stance for many surgeons and consequently many junior surgeons lack expertise in that region. Others from an earlier radical training and surgical philosophy retained vestiges of the surgical practice predating 1965. Total mastectomy, quadrantectomy and segmental mastectomy were, therefore, accompanied by axillary dissection. Radical apologists opted for the 'Patey' procedure (Patey and Dyson, 1948) with or without removal of pectoralis minor. Many surgeons, however, were content with a full level 1 and 2 dissection and were unimpressed with any value from extension to level 3 (above pectoralis minor). But because of the need for careful and supervised shoulder mobilization, increased hospitalization and a risk of arm oedema (15% quoted), axillary dissection is not popular (Cady, 1990). For some, axillary dissection has become more refined. Level 1 and 2 clearance leaving fascia and fat over the axillary vein (non-skimming) with preservation of the intercostobrachial nerve is quite feasible. The critical element is that such a cleared axilla is spared radiotherapy. The combination of surgery and radiotherapy leads to a much higher risk of arm oedema (40–50%).

The idea that axillary dissection is necessary for the informed management of breast cancer rests on two principles (Kissin et al., 1982). First, detailed examination of the nodes (between 10 and 20 nodes should be harvested by the histopathologist) will provide information on whether adjuvant treatment should be offered. Secondly, metastatic nodes are most effectively treated by surgical excision (block dissection). This approach has been forcibly restated by Fentiman and Mansell (1991) and supported by others (Ball et al., 1990). Surgeons who had initially preferred node biopsy have reverted to axillary clearance (Aitken et al., 1989).

Axillary node status associated with DCIS has been considered, but within this heterogeneous entity 1–5% could be node positive (Wong et al., 1990). Perhaps a reasonable compromise would be to dissect four low axillary nodes from the central pad. This can be achieved without morbidity. Future treatment trials for DCIS and FCIS will attract more credence if nodal status is known.

9. Currently there is a hope that refined analysis of the primary tumour will see the emergence of reliable prognostic markers which will guide selective therapy (Baildam et al., 1989). Several features are relevant:

(a) axillary node state
(b) tumour size – this is related to nodal involvement (Carter et al., 1989)
(c) Tumour type – good prognostic patterns being tubular, mucoid, intracystic papillary cancer, etc. (Greening, 1983).
(d) ploidy measurements of nuclear DNA content by flow cytometry – this measures the proportion of proliferating cells (Dowle et al., 1987)
(e) cell kinetics by radioactive thymidine studies
(f) cell steroid receptors, oestrogen (ER) and progestogen (PR)
(g) oncogene expression on chromosome 17, e.g. c-erb B-2
(h) epidermal growth factor elaboration (EGR) (Sainsbury et al., 1988)
(i) Serum markers, cathepsin D, CEA and others.

The major issue for all of the above is which, from such a diverse field, is accurate enough to correlate with long-term follow-up and which could become easily available and cost effective 1 or the large number of patients to be treated.

Naturally it would be hopeful to suggest that the relatively simple Nottingham prognostic index (Haybittle et al., 1982; Williams et al., 1986), which has stood the examination of long follow-up, holds much attraction. Epidermal growth factor is a particularly promising field for further investigation (Gullick, 1990).

ER and PR receptors have been in vogue for some years. Consistently the literature states that ER status of the primary tumour is an important guide to selecting adjuvant therapy. ER positivity is inversely related to EGF status.

The PR status is less certain and possibly not of independent prognostic value (Hawkins et al., 1987). It is relevant that the UK facilities for measuring receptor status are limited and the majority of women are managed without knowledge of their ER status. The histological grade and refined detail (lymphatic and vascular involvement, elastosis, etc.) is used instead.

10. The molecular biology of breast cancer is a rapidly advancing field. Certain genes and their protein products, known as oncogenes, may play a part in the development and progression of the disease. An example cited in several reports is c-erb B-2, a proto-oncogene which can be activated to become an oncogene's protein product, a membrane receptor very similar to the EGF receptor, has been linked by some gene's protein product, a membrane receptor very similar to the EGF receptor has been linked by some

research groups to poor prognosis in breast tumours. The protein product of tumour suppressor gene p53 located on the short arm of chromosome 17 has also been the subject of investigation. The research field is mobile and exciting, but it remains to be seen whether genetic probing, particularly in inherited and familial breast cancer, will be a discriminant of practical value.

11. Psychosocial and psychosexual aspects of breast cancer are of self-evident importance, but difficult to evaluate objectively (Collins, 1991). Cady (1990) has evaluated patient choice:

What a woman wants to do with her breast has become the paramount decision point in the treatment of breast cancer.

It is well accepted that between 20% and 25% of women suffer significant postoperative depression and psychosexual symptoms. Common knowledge supports the evidence that reaction also develops after conservation surgery, especially when recurrent disease develops (Fallowfield et al., 1986). The two factors which relate to minimizing psychological stress are participation by the woman in the treatment decisions and the degree of concern over recurrent disease. For some women, participation in major therapy decision is quite impossible for them to sustain (Morris and Royle, 1987; McArdle et al., 1990). There are probably four rules in this important aspect of cancer management. The surgeon should be professional and skilled in his approach, yet sensitive and sympathetic. He should be assisted by a trained breast counselling nurse and understanding, supportive relatives. There will be exceptions, but most women prefer an honest and direct approach coupled with the promise to maintain, wherever possible, personal, unfussed and confident follow-up.

It must be understood that some women will never come to terms with the existence and discovery of breast cancer, and mental torture will often be vented by unreasonable allegations against all who attempt to treat them. For each and every breast surgeon this cross has be to borne!

Taking all of these factors into account, a reasonable plan of management for breast cancer is shown in Figures 30.12–30.15.

Hormone therapy for breast cancer (Mansi and Smith, 1989)

The two principal roles for hormonal manipulation are in treatment of metastatic disease and as adjuvant therapy following primary surgery. There exists little controversy over the use of oral tamoxifen in a daily dose of 20 mg for post-menopausal women who are node positive (Wilson et al., 1985; Carbone et al., 1985; Ribiero and Swindell, 1988).

Benefit is reported in the incidence of relapse and for survival. At 7-year follow-up after 1 year of tamoxifen, a 25% improvement in relapse-free survival and 15% reduction in mortality is evident. Additional studies have led to increasing benefit from prolonging the adjuvant treatment for 5 years and beyond (B. Fisher, personal communication). Late menopausal women are treated in this manner. The long-term effects of tamoxifen are uncertain, but could include skeletal and cardiovascular effects. Its efficacy in some ER- and PR-negative tumours is unexplained. This agent is an attractive one because it is taken orally and is associated with few serious side effects. The cost for NHS hospitals is around 60p per tablet.

For metastatic disease, hormonal manipulation is a continuing and important chapter in surgical oncology. If a tumour is responsive, hormonal manipulation confers by far the 'kindest' and most prolonged relief. Its action is based upon the assumption that malignant breast tissue retains some of the growth and differentiation responses of normal breast tissue. Oestrogens direct proliferation of functioning breast elements and this action will presumably continue if breast cancer cells express oestrogen receptors (ERs).

Surgical ablation was the beginning. Bilateral oophorectomy was demonstrably effective in around 50% of pre-menopausal women suffering metastatic cancer. Adrenalectomy which became popular in the early 1950s was more suited to post-menopausal women to reduce oestrogen production from androstanedione. Some peri-menopausal women received oophorectomy and adrenalectomy at one surgical intervention. Pharmacological ablation is reversible and less invasive. It should be emphasized that, on some occasions, a pre-menopausal woman will prefer oophorectomy for therapy and sterility as opposed to long-term expensive drug manipulation. It can be associated with dramatic remission.

Treatment modes are designed to reduce oestrogen stimulation by removing the source: inhibiting oestrogen synthesis or blocking oestrogen receptor function at cellular level. Hypophysectomy or irradiation of the pituitary reduced FSH and LH stimulus to the ovarian follicle.

Currently, ovarian oestrogenic secretion, which may continue in post-menopausal women, is blocked at cellular level by oral tamoxifen. This interesting and complex substance binds with the oestrogen receptors of the cancer cell to result in a competing complex which reduces cell growth. This complex may inhibit tumour growth at other sites (Hamm and Allegra, 1988).

The end result is oestrogen deficiency and tumour cytostasis. A response rate of 50–60% is anticipated if both ER and PR receptors are present. High ER receptor levels may be associated with even greater benefit. Tumours which are ER and PR negative respond less, but between 5% and 10% do benefit.

Oral progestogens bind progestogen receptor (PR) sites and tumour growth is limited at rates which match those for tamoxifen. Megestrol acetate, 40 mg orally, three or four times a day, is the popular drug. It tends to be invoked as second-line (choice) hormonal treatment. Progestogens do unfortunately

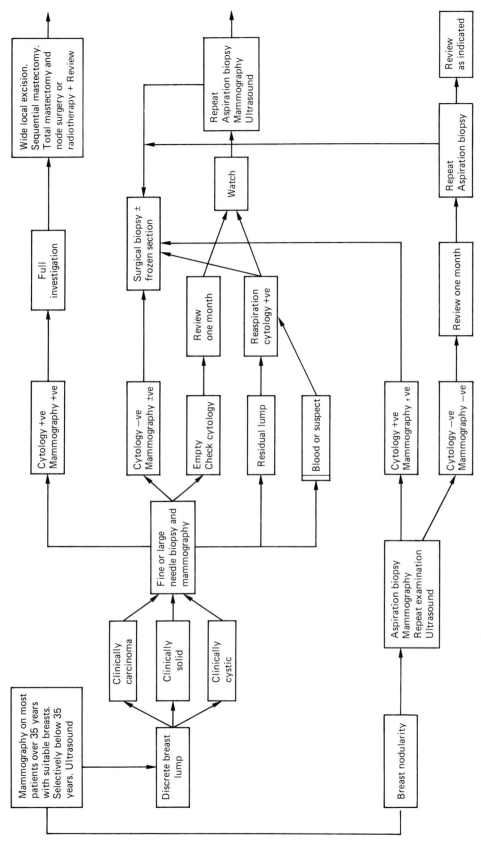

Figure 30.12 Plan for investigation of breast lump and nodularity

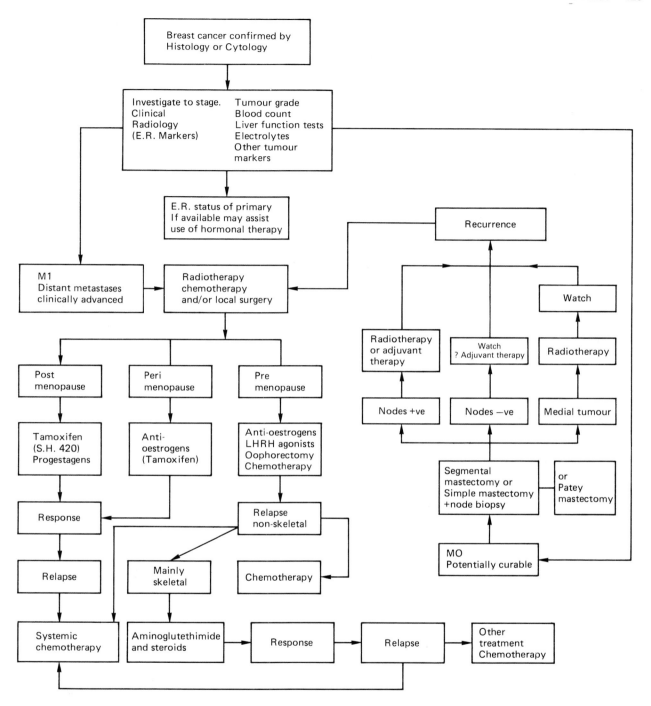

Figure 30.13 Scheme for the management of primary breast cancer

induce more side effects than tamoxifen (weight gain, hypertension, etc.). Gonadotrophin hormone release hormone agonists (LHRH agonists) were introduced during the 1980s. Their action is interesting. LHRH is normally released from the hypothalamus and stimulates the anterior pituitary lobe to secrete luteinizing hormone (LH) and follicle-stimulating hormone (FSH). In the female this stimulates oestrogen production. The normal secretory pattern of LHRH is pulsed or discontinuous. Paradoxically, continuous administration of an LHRH agonist by injection suppresses FSH and LH production and this is the basis of its therapeutic action. These agents are suitable for pre-menopausal women and response rates lie between 30% and 40%. Their action should be most predictable in receptor-positive tumours.

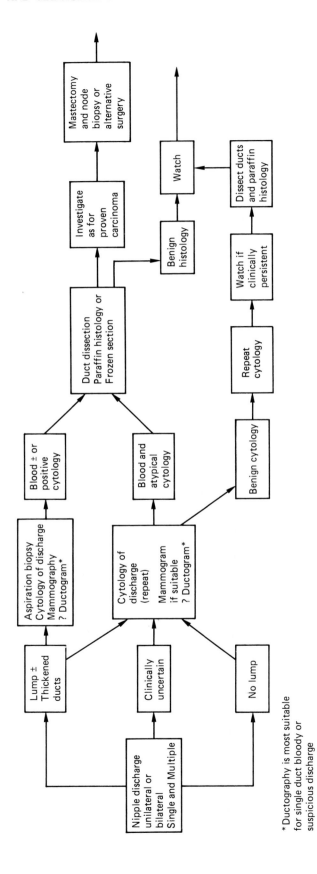

Figure 30.14 Investigation and management of nipple discharge – spontaneous or expressible

*Ductography is most suitable for single duct bloody or suspicious discharge

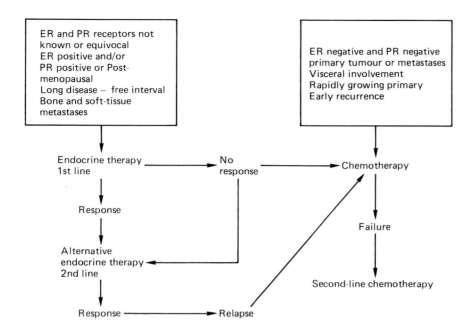

Figure 30.15 Scheme for therapeutic management of metastatic breast cancer.

The beneficial effects of adrenalectomy in post-menopausal women were related to the obliteration of adrenal androstanedione which after secretion was peripherally converted to oestrone by aromatization.

This effect is matched pharmacologically by amino glutethimide which blocks androstanedione and other steroid production. For receptor-positive patients it confers a 50% response rate and may be useful treatment at an interval when oophorectomy or other hormone manipulations have been effective but relapse has supervened. Oral cortisone acetate or hydrocortisone maintenance is necessary with amino-glutethimide treatment.

A further group of agents is the aromatase inhibitors which function in a manner similar to amino-glutethimide but interfere with peripheral oestrogen production. It is hoped that these inhibitors might be useful in post-menopausal women where tamoxifen benefit has been lost.

Loss of responsiveness to hormone manipulation is an all too familiar clinical observation and is presumably related to the heterogeneity of a tumour cell population. Synchronization–stimulation chemo-hormonal therapy has been investigated by several groups. This has included a sequence of anti-oestrogen followed by oestrogen priming and then a chemotherapy regimen (Allegra *et al.*, 1987; Lipton *et al.*, 1987).

The results are controversial and unlikely at present to induce an impact on UK clinical practice.

A scheme for therapy is set down in Figure 30.15.

Chemotherapy and breast cancer (Smith, 1987)

The first adjuvant trials began with single agents (melphalan) in the 1960s (Fisher *et al.*, 1968) with some benefit. Combination regimens followed in the 1970s and were applied to patients with advanced breast cancer. The possibility of chemotherapy attaining a place in adjuvant treatment developed from reports in the 1970s (Fisher *et al.*, 1975; Bonnadonna *et al.*, 1976).

The Fisher National Surgical Adjuvant Breast Project (NSABP) reported on two years of oral melphalan and the Milan (Bonnadonna) trial chose cyclophosphamide, methotrexate and 5-fluorouracil (CMF). Early results detected a delay in tumour recurrence, but no definite survival benefit for pre-menopausal node-positive women.

Ten-year follow-up from the NSABP trial (Fisher *et al.*, 1968) produced a statistically clear-cut 37% reduction in mortality for women under 50 years old (60% against 36% still alive). Women over 50 years did not benefit, with the caveat that a subgroup with poor prognostic features required more detailed study. The Milan trial's 10-year results reported a 35% reduction in mortality (59% against 45% alive at 10 years). This benefit was solely for pre-menopausal women. Some British studies failed to confirm those promising results (Padmanabhan *et al.*, 1986).

Comprehensive review of many thousands of women treated in chemotherapy trials has been undertaken (Peto, 1986). Combination therapy (CMF predominantly) reduced mortality by around 25–30%. How beneficial is a 25% reduction in mortality and what does it mean in clinical practice. Considering the Milan/CMF trial, 59% versus 45% alive at 10 years is a difference of 14%. The Peto review produced an overall figure of 10%. This means that for 100 women with recurrent breast cancer, 90 will derive no benefit from combination regimens of chemotherapy. The total lack of benefit in both disease recurrence and mortality for women over 50 and the small but definite benefit in the pre-menopausal group has led to the inevitable suggestion that chemotherapy produces its benefit by chemical castration. In fact, the success of oophorectomy was rather better, at 29% reduction in odds of mortality.

Disadvantages of chemotherapy are that current drugs are not very effective and they are associated with significant toxicity. Consequently, there is the need for a skilled team of medical oncologists and trained nurses within a fully equipped clinical environment to ensure maximum safety. An early study from the Royal Marsden Hospital (Palmer et al., 1980) concerned a small series of patients in whom 80% were seriously disturbed by side effects. For 29% of the women treated the verdict, in simple terms, was 'never again'! General experience since that time would be more reassuring. In particular, skilled and honest counselling is obligatory before a course of treatment is commenced. Benefit from treatment, despite some side effects, should be emphasized. Toxic symptoms are related, in part, to the length of treatment. Current research is directed towards potential benefit from shorter courses of treatment.

The Consensus Development Conference on Adjuvant Therapy (Fisher et al., 1986) recommended early postoperative chemotherapy for all pre-menopausal node-positive women. An alternative regimen has been investigated and reported (Smith et al., 1990). No decision was made then for pre-menopausal node-negative patients, but it was accepted that 25% show recurrent disease at 5 years and by 10 years the survival rate was around 70%. Node negativity was pronounced after axillary dissection and detailed examination of at least 15 nodes.

A 'Clinical Alert' (1988) heralded publication of four studies upon which it was proclaimed that node-negative pre-menopausal women should receive adjuvant therapy. Collins (1991), who analysed the papers, considered the 'Alert' ill-judged and ill-timed. Disease-free interval was prolonged in node-negative cases, but a clear difference in overall survival was absent. A similar view was adopted by Cady (1990) who found the 'Alert' message unproven. There is nevertheless no doubt that detailed assessment of node-negative cases is timely. Perhaps EGF, ploidy studies or other modes might in future identify subgroups who should receive chemotherapy. Apparently, steroid receptor status in these patients is a poor discriminator (Fisher et al., 1989; Mansour et al., 1989).

For advanced breast cancer 'de novo' Blamey suggests two important approaches (Wilson et al., 1979; Williams et al., 1986):

1. 'Soft' chemotherapeutic agents might be preferable as first-line treatment because 70% of women will be hormone resistant and half of these will be dead by 6 months! Why not therefore exhibit chemotherapy at the outset?
2. Select patients with metastatic disease who will bear no chance of response to hormone measures. This is discussed from an index of prognosis (I) formulated from multivariate analysis. The formula is: 4.0 × Grade of primary tumour (Bloom and Richardson)

   − 6.0 × ER status + 0.40 × Tissue of metastases − (0.1 × Disease-free interval in months)

Codes: ER positive = 1, negative = nil; tumour grades 1–3; tissue scores – bone (1), lung (2), bone and lung (3), hepatic (4).

From this rather contrived but seemingly valuable and tested index, the following treatment guide has been suggested:

(A) Lymphangitis carcinomatosa and/or solid lung metastases presenting as symptoms of dyspnoea are treated by broad-spectrum antibiotics and prednisolone with mucolytics. Chemotherapy should follow if rapid improvement is not achieved.
(B) I values > 16.5 (poor prognosis group) require cytotoxic therapy.
(C) I values < 16.5 are suitable for a trial of hormonal manipulation. First-line therapy is tamoxifen for post-menopausal women, and Zoladex (ICI, Macclesfield, an LHRH agonist) for pre-menopausal women. It should be added that second-line hormonal therapy might be megestrol acetate. The first- and second-line cytotoxic combinations are a matter of choice – mitozantrone, methotrexate and mitomycin C (the 3 Ms) is a current favourite in some units.

Progress or otherwise in adjuvant chemotherapy since 1985 has been reviewed by Abeloff and Beveridge (1988). Carbone (1988) appraised the review and stressed the importance of basic biological principles in breast cancer management. This involves the recognition of tumour heterogeneity and the need for future work to address the biological characteristics of the primary tumour.

It will be salutary if refined analysis of the simple histopathology and cytology of the cancer unlocks the keep to biology and thence prognosis.

Future developments

In respect of breast surgery there is no shortage of questions which need to be answered (Baum, 1982; Veronesi, 1984).

Some of the outstanding problems have been dealt with in the previous text. An overall view with comment on the worsening medico-legal scene and other aspects is considered by Cady (1990). Breast screening errors of both omission and commission will tax surgical wisdom and practical ethics to the limit.

For a volume on many aspects of breast cancer the reader is referred to that edited by Bonnadonna (1984). The incorporated bibliography is exhaustive.

Diseases of the male breast

The commonest lesion encountered in general surgical practice is gynaecomastia, which is enlargement of the ductal and stromal tissue of the male breast. From autopsy studies (Sandison, 1962) gynaecomastia is recognizable in around 5% of subjects. Gynaecomastia proper must be distinguished from pseudo-gynaecomastia which is purely fatty replacement without any palpable breast disc. The physical signs may be difficult to define. In gynaecomastia, breast tissue should be evident and should lie concentrically behind the mamilla. Any gross eccentricity or irregularity of the breast disc should lead to the suspicion of malignancy.

Important diagnostic steps include fine-needle aspiration cytology (Martin-Bates et al., 1990) and mammography. Soft-tissue radiology of the male breast can be a most useful diagnostic mode (Dershaw, 1986). The hormonal basis for and aetiological factors suggested for this fascinating pathology have been extensively reviewed (Hall, 1959; Hall et al., 1980; Hughes et al., 1989).

Puberty and a proportion of post-puberty breast enlargements will often resolve in time (Nydick et al., 1961), but persisting gynaecomastia becomes a significant cosmetic blemish.

Many cases of middle- and old-age gynaecomastia are seemingly idiopathic, but secondary enlargement must always be considered. These include hormonal imbalance due to hepatic impairment, Klinefelter's syndrome, cryptorchidism, testicular atrophy, testicular and lung carcinoma. Alternatively, drugs which exert their action in a variety of ways (anti-androgens, oestrogen receptor binding, gonadotrophin interference) disturb the androgen : oestrogen ratio and bilateral gynaecomastia results.

In clinical assessment, a careful check on hepatic enlargement, stigmata of cirrhosis, testicular state, and pathological lymphadenopathy, should be supplemented by a chest radiography. It is rare in surgical outpatient clinical practice to discover a cause for gynaecomastia.

Conservative treatment

Drug therapy has been proposed, with anti-oestrogens (clomiphene tamoxifen), anti-gonadotrophins (danazol) and anabolic steroids (nandrolone). The results of treatment are variable and surgical excision is often requested by the patient.

Surgical treatment

Once malignancy has been excluded, then surgery is basically a debulking procedure, with careful attention being paid to the eventual shape and preservation of a uniform subcutaneous fatty layer.

Small and moderate sized breasts can be approached through a peri-areolar incision. The excision can be exacting, as tissue planes are ill-defined. It is possible to bisect or quadrisect the breast disc to facilitate dissection (Hughes et al., 1989). Haemostasis can be difficult to secure because of local access, and lateral extension of the peri-areolar incision is sometimes a help. Large breasts can be tidily removed through a submammary incision. Again, a rather tedious dissection is required for a pleasing cosmetic result. In bilateral cases, the patient needs to be specifically warned of the surgical problems.

The complex bilateral gynaecomastia resulting from spironolactone treatment is particularly awkward because of cystic change, duct ectasia and abscess formation. Following simple drainage of sepsis, the inflammation should settle and, subsequently, excision of the breast disc, associated fibrosis and all ducts is undertaken.

Carcinoma of the male breast (Holleb, 1970)

This is a rare disease which accounts for 0.7% of all male cancers and between 0.5% and 1% of all breast cancers. Histopathologically the majority (62–70%) are infiltrating duct cancers. The mean age of presentation lies around 60 years. A major clinical feature is the delay in presentation, so that disease tends to be advanced and 25–30% of patients are inoperable when first seen.

The disease must be suspected in all cases of breast enlargement beyond the age of 30 years and certainly in middle age.

Most cases show undeniable clinical signs of malignancy. Confirmation is by some form of needle biopsy or total excision of the total mamma and frozen section diagnosis.

A recent long-term retrospective study of 41 men (Digenis et al., 1990) reported that a surgical clearance by a Patey-style mastectomy and axillary (level 1–3) dissection produced acceptable results. Skin grafting is sometimes necessary. Tamoxifen therapy was regarded as a promising development (Ribiero, 1983), especially for stages 2 and 3 tumours. Radiotherapy and chemotherapy were disappointing modes of treatment.

Compared stage by stage with female breast cancer, the survival rates were similar. Interestingly, male breast cancers may possess a dominance of oestrogen receptor positivity. The important message for patients and surgeons alike is early detection before lymph node metastases develop, and an adequate local procedure should be performed.

References

Abeloff, M. D. and Beveridge, R. A. (1988) Adjuvant chemotherapy of breast cancer. The consensus development conference revisited. *Oncology*, 2, 21

Adair, F., Berg, J., Joubert, L. *et al.* (1984) Long term follow up of breast cancer patients. The 30 year report. *Cancer*, **33**, 1145

Aitken, R. J., Gaze, M. N., Rodger, A. *et al.* (1989) Arm morbidity within a trial of mastectomy and either node sample with selective radiotherapy or axillary clearance. *Br. J. Surg.*, **76**, 568

Allegra, J. C., Woodcock, T. M., Seeger, J. *et al.* (1987). A phase II trial of tamoxifen, premarin, methotrexate and 5 fluorouracil in metastatic breast cancer. In *Hormonal Manipulation of Cancer* (ed. J. G. M. Klign), Raven Press, New York, p. 485

Baildam, A. D., Turnbull, L., Howell, A. *et al.* (1989). Extended role for needle biopsy in the management of carcinoma of the breast. *Br. J. Surg.*, **76**, 553

Baker, R. (ed.) (1977) *Current Trends in the Management of Breast Cancer*, Baillière Tindall, London

Ball, A. B. S., Waters, J. and Thomas, J. M. (1990) Formal axillary dissection. *Br. J. Hosp. Med.*, **44**, 396

Banerjee, A. K. (1990) In situ breast carcinoma – recent advances. *Surgery*, **76**, 1815a (The Medicine Group)

Baum, M. (1981) *Breast Cancer, The Facts*, Oxford Medical Publications, Oxford

Baum, M. (1982) Will breast self examination save lives? Editorial. *Br. Med. J. (Clin. Res.)*, **284**, 142

Berna, J. D., Madrigal, M., Guirao, J. *et al.* (1990) Microdochectomy: the precise identification of the suspicious duct. *Br. J. Surg.*, **77**, 1217

Blamey, R. W., Davies, C. J., Elston, C. W. *et al.* (1979) Prognostic factors in breast cancer – the formation of a prognostic index. *Clin. Oncol.* **5**, 227

Bloom, H. J. G. and Richardson, W. W. (1957) Histological grading and prognosis. *Br. J. Cancer*, **4**, 359

Bonnadona, G. (1984) *Cancer Investigation and Management*, Vol 1, *Breast Cancer: Diagnosis and Management*, Wiley, New York

Bonnadonna, G., Brusamolion, E., Valagussa, P. *et al.* (1976) Combination chemotherapy as an adjuvant treatment in operable breast cancer. *N. Engl. J. Med.*, **292**, 117

Bonnadona, G. and Valagussa, P. (1984) Combined modality approach. In *Breast Cancer: Diagnosis and Management* (ed. G. Bonnadonna), Wiley, New York, p. 281

Bonnadonna, G., Valagussa, P. and Veronesi, U. (1976) Results of ongoing clinical trials with adjuvant chemotherapy in operable breast cancer. In *Breast Cancer: Trends in Research and Treatment* (eds J. C. Heusen, W. H. Mattheiem and M. Rozenweig) European Organization for Research on Treatment of Cancer Monographs, Raven Press, New York, p. 239

Bostwick, J. III (1990) Reconstruction after mastectomy. *Surg. Clin. N. Am.*, **70**, 1125

Bostwick, J., Vasconex, L. O and Jurkiewicz, M. J. (1978) Breast reconstruction after radical mastectomy. *Plast. Reconstr. Surg.*, **61**, 682.

Brady, L. W. and Bedwinek, J. M. (1984) The changing role of radiotherapy. In *Breast Cancer Diagnosis and Management* (ed. G. Bonnadonna), Wiley, Chichester, UK, p. 205

Breast Cancer Screening (1986). *Report to the Health Ministers of England, Wales, Scotland and Northern Ireland*, by a Working Group chaired by Professor Sir Patrick Forrest, HMSO, London

Breast Cancer Screening (1991a). *Evidence and Experience since the Forrest Report*, NHS Breast Screening Programme (Chairman, M. Vessey)

Breast Cancer Screening (1991b) Letter to all doctors in England, from Sir Donald Acheson, 20 February (PL/CMO/91)2

Burn, J. I. (1973) Biopsy. In *Recent Advances in Surgery* (ed. S. Taylor), Churchill Livingstone, Edinburgh, p. 442

Burn, J. I., Deeley, T. J. and Malaker, K. (1968) Drill biopsy and the dissemination of cancer. *Br. J. Surg.*, **55**, 628

Cady, B. (1989) New diagnostic, staging and therapeutic aspects of early breast cancer. *Cancer*, **65**, 634

Cady, B. (1990) The Society of Surgical Oncology at a crossroads: thoughts for the future. Presidential address. *Arch. Surg.*, **125**, 153

Carbone, P. P. (1988) The article reviewed. *Oncology*, **2**, 30–32

Carbone, P. P., Gray, R., Tormey, D. C. *et al.* (1985) Adjuvant treatment with tamoxifen: the Eastern Cooperative Group (ECOG) experience. In *Reviews of Endocrine Related Cancer*, Suppl. 17, *Antihormones in Primary Breast Cancer*, Nov., 65

Carpenter, R., Boulter, P. S., Cooke, T. *et al.* (1989) The surgical treatment of ductal carcinoma of the breast. *Br. J. Surg.*, **76**, 564

Carter, C. L., Allen, C. and Hensen, D. E. (1989) Relation of tumour size, lymph node status and survival in 24,740 breast cancer cases. *Cancer*, **63**, 181

Chamberlain, J., Coleman, D., Ellman, R. *et al.* (1988) (Trial Coordinating Centre) First results on mortality reduction in the UK trial of early detection of breast cancer. *Lancet*, **ii**, 411

Coleman, D. V. (1982) Fine needle aspiration of solid tumours. In *Rob and Smith's Operative Surgery*, 4th edn (eds H. Dudley and W. Pories), Butterworths, London, p. 254.

Collins, J. A. (1991) Overview of surgery 1991. In *Surgery Annual*, Pt 1. (ed. L. M. Nyhus), Appleton and Lange, Norwalk, Conn., p. 1.

Coombs, R. C., Powles, T. J., Berger, U. *et al.* (1987) Immunocytochemical detection of ER in fine needle aspirates. *Lancet*, **ii**, 701.

Cronin, T. D. and Gerow, F. J. (1964) Augmentation mammoplasty: a new 'natural feel' prosthesis. *Transactions of the International Society of Plastic Surgeons, 3rd Congress, 1963*, Excerpta Medica, Amsterdam, p. 41

Davies, C. J., Elston, C. W., Cotton, R. E. *et al.* (1977). Preoperative diagnosis in carcinoma of the breast. *Br. J. Surg.*, **64**, 326

Dean, C., Chetty, U. and Forrest, A. P. M. (1983) Effects of immediate breast reconstruction on psychosocial morbidity after mastectomy. *Lancet*, **ii**, 459

Dershaw, D. D. (1986) Male mammography. *Am. J. Roentgenology*, **146**, 127

Digenis, A. G., Ross, C. B., Morrison, J. D. *et al.* (1990) Carcinoma of the male breast: a review of 41 cases. *South. Med. J.*, **83**, 1162

Dixon, J. M., Anderson, J. M., Lamb, J. *et al.* (1984) Fine needle aspiration cytology in relationship to clinical examination and mammography in the diagnosis of a solid breast mass. *Br. J. Surg.*, **71**, 593

Dixon, J. M. Anderson, T. J., Lumsden, A. B. *et al.* (1983) Mammary duct ectasia. *Br. J. Surg.*, **70**, 601

Dixon, J. M., Clark, P. J., Crucioli, V. *et al.* (1987) Reduction of the surgical excision rate in benign breast disease using fine needle aspiration cytology with immediate reporting. *Br. J. Surg.*, **74**, 1014

Dowden, R. V. and Dinner, M. I. (1984) Breast reconstruction without skin flaps. *Clin. Plast. Surg.*, **11**, 265,

Dowle, C. S., Owainati, A., Robins, A. *et al.* (1987) Prognostic significance of the DNA content of human breast cancer. *Br. J. Surg.*, **74**, 133

Dudley, H. (1977) In *Operative Surgery*, 3rd edn, *General Principles, Breast and Hernia* (eds H. Dudley, C. Rob and Sir R. Smith), Butterworths, London, p. 113

Editorial (1977) Pinning down the diagnosis in breast cancer. *Br. Med. J.*, **2**, 282

Fallowfield, L. F., Baum, M. and Maguire, G. P (1986) Aspects of breast conservation and psychological morbidity associated with diagnoses and treatment of early breast cancer. *Br. Med. J.*, **293**, 1331-1334

Fentiman, I. S. and Mansell, R. E (1991) The axilla: not a no-go zone. *Lancet*, **i**, 221

Fisher, B., Bauer, M., Margolese, R. *et al.* (1985) Five year results of a randomised clinical trial comparing total mastectomy and simple mastectomy with or without radiation in the treatment of breast cancer. *N. Engl. J. Med.*, **312**, 665

Fisher, B., Carbone, P., Economon, S. G. *et al.* (1975) L phenyl alanine mustard (L-PAM) in the management of primary breast cancer: a report of early findings. *N. Engl. J. Med.*, **292**, 117

Fisher, B., Ravdin, R. G., Ausman, R. K. *et al.* (1968) Surgical adjuvant chemotherapy in cancer of the breast: results of a decade of cooperative investigation. *Ann. Surg.*, **168**, 337

Fisher, B. Redmond, C., Poisson, R. *et al.* (1989) Eight year results of a randomised clinical trial comparing total mastectomy and lumpectomy with or without irradiation in the treatment of breast cancer. *N. Engl. J. Med.*, **320**, 822

Fisher, E. R., Sass, R., Fisher, B. *et al.* (1986) Pathologic findings from the national surgical adjuvant breast project protocol (6) Intraduct carcinoma (DCIS). *Cancer*, **57**, 197

Forrest, A. P. M. (1974) Primary cancer of the breast: indications for therapy. In *The Treatment of Breast Cancer* (ed. Sir H. Atkins), MTP, Lancaster, p. 9

Forrest, A. P. M. (1982) Total mastectomy and axillary node sample. In *Rob and Smith's Operative Surgery, General Principles, Breast and Intracranial Endocrines* (eds. H. Dudley and W. J. Pories), 4th edn, Butterworths, London, p. 284

Fox, M. S. (1979) On the diagnosis and treatment of breast cancer. *J. Am. Med. Ass.*, **241**, 489

Freeman, B. S. (1972) Whither subcutaneous mastectomy? *Plast. Reconstr. Surg.*, **49**, 654

Fung, A., Rayter, Z., Fisher, C. *et al.* (1990) Preoperative cytology and mammography in patients with single duct nipple discharge treated by surgery. *Br. J. Surg.*, **77**, 1211

Georgiade, N. G. (1977) Reconstructive surgery of the breast. In *Davis–Christopher Textbook of Surgery*, 11th edn (ed. D. C. Sabiston), Saunders, Philadelphia, p. 666

Grant, E. C. G. (1989) Why women should not be given hormone replacement therapy. *Br. J. Hosp. Med.*, **42**, 159

Greening, W. P. (1983) Avoiding mastectomy. *Br. J. Hosp. Med.*, **2**, 334

Grubb, C. (1981) *Colour Atlas of Breast Cytopathology*, HM & M, England

Gullick, W. J. (1990) New developments in the molecular biology of breast cancer. *Eur. J. Cancer*, **26**, 509

Haagensen, C. D. (1971) *Diseases of the Breast*, 2nd edn, Saunders, Philadelphia

Hadfield, G. J. (1960) Excision of the major duct for benign disease of the breast. *Br. J. Surg.*, **47**, 472

Hadfield, G. J. (1968) Further experience of the operation for excision of the major duct system of the breast. *Br. J. Surg.*, **55**, 530

Hall, P. F. (1959) *Gynaecomastia*, Monographs of the Federal Council of the BMA, Australia

Hall, R., Anderson, J., Smart, G. A. and Besser, M. (1980) *Fundamentals of Clinical Endocrinology*, Pitman Medical, London

Hamilton, C. R. and Buchanan, R. B. (1990) Radiotherapy for ductal carcinoma in situ detected by screening. *Br. Med. J.*, **301**, 224

Hamm, J. T. and Allegra, J. C. (1988) Advances in the hormonal therapy of metastatic breast cancer. *Adv. Oncol.*, **4**, 22. Cligott Publishing, Bristol

Handley, R. S. (1964) Benign breast disease. In *Clinical Surgery: General Principles and Breast* (eds C. Rob and Sir R. Smith), Vol 1, Ch. 33, London, Butterworths p. 349

Handley, R. S. (1974) Techniques of surgical treatment. In *The Treatment of Breast Cancer* (ed. Sir H. Atkins), MTP, Lancaster, p. 49.

Harris, J. R., Botnick, L., Bloomer, W. B. *et al.* (1981) Primary radiation therapy for early breast cancer: the experience at the Joint Centre of Radiation Therapy. *Int. J. Radiat. Oncol. Biol. Phys.*, **7**, 1549

Hawkins, R. A., White, G., Bundred, N. J. *et al.* (1987) Prognostic significance of oestrogen and progestogen receptor activities in breast cancer. *Br. J. Surg.*, **74**, 1009

Haybittle, J. L., Blamey, R. W., Elston, C. W. *et al.* (1982) A prognostic index in primary breast cancer. *Br. J. Cancer*, **54**, 301

Henderson, B. E., Pike, M. C. and Ross, R. K. (1984) Epidemiology and risk factors. In *Cancer: Diagnosis and Management* (ed. G. Bonnadonna), Wiley, Chichester, UK, p. 15

Hermann, R. E. and Esselstyn, J. R. C. B. (1982) Partial mastectomy for carcinoma of the breast. In *Rob and Smith's Operative Surgery, General Principles, Breast and Intracranial Endocrines* (eds H. Dudley and W. J. Pories), 4th edn, Butterworths, London, p. 287

Holleb, A. I. (1970) Cancer of the male breast. In *Breast Cancer: Early and Late*, Proceedings of the 13th Annual Clinical Conference on Cancer, Houston, Texas, 1968, Year Book Medical Publishers, Chicago, p. 245

Hughes, L. E. (1982) Operations for benign breast disease. In *Rob and Smith's Operative Surgery*, 4th edn (eds H. Dudley and W. Pories) Butterworths, London, p. 239

Hughes, L. E. (1984) Breast reconstruction after mastectomy. *Surgery* (Medical Education International Ltd, p. 165

Hughes, L. E., Mansell, R. E. and Webster, D. J. T. (1989) *Benign Disorders and Diseases of the Breast*, Baillière Tindall, London

Kissin, M. W., Thompson, E. M., Price, A. B. *et al.* (1982) The inadequacy of axillary sampling in breast cancer. *Lancet*, **i**, 1210

Koelmeyer, T. D. and MacCormick, D. E. M. (1976) Granulomatous mastitis. *Aust. NZ J. Surg.*, **46**, 173

Lagios, M. D., Margolin, F. R., Westdahl, P. R. *et al.* (1989) Mammographically detected ductal carcinoma in situ: frequency of local recurrence following tylectomy and prognostic effect of nuclear grade on local recurrence. *Cancer*, **63**, 618

Lagios, M. D., Westdahl, P. R., Margolin, F. R. *et al.* (1982) Duct carcinoma in situ. Relationship of extent of non-invasive disease to the frequency of occult invasion multicentricity, lymph node metastases and short term treatment failure. *Cancer*, **50**, 1309

Levit, F. (1977) Jogger's nipples. *N. Engl. J. Med.*, **297**, 1197

Lipton, A., Santen, R. J., Harvey, H. A. *et al.* (1987) A randomised trial of aminoglutethimide and oestrogen before chemotherapy in advanced breast cancer. *Am. J. Clin. Oncol.*, **10**, 65

Lundy, J., Lozowski, M. S., Darvy, A. S. *et al.* (1990) The use of fine needle aspirates of breast cancers to evaluate hormone receptor status. *Arch. Surg.*, **125**, 174

Lynch, H. T. (1990) The family history and control of hereditary breast cancer. *Arch. Surg.*, **125**, 151

McArdle, J. M., Hughson, A. V. M. and McArdle, C. S. (1990) Reduced psychological morbidity after breast conservation. *Br. J. Surg.*, **77**, 1221

McKinna, J. (1983) Clinical examination. In: *Diagnosis of Breast Disease* (ed. C. A. Parsons), Chapman and Hall, London, p. 26

McKissock, P. K. (1972) Reduction mammoplasty with a vertical dermal flap. *Plast. Reconstr. Surg.*, **49**, 245

Magarey, C. J. and Watson, W. J. (1976) The outpatient diagnosis of breast lumps. *Aust. NZ J. Surg.*, **46**, 344

Maguire, P. (1984) Psychological reactions to breast cancer and its treatment. In *Breast Cancer: Diagnosis and Management* (ed. G. Bonnadonna), Wiley, Chichester, p. 303

Mansi, J. L. and Smith, I. E. (1989) Endocrine therapy for breast cancer: mechanisms and new approaches. *Cancer Topics*, **7**, **57**, Media Medica, Chichester, UK/Lederle Laboratories

Mansour, E. G., Gray, R., Shatila, A. *et al.* (1989) Efficacy of adjuvant chemotherapy in high risk node negative breast cancer. *N. Engl. J. Med.*, **320**, 485

Martin-Bates, E., Krausz, T. and Phillips, I. (1990) Evaluation of fine needle aspiration of the male breast for the diagnosis of gynaecomastia. *Cytopathology*, **i**, 79

Masood, S., Frykberg, E. R., McLellan, G. L. *et al.* (1990) Prospective evaluation of radiologically detected fine needle aspiration biopsy of non-palpable breast lesions. *Cancer*, **66**, 1480

Melcher, D., Lineham, J. and Smith R. (1984) The breast. In *Practical Aspiration Cytology*, Churchill Livingstone, Edinburgh, p. 10

Michell, M. J. and Ebbs, S. R. (1989) Needle localisation of impalpable breast lesions. *Surgery*, **67**, 1588, The Medicine Group, Abingdon, UK

Millis, R. R. and Thynne, G. S. J. (1975) In situ intraduct carcinoma of the breast: a long term follow up study. *Br. J. Surg.*, **62**, 957

Morgan, B. D. G. (1987) Skin cover. In *Current Surgical Practice* (eds J. Hadfield and M. Hobsley), Vol. 4, Edward Arnold, London, p. 80

Morris, J. and Royle, G. T. (1987) Choice of surgery for early breast cancer: pre and post operative levels of clinical anxiety and depression in patients and their husbands. *Br. J. Surg.*, **74**, 1017

Morrison, R. and Deeley, T. J. (1955) Drill biopsy: technique using high-speed drill. *J. Fac. Radiol.*, **6**, 287

Nash, A. G. and Hurst, P. A. E. (1983) Central breast carcinoma treated by simultaneous mastectomy and latissimus dorsi flap reconstruction. *Br. J. Surg.*, **70**, 654

Nicholson, S., Sainsbury, J. R. C., Wadhera, V. *et al.* (1988) Use of fine needle aspiration cytology with immediate reporting in the diagnosis of breast disease. *Br. J. Surg.*, **75**, 847

Nydick, M., Bustos, J., Dale, J. H. *et al.* (1961) Gynaecomastia in adolescent boys. *J. Am. Med. Ass.*, **178**, 449–457

Osborne, M. P. and Borgen, P. J. (1990) Role of mastectomy in breast cancer. *Surg. Clin. N. Am.*, **70**, 1023 Mechanism of action of adjuvant chemotherapy in early breast cancer. *Lancet*, **ii**, 411

Page, D. L. and Anderson, T. J. (1987) *Diagnostic Histopathology of the Breast*, Churchill Livingstone, Edinburgh, pp. 89–103

Palmer, B. V., Walsh, G. A., McKinn, A. J. A. *et al.* (1980) Adjuvant chemotherapy for breast cancer: side effects and quality of life. *Br. Med. J.*, **2**, 1594

Patey, D. H. and Dyson, W. H. (1948) The prognosis of carcinoma of the breast in relation to the type of operation performed. *Br. J. Cancer*, **2**, 7

Peto, R. (1986) Data presented at King's Fund Forum on treatment of primary breast cancer, London, October 1986, quoted by Smith, I. E. (1987)

Phipps, R. F. and Rayter, Z (1990) In situ carcinoma of the breast. *Br. J. Hosp. Med.*, **44**, 168

Radovan C. (1982) Breast reconstruction after mastectomy using the temporary expander. *Plast. Reconstr. Surg.*, **69**, 195

Ribiero, G. G. (1983) Tamoxifen in the treatment of male breast carcinoma. *Clin. Radiol.*, **34**, 625

Ribiero, G. and Swindell, R. (1985) The Christie Hospital tamoxifen (Nolvadex) adjuvant trial for operable breast cancer, 7 year results. *Eur. J. Cancer. Clin. Oncol.*, **21**, 897

Ribiero, G. and Swindell, R. (1988) Adjuvant tamoxifen therapy. *Br. J. Cancer*, **57**, 601

Riddell, V. H. (1954) Carcinoma of the breast: a review of the treatment. *Ann. R. Coll. Surg. Engl.*, **14**, 215

Rilke, F. (1984) Influence of pathologic factors on management. In *Breast Cancer: Diagnosis and Management* (ed. G. Bonnadonna), Wiley, New York, p. 50

Roberts, J. G., Preece, P. E., Bolton, P. M. *et al.* (1975) The 'Tru-cut' biopsy in breast cancer. *Clin. Oncol.*, **1**, 297

Roberts, M. M. (1989) Breast screening: time for a rethink. *Br. Med. J.*, **299**, 1153

Rodgers, A. (1990) To tell or to sell. Informed consent in breast screening. *Cancer Topics*, **8**, 27. Media Medica, Chichester, UK/Lederle Laboratories

Rosen, P. P., Lieberman, P. H., Braunn, D. W. *et al.* (1978) Lobular carcinoma in situ of the breast. *Am. J. Surg. Path.*, **2**, 225

Rosen, P. P., Saigo, P. E., Braunn, D. W. *et al.* (1981) Predictors of recurrence in Stage 1 (T_1 N_0 M_0) breast carcinoma. *Ann. Surg.*, **193**, 15

Rosen, P. P., Servie, R. Schottenfeld, D. *et al.* (1979) Non invasive breast cancer. Frequency of unsuspected invasion and implications for treatment. *Ann. Surg.*, **189**, 377

Rosner, D. (1980) Non invasive breast cancer. Results of a national survey by the American College of Surgeons. *Ann. Surg.*, **192**, 139

Sainsbury, J. R. C., Nicholson, S., Angus, B. *et al.* (1988) Epidermal growth factor receptor status of histological subtypes of breast cancer. *Br. J. Cancer*, **58**, 458

Sandison, A. T. (1962) *An Autopsy Study of the Human Breast*, Monograph No. 8, National Cancer Institute/ US Dept. Health Education and Welfare

Silverstein, M. J., Gierson, E. D., Gamagami, P. *et al.* (1990) Breast cancer diagnosis and prognosis in women augmented with silicone gel filled implants. *Cancer*, **66**, 97

Silverstein, M. J., Waisman, J. R., Gamagami, P. *et al.* (1990) Intraductal carcinoma of the breast, 208 cases. Clinical factors influencing treatment choice. *Cancer*, **66**, 102

Skrabanek, P. (1988) The debate over mass mammography in Britain. *Br. Med. J.* **297**, 970

Smallwood, J., Herbert, A., Guyer, P. *et al.* (1985) Accuracy of aspiration cytology in the diagnosis of breast disease. *Br. J. Surg.*, **72**, 841

Smith, D., Dewar, J. A., Horobin, J. M. *et al.* (1990) Meakin adjuvant regimen in premenopausal patients with breast cancer. *Br. J. Surg.*, **77**, 129

Smith, I. E. (1987) *Adjuvant Chemotherapy in Early Breast Cancer. Focus: Breast Cancer; a Changing Scene*, Medicom (UK) Ltd

Tabar L. and Dean, P. B. (1984) Risks and benefits of mammography in population screening for Breast Cancer. In *Breast Cancer: Diagnosis and Management* (ed. G. Bonnadonna), Wiley, Chichester, UK, p. 63

Thomas, B. A. and Boulter, P. S. (1984) Clinical examination and investigation of the breast. *Surgery* (Medical Education International Ltd), **1** (4), 86

Thomas, W. G., Williamson, R. C. N. Davies, J. D. *et al.* (1982) The clinical syndrome of mammary duct ectasia. *Br. J. Surg.*, **69**, 423

Trott, P. A. (1983) Cytological investigation. In *Diagnosis of Breast Disease* (ed. C. A. Parsons), Chapman and Hall, London, p. 203

Veronesi, U. (1984) Current status of primary surgery in the management of breast cancer. In *Breast Cancer: Diagnosis and Management* (ed. G. Bonnadonna), Wiley, Chichester, UK, p. 169

Veronesi, U., Banfi, A., Salvadori, B. *et al.* (1990) Breast conservation as the treatment of choice in small breast cancers. *Eur. J. Cancer*, **26**, 668

Veronesi, U., Saccozzi, R., Del Vecchio, M. *et al.* (1981) Comparing radical mastectomy with quadrantectomy, a dissection and radiotherapy in patients with small cancers of the breast. *N. Engl. J. Med.*, **305**, 6

Vinton, A. L., Traverso, W. and Zehring, R. D. (1990) Immediate breast reconstruction following mastectomy is as safe as mastectomy alone. *Arch. Surg.*, **125**, 1303 (paper and discussion by several contributors)

Wanebo, H. J., Huvos, W. D. and Urban, J. A. (1974) Treatment of minimal breast cancer. *Cancer*, **33**, 349

Ward, D. C. and Edwards, M. H. (1983) Early results of subcutaneous mastectomy with immediate silicone prosthetic implant for carcinoma of the breast. *Br. J. Surg.*, **70**, 651

Watts, G. T. (1977) In *Operative Surgery*, 3rd edn, *General Principles, Breast and Hernia* (eds H. Dudley, C. Rob and Sir R. Smith), Butterworths, London, p. 86

Webb, A. J. (1970) The diagnostic cytology of breast carcinoma. *Br. J. Surg.*, **57**, 259

Webb, A. J. (1975) A cytological study of mammary disease. *Ann. R. Coll. Surg. Engl.*, **56**, 181.

Webb, A. J. (1982) Surgical aspects of aspiration biopsy cytology. In *Recent Advances in Surgery* (ed. R. C. G. Russell), Churchill Livingstone, Edinburgh

Webster, D. J. T. and Hughes, L. E. (1983) The rectus abdominis myocutaneous island flap in breast cancer. *Br. J. Surg.*, **70**, 71

Weiner, D. L. (1972) On subcutaneous mastectomy. *Plast. Reconstr. Surg.*, **49**, 654

Welch, M., Durrans, D., Gonzalez, J. *et al.* (1990) Microdochectomy for discharge from a single lactiferous duct. *Br. J. Surg.*, **77**, 1213

Wellings, S. R. (1980) development of breast cancer. *Adv. Cancer Res.*, **31**, 287

Wellings, S. R., Jensen, H. M. and Marcum, R. G. (1975) An atlas of subgross pathology of the human breast with reference to possible precancerous lesions. *J. Nat. Cancer Inst.*, **55**, 231

Widow, W. (1968) *Atlas on the Clinical Diagnosis of Mammary Carcinoma*, Akademie Verlag, Berlin

Williams, J. E. (1972) Experiences with a large series of silastic breast implants. *Plast. Reconstr. Surg.*, **49**, 253

Williams, M. R., Todd, J. H., Nicholson, R. I. *et al.* (1986) Survival patterns in hormone treated advanced breast cancer. *Br. J. Surg.*, **73**, 752

Wilson, A. J., Baum, M., Brinkley, D. M. *et al.* (1985) Six year results of a controlled trial of tamoxifen as a single adjuvant agent in the management of early breast cancer. *Wld J. Surg.*, **9**, 756

Wilson, R. G., Blamey, R. W., Benton, F. M. *et al.* (1979) Combination chemotherapy in breast cancer: response rate and attempts to predict response. *Clin. Oncol.*, **5**, 169

Wong, J. H., Kopald, K. H. and Morton, D. L. (1990) Impact of microinvasion on axillary node metastases and survival in patients with intraductal breast cancer. *Arch. Surg.*, **125**, 1298

Further reading

Atkins, Sir H. (ed.) (1974) *The Treatment of Breast Cancer*, MTP, Lancaster

Breast Cancer: Early and Late, Proceedings of the 13th Annual Clinical Conference on Cancer, Houston, Texas, 1968, Year Book Medical Publishers, Chicago

Dudley, H., Rob, C. and Smith, Sir R. (eds) (1976-1978) *Operative Surgery*, 3rd edn, *General Principles, Breast and Hernia*, London, Butterworths

Johnston, G. S. and Jones, A. E. (1975) *Breast Cancer Diagnosis*, Plenum, New York

Joslin, C. A. (ed.) (1978) *Aspects of Cancer Management: Carcinoma of the Breast*, Proceedings of a Symposium held at the University of York, 13 April 1977, Medical Congresses and Symposia Consultants, Tunbridge Wells, UK

Voeth, J. M. (ed.) (1976) *Frontiers of Radiation Therapy and Oncology*, Vol. 2, *Breast Cancer*, Karger, Basel

31

Microsurgical techniques in reconstructive surgery

P. L. G. Townsend

The introduction of the operating microscope has facilitated surgery on smaller structures than would be possible without the aid of such magnification.

In hand surgery its value has been established in nerve repair but the main advances have occurred in microvascular work where it is now possible to repair small vessels of diameter 0.5–3 mm. This has enabled replantation of digits to take place and has allowed reconstructive procedures with tissue transfer from one area of the body to another. The blood supply is reconnected, flow restored and living grafts established.

Microsurgical techniques require training as under the limited field of the microscope, specialized instruments such as fine jeweller's forceps, needle holders and small, non-crushing vascular clamps are manipulated. A bipolar electrocautery is necessary as this allows coagulation only between the tips of its fine forceps. Diamond knives or disposable micro-knives are used for dissecting nerve fasciculi or opening up small vessels to facilitate end-to-side anastomosis. Fine vessel cutters, micro-scissors, micro-irrigation and suction devices and, lastly, coloured background to provide contrast (blue behind vessels and yellow behind nerves) are all essential.

Microscopes developed for plastic surgery have beam splitters, allowing the surgeon and the assistant to sit opposite each other, which enables them to have an identical operative visual field with stereoscopic vision. The assistant is able to assist the surgeon in, for example, counter-traction or cutting fine sutures and irrigation. A microscope with magnification 25–40 times allows visualization of the connective tissue layer on a nerve 0.1 mm in thickness.

Nerve repair

The results of nerve repair, whether primary or secondary, depend on the ability to bring nerve ends together with minimal tension, carrying out accurate placement of sutures as atraumatically as possible. If after debridement of the ends of the nerve there is a gap, in some situations it may be possible to reroute the nerve, shortening its course as occurs in anterior translocation of the ulnar nerve, but usually a nerve graft is required. The sural nerve is the usual donor site for a nerve graft.

The blood supply to a peripheral nerve is usually via the mesoneurium or suspending mesentery. Within the nerve trunk itself there is a longitudinal system of vessels which allows circulation to continue even after some freeing of the surrounding tissue. If after repair the nerve is elongated more than 15%, there is evidence that this intraneural flow ceases. Continuous circumferential sutures are not advised as sutures are placed to provide correct alignment and not to provide a watertight seal. It is important during nerve repair to keep the ends moist.

Epineurial repair (Figure 31.1)

This is the repair of the outer sheath of the divided nerve. Although it may be carried out without magnification, even simple enlargement by the use of loupes can help to visualize longitudinal vessels which can then be matched. Results are best where the nerves are either purely sensory or purely motor and where the intraneural connective tissue component is small (this can vary from 22% to 80%).

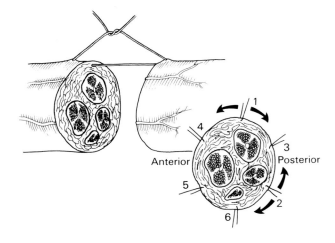

Figure 31.1 Epineurial nerve repair

After looking at the longitudinal vessels the epineurium is picked up with jeweller's forceps about 1 cm from the ends, and traction gently decreases the nerve gap. A microsuture (usually 8/0–10/0 Ethicon) is placed through the epineurium about 1 mm from one cut end, starting at the top end or 12 o'clock. This suture passes longitudinally down the axis of the nerve and out of the divided end and then through the equivalent position on the other nerve stump, with the needle bites in the same location in both stumps. The suture is tied relatively loosely and left long to allow rotation of the nerve by traction. A second suture is placed at 120° to the first behind the nerve, and this is also left long. Repair can then be completed and six sutures placed symmetrically may be required. If, after completion, fasciculi are herniating out, further sutures must be placed to prevent a lateral neuroma forming.

Perineurial or fascicular repair (Figure 31.2)

The perineurium is the connective tissue condensation around the individual nerve fasciculi, the larger the fasciculus the thicker the layer.

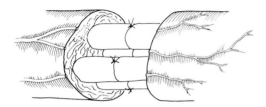

Figure 31.2 Perineurial or fascicular repair

With large or mixed nerves where there are a number of fasciculi, accurate alignment of the equivalent ends undoubtedly improves the quality of the result. Within the more distal part of the peripheral nerve, there is less reshuffling of the axons. With more accurate fascicular orientation more peripheral divisions of the nerves should, and usually do, provide the best results following repair. More proximally each fasciculus contains a mixture of components and with even the more accurate reapposition results may be inadequate as it is impossible to align individual axons.

The number of sutures used in fascicular repair must be a balance between accurate alignment and increase in the amount of foreign material introduced.

Perineurial repair is difficult without magnification. Initially, the epineurium is stripped off for about 1 cm as it is believed that this layer is primarily responsible for connective tissue proliferation, and this stripping can be aided by blowing up this outer layer using saline injected via a blunt-ended needle. A cuff of this tissue is resected and allowed to retract, and the fasciculi can then be separated using micro-scissors and knives. It is best to divide these cleanly at different levels to prevent superimposition of the joins. Sutures (10/0 Ethicon) are placed within the connective tissue layer to prevent damage to the axons.

Usually one suture per fasciculus is required but in some mixed nerves, such as the median, which has about 30 fasciculi, only the larger ones may be aligned.

Alternative techniques using epineurial – perineurial sutures can provide the advantages of both methods. The epineurium is picked up accurately, the suture passed more deeply between the fasciculi picking up equivalent ends and not all of these need to be tied since they act as guides.

Nerve grafts

In secondary nerve repair, where there has been a traumatic deficit, or after resection of the ends including neuromas, there may be a deficit which cannot be closed without tension. In this situation a nerve graft is indicated.

In larger nerves, several cables of donor nerve are required, usually from the sural, and these are taken slightly longer than the deficit, to allow for contraction. The epineurium is transected from both ends of the nerve to be repaired. In the nerve graft the epineurium is left intact, partly for placement of sutures but also because the vascular network here needs to pick up a new blood supply from the bed.

Vascularized nerve grafts

Long nerve grafts, over 8 cm, and grafts placed in poor vascular beds which are heavily scarred, function badly and for this reason techniques are being developed to vascularize nerves.

Microvascular repair

The technique of learning microvascular anastomosis must be acquired in the laboratory. Although some expertise can be obtained by practising on pieces of rubber glove, silicone tubing or leaves, it is only on blood vessels that the technique may be perfected. Although there is some value in practising on vessels from cadavers or dead animals, it is only in those vessels with blood flow that a real judgement of anastomotic success can be applied. This is usually carried out on animals, such as rats or rabbits.

With nerve repair accurate placement of sutures is required, but the only assessment is in the long term, and even then other factors such as infection, haematoma or a poor vascular bed may influence the result.

In microvascular anastomosis poor technique will restrict or terminate blood flow: a single incorrect suture may produce thrombosis at the anastomotic site. The beam splitter enables the assistant to pass judgement on suture placement, tension and numbers required. After removal of the clamps any leaks are immediately apparent.

Microvascular anastomosis (Figure 31.3)

It is neccessary to resect damaged vessels back until they look normal; this pathology may have been due to trauma, irradiation or atherosclerosis. The vessel can then be cleanly resected, either with a vessel cutter or sharp micro-scissors. In the case of the proximal end of the artery, demonstration that a free flow of blood occurs is advisable. If there is vessel disparity, the smaller vessel may be cut obliquely to increase the circumference of the lumen.

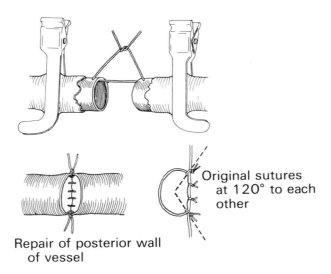

Repair of posterior wall of vessel

Original sutures at 120° to each other

Figure 31.3 End-to-end anastomosis of small blood vessel using microsurgical techniques

The ends of the vessels to be anastomosed are then clamped with non-crushing micro-clamps, which are either individual or special approximating clamps. The adventitia on the outside of the vessels (which contributes to thrombosis) is cleaned off the ends using micro-scissors and jeweller's forceps. With an artery it is often possible to pull a sleeve of adventitia over the end and then transect it. The adventitia then retracts beyond the media and intima.

The adventitial resection should be at least 2–3 mm. The vessels often go into spasm and the ends of a micro-dilator can then be inserted into the lumen and allowed to separate without force. The tips of these dilators are machined smooth to minimize intimal damage and should be the only instruments placed on the inside of the vessels. Blood or clots are then washed out using a fine cannula and heparinized saline, and after both vessel ends are so treated they are approximated. Coloured background is placed behind the vessels, to provide contrast and to keep blood out of the lumen.

End-to-end anastomosis

Sutures, usually 9/0/ or 10/0 non-absorbable mono-

filament, are used. The first suture is applied to the posterior wall passing through the media and intima, taking a small bite of the latter. As a separate bite, the suture is then passed through the open end of the other vessel through the intima and then through the equivalent spot on the media. Symmetry is all important. The suture is then tied, more snugly with an artery than with a vein or a nerve. A surgeon's knot is used with the double throw placed squarely so that there is less likelihood of it breaking. The end of this first suture is left long to allow it to be held by forceps.

A second suture is then placed at 120° to the first on the posterior wall. When this is tied the opening on the front of the vessel tends to pout and it is easier to check from the intimal aspect the effect of the sutures placed on the posterior wall. The second suture is also left long so these ends may be grasped and the vessel rotated by the assistant. The repair of the posterior wall is then completed by two or three more sutures depending on the size and type of the vessel. Veins require fewer sutures as the blood pressure is lower.

The long-stay sutures are released and inspection again made of the lumen to make sure the initial sutures have not accidentally picked up the anterior wall. A suture is then placed in the front of the vessel at 120° to the first suture and each of the remaining sections then separately sutured. During suturing it is often necessary to irrigate with heparinized saline to remove blood seeping into the vessel ends. Placement of the final sutures may be difficult, for when these are tied it may be impossible to visualize the lumen adequately and to ensure that the posterior wall has not been picked up by the needle. A method which avoids this is to pass several sutures through the appropriate layers and divide them, leaving the ends long. A final inspection of the lumen is then carried out with irrigation and these remaining sutures are then tied.

After anastomosis of vein and artery is complete the clamps are removed; venous clamps are usually released before the arterial, and distal before the proximal arterial clamp. Blood should then be seen to cross the anastomosis. Usually there is some seepage of blood in the gaps between the sutures which should stop, but if there is free bleeding further sutures may be necessary.

Should the vessels go into spasm, lignocaine or Praxilene Forte (naftidrofuryl) is squirted on and a warm, moist pack placed over the anastomosis for a few minutes. Assessment of flow can then be made either clinically by obvious perfusion of the replant or flap or by direct vision. The Ackland test is useful. The tips of two micro-forceps are placed beyond the anastomosis occluding the lumen. The forceps downstream are then used to milk the blood out of the lumen so a segment of vessel between the two forceps is collapsed. The forceps adjacent to the anastomosis are then released and blood flow into the collapsed segment indicates a patent anastomosis (Figure 31.4).

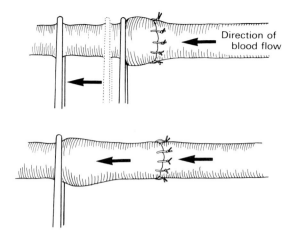

Figure 31.4 Ackland patency test following microvascular anastomosis

The technique for artery and vein anastomosis is essentially the same, although fewer sutures are required for the vein. Vein walls may be very thin and slightly larger bites may be required, and sutures are tied less tightly. It may be of help with thin-walled veins to float the vessel ends in fluid which helps to separate the walls.

End-to-side anastomosis

One of the problems of end-to-end anastomosis is the tendency for the vessel to go into spasm occluding the lumen. In a vessel which is partially divided the opening tends to retract which enhances blood flow, a situation well known clinically where a completely transected vessel usually stops bleeding, whereas a vessel which has been nicked tends to bleed profusely.

Advantage is taken of this observation by anastomosing the donor artery in, for example, a free flap into the side of the recipient artery.

The end of the donor vessel and a section of the side of the recipient vessel are prepared by removing adventitia. An appropriate sized stoma comparable to the lumen of the donor artery is made either by a clean longitudinal cut or by picking up the media and intima with forceps and cutting this with curved sharp scissors, although this latter manoeuvre may be difficult. The anastomosis is then carried out, the posterior wall first. It is not usually possible to rotate the vessel by this method, so technically this T anastomosis can be more difficult to accomplish although undoubtedly there is an improved patency rate.

Replantation

The first indications for microvascular surgery were for replantation of digits, limbs, scalps or ears although the majority are digital replantations. Amputation may be partial or complete.

In partial amputation the blood supply has been interrupted and necrosis of the end will occur unless this supply is re-established. The connection remaining may be tendon or even a small skin bridge, and the latter may contain valuable veins. If the connection is badly crushed, then debridement may require excision producing a complete amputation.

Complete amputation may be a clean-cut guillotine-type amputation or associated with crushing or avulsion or a combination of these factors.

Treatment of the severed part

The amputated part should be placed in an isotonic saline soaked sterile gauze, which may be placed in a plastic bag which is then placed into an outer plastic bag containing ice from a domestic refrigerator. On no account should the digit be allowed to freeze as ice particles will form and the success rate will fall. The bag should not, therefore, be placed in a Thermos or insulated box.

If revascularization is achieved within 8 h of cold ischaemia time, the success rate is as high as 90%, depending on the type of amputation. Particularly successful with guillotine amputations, this success rate falls rapidly after this time. For this reason prior warning to the replantation centre and a two-team approach can improve results. One team identifies the structures on the amputated part and excises traumatized tissue and the other team works in a similar way on the stump.

Indications for replantation surgery

Not every patient is suitable for surgery and consideration has to be given to the type and level of the injury. Multiplicity of digital loss, dominance of the hand, social factors, job requirement, age and the likelihood of long-term use all need careful thought. Absolute indications for replantation are where there is loss of more than one finger, a thumb or whole hand amputation. The presence of severe crushing may be a contraindication depending on how much shortening is necessary to obtain apposition of undamaged vessels, although vein grafts can reduce the lengths needing resection. Undoubtedly avulsion causes skip lesions in the vessels and reduces the success rate, but an attempt at replantation could still be indicated in, for example, complete thumb amputation. Single digit replantations, except in children, are usually unrewarding, often leading to stiff fingers, and the patient ultimately may request the offending digit to be removed.

Clean-cut amputations from distal palm up to distal forearm, are very rewarding when replanted. There is relatively little muscle bulk here and, therefore, more tolerance to ischaemia. Repairs are mainly of tendons rather than muscle and return of sensation to fingers and thumb is usually very adequate.

More proximal amputations involve an increasing

amount of muscle bulk in the specimen and with it, after circulation has been restored, a definite risk of renal failure with distribution of toxins into the general circulation. In upper arm amputations, vessels are large and relatively easy to repair. Nerve repair is, however, disappointing at this level, not only because of the long delay before nerve regeneration reaches the hand but also due to the intermixing of sensory and motor modalities at a higher level. Following replantation at a proximal level on the upper limb, some movement of flexion and extension of the elbow may be achieved with some poor protective sensation in the hand, but little else can be expected. In China, better functional results have been achieved by shortening the upper arm but this technique is probably unacceptable in the Western world.

Technique

Debridement

The full extent of the injury may only be perceived under magnification. There may be damage at several levels making revascularization, even with the aid of vein grafts, unlikely, and a decision may be made at this late stage not to proceed. Trimming back the vessels until they look normal is essential, and skin-releasing incisions on the side and back may be required to identify arteries and veins.

Bony fixation

This may be achieved by wires, plates or pins, and may be done after trimming, but shortening digits should be restricted to 2 cm.

Tendon and muscle repair

Those structures lying deep to the vessels should be repaired first since after the circulation is restored great difficulty may be had in achieving this without damaging the reconstructed vessels. Accurate repair should be carried out in the primary situation as secondary repair is more hazardous.

Nerve repair

This is usually carried out prior to vessel repair by the techniques described earlier.

Restoring circulation

The more distal the amputation of a digit the more difficult it is to find suitable veins, in which case arterial repair is carried out first, clamps released and veins allowed to dilate up to enable them to be visualized. In amputation of finger tips, arterial anastomosis alone may be sufficient if leeches are used or the patient heparinized. After 48 h the microcirculation is usually restored.

However, both arteries and veins are usually repaired to prevent congestion, more veins being anastomosed than arteries. Thus if both digital arteries are repaired, the aim should be to reanastomose three veins. If there is a deficit a vein graft, reversed in the case of the artery, needs to be interposed to produce end-to-end anastomosis. In the case of the thumb, opportunity may be taken for a long vein graft to be attached and carried down to anastomose end to side onto the radial artery.

Skin

Suturing should be achieved without tension, allowing for postoperative swelling. Skin grafts may be required or even cross-finger flaps from adjacent undamaged fingers.

Postoperative care

Clinical observation is satisfactory, but monitoring may be of help to assess the circulation and to compare, for example, the temperature of the tip of the replanted digit with equivalent tip of a healthy finger. This may give early indication should the circulation become impaired, when re-exploration is indicated. The use of heparin or other anticoagulants may produce more problems than they solve in the form of haematomas but may be useful in fingertip injuries.

Digital reconstruction

The techniques used for replantation may be used in reconstruction. In the hand, loss of thumb or digits may be either congenital or traumatic. In traumatic cases, proximal to the site of amputation, the end of the nerves and tendons are all present, as is the case in congenital amputations secondary to amniotic bands. In transverse metatarsal arrest the digits are missing but the equivalent tendons and nerves are absent.

Reconstruction of these digits may be achieved by transferring a toe or toes to replace the missing digits, either to provide a pinch grip between the reconstructed thumb and remaining fingers or between the thumb and reconstructed finger. In the latter case two toes may be taken up to provide a tripod grip.

Dissection of the toe

The toe, usually the second, is mobilized, together with its metatarsophalangeal joint and metatarsal. The blood supply is usually from the dorsalis pedis and its first dorsal metatarsal artery. This superficial arterial system is connected via a communicating artery with the plantar arch and occasionally it is necessary to anastomose this vessel rather than the dorsalis pedis.

A superficial drainage vein from the dorsum of the foot is mobilized for venous drainage. The plantar nerve branches in the first and second web space are mobilized to provide sensory reconstruction, flexor and extensor tendons to the second toe are traced back as far proximal as possible prior to division.

On the hand the appropriate vessels, nerves and tendons are exposed, and in the case of congenital absence equivalent tendons such as the flexor carpi ulnaris may be used. After separation of the vessels and other structures from the foot the second toe, toes or even big toe are transferred to the hand. After fixing the bone in a suitable position the nerves and tendons are repaired. The dorsalis pedis or plantar artery is anastomosed either to the palmar arch or the radial or ulnar artery, and the vein is anastomosed to a dorsal vein on the hand. After release of the micro-clamps circulation is restored.

If a big toe is used, to reduce donor skin deficit and to create a smaller transferred nail, a wrap-around flap has been devised taking the tissue off the tip and lateral aspect of the toe. The donor deficit is then skin grafted. The flap is mobilized with its vessels and nerve supply and is transferred to the hand where the flap is wrapped around a bone graft. As the bone is not vascularized primarily there is an increased tendency for bone absorption. This latter technique is useful in reconstruction for deficits distal to the metacarpophalangeal joint

Free skin flap transfers

Skin grafts will take where there is a vascularized bed. Where there is no such bed, for example following injury where tendons are exposed without paratendon or bone without periosteum or an exposed joint, alternatives are required to maintain the viability of these structures.

Local flaps may be possible or even distant flaps, bringing the affected limb up to the flap as in a groin flap to cover the dorsum of the hand, or in a cross-leg flap. In both these cases the flap is still nourished by its attached blood supply. These then have to be divided at the base of the flap, usually after 3 weeks.

In certain cases such flaps are difficult or impossible to achieve without multiple stages. In the groin flap mentioned above, the skin and subcutaneous fat of the lateral groin can be mobilized, leaving the flap attached by its arterial supply and venous drainage only. The flap remains viable. These vessels may then be divided and transferred to the lower leg, for example to cover exposed bone in a compound injury. The artery to the 'free flap', either the superficial circumflex iliac or epigastric artery, is then anastomosed under the microscope to a suitable undamaged vessel on the lower leg, either the anterior or posterior tibial artery. A superficial draining vein from the groin flap is also anastomosed with an equivalent vein in the leg. After removal of the micro-clamps, flow is restored, producing vascularized skin and subcutaneous fat to cover the exposed area.

The advantages of such free flaps are clear. It is possible, for example, to resurface a lower tibia in a compound injury in one stage where earlier, using a tube pedicle, five stages and about 6 months in hospital were required. Early cover of exposed bone may also prevent it drying out and dying. The aim is now to cover exposed bone either as an emergency or as a secondary procedure after initial debridement within 24 h.

The free groin flap described above was the first such flap to be used. The disadvantage of this particular flap was the variability of its blood supply, a fairly small calibre artery (range 0.8–3 mm) and a short pedicle.

Latissimus dorsi flap

Following development of the groin flap, other sites have been explored to obtain more reliable anatomy, longer pedicles and larger vessels. The latissimus dorsi flap is such a vascularized myocutaneous flap, and flaps from this area are used by translocation to aid breast reconstruction after mastectomy. When dissecting the flap an ellipse of skin is marked out, usually aligned parallel to the direction of the muscle, the anterior edge lying about 3 cm anterior to it. The skin is nourished by the thoracodorsal branch of the subscapular artery and the vessels may be traced proximally into the axilla. Distally the artery and vein run just beneath the free border of the muscle, sending perforating vessels into the overlying skin. Providing this segment of muscle is maintained in the flap, a large portion of skin may be taken with only a relatively small amount of muscle. The advantages of this flap are a long pedicle (about 10 cm) and a large diameter artery (2–3 mm). With a smaller skin flap about 10 cm wide by 15 cm it is possible usually to close the donor defect directly, but if a large flap is required the donor area may require skin grafting. The donor skin ellipse may be orientated horizontally producing a better cosmetic result on closure. The disadvantages of this otherwise very reliable flap are its bulk and the need to sacrifice the nerve supply to the latissimus dorsi. The latissimus dorsi muscle alone can be taken and skin grafted, providing a more rigid surface. This is probably the commonest free flap used in lower limb injuries. In the hand and forearm, the lateral arm flap from the upper arm can be used, taking a skin paddle nourished by the perforating septal vessels originating from the terminal branches of the profunda brachii artery.

Other flaps like the latter have been developed to provide vascularized skin without sacrificing valuable muscle, such as the scapular flap based on the cutaneous scapular artery originating from the circumflex scapular artery. The skin flap is taken just lateral to the scapula and the vessels are traced through the triangular space.

Innervated skin flap transfers

The free skin flap transfers outlined above do not regain a significant return of sensation. In certain situations such as loss of skin from the heel or weight-bearing area of the foot, attempts should be made to reinnervate the skin otherwise trophic ulceration will occur. In reconstruction of the hand following extensive injuries, a 'sensory' flap will help in regaining use, the nerve supply of the free flap being attached to the divided sensory nerve supplying this area.

Dorsalis pedis or dorsal foot flap

In this flap the skin on the dorsum of the foot is mobilized, together with the dorsalis pedis artery and a superficial vein. This area is supplied by the terminal branches of the peroneal nerve which may be identified and reanastomosed to the appropriate nerve.

The advantage of this flap includes the possibility of incorporating tendons of the extensor digitorum brevis which are then used to reconstruct, for example, extensor tendons on the dorsum of the hand lost after an abrasion injury. This tendon reconstruction can, therefore, be carried out in one stage using vascularized tendons.

The disadvantage of this flap is the rather precarious blood supply to the skin from the dorsalis pedis vessels which is also a rather poor donor site. A smaller but better innervated flap may be taken from the web space between the big toe and the second toe, the skin being innervated by branches from the medial plantar nerve and terminal branches of the peroneal nerve.

Other innervated flaps are now being developed, such as the lateral arm flap mentioned earlier, innervated by the lateral cutaneous nerve of the arm, or the ulnar artery forearm flap, the latter being innervated by the medial cutaneous nerve of the forearm which runs with the basilic vein.

Vascularized bone grafts

Where there has been a large segment of bone loss or where extensive resection is required, as in lower jaw malignancies, free non-vascularized segments of bone tend to be absorbed or become infected, and this is especially likely to occur after radiotherapy.

Initial attempts at using vascularized bone were carried out with ribs using the intercostal vessels, but the pedicle is very short and potentially hazardous if the posterior intercostal vessels are used. Vascularized ribs may be raised with the latissimus dorsi flap taking the overlying serratus anterior and arterial supply, which is a branch of the thoracodorsal, so that it is possible to provide skin cover as well as vascularized ribs through a composite latissimus dorsi flap. In this situation, the blood supply to the ribs is via the muscular attachment and only indirectly to the periosteum.

Radial forearm flap

In lower jaw reconstructions, bone and skin are often required, as a thin hairless flap which is pliable and taken with a segment of bone. This may often be provided by the radial forearm flap based on the radial artery. A very long vessel pedicle usually enables vascular anastomosis to be carried out well away from the irradiated area, although only part of the radius can be taken so there is a limit to the amount of mandible which can be reconstructed this way. Prior to surgery it should be demonstrated that the circulation of the hand can be maintained by the ulnar artery. An attempt should be made to restore the original circulation by inserting a long vein graft into the radial artery defect.

Deep circumflex iliac artery flap (DCIA) (Figure 31.5)

Injuries of the lower leg with skin and bone loss are on the increase, occurring especially following motor-cycle accidents. Amputation rates of up to 80% have been reported, indicating the difficulty in reconstruction.

For cases where there is bone loss of less than 12 cm, the deep circumflex iliac artery flap is probably the flap of choice, giving good blood supply to the overlying skin in addition to using the whole iliac crest in reconstruction.

Dissection of deep circumflex iliac artery flap

The artery (1.5–3 mm in diameter) arises from the external iliac artery and the venae comitans which accompany it usually join to form one draining vein which passes either in front of or behind the external iliac artery to drain into the external iliac vein.

Dissection to find the vessels is through the posterior wall of the inguinal canal beneath the fascia transversalis. The vessels are traced laterally: an ascending branch is given off at a variable distance from the anterior superior iliac spine. This vessel does not provide musculocutaneous perforators. As the anterior superior iliac spine is approached, anastomosis with the cruciate anastomosis is noted and carefully tied. The deep circumflex iliac vessels pierce the fascia transversalis and transversus abdominis to run under the internal oblique muscle just beneath the rim of the pelvis. The skin supplied by this artery is centred just above the iliac crest and is nourished by musculocutaneous perforators given off as the artery passes adjacent to the inner lip of the iliac crest.

To reduce the bulk of flap only a cuff of external and internal oblique and transversus muscles are required to protect the vessels. The tensor fascia lata can be divided directly off the lower border of the

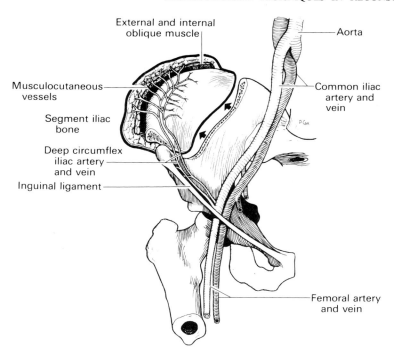

Figure 31.5 Mobilization and raising of deep circumflex iliac artery flap

ilium as there is no contribution to the flap's blood supply from this source.

The size of the bone and skin of the flap depends on the defect being reconstructed. To provide stability afterwards the anterior superior iliac spine and attached inguinal ligament are left behind. The ilium can then be taken as necessary using a power saw. After the composite flap (skin/muscle/bone) (Figure 31.6) has been isolated on its vessels it should be left attached for about 1 h to allow any vessel spasm to be rectified and for the circulation to re-establish itself. Free bleeding should be noted from the cancellous bone.

In this form of microvascular surgery two teams work simultaneously, one raising the flap, the other identifying suitable undamaged recipient vessels, usually the anterior or posterior tibial. Bone ends are freshened, making certain all devitalized tibia is removed. Bony fixation above and below the defect is provided by external fixators. Normally Hoffmann apparatus is adaptable enough to be positioned to allow access to suitable recipient vessels and to provide visibility for the microvascular anastomosis (Figure 31.6).

Only when these recipient vessels are prepared is the deep circumflex iliac artery flap detached. The bone in the flap is fixed in position and microvascular anastomoses are then carried out, usually end to side for the deep circumflex iliac artery and end to end for the deep circumflex iliac vein, the latter usually to a vena comitans (Figure 31.7). Often a superficial vein is also raised with this flap to anastomose to a

superficial vein of the leg which reduces postoperative swelling and makes the flap safer.

In extensively damaged limbs long vein grafts may be required to allow anastomosis to the popliteal artery. In multiple and extensive leg injuries it may be necessary to anastomose the flap vessels to undamaged vessels in the opposite leg (Figure 31.7), the legs being held rigidly together by external fixation. After 5 weeks the vessels may be safely divided and after 6 weeks the skin bridge also.

Experience shows that the rate of bony union at both ends, with full weight-bearing, is on average 6 months using the DCIA flap to reconstitute the bony defect. This is similar to that achieved by a double fracture, showing that free vascularized bone grafts behave like ordinary living bone.

Following replacement of a bony defect with vascularized ilium there is an incidence of non-union in one end of the vascularized bone graft. The situation is similar to a double fracture of the tibia which this deep circumflex iliac artery free flap reconstruction clinically reproduces. It is then necessary to freshen up the appropriate end and insert cancellous bone chips. In chronic non-union of the tibia with poor overlying skin, the deep circumflex iliac artery flap can be raised taking skin and periosteum only. The ends of the tibia may then be freshened and cancellous bone chips inserted, the area then covered with this vascularized periosteum and skin.

In a successful case of reconstruction of the tibia using vascularized ilium, the living bone graft undergoes remodelling with resorption of the non-stress

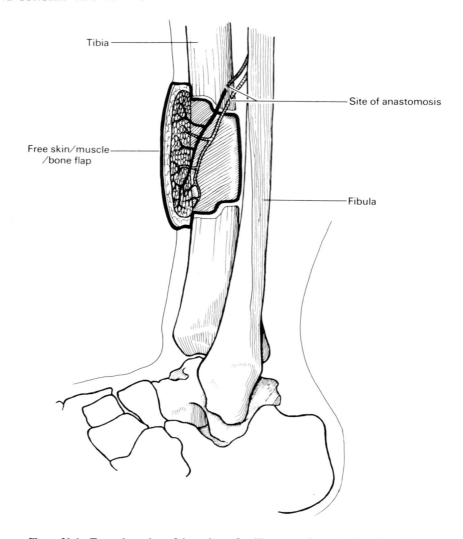

Figure 31.6 Transplantation of deep circumflex iliac artery flap to bridge tibial defect

areas and hypertrophy of the stress lines so that after 2 or 3 years it is often difficult to visualize the original graft.

Following an extended hemimandibulectomy for malignancy the deep circumflex iliac artery flap may be used in reconstruction. The iliac crest is cut to shape and the muscular and tendinous attachments to the iliac crest are then used to reconstruct the temporomandibular joint, and to reattach the temporalis and masseteric muscles.

It is possible to use the bone alone in this situation, but the skin in the composite flap may be used to provide cover, especially externally.

Vascularized fibula

When a bone defect is greater than 12 cm the deep circumflex iliac artery flap is not used, for fear of shortening of the limb. This is one of the indications

for use of vascularized fibula based on the peroneal artery and veins. Provided that about 6 cm of fibula are left at the upper and lower ends, stability is maintained at the ankle and knee joint, and this stability may be enhanced by a screw placed between the lower fibula and tibia.

The nutrient artery to the fibula lies in the middle third, so this central segment may be taken alone with the peroneal vessels.

Vascularized shorter segments have been utilized in avascular necrosis of the head of the femur prior to its collapse, but a more specific indication is in pseudoarthrosis of the tibia where the fibula may be passed up and down within the shaft of the remaining normal tibia, as ordinary bone-grafting techniques in this latter situation have a very high failure rate. Larger segments of fibula have been used in reconstruction of long bone loss in the tibia, femur and humerus, either following traumatic loss or after

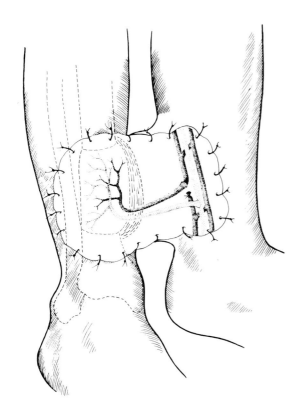

Figure 31.7 Anastomosis of deep circumflex iliac artery flap to undamaged vessels in opposite leg where there has been extensive leg injury

tumour excision where prosthetic replacement may not be suitable such as in young people. In the forearm where there has been loss of both radius and ulnar bones, it has been used to reconstruct the forearm. In this situation the fibula may be double-barrelled. After dividing it in the centre, both halves are still attached to the peroneal vessels; the proximal half is nourished by periosteal and endosteal circulation and the distal half by periosteal circulation. This allows reconstruction of both bones. Unlike the deep circumflex iliac artery flap the fibula does not have the same structural strength and in the lower limb especially some form of extra support is required while the fibula hypertrophies, often up to 18 months. As indicated previously, this hypertrophy is a function of vascularized bone graft and does not occur with traditional free bone grafts. It is of interest that if the fibular graft fractures, extensive callus is thrown up and this remodelling is often speeded up.

The dissection of the fibula is best carried out by a direct lateral incision. There are musculocutaneous branches given off from the peroneal artery, also direct cutaneous branches usually between the soleus and peroneal muscles. It is, therefore, possible to take skin as well as bone if this is wished. Dissection of the fibula at the upper and lower ends is carried out and

is divided, usually with a Gigli saw, which allows the isolated segment to be retracted laterally. The interosseous membrane is then identified and carefully released, commencing at the lower end. The peroneal vessels lie just behind this and should be divided and tied at the lower end. The fibula with a small cuff of muscle on the medial side can then be dissected free. The peroneal artery and veins are then traced, providing a pedicle of about 5 cm.

If a short segment only of fibula is required this pedicle can be lengthened by subperiosteal dissection of the fibula at the upper end and excess bone removed, maintaining carefully undisturbed the site of the nutrient artery. An extra advantage is that there is now an additional cuff of vascularized periosteum which may be draped around the bone end and may help with final bony union.

The omentum

It has been known for a considerable time that the omentum may be mobilized by dividing one or other gastro-epiploic vessels and then lengthened by dividing some of the interconnecting vessels but preserving the peripheral arcade. This pedicle flap which is still attached by one of the gastro-epiploic vessels can be brought up subcutaneously on to the chest wall to reconstruct, for example, an area of radionecrosis. Skin grafts can then be applied and these take well on the surface of the omentum.

There are certain areas of the body where such a pedicle flap cannot reach, but the omentum may then be transplanted for microvascular reconstruction. In extensive scalp loss where there is exposed bone denuded of periosteum the area can be covered using omentum, which tends to mould over the area required. Anastomoses can then be carried out between the gastro-epiploic vessels and the superficial temporal vessels, although vein grafts may be required to provide anastomosis to the larger facial vessels. The gastro-epiploic artery diameter is a good size, at least 2–3 mm. The veins, however, are very friable and require careful handling.

Another indication for the use of vascularized omentum is in cases of extensive fat atrophy, as in Romberg's disease where the fat on one side of the face may be lost. The omentum may be separated into various fingers and passed subcutaneously onto the forehead, around the eyes and over the cheek and mandible. The omentum is then vascularized.

Previous abdominal surgery or history of pelvic inflammation or obesity may make it impossible to use the omentum.

Vascularized muscles

Using microneurovascular anastomosis it is possible to transfer muscles as free vascularized grafts and expect return of motor function. There are two main indications. Benefit has been achieved after

Volkmann's contracture where there has been extensive necrosis and subsequent fibrosis of the flexor muscles of the forearm. The second indication is in the management of facial paralysis.

Both pectoralis major and latissimus dorsi muscles have been used in the forearm to try to re-establish mass flexor movements of the fingers. If the blood supply of the forearm has been partially disrupted this can be repaired at the same time, using in the case of latissimus dorsi the distal end of the thoracodorsal vessels.

In facial paralysis cross-facial nerve grafting has been attempted. Nerve grafts are taken, connecting some of the more distal branches of the normal side which may be sacrificed with minimal functional loss due to interconnection. The graft or grafts are then anastomosed on the paralysed side to the distal ends of the facial nerve. During the long delay before nerve regeneration occurs down these long grafts the facial muscles atrophy and the results have been rather disappointing. This technique may be carried out in two stages, the nerve anastomosis on the paralysed side being carried out after the axons have grown across. To reduce this problem of muscle atrophy, vascularized muscle grafts can be carried out as a secondary procedure using either the extensor digitorum brevis muscle of the foot gracilis muscle or pectoralis minor muscle. The transplanted muscle therefore undergoes earlier reinnervation and does not undergo such excessive degeneration, although it seems some allowance should be made for this and a bulkier muscle preferably used.

Vascularized tendons

As indicated earlier, it is possible to take the dorsalis pedis flap with tendons of extensor digitorum brevis and maintain their blood supply. Results are very encouraging, for example in abrasion injuries to the back of the hand where there is loss of both skin and tendons.

Tendon-like structures such as the external oblique aponeurosis are also used and can be incorporated in a groin flap. The strip of aponeurosis taken is rolled up to reproduce the tendon, for example the Achilles tendon, in its reconstruction after skin and tendon loss.

Jejenum or colon

In patients with hypopharyngeal carcinoma who have had pharyngolaryngectomy with partial or complete resection of the cervical oesophagus, vascularized jejunum or colon can be considered to restore continuity.

Reconstruction of the upper pharyngeal end is fraught with complications using traditional methods such as mobilizing the stomach or colon and elevating them through the chest or subcutaneously. Anastomotic breakdown often occurs at this upper end at the limit of the vascular supply. To reduce the incidence of this complication, anastomosis may be undertaken between the colonic or gastric vessels, preferably with non-irradiated vessels in the neck. This technique may also be used in reconstruction after excision of the thoracic oesophagus.

In reconstruction using microvascular anastomosis, sections of jejunum or colon are taken isolating a single branch of the mesenteric vessels, as these vessel diameters match well with the superior thyroid artery and external jugular vein. After resection, jejunal or colonic oesophageal reanastomosis is carried out in the neck, the lower end first, either with sutures or a stapling gun. By the latter technique the lower anastomosis can be carried out at an intrathoracic level and the upper bowel segment anastomosis to the oropharynx is then fairly easily accomplished. After the microvascular anastomoses are carried out, peristalsis may return almost at once; it is important to ensure that the bowel segment is placed isoperistaltically or there may be constant regurgitation of mucus.

The use of vascularized bowel allows a single-stage reconstruction and although it requires resection of a section of the bowel, there is far less dissection and morbidity associated with this than with the usual alternatives and should the vascular anastomoses fail, the consequences are not nearly so catastrophic. However, the success rate world wide is high and as an added bonus it is also possible for the patients to develop oesophageal speech.

Autotransplantation of the testis
(Figure 31.8)

In up to 5% of cryptorchid testes the testicles are so high that it is necessary to divide the spermatic vessels to allow the testis to be relocated in the scrotum. The blood supply then consists only of collaterals from the vas deferens and cremasteric muscle, with a significant incidence of testicular atrophy. In bilateral cases an attempt should usually be made on one side as it is a relatively simple procedure. If this fails and because of the risk of malignancy, the other testis will be considered for removal. However, the blood supply to the testis can be enhanced by microvascular techniques with prospects of a higher success rate of normal testicular development.

To obtain this renewed blood supply to the testis the testicular vessels are identified close to their origin to achieve as long a pedicle as possible. After division, microvascular anastomosis is then carried out. The recipient vessels are usually the inferior epigastric and a superficial vein which have been prepared prior to division of the testicular vessels. This is usually achieved using end-to-side anastomosis for the testicular artery to the inferior epigastric artery and end-to-end for the testicular vein to a more superficial vein.

Preservation of the stroma of the testis has been

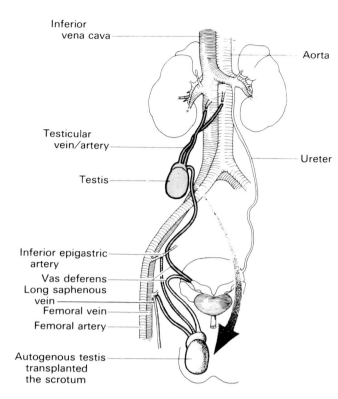

Inferior vena cava

Aorta

Testicular vein/artery

Testis

Ureter

Inferior epigastric artery

Vas deferens

Long saphenous vein

Femoral vein

Femoral artery

Autogenous testis transplanted the scrotum

Figure 31.8 Autotransplantation of the testis

demonstrated experimentally using this microvascular anastomosis by the ability to regain spermatogenesis. The operation is, however, best done before 6 years of age. In older patients, even if there is a failure of spermatogenesis, testosterone levels in a successful case can be maintained, thus making it unnecessary for the patients to have testosterone implants indefinitely. In these older patients at a later stage there may still be an increased risk from malignancy and testicular biopsies may be indicated. In vasculogenic impotence, re-creation of an erection may be achieved by anastomosis of the epigastric artery to the deep dorsal vein of the penis.

Conclusions

This summary of microvascular procedures is by no means exhaustive and new indications and methods are being developed. Undoubtedly the long operations and specialized training are very demanding but the operations are usually performed as single-stage techniques reducing hospital stay and allowing earlier mobilization.

The best results are achieved using a team approach and if a flap, for example, develops congestion or becomes ischaemic, then re-exploration of the anastomosis must be carried out at once. This requires some depth of skilled surgical personnel cover and with it the implication that these cases are best undertaken in an appropriate unit.

Urogenital and adrenal glands

32

The open approach to the kidney and ureter

C. A. C. Charlton

Introduction

Although endoscopic and non-invasive procedures are developing at a rapid pace, and in part replacing open operations, there is a need for the surgeon to be familiar with alternative approaches for managing renal and ureteric pathology. This necessity applies not only to the treatment of malignant disease, undertaking reconstructive plastic procedures and urinary diversions, but it is also sometimes necessary in the management of stone disease, when large and impacted calculi are present which lead to unrelieved pain, obstruction and infection, and fail to respond to those manoeuvres introduced in the last couple of decades.

Incisions and approach to the kidney

The surgical approach to the kidneys is conditioned by their position as retroperitoneal structures, with their upper poles protected in part by the lower ribs, and the fact that the artery and vein (occasionally multiple) are situated high up at the back of the abdominal cavity. Surrounding the perinephric fat is Gerota's fascia which resembles a sac with the open end facing inferiorly (towards the bony pelvis).

There are many incisions used for approaching the kidney, and the decision as to which one is employed depends on the pathological process which has determined the need for operation. Since the kidney is a retroperitoneal structure, it is preferable if the surgical procedure remains exclusively located to that compartment, i.e. is extrapleural and extraperitoneal. The advantages of not opening the pleural cavity are that it diminishes the risk of postoperative atelectasis and pneumonia, the development of pleural effusions or pneumothorax, and the possible need for underwater seals and drains. Similarly, opening the peritoneal cavity is more likely to be followed by intestinal ileus, gastric dilatation and the development of peritoneal adhesions than if the surgical manoeuvres are wholly extraperitoneal. Obviously, the need for a nasogastric tube and intravenous feeding is more likely in these circumstances.

However, good access is an important maxim in safe surgery and if it is apparent that the operation would be difficult by confining the operative field to the retroperitoneal space, as might occur with a large upper pole tumour, then there should be no hesitation in opening the pleural and peritoneal cavities.

With these principles in mind, the majority of kidney operations undertaken by the author are by the lumbar route along the line of the 12th rib. If, due to unforeseen circumstances, the access obtained proves unsatisfactory, the incision is extended dorsally into the dorsolumbar approach of Nagamatsu (1950). In the case of large tumours in which it may be expected to find involvement of abdominal viscera (e.g. the spleen or colon) or the diaphragm, or when access to the renal blood vessels from behind can be predicted to be difficult, then a thoraco-abdominal approach along the interspace between the 9th and 10th ribs is employed. Finally, in a selected group, namely thin patients in whom exposure of the renal pelvis is the only consideration, the lumbotomy incision (which is a vertical paravertebral one) is preferred since it does not involve division of the abdominal wall muscles, and so reduces postoperative pain.

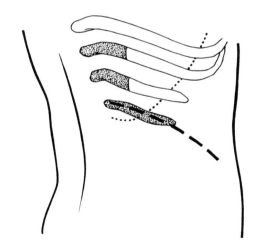

Figure 32.1 Exposure of kidney via loin incision incorporating resection of the 12th rib. Note the reflexion of the pleura

Twelfth rib resection incision (Figure 32.1)

Correct positioning of the patient on the operating table is important. The lateral decubitus position is adopted, the patient being so placed that the space between the iliac crest and the 12th rib on the non-operative side is at the level of the 'break' in the table. Two table supports are used along the back of the patient, one at the level of the scapula and the lower one supports the ischial tuberosity. A further support for the forearm of the uppermost arm is positioned, such that the humerus is at right angles to the line of the patient's torso (i.e. the shoulder is flexed to 90°), and the elbow is flexed to 90°. The lower leg is slightly flexed, and the uppermost one is straight. Pillows or Sorbo pads are placed between the knees and ankles of the two limbs.

The table is then tilted laterally towards the surgeon (who is standing facing the patient's back) so causing the patient to lean backwards against the supports which places him or her in a steady and stable position. The table is now 'broken' so that the dip of the patient's waist (on the side to be operated on) is eliminated or straightened out. If the surgeon feels that the patient's position is not stable, a strap encircling the table and the patient's pelvis can be applied at this juncture.

The incision is made along the line of the 12th rib from the angle (i.e. posterior axillary line) to the lateral edge of the rectus sheath. The underlying muscles (i.e. those covering that part of the rib exposed by the incision) are divided. The intercostal muscles attached to the upper border of this part of the rib are detached. Similarly, by keeping the knife blade close to the lower edge of the 12th rib, the attached muscles are divided, avoiding the subcostal blood vessels and nerve. The structures attached to the tip of the rib are also divided, and so the anterior part of the rib (the length of this varies with the length of the 12th rib) is free of any attachments. This protruding portion of the rib is now cut with the costotome. The pleura may now come into view but, with this relatively anteriorly placed incision, should not intrude into the operating field. By introducing a finger into the anterior part of the space made by removing the rib, it is a simple matter to displace the peritoneum anteriorly, by stripping it off the undersurface of the transversus abdominis muscle. Consequently, the external and internal oblique muscles, and the transversus abdominis can be divided without inadvertently opening the peritoneum. At this juncture a self-retaining retractor can be introduced or this can be reserved until the kidney has been mobilized.

Returning to the posterior aspect of the wound, Gerota's fascia is incised for 8 cm or so, as is the underlying perinephric fat. The anterior flap of fat is grasped by a Duval's forceps and the separation of the fat from the kidney capsule is undertaken, preferably with scissors. The capsule should not be breeched since this leads to bleeding.

Subcapsular dissection is to be deprecated, not only because of bleeding, but it also makes access to the renal blood vessels difficult, and, furthermore, in some operations (e.g. partial nephrectomy and nephrolithotomy) the capsule is useful for closing incisions made in the renal cortex. In addition, any subsequent operation on the kidney is made difficult by the absence of the capsule. In the case of reoperation, it may be time consuming, difficult and tedious to aim at preserving the capsule intact, since separation of the perinephric fat and fibrous tissue from the underlying kidney involves sharp dissection, but the surgeon will be rewarded by the resulting decrease in blood loss and improved view which results. When the perinephric tissues are directly adherent to the renal cortex, operating on a kidney subsequently is hazardous, since the dividing line is not apparent and brisk bleeding ensues from incising the renal parenchyma.

Mobilization of the upper pole should also be undertaken with scissors so as to separate the suprarenal from the kidney. This manoeuvre allows the kidney a considerable increase in movement, and it can then be gently retracted downwards into the wound. At this juncture, it is relatively easy to feel the renal artery. In many kidney operations it is desirable to identify the renal artery and dissect it free so that, if at any time bleeding becomes troublesome, a bulldog clamp or digital pressure can be accurately and rapidly applied. By drawing the upper pole of the kidney up towards the surface of the wound, the artery will be found in the angle between the medial aspect of the upper pole and the posterior abdominal wall. Dividing the sympathetic fibres and fascial layers will expose the artery.

Closure of the wound is by interrupted chromic catgut sutures, which pass through all the muscle layers of the abdominal wall, but which are left untied until all the sutures have been placed along the length of the wound. Once all these have been inserted, the 'break' in the table is closed, and the sutures are tied. The fascia overlying the external oblique muscle is closed with a continuous catgut suture.

Dorsolumbar approach (Nagamatsu) (Figure 32.2)

This approach is used if it is not possible to obtain adequate access to the upper pole of the kidney or the renal blood vessels by the technique described above. It is a relatively simple matter to adapt the 12th rib resection to the osteoblastic flap technique of Nagamatsu by extending the incision backwards along the length of the 12th rib, to the lateral border of the sacrospinalis group of muscles. The incision is then taken through a right-angle turn to run parallel to the edge of the paravertebral muscles across the 11th and 10th ribs dividing the underlying latissimus dorsi muscle. Some 4 cm of the 10th and 11th ribs are exposed and the muscles attached to the upper and lower borders of these ribs are detached. The remainder of the 12th rib is removed, and some 2 cm of the 10th and 11th ribs are excised with care, so as to preserve the integrity of the pleura. The ligaments tethering the remaining stump of the 12th rib to the transverse process of the first lumbar vertebra (lumbocostal and lateral arcuate) are divided, and the resulting flap is turned up and the large Finochetto retractor can be introduced into the wound. Mobilization of the kidney then proceeds in the manner previously described.

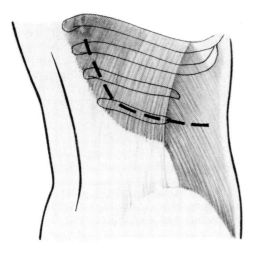

Figure 32.2   Dorsolumbar approach to the kidney (Nagamatsu)

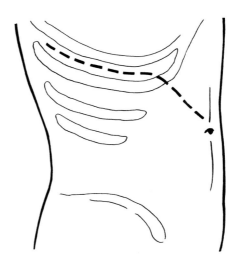

Figure 32.3   Thoraco-abdominal approach to the right kidney

The thoraco-abdominal incision

This approach is reserved for extensive malignant disease of the kidney, when it seems likely that the spleen, tail of the pancreas, colon, diaphragm or liver are likely to be involved. The major advantage of such an incision is that with the pleural and peritoneal cavities opened, it is easier to assess the extent of the spread of the tumour, and to remove adjacent involved structures. In addition, for those surgeons who believe in the value of excision of diseased lymph nodes, this incision offers an excellent operative field. Furthermore, rapid access to the aorta or inferior vena cava is possible if troublesome haemorrhage ensues.

The patient is positioned in a semi-recumbent position, with sandbags placed under the scapula and the buttocks so that the patient leans at 25° to the horizontal. The incision extends from the anterior axillary line along the interspace between the 9th and 10th ribs across the costal margin to the level of the umbilicus (Figure 32.3). The intercostal muscles attached to the upper border of the 10th rib are divided, as are the costal cartilage and the abdominal wall muscles (Figure 32.4). The pleura, peripheral part of the diaphragm and peritoneum are opened in the same line (Figure 32.5), and a large retractor is introduced into the wound. On either side, the colon is mobilized by incising the peritoneum on the lateral aspect. On the right side, the duodenum is reflected medially by Kocher's manoeuvre of incising the posterior layer of the peritoneum along the lateral aspect of the second part of the duodenum. On the left side, the attachments of the splenic flexure of the colon (the phrenicocolic ligaments) are divided. By these manoeuvres, the kidneys and the renal blood vessels are exposed.

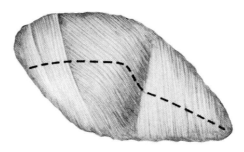

Figure 32.4   Thoraco-abdominal approach to the right kidney. The skin and subcutaneous fascia have been divided and the abdominal and lateral muscles are incised

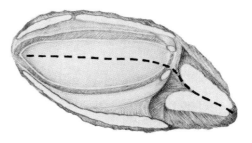

Figure 32.5   Thoraco-abdominal approach to the kidney. The pleural cavity and the peritoneal cavity have been opened

The lumbotomy incision

The main advantage of this approach is that the large muscles of the abdominal wall (the transversus and oblique muscles) are not cut and so pain in the post-operative period is considerably reduced. However, it has to be admitted that access to the anteromedial aspect of the kidney can be difficult. Consequently the author reserves this incision for simple pyelolithotomies.

The patient lies on the non-operative side with the waist at the level of the 'break' in the table. The patient is rolled forwards away from the surgeon, with the lowermost leg flexed at the hip and knee and the uppermost leg stretched out. A sandbag is firmly placed up against the abdomen, so pushing the viscera against the posterior abdominal wall. The shoulder of the uppermost arm is rolled forward and flexed to 90°, as is the elbow. The patient may be secured to the table by encircling the pelvis and table with a strap.

The incision is made along a line 2.5 cm lateral to the edge of the paravertebral muscles extending from the iliac crest to the level of the 12th rib. The underlying latissimus dorsi and serratus posterior inferior are divided in the line of the incision. A 2 cm segment of the 12th rib is removed, as described in the dorsolumbar approach. In the centre of the wound, running in a longitudinal direction, from the 12th rib to the iliac crest, is seen the fused margin of the three layers of lumbar fascia which enclose the sacrospinalis muscle. From the front edge of this conjoint lamellae of lumbar fascia arise the internal oblique and transversus abdominis muscles. Incising the fascia along this line leads directly into the retroperitoneal space. An opening is made in Gerota's fascia, and the kidney displaced forwards and the posterior surface of the kidney and pelvis exposed by dissecting off the perinephric fat.

A further advantage of the lumbotomy incision is that if it is intended to operate on both kidneys in one session (e.g. bilateral nephrectomy as a prelude to renal transplantation, or for bilateral renal pelvic stones), this is possible by positioning the patient prone, i.e. face-down on the table, and breaking it so as to put the patient in the 'jack-knife' position.

Renal surgery for calculous disease

One of the main objectives of urological practice is the preservation of renal function, and in the last analysis this is related to the number of surviving nephrons. Nephrons may be damaged or destroyed by infection or obstruction (and of course by malignant disease). Stones which are causing obstruction, whether to the whole or part of a kidney, will need removing, and so will those which are the cause of recurrent pyelonephritis (i.e. a systemic illness with loin pain). On the other hand, recurring bacteriuria in the absence of pyelonephritis does not necessarily demand the same strict adherence to the principle of elimination of calculous material from the urinary tract.

In the majority of cases with stones located in the kidney, by employing either percutaneous nephrolithotomy (PCNL) or extracorporeal shock wave lithotripsy (ESWL) or a combination of the two modalities, it is possible to clear the kidney of calculi. However, there are occasions when these two techniques are not possible; for example, if the renal stone is in a very bulky patient, ESWL is ineffective due to the fact that the stone is too distant from both the surface of the patient and to the focus of where the wave form is generated. Furthermore, some very hard stones, such as those made of cysteine and some types of oxalate, are resistant to fragmentation.

To establish a nephrostomy tract, the collecting system must be opacified, and commonly this is done by introducing dye through a ureteric catheter. On occasion it proves difficult or technically impossible to get the retrograde catheter up the ureter, and so the collecting system is not visualized. In addition, on some occasions puncturing the collecting system at a satisfactory entry site is unsuccessful. In rare circumstances, the bulk of the stone in the kidney is so considerable that the logistics of repeated PCNL and ESWL sessions to break up and extract the stones is inferior to clearing the collecting system of stones at one open operation.

It is not every hospital that possesses all the endoscopic instruments, image intensifier and other equipment necessary to undertake the establishment of a nephrostomy tract, visualize collecting system and stones, undertake lithotripsy and remove the fragments. Extracorporeal lithotriptors are limited to a dozen or so centres in the UK, and there are the usual problems of dealing with patients who have their treatment at one hospital and have to have the supervision and complications of the treatment dealt with at a distant hospital. For these and other reasons the need for open renal surgery for calculus disease will continue to be a factor of life.

In planning surgery for stone disease, a guiding principle is that relief of obstruction is a primary requirement. Hence if one kidney is obstructed by a stone at the pelvi-ureteric junction, while the other has a staghorn calculus in the lower half of the kidney which appears to be functioning reasonably well, then a pyelolithotomy on the first kidney should take precedence over surgery for the staghorn calculus.

Prior to any form of renal surgery, an intravenous urogram (IVU) is essential. It will depict the position, shape, size and to some extent the function of the kidneys. An IVU can be used for comparing the function of one kidney with its fellow, but should not be used to assess overall renal function, since such variables as dehydration, size of the bolus of the dye given and its concentration, and technical radiological factors all determine the quality of the pictures which may (if due allowances are not made for these many factors) give a false impression of renal function.

To establish the percentage of overall renal function attributable to each kidney, an isotope renogram is necessary. The isotope is attached to a chemical compound (e.g. *di* amino *tetra* ethyl *penta* *a*cetate), which is delivered to the kidney via the systemic circulation and filtered through the glomerulus. The labelled compound mixes with the urine and drains down the ureter, the radiation being measured by a gamma camera and interpreted by a recorder which prints out a tracing.

Other tests of renal function such as blood urea and serum creatinine with associated electrolyte levels should be done, and a measurement of glomerular filtration rate (by creatinine clearance) is indicated. The haemoglobin level should always be known. Urine cultures and appropriate treatment are indicated. The various metabolic investigations customary in patients with calculus disease are best undertaken on an outpatient basis, since the urinary calcium levels for an individual leading a normal active life are very different to those obtained in the same patient recumbent in bed and taking a hospital diet.

Pyelolithotomy

Removal of a calculus from the renal pelvis is most commonly undertaken by the lumbar approach, using the 12th rib resection previously described. In a thin patient, in whom there is a reasonable distance (15 cm or so) between the iliac crest and the lower border of the 12th rib (at the lateral edge of the paravertebral muscles), the lumbotomy incision has much to recommend it. This approach has been described earlier in this chapter. Routine mobilization of the kidney is undertaken, so making it possible to lift the kidney 'out' of the wound. It is an advantage to envelop the kidney in a length of Netelast (size B) gauze elastic bandage which provides an atraumatic sling held by the assistant, and prevents bruising from the handling of the kidney which often results from the fingers acting as forceps or tongs in trying to grasp the slippery organ. If the renal pelvis is intrarenal and particularly if it is not dilated, the extended sinus approach of Gil-Vernet (1965) is recommended. A pair of scissors is inserted into the renal sinus and a small curved retractor (the cross-section of which is C shaped) is then so positioned that the blood vessels coursing over the pelvis are lifted free with the renal parenchyma from the renal pelvis proper. This plane is bloodless and leads to the exposure of the intrarenal part of the renal pelvis. The renal pelvis is incised vertically between 4/0 chromic catgut stay sutures and the stone removed. A bougie is passed down the ureter, to ensure that no fragments are occluding the lumen, which would encourage a postoperative urinary fistula. Closure of the pelvis is with interrupted 4/0 chromic catgut sutures. It is advisable to drain the renal fossa.

Nephrolithotomy

Removal of stones from dilated calyces is simply an extension of the pyelolithotomy described above, and it is a simple matter to extract stones through the dilated calyceal necks. If, however, the calyces are of a normal size, the above procedure is often not technically possible; and if there has been previous surgery to the kidney in question, then the renal sinus may be difficult to identify. In these instances, incision of the renal parenchyma (nephrotomy) overlying the appropriate calyx is necessary. This may well result in brisk bleeding, and it is the author's practice to use renal artery occlusion for this type of surgery. The renal artery is dissected out (as previously described) and occluded with a small bulldog clamp (Figure 32.6). The kidney then becomes smaller and softer and it is far easier to feel the stone in a calyx. An incision is made in a radial direction (i.e. in the line of the calyceal necks and major intrarenal blood vessels) and using the blades of the stone forceps, the walls of the nephrotomy are gently parted, when the lining of the collecting system is visualized and incised, and so the calyx entered. In this dry field, the stone can be seen and picked out of the calyx. The renal capsule is closed with 4/0 chromic catgut and the bulldog clamp removed and virtually no bleeding occurs.

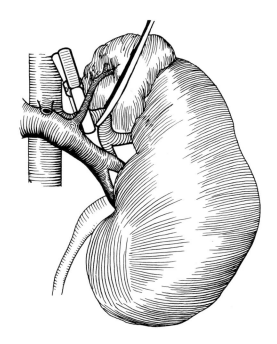

Figure 32.6 Nephrolithotomy. The renal artery is controlled to reduce bleeding and so improve vision

If it is envisaged that occlusion of the renal artery will last for more than 10 min, i.e. that multiple nephrotomies are necessary, then measures must be taken to protect the kidney from ischaemic damage.

A simple method of preserving renal function with renal ischaemia is by the intravenous injection of 2 g of inosine (Trophycardyl) (Wickham et al., 1979). This latter is a purine nucleotide and its mode of action is not totally understood. It appears that it preserves the integrity of the capsule or envelope of the red cell corpuscle during anoxia, and so prevents the lysis and sludging of red cells which are important factors in the development of acute tubular necrosis. This compound may also be concerned with preserving the brush borders of the renal tubular cell. Two minutes after the intravenous injection (in the antecubital vein), the renal artery is occluded and the removal of calculi is undertaken in a dry field. The period of ischaemia should not exceed $1\frac{1}{4}$ hours.

The calyces are opened and the stones removed as described above. To wash out any debris a high-pressure flush is employed, using 1-litre bags of sterile normal saline which have been kept in a domestic refrigerator (4°C). The bags are in a Fenwall bag compressor (used by anaesthetists for rapid blood infusions) and connected to an intravenous drip set. To the end of the tubing, a malleable antral catheter is attached, and by introducing it through the multiple nephrotomies, the calyces are flushed with saline delivered as a forceful stream. To ensure that all the stone fragments have been removed, close-contact radiographs are taken. Localization of the fragments is facilitated by using Cushing silver clip markers fixed to the Netelast gauze. Once all the calculous material has been removed, the nephrotomies are sutured as described above, and a no. 12 Fr. nephrostomy tube placed in the lowermost calyx. The bulldog clamp is then removed, the pyelotomy sutured and the wound drained as before.

Partial nephrectomy

The removal of the lower pole of the kidney in calculus disease can only be justified if, after removal of the stone, there remains a thin-walled sump containing a pool of stagnant urine, which readily becomes infected, so providing the conditions necessary for further calculus formation. If the sump is surrounded by a good thickness of renal parenchyma, drainage can be improved and kidney tissue preserved by doing a pyelocalycotomy (see below).

In the operation of partial nephrectomy, the kidney must be fully mobilized and the renal artery and its major branches are displayed. The arterial branch supplying that part of the kidney to be removed can be positively identified by injecting methylene blue into the isolated artery and noting the discoloration of the area it supplies. The renal capsule is preserved by incising it along the margin of the kidney and stripping it off that part of the kidney which is to be removed. The identified branch of the renal artery is ligated and divided and the renal parenchyma incised along the line demarcating the discoloured and ischaemic cortex from the normally perfused tissue. If, however, the areas of blood supply of the branches of the renal artery do not match the diseased portion of kidney to be removed, then the author employs the hypothermic technique described in the nephro-lithotomy operation. Having arrested the circulation, cooled the kidney and stripped off the renal capsule, the relevant portion of kidney is excised and the larger intrarenal blood vessels (which can be clearly seen in this dry field) are underrun with 4/0 chromic catgut. Defects in the collecting system are repaired with 4/0 chromic catgut and the bulldog clamp is then removed. Any blood vessels which were not secured will now bleed and are now identified and ligated. If bleeding is profuse the clamp can be reapplied while haemostasis is obtained.

The exposed renal tissue is covered with the preserved capsule, which is sutured with chromic catgut. Drainage of the renal fossa is advised.

Pyelocalycotomy

Removal of a large amount of calculous material in the lower calyces may be difficult, and it may leave a fair-sized cavity bounded by an adequate thickness of renal parenchyma. To ensure that thereafter there is adequate drainage of urine from the lower pole, a side-to-side anastomosis is made between the opened lower pole calyx and lower major calyx on the one side and the opened upper ureter and lower renal pelvis on the other side so as to form a large continuous cavity.

Initially the lower medial aspect of the renal pelvis is opened between stay sutures. The line of incision along the medial aspect of the lower pole of the kidney is determined by passing a probe through the pyelotomy into the lower calyx which is made to protrude on to the surface. The kidney tissue is cut between the point of the probe and the pyelotomy (Figure 32.7). To avoid the anastomosis being surrounded by renal parenchyma which may lead to an encircling of fibrous tissue with obstruction, the excess kidney tissue is trimmed off. Any bleeding vessels on the incised parenchyma are dealt with by full-thickness calycocapsular sutures.

A Cummings rat-tailed nephrostomy tube is passed down the ureter before the inferior pyelocalycotomy is anastomosed to the pyelo-ureterotomy, and the larger end of the tube passes through a stab incision in the pelvis to the skin (Figures 32.8 and 32.9).

Management of upper urinary tract obstruction

Obstruction to the free drainage of urine leads to impairment of function of the affected part of the

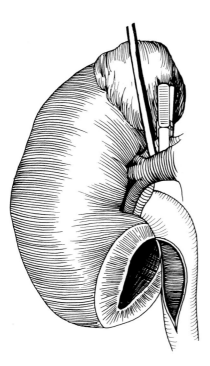

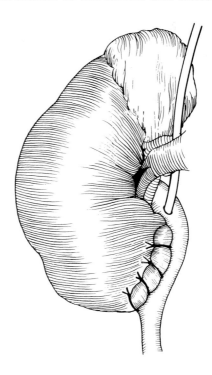

Figure 32.7 Pyelocalycotomy. The lower medial aspect of the renal pelvis is opened between stay sutures and the line of incision along the medial aspect of the lower pole of the kidney is determined by passing a probe through the pyelotomy into the lower calyx which is then made to protrude on to the surface. The kidney tissue is then cut between the point of the probe and the pyelotomy

Figure 32.9 Pyelocalycotomy. A pyelostomy tube is passed down the ureter before the inferior pyelocalycotomy is anastomosed to the pyelo-ureterotomy and the larger end of the pyelostomy tube passes through a stab incision in the pelvis and through the skin

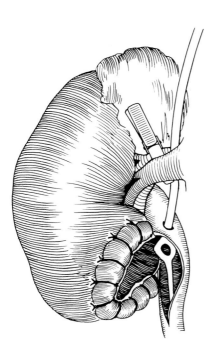

Figure 32.8 Pyelocalycotomy. Bleeding vessels of the incised kidney substance are dealt with by the use of full-thickness sutures

kidney, which if maintained may end with irreversible damage, so decreasing the overall renal function.

Obstruction leads to dilatation, and this latter can be identified by the non-invasive technique of ultrasound, but it is important to remember that this does not provide any information on the function of the kidney.

The diagnosis of upper urinary tract obstruction is commonly made by means of the IVU. A totally non-functioning kidney (e.g. due to arterial occlusion or to very long-standing obstruction with the contralateral kidney having hypertrophied to the extent that the blood urea is normal) will not show any renal opacification despite the injection of large amounts of dye. In the case of a functioning kidney, the dye is first seen as a kidney-shaped shadow due to its distribution through the arterial system which supplies the renal parenchyma. In a kidney with a satisfactory renal blood flow, this opacification will be seen within a minute of injecting the dye, and if the obstruction to urine flow is severe, the dye will continue to accumulate in the renal parenchyma to give a progressively denser shadow. As it emerges from the nephrons into the collecting system, so the calyces and renal pelvis will be seen and the renal shadow will fade. If, due to atrophy of the parenchyma (which may be due to long-standing obstruction) the renal arterial inflow is small, then it may take some hours for enough dye to diffuse through the residual renal tissue in sufficient quantity to outline this kidney; which is the reason for taking delayed (even up to 1 or 2 days) radiographs in this situation.

It follows from the above that the definition of the level of an obstructive lesion by an IVU depends on the amount of dye which will be excreted by the kidney into the collecting system; and this in turn depends not only on the quantity of dye injected and the taking of delayed radiographs, but also on the quality or potential function of the renal tissue. In most instances, the collecting system and ureter are sufficiently well outlined as to permit accurate localization of the level of the obstruction, but if this is not possible, alternative means of outlining the collecting system are necessary, if correctly planned surgery is to be undertaken. In the majority of cases, a retrograde ureterogram and pyelogram will serve this purpose. This is undertaken using a bulb or Chevassau catheter which plugs the uretic orifice. Although it is preferable to visualize the ascent of the injected dye using an image intensifier, a satisfactory series of pictures can be obtained by taking the radiographs as the dye is injected. If it is not possible to do a retrograde examination (e.g. the ureter has previously been implanted in the colon or ileum, or access to the ureteric orifice is technically difficult due to a urethral stricture or prostatic projection, etc.), then the radiologists are often able to puncture the dilated renal pelvis through the loin with a long flexible needle, through which is threaded a narrow catheter and dye is injected. The resulting pro- or antegrade ureterogram will clearly define the level of the obstruction and so the correct operation can be planned.

It should be realized that a dilated ureter as seen on the IVU does not necessarily mean obstruction. A ureter which has been damaged by infection may thereafter be wider and is certainly more distensible than the contralateral ureter. Similarly, certain developmental anomalies lead to a ureter being larger than usual, yet these are not obstructed. To establish whether the ureteric dilatation is due to urinary obstruction as opposed to atony and/or reflux, a DTPA renogram (see page 452) is undertaken. If obstructed, the isotope will not drain away from the kidney and the third part of the tracing will record a rising radiation count, as opposed to a declining value as is seen in the normal situation, as the isotope drains from the kidney to the lower urinary tract. If vesico-ureteric reflux is marked, a ureter may appear quite dilated on the IVU. This appearance is further exaggerated if the vesico-ureteric reflux is associated with infection.

Renal surgery for obstructive disease

The pelvi-ureteric junction is probably the commonest site above the level of the bladder neck at which obstruction to urine flow occurs. In the majority of cases, the diagnosis is made on the IVU, there being blunting (to an equal extent) of all the renal papillae, which in the more extreme cases exhibit spherical calyces, a large renal pelvis and a normal ureter.

In the majority, the obstruction is believed to be due to a failure of the transmission of the peristaltic waves from the pelvis passing across the pelvi-ureteric junction and down the ureter so causing the urine to accumulate in a relatively static state. Hydronephrosis may also be due to a stone becoming impacted at the pelvi-ureteric junction, or occasionally due to a polypoid tumour sometimes seen at this site. Hydronephrosis due to stricturing at the pelvi-ureteric junction is seen in tuberculosis, but other stigmas of this disease should also be evident on the IVU. Obstruction of a more temporary nature occurs with a renal papilla or blood clot.

Pyeloplasty

It is the author's opinion that the objectives of a pyeloplasty should be not only to remove the obstruction to urine flow at the pelvi-ureteric junction, but to reduce the volume of the enlarged renal pelvis, so as to permit the rapid 'turnover' of urine in the hydronephrotic kidney and so decrease the liability of urinary infection becoming established in a relatively stagnant pool of urine. The only operation which fulfils these requirements is the Anderson–Hynes dismembered pyeloplasty.

The kidney is approached through the usual 12th rib incision. If complete mobility of the organ is required, the whole of the kidney is freed from the surrounding tissues. In many instances all of the pelvis can be exposed without having to mobilize the upper pole of the kidney. The ureter is identified and the adherent condensed layers of fascia covering the pelvis are dissected off, so that at the time of anastomosis, only the tissues of the pelvis and ureter are sewn together (Figure 32.10). Often the lower pole blood vessels are buried in the peripelvic tissue and these must be completely freed.

Although on occasions it may appear that the manoeuvre of separating the lower polar vessels from the pelvis results in relieving the obstructed collecting system, it is difficult to prove whether the same situation persists in a patient who is upright with a significant diuresis. Hence to ensure relief of obstruction, the pelviureteric junction must be reconstructed (Figure 32.11). The redundant portion of the pelvis is excised, demarking each end of the incision with 4/0 catgut (on an atraumatic curved cutting needle). The majority of the gaping renal pelvis is closed with a continuous suture, starting at the superior aspect. The lowermost 2 cm of the pelvis are left open and attached to the spatulated ureter, using once again a continuous suture of 4/0 catgut. This anastomosis is positioned in whichever site it seems best suited, which can be either in front of or behind the lower polar blood vessels (if present) (Figure 32.12). There is no need to use a stent or nephrostomy drainage. A corrugated drain is positioned by the anastomosis.

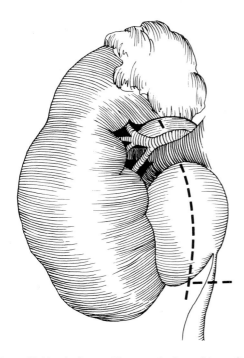

Figure 32.10 Anderson–Hynes pyeloplasty. Lines of excision

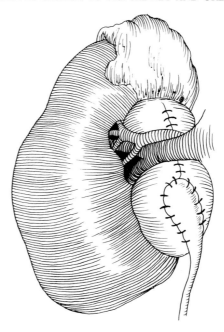

Figure 32.12 Anderson–Hynes pyeloplasty. Complete anastomosis and repair of pelvis

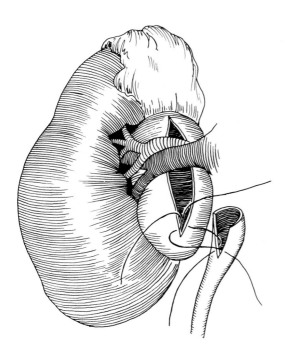

Figure 32.11 Anderson–Hynes pyeloplasty. Preparation for anastomosis of ureter to lower pelvis

In the unusual situation of the hydronephrosis being present in a horseshoe kidney, the bridge or isthmus joining the two halves of the kidney must be divided to ensure that there is no further obstruction below the reconstructed pelvi-ureteric junction.

Another advance, which is in its infancy, is the surgery of pelvic hydronephrosis. Access to the lumen of the upper urinary tract, by means of a nephrostomy tract, permits the passage of a urethrotome, and so incision of the mucosal and muscular layers of the pelvi-ureteric junction – a procedure described as pyelolysis.

Nephrostomy

The function of this operation is to:

1. Ensure urine drainage direct from the kidney so as to bypass an obstruction or protect a recently constructed anastomosis involving the upper urinary tract.
2. Drain from the kidney any blood which may be issuing forth after renal surgery or other trauma.

This is achieved by introducing a catheter or tube into the renal collecting system, and may be part of a more extensive operation or constitute the whole of the operation. In either case a definitive nephrotomy must be made and only then should the catheter be threaded through the renal substance. To ensure that the inner aspect of the nephrotomy is suitably placed, a pyelotomy is necessary. Through the opening in the renal pelvis, a finger is passed into the collecting system and the thickness of the renal cortex overlying an appropriate calyx (i.e. dilated, dependent or easily accessible) can be estimated. The end of a pair of curved nephrolithotomy forceps (e.g. Randall's) is passed through the pyelotomy into the chosen calyx.

If the overlying renal cortex is thin, a little pressure on the forceps will ensure its passage through the parenchyma, and so the end of the tube or catheter is grasped and withdrawn into the collecting system. If the thickness of the cortex is substantial, then the nephrotomy is made by cutting down with a scalpel onto the forceps positioned in the appropriate calyx.

One variety of catheter which may be used is a rat-tailed Cummings nephrostomy tube, the tail of which acts as a splint (no. 8 Fr. gauge) for intubating the upper ureter. This is necessary after doing a ureterotomy, whereby a longitudinal incision is made along a strictured ureter (Figure 32.13) (as occurs in tuberculosis). Alternatively, if the nephrostomy is being used to drain blood after multiple nephrotomies for stone disease, then a tube (of no. 12–18 Fr. gauge) with a number of openings is necessary. It is rare to envisage long-term catheter drainage from the kidney, but provided that the renal pelvis is of an adequate size retaining balloon catheters may be appropriate.

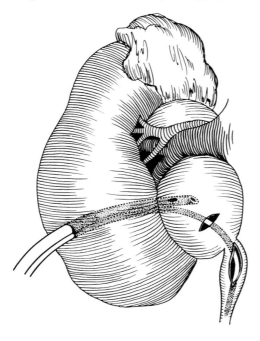

Figure 32.13 Nephrostomy and intubated ureterostomy

Where possible, the nephrostomy should be sited so that it emerges on the anterolateral aspect of the abdominal wall. This facilitates dressings and care of the tube and also enables the patient to lie on his or her back. Usually a belt with a flange is used to stabilize the position of the catheter.

Ureteric surgery for obstructive disease

As in the case of the kidney, it is preferable if surgical procedures on the ureter are kept in the extraperi-toneal space. Naturally this is not possible if an intra-peritoneal anastomosis with bowel is necessary, or in dealing with difficult ureterovaginal fistulas; but the incidence of intestinal ileus and peritoneal infection (which may be secondary to the extravasation of infected urine leaking from an anastomosis or ureter-otomy) prolongs convalescence and the need for par-enteral feeding. In addition, extraperitoneal surgery offers the technical advantages of excluding from the operating field the irritation of obtruding loops of bowel.

The surgical approach to the ureter is conditioned by the nature of the disease process involved. In the case of stone disease, different incisions are used for exposure of the upper, middle and lower thirds of the ureter. In the case of bilateral and advanced retro-peritoneal fibrosis, the ureterolysis and biopsy are best undertaken by a transperitoneal surgical exposure.

UPPER THIRD OF THE URETER

The commonest indication for approaching the upper third of the ureter is for removal of a calculus which is causing appreciable urinary obstruction or pain. A stone which lies within 4 cm or so of the pelvi-ureteric junction may, as a result of the dissection, slip back into the renal pelvis, and hence it is the author's practice to use an oblique lumbar incision with the patient on his or her side (see page 449) so that easy exposure of the kidney is possible if a pyelotomy should prove necessary to recover the stone. Satisfactory exposure of the renal pelvis and upper ureter can also be obtained through the lumbotomy incision (see page 451). In either case the upper ureter is identified, and an encircling tape placed round the ureter above the level of the stone. In these circumstances there is no need to undertake any dissection in the renal fossa, but if the stone should slip back into the renal pelvis, then this organ will have to be identified and opened to remove the stone.

Once the ureter has been secured and the site of the stone isolated, two stay sutures of 4/0 catgut are placed on the anterior aspect of the ureter overlying the calculus. The ureter is incised longitudinally between the stay sutures. With a blunt (McDonald's) dissector the stone is freed from the adherent ureteric mucosa and removed with stone forceps. Releasing the tape above the ureterotomy should result in a copious flow of urine, which proves that there is no proximal obstruction. To ensure that there is no distal obstruction from a fragment or unidentified lower stone, a ureteric catheter or bougie is passed down the length of the lower ureter. The ureterotomy is closed with a 4/0 catgut suture which passes through the muscle layer of the ureter. A corrugated drain is placed adjacent to the operation site and brought out through the abdominal wall with a stab wound which is separate from the main incision. The muscle layers are closed with interrupted catgut.

MIDDLE THIRD OF THE URETER

The approach to the middle third of the ureter is by means of a muscle-splitting (gridiron) incision of the anterior abdominal wall. The patient lies supine and the incision can be either transversely positioned or in the iliac fossa. If the part of the ureter to be approached is at the mid-lumbar spine level, then a transverse incision is used. Laterally it starts at the anterior axillary line, positioned at the midpoint between the tip of the 12th rib and the iliac crest — passing medially to the lateral border of the rectus sheath. The oblique and transverse abdominal muscles are split along the line of their respective fibres, and it is often an advantage to open the anterior and posterior layers of the rectus sheath for 2 cm to allow for an improved exposure. The peritoneum is stripped off the posterior abdominal muscles towards the midline and with the ureter will be found the gonadal vessels. The removal of the stone and subsequent manoeuvres are as described in the previous section.

To isolate the ureter at the level of the bifurcation of the common iliac artery or slightly lower down, an oblique iliac fossa incision is made and the ureter is approached retroperitoneally.

LOWER THIRD OF THE URETER

The pararectal incision immediately overlies the lower part of the ureter, and is made so that it traces the lateral edge of the rectus muscle. The fascia which is immediately lateral to the rectus muscle (formed as a result of the fusion into one layer of the muscles of the abdominal wall) is incised. This exposes the extraperitoneal space from the superior ramus of the pubis to the level of the semilunar line of Douglas (i.e. the lower edge of the posterior rectus sheath). The inferior epigastric blood vessels have to be divided and the peritoneum is stripped medially. If the ureter is not readily identified because of excess fat, it is best to extend the incision superiorly for another 3 cm and carefully separate the peritoneum off the rectus sheath, so that the bifurcation of the common iliac artery can be palpated. The ureter is here identified and traced down into the pelvis.

Mobilization of the ureter to within 3 cm of the bladder is unhindered by any structure until the superior vesical artery and vein are noted to be passing from the lateral wall of the pelvis towards the bladder and are intimately adherent to the ureter. These blood vessels must be divided between Moynihan clamps and securely tied, if access is to be obtained to the lowermost portion of the ureter. Thereafter the muscle fibres of the detrusor will become apparent. Removal of a stone is as previously described.

Drainage of this wound is with a corrugated rubber drain brought out through a stab wound, 5 cm from the lateral edge of the incision. Closure requires one layer of continuous unabsorbable material, since using absorbable material often results in an incisional hernia.

Ureterolysis

The condition of retroperitoneal fibrosis is becoming more readily diagnosed prior to operation, as a result of the increasing awareness of this disease as a cause of upper urinary tract obstruction. We need not concern ourselves with the symptomatology, but the IVU will show some significant features. The disease may involve one or both ureters, and since the obstruction is extramural, the lower limit of the dilated ureter shows a characteristic tapering or spindle-shaped appearance. There may be other evidence of the cause of the obstruction, e.g. the linear calcification seen in the wall of an aortic aneurysm, which then leaks some blood, and as a result of organization of the haematoma goes on to fibrosis with compression of the ureter.

In so-called 'idiopathic retroperitoneal fibrosis', whereby the disease spreads from the midline laterally, the ureter may occasionally be pulled medially. In this disease and also in that due to spreading carcinoma from the rectum, uterus or prostate, the pelvic portion of the ureter is commonly involved. Retroperitoneal tumours originating in carcinoma of the stomach, pancreas, ovary and breast are other extramural causes of the ureteric obstruction.

It is often necessary to undertake a retrograde ureterogram to define the extent of the ureteric compression, and so plan the correct incision for the operation. A retroperitoneal exposure of the ureter is the best approach if only one ureter is involved, but if both ureters are shown to be obstructed, then a transperitoneal approach may be preferable. The object of the operation is to obtain a biopsy of the material and to free the ureter from the enveloping tissues without making a hole in the ureter. The ureterolysis is best undertaken by identifying the normal ureter below the obstruction, and then by careful dissection establishing the plane which preserves the integrity of the ureter and strips it free from the enveloping tissues. It is important to ensure that the obstruction to the ureter is relieved, which will only occur if the ureter is pared down to the muscle layers. The whole length of the involved ureter must be dealt with in this manner. The vascularity of the ureteric wall is considerably reduced as a result of this peri-ureteric activity, and if the integrity of the mucosa is breached, it may lead to a persistent fistula, despite proximal urinary diversion. In these circumstances, a nephrostomy is to be preferred to the use of a ureterostomy, because of the uncertainty of the nature of the disease process surrounding the ureter (until a histological report becomes available) and subsequent healing.

The exposed ureter should be positioned away from the pathological tissue, and if convenient can be placed in the peritoneal cavity. The biopsy report is important in the further management of these patients. If the patient has bilateral obstruction due to malignant peri-ureteric fibrosis, it is probably inadvisable to undertake proximal urinary diversions. Failure to respond to carcino-chemotherapy will lead to uraemia as a terminal event, which is often preferable to a protracted and miserable terminal illness. If the biopsy shows the obstruction to be due to periureteric fibrosis, corticosteroid therapy is necessary to arrest the disease (the duration of drug therapy is judged by the response to the blood sedimentation rate and degree of ureteric obstruction).

Nephrectomy and other renal operations

As previously indicated, the removal of functioning nephrons should not be lightly undertaken. Hence renal surgery should be as conservative as possible, provided that this in no way limits the effectiveness of the treatment.

The more common indications for the removal of a kidney vary from malignant disease to that for a severely traumatized organ, or for a kidney virtually destroyed by infection or obstruction (with or without accompanying stone disease). Nephrectomy in vascular disease, e.g. renal hypertension and arteriovenous malformations, should only be considered if other modalities have proved ineffective, i.e. the failure of reconstructive surgery or drug therapy in the case of hypertension.

There are two overriding prerequisites before contemplating nephrectomy. First, a preoperative diagnosis should have been made, since exploratory operations of the kidney are a very poor investigative tool (the investigations relevant to a disease process are described earlier). Secondly, the surgeon must be informed of the total renal function and in particular the function of the contralateral kidney. The value of the IVU and blood tests have already been described (page 456).

Before embarking on a nephrectomy, the haemoglobin level must be known, and blood should have been cross-matched for transfusion purposes. The technique now to be described is that commonly performed by the author when removing the kidney, but when dealing with malignant disease there are some additional features which are mentioned later in this chapter.

The incision and approach to the kidney are determined by the condition of the underlying kidney pathology. The renal artery will be found in the angle between the upper medial border of the kidney and the posterior abdominal wall. It should be traced towards its origin, as far as is possible, to ensure that it is the stem of the artery and not its major branches (which, due to early division, originate close to the aorta) which has been dissected out. Care is taken to ensure that the artery and vein are sufficiently separ-

ate to make it possible to put three Moynihan clamps on the artery, without involving the vein in any way. The artery is divided in the space between the clamp nearest to the kidney and that of the adjoining clamp, so that after division there are two clamps on the stump of that part of the renal artery in continuity with the aorta. Using 5 metric (1) chromic catgut, the artery is first ligated behind the furthermost clamp, i.e. the one nearest the aorta, and after removal of that clamp, a second ligature is tied behind the remaining clamp. Finally, the stump of artery attached to the kidney is tied. This procedure is repeated for the renal vein.

Securing and ligating the artery and vein separately ensure good visualization of the blood vessels. 'Blind' clamping of the renal pedicle may be associated with inadvertently including unwanted structures in the tip of the forceps. On the right side the inferior vena cava is particularly at risk. Furthermore, ligating the major vessels together may lead to the formation of an arteriovenous fistula. Catgut is used in preference to non-absorbable material, to avoid the possibility of sinus formation, which does occur if the wound and renal bed become infected. It is advisable to drain the renal fossa, since there is often some oozing from the smaller blood vessels of the surrounding tissues.

Nephrectomy for malignant disease

The commonest condition for which a nephrectomy is undertaken is a hypernephroma (or carcinoma of the renal tubular epithelium). The diagnosis should be firmly established before embarking on the removal of the kidney. If on the IVU the space-occupying lesion looks more like a renal cyst than a tumour, an ultrasound examination is recommended. If this latter demonstrates that the space-occupying lesion is of a fluid nature, aspiration of this by the radiologist using the image intensifier will often resolve the problem. It is of further help if the fluid obtained is examined by a cytologist for malignant cells. This approach to the treatment of a renal cyst spares the patient an unnecessary kidney exploration.

If the ultrasound shows a solid lesion to be present, then the differential diagnosis lies between a hypernephroma, angiomyolipoma which may be associated with tuberous sclerosis or rarely a nephroblastoma. With appropriate apparatus, ultrasound may demonstrate extension of tumour in the renal vein and the inferior vena cava. In hamartomas with a significant amount of fat, the ultrasound will clearly demonstrate this fact which indicates non-operative treatment.

If doubt remains as to the diagnosis, then a CT scan will delineate the features described above and noted on ultrasound, and also demonstrate lymph node involvement and attachment of any tumour to the related viscera or muscle wall. Nuclear magnetic resonance has little to offer beyond that described above and the place of an invasive investigation like angiography has been considerably diminished, although it has the advantage of outlining the number of renal arteries present.

Prior to nephrectomy for malignant disease, a chest radiograph is mandatory. Urinary cytology is particularly useful if seeking to establish a diagnosis of a transitional cell carcinoma of the kidney. This information is important, since a nephro-ureterectomy may be indicated.

It should be realized that total nephrectomy is not the only renal operation undertaken for malignant diseases. Transitional cell carcinoma has a multifocal origin, and when this disease is localized to one of the poles of the kidney, it may be justified, particularly in a relatively young individual with similar disease in the bladder, to limit the renal surgery to a partial nephrectomy (this operation is described in the previous section). It is of course incumbent on the surgeon to examine the ureter (by retrograde ureterography) particularly carefully for evidence of tumour in that organ before planning renal surgery. Partial nephrectomy is also indicated when the tumour occurs in a solitary kidney, or sometimes in bilateral renal tumours.

Nephrectomy is in part being replaced by extensive embolization of the renal artery and its tributaries. In the future it is hoped that the infarcted kidney will be macerated and aspirated by instruments which enter the renal fossa through a loin puncture wound.

Surgery for renal trauma

The majority of traumatized kidneys are managed conservatively. Immediate operative interference for an injured kidney is restricted to those cases where continuing significant bleeding persists, or where the IVU shows total absence of function on the side of the injured kidney.

The criteria which indicate continuing significant bleeding from a kidney are a falling blood pressure, rising pulse rate and a progressively enlarging mass in the renal fossa. Haematuria is not a helpful pointer as to the need for surgery, even if it be prolonged for weeks. An IVU is mandatory. It will give valuable information in respect of the number of kidneys and their function. Marked extravasation of dye and urine is not an indication for immediate surgery, although operation may subsequently be required.

Total absence of function on the side of the supposedly injured kidney should be followed by an emergency renal arteriogram. This will give information which is vital to the correct management of the patient. If the angiogram indicates a contusion with thrombosis (or avulsion) of the renal artery, then immediate operation is indicated, and the operator should be prepared to undertake reconstructive arterial surgery. However, complete absence of a kidney on the urogram may be due to a relatively minor injury to a previously poorly functioning kidney, as would be seen in a long-standing pathological con-

dition (e.g. a grossly hydronephrotic kidney) or congenital abnormality (e.g. a hypoplastic kidney). In these cases the treatment of choice is conservative management, provided that there is no continuing significant bleeding occurring.

Immediate surgery to arrest severe bleeding from a lacerated kidney leads more often than not to nephrectomy. Obviously a more conservative approach is to be preferred, and this may be possible if the damage is localized (as judged by a urogram) to one or other of the poles. Similarly, severe bleeding from a solitary kidney is a fairly desperate situation, and conservative surgery should be attempted. Preferably this requires isolation of the renal pedicle, so as to be able to use bulldog clamps for arresting the haemorrhage. Usually the 12th rib lumbar approach is satisfactory, unless intraperitoneal manoeuvres are also contemplated. Mobilization of the kidney in these circumstances usually means evacuation of clot, and, as indicated above, isolation of the renal artery may be difficult and a pedicle clamp may have to be placed across both the artery and vein for the purposes of controlling the bleeding.

In the less severely injured kidney, soon after the haematuria has ceased, the IVU should be repeated. If there is evidence of persisting extravasation, this may lead to fibrosis with compression of the ureter and/or vascular pedicle. If surgery is delayed until organization of the extravasated blood has occurred, the procedure is difficult. Therefore, operation should not be long delayed, and evacuation and drainage of extravasated fluid and blood are undertaken, with resuturing of torn collecting system and debridement of necrotic tissue with possible extension to partial nephrectomy (as described in the appropriate section).

Ureteric excision, repair and substitution

Ureterectomy

Removal of a ureter is usually total, and commonly part of a larger operation, namely a nephro-ureterectomy, which may be necessary with tuberculous disease or a transitional-cell carcinoma of the upper urinary tract.

In the case of a carcinoma of the ureter, it may be possible to do a segmental ureterectomy by excising the tumour with a 1 cm margin, and still permit a primary anastomosis. This approach is justified on the grounds that this disease is multifocal in origin, and extirpation of the upper urinary tract for a well-circumscribed lesion of the renal pelvis or ureter may be considered excessive, since recurrent disease can be expected in the bladder or in the contralateral kidney and ureter. Following local removal of a tumour, careful follow-up examinations with urinary cytology, IVU and urethrocystoscopy are mandatory.

Excision of the ureter is also undertaken if a kidney

has to be removed due to extensive destruction by tuberculosis, since removal of a kidney alone does not guarantee eradication of the tuberculosis from the residual ureter. To combat active ureteric disease, either the circulating antituberculous drugs must be able to get at the bacillus (which is limited by the blood supply to the ureter) or, alternatively, the drug must come in contact with the ureter by means of its urinary content, and this is only possible if there is a significant degree of vesico-ureteric reflux in the remaining stump.

The operation of nephro-ureterectomy is best undertaken through two incisions. The 12th rib lumbar incision is employed and the routine operation of nephrectomy is undertaken except that the ureter is not divided. Through the lower regions of the incision, the peritoneum is stripped off the abdominal parieties and the kidney is placed in the iliac fossa. The lumbar incision is closed in the usual manner. The patient is then repositioned and laid supine and retowelled. The incision and approach are as described for the lower third of the ureter. Having dissected the ureter within 3 cm or so of its termination, the superior vesical pedicle is divided which allows the ureter to be followed to the bladder wall. Traction on the ureter makes it possible to put a Moynihan clamp on the tented-up portion of the bladder; and a ligature is applied to the bladder side of the clamp. This clamp is then loosened and repositioned 2 cm up the ureter. The crushed segment is divided and the specimen removed includes a cuff of the bladder.

Primary ureteric anastomosis

The ureter may be damaged by trauma, as occurs in penetrating and crushing wounds, or during surgery or by inflammatory and neoplastic disease and other rarer pathological entities. This may result in extravasation of urine, often associated with infection which in turn is followed by upper urinary tract obstruction, intestinal ileus, etc. The defect in the ureter must be repaired or bypassed, if the serious complications of urinary extravasation are to be eliminated.

If the ureter is injured at the time of a surgical procedure, then identification and repair of the defect should be undertaken immediately. Immediate surgery is also recommended following a road traffic accident or other traumatic injuries such as a stab injury. In these circumstances, an IVU should be undertaken before the patient is submitted to surgery, in order to identify the site of the injury and establish the presence of two functioning kidneys.

Factors which determine the type of repair to be undertaken are how recent the injury is, its site and whether there has been any significant loss of ureteric length. If the ureteric injury was not identified at the time of operation, or the defect developed as a complication of other pathology, then it may be wise to deal first with the complications of the ureteric injury,

namely infection and fistula formation, by using a proximal urinary diversion, e.g. a nephrostomy. In these circumstances, it will be necessary later to localize the site of the damage by means of an IVU and possibly a retrograde ureterogram.

On those rare occasions that a localized injury occurs to the upper three-quarters of the ureter, local excision of that part of the ureter which may have been devitalized by the inadvertent application of an artery clamp or ligation with a suture is undertaken. The ureteric ends are then spatulated and sutured with interrupted 4/0 catgut material. When healthy ureter is repaired, there is no advantage in intubating the ureter or using a proximal urinary diversion. A corrugated drain is placed down to the site of the ureteric repair.

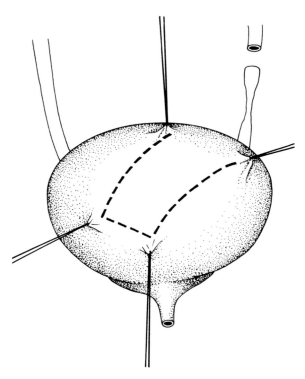

Figure 32.14 Boari flap for reconstruction of lower ureter. Demarcation of flap

Ureteroneocystostomy (and Boari flap) (Figures 32.14–32.18)

An end-to-end anastomosis as described above is technically difficult in the lower quarter of the ureter. If the damage to the ureter is within 5 cm of the ureteric orifice, a simple reimplantation of the ureter is done. The bladder is opened and a Leadbetter–Politano type of reimplantation which avoids vesicoureteric reflux (see Figures 32.16 and 32.17) is used. If the cut end of the ureter will not reach the intact bladder without tension, then a bladder flap is raised.

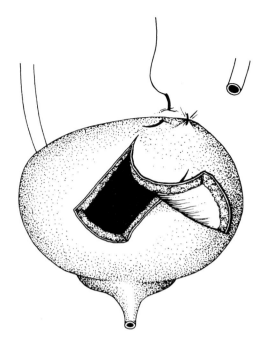

Figure 32.15   Boari flap. Incision and elevation of flap and psoas hitch sutures

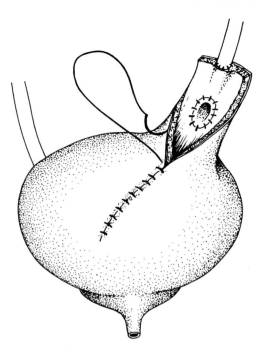

Figure 32.17   Boari flap. Closure of bladder

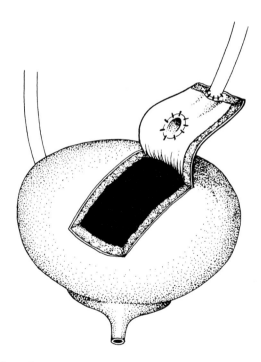

Figure 32.16   Boari flap. Intramural implantation of ureter

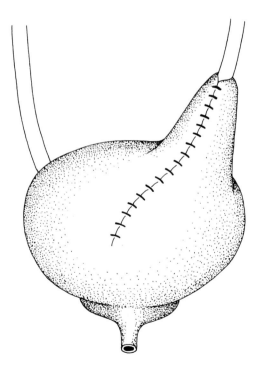

Figure 32.18   Boari flap. Completed

Construction of a Boari flap implies adequate access to the bladder with ligation of the superior vesical blood vessels on the affected side, so as to be able to mobilize the bladder to a significant extent. The flap is constructed on the superior aspect of the bladder with the base posteriorly. At the level of the hinge flap, the bladder is anchored to the psoas minor muscle at the pelvic brim. The flap is turned up towards the cut end of the ureter and a submucosal reimplantation of this ureter is undertaken, using the tunnel technique as for a Leadbetter–Politano operation. If the anastomosis appears to be under tension, then a ureteric splint is passed up the ureter, and brought out through the bladder wall and abdominal wall attached to a pointed trocar needle as used with Redivac drains. The bladder flap and cystostomy wound are closed with two continuous layers of catgut. A corrugated drain should be put down to the anastomosis, and urethral catheter drainage maintained for 10 days.

If it is not possible to anastomose the damaged ureter directly to the bladder due to pelvic trauma or disease, or loss of a considerable length of ureter, then the injured ureter should be anastomosed to the contralateral ureter above the level of the pelvic brim – this is known as a transuretero-ureterostomy.

Transuretero-ureterostomy (Figures 32.19 and 32.20)

To undertake an anastomosis of the shortened damaged ureter to the contralateral intact ureter, a paramedian incision is used and the peritoneal cavity is opened. The divided ureter is identified and mobilized retroperitoneally to the mid-lumbar spine level, and a length of 4/0 catgut is attached to the cut end, as a stay suture. The intact ureter is identified at the level where it crosses the common iliac artery, and the peritoneum is incised, the ureter mobilized and isolated between two tapes.

A finger is introduced through the peritoneal opening made over the intact ureter, and passed medially anterior to the aorta and vena cava, but behind the inferior mesenteric blood vessels and mesocolon to emerge at the site where the divided ureter is situated. A pair of artery forceps is now guided along the length of the tunnel created by the exploring finger and the stay suture attached to the cut ureter is grasped and withdrawn across the midline so as to bring it out by the side of the exposed intact ureter. A 4/0 catgut suture is placed either side of the midline of the intact ureter, and a 1.5–2 cm longitudinal incision is made between these two markers. The cut end of the ureter is spatulated by incising it for 1.5 cm.

The anastomosis of the divided ureter to the intact ureter is done with interrupted 4/0 catgut sutures. The peritoneum overlying the incision is not closed, and a corrugated drain is positioned at the site of the anastomosis and brought out through a separate stab incision. The paramedian incision is closed with continuous catgut for the peritoneum and continuous non-absorbable material for the anterior rectus sheath. The peritoneal drain is removed on the 4th postoperative day if there is no urinary leakage occurring. If there is any leakage, then it should be left in place for 1 week, by which time a well-established drainage track is formed.

Ureteral substitution

If a transuretero-ureterostomy is not possible because the contralateral ureter is inaccessible (due to previous surgery or other pathology) or absent (due to previous removal or congenital absence), then the

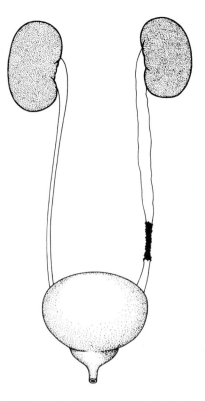

Figure 32.19   Ureteric stricture following injury

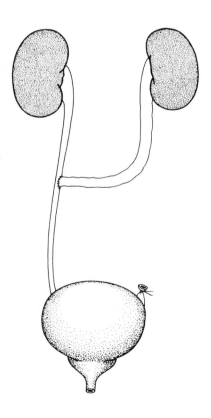

Figure 32.20   Transuretero-ureterostomy

choice lies between a cutaneous ureterostomy or the use of a segment of ileum to re-establish continuity between the ureter and the bladder. A cutaneous ureterostomy in the adult is on the whole an unsatisfactory procedure. In the first place the length of residual ureter is usually short and so the stoma is often situated in the flank, and there is difficulty in conveniently attaching a collecting bag. In a ureter of a normal calibre, the stoma tends to stenose, despite plastic procedures for increasing the lumen and the size of the ureterocutaneous anastomosis.

It is therefore preferable to use a length of bowel to replace the missing part of the ureter, and a segment of ileum is isolated in the same way as described for an ileal conduit. The ureter is implanted into the proximal end of the ileum, some 2 cm from the cut end of the bowel using the nipple technique. To prevent the nipple coming undone, a 4/0 catgut stitch is used to fix the turn-backed flap of ureter on to itself. A splint is secured in position by transfixing (with 4/0 catgut on an atraumatic cutting needle) a suture through both the tube and the ureter at the apex of the nipple. The splint is threaded down the whole length of the ileal segment. The proximal end of the ileum is closed. The bladder is opened between stay sutures. The end of the ureteric splint is attached to a Redivac needle, and this latter is brought from within the bladder through the detrusor and abdominal wall, and the splint is securely fixed onto the anterior surface of the abdomen with a non-absorbable suture. The anastomosis between the bladder and distal end of the ileal segment is done with one layer of interrupted catgut sutures, passing through all layers of gut and bladder. A peritoneal corrugated drain is placed at the site of this lower anastomosis. Urethral catheter drainage is instituted for 14 days. If there is any hint of bladder outflow obstruction, this should have been dealt with prior to the ureteric reconstruction. The splint is removed by gentle traction 10 days after the operation.

References

Gil-Vernet, J. (1965) New surgical concepts in removing renal calculi. *Urol. Int.*, **20**, 255–288

Nagamatsu, G. R. (1950) Dorso-lumbar approach to the kidney and adrenal with osteoplastic flap. *J. Urol.*, **63**, 569–571

Wickham, J. E. A. (1968) A simple method for regional renal hypothermia. *J. Urol.*, **99**, 246–247

Wickham, J. E. A., Fernando, A. R., Hendry, W. F. *et al.* (1979) I. V. inosine for ischaemic renal surgery. *Br. J. Urol.*, **51**, 437–439

Further reading

Glen, J. (ed.) (1975) *Urologic Surgery*, 2nd edn, Harper and Row, New York

Wickham, J. E. A. (ed.) (1979) *Urinary Calculous Disease*, Churchill Livingstone, Edinburgh

Wickham, J. E. A. and Miller, R. A. (eds) (1983) *Percutaneous Renal Surgery*, Churchill Livingstone, Edinburgh

Williams, D. I. (1977) *Operative Surgery: Urology*, 3rd edn, Butterworths, London

33

Functional assessment of the lower urinary tract

R. C. L. Feneley and J. A. Massey

Introduction

A disturbance of the normal pattern of micturition can be the presenting symptom of a wide spectrum of conditions that includes inflammatory, neoplastic, endocrine, neurological, degenerative and psychogenic disorders. Assessment needs to be comprehensive; the traditional approach follows a methodical course that starts with the history, clinical examination and routine pathological tests, and proceeds to appropriate radiological and endoscopic investigations in selected cases such as those with haematuria. This regimen identifies pathology and localizes it anatomically within the urinary tract, but fails to demonstrate any cause for the symptoms in many cases; 50% of women with symptoms of cystitis have no evidence of bacteriuria (Gallagher et al., 1965).

Urodynamic studies introduced objective criteria by which the functional disorders could be evaluated. The results challenged the validity of traditional concepts such as the relevance of prostatic size or bladder trabeculation, and highlighted factors such as the unstable and the hypersensitive bladder. Reliable criteria are essential for accurate diagnosis, selecting appropriate treatment and monitoring therapeutic response; in a study of men with suspected prostatic obstruction, 30% had no urodynamic evidence of obstructed micturition (Abrams and Feneley, 1978). Urodynamic studies have answered some questions and stimulated many more, but they have introduced better patient selection for operative treatment and a more critical analysis of the results. This chapter introduces urodynamic techniques and concepts, and their application in clinical practice. The terminology and definitions are those recommended by the International Continence Society (ICS) (Abrams et al., 1988).

Urodynamic techniques

Flowmetry

Direct observation and timing of the flow are time-honoured methods of assessing micturition. However, modern electronic equipment is more accurate and produces a graphic display for measurement and comparison. A number of principles are employed – weight transducers, the decrease in capacitance as urine rises up a metal strip capacitor or the inertia of urine falling on a spinning disc. Electronic differentiation provides a measure of the volume and the rate of change of flow. The test is further enhanced by ultrasonically determining the post-void residual.

Cystometry

Access to the bladder may be either per urethram or suprapubically; the latter is especially useful in children. The intravesical pressure is transmitted through fine tubes, e.g. an epidural catheter attached via manometer tubing, to an external pressure transducer. The whole system is water-filled. A similar arrangement may be employed for measuring the rectal pressure. In the female the proximal vagina has been shown to be a suitable alternative site for the estimation of 'intra-abdominal' pressure. Instead of external transducers, it is possible to use microtransducers mounted on catheters in bladder, urethra or rectum.

For filling the bladder, a small catheter (10 Fr. gauge) is used, but this must be removed before pressure/flow studies since it will produce obstruction to the flow.

Saline is the commonly used filling medium in the UK and has been shown to be more physiological than the CO_2 employed in gas cystometry. Infusion may be gravity fed or by use of a peristaltic pump to give greater control of the filling rate.

Videocystometry

In order to record pressure changes and the appearance of bladder and urethra synchronously, an image intensifier and videomixer are required. The filling medium contains radiological contrast so that cine X-ray pictures and pressure traces are recorded on videotape for later perusal.

Urethral profilometry

Profilometry may be performed directly using catheter-mounted microtransducers by withdrawing the catheter from the bladder through the urethra. The withdrawal mechanism is usually synchronized with chart speed to allow direct measurement of urethral length. By mounting two microtip transducers 5 cm apart, simultaneous recording of intravesical and urethral pressures can be performed. Water profilometry cannot be performed directly. Fluid is infused at a constant rate by a syringe pump through a small catheter. The occlusive pressure of the urethral wall is measured indirectly by a manometer attached to a side channel. Gas perfusion or small intraluminal balloons may also be used.

Urodynamic concepts

Urodynamic studies started when suitable equipment and methods became available to record accurately events during the micturition cycle such as the flow rate and hydrodynamic changes that occur in the bladder and urethra during filling and emptying. The concept is simple; urine is stored in the lower urinary tract and continence maintained so long as the total bladder or intravesical pressure (P_{ves}) remains lower than the maximum urethral intraluminal pressure (P_{ura}). The difference between these pressures is termed the maximum urethral closure pressure (MUCP = $P_{ura} - P_{ves}$).

The bladder normally empties completely on voiding, which occurs when the pressure gradient is reversed and is sustained throughout micturition. The whole cycle of filling and voiding can thus be analysed using these parameters and the flow rate.

The storage phase

Intravesical pressure

The total bladder pressure is composed of two elements, intra-abdominal and detrusor pressures. Changes in abdominal pressure (P_{abd}) occurring on movement or exertion are transmitted directly to the bladder; detrusor pressure (P_{det}) is that component of intravesical pressure created by passive and active forces in the bladder wall. It is estimated by subtracting abdominal pressure from intravesical pressure ($P_{det} = P_{ves} - P_{abd}$), usually automatically calculated by the equipment.

Intravesical pressure during filling is normally within the range 30–55 cmH$_2$O but varies with posture, movement, straining and obesity. Detrusor pressure is usually less than 15 cmH$_2$O throughout filling; under normal circumstances, the detrusor does not contract during filling even under the most provocative and unphysiological conditions of cystometry with indwelling catheters, fast filling, changes in posture and coughing (Figure 33.1).

Cystometry is used to record the pressure/volume relationship of the bladder during filling and voiding; the response of the bladder to filling is described in terms of its capacity, compliance, contractility and sensation. When considering the capacity, it is necessary to differentiate between the structural, functional and cystometric capacity.

The structural bladder capacity refers to the amount of fluid the organ holds under general or regional anaesthesia. This volume should be recorded routinely at cystoscopy, particularly where the capacity is reduced as in interstitial cystitis, radiation fibrosis or malignant disease.

The functional bladder capacity is the volume the individual voids. Under normal conditions the bladder empties completely. Failure to do so is related to an obstructed outflow tract, detrusor failure or inefficient voiding due to detrusor instability.

The cystometric bladder capacity is the maximum volume held in comfort during cystometry and hence is related to bladder compliance and sensation. Its relation to functional capacity is a matter of debate. J. George and K. F. Lewis (personal communication, 1978) considered that cystometry underestimated the functional capacity by about 40%. However, in a study of 200 ambulatory incontinent women, Diokno et al. (1987) concluded that there was a significant positive correlation between the cystometric capacity and the largest voided volume recorded by the patient.

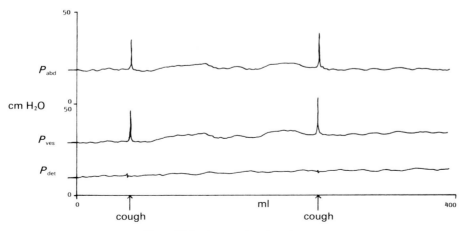

Figure 33.1 A normal cystometrogram

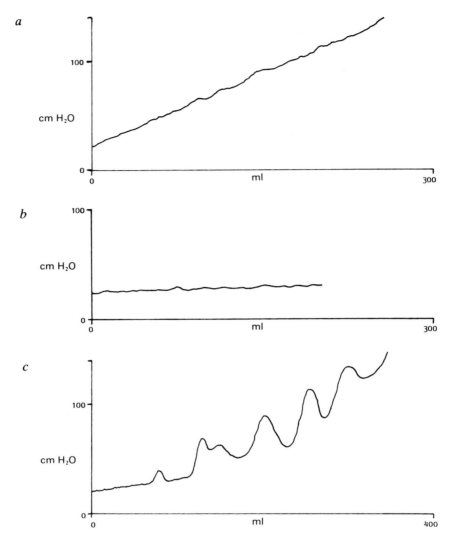

Figure 33.2 Cystometrograms showing low compliance (*a*), hypersensitivity (*b*) and detrusor instability (*c*)

Bladder compliance is normally high: an increase in the volume of the bladder is associated with minimal change in intravesical pressure (compliance = change in volume ÷ change in pressure). The elastic and viscoelastic properties of the bladder wall allow the expansion on filling to occur at low pressure. Factors influencing those properties such as detrusor hypertrophy or fibrosis will reduce the compliance. Increased sensitivity of the bladder will also influence the capacity; some patients experience a strong desire to void on filling to 50–150 ml and these are termed hypersensitive bladders.

The bladder does not normally contract during filling; the term 'detrusor instability' is applied to the condition wherein the bladder is shown to contract spontaneously or on provocation while the patient is attempting to inhibit micturition (Figure 33.2). It has been estimated that about 15% of the population experience detrusor instability associated with no overt neurological abnormality. The term 'detrusor hyperreflexia' is applied in those cases where there is a demonstrable neurological abnormality.

Urethral pressure

The sphincter active zone of the urethra lies between the bladder neck and the pelvic floor muscle. Radiological studies show that the bladder neck or proximal sphincter mechanism normally, but not invariably, remains closed throughout filling, even on coughing and straining, despite sudden rises in intravesical pressure. The site of the maximum urethral pressure lies at the level of the external urethral sphincter muscle and pelvic floor, together constituting the distal sphincter mechanism (Figure 33.3). Gosling (1979) has described the complex arrangement of the striated musculature at this level with its intramural and peri-urethral components. The intra-

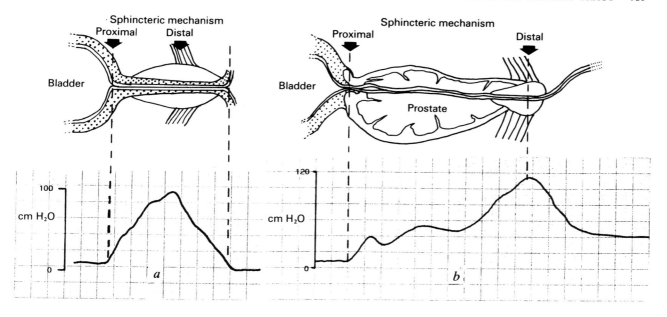

Figure 33.3   Static urethral pressure profiles in the female (*a*) and male (*b*)

mural muscle appears to be unique, consisting only of slow-twitch fibres without muscle spindles and supplied by pelvic parasympathetic nerves. The peri-urethral component is derived from the pubococcygeus part of the pelvic floor muscle and consists of a mixture of fast- and slow-twitch fibres, with associated muscle spindles. Nerve supply is by the pudendal nerve.

The maximum urethral pressure at the level of the distal sphincter mechanism can be raised by voluntary contraction of the muscle. The intramural muscle is considered to maintain long-term occlusion of the urethra without fatigue, while the peri-urethral component responds to a sudden rise in intra-abdominal pressure by a rapid contraction.

In men, the maximum urethral pressure shows minimal variation with age, being of the order of 70–80 cmH$_2$O. In women, there is a steady reduction with age from about 80 cmH$_2$O in the 20s to 65 cmH$_2$O in those over 65.

The stress urethral pressure profile

Enhorning (1961) confirmed that the proximal urethra above the pelvic floor is subject to the same variations in pressure as any other abdominal viscus. A stress urethral pressure profile is performed by asking the subject to cough during the recording of a static urethral pressure profile as the catheter is withdrawn along the urethra. In normal subjects the closure pressures on coughing should show a positive response (Figure 33.4a). Negative closure pressures on coughing are associated with genuine stress incontinence (Figure 33.4b).

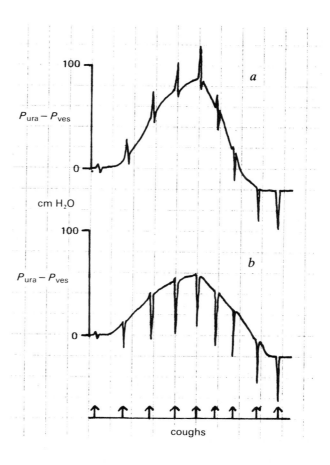

Figure 33.4   Stress urethral profiles. *a*, Maintenance of positive closure pressure. *b*, Negative closure pressure on coughing

Urinary incontinence

Urinary incontinence has been defined by the ICS as the involuntary loss of urine causing a social or hygienic problem and is objectively demonstrable. Incontinence occurs when intravesical pressure rises above urethral pressure unless the loss is through some channel other than the urethra (extra-urethral incontinence, e.g. fistula or ectopic ureter).

Stress incontinence describes a symptom, a sign and a condition. The symptom is the patient's report of involuntary loss of urine when exercising physically or coughing. The sign denotes the observation of involuntary urine leakage when intravesical pressure exceeds maximum urethral pressure in the absence of detrusor activity. The condition, termed genuine stress incontinence (GSI), applies when the above has been demonstrated urodynamically.

Urge incontinence is involuntary loss of urine associated with a strong desire to void. It may be subdivided into motor urge incontinence which is associated with uninhibited detrusor contractions and sensory urge incontinence where no such contractions occur.

Reflex incontinence refers to the loss of urine due to abnormal reflex activity in the spinal cord, in the absence of the sensation usually associated with the desire to micturate.

Overflow incontinence occurs when the intravesical pressure exceeds the urethral pressure due to passive elevation associated with bladder distension.

The voiding phase

Synchronous videocystometry and EMG recording of the pelvic floor muscle has demonstrated the sequence of events that initiate voiding. In the majority of cases there is an initial decrease in the maximum urethral pressure at the level of the pelvic floor, with a reduction in EMG activity and descent of the bladder base. There follows a rise in detrusor pressure from active detrusor contraction, opening of the bladder neck and a complete cessation of EMG activity. Urine flow commences and the raised detrusor pressure is sustained until bladder emptying is complete. Thereafter the urethral pressure rises and the detrusor pressure falls simultaneously to a low level.

The normal urinary flow trace shows a rapid rise to peak value within 5 s of the commencement of voiding (Figure 33.5). The flow rate is related to the sex and age of the individual and to the volume voided. Women tend to void at a faster rate than men, with a mean flow of 25–30 ml/s and with a lower detrusor pressure of 50 cmH$_2$O or less. Some women void by relaxation of the urethral sphincter or by increasing abdominal pressure with minimal evidence of detrusor contraction.

In men, the urine flow rate shows greater variation with age owing to prostatic hypertrophy. Men under 45 void at rates of around 20–25 ml/s. This decreases to 10–15 ml/s in men over 65.

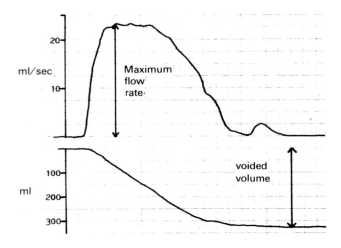

Figure 33.5 A normal flow trace

Voiding detrusor pressures in men are normally of the order of 70–80 cmH$_2$O. Measurement of the detrusor pressure does not necessarily correspond to the strength of the detrusor contraction; in the presence of a large bladder diverticulum or gross ureteric reflux, the interpretation of the detrusor pressure can be misleading.

The strength of detrusor contraction and voluntary sphincter control can be estimated by asking the patient to stop voiding suddenly during micturition. Contraction of the distal sphincter mechanism is followed by an isometric rise in detrusor pressure (P_{det} iso) and the fluid remaining in the proximal urethra is milked back into the bladder.

Outflow obstruction

In voiding studies, the flow rate and the detrusor pressure are the two critical factors. A reduced urine flow rate and a raised detrusor pressure (above 100 cmH$_2$O in the male) are indicative of obstruction (Figure 33.6). The shape of the flow curve is as important as the recorded values. A plateau may indicate a urethral stricture. Fluctuating or interrupted flow may be due to an unsustained detrusor contraction associated with outflow obstruction or neuropathy. Both storage and voiding disorders may be complex in the neuropathic bladder. Detrusor–bladder neck or detrusor–sphincter dyssynergia are more precisely defined by video studies.

Applications and controversies in clinical practice

History and examination

Analysis of lower urinary tract symptoms has been influenced by the results of urodynamic studies. Fre-

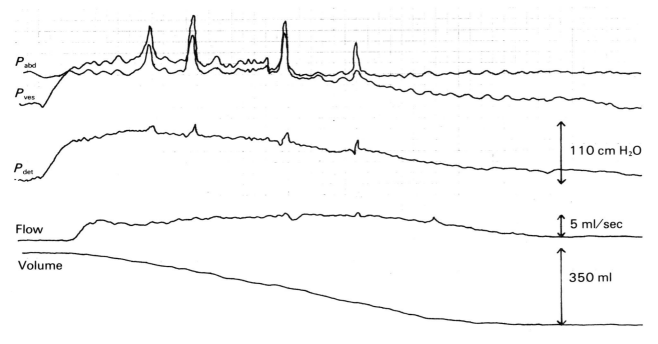

P_{abd}

P_{ves}

P_{det}

110 cm H₂O

Flow

5 ml/sec

Volume

350 ml

Figure 33.6 An obstructed cystometrogram

quency, urgency and nocturia are considered irritative symptoms, associated with an unstable bladder, whereas hesitancy and a poor stream suggest obstructed micturition. The term 'prostatism' is misleading both to the clinician and the patient and should be avoided. However, the possibility of underlying pathology should not be forgotten in the search for a label for the functional disorder. A full history and examination, including the neurology of the lower limbs and perineum, is mandatory and haematuria and infection investigated fully. Bladder tumours and cystitis may mimic detrusor instability or hypersensitivity, obstruction may be due to a malignant prostate and a voiding disorder may be the first symptom of a condition such as multiple sclerosis.

On the other hand, neither are symptoms and signs alone a sufficient guide in incontinence. Clinically GSI can be indistinguishable from provoked instability and is often accompanied by frequency and urgency. The former may be 'preventive' and the latter provoked by the presence of urine in the proximal urethra.

Frequency and volume chart

Such a chart recorded by the patient provides an invaluable supplement to the history. The time and volume of each void over a 5–7-day period is noted.

The frequency of micturition is related to the capacity of the bladder and to the rate of urine production. The maximum functional bladder capacity varies from 350 to 600 ml and the normal output from 1200 to 1800 ml per 24 h. In a normal healthy population the frequency of voiding ranges from 4 to 8 times a day; 10–15% regularly pass urine once at night.

A well-kept chart identifies the following: maximum functional bladder capacity; average functional bladder capacity; total urine output, by day and night; patient motivation.

A functional bladder capacity consistently less than 200 ml may be indicative of a hypersensitive bladder, but a cystoscopy is essential to exclude local pathology.

Widely variable volumes, e.g. from 50 to 450 ml, suggest an unstable detrusor. Nocturia may be caused by reversal of the diurnal rhythm; some elderly produce more urine at night than by day. Nocturnal polyuria may occur in some enuretics. There is rarely a place for urodynamics in enuretic children. Those with daytime frequency and urgency may be assumed to have instability. Those without may be treated with synthetic antidiuretic hormone, e.g. desmopressin, at night.

Urine flow rate

This is the simplest urodynamic investigation, but consideration needs to be given to the manner in which the test is conducted. If the volume voided is less than 150 ml, the measurement is unreliable. Thus it is not satisfactory to perform a single flow at the patient's first attendance at clinic after the routine mid-stream specimen of urine has been collected. The patient should be asked to arrive for the test with a reasonably full bladder and two further flows performed in a comfortable, private environment. The urine flow/residual study provides an indication of outflow tract obstruction, although the correlation between flow rate and the diagnosis of obstruction has been questioned (Neal *et al.*, 1987). It may be more indicative of detrusor decompensation.

Voiding difficulty in the female is a rare problem and should be investigated by pressure-flow cystometry (Massey and Abrams, 1988).

Cystometry

Cystometry is essential to differentiate the stable from the unstable bladder, particularly when assessing women with mixed symptoms of stress and urge. Obstruction, detrusor instability or underactivity can adversely affect the outcome of surgery for GSI. Since most operative procedures for the condition are to some degree obstructive, it is helpful to have some idea of the detrusor power, if only to warn the patient that self-catheterization may be required postoperatively. This is the value of the 'stop test'. Problems arise in those women who are only able to interrupt micturition by inhibiting the detrusor contraction. An alternative that has achieved varying degrees of success is to attempt to have the patient void through a catheter and then occlude the catheter.

Cystometry is indicated in men when the screening investigations are inconclusive. Not infrequently men present with both irritative and obstructive symptoms; if they are passing only small volumes of urine, it is not possible to assess the obstructive element on flow rate alone.

It has been mentioned that instability may occur only on provocation. The test should, therefore, incorporate change of posture, movement, coughing, straining and running water. Some immerse the hands in cold water.

Full details of the above should be recorded in the report along with all other parameters such as the filling rate. Some practitioners consider that fast filling is essential to uncover all cases of instability; others feel a slow fill rate is more physiological. The majority compromise on a medium fill of 50–60 ml/min, except in neuropathic disorders when a very slow infusion without prior removal of any residual is important in order to approximate the 'normal' functional parameters of the disordered vesico-urethral activity. This may have repercussions on retention pressure, reflux and suitability for insertion of artificial sphincters. Of course, if self-catheterization is an option, the residual should be drained.

Synchronous video-urodynamics

The additional information provided by video-urodynamics is invaluable in the neuropathic bladder, providing evidence of detrusor–bladder neck or detrusor–sphincter dyssynergia, and the presence of diverticula and vesico-ureteric reflux. It is also worth considering in children when the need arises; reflux has been demonstrated in some children as a result of dysfunctional voiding – the 'voluntary' interruption of urine flow during micturition. Biofeedback techniques using urodynamic parameters may be employed in this and several other problems, including detrusor instability.

Any complicated case such as incontinence after prostatic surgery, or persisting following gynaecological procedures, will benefit from the enhanced information obtainable by video-urodynamics.

Urethral profilometry

Static or stress urethral profilometry are additional confirmatory tests for those patients in whom the diagnosis of stress incontinence is in any doubt. On their own, there is such a wide variation in normal parameters such as the MUCP or even the shape of the profile, that they are inadequate criteria. The stress profile has been criticized on the grounds that the urethra may be moving considerably on coughing, in relation to the catheter, so that one is not measuring where one thinks. In addition, many women can be shown to have an incompetent bladder neck on coughing or straining, yet remain dry; in a study of 98 climacteric women, Versi *et al.* (1986) demonstrated such incompetence on coughing in 50.

Ambulatory urodynamics

With miniaturization and the use of telemetric techniques it has become possible to perform bladder pressure studies in the ambulatory patient within their normal environment. Despite still being in some degree invasive, this is the nearest approach to physiological normality that we can achieve. Events in the bladder can be correlated with episodes of urgency, incontinence and voiding as noted by the patient in their daily round. As yet the complications and cost involved preclude their regular employment, but care in the performance and interpretation of routine studies leave few undefined problems.

Summary

Urodynamic studies should be a routine part of the structured investigation of patients with lower urinary tract symptoms. The initial protocol should identify those patients with significant uropathology, invariably requiring urographic and endoscopic procedures. Whereas formerly the diagnosis and treatment of disorders lacking such evidence was largely empirical, urodynamic studies have provided a scientific basis for diagnosis, management, the evaluation of response to treatment, and even the design of operative procedures.

References

Abrams, P., Blaivas, J. and Stanton, S. L. (1988) Standardisation of terminology of lower urinary tract function. *Scand. J. Urol. Nephrol.* (Suppl.), **114**, 5–19

Abrams, P. H. and Feneley, R. C. L. (1978) The significance of the symptoms associated with bladder outflow obstruction. *Urol. Int.*, **33**, 171

Diokno, A. C., Wells, T. J. and Brink, C. A. (1987) Comparison of self-reported voided volume with cystometric bladder capacity. *J. Urol.*, **137**, 698–700

Enhorning, G. (1961) Simultaneous recording of intravesical and intraurethral pressure. *Acta Chir. Scand.* (Suppl.), **276**, 1–68

Gallagher, D. J., Montgomerie, J. L. and North, J. D. K. (1965) Acute infections of the urinary tract and the urethral syndrome in general practice. *Br. Med. J.*, **i**, 622–626

Gosling, J. A. (1979) The structure of the bladder and urethra in relation to function. *Urol. Clin. North Am.*, **6**, 31–38

Massey, J. A. and Abrams, P. H. (1988) Obstructed voiding in the female. *Br. J. Urol.*, **61**, 36–39

Neal, D. E., Styles, R. A., Ng, T. *et al.* (1987) Relationship between voiding pressures, symptoms and urodynamic findings in 253 men undergoing prostatectomy. *Br. J. Urol.*, **60**, 554–559

Versi, E., Cardozo, L. D., Studd, J. W. *et al.* (1986) Internal urinary sphincter in maintenance of female continence. *Br. Med. J.*, **292**, 166–167

Further reading

Abrams, P., Feneley, R. and Torrens, M. (1983) *Urodynamics: Clinical Practice in Urology*, Springer-Verlag, Berlin

Mundy, A. R., Stephenson, T. P. and Wein, A. J. (1984) *Urodynamics: Principles, Practice and Application*, Churchill Livingstone, Edinburgh

Turner-Warwick, R. and Whiteside, C. G. (1979) *The Urologic Clinics of North America*, Vol. 6, part 1, W. B. Saunders, Philadelphia

34

The bladder and prostate

C. G. Fowler

Introduction

The development of endoscopic surgery of the bladder and the prostate and the need for special skills to perform it safely were the main stimuli for the separation of urology as a distinct speciality. By the 1990s the range of urological endoscopy has increased with advances in ureteroscopy and nephroscopy, but endoscopic surgery of the lower urinary tract (Figure 34.1) remains at the heart of urological practice. Open operations on the bladder and prostate are now comparatively rare and largely confined to radical surgery for cancer and relatively major procedures to reconstruct or replace the bladder. These are operations which even a fully-trained urologist can find taxing and there are relatively few of the less complex procedures on which the beginner might expect to cut his or her teeth. Becoming a urologist is therefore a challenge, but a worthwhile one.

Endoscopic surgery uses skills which are not necessarily those that come easily to a good open surgeon. While most able surgical trainees can be taught to perform safe transurethral surgery, there is no doubt that some are naturally more endoscopically adept than others. In any case, it takes time to become a good endoscopic surgeon. The ideal trainee is patient, able to think in three dimensions and willing to stop and ask advice when, as is inevitable, he or she becomes lost or confused. There is no substitute for hands-on experience because although the most common endoscopic abnormalities are soon recognized, the variety of possible appearances is such that surprises and puzzles in the lower urinary tract are quite common. In particular, there is a shadowy area between the normal and abnormal where only a biopsy will give the answer. The surgeon must have sufficient awareness of the possibilities to be suspicious and this can only come by accumulating a large experience of normal cystourethroscopy.

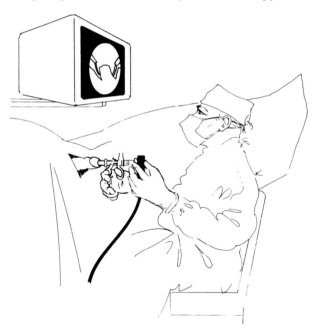

Figure 34.2 Modern endoscopic television and videoresection

It has become much easier to teach and learn endoscopic surgery because of the miniaturization of television cameras which can now be attached directly

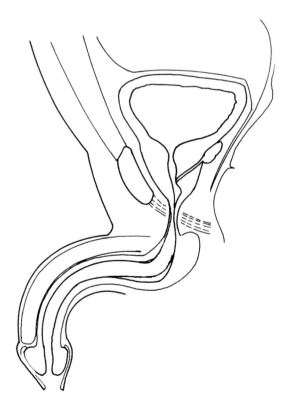

Figure 34.1 General anatomy of the lower urinary tract

to the eyepiece of an endoscope and are so small and light that they do not inconvenience the operator (Figure 34.2). This allows the trainee to learn by watching others operate and also permits proper supervision of his or her own work. This is a great improvement over the older teaching attachments which were much more cumbersome to use.

Catheterization

Catheterization of the bladder is the most common instrumentation of the lower urinary tract, often performed by a junior member of the medical team. Short-term drainage of the bladder by Foley balloon catheter may be needed in acute or chronic retention of urine, to monitor urine output in the critically ill or to keep the bladder empty during pelvic surgery. A three-way Foley catheter is commonly used after surgery to the bladder and prostate; the third channel allows irrigation to wash blood away before it can clot. Intermittent catheterization using a simple Nelaton catheter is used to administer drugs intravesically and to drain the bladder in some patients with a neurological cause for failure of bladder emptying. Such patients may often be taught to catheterize themselves, and clean intermittent self-catheterization (CISC) can help them to avoid the many potential complications of long-term catheterization. Indeed, permanent catheterization is best regarded as a last resort to be recommended with reluctance.

Method

Urethral catheterization is performed under aseptic conditions, usually with the patient in a comfortable supine position with hips slightly abducted. Unless the patient is already unconscious, the urethra must be lubricated and anaesthetized by a gel containing 1% or 2% lignocaine. Local anaesthetic takes at least 5 minutes to work and there is a danger that impatience will lead the busy doctor waiting beside the patient to start catheterization before this time has elapsed. Fifteen ml of local anaesthetic gel is gently instilled into the external meatus and massaged towards the sphincter by firmly stroking the ventral surface of the penis. An able-bodied man can then be asked to hold the glans penis between finger and thumb to stop the gel escaping during the time it takes for the anaesthetic to take effect, thus avoiding the use of an uncomfortable penile clamp. The female urethra, though shorter and less tortuous than the male, is just as sensitive and should always be anaesthetized with lignocaine gel before instrumentation.

While the anaesthetic is taking effect there is time to open a catheterization pack and choose the catheter (Figure 34.3). If it is to remain in place for more than a few days, a less irritant but more expensive Silastic catheter should be used. Large catheters tend to block

the para-urethral glands and cause urethral damage by pressure necrosis. Very small calibre catheters can easily become blocked by debris and are difficult to insert. For most purposes a middle-sized tube of 14 or 16 Charrière is about right.

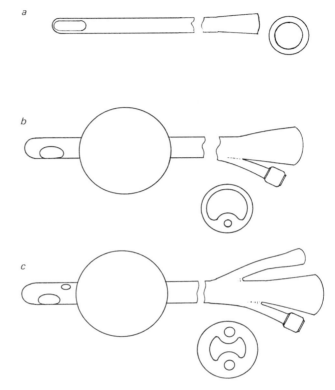

Figure 34.3 Three commonly-used catheters: *a*, Nelaton. *b*, Two-way Foley. *c*, Three-way Foley

Urethral catheterization in the male

When the local anaesthetic has taken effect the genitals are swabbed with aqueous chlorhexidine and the area draped by a single sheet with a central hole through which the penis protrudes. As with all procedures performed under local anaesthesia, the cooperation of the patient can make the difference between success and failure. In urethral catheterization, relaxation, particularly of the sphincter muscle, is important and reassurance throughout the insertion will help to achieve this.

While holding the glans penis between gloved finger and thumb, the penis is lifted until it is vertical. In this position the penile urethra is straightened and the catheter can be inserted into the external urethral meatus and passed smoothly towards the urethral sphincter. The sphincter presents an obstruction to the further passage of the catheter and there is a danger that a ham-fisted attempt to negotiate it will cause reflex spasm. Before trying to pass the sphincter, the penis should be pulled caudally between the man's legs until its axis is horizontal. This brings the catheter more in line with the prostatic urethra. If the patient is then asked to attempt to void, the sphincter should relax and by gentle but firm pressure, the catheter will advance into the bladder.

The balloon of a Foley catheter should not be inflated until a flow of urine confirms that the catheter is within the bladder lumen. Sometimes the catheter may be blocked by gel during insertion and will need to be cleared by gentle irrigation with sterile water from a bladder syringe. Inflation of the balloon within the urethra will cause pain and damage and if there is doubt the catheter should be withdrawn and reinserted.

Urethral catheterization in women

Because the female urethra is straight and short, catheterization in women is usually relatively easy. With the patient lying with knees flexed and hips in moderate abduction and flexion, the labia are parted by the operator's gloved finger and thumb. This exposes the external urethral meatus which is guarded by a frill of soft tissue and lies between the clitoris anteriorly and the vagina behind.

In some women the urethral meatus is difficult to identify because of senile atrophy or surgical scarring of the vulva, urethral prolapse, or because extreme obesity makes it impossible to get a good view. In these women and in those whose urethral meatus lies further back almost in the anterior wall of the vagina, it can help to catheterize them from behind as they lie in the left lateral position or to have them in the lithotomy position.

Complications

Closed catheter drainage

The commonest complication of urinary catheterization is ascending infection which is almost inevitable if the catheter is indwelling for more than a day or so. This is particularly undesirable in hospital where resistant organisms are rife. The development of such infection is delayed and may be prevented by the use of a closed system of drainage. The catheter is connected via a non-return valve to a plastic drainage bag immediately after insertion and the closed system is routinely opened only to drain the bag by a tap set in its dependent lower edge. If debris accumulates in the tubing it can usually be cleared by using a roller device to massage the tube. If there is reason to open the system to clear a catheter blockage or wash out the bladder, this is done under strict aseptic conditions.

CATHETER CARE

The presence of the catheter in the urethra leads to irritation and there is often a mucoid discharge even if there is no infection. Strapping the catheter to the thigh may help to minimize the physical trauma to the meatus, reducing the risk of later stenosis. Gentle swabbing with normal saline to remove accumulated discharge is soothing and may perhaps delay the onset of infection. A good flow of urine is desirable and should be promoted by encouraging fluid intake.

Trouble-shooting

Failure to pass a catheter beyond the penile urethra in a man may be due to the presence of a urethral stricture. If a stricture is present, further attempts to advance the catheter will lead to the development of a false passage which will inevitably make the stricture very much worse. The appearance of blood at the external urethral meatus during catheterization suggests that there is trauma, possibly due to a stricture. If it is not possible to deal with the stricture by dilatation or urethrotomy, the attempt at urethral catheterization should be abandoned and a suprapubic tube inserted instead.

More commonly, the passage of the catheter is obstructed within the prostatic urethra. If this happens, it often helps to use a larger, slightly stiffer catheter which will prise apart the fleshy lobes of adenoma where they meet in the midline. The more rounded tip of a larger catheter is less likely to make a false passage. An experienced urologist may choose to stiffen the catheter even further by using a catheter introducer, but the danger of trauma to the urethra is such that this device should not be used by a trainee. In no circumstances should excessive force be used and if urethral catheterization fails, it is almost always safest to proceed to suprapubic puncture.

Bladder spasms and bypassing can be caused by blockage of the catheter, but are usually due to uncontrolled contractions of the bladder detrusor caused by irritation by the balloon. Certainly, it is useless to put in a larger catheter. Instead, the volume of fluid in the balloon should be reduced and it may be worth trying anticholinergic drugs. Some neurological patients in whom the bladder spasms are sufficient to extrude the catheter, balloon and all, should be considered for suprapubic catheterization.

SUPRAPUBIC CATHETERIZATION

Suprapubic catheterization (Figure 34.4) is indicated when the bladder must be drained and urethral catheterization is undesirable. If, as is usual, this is to be a temporary measure, a fine-gauge (10–12 Charrière) catheter can be inserted percutaneously. For long-term suprapubic diversion, a formal operative suprapubic cystostomy will allow a larger catheter to be inserted. In either case, it is essential that the bladder should be full at the start of the procedure and this may have to be checked by ultrasound scanning. Special care is needed when there is a previous lower

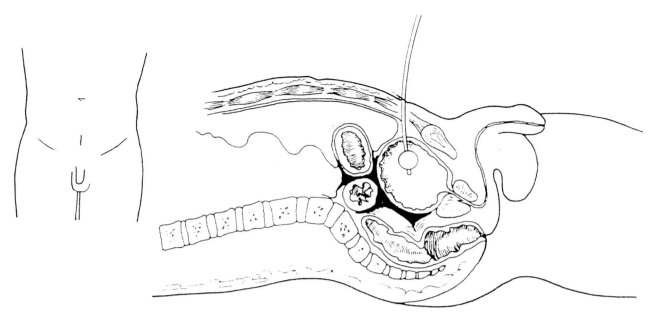

Figure 34.4 Suprapubic cystotomy and bladder drainage. It is important that the bladder is distended preoperatively

abdominal incision which may have caused a loop of bowel to become fixed to the bladder dome.

PERCUTANEOUS SUPRAPUBIC CATHETERIZATION

With the patient supine, the pubic hair is shaved in the midline to expose a point 1 cm above the symphysis pubis where the catheter is to be inserted. After appropriate skin disinfection and draping, the puncture site is infiltrated with 1% or 2% lignocaine with or without adrenaline, in the usual manner, with a series of needles of increasing length to infiltrate the deeper layers of the anterior abdominal wall. When the largest needle passes through the linea alba, a distinct 'give' will be felt as the needle reaches the soft tissues beyond. Aspiration of urine will confirm that the bladder is full enough for puncture.

Some suprapubic catheters are threaded on a spiked central introducer. Others are introduced through the lumen of a tubular trocar. When the anaesthetic has taken effect, a tiny incision in the skin is necessary to allow the catheter and its trocar to be inserted into the subcutaneous layers. The line of insertion is directly downwards at right angles to the bed. To get the catheter through the linea alba often takes a surprising amount of force and there is a real danger of skewering the patient when the tip of the trocar eventually gets through into the bladder. With proper care, the catheter enters the bladder under control and when it does so urine comes out under pressure. The tube can then be advanced beyond the end of the trocar. Whether the catheter has a balloon or a pigtail arrangement to keep it in the bladder, it is worth securing it to the skin with a suture.

FORMAL OPERATIVE SUPRAPUBIC CYSTOTOMY

This simple procedure can be performed under general, regional or local anaesthesia. A small midline or 'mini' Pfannenstiel incision about 4 cm long is used to expose the bladder. The bladder wall is opened between catgut stay sutures, and a suitable self-retaining catheter (usually a large Foley) is inserted.

Retained balloon catheter

Occasionally, the balloon of a Foley catheter fails to deflate when the time comes to remove it. Cutting the catheter across and advancing a fine-wire stilette (from a ureteric catheter) down the balloon channel usually lets the fluid out. If this fails, the balloon can be burst by suprapubic puncture using a spinal needle under ultrasound control. If the balloon has burst, a cystoscopy is necessary to check for bits of rubber left in the bladder. Misguided instillation of ether or an attempt to burst the balloon by over-inflating it are likely to end in disaster.

Endoscopic instruments

Both rigid rod-lens instruments and flexible fibrescopes have a place in the endoscopy of the lower urinary tract. The flexible cystoscope with its granular image and relatively limited operative potential is predominantly an instrument to inspect the urethra and bladder. Its ability to adapt to the sigmoid anatomy of the male urethra makes it easy and painless to pass under topical urethral anaesthesia. It is the ideal instrument to rule out bladder pathology.

By contrast, the more established rigid rod-lens instruments give a view of the lower urinary tract of unparalleled clarity. They tend to be passed with the patient under general or spinal anaesthesia, allowing the use of diathermy to cut, coagulate and resect lesions.

Flexible cystoscopy

The flexible cystoscope is passed with the patient lying supine, the urethra prepared with topical lignocaine anaesthesia and the genitals disinfected and draped as for urethral catheterization (Figure 34.5). Indeed, flexible cystoscopy can be performed anywhere appropriate for urethral catheterization, making it suitable for use in the outpatient clinic. The fibrescope is too delicate to be sterilized by low-pressure steam and has to be disinfected by immersion in activated 2% glutaraldehyde or its equivalent. Before the examination starts, the chemical must be rinsed from the surface of the instrument and flushed from the irrigation channel with sterile water.

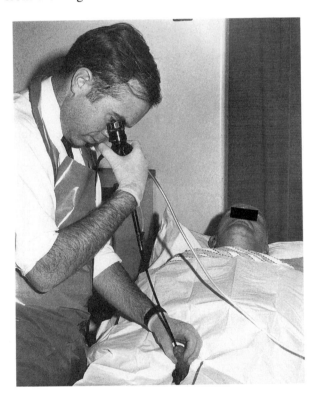

Figure 34.5 Flexible fibreoptic cystourethroscopy

The patient voids urine before flexible cystoscopy starts. In a man, the examination begins with an inspection of the urethra. With sterile water or saline running through the irrigation channel, the tip of the flexible cystoscope is inserted into the urethral meatus and passed under vision to the urethral sphincter.

The patient is fully conscious and so a continuous explanatory commentary is maintained throughout. When the objective of the fibrescope is touching the sphincter, the man tries to void, the sphincter relaxes and the fibrescope enters the prostatic urethra and thence the bladder. In a female patient, the flexible cystoscope is introduced just as if it were a urethral catheter. However, once the instrument is inserted, the hips can be fully extended and adducted so that the woman lies in a completely decorous supine position for the examination.

Flexible endoscopy of the bladder itself proceeds according to a routine, so that no part of the urothelium is missed. With the objective at the bladder neck, the wide angle of the lens gives a panoramic view of the interior of the bladder which often reveals any abnormalities which are present. The trigone is examined and one ureteric orifice is sought to give orientation. The urothelium is then systematically scanned by rotating the instrument and flexing its angulating tip by means of the thumb lever until the other orifice comes into view. Finally, the whole length of the insertion tube is passed into the bladder so that it is deflected from the bladder wall opposite. This allows an antegrade view of the bladder neck region which completes the examination. The instrument is removed and the patient asked to void the small volume of irrigation fluid which has been instilled into the bladder to clear the view.

The operative potential of the flexible cystoscope is limited by the narrow instrumentation channel and the requirement that any intervention should be painless or nearly so. Urothelial biopsies can be taken using flexible cup biopsy forceps, the ureteric orifices can be cannulated and small bladder tumours can be coagulated with the Nd YAG laser. Flexible cystoscopy is indicated as a means of screening the bladder when the presence of a lesion requiring surgery is relatively unlikely and when a full bimanual pelvic examination is not needed. For more extensive endoscopic procedures, it is necessary to use rigid instruments.

Rigid cystoscopy

Although rigid endoscopy under topical urethral anaesthesia is possible, it is somewhat uncomfortable for the male patient and has become redundant since the development of flexible cystoscopy. The procedure will usually be performed under general or spinal anaesthesia in an operating theatre with full aseptic precautions. With the patient lying in a modified lithotomy position with the lower limbs supported in stirrups, the examination in a man begins with an inspection of the urethra (Figure 34.6).

The standard cystourethroscope is a tubular metal sheath with a series of interchangeable rod-lens telescopes which fit within it. For urethroscopy a straight ahead (0°) or fore-oblique (12° or 30°) optic is used. The penis is drawn upward as the instrument is inserted and a clear view is obtained by instilling sterile irrigating fluid to distend the urethra as the endoscope is advanced. Urethral pathology may be assessed and dealt with appropriately. When the instrument has negotiated the angle at the peno-scrotal junction, the outer end of the cystoscope is

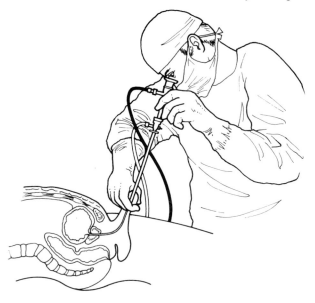

Figure 34.6 Rigid urethrocystoscopy with a rod-lens telescope

gently depressed between the patient's thighs so that its axis is aligned with that of the prostatic urethra. The objective can then be advanced into the bladder. Routine antegrade endoscopy of the female urethra is unrewarding and the cystoscope sheath is usually inserted 'blindly' with an obturator in place.

Once inside the bladder, it is sometimes possible to make a full inspection with the fore-oblique telescope. If necessary, however, it can be replaced with a 70° optic which makes it easier to examine the region of the bladder neck. The object is to examine the whole internal surface of the lower urinary tract in a systematic manner. The ureteric orifices should be found and inspected, an apparently simple task which sometimes eludes even an experienced endoscopist. The shape of the orifice is very variable and it should be stressed again that the student endoscopist should seize every opportunity to experience the range of normality of lower tract anatomy. By advancing and withdrawing the cystoscope and steadily rotating it through 360°, the whole of the urothelium is scanned for evidence of abnormality (Figures 34.7 and 34.8). Inflammation is characterized by redness, increased vascularity, cystic changes or bleeding on distension. The presence of tumour, stone or foreign body is obviously a major discovery, while the trabeculation of the detrusor muscle and bladder saccules or diverticula give useful evidence of bladder outflow obstruction. The examination is completed with a careful

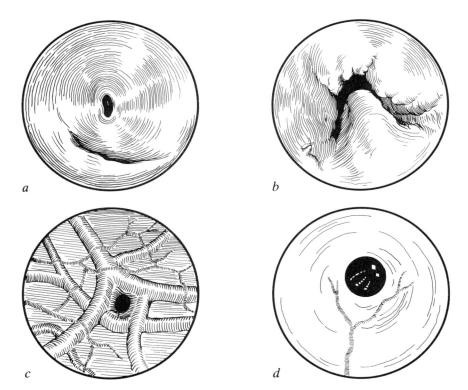

a *b*

c *d*

Figure 34.7 Typical endoscopic appearances. *a*, Urethral stricture. *b*, Veru montanum. *c*, Trabeculation with mouth of small diverticulum. *d*, Air bubble in bladder dome

inspection of the anterior wall and bladder neck region and, in a man, the prostate. A 120° lens is available to examine this part of the bladder but is rarely used.

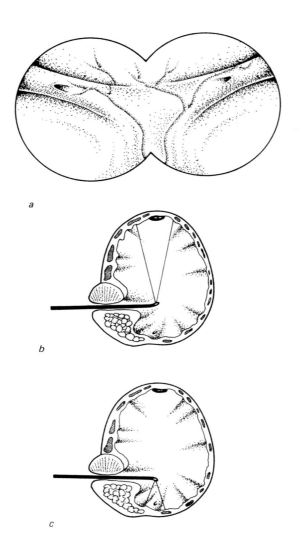

Figure 34.8 Rigid rod-lens cystoscopy. *a*, Typical appearance of trigone with ureteric orifices. *b*, Air bubble in bladder dome located with 70° optic. *c*, 70° optic rotated through 180° to locate the trigone

Retrograde ureterography

With the high quality of intravenous urography and the range of more modern imaging now available, retrograde ureterography is rarely necessary simply to visualize the upper urinary tract. The study can if necessary be performed under urethral anaesthesia with the flexible cystoscope. More commonly, ureterography is a prelude to ureteroscopy, ureteric stone manipulation or the insertion of self-retaining ureteric stents. With a catheterizing cystoscope, a ureteric catheter can be guided into a ureteric orifice using an Albarran deflecting lever. A Chevassu catheter has an expanded end which can be lodged in the orifice, while many urologists prefer to use a straight-tipped catheter to cannulate the ureter (Figure 34.9). A retrograde ureterogram is performed by injecting liquid contrast medium via a ureteric catheter, taking care not to cause extravasation by overdistending the system. Radiographs are most conveniently taken by image intensifier, but if this is not available, the ureteric catheter can be secured by tying it to a urethral catheter while the patient is moved to the radiology department.

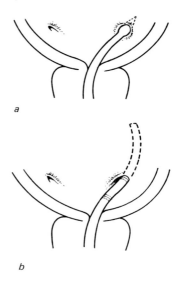

Figure 34.9 Retrograde ureterography. *a*, Chevassu catheter lodged in ureteric orifice. *b*, Straight catheter passed up ureter

The most common indications for cystourethroscopy are the investigation of haematuria and the follow-up of patients with a history of bladder cancer. All instrumentation of the urinary tract runs the risk of inadvertent trauma and urinary infection and should be avoided where possible. The appreciable morbidity along with the relative unpleasantness of even fibreoptic cystoscopy should limit the number of patients who are endoscoped for irritative or obstructive symptoms in which positive findings are rare or difficult to interpret.

Bladder tumours

Nearly all bladder tumours are transitional cell carcinomas of varying malignancy and truly benign papillomas are rare. Squamous cell carcinoma may occur in areas of squamous metaplasia associated with bladder stone or Bilharzia and adenocarcinoma may arise from a urachal remnant or secondary spread. Bladder cancer has a male predominance of 3:1 and usually presents after the age of 40. However, it may

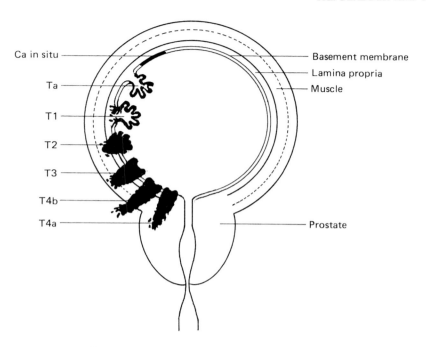

Figure 34.10 Staging bladder cancer

occur at a much earlier age and there are well-documented examples in teenagers. Cytological screening of workers exposed to carcinogenic industrial chemicals such as beta-naphthylamine, auramine and magenta yields an incidence of up to 20 times that of the general population. Most patients with bladder tumours have no history of industrial exposure, but most of them smoke.

Carcinoma of the bladder usually presents with haematuria and this may be the only indication that a tumour is present. The symptoms of cystitis are less common. Assessment includes examination of the urine to confirm the presence of red blood cells and to detect infection. Papanicolaou staining of the urinary sediment may reveal clusters of malignant cells: urine cytology is most likely to be positive when the tumour is poorly differentiated. Imaging of the upper urinary tract by ultrasound scanning or more often by intravenous urography will demonstrate alternative causes for haematuria such as upper tract tumours or stones and will show the ureteric dilatation which is associated with malignant infiltration of a ureteric orifice. Larger bladder tumours (diameter greater than 1 cm) will show up on ultrasound or appear as a filling defect on the bladder films of the urogram. When the tumour fails to declare itself on imaging or by positive urinary cytology, it may become apparent on flexible cystoscopy under local anaesthesia.

Carcinoma of the bladder is classified and treated according to its histological grade and clinical stage. Whatever means are used to identify the presence of tumour, confirmation of the diagnosis and assessment need a full staging cystoscopy, biopsy and bimanual pelvic examination under anaesthesia.

Management of carcinoma of the bladder

Transitional cell bladder tumours range in biological activity from the rare and truly benign papilloma to very aggressive anaplastic tumours of high malignancy. The staging cystoscopy is essential to obtain representative biopsies to assess the histological grade of the tumour (G1 – well differentiated to G3 – poorly differentiated) and to stage the tumour according to the depth to which it has infiltrated the bladder wall (Figure 34.10).

Well-differentiated superficial tumour

Superficial tumours (T1) are impalpable on bimanual examination and biopsies taken from the tumour base confirm that the detrusor muscle is not invaded. They are usually managed by transurethral diathermy resection. Though the bladder should be cleared of tumour at the staging cystoscopy, more than half of those who have a superficial tumour will develop a recurrence in time.

Transurethral resection of bladder tumours is not without its problems. It is important to remove the base of the tumour completely and there is a risk of perforation, particularly of the very thin elderly female bladder. The other cause of substantial perforation is the 'obturator kick', a spasm of the obturator muscles induced by secondary electrical effects of the diathermy used in the region of the ureteric orifice. Obturator spasm can be countered by profound curarization of the patient. Small bladder perforations usually cause little trouble, but larger ones require a prolonged period of bladder drainage with a urethral catheter. If there is a huge tear or an intraperitoneal leak, open repair and extravesical drainage may be necessary. Persistent bleeding after bladder tumour resection can be difficult to handle. Careful intra-operative haemostasis is essential and can at times be extremely difficult and time-consuming.

Most bladder tumours are easy to recognize, but occasionally an area of mossy roughness is all that can be seen.

Carcinoma in situ is a high-grade malignant change in the urothelium without exophytic tumour. It may be very difficult to detect visually and if there is any doubt an endoscopic cup biopsy must be taken. Most urologists take random sample biopsies at the staging cystoscopy. These may reveal unexpected dysplasia of the urothelium or frank malignancy secondary to the main tumour. Such changes are important because they give an indication of malignant potential in the urothelium which may alter the prognosis. Carcinoma in situ is particularly ominous because of its tendency to change to invasive cancer.

Sometimes superficial tumours are too numerous or bulky to be removed easily by transurethral resection alone. In these circumstances chemotherapy with agents such as mitomycin or thiotepa or immunotherapy with bacille Calmette-Guérin (BCG) can help to discourage tumour growth. These agents are commonly given by the intravesical route through a urethral catheter. Typically, repeated courses of treatment will be needed for success. Helmstein described the use of prolonged hydrostatic distension of the bladder under epidural anaesthesia. The Helmstein balloon is inflated to a pressure higher than the systemic blood pressure which has itself been lowered by the epidural. Four or more hours of compression can cause dramatic necrosis of extensive or bulky tumour, leaving relatively small areas for resection. Total cystectomy for superficial tumours may very occasionally be necessary when all else fails.

FOLLOW-UP

Superficial tumours tend to recur and there is a possibility that the recurrent tumours may show progression in stage or grade from the original growth. Every diagnosis of superficial bladder tumour commits both the surgeon and the patient to a programme of follow-up to detect recurrence. This imposes an enormous burden on both which can be minimized by using the least invasive means of surveillance available and by relating the frequency of the checks to the activity of the tumour. Thus the patient with a small solitary well-differentiated tumour with no associated urothelial dysplasia can be quickly assigned to a regimen of yearly flexible cystoscopies. On the other hand, the bladder which is growing multiple moderately differentiated cancers must be examined endoscopically at much more frequent intervals. Because the chance of finding a lesion is much greater, it may be sensible to check these people with rigid equipment under general anaesthesia so that recurrent tumour can be resected and full urothelial biopsies taken if appropriate. Only when the urothelium has confirmed its relative inactivity by consecutive clear check cystoscopies will the patient be transferred to a less intensive regimen of fibre-optic-check cystoscopies.

Papanicolaou staining of the urinary sediment, urine cytology, is effective in detecting the presence of poorly differentiated tumours in the bladder, but well-differentiated tumours may be missed if this is used as the only means of follow-up. Advances in ultrasound imaging of the bladder wall mean that all but the tiniest of tumours can be detected without endoscopy, and ultrasound follow-up of bladder cancer with urine cytology may offer a less invasive alternative to check cystoscopy.

Because bladder cancer is a malignant change in an epithelium extending from the renal pelves to the urethra, there is a possibility of upper tract tumours growing against a background of bladder disease. However, transitional cell tumours of the ureter and renal pelvis are much less likely after a bladder cancer than is a bladder cancer after an upper tract tumour. Routine intravenous urograms are frequently advocated but rarely performed, most urologists confining upper tract studies to those patients in whom there is haematuria without apparent bladder disease or unexplained positive urine cytology. Positive urine cytology in the absence of exophytic tumour should also provoke a search for carcinoma in situ by biopsies which should include resection biopsies of the prostate to detect carcinoma in situ of the prostatic ducts.

Invasive bladder tumours

When tissue taken from the tumour base at the staging cystoscopy shows muscle invasion, the outlook is much less good and the presence of a mass after resection (T3) is extremely sinister, especially when it is fixed (T4). A small invasive tumour may be completely cleared by transurethral resection and such patients can reasonably be checked by resection biopsy of the tumour site at 3 months. However, most patients will need some more radical treatment and the choice of this treatment is subject to controversy. Central to this dispute is the fact that between one-third and one-half of patients with invasive bladder tumour will be dead of their disease within five years *whatever the treatment*. No radical treatment is without morbidity and the arguments hinge on the balance between the unpleasantness of the various treatment options and the marginal differences in survival which they appear to produce. This question will not easily be resolved. The choices include:

1. Radical radiotherapy with cystectomy considered for those who fail to respond (salvage cystectomy).

2. Limited radiotherapy with early cystectomy and urinary diversion.
3. Total cystectomy and urinary diversion without radiotherapy.
4. Chemotherapy with or without surgery.

TOTAL CYSTECTOMY

This is a major prolonged procedure (Figure 34.11) with a significant morbidity and perioperative mortality (3–10%). It is indicated either as the first line of treatment for invasive bladder tumour or when radiotherapy has failed. It is also indicated where conservative means have failed to control carcinoma in situ and to palliate symptoms of the growth itself or of the radiotherapy used to treat it. A very few patients whose superficial bladder tumours are uncontrollable by resection and other adjuvant measures may also come to cystectomy. Cystectomy is more tricky and dangerous after radiotherapy which tends to obliterate the tissue planes which make for easy surgery. The operation is usually preceded by a CT scan to rule out extensive extravesical spread which would make removal of the bladder difficult and local tumour clearance impossible. However, cystectomy in the presence of extravesical spread may be needed as a palliative measure, in which case the operation is likely to be fraught. Disease confined to the dome of the bladder may sometimes be cleared by partial cystectomy, but most patients in whom the procedure is considered worth while will need a radical operation with removal of the bladder along with the urethra and, in a man, the prostate and seminal vesicles.

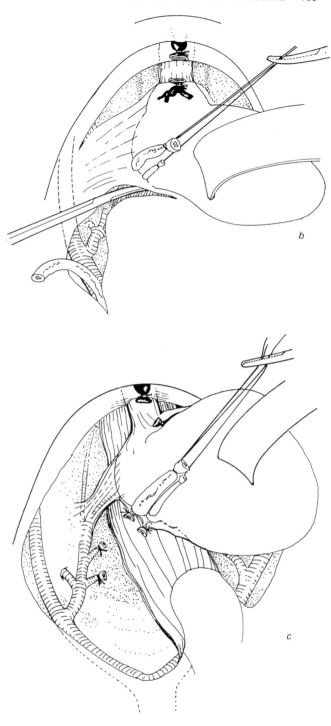

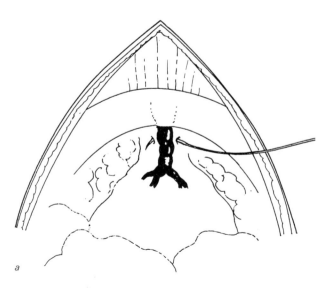

Figure 34.11 Stages in total cystectomy. *a*, Retropubic venous plexus ligated and divided exposing retropubic space. *b*, Ureter and vas divided and used to retract bladder medially. *c*, Vascular pedicle approaching the bladder posterolaterally ligated and divided in turn

With the patient anaesthetized on the operating table, a little Trendelenburg tilt helps to move the bowel out of the pelvis. A urethral catheter is inserted. If the urethra is to be removed in a man, the legs should be supported in stirrups and the perineum exposed. In any case the lithotomy position is helpful because it allows a place between the legs for another assistant. Bleeding from the long midline incision which is needed for full exposure may be minimized by judicious subcutaneous infiltration with 1:200 000 adrenaline. In any case, careful haemostasis of the wound edges prevents annoying superficial bleeding which can obscure the view during a procedure which is likely to last for 3 hours or more.

When the peritoneum has been opened, a thorough exploratory laparotomy will confirm whether the tumour is mobile and operable and whether there is obvious intra-abdominal metastasis, particularly to the liver.

The blood supply to the bladder comes from three reasonably well-defined leashes of vessels which originate mostly from the internal iliac vessels. The initial dissection is aimed at defining these pedicles so that they can be divided safely. A useful first step is to develop the plane between the bladder and the pubic bone. In a man there are some large veins just in front of the prostate which need careful clipping or suture ligature. Usually, however, the dissection is straightforward and the plane can be developed around the sides of the bladder and prostate. The separation of the bladder and prostate from the rectum posteriorly will then define the strips of tissue which attach posterolaterally to the pelvis on each side and which contain the vascular pedicles. The posterior dissection is made easier if the ureters are exposed by reflecting the sigmoid colon and caecum medially. The ureters can then be divided. Stay sutures in the proximal cut ends help to mark them so they are easy to find later. A tie on the distal end is useful to pull up to expose the posterior plane as it is entered through a transverse incision through the peritoneum of the rectovesical or uterovesical pouch. By angling the scissors anteriorly, this incision is carried through the fascia of Denonvilliers. There is usually a good plane between the leaves of this fascia which also offers some protection against inadvertently entering the rectal lumen, a disaster which almost always leads to postoperative complications through infection and fistula formation. The final step in exposing the vascular supply of the bladder is to incise the peritoneum on each side down the back of the bladder towards each end of the incision made in the rectovesical pouch. The vasa are encountered during this dissection and should be ligatured and divided. Traction on the tie on the distal end of the vas also helps increase exposure.

The bladder and prostate are then free front and back with the anterior and posterior dissections separated by the posterolateral bands of tissue which contain the main bladder vessels. The superior leash of vessels in the band contains the superior vesical artery which is a relatively large branch of the internal iliac. In radical cystectomy, the internal iliac is stripped of adjacent lymphatic tissue and the superior vesical pedicle is ligated and divided as part of this process. When the upper vessels have been tied, the middle and inferior bunches, which are much less well-defined anatomically, are made more obvious by gentle finger dissection. Division of these pedicles leaves the bladder attached only by the urethra.

In a woman, the posterior dissection is easier and safer because the uterus and vagina intervene between the surgeon and the rectum. It is usual to take a strip of anterior vagina wall with the specimen. The bladder is removed by circumcising the external urethral meatus. In a man, the urethra must be dissected through a separate midline perineal incision behind the scrotum. A tape around the urethral bulb is used to invert the penis as the dissection is continued up the penile shaft. The anterior end of the urethra is freed by cutting around the external meatus and when the urethra has been fully separated, it can be removed *en bloc* with the prostate and bladder.

The pelvic organs have a good vascular supply and there is considerable potential for bleeding during a cystectomy. A close watch must be kept on blood losses which must be replaced appropriately. When haemostasis has been achieved, a pack left in the pelvis while the urinary diversion is fashioned will help to discourage any remaining bleeders. At the end of the procedure, a 28 Charrière Foley catheter passed along the track of the urethral dissection acts as a good pelvic drain. If the balloon is over-inflated to 50 ml, it will tamponade the cavity left in the pelvis.

URINARY DIVERSION

Elaborate surgery to make a continent urinary reservoir is a possibility if radiotherapy has not been given. The urine is diverted into a pouch tailored from loops of small bowel. Valves have to be constructed to prevent urinary reflux and the finished reservoir is emptied by catheterization of a continent stoma on the anterior abdominal wall. In suitable cases where the urethra and the external urethral sphincter can be safely preserved, it may even be possible to re-establish micturition via the natural route by making a neo-bladder from bowel, as in a substitution cystoplasty. Unfortunately, these ingenious efforts have their problems. The design of the continent pouch is still subject to experiment and some patients need reoperation because of stone formation and malfunction. Patients with a neo-bladder are subject to incontinence due to sphincter weakness and spontaneous contractions of the muscle of the bowel segment. Making a neo-bladder adds considerably to the duration of the operation and is impossible in the presence of the inevitable damage to bowel microvasculature caused by radiotherapy. For most patients, simple ileal loop diversion is the answer.

A prolonged and destructive operation like cystectomy is bound to result in postoperative problems with fluid balance, even when haemostasis and intraoperative replacement of blood loss has been adequate. There will be a prolonged ileus which usually needs nasogastric suction for a day or so. Many patients with bladder cancer are relatively old and frail and it may be difficult to encourage them to mobilize as early as would be ideal. Indeed, this operation carries a high risk of deep venous thrombosis and appropriate precautions such as subcutaneous heparin, supportive stockings and early mobilization are advisable. A particularly ominous complication is signalled by discharge of faecal material from the wound. This is due either to unnoticed damage to the rectum or to failure of the ileo-ileal anastomosis used to re-establish bowel continuity. In either case, radiotherapy damage compromises bowel healing and the fistula rarely closes spontaneously. Preoperative bowel preparation is an obvious and sensible precaution.

PARTIAL CYSTECTOMY

Partial cystectomy is reserved for tumours which are confined to the dome of the bladder and is rarely performed except for urachal tumours. The remaining bladder wall will stretch remarkably and augmentation is rarely needed, even if a large section of the bladder vault is excised. It is a good thing to place catheters in both ureters to mark and protect them during the operation. The bladder is closed using sutures which should be absorbable to avoid stones forming on them.

Bladder diverticulum

Most bladder diverticula are pulsion diverticula which result from a sustained increase in intravesical pressure due to bladder outflow obstruction from prostatic disease. As long as the outflow obstruction is properly treated, the diverticula usually give little trouble and can be left alone. There are also rare congenital diverticula which are not due to outflow problems and para-ureteric diverticula are not infrequently seen with gross ureteric reflux. Diverticula cause trouble by acting as a reservoir in which urine stagnates with a risk of infection and stone formation. Tumours within diverticula may be difficult to see with a cystoscope and the thin wall is more easily breached by tumour growth than that of the normal bladder.

A true diverticulum of the bladder may be caused by traction into a femoral or inguinal hernia and is at risk during hernia repair when the bladder may be opened during excision of the sac. This mishap will be followed by a urine leak from the wound, into the peritoneum, or both, unless the problem is recognized at the time. Closure of the bladder wall with absorbable sutures and catheter drainage for 3–5 days will usually prevent any unfortunate consequences.

Bladder diverticula may be suspected on clinical grounds or be evident on ultrasound, the bladder films of the urogram or on cystoscopy. Excision is rarely indicated, except when the diverticulum is huge and producing symptoms or is complicated by persistent infection, stone formation or tumour. Most diverticula are close to a ureteric orifice and it is wise to begin the procedure with a cystoscopy and insertion of ureteric catheters. Marking the ureters in this way helps to preserve them from damage later.

With the patient in the Trendelenburg position, the bladder is exposed extraperitoneally and opened between stay sutures. The orifice of the diverticulum is identified and the cavity packed with gauze to make it easier to identify the extent of the diverticulum during the extraperitoneal dissection which follows. When the diverticulum has been excised, the defect in the bladder wall is closed in one or two layers with absorbable sutures and a catheter left in place for 5 days or so.

In some patients, dissection and excision of the diverticulum are simple, but where there has been infection and fibrosis there may be considerable risk to the ureter, even if it had been made easy to identify by a catheter within it. In such cases, it may be justifiable to circumcise the neck of the diverticulum to divide it from the bladder. The bladder wall is closed and the diverticulum left *in situ* with a drain run down to its lumen and left in place for one or two weeks.

Bladder stone

Bladder stones are usually secondary to urine stasis and infection associated with outflow obstruction. Occasionally they result from incrustation of a foreign body in the bladder or from the arrival of a calculus from the upper urinary tract. The composition of a bladder calculus is usually mixed: oxalate, urate and cystine may be present as well as a marked mucoprotein component. When the patient sits or stands, the stone irritates the trigone causing suprapubic discomfort and pain referred to the tip of the penis. There may be irritative symptoms of urgency and frequency, terminal haematuria or intermittent urinary obstruction due to the stone blocking the bladder neck. The diagnosis is confirmed by ultrasound, X-ray or cystoscopy.

Stones less than 3 cm or so in diameter can usually be crushed under vision using a cystoscopic lithotrite. These instruments have a punch mechanism or crushing jaws. Unfortunately bladder stones can be very hard and the instrument may break before the stones. The classical lithotrite still has a place in the treatment of bladder stones, but it is used 'blind' and considerable experience and skill is needed to avoid serious damage to the bladder wall. For bigger stones and when suitable lithotrites or the skills to use them are unavailable, a simple suprapubic cystotomy, performed if necessary under local anaesthesia, is a simple and safe alternative. If the stone is caused by outflow obstruction, correction of this will of course be necessary to avoid recurrence.

Permanent urinary diversion

Diversion of urine with transplantation of the ureters is indicated in total cystectomy. Patients with profound bladder dysfunction due to neurological disease are managed by conservative means wherever possible, but some of those with congenital or traumatic spinal cord disease or multiple sclerosis are better off with a urostomy. The physical and psychological implications must be considered carefully with each patient and surgery planned where possible with the assistance of an experienced stoma therapist.

A wide range of diversions are possible. They range from simple suprapubic cystostomy and cutaneous ureterostomy to complex continent reservoir diversion. The classical Mitrofanoff procedure uses the appendix to form a continent catheterizable conduit between the bladder and the skin. A continent conduit can also be made by doing a transuretero-ureterostomy and using the free distal end of the divided ureter. In some specially selected patients, implantation of the ureters into the sigmoid colon (ureterosigmoidostomy) may be considered, although careful follow-up is mandatory to detect the onset of metabolic problems or the development of bowel cancers which are well-recognized complications of all types of 'rectal bladder'. These are operations which are likely to be advised for individual patients under the care of a superspecialist. For the majority, an ileal loop diversion is the best option.

Uretero-ileostomy (ileal bladder, ileal conduit)

The patient should experiment with the urostomy appliance preoperatively to find the most comfortable site for the stoma. This will vary with body shape, the presence of surgical scars and whether the patient is able-bodied or confined to the sitting or lying position. It should be marked with indelible ink before the patient goes for surgery.

With the patient supine and a little head down to encourage the bowel out of the pelvis, the operation can be performed through a midline, paramedian or transverse incision. The ureters are identified where they cross the bifurcation of the common iliac arteries. They are divided, the distal end tied with absorbable thread and the proximal end marked with a stay suture. It is usual to perform an incidental appendicectomy to avoid the possibility of diagnostic and surgical difficulties with appendicitis in the future.

The theatre lights are dimmed and the vascular supply of the terminal ileum displayed by shining a theatre spotlight through the mesentery. A 30–35 cm length of ileum based on a suitable arterial arcade is isolated on its vascular pedicle and intestinal continuity re-established by an end-to-end ileo-ileal anastomosis.

The left ureter is brought across the midline without tension through a window made in the pelvic mesocolon. The ends of the ureters are spatulated and brought side to side to form a Wallace anastomosis with the proximal end of the prepared ileal segment (Figure 34.12). The other end of the loop is brought

out as a spouted stoma at the planned site. Stenting the uretero-ileal anastomosis with suitably sized infant feeding tubes gives added security. A tube drain is left to the site of the anastomoses.

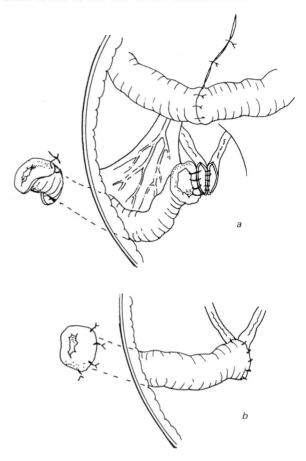

Figure 34.12 Ileal loop diversion. *a*, The ends of the ureters are spatulated and brought together to form a Wallace 1 uretero-ileal anastomosis. *b*, The distal end of the ileal loop is brought through the skin to form a urostomy

Provided that care is taken to ensure an adequate blood supply to the isolated ileal segment and to the ureters by keeping mobilization to a minimum, there should be no problems with healing or stenosis. Abdominal wall skin is at risk from ammoniacal dermatitis, but this can be controlled by proper stoma care. Hernia, retraction and stenosis of the stoma are all avoidable technical failures. As the conduit is not a reservoir, reflux should not be a problem but there is often dilatation of the upper tracts after a diversion even when there is no obstruction. Stone formation is relatively common due to infection, dehydration and an abnormality in uric acid metabolism which results from shortening the ileum. Hyperchloraemic acidosis is much less likely with an ileal loop than with ureterocolic anastomosis, although an excessively long conduit may predispose to this complication.

Vesicocolic and vesicovaginal fistula

Vesicocolic fistula

A fistula between the rectosigmoid and the bladder is usually due to colonic diverticular disease. Crohn's disease of the colon or small bowel or malignancy of either the colon or bladder are possible but much less frequent causes. The clinical result is intractable cystitis and pneumaturia, the passage of gas in the urine. This unusual symptom, which is also seen when diabetic urine is infected with gas-forming organisms, is best recognized if the patient is invited to pass urine while sitting in the bath. The tell-tale appearance of bubbles from the urethra is unmistakable and the diagnosis of fistula with the bowel can be confirmed by urine microscopy which should show the presence of meat and vegetable fibres from the faeces. It may be difficult to demonstrate the communication by contrast enema or cystography, and the intense cystitis causes oedema which may hide the hole at cystoscopy. On bimanual examination, a mass is palpable at the site of the fistula and may be confirmed by ultrasound or CT imaging. Such fistulae rarely close spontaneously and surgery is required to separate the bowel from the bladder. At operation, the bladder defect is closed and the diseased bowel resected. A temporary colostomy to defunction the bowel while it heals may be wise if there is extensive inflammatory tissue destruction around the fistula. If there is sufficient omentum available it can be brought down to separate the recently repaired bladder and bowel. A catheter is left in the bladder for 7–10 days.

Vesicovaginal fistula

Vesicovaginal fistula can result from obstetric trauma, irradiation of the cervix or follow operative injury during gynaecological surgery. The cases which follow childbirth are thought to be caused by prolonged pressure of the fetal head on the anterior vaginal wall and are more common in those countries where obstetric care is deficient.

Vesicovaginal fistula presents as a continuous leakage of urine from the vagina which follows the trauma that has caused the injury. The nature of the fluid loss can be confirmed by testing its urea content which will be higher than that of the blood. In cases where the fistula follows pelvic surgery, it is important to perform an intravenous urogram to rule out ureteric injury because a ureterovaginal fistula also causes a continuous urine leak and may be present instead of or as well as the vesical injury. The bladder films of the urogram occasionally demonstrate the fistula.

Because of the circumstances in which the injury occurs and the unpleasantness of the symptoms it produces, the patient with a vesicovaginal fistula is often depressed and demoralized. Although some very tiny fistulae may close with a period of catheter

drainage, this is the exception and unless there has been massive tissue destruction, early intervention to perform a definitive repair is usually desirable.

Because of the possibility of injury to other parts of the urinary tract, the repair should begin with cystoscopy and bilateral retrograde ureterography. The fistula is usually evident as a punched-out hole at or near the midline of the trigone or the posterior bladder wall close to the interureteric bar. The choice of surgical approach to the repair will depend upon the size of the defect and the presence of associated ureteric injury. The overriding aim should be to make a secure repair to avoid further surgery.

Abdominal repair of vesicovaginal fistula

An abdominal approach to the repair of vesicovaginal fistula gives the most certain results and is certainly indicated when the fistula is large and usually indicated when a recent lower abdominal operation is the cause of the trouble (Figure 34.13). When the assessment cystoscopy is complete, bilateral ureteric catheters are left in place. These are to mark the ureters so that they can be more easily recognized later.

The operation is performed with the patient supine. A general anaesthetic is usual. If a lower abdominal incision is present, it is reopened. Otherwise a lower midline or Pfannenstiel incision gives good access to the bladder which is approached transperitoneally. The dome of the bladder is opened between stay sutures and the bladder wall incision continued posteriorly in the midline. As the incision in the bladder is enlarged, the internal opening of the fistula comes into view between the two catheters marking the ureters. The incision is then continued down the back of the bladder until it reaches the site of the fistula. The effect is to bisect the bladder so that the two halves fall apart like shells of a mollusc. Because the detrusor is very vascular, cutting the bladder wall causes a lot of bleeding which is best controlled by a running haemostatic suture along the cut edges or individual suture ligature of the main vessels. Coagulation diathermy is usually disappointing.

When the bladder incision reaches the fistula, the vagina can be dissected away from the bladder so that the defect in its wall can be closed by interrupted absorbable sutures. If omentum is available, a plug brought down and sutured so that it is interposed between the vaginal and bladder wound seems to add security to the repair. The bladder incision is then closed in one or two layers with absorbable sutures. The ureteric catheters help to mark the ureters during the repair and are particularly reassuring when there has been extensive tissue destruction around the bladder base. They may be brought out suprapubically to stent the ureters postoperatively. In any case, a suprapubic tube drain to the bladder incision is wise and a urethral catheter should be left in place for 7–10 days after the repair.

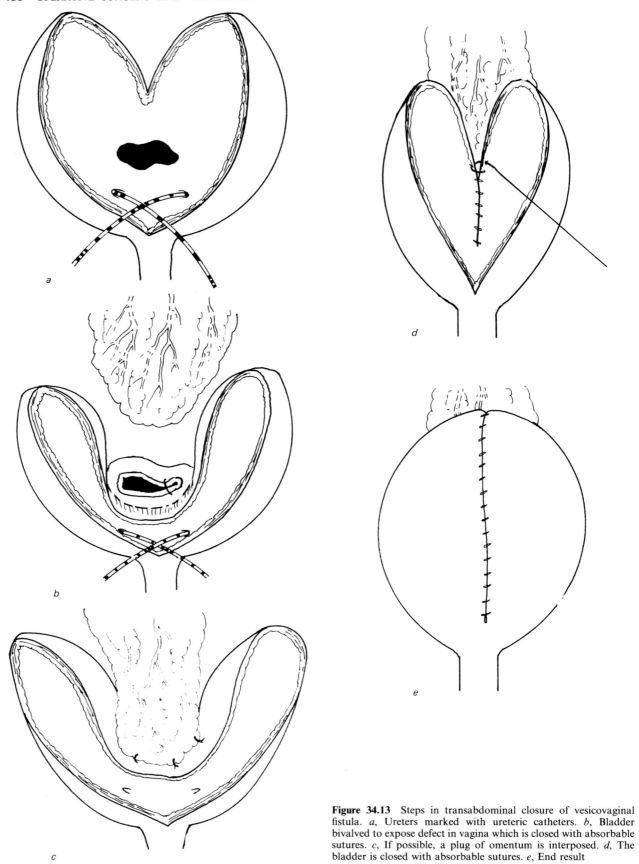

Figure 34.13 Steps in transabdominal closure of vesicovaginal fistula. *a*, Ureters marked with ureteric catheters. *b*, Bladder bivalved to expose defect in vagina which is closed with absorbable sutures. *c*, If possible, a plug of omentum is interposed. *d*, The bladder is closed with absorbable sutures. *e*, End result

Transvaginal repair

Surgical repair of a low fistula may be possible through the vaginal route. The fistula and its surrounding scar tissue are excised, leaving defects in both the bladder and the vaginal wall which have to be meticulously sutured in separate layers. If the hole in the bladder is large, mobilization of the bladder from above may still be needed to get satisfactory closure.

Bladder outflow obstruction

Bladder outflow obstruction is most commonly due to enlargement of the prostate, although a large prostate does not necessarily cause obstruction and a small prostate is not necessarily blameless. The obstruction to urine flow causes the same symptoms whether, as most frequently, the enlargement is benign or if there is a carcinoma of the prostate. Indeed, the same symptoms occur with stenosis of the bladder neck due to postoperative fibrosis, a stone lodged in the prostatic urethra or urethral obstruction due to stricture or congenital valves.

Benign prostatic hypertrophy

The exact mechanism by which the enlarged prostate causes outflow obstruction is somewhat mysterious. The gland has been likened to a thick collar wrapped around the bladder neck and open at the front. Enlargement has produced bulky masses of tissue bilaterally and in the midline. These appear as right and left lateral lobes and a middle lobe when the prostatic urethra is examined endoscopically. In some patients, the main hypertrophy seems to affect the middle lobe which may enlarge into the bladder giving the impression of a ball-valve in the bladder neck. In others it is one or, more usually, both of the lateral lobes which are prominent, pushing towards each other in the midline, occluding the prostatic urethra until it looks like a tight slit. These changes seem to be compounded by a loss of elastic tissue from the bladder neck and together they inhibit the normal opening of the bladder neck when the man tries to void. A reactive hypertrophy of the bladder muscle leaves it thickened in irregular bundles crisscrossing the bladder wall, giving the cystoscopic appearance of trabeculation. In long-standing cases where there is distension of the bladder due to decompensation of the detrusor, the trabeculation progresses to sacculation and the formation of diverticula. The pool of stagnant urine which remains in the bladder after micturition is liable to become infected and bladder stones may form. In chronic retention, back-pressure effects on the ureters may lead to hydronephrosis and varying degrees of renal failure. If the patient does not present with symptoms resulting from these changes, acute retention of urine may precipitate emergency treatment.

Clinical presentation may therefore be with symptoms of obstruction such as hesitancy, poor urinary stream and a feeling of incomplete emptying. Detrusor hypertrophy is associated with bladder instability causing urgency, frequency and nocturia. Haematuria may be due to infection, bladder stones or from suburothelial veins at the bladder neck. On the other hand, the first presentation may be with retention of urine or indeed the symptoms of uraemia without any direct complaint of urinary symptoms.

Management of bladder outflow obstruction

Acute retention of urine is relieved by a urethral or suprapubic catheter. Further investigations are usually unnecessary, especially when there is a good history of bladder outflow symptoms before the acute event. When acute obstruction has not been foreshadowed in this way, a trial without catheter is worth while because in some men normal voiding is re-established after a short period of bladder drainage. When the patient presents with symptoms other than acute retention, the decision to proceed to prostatectomy is less clear-cut. It is dependent upon the severity of the symptoms, and on an assessment of the degree to which the untoward secondary effects of obstruction have developed and on the patient's fitness for major surgery.

Rectal examination may reveal a craggy malignant prostate which will tip the scales towards prostatectomy after appropriate investigation. The presence of a distended bladder on palpation or suprapubic percussion will be evidence of chronic retention which can be confirmed by ultrasound scanning. When the ultrasound scan shows dilatation of the upper urinary tracts and there is biochemical evidence of post-renal renal failure, there is a very real risk of a massive diuresis when the obstruction is relieved. Preoperative urethral catheterization allows the metabolic consequences of this diuresis to be managed so that renal function has stabilized by the time the patient comes to surgery. In addition to identifying chronic retention, the aim of preoperative investigation is to alert the surgeon to the presence of calculi or metastases. Intravenous urography is an alternative to investigation by plain abdominal X-ray and ultrasonography, but rarely gives extra information to justify the additional expense. Cystometry is reserved for those patients in whom an alternative, usually neurological, cause of their symptoms is suspected and in those few patients in which frequency and urgency appear without a diminution of urine flow rate.

Prostatectomy

The most common operation on the prostate is transurethral resection which, despite recent questioning, remains the safest means of correcting bladder outflow obstruction due to prostatic disease. Open prostatectomy, usually by the Millin retropubic approach, is a rare operation for the specialist urologist capable of performing a skilled transurethral resection. Retropubic prostatectomy may be appropriate when the gland is truly enormous or when the surgeon is more at home with open surgery. Transvesical prostatectomy is virtually obsolete and will not be described here. More modern non-operative treatments such as stent insertion, drug treatment and prostatic hyperthermia have yet to prove their worth.

Transurethral resection of the prostate

Transurethral resection of the prostate (Figure 34.14) is a major operation and the patient needs appropriate preparation. Each patient should be warned that an open procedure may be necessary if endoscopic surgery proves impossible for some reason. He should be warned of the likelihood of retrograde ejaculation and, where appropriate, some mention should be made of the small incidence of postoperative erectile failure. Many of these patients are elderly and will need full medical work-up before anaesthesia. Where there is evidence of post-renal renal impairment with high serum creatinine and dilatation of the upper tracts, a period of preoperative catheter drainage is mandatory to avoid the onset of polyuria in the immediate postoperative period. Blood loss in transurethral prostatectomy is variable and all patients should have blood grouped and serum saved. The less experienced operator may feel reassured to have blood ready cross-matched. Preoperative shaving of the pubic hair is unnecessary.

The choice of anaesthesia for transurethral resection can usually be left to the anaesthetist: general anaesthesia or spinal anaesthesia are equally acceptable to most surgeons. Some urologists prefer some degree of hypotension. Others fear that this may inhibit bleeding during the operation, with a risk of reactionary haemorrhage from inadequately coagulated vessels. When he has been anaesthetized, the patient is positioned with his legs supported in stirrups so that flexion of hip and knee joints is less extreme than in the full lithotomy position. The genitals are cleaned with antiseptic and the patient is towelled so that only the penis is exposed. A rubber finger cot incorporated into the drapes allows the surgeon to insert a finger into the rectum during the procedure and it helps to lubricate the finger cot on both sides before draping the patient.

Every transurethral resection of the prostate is preceded by a thorough cystourethroscopy as described above. This precaution ensures that coincidental conditions such as transitional cell cancer or stone are not missed. Urethral strictures may mimic the symptoms of prostatic disease and if present may lead the unsuspecting surgeon to make a false passage if he attempts 'blind' instrumentation of the urethra. If a stricture is seen, it can be treated by dilatation or optical urethrotomy, while a decision has to be made whether to continue with the resection. In many cases, it is wise to wait to see whether curing the stricture is enough to cure the symptoms. If the urethra is normal and there is no urothelial abnormality, some attempt can be made to estimate the prostatic size both endoscopically and by bimanual examination. If the gland is enormous, it may be best to opt for open surgery at this stage. Appreciable trabeculation of the bladder is usually taken to confirm the presence of significant outflow obstruction.

The rigid cystourethroscope is 19 Charrière or less and it does not follow that the much larger 24 or 27 Charrière resectoscope sheath will pass easily when cystourethroscopy is complete. Certainly, the urethra must be lubricated with suitable gel which may contain an antiseptic such as chlorhexidine. The sheath is usually inserted with the obturator in place and a good deal of skill is needed to pass the instrument down the urethra by 'feel' without causing trauma. Any sensation of tightness is a signal that the urethra needs to be enlarged by judicious dilatation or by urethrotomy with the Otis urethrotome before the resectoscope can be passed with safety. An optical obturator which allows the resectoscope to be inserted under vision may be useful in some circumstances.

Transurethral resection of the prostate is simple in principle. The gland is cut away from within the prostatic urethra using a diathermy cutting loop. The strips of tissue removed, the prostatic chips, are small enough to be evacuated through the resectoscope sheath from the bladder where they collect during the resection. Bleeding vessels are controlled by touching them with the diathermy loop and applying the coagulation current.

Sadly, things are not quite so straightforward in practice. The removal of the prostate involves the inevitable sacrifice of the continence mechanism at the bladder neck, so that after the operation the man is wholly dependent on the external urethral sphincter mechanism to maintain continence. Damage to the sphincter during resection is an ever-present danger and even the most experienced resectionist has to take care to avoid making the man wet postoperatively. The key is to limit the resection to tissue which is proximal to the veru montanum, an organ of obscure function other than to signpost the external sphincter for the urologist. Even with the help of the veru, things can still go wrong because the prostate is a relatively vascular organ which may bleed profusely during the resection. It is then easy to become lost. Every resectionist needs a system of resection to help keep orientation and a selection of tricks to get out of trouble when he or she loses it.

Another potential problem results from the inflow of irrigant fluid which is used to clear the view during

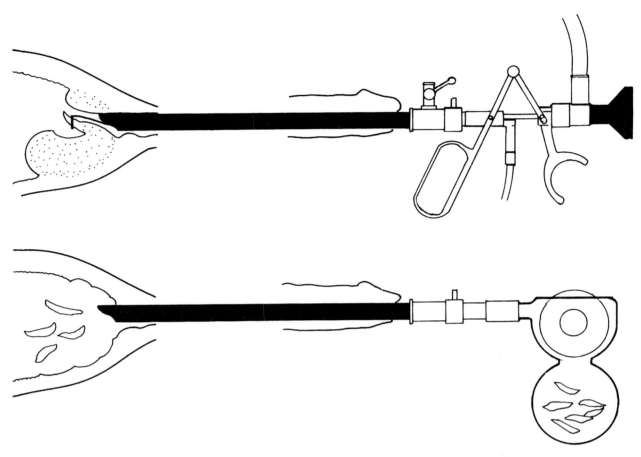

Figure 34.14 Transurethral resection of the prostate. The prostate is cut into chips small enough to be evacuated through the sheath

resection. If the venous sinuses which surround and pervade the prostate are opened and intravesical pressure rises, considerable volumes of this irrigant flow directly into the circulation causing a metabolic upset. If the volumes are large enough, the much-feared 'transurethral resection (TUR) syndrome' may result, with massive fluid overload, hyponatraemia, cerebral oedema and considerable danger of death. The use of isotonic irrigant fluid (often 1.5% glycine) for resection and restricting the total operating time to an hour or less are essential precautions to avoid this danger. Some urologists use a continuous flow irrigating system or a suprapubic trocar to allow sufficient irrigant flow to clear the view without a rise in intravesical pressure. The 'TUR syndrome' is relatively rare, but sufficiently unpleasant to require continual vigilance.

The aim of transurethral resection for benign disease is to resect all the adenomatous tissue to expose a layer of compressed normal prostate known misleadingly as the prostatic capsule. If the gland is very large, a complete resection may not be necessary and, in truth, most patients will do well even with a partial resection. Indeed, the much lesser operation of prostatic incision has been shown to give good results in many patients. In this operation, one or more deep cuts are made through the prostate with a Collings diathermy knife passed through the resectoscope sheath. Although there may be advantages in limiting the extent of the operation, incomplete removal of the adenoma leaves an increased likelihood of recurrent problems in the future.

If the prostate is clearly malignant on clinical grounds or shown to be so by biopsy, it is customary to perform a much more limited resection on the grounds that further growth of the cancer may threaten the competence of the external sphincter which has been carefully preserved during the operation. In these circumstances it is usual to resect a channel in the midline from the bladder neck to the veru montanum. If outflow symptoms recur after conservative resection for prostate cancer, there is a choice between further resection and measures aimed at discouraging growth of the tumour such as local radiotherapy or hormonal therapy.

When the transurethral resection is complete and haemostasis is satisfactory, a catheter is inserted using an introducer to lift the catheter tip safely over the resected bladder neck. A three-way catheter allows continuous irrigation to avoid the accumulation of clots in the bladder lumen. A similar diluting effect can be achieved by fluid loading the patient and administering a diuretic, in which case a simple two-way Foley catheter is all that is needed. Gentle traction on the catheter will bring the balloon down into the bladder neck and can be used to apply useful tamponade to discourage venous bleeding from the prostatic cavity. Perforation of the capsule is common during transurethral resection and usually of no importance. However, large tears can lead to massive leakage of irrigant fluid and on occasion formal retropubic exploration, suture and drainage is essential. Certainly, any suspicion that there is a tear in the anterior part of the capsule which connects with the peritoneal cavity merits immediate open exploration.

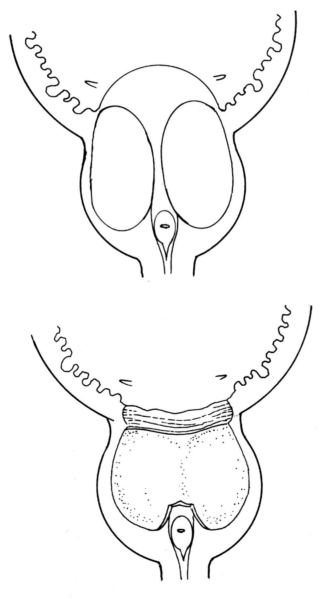

Figure 34.15 Millin's retropubic prostatectomy. The adenoma is 'shelled out', leaving a smooth prostatic cavity

Retropubic prostatectomy (Millin) (Figure 34.15)

Preliminary cystourethroscopy is essential because the bladder is not opened at operation and coincidental stone or tumour might otherwise be missed. Under general, epidural or spinal anaesthesia, a vertical lower midline or Pfannenstiel incision is made. Retropubic dissection reveals the preprostatic veins which are secured with suture ligatures. A transverse incision is made in the prostatic capsule just wide enough to allow removal of the enucleated prostate. The plane of enucleation is readily entered by inserting curved scissors and opening the blades in a plane parallel to the capsule. The lateral lobes are freed by digital dissection and the urethra immediately distal to the prostate is divided by scissors. Both lateral lobes are dislocated and the proximal attachment of the gland divided. A very large middle lobe may be removed separately.

When haemostasis has been secured and care taken to identify and avoid the ureters, a wedge is cut from the bladder neck to discourage postoperative bladder neck stenosis. The cut edge of the trigone is sutured down into the prostatic cavity. The prostatic capsule is then closed over a three-way Foley catheter and the suture line is tested by irrigation through it. Any clots are evacuated and continuous irrigation set up. The retropubic space is drained.

Complications

Infection and haemorrhage are the most common postoperative complications of prostatic surgery. All instrumentation of the urinary tract carries the risk of sepsis and this risk continues during the period of catheterization which follows. A system of *closed* catheter drainage, in which the connections between the catheter remain unbroken, can minimize the danger but inevitably some patients will suffer urinary infection and some will become very ill with septicaemia. A constant awareness of the rapidity with which overwhelming systemic infection can develop and a readiness to begin appropriate treatment on suspicion are essential if tragedy is to be avoided. Bleeding from the prostatic bed is inevitable after all methods of prostatectomy, despite careful intraoperative haemostasis. Some form of postoperative irrigation is almost always needed and if this is kept running, clot retention should not occur. In reality, excessive bleeding or neglect of the irrigation result in catheter blockage by clots in a few patients. These can usually be cleared by bladder washout through the catheter, but some more tenacious clots can only be removed by formal evacuation through a resectoscope sheath in theatre. In a tiny minority with intractable bleeding it may even be necessary to open the prostatic cavity through a retropubic approach to secure the vessels responsible.

Secondary haemorrhage occurring around 2 weeks from surgery is often associated with sepsis. Increased fluid intake to ensure a good urine flow and antibiotics will usually be all that is needed, but in some patients massive bleeding leads to clot retention.

Other complications are less common. Clinically important deep venous thrombosis is rare after transurethral prostatectomy, but much less so after the retropubic operation. Urinary incontinence is usually temporary after surgery and associated with persisting bladder instability. Even where there has been some damage to the urethral sphincter, time and pelvic floor exercises cure most patients and only a tiny number will be permanently and disastrously wet. These may need to be considered for an artificial urethral sphincter. Recurrent outflow symptoms may be due to regrowth of the incompletely removed gland or the development of strictures at the external urethral meatus, the bulbar urethra or the bladder neck. All patients should be warned before surgery that they are likely to have retrograde ejaculation, making them infertile. Surgeons are divided on the wisdom of advising men of the small risk of impotence after prostatectomy – the psychological effect of the warning may be enough to fulfil it!

Carcinoma of the prostate

Carcinoma of the prostate is the third most common malignancy in men and accounts for 1 in 10 cases of retention. Carcinoma may be detected histologically after removal of a clinically benign gland or may be suspected on rectal examination. Most patients present with bladder outflow symptoms, but a significant minority come with symptoms of metastatic disease. An increasing number of prostate cancers are discovered at an early stage as a result of routine health screening in men. The cancer which is commonly found in the prostates of very elderly men is of dubious clinical importance but, in general, carcinoma of the prostate is an extremely dangerous disease.

Diagnosis of prostate cancer suspected on rectal examination can usually be confirmed by transperineal Tru-cut biopsy or transrectal Franzen needle aspiration for cytology. The latter has the advantage of not requiring a general anaesthetic. The presence of extensive disease and particularly of metastases is associated with an elevated serum acid phosphatase, an estimation which is likely to be replaced by the more sensitive test for prostate specific antigen (PSA). Isotope bone scanning is the most effective way of demonstrating hot spots which can be confirmed as metastases by X-ray.

Argument rages about almost every aspect of the management of carcinoma of the prostate. Most prostate cancers have androgen receptors and the mainstay of treatment of metastatic disease is hormonal manipulation. The timing of hormonal therapy and whether it should be by orchidectomy, stilboestrol, antiandrogens or by injections of luteinizing hormone releasing hormone analogues is a matter of dispute. Outflow obstruction due to local disease is well treated by conservative transurethral resection, but the treatment of unsuspected cancer found in the prostatectomy specimen and the treatment of early stage disease are equally controversial. In the UK, supervoltage radiotherapy is most commonly used to treat local disease, although there is little indisputable evidence for its effectiveness. In the USA and mainland Europe, many surgeons treat early stage disease by total (radical) prostatectomy.

Total prostatectomy; radical prostatectomy

All patients must be fully informed of the risk of impotence following this operation and the possibility of incontinence. The patient is anaesthetized and positioned as for retropubic prostatectomy, and the first part of the operation with development of the retropubic space and ligation of the preprostatic veins is just like a Millin's operation. The urethra is then separated from its posterior and lateral attachments so that a sling can be passed around it just distal to the apex of the prostate. The urethra can then be divided between stay sutures at this level so that the prostate can be pulled up into the wound. The tissue plane between the layers of Denonvilliers' fascia is then developed, taking care to keep the dissecting scissors close to the prostate. This posterior dissection is complete when the top edge of the prostate and the seminal vesicles come into view.

The bladder is then opened through a transverse incision at its junction with the prostate anteriorly. Haemostasis of the cut edge of bladder is secured by a running suture ligature. The bladder interior is exposed and the ureteric orifices identified and marked with ureteric catheters. It is then safe to continue circumcising the bladder–prostate junction, picking up the large leashes of vessels which accompany the vasa when they come into view posterolaterally. The prostate and seminal vesicles can then be removed. Unless special attention is given to them during the dissection, the sacral parasympathetic nerves crucial to penile erection will be sacrificed and impotence is inevitable. In a 'nerve-sparing' radical prostatectomy, these nerves are carefully identified and conserved.

The operation is completed by suturing the bladder directly to the cut end of the urethra, taking care to avoid ureteric injury. If there is likely to be tension in this anastomosis, the gap between bladder and urethra can be bridged by fashioning a tube from a flap taken from the bladder wall. In any case, a urethral catheter and a suprapubic drain are left to protect the anastomosis.

Trauma to the bladder

Pelvic surgery and lower urinary tract endoscopy are the most common causes of accidental injury to the bladder. Blunt and penetrating trauma is comparatively infrequent but requires prompt recognition and treatment.

Blunt injury

When the bladder is full, a direct blow to the lower abdomen is liable to cause an intraperitoneal rupture. Crushing injury to the pelvis may be expected to cause extraperitoneal extravasation from rupture of the bladder or posterior urethra.

Urine leakage into the peritoneal cavity typically causes severe lower abdominal pain which later passes off. There is no desire to micturate and the bladder is impalpable. The presence of lower abdominal pain and a failure to obtain urine on urethral catheterization are indications for intravenous urography followed by laparotomy to close the rent in the bladder. The injury is treated by simple suture in one or two layers using catgut, followed by catheter drainage for 4–5 days or more.

Extraperitoneal rupture of the bladder usually occurs against a background of severe pelvic injury and may be very difficult to distinguish from urethral disruption caused by dislocation of the prostate. If there is any doubt, the patient should be treated as if he had a urethral injury. Extravasation of urine into the perivesical tissue occurs relatively slowly and a boggy swelling of the perineum and suprapubic region develops over 24 h or so. The attachments of Colles fascia prevent urine from tracking into the thighs or the posterior perineum. At laparotomy, extravasated blood and urine are obvious when the linea alba is opened. An anterior rupture can easily be treated by direct suture, but exploration of the bladder base is hazardous and should be avoided if possible. A suprapubic or urethral catheter and a retropubic drain are usually sufficient in this case. Occasionally so much tissue has been lost or traumatized that debridement and formal closure are unavoidable. Prophylactic broad-spectrum antibiotics should be considered in all cases.

Penetrating trauma

When the bladder has been injured by penetrating trauma it is difficult to exclude injury to other pelvic organs and emergency laparotomy is almost always necessary. The bladder wound is closed over a urethral catheter after debridement and a suprapubic drain left in place. Prophylactic antibiotics are essential.

Surgical injury

Damage to the bladder recognized during pelvic surgery can be treated by immediate suture and bladder drainage for 4–5 days. Little harm usually results. More serious is an injury which goes undetected until it causes unexpected lower abdominal symptoms and ileus in the postoperative period. A cystogram will confirm the diagnosis and all but the smallest tears merit laparotomy and closure. Lacerations of the bladder during endoscopic surgery can usually be treated conservatively by catheter drainage unless the hole is large or an intraperitoneal rupture is a possibility. In the latter case, the bowel should be carefully examined for unsuspected injury when the bladder has been sutured.

Operations for bladder dysfunction

Cystoplasty: bladder augmentation and substitution

Cystoplasty may be considered when the bladder fails to function as a reservoir. The most extreme case is when the bladder has been removed for cancer but scarring due to the ravages of radiotherapy, intravesical chemotherapy or surgical trauma may also make the bladder useless in this role. Extreme detrusor instability or hyperreflexia (in neurological disease) may be unresponsive to drug treatment and the intractable frequency of interstitial cystitis may resist all conservative management. Patients with these conditions, carefully selected, may benefit from replacement of the bladder (substitution cystoplasty) or increase of its capacity (augmentation cystoplasty).

Substitution cystoplasty

Replacement of the bladder with artificial materials has been unsuccessful and segments of bowel are used in operations to substitute the bladder. In caecocystoplasty, the caecum and a short length of terminal ileum are mobilized on the ileocolic artery and prepared as an isolated intestinal loop. If the bladder has been excised with preservation of the trigone, the open end of the caecum is sutured to the bladder base with an absorbable suture (Figure 34.16). The ileum is oversewn to occlude its lumen. If the whole bladder has been removed, the caecum is sutured to the proximal end of the urethra and the ureters must be anastomosed separately, if possible into the ileal part of the loop (with a Wallace anastomosis). The ileocaecal valve then acts as an anti-reflux device.

Despite the absence of a detrusor, bladder substitutes of this sort usually empty well by abdominal straining and suprapubic manual compression (Credé's manoeuvre). Besides the metabolic problems which occasionally ensue when a bowel segment is incorporated into the urinary tract, the main complications of substitution cystoplasty are reflux and incontinence. The latter is particularly troublesome when, as is common, there is weakness of the sphincter due to damage to its innervation when the bladder is removed. Peristaltic waves in tubular sections of bowel generate enough pressure to force urine past the weakened sphincter and stress incontinence and incontinence at night are common. Various ingenious surgical manoeuvres designed to detubular-ize the bowel have gone some way to overcome this problem.

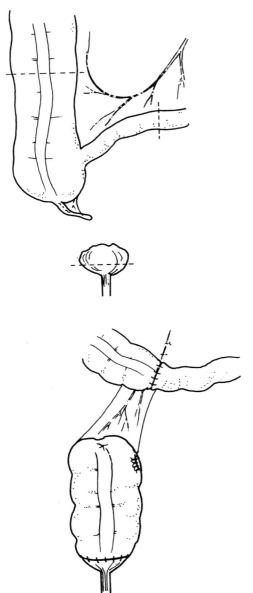

Figure 34.16 Substitution cystoplasty. The shrivelled bladder is excised and the isolated caecum sutured in its place

Augmentation cystoplasty

In augmentation cystoplasty, the aim is not to remove the bladder but to increase the volume of urine which it will hold. A scarred, shrunken bladder can be augmented by a caecocystoplasty. When the problem is of uncontrolled detrusor contraction as in insta-bility or hyperreflexia, a different approach can be used. The 'clam' cystoplasty is a simple operation which is very effective in dissipating the pressure generated by unwanted detrusor activity. In the clam operation (Figure 34.17), the bladder is bisected in the coronal plane, taking care to protect the ureters as the incision is taken to within a centimetre of the trigone. An isolated tube of ileum is opened along its anti-mesenteric border and the resulting sheet of small bowel is sewn as a gusset into the defect in the bladder. Detrusor–sphincter dyssynergia, a failure of appropriate sphincter relaxation during voiding, often accompanies hyperreflexia and may interfere with voiding postoperatively. Some patients will need to empty the augmented bladder by clean intermittent self-catheterization.

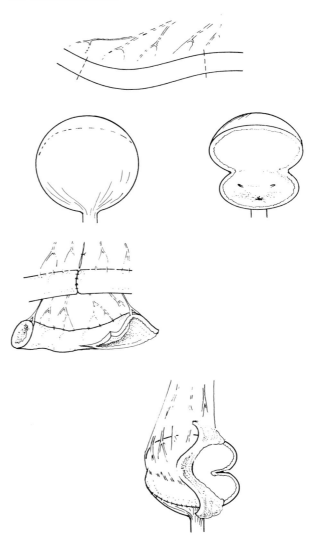

Figure 34.17 Augmentation ('clam') cystoplasty. The bladder is bivalved in the coronal plane and a patch made of mobilized ileum is inserted in the defect

Operations for stress incontinence

Stress incontinence occurs as a result of weakness of the normal mechanism which shuts the bladder outlet when intravesical pressure rises with intra-abdominal straining. It is uncommon in men, in whom it is almost always due to lower motor neuron damage to the innervation to the external urethral sphincter or surgical damage to the sphincter itself. In women, it is usually a late result of neuromuscular injury probably sustained in childbirth.

The patient gives a typical history and the stress test (demonstrable leakage of urine on abdominal straining) is often positive. The diagnosis of genuine stress incontinence is made on the basis of a filling cystometrogram which shows no evidence of detrusor instability and videocystographic evidence of bladder neck descent, 'beaking' of contrast at the bladder neck or frank incontinence when intra-abdominal pressure rises. Some patients with stress incontinence may respond to pelvic floor physiotherapy, but many of them can only be cured by surgery.

Anterior colposuspension

Many operations have been devised to cure stress incontinence in women by supporting the bladder neck. An anterior colposuspension is performed through a Pfannenstiel incision under spinal or general anaesthesia. The patient is in the lithotomy position and draped and prepared so that an assistant can have access to the vagina. A urethral catheter is inserted.

By blunt dissection in the retropubic space, the tissue on either side of the bladder neck is swept laterally until the vagina is exposed in the depths of the wound to each side of the urethra. At this stage the assistant inserts fingers into the vagina and flexes them to push the anterior vaginal wall towards the pubis on either side of the urethral catheter. Strong absorbable sutures are then placed in the vaginal wall and taken through a convenient part of the fascia on the back of the pubis. Tightening these sutures pulls the vagina forwards as a sling supporting the bladder neck.

Endoscopic bladder neck suspension

Anterior colposuspension is an effective operation, but it involves a major surgical incision, and a period of up to 10 days of postoperative urethral catheterization is usually recommended. Endoscopic bladder neck incision, usually a modification of the operation described by Stamey, is a much lesser procedure which seems to give broadly similar results (Figure 34.18).

After a preliminary cystoscopy, a urethral catheter is inserted and the balloon inflated. A tiny suprapubic incision is made and special long-eyed needle is passed 'blindly' through the rectus muscle in its sheath, behind the pubic bone and onwards until the tip of the needle penetrates the anterior wall of the vagina. This rather alarming puncture is guided by 'feel' with the aid of two fingers placed in the vagina

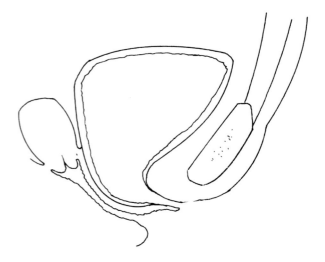

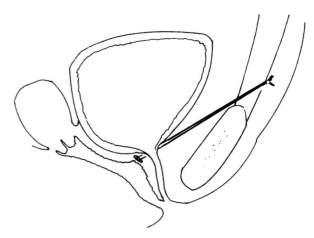

Figure 34.18 In the Stamey endoscopic bladder neck suspension, non-absorbable sutures pull the anterior vaginal wall forward to support the bladder neck

and flexed anteriorly to either side of the urethral catheter. A strong nylon suture is then inserted into the eye of the needle and drawn back along the track as the needle is withdrawn. The suture is then secured in the vagina according to the preference of the surgeon. In the Stamey operation, the vaginal suture is buttressed with a short length of Teflon tubing and buried beneath the epithelium through a separate vaginal incision. In later and simpler modifications of the operation, the suture is simply taken through all layers of the vaginal wall as a mattress suture. In either case the free end of the nylon suture is picked up by a separate pass of the eyed needle and withdrawn onto the anterior abdominal wall. The same procedure is repeated on both sides of the bladder neck. When both sutures are in place, the catheter is taken out and the bladder inspected to check that neither of them has inadvertently been passed through it. The sutures are then carefully tightened while the bladder neck is viewed endoscopically as it is pulled anteriorly by the sling of vaginal wall behind it. The tension to be used in tightening the sutures is a matter of judgement. If they are too loose, the operation will fail; if too tight, there is a danger of postoperative retention. It is usual to leave a suprapubic catheter which is clamped two or three days after the operation. If the woman fails to void, a more prolonged period of catheterization may be needed. In a few patients the urethra may need to be dilated or the tension of the sutures slackened.

Acknowledgement

The author would like to thank Professor John Blandy for his help with the figures.

Further reading

Blandy, J. P. (1984) *Operative Urology*, 2nd edn, Blackwell, Oxford

Gingell, J. C. and Abrams, P. H. (eds) (1988) *Controversies and Innovations in Urological Surgery*, Springer, London

Whitfield, H. N. and Hendry, W. F. (eds) (1985) *Textbook of Genito-urinary Surgery*, Churchill Livingstone, London

35

The scrotum, testes and penis

P. J. B. Smith

The scrotum

The scrotum is a musculocutaneous sac containing the testes and the distal ends of the spermatic cords. Beneath the rugose layer of skin is an area of loose connective tissue richly endowed with vascular tissue and containing an attendant layer of muscle known as the 'dartos'. This represents a portion of the subcutaneous muscle that covers many animals, but in man is only represented here, in the platysma and in certain facial muscles. In the midline the dartos extends backwards to form a septum which divides the cavity of the scrotum into two parts. Beneath the scrotum lie the fascial tissues that invest the testis and cord. These layers fuse at the triangular ligament and perineum below and above and are continuous with the subcutaneous fascia of the abdominal wall and upper anterior extent of the thigh.

Because of its excellent blood supply and the presence of a cutaneous contractile muscle in the dartos, the scrotum has excellent healing properties. Lacerations usually require no sutures, the main indication for stitching being to control bleeding.

By far the most important surgical manoeuvre relating to the scrotum is the formal incision and subsequent closure required for operations on its contents. These procedures can be done under local anaesthetic, the loose subcutaneous connective tissue being particularly easy to infiltrate. After cleaning the skin with spirit the scrotum is towelled up, particular care being taken to exclude the perianal area. The scrotum is then held on stretch and, with one hand steadying it behind, a transverse incision is made so as to expose the contents of one or both compartments. The incision is made through all layers including the dartos which is seen to fall back against the tension of the cut tissues. Further dissection will depend on the precise procedure involved.

To close this incision it is important to remember the vascular nature of the tissues. If such closure is done inadequately an extensive scrotal haematoma will occur. The incisions are closed with 2/0 chromic catgut on a cutting or tapered needle. Non-absorbable stitches are not indicated as they must be removed subsequently, often a more difficult procedure than the original operation. Although catgut stitches do produce a local reaction this soon disappears as surface catgut disintegrates within a week or so, particularly if the patient bathes daily in saline. The stitches should take all layers of the scrotum.

Two or three horizontal stitches are inserted so as to 'keel up' the scrotal skin. This layer is now closed with individual catgut stitches. With careful closure it should be possible to minimize the risk of haematoma.

Sebaceous cysts are common in the scrotum and, as elsewhere, can be nucleated with minimal dissection. The rarely encountered squamous cell carcinoma of scrotum is treated by wide excision. Such is the extent of scrotal tissue that primary closure is seldom difficult in these cases.

The testes

Epididymal cyst

The differential diagnosis of epididymal cyst and hydrocele is rarely of clinical importance. It lies in the fact that the epididymal cyst is separate from the testicle which, unlike in a hydrocele, can easily be felt. The differentiation of epididymal cyst into clear cyst and spermatocele has no clinical relevance. As with a hydrocele, the indications for surgery are cosmetic stress and local discomfort.

Treatment by aspiration and sclerosant therapy is not as easy or as effective as in hydrocele treatment. This is because an epididymal cyst is multilocular and hence difficult to drain properly. A cure is therefore best achieved by formal excision.

Excision of the cyst is achieved by careful dissection under general or regional anaesthesia. Following a transverse incision through the scrotal wall, the cyst and attached testicle are delivered. The epididymal cyst is seen to be covered with layers of thin fascia rich in blood vessels. All these layers need to be carefully incised using a scalpel for establishing the plane and scissors for its development (Figure 35.1a).

By holding the cyst firmly from behind, these layers are put on tension – facilitating their dissection. If by mischance one of the cysts is ruptured a tissue forceps (Duval or Babcock) can be used to close the leak and keep the remainder of the cyst as distended as possible. Eventually a plane is reached in which there are no blood vessels – the outer wall of the epididymal cyst. Using scissors and gentle dissection with a gauze pledget, the cyst is mobilized until its base on the epididymis is reached (Figure 35.1b). This, though small, is often adherent and may need to be formally excised, occasionally with a small amount of adjacent

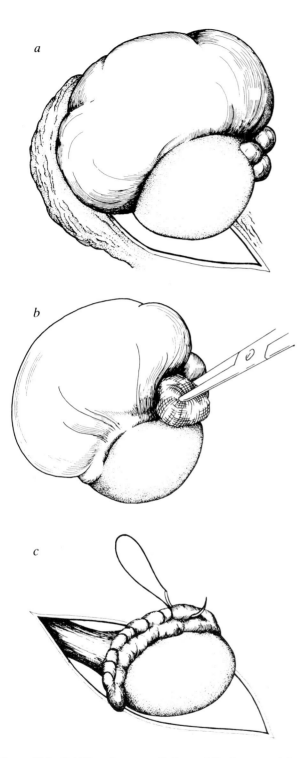

Figure 35.1 Epididymal cyst. *a*, Delivery following scrotal incision. *b*, Dissection of the cyst from the epididymis and testis. *c*, Following removal of the cyst wall its layers are obliterated using haemostatic suture

normal epididymal tissue (Figure 35.1c). Any bleeding points are coagulated and the tissue spaces and scrotum closed (Figure 35.2). No drain is required.

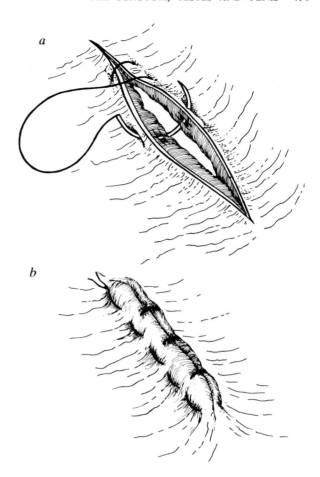

Figure 35.2 Closure of the scrotum should be undertaken carefully to ensure haemostasis

Hydrocele

A hydrocele is a cystic swelling of the sac surrounding the testes. This sac which persists after closure of the processus vaginalis, along which the testicle migrates from an abdominal to a scrotal position, invests the greater part of the testis. Hydroceles are common in the elderly male where they represent an acquired failure of reabsorption of hydrocele fluid. This may be associated with degenerative changes or chronic inflammation in the lining of the hydrocele. In the young male a hydrocele may arise as a reaction to trauma, infection or rarely, but importantly, testicular tumour. Hydroceles in infants and children usually relate to failure or closure of the processus vaginalis and as such are normally combined with an inguinoscrotal hernia.

A hydrocele is generally speaking a benign condition. When doubt exists about a possible underlying malignant testis, as in a young man with a lax hydrocele, scrotal ultrasound is required to prevent inappropriate treatment.

Surgery is usually required to relieve the symptoms of a hydrocele. These consist of the cosmetic distress caused by often quite large cysts, together with local discomfort and inconvenience. The surgical procedures available can be divided into aspiration of the hydrocele; installation of sclerosants; or the excision, plication or eversion of the greater part of the hydrocele sac.

Aspiration of a hydrocele is a time-honoured method of treatment. Although at one time it involved an impressive array of trocars and cannulas, the development of modern disposable materials now leaves a simple requirement of a Venflon needle, a three-way tap and a 50 ml Luer–Lok syringe. The hydrocele is steadied through the scrotum and a few millilitres of local anaesthetic infiltrated into the most prominent part of the stretched scrotal skin. Care must be taken to avoid the testicle which always lies below and behind the hydrocele sac. The Venflon needle is now inserted through the scrotal skin and the three-way tap applied. The hydrocele fluid is aspirated until the sac is empty. When installation of a sclerosant is used, this is now inserted along the Venflon needle prior to its removal. A variety of materials are used, including a dilute solution of tetracycline. Sclerosant therapy may be painful and it is best to use a cord block with 1% lignocaine in the event of its usage.

The fluid removed is traditionally described as 'straw-coloured'. It should normally be sent for microscopy, cytology and microbiology. If the hydrocele is associated with a chronic epididymitis, then consideration should be given to tuberculosis cultures. The main problem with aspiration alone is that it is not curative and the hydrocele may well re-form. This can occur too despite sclerosant therapy.

In general, then, the effective cure of a hydrocele is best achieved by direct surgery. The principles involved in this surgery are first the drainage of the hydrocele and then the elimination of the greater part of the hydrocele sac by its eversion, plication or direct excision. In this way the remaining portion of the sac invested in the testicle will communicate direct with the scrotal cavity through which absorption occurs readily.

Whichever technique is intended, the basic approach is the same. The hydrocele is delivered through a transverse all-layer scrotal incision. Often with a long-standing hydrocele there will be extensive adhesions with increased vascularity in the connective and fascial layers of the scrotum. Meticulous haemostasis using either diathermy or direct ligation is required. Excessive dissection and in particular blunt dissection with a gauze swab are to be discouraged. These manoeuvres increase the postoperative morbidity and predispose to haematoma and secondary sepsis. Although bipolar diathermy is best, monopolar currents can be used provided that the scrotal contents are kept in close contact with the body surface. In children, however, there is a risk, particularly if the cord or testis is on stretch, of coagulation of vessels due to the compression in the run-off of the current. In such situations bipolar diathermy alone should be used.

Having delivered the hydrocele through the scrotal incision, it is now incised longitudinally in its anterior surface (Figure 35.3). The hydrocele fluid is drained and the sac opened with scissors throughout its sagittal plane. The underlying testis is inspected to confirm its benign nature.

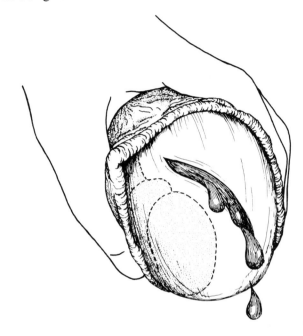

Figure 35.3 Hydrocele. An incision is made well anterior to the testis

Thin-walled hydroceles, as seen particularly in children, are treated effectively by the Jaboulay procedure in which the two halves of the sac are everted and sutured together across the back of the testis (Figure 35.4a). In adults with thin-walled hydroceles it is usually best to plicate the sac. A series of 2/0 catgut stitches on a cutting needle are inserted at 1 cm intervals from the sinus of the testis to the outward incised margin of the sac. These radial interrupted stitches are then tied so as to bunch up at the hydrocele leaving a ruff of tissue around the sinus of the testis (Figure 35.4b). In experienced hands it is possible to plicate the sac through a small scrotal incision without the need for excessive mobilization or even deliverance of the testis. The saving in dissection of this is, however, minimal and in most situations the technique described above is preferable.

In some, particularly long-standing hydroceles in the elderly, the sac is thick-walled and not suitable for plication. In these patients formal excision of the sac down to the testicular margin is required (Figure 35.4c). Care should be taken where the sac extends up on to the cord so as to prevent damage to the vessels of the testicle. Bleeding can be heavy in this excision technique and meticulous haemostasis with diathermy and underrunning catgut stitches are essential to prevent postoperative haematoma formation.

On completion of whatever surgery was used to the hydroceled sac, the testis is returned to the scrotum which is closed in the approved manner. Drainage is not required. Where dissection has been extensive and in particular where previous sepsis has been present, prophylaxis with a broad-spectrum antibiotic is indicated. Patients should be warned of the considerable local bruising and swelling that inevitably follows such scrotal surgery. A period of bed-rest for a few days should be followed by a period of convalescence using an appropriate scrotal support. Although the main effects of the surgery will have resolved within 2 weeks, it may be up to 2 months before the operation can be considered complete.

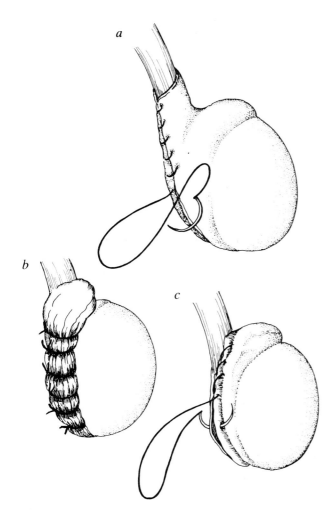

Figure 35.4 Hydrocele. *a*, The Jaboulay procedure of eversion and posterior suture of the hydrocele. *b*, Obliteration of hydrocele by plication. *c*, Obliteration by excision of redundant tissue and haemostatic suturing

Varicocele

This is a condition of varicosity in the pampiniform plexus of the testicle. It is usually confined to the left side where the left testicular vein drains directly into the left renal vein. Should valves not be present in the testicular vein there can be considerable back-pressure into the venous pampiniform plexus of the testicle producing the varicocele. Rarely this situation may arise in association with obstruction of the renal vein by carcinoma of the kidney.

Usually, though, a varicocele is an isolated benign condition. It requires surgical treatment only in relation to symptoms. The symptoms consist of local discomfort, traditionally a dragging sensation in the groin and scrotum or cosmetic distress from the so-called 'bag of worms' that arises in advanced cases.

In the past, varicocele was thought to be associated with male infertility. It was felt that in some way the varicocele reduced sperm motility. Despite the many and genuine 'clinical impressions' that ligation of a varicocele improved fertility, there has been no convincing evidence that this is so and no scientific proof produced to indicate the role of a varicocele in the pathology of infertility and sperm hypomotility in particular.

The operation for cure of a varicocele consists of ligation of the testicular veins draining the varicocele. This is best achieved by the so-called 'high operation' which involves identifying the testicular veins at or about the internal ring at the top of the inguinal canal. The patient under general anaesthetic is placed on a non-slip mattress. After cleaning the skin and towelling up, an inguinal incision is made. The inguinal canal is opened in the routine manner with care being taken to preserve the ilio-inguinal nerve as it passes through the external ring. The spermatic cord is identified at the internal ring either within the canal or by extraperitoneal dissection above. The dilated testicular veins, usually numbering two or three at this point, are dissected free. Intermittent reverse Trendelenburg tilt may be required to fill the veins for full identification. The cord is carefully dissected so as to free the vas and other tissues – in particular the testicular artery. This artery is difficult to see and feel. However, by isolating the veins it is protected from damage. The veins are divided with the excision of a segment of approximately 1 cm to prevent any risk of reanastomosis (Figure 35.5a–c).

Occasional varicose connections are seen at the lower end of the incision in the region of the pubic cubicle. These represent veins that pass into the obturator area whence they drain into the deep pelvic veins. These veins must also be divided, since if left they can prevent resolution of the varicocele. The incision is closed in layers with catgut to the deep tissues and nylon or subcuticular Dexon to the skin. No drain is required.

An alternative approach – the 'low operation' – makes a direct approach to the varicocele through

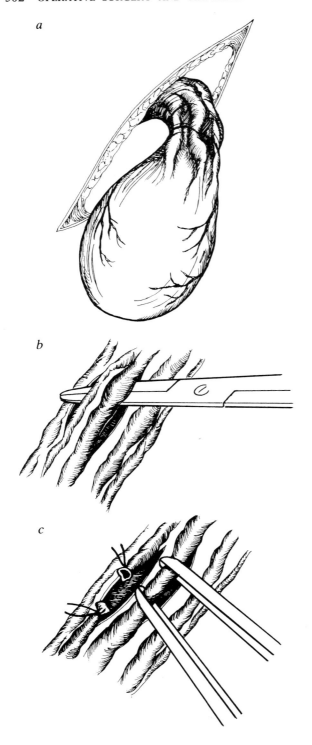

Figure 35.5 *a*, Delivery of spermatic cord and testis through scrotal incision. *b*, Identification of vas deferens and testicular artery. *c*, Varicocele. Division of veins and removal of varicosity

the scrotum itself. This is not nearly as easy a dissection since by this time the veins are many and multiple and closely associated with the varicocele itself. It may be difficult to see the other contents of the cord

and in particular the testicular artery. Ligation of every vein relating to the varicocele is difficult due to their multiplicity and tortuosity. Similarly, this exposure will not allow identification of the occasional retropubic venous connections mentioned above. The 'high operation' is therefore preferable in the majority of cases. Both procedures involve a 'defunctioning' of the varicocele rather than its formal excision. This means that for some time after the patient will still have the veins of the pampiniform plexus but not dilated. With time, usually 3–6 months, the remnants of the varicocele atrophy and both local pain and cosmetic distress are alleviated.

Undescended and ectopic testis

Maldescended, the testis presents either as an arrest of testicular migration in the inguinal canal – the undescended testis – or migration outside the normal line of descent – the ectopic testis. In both situations it is preferable to manoeuvre the testis into a scrotal position. This is required both for cosmetic and physiological reasons. With improvements in anaesthetic technique and infant care such surgery can be done in the neonatal period. However, it is generally best left till somewhere in the 2nd to 5th years for both medical and social reasons. Care must be taken in diagnosis, as some children have retractile testes which if left alone will occupy a normal scrotal position in due course. The use of hormone therapy to stimulate descent is generally viewed unfavourably.

The operation of repositioning of the testicle is known as orchidopexy. Under a general anaesthetic the groin is prepared with spirit and suitable towelling. An incision is made over the inguinal canal. The incision is deepened, taking care in the case of an ectopic testis which is superficial, to avoid damage to the cord. The ectopic testis is readily identified beneath the superficial layer of deep fascia from where it is put on stretch. This allows any remaining superficial fascial tissues to be dissected free. The testis and its cord are now held in three tissue layers which must be divided separately so as to steadily mobilize the cord and allow the testicle to reach the scrotum.

The same principle applies to the undescended testis which lies in some part of the inguinal canal. In both situations the inguinal canal is now opened by making a small incision in the aponeurosis of the external oblique muscle. This incision is extended upwards and laterally with scissors to reach the fibres of the internal oblique as they sweep upwards across the internal ring (Figure 35.6) Downward extension of the incision will open the external ring and at the same time divide the investing layer of external spermatic fascia. This is the first of the three holding layers. In the case of an ectopic testis this may be all that is required to achieve sufficient mobility and length to achieve a scrotal position. With an undescended testis, though, further mobilization is required.

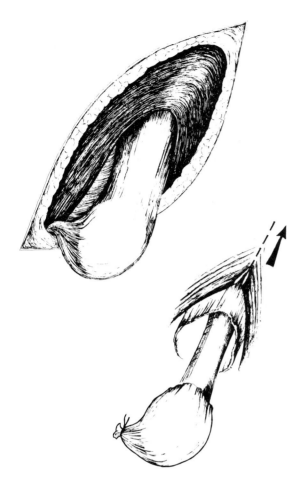

Figure 35.6 Orchidopexy. Exposure of the undescended testis and its investing layers. The investing layers are carefully divided, preserving the cord, following which proximal mobilization of the cord within the inguinal canal will allow the testis to be replaced within the scrotum

This involves dividing the two remaining tissue layers. The first of these is the internal spermatic fascia and its adjacent cremasteric muscle. By holding the testis on tension, this layer can be gently dissected off the cord using fine dissecting scissors or forceps. Although there is little bleeding at this point, coagulation diathermy is occasionally required. Bipolar diathermy is preferable.

This division of the cremasteric muscle and internal spermatic fascia exposes the cord down to the vascular pedicle and adjacent vas. On occasion, particularly in relation to an undescended testis, a small hernial sac (the remnants of the processus vaginalis) can be detected at this point. If present it should be dissected from the cord using scissors and ligated at the internal ring. Further mobilization of the cord at this point is achieved by division of the third and final layer of investing fascia. This is a layer of deep fascia which specifically surrounds the testicular vessels as

they pass from the retroperitoneal space through the internal ring. Under tension, this tissue is readily seen as it fans out. It is divided with scissors, care being taken to avoid damage to the vessels. This final manoeuvre is often the crucial step in achieving adequate mobilization of the cord in undescended testes. Once the cord has been fully mobilized, the hydrocele sac of the testis is opened and everted. This prevents any risk of hydrocele formation and encourages subsequent proper fixation of the testes and the scrotum.

The positioning of the testicle in the scrotum following this mobilization is achieved by the formation of a scrotal subcutaneous pouch. This is all that is required to hold the testis in its proper position. The previous crude manoeuvres of nylon stitch or, worse still, Keetley–Torek thigh stitch are no longer acceptable. Such a pouch is constructed by first opening up the inguinoscrotal canal by finger dissection from above. The index finger is pushed through into the scrotum and the scrotal skin stretched over it. A transverse incision is made in the most prominent point, as low as possible, about 1 cm in length. The incision should pass only through the scrotal skin. Scissor dissection is now performed with the finger still in place and the tissue still under tension. A subcutaneous space is opened up in all directions sufficient to take the testicle (Figure 35.7). The deeper dartos layer is now incised just sufficient to take the tip of an artery forceps. This is passed from below and with simultaneous withdrawal of the finger through the inguinoscrotal canal the forceps is presented through the neck of the scrotum into the inguinal wound. Here it is used to grasp the base of the testis which is then drawn back down into the scrotum and, with suitable encouragement using forceps, manipulated into the subcutaneous scrotal pouch (Figure 35.8). The dartos should sit snugly around the cord which should be checked to make sure it is not rotated or obstructed in any way. The scrotal incision is closed with interrupted 2/0 catgut stitches, one of which may be used to pick up a portion of the exposed tunica of the testis to complete fixation. The inguinal incision is closed with catgut and either nylon or subcuticular Dexon. No drains are required.

Rarely, with severe forms of undescended testis, sufficient mobilization of the cord cannot be achieved by the above methods. This is particularly true when the testis lies at the internal ring or even in an intra-abdominal position. In such situations where a normal contralateral testis is present in the scrotum, orchidectomy may be preferable. Where this is not possible, as in bilateral disease, complex peritoneal 'flap' techniques have been developed. Details of these methods are available in advanced paediatric urology textbooks.

The key to successful orchidopexy is not scrotal fixation but adequate mobilization of the cord.

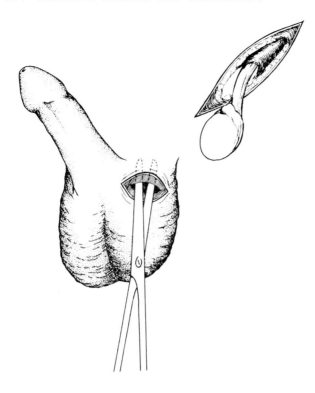

Figure 35.7 Orchidopexy. Following the creation of a scrotal pouch with the finger, the scrotum is opened

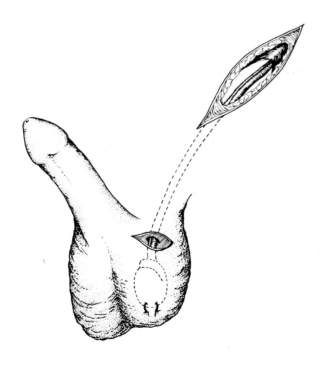

Figure 35.8 Orchidopexy. Through this opening the testis and the fully mobilized spermatic cord may be drawn into the most dependent part of the scrotum and held in place by sutures.

Torsion of testis

This is a condition of rotation of the testis about its cord, producing strangulation of its blood supply. Although it may be congenital or occur in the mature male, torsion most commonly is seen in young boys and adolescents. The sudden onset of pain, swelling and tenderness in the testicle in this age group, particularly if associated with exercise, should suggest torsion and indicate the need for urgent exploration.

Manipulation of the testis to reverse the rotation has been suggested. This may be worth attempting in the anaesthetic room immediately prior to surgery. Relief at this stage may give a few vital minutes of oxygenation to the testicle. At operation, the scrotum is opened through a standard transverse incision and the testis and cord delivered. The incision should include both halves of the scrotum so as to expose the contralateral healthy testis. The torted testicle is now untwisted. Even a dusky, congested testis is worth preserving. Even though it may have no further spermatogenic function, it may continue to contribute to hormone activity. Suggestions that torsion may contribute to subsequent problems of infertility have not been substantiated.

Only a clearly infarcted testicle should be removed since the loss of a testis may be psychologically damaging. If there is no sign of recovery of circulation following several minutes of exposure to warm saline swabs, this is achieved by simple ligation of the cord at the scrotal neck using catgut. If the testis is preserved it is necessary to fix both it and, either way, its companion to prevent further torsion. Synthetic (Vicryl) stitches are inserted through the base of each testicle and thence to the dartos muscle in the base of the scrotum. These are tied, thus fixing the testicle. This stitch, together with the local adhesions that follow surgery, should prevent further torsion. The wound is closed in the usual manner.

Testicular tumour

Testicular tumour is one of the commonest cancers affecting young men. It may be in the form of a relatively well-differentiated seminoma or an increasingly poorly differentiated teratoma. Tumour, particularly when teratomatous, is associated with widespread metastatic disease. This in turn is related to the development of tumour markers by way of serum hormone substances. A testicular tumour usually presents as a painless, or only mildly uncomfortable, progressive swelling of the testicle. It is sometimes associated with a lax hydrocele. The first and most important treatment for a testicular tumour is radical orchidectomy.

The surgical approach is through the groin because attempts to expose the tumour through a scrotal incision would run the slight risk of inducing tumour implantation in the incision, should the tumour capsule be breached during the exposure.

The inguinal incision is generous so as to expose the inguinal canal up to the internal ring. The canal is opened in the usual way, with preservation of the ilio-inguinal nerve. The cord is mobilized up to the internal ring (Figure 35.9). At this point a vascular compression clamp or constricting loop of a small catheter is applied to the cord, effectively obstructing both venous and lymphatic circulations. This minimizes any risk of tumour emboli extension during the subsequent handling of the testicle and its tumour. The testicle is now delivered through the neck of the scrotum by gentle traction from above and pressure from below.

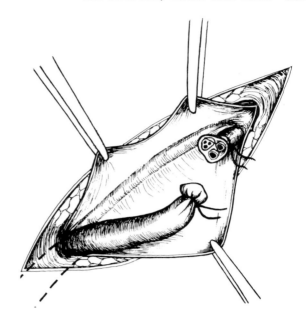

Figure 35.10 Orchidectomy. It is a good plan to divide the cord within the inguinal canal as early as possible and before delivery of the testis from the scrotum

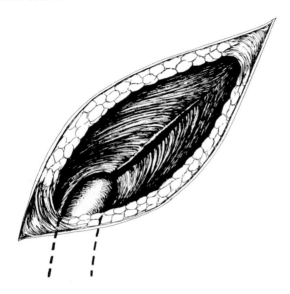

Figure 35.9 Orchidectomy. Exposure of the inguinal canal and spermatic cord

Confirmation of tumour presence is obtained by palpation and inspection. If necessary, any hydrocele may be drained so as to further confirm the diagnosis. Although in practice there is seldom any doubt about the presence of a testicular tumour, facilities do exist for biopsy and frozen section examination, or even incision and direct inspection of the cut surface (i.e. Chevassu manoeuvre).

Following confirmation of the presence of a tumour, the cord is fully mobilized up to the external ring where it is ligated (Figures 35.10 and 35.11). If necessary, the cord may be partially dissected so as to apply two ligatures. This is particularly helpful in the presence of a fatty cord. This minimizes any risk of the ligature slipping subsequently. The radical operation should remove all cord tissue as far as the internal ring, as well as the testis. Dissection of the cord at this point should also include a careful check to make certain that no hernial sac is involved. The incision is closed in layers with 2/0 catgut and nylon or subcuticular Dexon to the skin. No drainage is required.

There is no surgical, as opposed to diagnostic, urgency about orchidectomy for testicular tumour. In the preoperative period full assessment should be made and in particular serum samples obtained for measurement of gonadotrophin and alpha-fetoprotein estimations. Chest X-ray and CT scan of the abdomen are also required at this stage for staging the tumour. These measurements, together with the histology, and in particular microscopic examination of the cord, provide the basis for any subsequent treatment. Whereas in some early tumours, and in particular in seminoma, surgery alone by radical orchidectomy may be sufficient treatment, it is usual, however, that other patients, particularly with teratoma, may require adjunctive treatment. This is in the form of radiotherapy and/or chemotherapy. The management of this aspect of treatment is usually handed over to medical oncologists. The surgeon may, however, be subsequently requested to perform lymphadenectomy of residual tumour masses following successful localization and downgrading of para-aortic and occasionally pelvic lymph node metastases.

Subcapsular orchidectomy

Subcapsular orchidectomy is used in the management of metastatic and prostatic cancer. It is an operation whereby all the functioning testicular tissue, particularly the androgen-producing Leydig cells, are removed. The operation is simple and by leaving the outer shell of testicle behind, less psychologically debilitating to the patient than formal castration.

Through a transverse scrotal incision both testes are delivered. A sagittal incision in the tunica of each

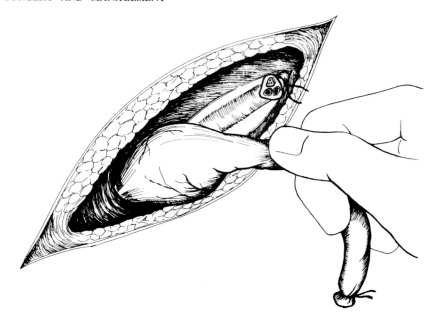

Figure 35.11 Orchidectomy. Removal of testis following ligation of cord

exposes the soft yellow homogeneous testicular tissue. This is now expressed by squeezing the testis around a dry gauze swab. The testis thus presented is removed by blunt dissection. Any residual tissue adherent to the posterior wall is coagulated. The empty shell of the testis is closed by suturing the incision in the tunica with 2/0 catgut. Any subsequent fluid or haematoma formation will serve to compensate for any cosmetic deficiency. The testicular remnants are returned to the scrotum which is closed in the usual manner. No drain is required.

Finally, a word about testicular prostheses. These are now readily available in a variety of sizes consistent with the patient's age. The prosthesis is made of a soft Silastic material. It has a flange at its lower border which can be sutured to the base of the dartos in the scrotum. This fixation ensures that it will occupy the correct anatomical plane. Such a prosthesis may compensate for any psychological distress caused by orchidectomy, particularly in those rare sad cases where this is bilateral. Not all patients, however, request such prostheses, preferring to rely on the single normal contralateral testis that remains to answer their psychological needs.

Vasectomy

The vas is a richly innervated muscular tube with an epithelial lining. It serves to conduct sperm from the epididymis to the ejaculatory duct. Its single and most important relationship to the surgeon is in the operation of vasectomy for male sterilization. Pre-operative counselling is an essential feature of any vasectomy service. Such counselling not only serves

to confirm the patient's suitability for the operation, but also provides the opportunity to give him full and frank details about the procedure itself. Such information is essential, since the vast majority of men undergoing this operation have no intrinsic medical defects and are usually being sterilized to protect the health of their wife or the socio-economic well-being of them both. Any complications or problems relating to vasectomy must be viewed in this light and it must be accepted that the man's attitude to any such complication will be different from that associated with normal surgical procedures for pathological disease.

The counselling must, in addition to details of the operation itself, also fully explain the potential failure rate associated with this method. Such failures are associated with spontaneous reanastomosis of the cut vas. This usually occurs across a granuloma formed from the proximal end. Spontaneous reversal can occur under any conditions and no one method of vasectomy is safe from this problem. Early spontaneous reversal will occur in the first 3 months. For this reason, though most men become sterile within a few weeks, the post-vasectomy semen analysis required to confirm this is deliberately postponed for 14 and 16 weeks. Only if sperm counts are negative at this stage can the operation be considered complete and the patient advised that he can rely on it as a contraceptive method. Furthermore, patients must be warned that, despite this apparent successful conclusion, cases have now been recorded where spontaneous reversal of vasectomy may occur some years later. However, the odds are extremely long: figures of 1 in 10 000 to 1 in 30 000 of such late spontaneous reversals have been described. There is no practical

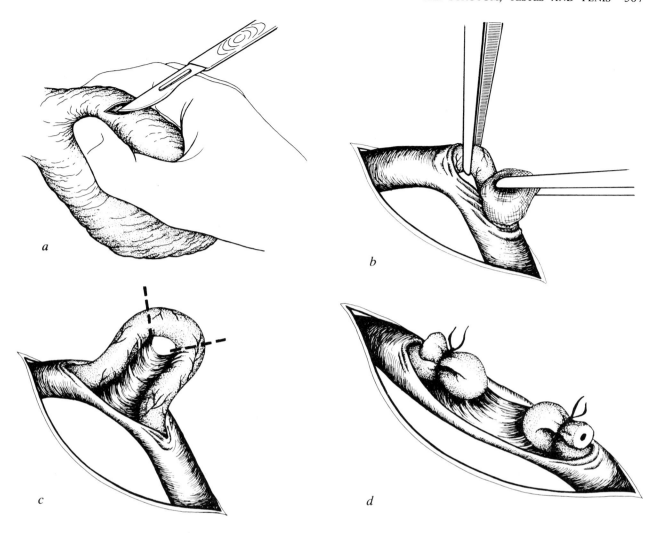

Figure 35.12 Vasectomy. *a*, The vas is displaced subcutaneously and the scrotal skin is divided over its prominence. *b*, The delivered vas is held with tissue forceps and dissected by sharp and blunt dissection. *c, d*. A short length of vas is removed (*c*) and the end carefully tied, or folded and tied (*d*)

method of detecting such late reversals, but at least should a pregnancy arise in this remote eventuality the couple will be reassured that the pregnancy is theirs and not due to any infidelity on the part of the female partner. Vasectomy carries a high litigation index and all surgeons involved in this operation must exercise the greatest care in counselling and advising the patients before allowing surgery to occur.

The operation itself is ideally performed under local anaesthetic. It involves the division, ligation and repositioning of the cut ends of the vas to prevent reanastomosis. Excision of excessive lengths of vas is meddlesome and unnecessary. Such extensive surgery may cause trauma to the distal end where it joins the ejaculatory ducts. Various extra techniques of banding, metal clipping and cauterizing the cut ends of the vas have been employed. While these may have their advocates, the basis of a successful vasectomy still

remains the careful dissection, ligation and transposition of the vas.

Having bathed and shaved the scrotal tissues the night before, the patient lies on the operating table. The genitalia are cleaned with Savlon. Suitable towelling is now applied to the scrotum. The testis is held between the finger and thumb of the hand and gently but firmly brought down. Through the tensed scrotum the vas can now be palpated with the fingers and thumb of the other hand. It is usually easily felt as a firm structure separate from the cord and usually medial to the testis. The testis is released but the finger and thumb holding the vas remain in position. The skin is infiltrated with local anaesthetic (1% lignocaine with or without adrenaline) and a 1 cm transverse incision is made through the scrotal wall (Figure 35.12a). The incision is stretched with artery forceps so as to divide the underlying connective tissue. The vas is now directly infiltrated with more local anaesthetic. This is in order to provide proximal anaesthesia into the cord proper. The exposed area of vas is now picked up between the jaws of a pair of tissue forceps (Allis).

The tissue forceps and their contained vas are now angled upwards to throw the loop of vas under tension. The vas will still be covered by fascial planes which may be extensive. It is vital to dissect away these layers to reveal an entirely naked vas. This is achieved by vertical incision of the tissues along the vas which itself gradually protrudes into the wound as the cut tissues retract. The vas has an unmistakable pearly-white appearance. Final freeing of the vas can be achieved with a gentle sweep of the loop of vas using a gauze swab (Figure 35.12b). The mesentery of the vas, with branches of its vessels, are seen and preserved. Using fine forceps the mesentery is opened and two artery forceps placed across the vas so as to leave 1–2 cm of vas exposed. This is then divided so as to produce two cut ends (Figure 35.12c). There is no need to excise a segment of vas – histology having no medical or indeed legal significance in this operation.

The cut ends of the vas are ligated with thread or Vicryl. Ligation is done in such as way as to ligate the main body of the vas initially and then, with a second knot, incorporate the cut end so as to bend back the divided vas (Figure 35.12d). The two ligated cut ends of the vas are then returned to the scrotum. The scrotal incision is closed with 2/0 catgut. No drainage is required.

It is best to divide both vasa through separate incisions. This prevents any chance of the same vas being ligated twice. Following vasectomy, simple gauze dressing is all that is required. The patient should be advised to commence daily salt baths the next day and to maintain these until the skin stitches have dissolved (7–10 days usually). He is again warned that the operation is not successful until he has had two negative sperm counts. This reinforces the advice given during the preoperative counselling. Sperm tests are designed for 14 and 16 weeks. Occasionally, even in successful procedures, a few sperm cells may linger. It is, however, essential to maintain repeated tests until two consecutive negative counts have been achieved. Regular ejaculation should be commenced as soon as possible. Most men find this can occur within a matter of days, although some may have a temporary psychological impotence in association with the discomfort relating to the operation

No vasectomy procedure is exempt from complications and a proportion of men will complain of pain and discomfort for some weeks after. Most, however, are able to return to work within a matter of 2–3 days. There is no firm rule on this, and all patients must be warned of the unpredictable nature of this operation. In some cases quite marked discomfort may persist or occur some months later. This problem of post-vasectomy pain is little understood.

It appears to be a form of causalgia and may relate to damage to the fine nerves associated with the vas or possibly due to trauma to the upper or proximal end of vas as it lies within the ejaculatory apparatus. Treatment for this post-vasectomy pain syndrome is difficult.

Reanastomosis of the vas

The proper care of the vas and its mesentery during vasectomy is essential not only for reasons of good surgical practice but also to give maximum assistance to the surgeon if subsequently a reanastomosis operation is requested. This technique is simple and carries a high success rate, provided that the vas was not divided too close to the epididymis and provided that only a minimum of vas and mesentery were removed during the original operation. Reanastomosis, though possible under a local anaesthetic, is best performed under general anaesthetic. Both vasa are mobilized through separate scrotal incisions and the area of vasectomy identified. This is readily seen, as there is a distinct area of fibrous swelling into which go the proximal and distal ends of each vas. Each segment of vas is carefully dissected, preserving its mesentery down to the scar tissue, and is then divided with scissors to expose a healthy cut surface with a readily identifiable lumen. Microsurgical techniques have been employed for this, but are not essential and, for those not used to the operating microscope, may prove to be a positive disadvantage. The two cut ends are now further dissected to ensure complete freedom and mobilization from the scarred area. The scar itself can be excised but this is not essential.

A 2/0 nylon ligature is now threaded down the lumen of the distal vas for 10 cm or so, in order to confirm its patency. With fine forceps and using 6/0 Dexon, four quadrant stitches are inserted through adjoining parts of both cut ends of the vas. After inserting all four stitches, each is tied. As these stitches are knotted, the two ends of the vas are drawn together and after withdrawal of the nylon splint the walls of the vas are brought into apposition. Several interrupted holding stitches are now placed in the surrounding fascia and are used to buttress the anastomosis.

The single, most important feature of reanastomosis is to have an adequate length of well-vascularized vas which again is dependent on the technique of the original vasectomy.

It is the case that where reanastomosis is technically successful, fertility may not necessarily follow, as the sperm in the ejaculate may be of poor quality. Nevertheless, with time there may be an improvement in sperm quality and an optimistic approach can be justified.

The penis

The penis is essentially a vascular organ. It consists of

two corpora cavernosa lying on either side of a central and underlying corpus spongiosum. Within the spongiosum lies the extension of the urethra – the penile urethra. The tip of the spongiosum dilates into the glans penis on the surface of which the urethra opens at the external meatus. Surrounding both corpora is a dense layer of fascia – Buck's fascia. Within the fascial planes and deep in the corpora lie the blood vessels and nerves relating to the erectile function of the penis. On the ventral surface similar vessels and nerves supply the urethra with one vascular bundle in particular – the frenular vessels – providing the blood supply of the glans itself. The terminal portion of penile skin surrounding the organ – the prepuce – is reflected back on itself so as to connect with the epithelium around the glans. Removal of this hood of skin is known as circumcision.

Circumcision

Ritual circumcision for religious reasons is one of the oldest and probably still most commonly performed of operations. In these circumstances it is performed either at birth or at the commencement of adolescence. The technique used is usually that of a simple guillotining of the skin. In proper surgical practice neither this method, nor indeed its indication, should be accepted practice. Circumcision, like any operation, is not without its complications or indeed, in the case of neonates, its potential mortality. It should be restricted to those situations in which disease of the foreskin warrants its removal. The commonest of these conditions is recurrent balanitis due to an underlying dermatological problem – balanitis xerotica obliterans.

Circumcision requires formal dissection together with adequate excision. Under general anaesthetic and after cleaning with aqueous Hibitane, the penis is towelled up. The line of excision should be indicated with skin ink so as to ensure a subsequent satisfactory cosmetic appearance. The edges of the foreskin are seized with the tips of two small forceps at 2 and 10 o'clock, respectively. A fine curved scissors is used to dilate any phimosis. The scissors are then used to break down adhesions between the glans and the inner surface of the foreskin. The scissors are advanced anteriorly until it is estimated that the coronal sulcus of the glans has been reached. A dorsal incision at 12 o'clock is then made with scissors to divide the foreskin down to the level of the sulcus (Figure 35.13 a,b). On peeling back the two sides of foreskin thus produced, further adhesions between the inner skin layer and glans are divided. Any smegma secretions are removed and the junction between the prepuce and the glans accurately defined.

With the two forceps still holding the distal rim of the divided foreskin, sharp scissor dissection of the 'ears' of foreskin is performed, starting at the tip of the dorsal incision and coming round in an oblique curve using the skin ink marking for guidance (Figure 35.13c). In this way the foreskin is completely removed, the final 'snip' dividing the frenulum on the ventral surface.

Bleeding points, including frenular vessels, are now ligated or coagulated with diathermy. Ligation should use fine plain catgut (3/0). Diathermy should be bipolar since monopolar techniques, particularly in children, run the risk of deep coagulation of the penile vessels proper or diathermy damage to the urethra. Any excess of inner mucosal layer can be trimmed so as to leave a clean rim of tissue around the coronal sulcus. This layer and that of the skin are now sutured together using 3/0 plain catgut on a cutting needle (Figure 35.13d). Attention is required at the frenulum to underrun any bleeding vessels, but special stitches in this area are not necessary and indeed, if used, can cause a less than satisfactory cosmetic appearance. Care should be taken to line up

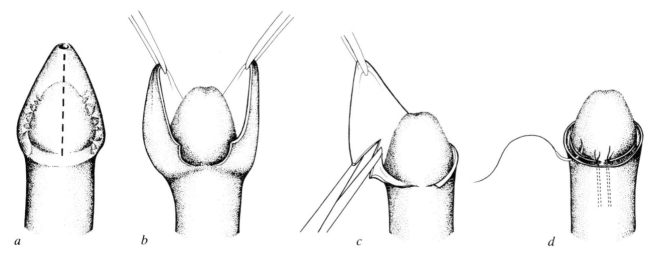

Figure 35.13 Circumcision. Initial dorsal slit (*a*) followed by separation from the glans (*b*). The foreskin is carefully removed (*c*), leaving a 2–4 mm rim of tissue which is then carefully sutured (*d*)

the skin prior to closure by inserting stitches at 12 and 6 o'clock, respectively. Traction on these stitches will present an even presentation of the two layers. Interrupted stitches are used commonly, but a continuous subcuticular stitch can be used if time permits. The operation site is finally cleaned with Hibitane and a simple dressing applied. In most cases this operation is on a day-case basis with the majority of patients being back to normal within 7–10 days following dissolution of the catgut stitches. The procedure is painful and adequate analgesia is required in the postoperative period. In addition, the use of a penile block using 1% plain lignocaine into the root of the penis gives useful postoperative pain control.

Peyronie's disease

This is a rare and little understood condition. It consists of a non-specific inflammatory reaction in one or both corpora cavernosa of the penis. Initial symptoms are of pain and discomfort, particularly on erection. This usually settles in the first few months, but is then replaced by a variable and progressive degree of distortion of the penis on erection. This is known as chordee. In the early stages, reassurance and analgesia are all that is required. The subsequent chordee may, however, cause significant difficulty with erection and intercourse. A minimum period of 12 months is required to allow for spontaneous resolution of this. In the event of it not occurring, then surgical correction can be performed using a technique known as Nesbitt's procedure. This technique in effect takes a 'tuck' from the contralateral healthy corpora which produces a mirror image of the fibrosis caused by the disease. Although complete straightening can never be guaranteed, it is usually possible to correct the chordee sufficient for satisfactory intercourse. The technique does inevitably cause some overall shortening of the penis and the patient should be warned of this beforehand. In extensive cases where considerable amounts of healthy corpora must be excised to produce straightening, this foreshortening can be a problem. Finally, in some patients the fibrosis may extend into both corpora and though a straight penis may be produced, the poor distal filling associated with the underlying disease may prevent the return of satisfactory intercourse. In these situations the use of a penile prosthesis may be considered (see below).

The operation of Nesbitt's procedure is performed under general anaesthesia following careful skin cleaning and towelling up. If the patient has already had a circumcision, then a simple coronal incision is made immediately behind the glans. Where the foreskin is still present it is necessary to perform a circumcision – the patient being warned of this beforehand. The penile skin is now dissected backwards so as to 'de-glove' the penis. A rubber tourniquet (fine catheter) is applied to the root of the penis. Saline under pressure is now injected via a Venflon (no. 21) needle

inserted into an area of corpora remote from the Peyronie's disease. In this way an artificial erection is produced. This demonstrates the extent and position of the Peyronie's disease and its consequent chordee. An area of healthy corpora diametrically opposite to the point of maximum tethering is now identified. If this involves the dorsum of the penis, care must be taken to isolate the dorsal nerves and the blood vessels. Careful dissection and the insertion of a 'marker' stitch is required. Where this dissection is required on the ventral surface, equally careful dissection must be made of the urethra and spongiosum. If necessary, the urethra may need to be mobilized off the corpora. Once the field is clear, a diamond-shaped excision is made of the corporal wall. This is now closed with 3/0 Vicryl interrupted stitches. A further artificial saline erection is produced to check on the degree of correction. This second saline erection is usually not as impressive due to inevitable leakage of some saline from the line of excision in the healthy corpora. However, a good idea can be achieved and if necessary further segments of corpora removed until a reasonably straight penis can be seen. Following this the fascial layers are closed and the skin reanastomosed as in a circumcision. The penis should be bandaged using wool and crepe in order to reduce postoperative swelling. Catheter drainage is not required.

Surgery for impotence

Erectile impotence may arise as a result of psychogenic, neurogenic or vasculogenic causes. Whatever the cause, the effect is a failure either to initiate or maintain a satisfactory erection for intercourse. Nonsurgical treatments are available for this problem. They include psychotherapy for those with predominantly psychogenic causes. In others the use of vacuum suction devices have proved helpful. The majority of patients with erectile impotence are, however, nowadays treated by intra-penile papaverine or prostaglandin injections. These drugs have the effect of altering the penile vascular flow so as to engorge the corpora and maintain an erection. The disadvantage is that these drugs have to be self-administered and many men, particularly elderly patients, find this difficult. In place of this so-call 'chemical' prosthesis, therefore, some men will occasionally opt for a penile prosthesis.

These come in either rigid or inflatable varieties. The inflatable varieties are inevitably more complex, more prone to complications and, of course, more expensive. Both types of prosthesis require similar surgical procedure for their insertion. In those inflatable prostheses with a remote pump, a separate incision is required to place this either in the lower abdominal wall or, more usually, in the scrotum in place of a testicle.

The insertion of the prosthesis itself into the penis is the same in all cases. The corpora are exposed, as described above, by either releasing the skin at the coronal sulcus or by formal circumcision or through an incision at the penis–scrotal junction. The subsequently de-gloved penis is dissected so as to show the corporal margins. A transverse incision is made behind the glans through the corpora on each side. Stay stitches are used to protect this incision. The corporal contents are now dilated using Hegar dilators, starting at no. 6 and increasing up to no. 13. Some bleeding occurs at this point and in between dilatations compression of the penis is required. A specially designed 'sizing' instrument is now inserted so as to measure the length of each corpora. A suitably selected prosthesis is now inserted, first upwards to the root of the penis and then by bending and 'shoe-horning' into the distal tip. Following insertion of the prosthesis any additional inflatable mechanisms are suitably implanted. For the simple rigid prosthesis nothing further need be done. The incision in the corpora is closed with 3/0 Vicryl. Care is taken to prevent any damage, particularly in the inflatable variety, to the underlying prosthesis. Special protective guards are provided by the prosthesis manufacturers for this. The incision is finally closed with Vicryl to the skin. As with all prostheses, prophylactic antibiotics and meticulous haemostasis are required to prevent secondary sepsis and prosthesis rejection.

Carcinoma of the penis

This is a rare squamous cell carcinoma. It never occurs in men circumcized at birth. It is often associated with chronic balanitis and phimosis, sometimes making its early diagnosis difficult. It spreads by local extension into the penis and by lymphatic extension into the superficial inguinal lymph nodes. Prognosis, as in most situations, is related to the grade and stage of the presenting tumour.

In early clinically localized disease, particularly in the elderly, a local excision can be performed. This should involve as wide a margin as possible away from the tumour site but leaving a reasonable stump of penile tissue so as to support an opening for the urethra. Where the external penis proper has to be excised, a perineal urethrostomy can be constructed. Wherever possible though, limited surgery in these situations will give the patient a better chance to cope with the emotional, and often sexual, frustrations that this surgery inevitably causes.

Under general anaesthesia and with a rubber catheter applied as a tourniquet to the base of the penis, an oblique incision is made on the penis proximal to the tumour. This incision should provide adequate clearance of the tumour and at the same time an adequate stump of penis. Superficial vessels, especially the dorsal vein, are ligated with 3/0 catgut and divided. The two corpora are now boldly divided in the same line as the skin incision, starting dorsally and extending the incision downwards on each side. This incision should not go through the spongiosum

and urethra at this time. The deep vessels in the corpora cavernosa are identified and ligated. Troublesome oozing can be treated by a 'figure-of-eight' stitch placed across the cavity of each corpora. Following this, the spongiosum and urethra are carefully dissected forwards for at least 1 cm beyond the line of division of the corpora. Following amputation of the penile tumour, this will leave a spout of urethra projecting. The skin flap previously constructed is now brought down over the raw corporal area and a slit cut to allow the urethral stump to project through. Any excess skin is trimmed and the flap now sewn across the penile stump using interrupted 3/0 catgut.

The urethral stump is left projecting. It will remodel itself back to the skin line over the next few weeks. No catheter or drain is required. This technique provides a better urethral opening than more formal skin-to-mucosa stitches.

In many cases, however, the carcinoma may be extensive. In these cases radiotherapy is the treatment of choice. Surgery can be kept for palliative treatment, particularly if meatal strictures occur following radiotherapy. Any lymphadenopathy at the time of presentation should be investigated by needle aspirate or direct biopsy. In the event of lymph node spread the radiotherapy field can be expanded or consideration given to local lymphadenectomy.

The use of radical penile surgery with total amputation and simultaneous block dissection of inguinal lymph nodes has little to recommend it. The emotional effects on patients of such mutilating surgery is immense. Postoperative depression and even suicide is well recognized in patients following such surgery. The lymph node dissection has a significant morbidity in relation to lymph discharge and lymphoedema of the lower limbs. Carcinoma of the penis, particularly advanced disease, has a bad prognosis and care must be taken that any surgical treatment should not worsen the situation for the patient without providing any long-term benefit.

The male urethra

Though strictly speaking a urinary structure and hence not part of a chapter on external genitalia, the male urethra is nevertheless part of the penile apparatus and certain aspects of its surgical management can be included in this section. The male urethra commences at the bladder neck where its first section is known as the prostatic or posterior urethra. This contains the opening of the ejaculatory ducts and the adjoining prostate gland. Below this lies the external sphincter which is the main urinary sphincter of the male. The bladder neck sphincter above is essentially a sexual sphincter and is used, in addition to its role in urinary continence, as a mechanism for closing off the bladder during ejaculation. The external sphincter lies in the area of the membranous urethra which then passes into the bulb of the urethra from whence it

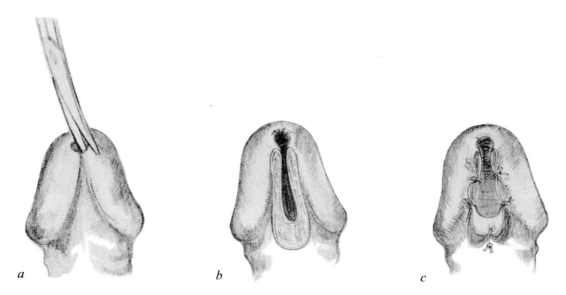

a　　　　　　　　*b*　　　　　　　　*c*

Figure 35.14 Meatoplasty. The stricture is opened boldly on its ventral aspect, following which a plastic mucocutaneous repair is undertaken

leads forwards into the corpora spongiosum to become the penile or anterior urethra. This opens onto the surface of the glans penis as the external meatus.

Meatal stenosis

Meatal stenosis may arise from a variety of causes, of which by far the commonest is urethral instrumentation and, in particular, catheterization. It may be symptomless, only presenting problems in relation to the insertion of urethral instruments. In this situation a simple meatotomy is all that is required. Under general anaesthesia, one blade of a pair of scissors is inserted into the urethra, with the other on the outside. The scissors are then closed so as to divide the external meatus from mucosa to the skin of the ventral aspect of the penis. The area of stenosis is usually short and one cut (less than 0.5 cm) is all that is required. Instruments may now pass easily. Any troublesome bleeding from the urethral edge can be managed by 3/0 chromic catgut stitches.

When a more troublesome meatal stenosis arises, a formal meatoplasty is required. Under general anaesthesia a flap of skin is raised over the ventral aspect of the penis using either preputial or penile skin (depending on whether circumcision has been performed previously). The skin flap is elevated and, again using scissors, the urethra is opened from the external meatus downwards so as to divide the whole area of stenosis (Figure 35.14a). It is essential to cut through all fibrous tissue and then into healthy urethra (Figure 35.14b). At this stage the apex of the skin flap is sewn down to the apex of the opened urethra. The edges of the flap are now sewn to the urethral edges so as to bring the whole skin flap down as a new floor to the distal urethra (Figure 35.14c). The opening of the new meatus should be constructed so as to provide an adequate, but not too great, opening. In the event of the latter, a spraying urinary stream may occur. Catheter drainage is not required.

Trauma of the urethra

The commonest trauma to the urethra arises during instrumentation, either with a catheter or metal endoscope sheath. Tears are produced in the delicate urethral epithelium. These, if associated with further clumsy manipulation, may give rise to false passages which are blind iatrogenic diverticulae in the urethral wall. All such trauma heals by fibrosis. If the fibrosis is stenosing, then a stricture is formed.

Damage to the urethra may also occur as a result of direct injuries to the perineum involving the bulb of the urethra. Indirect trauma to the posterior urethra may also arise as a result of 'shearing' effects associated with fractures of the bony pelvis or simple separation of the symphysis pubis. A traumatic rupture of the urethra is suggested by the presence of blood at the external meatus in association with such injuries. Similarly, either alone or in combination with such blood, urinary retention, under these circumstances of pelvic injury, should suggest the possibility of urethral damage. The important urological diagnosis in such situations, often complicated by other orthopaedic and abdominal injuries, is the establishment of whether such a urethral rupture is complete or incomplete. With complete rupture there is separation of the urethral ends, giving rise subsequently to extensive fibrosis with an impenetrable stricture. With an incomplete rupture, however, part of the urethral epithelium remains in continuity. In such cases, although stricture formation is still inevitable, it is usually of a less severe quality and, because of the continuity of the urethra, more easy to deal with.

The important feature of urological management of a suspected ruptured urethra is to attempt to preserve or recreate (depending on the degree of rupture) urethral continuity.

If a patient with a suspected urethral rupture subsequently passes urine spontaneously, then such an injury can be construed as either a minor contusion or an incomplete tear. In either event, healing can occur and surgical intervention is not required in the immediate phase. However, in these situations, the risk of subsequent stricture formation is such that follow-up is required for a period of at least 12 months.

Where a patient fails to void and a palpable bladder is detected, then drainage must be instituted. For patients with multiple injuries requiring intensive care, the simplest solution is to insert a suprapubic catheter. This relieves the immediate problem of management. At a subsequent period (a minimum of 3 weeks) the suprapubic catheter can be spigoted and attempts made to initiate normal voiding. If these are successful the suprapubic catheter can be removed. Unsuccessful voiding indicates a total urethral rupture which can then be confirmed by ascending and descending urethrogram views. A formal urethroplasty reconstruction can be performed at a later date. It is preferable to wait on average 6–12 months for the scar tissue to settle to provide optimum conditions for such, usually complicated surgical repairs.

While this suprapubic drainage approach does have the merit of simplicity in the initial stages, it may predispose to complicated and lengthy urological surgery at a later date. Therefore, provided that the patient's general condition is suitable, an earlier and more aggressive urological assessment can be considered in some patients. Thus, patients with signs and symptoms suggesting urethral rupture can be taken to theatre immediately. There in the anaesthetic room, prior to induction, an experienced urologist should attempt to pass a soft catheter (16 Fr. gauge) along the urethra into the bladder. This should be done under full aseptic conditions with the liberal use of lubricating jelly. If the catheter passes into the bladder and urine drains, no more need be done. The catheter is connected to a bag for continuous drainage and the patient returned to the ward. Here the catheter can be removed in 2–3 weeks, following which spontaneous voiding should occur. Again, though, follow-up is required to monitor the possibility of significant stricture formation.

If, however, in this situation the catheter cannot be made to enter the bladder, then it must be assumed that a complete rupture has occurred. Attempts should now be made to align the urethra so as to reduce the degree of postoperative fibrosis and hence

simplify the management of the inevitable stricture formation. A full general anaesthetic is given and the patient, in a modified lithotomy (Lloyd-Davies) position, has a lower midline incision to expose the distended bladder. This is opened between stay stitches. A bladder retractor is inserted and the internal meatus displayed. A metal sound is now passed along the penile urethra and attempts made to manoeuvre it into the bladder. If the urethral injury is mild (i.e. incomplete) the sound may enter the bladder. In that event a nylon ligature is tied to its tip, preferably one with a specially designed eye. The end of the ligature is then drawn back to the external meatus. Here it is tied to a catheter which is then pulled back, using the distal end of the same ligature, into the bladder.

If the sound cannot be advanced across the urethra into the bladder a second sound, the Hey Groves' sound, is now advanced progradely through the internal meatus across the bladder incision. The tips of the two sounds are engaged, an engagement detected via the sound by 'feel'. Then either sound, usually the Hey Groves', is advanced until a tip becomes visible. In the case of the Hey Groves' sound this will be at the external meatus. Here again, a ligature is tied and the nylon brought back into the bladder cavity. The catheter is tied to the external end and itself drawn through into the bladder (Figure 35.15a–c).

In both these methods, therefore, either the direct or the 'railroading' technique, the end result is to have a urethral catheter (22 gauge) lying across the damaged urethra maintaining the alignment of the urethra and draining the bladder cavity.

The patient is returned to the ward and again following a 2–3-week period of drainage the catheter is removed and normal voiding commenced. Inevitably with extensive fibrosis following such ruptures stricture formation is common and close follow-up is required.

Variations in the general principles of technique described above include the use of traction stitches inserted transabdominally through the pelvic floor onto the perineal skin. These are ligated across rubber bands where they assist in pulling the post-urethra down onto the perineal floor and hence helping to hold the urethra in alignment. Some surgeons prefer to cut fenestrations in the side wall of the draining urethral catheter roughly adjacent to the area of the stricture. These act by draining blood and debris from the site of the injury.

All cases of urethral injury require antibiotic cover in view of the inevitable urinary sepsis, both at the time of injury and subsequently in association with the catheter drainage. Such antibiotic cover is essential in view of the associated marked tissue trauma and haematoma formation in both pelvis and perineum. The key to management of urethral trauma is the constant awareness of its possibility, particularly in the presence of pelvic fractures. Both the simple

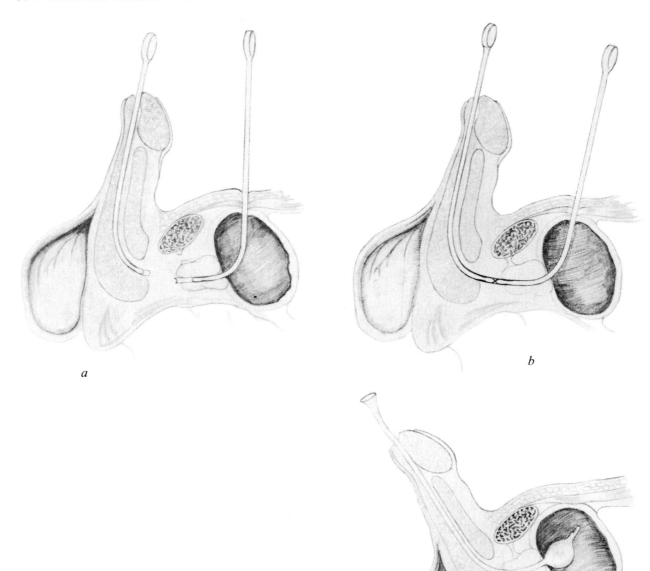

Figure 35.15 Rupture of the membranous urethra. *a*, The proximal and distal ends of the ruptured urethra are approximated using urethral and bladder sounds, the so-called 'railroading' technique. *b*, Approximation of sounds. *c*, Final position of catheter

suprapubic drainage and the more complex peroperative urethral drainage have their place in the management of the condition. Each should be available and each should be tailored to the particular needs of the patient, his general condition and any associated injuries.

Urethral stricture

A fibrosing stenosis of the urethra is termed a stricture. Such strictures arise as a result of inflammation or of trauma. Strictures associated with rupture of the urethra, as previously mentioned, provide the biggest problem, but the commonest source of strictures is following instrumentation and, in particular, catheterization. Stricture of the urethra is treated in one of three ways – regular dilatation, urethrotomy or urethroplasty.

Regular dilatation is a time-honoured method of dealing with strictures. Either curved metal sounds or soft rubber bougies are used. The metal sounds are shaped to engage the posterior urethra and bladder neck. The name indicates their original use which was to detect bladder stones by listening to the sound made by the metal against the stone. Bougies are easier to manipulate in the anterior urethra and patients are often nowadays encouraged and trained to use such soft dilators on themselves.

The use of a metal sound requires considerable skill on the part of the urologist and considerable patience on the part of the patient. It also requires a thorough understanding of the anatomy and 'feel' of the urethra.

In the majority of cases sounds are passed on the conscious patient in the supine position. Following meticulous aseptic techniques an anaesthetic gel is instilled into the urethra. It is preferable to wait at least 10 min after this in order to obtain adequate surface anaesthesia. Each sound, fully lubricated, is then passed in a series of ascending sizes. These sizes are traditionally in the Charrière scale, so named after the original French manufacturer. The size indicates the range of circumference of each sound measured in millimetres. These sounds should be passed up to the maximum size acceptable to the urethra.

Dilating a stricture in this way is, however, an unpleasant procedure for the patient. It never cures the stricture, the dilatation needing to be repeated at regular intervals. The effects of such dilatations rarely last more than 2–3 weeks. For this reason, urethrotomy or formal incision of the stricture was developed as an alternative. In the earlier instruments a so-called 'blind' technique was used. The Otis urethrotome is the best example of this type of instrument. The 'blind' nature, however, made its use difficult and bleeding was a significant complication of treatment.

The development of an optical urethrotome has now made urethrotomy the treatment of choice for the vast majority of strictures, and in particular those related to post-instrumentation trauma. This instrument consists of a standard panendoscope sheath using a 0° viewing lens. Within the sheath, using an electrotome action, a cold knife can be operated in the visual field. This knife is extended into the stricture and, in a series of upward cutting movements, using the whole instrument, the encircling fibrous bands of the stricture are divided. With each cut the fibres spring back. The incision is continued until the whole length and depth of the stricture has been divided. This means that bleeding will occur towards the terminal stage of the incision as healthy tissue is reached. This incision beyond the scar of the stricture is essential to prevent reformation of the stricture. Any bleeding is readily controlled by the insertion of a catheter which can be left in place for 48 h. Strictures with small openings can be displayed initially by the insertion of a fine ureteric catheter down a side arm on the instrument. This is threaded through the aperture of the stricture and along the urethra beyond. By cutting along the line of this catheter, the incision can be maintained within the urethral lumen, thus preventing the development of a false passage.

In the postoperative period, following antibiotic cover, the catheter can be removed. For the majority of patients a single incision is all that is required to cure the stricture permanently. In some cases, however, the treatment is supported by additional measures including hydraulic self-dilatation, in which the patient squeezes the distal urethra during micturition to dilate the previously strictured area. In other cases patients are taught, using soft catheters, to perform regular self-dilatation. Such adjunctive treatments rarely need to be performed for more than 3 months following initial treatment.

However, there are still some strictures which do not respond to either dilatation or urethrotomy. These are usually dense strictures associated with urethral trauma. In these situations much of the fibrosis is outside the urethral wall and hence beyond the reach of the cutting blade of the urethrotome. In these situations, formal open corrective surgery in the form of urethral reconstruction or urethroplasty is required.

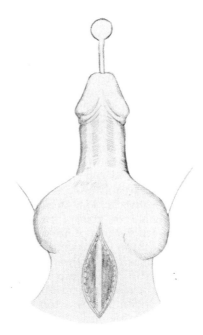

Figure 35.16 Perineal approach for excision of urethral stricture

These procedures are of two types, either formal excision of the stricture with a direct end-to-end anastomosis, or incision of the stricture with an inlay of skin (from prepuce or scrotum) to provide a graft to cover the area of urethra opened thereby. The variations in these techniques are considerable indicating, as is usual in surgery, the less than perfect results obtained overall. Considerable surgical skill is required, the operating field high in the perineum being extremely difficult to work in. Hence the more distal the stricture in the urethra, the easier the techniques. Those strictures lying at or above the

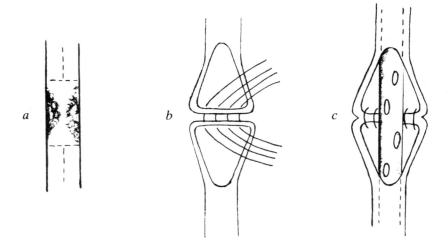

Figure 35.17   Urethral stricture. The stricture is excised, the healthy urethra is spatulated and carefully sutured on its dorsal aspect only over a fenestrated catheter

membranous urethra often require exposure via the retropubic as well as the perineal routes for their completion.

Excision and primary anastomosis requires first the full dissection of the area of stricture. This should be defined by preoperative ascending and descending urethrograms and peroperative panendoscopy. A curved metal sound is placed in the urethra until its tip reaches the distal end of the stricture. The patient, now in a lithotomy position, undergoes a midline perineal incision. This incision is developed until the urethra is revealed. At this point it is covered by the bulbospongiosum muscle. This muscle is divided in the midline, exposing the urethra itself. Dissection is now continued until the area of normal distal urethra immediately adjacent to the stricture is fully exposed. Between stay stitches the urethra is opened at this point (Figure 35.16). Troublesome bleeding may occur from the associated spongiosal vessels. This can be controlled by a continuous nylon stitch which is removed at the end of the procedure. On opening the urethra the sound is withdrawn and the stricture seen directly. Using, if necessary, a metal probe, the area of strictured urethra is opened until healthy proximal urethra is detected. Further mobilization of this urethra is performed, if necessary through a synchronous suprapubic or transpubic exposure. The area of strictured urethra is divided, care being taken on the dorsal surface to prevent damage to the associated bulbospongiosum. The cut ends are spatulated and the urethral mucosa anastomosed using interrupted 3/0 Dexon or Vicryl sutures (Figure 35.17). A no. 18 gauge catheter is passed into the bladder. The bulbos-

pongiosum and its attached muscles are closed. A Redivac drain is placed in the subcutaneous tissues and the skin closed with subcuticular Dexon. The catheter is removed on the tenth day. Antibiotic prophylaxis is essential.

This type of urethroplasty is very effective for small circumscribed strictures, particularly in the area of the bulb. It is, however, difficult for strictures in the membranous urethra above. In such cases, particularly where the stricture is lengthy, a skin inlay is required. The stricture is exposed in the same manner, but instead of excision, the incised area is grafted with skin. This may be in the form of a free graft, traditionally from the preputial skin, or a pedicle graft brought down again from the prepuce or from the scrotal skin. The grafts are sutured so that the epithelial surface is on the urethral side. 3/0 Dexon or Vicryl stitches are used. Again, catheter drainage is maintained for 10 days.

Skin inlay techniques do result in some laxity of that segment of the urethra, causing pooling and occasional problems with post-micturition dribbling. They may also cause difficulties in relation to ejaculatory function. Those inlays using scrotal or perineal skin can be complicated by the development of hair balls associated with the skin used.

In summary, therefore, although urethral strictures may be managed by regular dilatation, the best treatment by far is optical urethrotomy with its high curative rate. Urethroplasty procedures should be reserved for those patients in whom dilatation or urethrotomy are inappropriate or unsuccessful.

36

The adrenal gland

J. R. Farndon

The advent of drugs, such as aminoglutethimide, which produce 'medical adrenalectomy', has meant that the requirement for bilateral adrenalectomy in the treatment of endocrine-responsive metastatic cancer has decreased. In its place has developed a new phenomenon – the 'incidentaloma' – which requires special investigations and treatment and which will be described below. Surgery is still required for the treatment of functioning adrenal adenomas and carcinomas and occasionally for patients with pituitary-driven bilateral adrenal hyperplasia. Patient management is often coordinated between surgeon, physician and radiologist, with investigations describing the location, size and endocrine effects of the abnormal adrenal pathology. With informed pre-, per- and postoperative management and the appropriate surgical approach, the operative mortality should be less than 1%. Long-term results of surgery for benign tumours are excellent, with reversal of abnormal endocrine effects. Malignant adrenal tumours are difficult to treat and metastatic disease frequently ensues, causing the death of the patient within a few years.

Surgical anatomy

The triangular-shaped right adrenal gland lies posterior and lateral to the vena cava and above the kidney. The crescent-shaped left adrenal gland lies medial to the upper pole of the kidney and lateral to the aorta. The adrenal glands are readily identified from the surrounding fat by their characteristic orange-yellow coloration and more firm, granular consistency.

The arterial blood supply is variable and small arteries enter the glands from the inferior phrenic artery, the abdominal aorta and the renal arteries. There is usually a single draining adrenal vein on each side. On the left side the adrenal vein usually drains into the renal vein and is readily dealt with at surgery. On the right side, however, the adrenal vein is short and wide and usually drains directly into the postero-lateral aspect of the vena cava. The point of entry of the right adrenal vein is usually close to where the inferior vena cava disappears into the substance of the liver. At this point the adrenal vein and cava are vulnerable to injury and this element of surgical dissection must be carried out with particular care.

There are very few vessels entering the gland from laterally and posteriorly. Embryologically the glands are derived from two sources: the cortex is derived from coelomic mesoderm and the medulla from neural crest ectoderm. The cortex produces adrenal steroids (glucocorticoids, mineralocorticoids and sex steroids) and the medulla, as part of the 'APUD series' (Amine Precursor Uptake and Decarboxylation) produces catecholamines (dopamine, adrenaline and noradrenaline).

Cushing's syndrome

Clinical features

The clinical features of Cushing's syndrome are due to supraphysiological circulating levels of glucocorticoids. These produce weakness, obesity (particularly affecting the face, abdomen and neck – producing 'moonface' and 'buffalo hump'), hirsutism, acne, purple striae of the abdomen, capillary fragility and skin bruising. Osteoporosis occurs and there may be loss of height. Hypertension, oligomenorrhoea, mild diabetes and mental disturbance may occur. Cushing's syndrome occurs four times more commonly in females and, if untreated, the effects of excess cortisol are progressive and very debilitating.

Pathophysiology

In 50% of patients the cause of excessive cortisol is due to a small ACTH-secreting adenoma of the anterior pituitary driving both adrenal glands and producing diffuse cortical hyperplasia. This syndrome was first described by Harvey Cushing and is referred to eponymously as Cushing's disease or pituitary-dependent disease. Oat cell carcinoma of the bronchus or thymic carcinoid tumours may produce ectopic ACTH. This also produces adrenal hyperplasia, hypercortisolism which is often associated with marked muscle weakness, hyperpigmentation, electrolyte disturbance and oedema which is not typically seen in Cushing's disease. This is the ectopic ACTH syndrome. Cushing's syndrome may be caused by functioning adenomas of the adrenal cortex or by an adrenocortical carcinoma, and virilization may be a feature of these latter tumours.

Investigations

Diagnosis of Cushing's syndrome is dependent upon

a demonstration of excess cortisol production with loss of the normal diurnal variation. This is determined by measuring plasma cortisol levels at several time points during the day and measuring the urinary free cortisol production over a 24-hour period. Pituitary-dependent disease can be suppressed by giving patients a high dose of dexamethasone. Adrenal adenomas and tumours producing the ectopic ACTH syndrome are usually unresponsive to dexamethasone. The combination of an enlarged pituitary fossa on CT scan and a normal or raised plasma ACTH level favours the diagnosis of pituitary-dependent disease. Undetectably low plasma ACTH (suppressed) and a visible abnormality in one adrenal gland (CT scan or MRI scan) suggest an autonomous functioning adrenal tumour. Very high ACTH levels are usually produced from ectopic ACTH-producing neoplasms. Thymic or pancreatic carcinoids and bronchial tumours producing ACTH may be so small that they may not be seen on CT or MRI scan.

Pituitary-dependent disease

Mild forms of the disease, with bilateral adrenal cortical hyperplasia may be treated medically with metyrapone and aminoglutethimide which block cortisol synthesis. The pituitary tumour may be treated directly by surgical removal through a transphenoidal route. Some centres continue to treat pituitary tumours by external beam irradiation or by implantation of radioactive seeds such as yttrium. Panhypopituitarism may result. Pituitary tumour recurrence may occur.

In patients where medical or pituitary surgical treatment is not effective, bilateral total adrenalectomy may be carried out. Lifelong steroid replacement therapy (hydrocortisone and fludrocortisone) will be required, with recommendations about appropriate increase in therapy should there be excess stress or intercurrent illness. Up to 30% of patients develop a more rapidly enlarging pituitary tumour associated with hyperpigmentation (Nelson's syndrome) and this is often difficult to treat. Surveillance for Nelson's syndrome includes CT scan of the pituitary fossa and measurement of plasma ACTH at regular intervals.

Unilateral adrenal disease

Large adrenal tumours (10 cm or more) may be palpable on bimanual abdominal examination. A soft-tissue mass may be seen on plain abdominal radiography and there may be calcification in large tumours with degeneration. Ultrasonography of the adrenal glands is able to detect lesions of about 2 cm in diameter. The current investigations of choice are computed tomographic (CT) scanning or magnetic resonance imaging (MRI) of the adrenal glands. Small functioning adenomas of 1 cm or less may be detected by these modalities. The weighting of the

image on MRI scanning may give some indication of the nature of the adrenal lesion.

Intravenous urography with tomograms, arteriograms and selective venous sampling are rarely required in current practice.

Small tumours (less than 5 cm) are best removed through a posterior approach and larger tumours through a lateral, retroperitoneal approach.

Bilateral nodular adrenal hyperplasia

Bilateral total adrenalectomy may be indicated for disease due to pituitary-dependent or autonomous hyperplasia. Synchronous bilateral posterior adrenalectomy is the procedure of choice rather than the anterior transperitoneal approach.

Perioperative care

The preoperative condition of the patient may be improved by blocking excess cortisol production by the use of metyrapone, a competitive inhibitor of 11β-hydroxylase enzymes within the adrenal cortex. Muscle strength may thereby be improved and this may reduce postoperative morbidity such as the incidence of chest infections. Postoperatively, glucocorticoid support is required after either unilateral adrenalectomy (grossly suppressed normal gland on the opposite side) or after total adrenalectomy. A suggested regimen in the postoperative period would be: postoperative day one, 100 mg hydrocortisone t.d.s. intravenously; postoperative day two, 50 mg hydrocortisone t.d.s. intravenously; postoperative day three, 25 mg hydrocortisone t.d.s. intravenously; postoperative day four, as day three but medication orally; postoperative day five, 20 mg hydrocortisone in the morning and 10 mg in the evening, with the introduction of 0.1 mg of fludrocortisone as required to maintain normokalaemia. Fludrocortisone 0.1 mg each day or alternate days is a usual adult dose.

After removal of an adrenal adenoma the remaining suppressed gland frequently takes a long period of time to recover. Biochemical tests of a normal hypothalamopituitary–adrenal axis must be obtained before reduction of exogenous cortisol replacement.

Primary aldosteronism (Conn's syndrome)

Pathophysiology

Aldosterone is released by the outermost layer of cells of the adrenal cortex, the zona glomerulosa, and acts to maintain normal concentrations of sodium and potassium by its action on the distal renal tubule. The main stimulus to aldosterone production is sodium depletion, resulting in a fall in the circulating blood volume, which in turn stimulates the kidney to release renin. Renin causes aldosterone to be secreted via the renin–angiotensin system and aldosterone acts to restore the circulating blood volume by causing sodium retention. In Conn's syndrome the autonomous hypersecretion of aldosterone produces excessive sodium retention and hypertension and hypokalaemic alkalosis secondary to potassium loss.

The condition is due to a cortical adenoma in 60–70% of patients and in others to bilateral cortical hyperplasia of the zona glomerulosa. Females are affected two to three times more frequently than males.

Clinical features

Most patients with Conn's syndrome present with essential hypertension and are found to have persistent hypokalaemia. Occasionally the presenting features are those of hypokalaemia, e.g. polyuria, muscle weakness or tetany. Rarely, carpal spasm is produced by the sphygmomanometer cuff when the blood pressure is being recorded.

Investigations

In patients with persistent hypokalaemia in whom Conn's syndrome is suspected, causes of secondary aldosteronism such as malignant hypertension, cirrhosis, nephrotic syndrome and severe cardiac failure should be excluded.

Hypokalaemia (less than 3.5 mmol/litre) should be confirmed and this will usually be associated with a raised bicarbonate and a plasma sodium over 140 mmol/litre. Hyperkaluria (greater than 10 mmol/day in the face of hypokalaemia) with an elevated plasma aldosterone and a decreased or suppressed plasma renin is indicative of Conn's syndrome. In secondary hyperaldosteronism the plasma renin and aldosterone are both raised.

Management

Spironolactone is a competitive antagonist to aldosterone and treatment for 2–3 weeks (200–400 mg/day) will correct the metabolic alkalosis and restore the blood pressure towards normal. Bilateral adrenal hyperplasia is best treated in this way. Three weeks of medical treatment allows replacement and correction of the potassium deficit and decreases the risk of cardiac arrhythmia. Muscle strength is improved and the hypertension resolves, making surgery safer.

Surgical treatment is recommended for those patients with unilateral adrenal cortical adenomas. These tumours are best demonstrated by ^{75}Selenium iodocholesterol imaging (Figure 36.1), ultrasonography, CT scanning or MRI scans. These latter two scans are able to demonstrate tumours of 1 cm or less.

Surgical treatment

A solitary tumour (Figure 36.2) is best removed by unilateral adrenalectomy through the posterior approach. In patients who are unfit, medical therapy or infarction of the tumour by retrograde venous injection of the adrenal vein may produce therapeutic benefit.

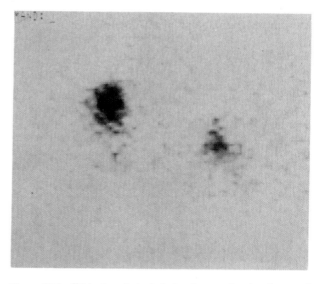

Figure 36.1 ^{75}Selenium iodocholesterol scan showing increased uptake from a functioning adrenal tumour (left) in Conn's syndrome, compared with normal adrenal (right)

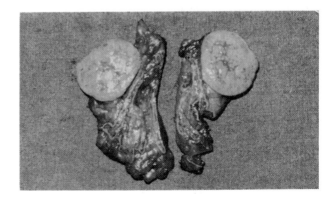

Figure 36.2 Operative adrenalectomy specimen in Conn's syndrome showing an adrenal adenoma

Virilizing and feminizing syndromes

The development of masculine features in an adult woman is occasionally due to a functioning benign adrenal tumour, removal of which results in the long-term restoration of the patient's female characteristics. These adrenal tumours, however, are usually large and malignant with a poor prognosis following surgical excision. Functioning adrenocortical tumours which cause feminization in males are exceedingly rare. Masculinization is more commonly caused by congenital adrenal hyperplasia (the adrenogenital syndromes), or the exogenous administration of androgens or by functioning tumours of the ovary, testis or placenta.

Adrenalectomy for metastatic breast cancer

Aminoglutethimide has replaced adrenalectomy in post-menopausal women with metastatic breast cancer. The drug acts predominantly by inhibiting the conversion of androgens to oestrogens in peripheral tissues. Corticosteroid replacement therapy is necessary.

Adrenocortical carcinoma

Ten per cent of adrenocortical tumours are carcinomas. The disease is usually advanced on presentation. Although the tumours may remain functional, they are often greater than 5 cm in diameter and patients frequently have pulmonary metastases on presentation. The outlook is not good. Mitotane (o,p'-DDD) inhibits biosynthesis of corticosteroids and destroys adrenocortical cells which secrete cortisol. This drug may be used in the treatment of patients with adrenocortical carcinoma, especially if this is producing Cushing's syndrome. Hydrocortisone replacement therapy is required.

Phaeochromocytoma

Clinical features

Patients with catecholamine-secreting tumours of the adrenal medulla characteristically present with symptoms of headache, excessive sweating and palpitations. They often have feelings of impending doom. On examination the blood pressure is raised, may fluctuate widely and is associated with alternate blanching and flushing of the face. These symptoms and signs are due to the release of excessive amounts of dopamine, adrenaline and noradrenaline. In the absence of severe paroxysms of hypertension, there may be a variety of other features such as tremor, nausea, weakness, dyspnoea and weight loss. Phaeochromocytomas produce symptoms which may mimic many other conditions and the true cause may not be uncovered for some time.

In a few patients, the first indication of a phaeochromocytoma is a sudden escalation in blood pressure during a general anaesthetic given for some other condition such as a hernia repair or manipulation of a fracture.

Phaeochromocytomas are particularly hazardous when they occur in children, in pregnancy and when located extra-adrenally, such as in the wall of the urinary bladder. The tumour may be familial, as in multiple endocrine neoplasia type II when patients also have medullary thyroid carcinoma and hyperparathyroidism. This condition is inherited as an autosomal dominant and screening of affected families is required.

Investigations and initial management

Diagnosis is confirmed by the finding of raised HMMA (4-hydroxy-3-methoxymandelic acid) or metadrenaline levels in 24-hour collections of urine. Urinary free catecholamines and plasma catecholamines may be measured. Non-specific elevations of catecholamines and their metabolites, for example in anxiety states, can be blocked by the use of a ganglion blocking agent such as pentolinium.

If raised levels are detected, then adrenergic blockade should be instituted to render the patient asymptomatic and safe. Sudden surges of amines can precipitate fatal arrhythmias or paroxysms of hypertension which may lead to cerebrovascular accidents or acute, severe heart failure. Phenoxybenzamine in a starting dose of 10 mg three times each day will begin alpha-adrenergic blockade. The dose is increased until mild orthostatic hypotension is noted. The blood volume will expand and anaemia may be noted. Tachycardia may be exposed due to unopposed beta-adrenergic effects, and beta-adrenergic blockade would then be indicated with propranolol in increasing dosage beginning with 10 mg t.d.s. The dose is increased until tachycardia is controlled.

Beta-blockade will be required if the tumour secretes predominantly adrenaline. It is probably safer to institute alpha-blockade before beta-blockade to avoid the consequences of unopposed agonist, pressor alpha effects.

Preoperative blockade restores the blood pressure to normal, allows the patient to feel better, often restores euglycaemia and reduces the incidence of cardiac arrhythmias. Preoperative preparation is usually carried out over a period of 2–4 weeks. Such careful preparation has been one of the factors which has led to significant reductions in morbidity and mortality in the treatment of patients with phaeochromocytoma.

Localization

Ten per cent of phaeochromocytomas are bilateral and 10% occur outside the adrenal glands. Ultrasonography may show the location of a phaeochromocytoma, but most patients undergo CT or MRI scanning as the localization investigation of first choice (Figure 36.3). [131]Iodine-metaiodobenzylguanidine (IMIBG) is a substance taken up specifically by catecholamine granules and this isotopically-labelled compound will localize small, bilateral and ectopic tumours. It will also localize functional metastases in patients with malignant phaeochromocytoma.

Phaeochromocytomas may be found in any of the paraganglionic sites, on or around the aorta, between the inferior mesenteric artery and the aortic bifurcation (the organ of Zuckerkandl). The tumour may occur in the hilum of the kidney, in the thorax or neck, and may occur in the bladder wall. Patients with this latter tumour location develop hypertension

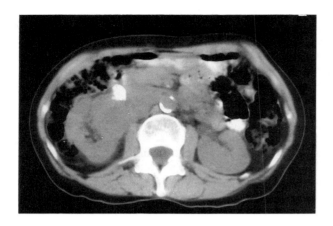

Figure 36.3 CT scan showing a phaeochromocytoma arising in the pelvis of the right kidney. The tumour is calcified and is invading the inferior vena cava. The inferior vena cava is seen alongside the calcified aorta

Phaeochromocytoma during pregnancy

Mild signs and symptoms of the effects of catecholamine excess can be seen in normal pregnancy with degrees of hypertension, but raised catecholamines in the urine or plasma must mean a diagnosis of phaeochromocytoma until proved otherwise. If left untreated, phaeochromocytoma in pregnancy is associated with significant morbidity and mortality of mother and baby. Establishment of blockade can be achieved during pregnancy and caesarian section and excision of phaeochromocytoma carried out at the earliest possible time compatible with delivery of a viable fetus.

and headache on micturition. Diagnosis is confirmed on cystoscopy and treatment is by partial cystectomy.

Operative management

Premedication is by tranquillizers, as opiate narcotics may stimulate catecholamine release. Continuous monitoring of ECG, CVP and arterial pressure is established and intravenous lignocaine, propranolol, sodium nitroprusside and phentolamine are available to treat dysrhythmias and fluctuations in blood pressure as required. Prompt replacement of measured blood loss is important and additional fluid replacement by crystalloid and colloid solution may be required to correct any residual preoperative deficit in plasma volume.

Current localization procedures allow a degree of confident identification of the site and location of phaeochromocytomas and therefore the surgical approach can be directed. An anterior transabdominal approach should be avoided whenever possible and it should no longer be required to carry out direct inspection and palpation of potential sites of phaeochromocytoma development. If at all possible, the venous drainage should be divided at an early stage to minimize potential huge surges of catecholamines into the circulation.

After tumour removal, the blood pressure may fall and volume replacement will be required. Since most phaeochromocytomas are usually of the order of 4–5 cm in diameter, a lateral approach is recommended. In the multiple endocrine neoplasia type II syndrome the tumours are frequently bilateral, although asynchrony in tumour development can occur. The differential can often be detected by IMIBG scan and since the tumours are usually uncovered by screening they can be removed when small through a posterior approach.

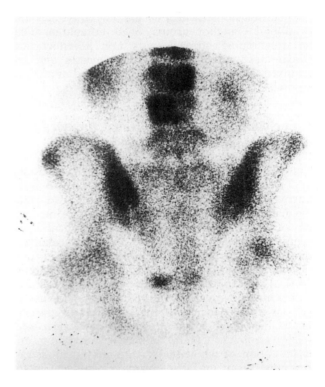

Figure 36.4 IMIBG scan of a patient with a malignant phaeochromocytoma and metastatic disease to bone. The isotopically labelled IMIBG localizes functional metastases in the axial skeleton and pelvis

Prognosis

Residual hypertension (presumably due to prolonged exposure of the vascular circuit to catecholamines) will be found in 30% of patients, who will require some form of medication or hypertension control.

Seventy per cent of patients can be reassured that their hypertension should be cured. There are no preoperative markers which clearly delineate those patients who will have postoperative normotension.

Malignancy is difficult to define using normal histopathology criteria. Nuclear pleomorphism, mitoses and capsular invasion can be seen in tumours which behave in a totally benign fashion. Patients with tumours which appear bereft of features associated with malignancy can surprisingly return with metastatic disease within one or two years. Metastases grow slowly and may not respond to radiotherapy, but alpha-methyl tyrosine, which inhibits catecholamine synthesis, with or without alpha- and beta-blockade, can provide symptomatic relief. Loading of therapeutic doses of radio-iodine onto MIBG may provide localized targeted radiotherapy (Figure 36.4).

Non-endocrine tumours of the adrenal gland

The most common non-endocrine adrenal tumour is the neuroblastoma, which occurs only in infancy and childhood. Ganglioneuromas of the adrenal medulla, non-functioning adrenal cysts and adrenocortical carcinomas present as abdominal masses and are removed through a lateral thoraco-abdominal incision.

Coincidentally detected adrenal tumours – 'incidentalomas'

The greater application of CT and MRI scanning and, to a lesser extent, ultrasonography has led to the uncovering of unexpected adrenal masses – so-called incidental tumours or 'incidentalomas'. Sometimes no evidence of biochemical hyperfunction or symptoms can be ascribed to these coincidentally uncovered tumours. They might be benign, non-functioning cortical adenomas, but could be adrenocortical carcinomas or represent metastases from occult primary neoplasms. In the first instance, investigations should focus on the detection of possible biochemical hyperfunction of either cortical or medullary tumours. Careful clinical examination and examination of whole-body scans may demonstrate the presence of an occult primary neoplasm in the breast, pancreas or ovary, for example, which has metastasized to the adrenal glands. Diagnosis can be confirmed by fine needle biopsy. Surgery is indicated for functioning incidentalomas, but is not required if the glands are affected by metastatic disease. If the diameter of the lesion is over 5 cm, a greater proportion are malignant. Some advise a conservative and observational policy for tumours less than 5 cm in diameter.

Operative techniques

Lateral approach

The lateral approach is required for large adrenal tumours, for example greater than 5 cm in diameter. The patient lies on the side opposite the affected

adrenal gland with anterior and posterior supporting sandbags or pillows. The arm resting on the table is usually placed behind the line of the body and the superior arm placed in an appropriate armrest. The operating table is tilted and broken to make tense the skin and fascia over the affected adrenal gland.

Right side (Figure 36.5)

It is possible to reach the adrenal gland without breaching the pleura or peritoneum. The higher the rib which is excised, the more risk there is of entering the pleural space. It is possible to excise the 10th rib subperiosteally and not enter the right pleural space, but in the posterior half of a subperiosteal resection the pleural recess will be encountered and needs to be dissected and swept superiorly. It is very easy to tear and breach the pleura at this point. If the 11th rib is excised, then the overhang of the 9th and 10th ribs makes exposure and dissection more difficult, but there is less chance of breaching the pleura. The peritoneum anteriorly can be identified and swept forwards. If there is a likelihood of the lesion being malignant and/or that the lesion is large (say 10 cm) a thoraco-abdominal approach is required with division of the diaphragm (Figure 36.6).

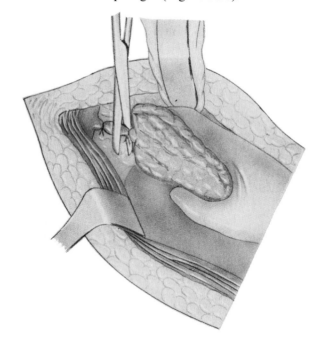

Figure 36.5 The right adrenal gland is carefully dissected until the adrenal vein is identified and ligated

On the right side the adrenal vein is short and broad, and if it is important to gain control of the vein early, as in a patient with a phaeochromocytoma, then adequate careful dissection is required so that, should bleeding occur, appropriate clamps might be applied to arrest venous bleeding. A backward-leaning Satinsky clamp is ideal for this situation, since the cava need not be totally occluded. If the vein is particularly short and broad it is often safer to side-clamp the cava at the confluence of the adrenal vein and oversew the stump as a separate procedure. A 5/0 prolene suture should be used.

Feeding arteries and draining veins will be encountered superiorly (coming from the inferior phrenic vessels), medially (mainly small arteries from the aorta) and from inferiorly (from the renal artery and vein). These can be divided between ligatures or, if small enough, after diathermy. With benign adenomas, dissection should occur close to the adrenal gland. Straying away from the adrenal gland into the perirenal and retroperitoneal fat produces significant bleeding.

If a carcinoma is expected, it may be necessary to excise the kidney *en bloc* with the adrenal gland.

forwards. The kidney is retracted inferiorly and the adrenal gland should come into view after dissection in the retroperitoneal fat. The left adrenal vein is usually longer and narrower than on the right side and usually enters the left renal vein. As on the right side, for very large tumours and those in which malignancy is suspected, it may be necessary to enter the peritoneum and remove the adrenal tumour with the spleen and tail of the pancreas.

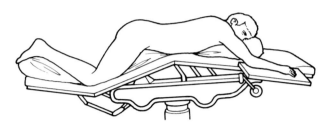

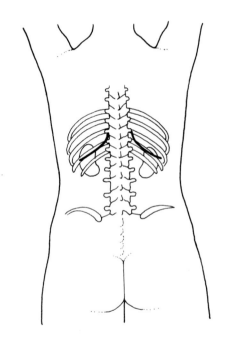

Figure 36.7 The posterior approach. Careful positioning of the patient is important. On either side, extraperitoneal access is gained via the bed of the 11th or 12th rib

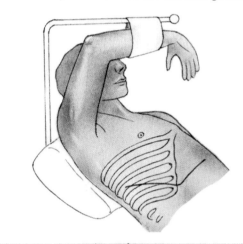

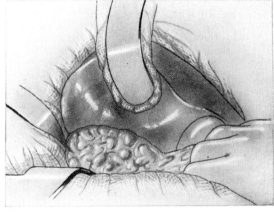

Figure 36.6 Operative exposure of a large tumour of the right adrenal by a lateral thoraco-abdominal approach through the 9th rib

Left side

The 11th rib can be resected subperiosteally and the pleura protected superiorly. The peritoneum is swept

Posterior approach

The patient is placed prone on the operating table with support under the hips and shoulders so that the abdomen does not touch the operating table. Care must be taken with patients with Cushing's syndrome because the skin and bones are easily damaged. The table is broken until the skin and deep fascia become tense (Figure 36.7). A curved incision is made over the 11th or 12th rib. The kidney is retracted inferiorly and the adrenal gland sought until its characteristic colour is obvious. If the tumour is a benign adenoma, dissection is continued around the gland and the adrenal vein is ligated as before. As in the lateral approach, the right adrenal vein and adjacent vena cava must be dissected with care to avoid injury and torrential venous bleeding.

Anterior transperitoneal approach

This is mentioned for historical reasons only, and with the other two approaches and the confidence with which phaeochromocytomas can be located, there should be no need to broach the peritoneum with large transverse or vertical incisions which have been the cause of morbidity in the past.

Further reading

Ahmed, S. R., Shalet, S. M., Beardwell, C. G. et al. (1984) Treatment of Cushing's disease with low dose radiation therapy. Br. Med. J., 289, 643–646

Clarke, D., Wilkinson, R., Johnston, I. D. A. et al. (1979) Severe hypertension in primary aldosteronism and good response to surgery. Lancet, 1, 482–485

Edis, A. J., Ayala, L. A and Egdahl, R. H. (1975) Manual of Endocrine Surgery, Springer-Verlag, Berlin

Eriksson, B., Oberg, K., Curstedt, T. et al. (1987) Treatment of hormone producing adrenocortical cancer with o,p'-DDD and streptozotocin. Cancer, 59, 1398–1403

Ferris, J. B., Brown, J. J., Fraser, R. et al. (1975) Results of adrenal surgery in patients with hypertension, aldosterone excess and low plasma renin concentration. Br. Med. J., 1, 135–138

Friesen, S. R. (ed.) (1978) Surgical Endocrinology, Clinical Syndromes, Lippincott, Philadelphia

Hunt, T. K., Roisen, M. F., Tyrell, J. B. et al. (1984) Current achievements and challenges in adrenal surgery. Br. J. Surg., 71, 983–985

Leading Article (1977) Pituitary-dependent Cushing's disease. Br. Med. J., 1, 1049

Leading Article (1983) Primary aldosteronism: how hard should we look? Br. Med. J., 287, 702–703

Levine, S. N. and McDonald, J. C. (1984) The evaluation and management of phaeochromocytomas. Adv. Surg., 17, 281–313

Mathias, C. J., Peart, W. S., Carron, D. B. et al. (1984) Therapeutic venous infarction of an aldosterone producing adenoma (Conn's tumour). Br. Med. J., 288, 1416–1417

Moldin, I. M., Farndon, J. R., Shepard, A. et al. (1979) Phaeochromocytomas in 72 patients: clinical and diagnostic features, treatment and long-term results. Br. J. Surg., 66, 456–465

Montgomery, D. A. D. and Welbourn, R. B. (1975) Medical and Surgical Endocrinology, Arnold, London

Montgomery, D. A. D. and Welbourn, R. B. (1978) Cushing's syndrome: 20 years after adrenalectomy. Br. J. Surg., 65, 221–223

Scott, H. W., Liddle, G. W., Mullhevin, J. L. et al. (1977) Surgical experience with Cushing's disease. Ann. Surg., 185, 524–534

Thompson, N. W., Allo, M. D., Shapiro, B. et al. (1984) Extra-adrenal and metastatic phaeochromocytoma: the role of [131]Iodine-metaiodobenzylguanidine ([131]IMIBG) in localization and management. Wld J. Surg., 8, 605–611

Thompson, N. W. and Cheung, P. S. Y. (1987) Diagnosis and treatment of functioning and non-functioning adrenocortical neoplasms including incidentalomas. Surg. Clin. N. Am., 67, 423–436

Walker, R. M. (1964) Phaeochromocytoma in relation to pregnancy. Br. J. Surg., 51, 590–595

Watson, R. G. G., van Heerden, J. A., Northcutt, R. C. et al. (1986) Results of adrenal surgery for Cushing's syndrome: ten years' experience. Wld J. Surg., 10, 531–538

37

The management of renal stones

D. A. Tolley

Introduction

In the past decade the development of new operative techniques and collaboration between engineers and surgeons have resulted in dramatic changes in the management of urinary stone disease. As will be seen, these developments have altered the indications for surgical intervention and very high success rates from minimally invasive surgery can be achieved for stones which were previously regarded as inoperable.

In order to maximize the success rate, the urologist should have all tools in the armamentarium available to him, and the development of fully equipped Stone Centres for the management of complex stone disease should result in fewer than 1 in 100 patients requiring open surgery to treat their stones.

Although general comments can be made about the treatment of particular types of stones, it should be recognized that a plan of treatment must be tailored to the individual patient and his or her stone and there are times when the guidelines set up below will be inappropriate.

Indications for treatment

These fall into two groups. Absolute indications for intervention are the presence of upper urinary tract obstruction or infection. A combination of the two is an indication for urgent intervention since delay will almost certainly result in renal damage and/or septicaemia. In cases where the patient is already toxic, preliminary decompression of the kidney by percutaneous nephrostomy may be necessary before definitive treatment of the stone is undertaken. Staghorn calculi should always be treated irrespective of age, since there is a risk of the patient developing silent obstruction, infection or perinephric abscess.

Pain is not in itself an absolute indication for intervention since it will depend upon the frequency and severity of pain suffered by the individual. Clearly, a patient who is suffering recurrent bouts of renal pain will require earlier intervention than the elderly patient who has a mild attack of pain once a year. Stones which increase in size should be treated, irrespective of symptoms, because of the increasing risk of obstruction if the stone subsequently moves.

The presence of an asymptomatic stone (other than a staghorn calculus) is not necessarily an indication for treatment. However, if the patient is unable to follow his occupation until the stone has been treated (e.g. airline pilots, deep-sea divers) or is planning to travel extensively, treatment will be necessary. Occasionally, asymptomatic stones will be treated prophylactically in patients who have already suffered from ureteric colic due to the previous passage of a stone, and it is especially important to treat stones in solitary kidneys because of the risk of calculus anuria.

Contraindications

Less invasive procedures have reduced the contraindications for treatment. These will be discussed under the headings of individual treatments, but include the usual contraindications to surgery, a recent myocardial infarction, cardiac and respiratory problems and bleeding diatheses. The presence of renal impairment is not in itself a contraindication to stone surgery, since in patients with end-stage renal failure and recurrent urinary infections due to stone disease, the stones must be removed before transplantation is considered.

Preparation for treatment

Irrespective of the form of treatment chosen, some general principles are common to all forms of stone management.

A *contemporary* abdominal radiograph is required before embarking upon treatment, so that the current position of the stone can be assessed. This is in addition to a good-quality intravenous urogram which demonstrates the renal anatomy. It is quite acceptable to X-ray only the kidney and ureter containing the stone, since this will reduce both radiation dose to patient and cost.

A preoperative assessment of renal function by measurement of serum, urea, creatinine and electrolytes is required and the result of a recent urine culture must be available before commencing treatment.

Patients should be well hydrated, particularly if renal function is impaired or if open surgery is contemplated, and this may require an intravenous infusion to be started on the evening before surgery. Patients with impaired renal function may develop further renal damage if they become dehydrated.

Antibiotic prophylaxis is required for all patients undergoing surgery, but is only required for patients with infected urine or staghorn, i.e. (matrix) calculi when treated by lithotripsy.

When percutaneous surgery is contemplated, the patient's blood group should be determined and serum saved for possible cross-match and up to 4 units of blood should be cross-matched for patients undergoing open stone surgery or nephrectomy, depending upon the anticipated complexity of the procedure.

Radioisotope scan to determine the differential renal function is necessary in patients with staghorn calculi, since this may influence the decision to carry out conservative surgery or nephrectomy.

Treatment options

Open surgery

The sole indication for open surgery is nephrectomy for a non-functioning calculus containing kidney. Open surgery may occasionally be required in combination with pyelolithotomy or nephrolithotomy to correct an anatomical defect which cannot be corrected by an endo-urological procedure.

Ureterolithotomy may be required for very large stones in the mid third of the ureter or when endo-urological procedures have failed.

Pyelolithotomy

This procedure is carried out under general anaesthesia with the patient placed in the loin position. A supracostal incision is used, taking care to avoid the pleura and the intercostal vessels and nerves. The approach to the kidney is extraperitoneal and dissection may well prove to be difficult due to the presence of oedema, adhesions and scarring. The lower pole of the kidney is mobilized and the ureter identified and taped. The kidney is further mobilized and the renal pedicle identified anteriorly. The renal artery(ies) and vein(s) are identified and marked with silicone slings. A longitudinal incision is made in the renal pelvis between catgut stay sutures and the stone is extracted using Desjardin's cholecystectomy forceps. Access to the infundibulum of the calices can be achieved by gentle dissection and subsequent retraction of the renal sinus with a small retractor. Otherwise inaccessible fragments in the calices may be removed by radial nephrolithotomy (Figure 37.1). This is a blood-losing procedure and therefore it is necessary to clamp the renal artery after first cooling the kidney to 20°C. There is invariably some loss of renal function following this procedure which should therefore only be carried out if percutaneous nephrolithotomy is contraindicated.

The incisions in the renal pelvis and parenchyma are closed with interrupted catgut sutures and a nephrostomy tube inserted through one of the nephrotomy incisions. If part of the kidney is non-functioning or there is gross caliceal distortion and dilatation which is not correctable endo-urologically, then a partial nephrectomy will be carried out.

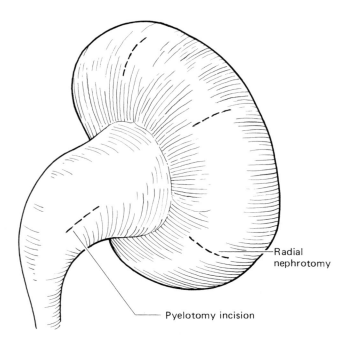

Figure 37.1 Pyelotomy incision and radial nephrotomy. Dissection of the renal sinus has exposed the infundibulum of the upper calices

It is necessary to check that there are no stone fragments remaining and this will be done by intraoperative X-rays or the use of an intraoperative ultrasound probe.

The wound is closed in layers of absorbable suture material. A silicone tube is used to drain the perinephric area.

Complications

Pneumothorax may develop due to inadvertent puncture of the pleura. This is generally recognized intraoperatively and it is only necessary to repair the hole in the pleura with catgut and to insert an intercostal drain if the pneumothorax is large. The drain is inserted in the mid-axillary line in the 9th intercostal space and the anaesthetist is then asked to inflate the lung and to keep it inflated while the hole in the pleura is repaired.

Intraoperative bleeding from the kidney may generally be controlled by a tamponade and blood transfusion, but occasionally dissection of the renal pelvis will result in tearing of small veins in the renal sinus which cannot be controlled by these means. Under these circumstances the only option available is nephrectomy. Lacerations of larger renal veins can be repaired by standard vascular techniques.

Occasionally, it may be impossible to locate any remaining stone fragments. These may be dealt with subsequently by extracorporeal shock wave lithotripsy (ESWL) or percutaneous nephrolithotomy (see below).

Postoperative complications

In addition to general postoperative complications such as pulmonary embolism, deep vein thrombosis and wound infection, patients undergoing renal surgery are more prone to postoperative chest infection and basal atelectasis since the large painful wound makes deep breathing difficult and, in addition, the frequently prolonged nature of the procedure encourages collection of secretions in the dependent lung. These problems will be minimized by preoperative and postoperative physiotherapy.

Urinary fistula sometimes occurs following removal of the nephrostomy tube due to ureteric obstruction caused by blood clot or stone fragments. This complication can be avoided by plain radiography and a nephrostogram prior to removal of the nephrostomy tube. However, if a fistula develops, retrograde removal of the obstruction by ureteroscopy or passage of a ureteric catheter usually results in resolution of the problem.

Ureterolithotomy

This operation is only required for ureteric stones (usually in the middle third) which are either too large to be disintegrated successfully by lithotripsy or an endo-urological procedure or where endo-urological access to the stone has failed. Ureterolithotomy should be required in less than 5% of all patients undergoing treatment of ureteric stones.

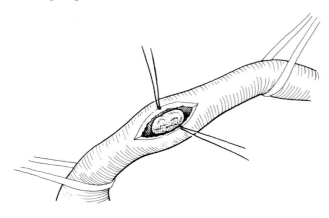

Figure 37.2 Ureterolithotomy. Silicone slings are used to prevent mobilization of the stone during dissection. The ureter has been opened over the stone between stay sutures

The approach to the ureter should be extraperitoneal. The incision will vary according to the position of the stone. For stones in the upper third of the ureter, a supracostal incision is best since this gives easy access to the kidney should the stone inadvertently move upwards during the procedure, and occasionally mobilization of the lower pole of the kidney will be necessary to identify the stone. A flank incision is best for stones in the mid third of the ureter

since this incision may be extended in either direction should difficulty be encountered in locating the stone. For stones in the lower third of the ureter, an oblique or hockey-stick incision in the iliac fossa affords optimum exposure. The bladder must be empty prior to embarking on a lower third ureterolithotomy because this greatly improves access in the pelvis.

A large stone may be palpated easily, but more often it will be too small to feel or be surrounded by fibrosis. Therefore it is better to identify the ureter at some distance above and below the suspected site of the stone and to occlude the ureteric lumen with silicone slings passed around the ureter (Figure 37.2). Once the stone has been identified in the ureter a longitudinal incision is made directly over it and the stone removed with a pair of stone forceps. Occasionally, a blunt dissector is required if the stone is embedded in the wall of the ureter.

Once the stone is removed it is essential to ensure that the ureter is not obstructed distally by a further stone as this may lead to a urinary fistula. Therefore, an umbilical catheter should be passed antegradely until it reaches the bladder. Aspiration of urine from the bladder by a syringe will confirm that the catheter has passed far enough and that there is no obstruction.

The ureterotomy is closed with two or three interrupted plain catgut sutures which are lightly tied.

A silicone tube drain is placed through a separate stab incision and the wound closed in layers with absorbable suture material.

Complications

If the stone is not identified during surgery, it may have slipped down into the bladder or returned to the kidney. An intraoperative abdominal X-ray is taken to try to locate the opacity and appropriate action is taken.

Persistent urinary leakage

If urine continues to leak from the drainage site for more than a week, an abdominal X-ray is taken to ensure that no stones remain. If a ureteric catheter or ureteric stent is inserted retrogradely, the fistula frequently dries up rapidly and the need for reoperation is most unusual.

Percutaneous nephrolithotomy

This is the treatment of choice for all renal stones greater than 3 cm in diameter or for smaller stones with associated anatomical abnormalities which can be corrected endo-urologically. It may be the preferred method of treatment for stones between 2 and 3 cm in diameter in certain individuals. A percutaneous approach may also be used to obtain access to the upper ureter. Occasionally, smaller stones may be removed in this way depending upon the non-availability of lithotripsy or patient's preference.

There are few contraindications to percutaneous nephrolithotomy; the operation may be restricted in very obese patients where the instruments are simply too short to allow adequate access to the collecting system, and in patients with bleeding diatheses, staged ESWL may be the treatment of choice.

There are five principal stages in the operation:

1. Access to the kidney.
2. Dilatation.
3. Endoscopy.
4. Stone fragmentation.
5. Extraction of fragments.

Choice of calix will be determined by the position of the stone(s) to be removed (Figure 37.3). Access through a lower pole calix enables stones in the lower calices and renal pelvis and occasionally upper calices to be removed. However, lower caliceal puncture precludes access to the mid-pole calices. Thus, for a stone occupying the mid-pole calices and renal pelvis or for access to the upper ureter, an approach through a middle calix is preferred. For complex staghorn calculi or multiple stones in different calices, multiple punctures or a 'Y' puncture will be required.

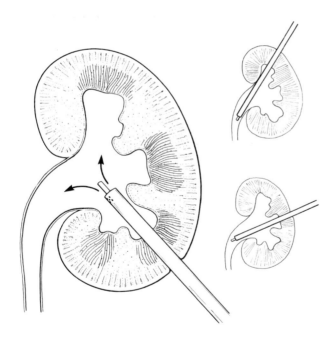

Figure 37.3 Access for percutaneous surgery. Access via a mid-pole or upper calix provides the best approach to the upper ureter. Access through a lower calix usually enables the upper calix to be visualized

A good-quality intravenous urogram and plain abdominal radiograph taken preoperatively are essential in order to plan the most appropriate approach. The patient is anaesthetized and lies in the prone position. The collecting system is opacified with radio-opaque contrast medium injected through a previously placed ureteric catheter. The use of a C-arm for fluoroscopic screening enables images to be checked in two planes, thus enabling more accurate puncture to be carried out. A caliceal puncture and track dilatation may be carried out either by a surgeon or radiologist, but in either case the technique used should minimize the amount of radiation exposure by the use of small fields, short exposure time and the use of a fluoroscope with a built-in memory. The operator must be protected by a lead apron, and additional protection to the thyroid by use of a neck collar and the eyes by radiation spectacles is required.

The combination of real time ultrasound monitoring and fluoroscopy will further reduce screening times and aid in insertion of the needle.

A fine-bore needle is placed vertically over the chosen calix and is then withdrawn for 6 or 7 cm in a line parallel with the lower border of the 12th rib (Figure 37.4). Puncture of the skin at 30° from the vertical and insertion of the needle for 6 or 7 cm will complete the equilateral triangle and enable easy puncture of the lower pole of the kidney. The tip of the needle is advanced into the calix and its position checked, if necessary, by biplane screening. One or 2 ml of air is injected through the hollow needle and the resultant stream of bubbles observed in the collecting system on fluoroscopy confirms that the needle is in the correct position.

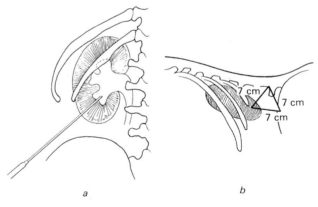

a   b

Figure 37.4 Percutaneous puncture. *a*, The track is made parallel to the lower border of the 12th rib. *b*, Initial vertical placement of the needle which is then withdrawn 7 cm inferolaterally and inserted through the skin at 30° to produce an equilateral triangle with the calix as the deepest point

The same principle is used to puncture an upper- or mid-pole calix, but it may prove necessary to create a track in the 11th or even 10th interspace. The needle puncture should be as lateral as possible to avoid puncturing the pleura.

If the collecting system cannot be opacified because of total obstruction, a double needle technique may help to manage difficult cases. The renal pelvis is punctured directly posteriorly with a fine needle and the collecting system filled with contrast medium. Definitive puncture for nephrostomy is then carried out through a second puncture.

Following correct placement, a J-tipped guidewire is advanced through the lumen of the needle until it comes to lie within the pelvis. The wire is then manipulated until it passes down the upper ureter, thus creating a stable track between collecting system and skin (Figure 37.5).

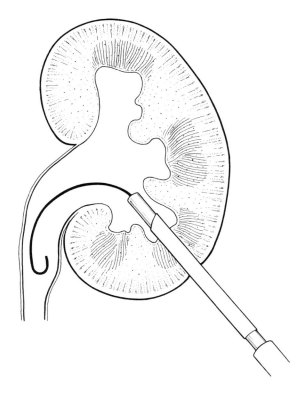

Figure 37.5 Percutaneous puncture. The J wire is passed into the upper ureter to produce a stable track

Track dilatation

Percutaneous nephrolithotomy requires dilatation of the nephrostomy track to 26 or 28 French. This may be accomplished in one of three ways: (a) graduated fascial Teflon dilators; (b) metal telescopic bougies; (c) balloon catheters.

Teflon dilators are semi-flexible and easily controlled, but are occasionally difficult to pass through scar tissues. Alken metal telescopic bougies are reusable and rigid. However, it is very easy, particularly for the inexperienced operator, to perforate the renal pelvis with this system. Balloon catheters are the most expensive and confer little advantage over the other methods of track dilatation (Figure 37.6).

Track dilatation for the novice can be taxing and occasionally the track between kidney and skin may

be lost, particularly in the presence of fibrosis. The use of a reserve or second guidewire ensures that the track can be re-entered if it is lost during track dilatation.

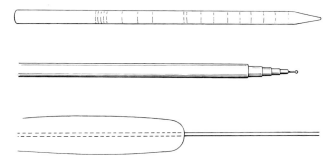

Figure 37.6 Track dilatation. This can be achieved using coaxial Teflon dilators (top), metal bougies (centre) or balloon dilatation (bottom)

Endoscopy

Both rigid and flexible endoscopes are available. The optics associated with rigid lens systems are far superior and afford a much better view of the collecting system, particularly when used in conjunction with CCD television. The surgeon has much more control over a rigid instrument, which is far more versatile as it allows the passage of both ultrasound and electrohydraulic probes for stone disintegration. In addition, the high flow of irrigant fluid through the instrument sheath optimizes the operator's view. Warm normal saline should be used for irrigation since this will cause least physiological disturbance in the event of hyperabsorption in the presence of perforation of the renal pelvis.

Flexible endoscopes have a theoretical benefit of being more manoeuvrable, but this has not been translated into surgical practice since the presence of an instrument in the instrument channel in practice reduces the manoeuvrability of the endoscope and both irrigation and optics are considerably inferior to those of rigid endoscopes.

Initial difficulties with orientation may be overcome by first identifying the ureteric catheter at the ureteropelvic junction and then following the medial wall of the renal pelvis superiorly towards the upper calices. All calices should be inspected if possible and an assessment of the size of the stone is made in order to ascertain whether the stone can be removed intact or whether it will require stone disintegration.

Stone fragmentation

Stones or stone fragments up to 10 mm diameter may be extracted percutaneously without fragmentation. Larger stones with a minimum diameter of less than 1 cm in one plane may also be removed without disintegration, although this may require intrarenal manipulation. Larger stones require fragmentation which can be accomplished mechanically using forceps or by more elaborate techniques:

1. Forceps.
2. Stone punch.
3. Electrohydraulic lithotriptor.
4. Ultrasound lithotriptor.
5. Laser lithotriptor.
6. Micro-explosives.

Small soft stones may be fragmented intrarenally using forceps or a smaller version of a Mauermeyer stone punch in a capacious collecting system. However, both of these methods are inferior to non-mechanical stone disintegration. The only advantage which they offer is one of cheapness.

Ultrasound waves (28 kHz) are produced by a small piezoelectric generator and transmitted via the hollow rigid metal probe which is brought into direct contact with the stone. This results in disintegration of the stone. Usually stress fractures occur, resulting in fragmentation. Suction is applied via the hollow probe and small stone fragments 'hoovered' up from the renal pelvis. *A liquid medium* facilitates the transmission of ultrasound. This process causes the development of heat at the tip of the probe which requires cooling by continuous irrigation with saline.

Electrohydraulic lithotripsy (EHL) is based on an electric spark discharge produced from a 2.5 kV generator between the two insulated electrodes at the tip of the probe. Multiple short impulses result in the formation of shock waves, leading to stone disintegration. This technique has the advantage of being quicker than ultrasound lithotripsy, but permits less controlled fragmentation of the stone.

LASER LITHOTRIPTORS

Transmission of pulsed dye laser energy via a quartz fibre measuring 320 μm diameter placed in contact with a stone results in fragmentation of the stone by absorption of the energy. A plasma forms between the surface of the stone and the tip of the fibre, resulting in stone disintegration. Laser systems are highly expensive and their main role is in the disintegration *in situ* of ureteric stones. The advantage of the small fibre is that it can be used through a flexible endoscope and may thus reach parts of the collecting system which would otherwise be inaccessible to rigid instrumentation without second puncture.

MICRO-EXPLOSION TECHNIQUE

These techniques, which require placement of minute quantities of lead azide inside a stone which is then detonated, are used only in Japan and the equipment, although commercially available, is not available in Europe or the USA.

Stone extraction

There is a variety of forceps available for stone extraction under vision. Three-arm forceps tend to be stronger and are useful for removing fairly large fragments from the kidney. However, they have the disadvantage of requiring a larger working space. Crocodile jaw forceps can be used for the smallest pieces of stone, but in the author's opinion the peanut type of forcep is by far the most versatile and has the advantage of requiring very little working space. Small stones in peripheral calices can be removed using helical or flat wire baskets, and occasionally irrigation fluid can be used to flush a stone out of an otherwise inaccessible calix (Figure 37.7).

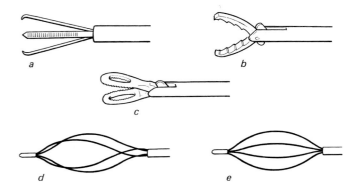

Figure 37.7 Stone extractors. *a*, Triradiate grabber. *b*, Crocodile jaw. *c*, Peanut forceps. *d*, Helical basket. *e*, Flat wire basket

Intraoperative screening and X-rays are performed as necessary and at the end of the operation a nephrostomy tube is inserted through the Amplatz sheath which is then removed. There are no hard-and-fast rules governing the choice of nephrostomy tubes. Many surgeons use a standard Foley catheter, but it is the author's preference to use a silicone Cope loop catheter which is very comfortable for the patient.

Intraoperative complications

These mainly relate to loss of the track which can be avoided if a second or reserve wire is used as a routine. Occasionally, excessive bleeding is encountered. This is usually due to tearing of a vein lying close to the infundibulum, and tamponade with the Amplatz sheath usually results in its control. Rarely, the main renal vein or even the vena cava may be entered when bleeding is of course brisk. The diagnosis is confirmed by insertion of a Foley catheter through the track and injection of contrast medium which effectively produces a venogram. Inflation of the balloon ensures haemostasis while the kidney is explored. It may be possible to repair the vein, but nephrectomy is usually necessary.

In general, intraoperative bleeding is minimized by the tamponade effect of the Amplatz sheath, but bleeding may occur from other parts of the collecting system, especially in the presence of inflammation. Under these circumstances a 'red out' occurs and there is no option but to terminate the procedure.

Adjacent organs may be penetrated by the dilators. In particular, the colon and spleen are at risk. Although punctures of the bowel will heal spontaneously, more major damage will require laparotomy and appropriate repair of the viscus.

Minor perforation of the renal pelvis occurs frequently during track formation and requires no special treatment other than the insertion of a nephrostomy tube for 48 h postoperatively.

Retained inaccessible fragments may be dealt with either by second puncture or by lithotripsy where appropriate.

Postoperative complications

In addition to general postoperative complications, continued bleeding from the parenchyma may occur resulting in a retroperitoneal haematoma. A small haematoma will resolve spontaneously, but prophylactic antibiotics should be prescribed. Larger haematomas are painful because of the irritant effect of the blood on the psoas muscle, producing spasm. Epidural anaesthesia is a reliable and simple way of obtaining analgesia. Therapeutic ultrasound aids dispersal of the haematoma and operative removal is generally not required. The only indication for surgical intervention is the same as for renal trauma, i.e. continuing bleeding which cannot be compensated for by blood transfusion. In cases where exploration is required, nephrectomy is usually the end result. Thus, it is better to try and control bleeding by a renal arteriogram and embolization of the bleeding vessel.

Arteriovenous fistula is an extremely rare complication which is characterized by intermittent (and usually late) bleeding which may on occasion be severe. It is diagnosed by angiography and is treated by embolization.

Persistent fistula after removal of the nephrostomy tube is dealt with in a similar fashion to persistent urine leak following pyelolithotomy or nephrolithotomy.

Postoperatively, antibiotics are required. Following radiographic demonstration of complete stone removal, and/or the absence of ureteric fragments, the nephrostomy tube is removed. Most patients can be discharged within 48 h of surgery.

Ureteroscopy

Indications

Endoscopic removal of ureteric stones is indicated primarily for stones in the lower third of the ureter. Unless some form of non-mechanical stone disintegration is available, endoscopic extraction of stones should be restricted to those stones which will comfortably pass through the ureteric orifice, i.e. less than 6 mm in diameter. The development of semi-rigid and steerable flexible ureteroscopes has broadened the indications for endoscopic extraction to include stones in the mid and upper third of the ureter. However, removal of stones in these sites can be technically very demanding and should not be undertaken by the inexperienced endoscopist.

At least five major instrument manufacturers make ureteroscopes which are available in different lengths and external diameters and with a choice of telescopes. Most rigid ureteroscopes use a rod-lens system which affords a clearer vision and each instrument has at least one instrument channel for the passage of wire baskets and other instruments. Semi-rigid instruments generally have a smaller diameter and are longer to enable them to reach the renal pelvis. Consequently the instrument channels are smaller, a factor which reduces the maximum rate of irrigation attainable through the sheath. A fibreoptic or quartz lens system is employed which reduces the clarity of the image obtained. The instrument channel is even smaller in flexible ureteroscopes; both the field of view and the procedures which can be undertaken with these instruments is extremely limited.

Contraindications

Ureteroscopic stone extraction is mainly contraindicated in patients where physical characteristics preclude access to the stone, e.g. gross obesity, hip or spinal deformity. Gross prostatic enlargement which obscures the ureteric orifice or prevents sufficient angulation of the ureteroscope to allow access is also a contraindication to ureteroscopy.

Preoperative assessment

It is particularly important that a contemporary plain radiograph of the abdomen is available immediately before surgery is undertaken. This should be performed on the way to the operating room. A full-length radiograph from the intravenous urogram series is also helpful to determine the ureteric anatomy.

There are five principles in the planning of endoscopic ureteric stone extraction

1. Access.
2. Stone identification.
3. Fragmentation.
4. Removal.
5. Postoperative care.

Access

As a general principle the narrower and shorter the ureteroscope, the easier it is to gain access to the ureter. Although it is possible to identify the ureteric orifice with the ureteroscope, without prior cysto-scopy, for the novice it is easier and safer to carry out a preliminary cystoscopy and to identify the ureteric orifice. Once this has been identified, a 0.038 guide-wire or 3 Fr. gauge ureteric catheter is inserted into the ureter and *cautiously* advanced for up to 10 cm in order to stabilize it (Figure 37.8). This procedure should be undertaken cautiously, since it is possible for the ureteric catheter to dislodge the stone which is then pushed up on the tip of the catheter. Beaked ureteroscopes of 8.5 Fr. gauge or less can be intro-duced through the ureterovesical junction without the need for dilatation of the orifice, but it is advisable to carry out preliminary dilatation of the ureteric orifice if larger instruments are used. This can be done very simply with the aid of a Fogarty balloon catheter which is placed through the instrument channel of the ureteroscope. The ureteric orifice is then inflated under vision and the tip of the deflated Fogarty balloon catheter is then used as a guide to show the way while the inverted ureteroscope is passed through the ureteric orifice.

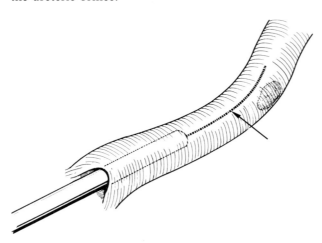

Figure 37.8 Ureteroscopy. A guidewire (arrowed) may facilitate ureteroscopy by straightening out the natural curves

The use of Teflon-coated plastic dilators passed over a guidewire is less satisfactory because the larger dilators frequently do little more than push the ure-teric orifice away from the tip of the advancing dilator rather than allowing it to dilate the ureter. However, the use of such dilators, together with a hollow Teflon sheath which remains in the lower few centimetres of the ureter, is usually necessary to allow passage of a flexible ureteroscope.

The use of a smaller instrument without dilatation is undoubtedly less traumatic for patient and surgeon, and failure to introduce a smaller instrument into the ureter is a rare event. Access to the ureter with a small ureteroscope is achieved simply by 'back-feeding' the catheter or guidewire through the instrument channel and out through the instrument port adjacent to the eyepiece. The tip of the catheter or wire is grasped in the left hand and the ureteroscope is advanced along the urethra and into the bladder over the guidewire. Once the ureteric orifice is identified, the instrument is inverted so that the beak lies in contact with the base of the bladder and ureteric orifice. The instrument then passes through the ureterovesical junction and is then rotated through 180° so that it assumes its normal position. This procedure should be entirely atraumatic and accomplished without causing ure-teric bleeding. Thus, the interior of the ureter should clearly be seen.

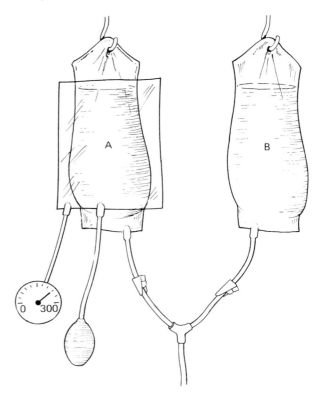

Figure 37.9 Irrigation system for ureteroscopy. In 'bag A' the pressure is maintained at 200 mmHg with a pressure cuff; in 'bag B' it is maintained by hydrostatic pressure. Use of a Y irrigation set allows the surgeon easily to switch between high and low pressure

Sometimes it is necessary to increase the irrigation rate through the scope in order to improve vision. Although there are products which are commercially available to achieve this, they are very expensive, and a simpler system using a bag of saline inserted into a pressure cuff which in inflated to 200 mmHg is just as effective. If the other limb of a double irrigation set is connected to a bag of saline to which pressure is not applied, the operator can switch between pressurized and non-pressurized irrigation very easily (Figure 37.9). High-pressure irrigation should be used very sparingly because of the risk of renal damage and infection caused by prolonged use of irrigant fluids under high pressure.

Stone identification

The guidewire should now be withdrawn to the tip of the ureteroscope which is then advanced proximally until the stone is identified. If the ureter is very tortuous, by advancing the tip of the guidewire or ureteroscope for a further 2 cm beyond the beak of the instrument, it can be used to negotiate the tortuosities quite safely without risk of perforation. Once the stone is identified, a further assessment of size is made and it should be remembered that the optics of a ureteroscope are such that gross magnification occurs when the stone is viewed close up. However, the size can be gauged both by reference to the preliminary radiograph and also by reference to the centimetre markers on the ureteric catheter.

If the stone is not identified in the expected site, a further search is required. The lower third of the ureter is quite bulbous, particularly in its distal part, and it is possible for the ureteroscope to pass over even quite large stones without them being observed. This is particularly so if the instrument is introduced over a guidewire. Therefore, the ureteroscope should be withdrawn to the level of the ureterovesical junction and the ureteroscopy recommenced. If the stone is not identified during this manoeuvre, then the ureteroscope should be advanced further since the stone may have become dislodged. Occasionally, a stone may be hidden in oedematous mucosa and, at the pelvic brim, the field of view is such that the stone simply lies out of the operator's vision. Rotation of the instrument through 360° will identify a stone which is not seen for this reason.

If the stone is still not identified, fluoroscopic screening will be necessary because occasionally the stone has passed retrogradely into the kidney. If this is the case, percutaneous extraction or lithotripsy, depending upon the armamentarium available, will be required.

Stone fragmentation

There is little point in attempting endoscopic removal of a stone that is too big to pass either down the ureter or through the ureteric orifice. This procedure is extremely traumatic and will, at best, result in temporary damage to the ureter. The risk of stricture formation and/or ureteric perforation is high and with the wide range of methods of stone disintegration available, the procedure is unnecessary.

There are three principal methods of stone disintegration available for use in the ureter: (a) ultrasound; (b) electrohydraulic lithotripsy; (c) laser lithotripsy.

ULTRASOUND

This method employs a narrower and longer probe than that used for ultrasound disintegration in the kidney. The probe is rigid and therefore a telescope with an offset eyepiece is essential, which may cause some difficulties for the inexperienced operator. Additionally, considerable heat is generated during ultrasound disintegration and, unless irrigation fluid is used under pressure, the flow of irrigant is generally not sufficient to cool the probe adequately and therefore thermal damage may result in stricture formation.

ELECTROHYDRAULIC LITHOTRIPSY

The principal problem associated with this method of stone disintegration is the risk of ureteric perforation if the tip of the probe is in contact with or in proximity to the ureteric mucosa when the spark is discharged. Thus, it is unsuitable for use when the view is obscured by blood or turbid urine, in an undilated ureter, or high in the ureter where a suboptimal view is obtained. The development of smaller electrohydraulic lithotripsy (EHL) probes of 3 or 1.9 Fr. gauge has widened the application of EHL for use with ureteric stones and, provided that the above precautions are observed, EHL provides a cheap, safe and effective alternative to laser lithotripsy.

LASER LITHOTRIPSY

The principal advantage of laser disintegration of stones in the ureter is that the small flexible fibre enables smaller and more flexible instruments to be used which in turn widens the indication for endoscopic extraction by allowing stones higher in the ureter to be reached. The principal drawback is, however, the very high cost of such units which, at the beginning of the 1990s, is £150 000. Thus the acquisition of this technology can only be justified by those centres carrying out large numbers of ureteric stone removals. The other advantage claimed for this technique is that ureteric damage does not occur even when the quartz fibre is placed directly in contact with ureteric mucosa and the laser discharge. This is because the laser wavelength of 502 nm is selectively absorbed by the stone. It is not absorbed by surrounding mucosa and therefore no damage ensues. Although this is true if the laser energy discharged is low (of the order of 60–80 mJ), ureteric damage certainly occurs when energy levels approximately double this level are generated.

Laser lithotripsy does, however, have distinct practical advantages. The tiny size of the fibre enables high irrigation flow rates to be obtained, with consequent clear vision. In addition, the characteristics of laser disintegration produce very fine fragments of stone which can be allowed to pass spontaneously and do not need to be removed directly, unlike the former two methods of stone disruption. The technique does take a little time to learn but, used correctly, laser lithotripsy is a highly efficient and safe means of stone disintegration.

Removal of stones

There is a wide range of baskets and forceps available for stone removal. Many different sizes and lengths of baskets are available, i.e. helical and flat, but there are principally two configurations of the basket itself (see Figure 37.7).

The helical wire basket with up to six wires is the safest. The basket is opened under vision in the ureter and then juggled until the stone fragment drops into the centre of the basket. The basket is then closed and both ureteroscope and basket are withdrawn. It may be necessary to repeat this procedure a number of times until larger fragments are removed, but any stone fragment which is 2 mm in diameter or less can be left safely to pass spontaneously.

In a healthy and dilated ureter, in which there is a lot of stone bulk after disintegration, the closed basket can be advanced beyond the stone and then opened out of sight, keeping the stone in view. The open basket is then pulled down into the field of view and used to 'trawl' the stone fragments by withdrawing both basket and ureteroscope. However, once the basket contains stone fragments, it is essential to keep it in view at all times.

Flat wire baskets are rather more precise and should be used to pick up fragments under vision which are then removed piecemeal.

If a stone is impacted in the lumen of the ureter, it is sometimes necessary to fragment the leading edge of the stone and then to remove fragments of stone with flexible grasping forceps before returning to the stone and carrying out further disintegration. It will be seen that it is impossible to use a wire basket for stone extraction unless it is possible to pass the tip of the basket beyond the stone.

Postoperative care

Ureteroscopy undoubtedly causes some ureteric oedema, with the resulting potential for obstruction. In addition, small stone fragments which have been left to pass spontaneously may come to lie in the mucosal oedema and cause obstruction. The routine use of a small ureteric catheter attached to a Foley urethral catheter is a cheap and effective means of reducing the risk of obstruction and minimizing postoperative discomfort. This catheter can be removed following a plain radiograph at 48 h.

Complications

Complications can be minimized by observing the simple rules outlined above, by the use of the smallest available ureteroscope and the availability of reliable stone fragmentation equipment.

Intraoperative complications

Perforation of the ureter by the ureteroscope, ultrasound or EHL probe is of little consequence, provided that it is recognized intraoperatively. If the perforation is small, temporary drainage of the ureter with a 3 Fr. gauge catheter, until the perforation has healed (usually within 72 h), is all that is required. If a larger perforation occurs, particularly in an already oedematous ureter, it is wise to insert a ureteric stent for 2 weeks or so. The ureter can then be examined at the time of stent removal to check that it has healed. Unrecognized perforation is characterized by *severe* loin pain, iliac fossa or loin tenderness, depending upon the site of perforation, and fever. The symptoms are caused by urinary extravasation and are relieved by insertion of percutaneous nephrostomy.

Haemorrhage is generally not a problem which requires transfusion, but even small smounts of bleeding from the ureteric mucosa can impair vision. If increase in irrigation flow does not improve the situation it may be necessary to insert a ureteric catheter, abandon the procedure and try again a few days later. Only the most clumsy operator will manage to perforate the ureter and peri-ureteric veins to cause major bleeding.

On rare occasions the size of the stone is misjudged and the basket and stone will become impacted in the ureter. This situation is overcome by removing the outer sheath of the basket. The resulting increase in capacity of the instrument channel will allow passage of an EHL or laser fibre. Further stone disintegration then takes place allowing the trapped basket to be removed. Occasionally, metal fatigue will cause the tip of the ultrasound probe to break off. This can be retrieved with forceps or a basket.

Removal of a stone from an obstructed or infected ureter may produce intraoperative bacteraemia. If this occurs, appropriate antibiotics and supportive measures are given, the obstruction should be relieved, the procedure abandoned and a second attempt made once the patient has become stable.

Late complications

A ureteric stricture will develop in a small but significant number of cases. Although many of these strictures are iatrogenic and caused by the use of too large an instrument or other mucosal damage, some strictures undoubtedly occur at the original site of the stone. Such strictures often respond to an endoscopic ureterotomy or to balloon dilatation, in contrast to those strictures caused by trauma which usually fail to respond to dilatation and require surgical correction.

Ureteric reflux secondary to ureteral dilatation occurs transiently and has been observed several months after ureteroscopy but does not appear to be a problem in clinical practice.

Other methods of ureteric stone removal

Stones impacted at the ureterovesical junction may be

removed by meatotomy with a Bee-sting electrode. The risk of ureterovesical reflux will be minimized if the incision in the bladder and ureteral mucosa is kept as short as possible. The stone then either falls into the bladder where it can be removed or grasping forceps can be applied to extract the stone from the ureter.

Basket extraction

For stones less than 5 mm in diameter and less than 5 cm up an unobstructed ureter, which have been present for a short time, it is possible to pass a helical wire basket 'blindly' up the ureter. With fluoroscopic screening as an aid, the basket is passed beyond the stone and opened in the ureter. It is then gently withdrawn and an attempt made to 'catch' the stone. The success rate of this procedure is around 50% and the indications for its safe use are extremely limited. This compares with a success rate of well over 90% for endoscopic removal of stones in all parts of the ureter.

Extracorporeal shock wave lithotripsy

The *in vitro* success of the application of shock wave technology as an effective method of fragmenting the urinary tract stones is both well known and well proven. In the mid-1970s, Dornier Medical Systems (an offshoot of the Dornier Aircraft Company) worked in collaboration with the Department of Urology of Munich University to develop a method to fragment renal calculi using extracorporeal shock wave lithotripsy (ESWL). The first patient was treated in February 1980 and there has since been a profusion of commercially available lithotriptors.

This section will present a brief overview of the principles of lithotripsy and the basic concept of ESWL.

A shock wave is a complex acoustic pulse that is formed from the sum of many sinusoidal waves of different frequencies. As the wave passes through a medium, a shock front is formed at which there is a sudden rise in pressure and density. If the pressure wave converges towards its geometric focus, the shape of the pressure wave is altered and a finite pressure is attained.

The physical characteristics of water and the soft tissues of the body are similar and it is thus possible to couple the focused shock wave to the body via a water–skin interface. Although some of the energy will be absorbed during this process, a significant amount of focused energy can be delivered to the surface of a stone.

When a shock wave hits the surface of a stone, some energy is reflected creating a compressive force on the front surface of the stone. A compression pulse will then travel through the stone faster than its originating shock front through tissue and this produces further stress on the sides of the stone. At its back surface a reflection of the compression pulse creates a tensile pulse travelling back through the stone which produces micro-cracks. Continued shock wave application will eventually produce fragmentation. The speed at which this occurs will depend upon the composition and tensile strength of the stone.

The basic components of a lithotriptor are: energy source, focusing system, and localization system. Each component will be combined with other components and 18 different configurations of lithotriptor are theoretically possible. At least 13 different machines are commercially available and there is at first sight a bewildering array of lithotriptor technology on the market. In practice, the choice of machine will be governed as much by local needs as the theoretical considerations and the claims of the manufacturers.

Energy source

Any physical mechanism which converts energy into its acoustic form can be used for ESWL. This will include lasers and micro-explosives which is the most efficient means of converting energy. However, technical problems have not been overcome using laser energy and only the Japanese have produced a commercial lithotriptor using lead azide pellets. Dornier initially produced a spark gap energy source in which two underwater metal electrodes are connected in series with a capacitor charged to a high voltage (15–22 kV). A conducting path forms between the electrodes, and the capacitor quickly discharges the electrical energy into the water which causes a rise in temperature with the formation of vapour bubbles. A compressive pressure pulse results from expansion of the heated gases. Rather like the spark plug of a motor car, high spark temperatures of the electrodes cause metal vaporization and erosion requiring regular adjustment and replacement of the spark plug.

The application of electrical energy across a piezo-electric crystal changes its external dimensions. Movement of the crystal produces a pressure wave and the use of multiple crystals will produce a wave of sufficient magnitude to allow stone disintegration to take place. In practice, some 3000 piezoelectric crystals are used as an energy source in some lithotriptors.

The application of an alternating current to a fixed helical coil will produce a fluctuating magnetic field which can be used to repel a flexible metallic membrane to create a pressure wave. The speed of the current rise through the coil and the properties of the membrane are critical in determining the characteristics of the acoustic impulse.

Focusing

The system may be self-focusing where the source is shaped so as to concentrate the energy at the focus. This system is used in the piezoelectric generators where the piezoelectric crystals are so arranged as to form part of a sphere with its focus at the centre (Figure 37.10).

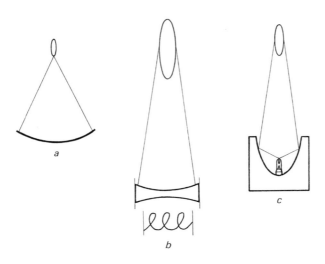

Figure 37.10 Shock wave production and focusing. *a*, Self-focusing system of piezoceramic generator. This produces a wide aperture and small focus. *b*, Acoustic lens focusing of electromagnetic system producing a long narrow focus. *c*, Geometric focusing of spark gap lithotriptor using ellipsoid reflector and cigar-shaped focus

An acoustic lens used in conjunction with electromagnetic generators can be used to focus the energy. Some energy is lost by reflection at the lens–water interface and absorption within the lens and the focusing action is controlled by the difference in acoustic properties between water and lens material and the shape of the lens.

The geometrical properties of an ellipsoidal reflector are used in the focusing systems of many spark gap lithotriptors. The electrode is centred at the primary focus of an ellipse (F1) and the shock waves are reflected to arrive simultaneously at the second focus (F2).

Localization

In order to maximize efficiency and to minimize damage to surrounding tissues, accurate localization during ESWL is crucial. The localization system must be extremely precise if the shock wave volume is small. X-rays or ultrasound may be used for stone positioning. Fluoroscopic localization is undoubtedly more versatile since it allows imaging of the ureter, but it is not suitable for visualization of radiolucent stones or stones overlying the pelvic brim. Radiation is an important factor and fluoroscopy cannot be used for constant monitoring of treatment. By contrast, ultrasound localization provides excellent visualization of stones in the kidney and to a lesser extent stones in the upper third of the ureter and within a

few centimetres of the bladder. Ultrasound is safe and there is, of course, no radiation risk, but one drawback is that the surgeon requires some training before becoming entirely proficient. Most manufacturers have now adopted a compromise and combine both fluoroscopic and ultrasound localization systems in the same machine.

Radiolucent stones are, of course, impossible to locate with X-rays unless intravenous or retrograde contrast medium is used to outline the collecting system. The ability to image stones with fluoroscopy is directly proportional to the quality of the X-ray equipment integrated into the lithotriptor. Occasionally, the fixed ultrasound probe which is mounted in the centre of an array of piezoceramic crystals may prove inadequate for visualization of stones which are hidden behind a rib structure. The robotic arm ultrasound principle used in other machines does not have this disadvantage, but in all cases identification of ureteric stones with ultrasound is not as easy as with fluoroscopy.

To assist in visualization and fragmentation of ureteric stones greater than 1 cm in diameter, retrograde flushing of the stones into the renal pelvis or calix is required.

The aperture of entry of the shock wave into the body with early lithotriptors was narrow and shock wave application was therefore painful, and general or epidural anaesthesia was required. However, it was discovered that by widening the aperture, application of shock waves became less painful and could be tolerated in the conscious patient with the aid of parenteral analgesics. Only one machine, using a piezoelectric generator, has a sufficiently wide aperture to permit treatment without any form of analgesia or sedation, but by increasing the diameter of the aperture the focus of the shock wave and therefore the pulse pressure contained within it is reduced, possibly reducing its efficiency.

In practice, all major manufacturers now produce machines which are virtually bespoke. Some machines are combined with an operating table facility for use with endo-urological procedures. Developments in this field are so rapid and a number of machines so large that it is impossible to discuss the advantages and disadvantages of each machine. However, the basic principles of lithotripsy treatment are outlined below.

The underlying principle of extracorporeal shock wave lithotripsy is the fragmentation of stones by shock waves and the consequent discharge of stone fragments from the upper urinary tract. Thus, it will be seen that the following factors must be taken into account in determining whether lithotripsy is optimum treatment for a stone:

Stone size.
Stone hardness.
Stone position.
Anatomical abnormalities.
Urine output.

STONE SIZE

It is self-evident that the larger the initial size of the stone, the greater the amount of stone bulk which must pass through the ureter. Thus, with increasing stone bulk there is a greater risk of ureteric obstruction due to stone fragments. This will also occur if fragmentation is inadequate, i.e. if fragments of stone 4 mm or greater remain after lithotripsy. Extensive studies show that irrespective of the type of lithotriptor, this risk becomes significantly greater once the initial stone size exceeds 2 cm. Therefore, lithotripsy as the *sole* treatment is contraindicated if the stone bulk exceeds 2 cm. Insertion of a ureteric stent which allows free drainage of urine and causes the ureter to dilate will reduce the risk of obstruction if stones larger than 2 cm are treated by lithotripsy.

Once the stone bulk exceeds 3 cm, the number of shock waves required to achieve adequate fragmentation is increased and with it the potential for long-term renal damage.

STONE HARDNESS

This is a very difficult factor to assess prior to treatment. However, it appears that stones which seem denser than the adjacent bone (i.e. whiter) are probably harder. Stone hardness is a factor which appears to be more important with smaller focus machines where the pulse energy is lower than that delivered by machines with a large focus. Cystine stones are particularly difficult to fragment by ESWL.

STONE POSITION

It is again self-evident that stones in a dependent portion of the kidney, i.e. lower or mid calix, are less likely to clear than stones elsewhere and this is particularly so in the presence of scarring or hydrocalicosis. Thus, although the lithotripsy may produce effective fragmentation, the fragments remain and ultimately coalesce to form a second stone.

ANATOMICAL ABNORMALITIES

Patients with a long infundibulum from the lower calix and the presence of hydrocalicosis or any form of outflow obstruction, e.g. caliceal neck stenosis, ureteropelvic junction obstruction, will experience a delay in discharging fragments. Obstruction will, at best, delay the passage of stone fragments and may in fact result in further obstruction due to retained stone fragments. In addition, the presence of a horseshoe kidney may well impair drainage and these factors must be taken into account when assessing a patient's suitability for lithotripsy.

URINE OUTPUT

The decision to undertake conservative management of a renal stone will depend upon an assessment of renal function. However, this determination of renal function is completely different from an assessment of urine output from an affected kidney, since some kidneys which function poorly continue to produce large urine volumes and it is the urine output which is important in these circumstances.

Indications

It will be seen from the above that the indications for lithotripsy are independent of the type of lithotriptor available. Thus, lithotripsy is ideal for stones less than 2 cm in diameter in anatomically normal and functioning kidneys. Stones between 2 and 3 cm can be treated adequately, provided that a JJ ureteric stent is inserted to minimize the risk of obstruction. Stones greater than 3 cm in diameter, for the reasons outlined above, should be treated by a combination of percutaneous debulking and lithotripsy 'mop up' for any residual fragments.

Small ureteric stones (i.e. less than 1 cm) in an unobstructed system which can be visualized can also be treated by lithotripsy, with an 80% chance of success, but this figure is reduced if the stone is greater than 1 cm in diameter or the ureter is obstructed. In such cases, depending upon the position of the stone, retrograde manipulation, or antegrade or retrograde endoscopic approaches, are preferable.

Contraindications

Physical size may be a contraindication if the patient's bulk is too big to permit focusing of the shock waves on the stone. Treatment of children, however, is *not* contraindicated. They frequently do very well as the stones are often much softer and fragment more readily.

Machines which have a larger focus have a greater potential for haematoma production and thus their use is contraindicated in patients with a bleeding diathesis. However, the small-focus machines, because of the lower incidence of haematoma, can be used with care in patients with coagulation disorders.

Anatomical deformities may also prove problematical, particularly in the presence of kyphoscoliosis. However, it may be possible to treat patients with these deformities in an alternative position, e.g. prone rather than supine.

Although radiolucent stones can be fragmented with lithotripsy, the use of ESWL in this group of patients is not recommended because of the difficulties involved with follow-up and assessment of stone-free status.

Operative technique

This will depend upon the shock wave generator and

the means of focusing. It is not possible to describe the operative technique in detail for each type of lithotriptor, but a few general points are outlined below.

PREOPERATIVE PREPARATION

A full-length film from the IVU series which shows the renal anatomy clearly and a plain radiograph taken immediately before treatment are *essential* prerequisites. Antibiotic therapy is only required for those patients with a history of infective stones or during ESWL 'mop up' treatment for staghorn calculi.

Intravenous sedation and/or analgesia is given immediately prior to treatment where necessary. This is generally required for all lithotriptors except those with a small (less than 1 cm long) focus.

The stone is localized with the aid of fluoroscopy or ultrasound and treatment is commenced. The number of shock waves administered will vary according to the size of the focus and the shock wave intensity and will range from 1500 to 4000 per treatment session. Unless continuous ultrasound monitoring is used, respiratory 'gating' can be used to trigger the shock wave only during the expiration phase to ensure that the majority of shock waves fall upon the targeted area. Electrocardiograph 'gating' is required for machines with a larger focus, since arrhythmias have been reported if shock waves are fired at an inappropriate time during the cardiac cycle. It is possible to monitor fragmentation throughout the treatment with ultrasound, but in those machines which use fluoroscopy as the only means of stone localization, a short period of screening can be used to determine progress of fragmentation.

Patients who have been given intravenous sedation should be given time to recover, whereas patients who do not require sedation may leave shortly after treatment has finished.

The success of stone fragmentation should be assessed by a plain abdominal radiograph. The timing of this film is controversial because some authorities believe that it is impossible to assess the degree of fragmentation immediately after treatment. However, all centres would agree that it is appropriate to carry out a check X-ray within 24 h of treatment.

Complications

The procedure is remarkably free of complications and there should be very few intraprocedural problems. However, particularly in a non-sedated patient, severe pain may develop either due to the application of shock waves or to passage of small fragments of stone. Nausea and occasionally vomiting will also occur. Temporary suspension of treatment and/or the prescription of analgesia will rectify the problem. Occasionally, patients will develop fever and rigor during treatment, in which case the treatment should

be suspended immediately and appropriate antibiotic therapy and other support given. A stone may suddenly become invisible during ultrasound monitoring, particularly if it is mobile, and if it cannot be found by further ultrasound examination it may be necessary to suspend treatment, obtain a plain radiograph and recommence localization.

Postoperative complications

Transient haematuria is a feature of lithotripsy and should not be regarded as a complication. However, perirenal haematoma can be observed in a significant number of patients undergoing lithotripsy who are followed up by renal ultrasonography or CT scanning. The haematoma may be of sufficient size to cause loin pain, but it usually resolves without further intervention.

Patients with staghorn or matrix calculi treated by lithotripsy are especially prone to develop postoperative urinary infections and this can be minimized by prophylactic antibiotic therapy. There are a few case reports of patients developing a perirenal abscess following lithotripsy; this is often not apparent until some weeks after treatment and may present as continuing loin pain, unexplained fever and weight loss. The condition is diagnosed by the characteristic appearances seen on an ultrasound scan.

The commonest postoperative complication is ureteric colic which occurs in up to 20% of patients. This is due to the passage of fragments of stone and should be treated expectantly. However, some stone fragments will jam in the ureter to produce obstruction and increasing pain. The presence of one fixed fragment causes other smaller fragments to build up proximal to the obstructing fragment forming a sort of log-jam or steinstrasse. Small-bulk steinstrasse with small fragments generally pass spontaneously, but large-bulk steinstrasse with large obstructing fragments require endoscopic fragmentation and removal. Occasionally it will be necessary to decompress the upper urinary tract by percutaneous nephrostomy, and often relief of the obstruction and resultant return in peristalsis enables the fragments to pass spontaneously.

The long-term effects of lithotripsy are not known. There are conflicting reports that lithotripsy will increase the incidence of hypertension, but this point has not been proven. Certainly, in the short term, parenchymal haematomas are formed and there is enzymatic evidence of temporary renal damage, but in experimental studies all of the acute changes seen in association with lithotripsy resolve.

Choice of treatment

It can be seen that there are many different treatment options and although it is possible to generalize about treatment for a particular type of stone, optimum results will be obtained by adopting a flexible approach to treatment and tailoring that treatment to the individual patient's requirements. A multidisciplinary approach and the use of more than one

Table 37.1 **Multidisciplinary approach to renal stone management**

Site	Type/size	Treatment*
Kidney	<1 cm	ESWL
Upper ureter	<1 cm	P-B/A.URS/ESWL
Mid ureter		P-B/laser
Lower ureter		Laser/ESWL
Kidney	1–2 cm	ESWL
Upper ureter	1–2 cm	A.URS/P-B
Mid ureter		P-B/open
Lower ureter		Laser
Kidney	2–3 cm	ESWL + stent
Kidney	>3 cm solitary	PCNL
	>3 cm staghorn	PCNL + ESWL
	>3 cm partial	
	staghorn	PCNL/ESWL

* ESWL, extracorporeal shock wave lithotripsy; P-B, push-bang (ESWL); A.URS, antegrade ureteroscopy; PCNL, percutaneous nephrolithotomy.

method of treatment should ensure the highest possible chance of rendering the patient stone free.

There are three major factors involved in determining the treatment. These relate to the patient, kidney and the stone.

The age, general health and fitness of the patient for surgery, together with size, may well be determining factors and although of lesser importance, occupation may have a role in deciding on the best treatment.

Account must be taken of anatomical abnormalities such as fusion, rotation and the presence of cysts and the degree of renal function present. The presence of kyphoscoliosis or other anatomical deformity such as a fixed hip will also influence treatment choice.

Recurrent infections and the presence of scarring must be taken into account, but stone size, likely composition and not least the position of the stone are a major influence in determining treatment. Thus it can be seen that a multidisciplinary approach to renal stone management, as summarized in Table 37.1, is essential if optimum results are to be obtained.

Arterial, cardiac and venous surgery

38

Arterial ischaemia

R. N. Baird

Introduction

In the past 50 years, surgical techniques have become available to repair arteries which have been damaged by injury and disease. Examples include the insertion of Dacron and vein conduits to bypass atherosclerotic occlusions of the leg arteries, and endarterectomy of the diseased internal carotid artery in the neck. Less invasive interventions have also become available; these include recanalization with balloon dilatation, and intra-arterial thrombolysis for acute-on-chronic ischaemia.

Procedures which are less commonly performed include balloon catheter embolectomy, the repair of arterial injuries, upper limb sympathectomy for hyperhidrosis, and bypass for mesenteric ischaemia. Balloon dilatation is the treatment of choice for renal artery stenosis causing hypertension and renal failure.

As already mentioned, atherosclerosis is the usual cause, and others are rare. Fibromuscular disease of the renal artery and cystic adventitial disease of the popliteal artery are occasionally encountered in young adults. The subclavian artery can be *externally compressed* by cervical and first ribs in the thoracic outlet syndrome, and the popliteal artery by the medial head of gastrocnemius, in claudicants under 40 years of age. *Large vessel arteritis*, radiation, giant cell and Takayasu, can affect the subclavian, axillary and temporal arteries.

Systemic disorders affecting small arteries of the extremities include Buerger's disease, also known as thrombo-angiitis obliterans, and connective tissue disorders including systemic sclerosis and scleroderma. Diabetes mellitus causes a *microangiopathy* which, in combination with atheroma and neuropathy, makes these patients *fifty* times more susceptible to ulceration, infection and gangrene of the feet than non-diabetics.

Neoplasia seldom invade arteries. Exceptions are sarcomas of the thigh, which sometimes involve the femoral vessels, and carotid body tumours.

The first part of this chapter covers basic principles and the conditions for which a surgical opinion is sought. This is followed by an outline of the procedures which are available to treat these conditions.

Surgical anatomy

The arteries conduct and distribute oxygen and other nutrients. The pulsatile output of the left ventricle is smoothed to streamlined, laminar flow sustained throughout diastole, by the *windkessel* or elastic reservoir of the walls of the main arteries (Figure 38.1). This is most effective in the cerebral circulation, because of its low peripheral resistance and also the elasticity of the carotid bulb which smooths flow in the internal carotid artery.

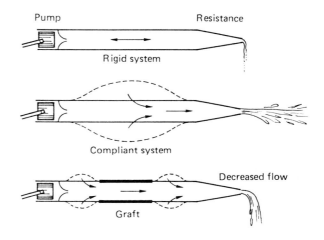

Figure 38.1 Effect of arterial wall compliance in sustaining distal perfusion during diastole, and of the adverse effect of inserting a rigid prosthetic replacement

Diastolic flow in the extremity vessels is often restricted by constriction of circular smooth muscle in the walls of small arteries and arterioles. This can be overcome, for a time, by vasodilators and sympathectomy. Central factors, mainly left ventricular function, also affect blood flow to the extremities. If symptomatic atheroma exists at multiple sites, as with myocardial ischaemia and claudication, strengthening of cardiac output by coronary artery bypass can improve the blood supply to the legs sufficiently so that claudication is less of a problem. Claudication is made worse by beta-blockers which are widely used to treat hypertension and angina, and alternatives with positive inotropic effects during exercise are better.

Atherosclerosis

Cholesterol is laid down by chylomicra as yellow fatty streaks. The posterior arterial wall is particularly affected during the low circulatory state of sleep.

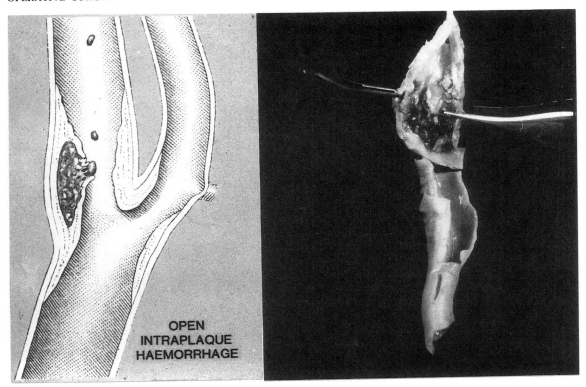

OPEN
INTRAPLAQUE
HAEMORRHAGE

Figure 38.2 Diagram (*left*) of intra-plaque haemorrhage with emboli from the carotid bulb and the operative specimen (*right*) at carotid endarterectomy

Smoking has a prolonged nicotine-related vasoconstrictor effect with every inhalation. Tobacco also causes *injury* to the arterial endothelium and *hypercoagulability* from secondary polycythaemia. This is a response to the loss of oxygen-carrying capacity when carbon monoxide in tobacco smoke is preferentially taken up by red blood cells.

As the diseased artery narrows, the volume of blood flow within it is reduced. However, the blood velocity is increased, similar to the effect of putting a thumb over the end of a garden hose. This jet effect causes the systolic murmur of an arterial stenosis. Examples include the aortic valve, coarctation of the aorta and carotid stenosis. The peak systolic velocity (normally less than 4 kHz) is increased, for example, to 7.5 kHz in a 75% stenosis of the internal carotid artery and this can be measured non-invasively by duplex ultrasound. Blood flow may enter fissures within a complicated atheromatous plaque, obstructing the vessel lumen and causing it to break away from the arterial wall (Figure 38.2). This haemorrhage into a plaque leads to a sudden worsening of symptoms.

In addition to their flow-reducing effects, irregular atherosclerotic plaques are the source of arterial emboli. These can be either fibrin/platelet thrombi which cause transient cerebral ischaemia, or calcific debris which is seen in the retinal arteries as a Hollenhorst plaque. This atheroembolism produces end-organ ischaemia in the presence of palpable pulses, as in the blue-toe syndrome. Straightforward arterial emboli are nowadays quite rare. Their source is usually the left side of the heart, either from the auricular appendage in atrial fibrillation or from the hypercoagulable left ventricular endothelium during the days after a large myocardial infarct

Risk factors

The main risk factors for atherosclerosis are lipid abnormalities, cigarette smoking, hypertension, diabetes mellitus, fibrinogen and haemostatic factors. Lack of exercise and physical activity, obesity and competitive and ambitious behaviour patterns in so-called type A personalities also carry risks, which are less sharply defined. Risk control and reversal will arrest the progression of atheroma, and there have been reports of regression. In practice, this means stopping smoking, reducing intake of total fat with cholesterol, some substitution with polyunsaturated fats, reduction to ideal weight, and review of lifestyle. Some younger patients, including those with familial (type III) hyperlipidaemia, should be considered for drug treatment by lipid-lowering agents. The majority are in the retired age group, and they should concentrate on abstinence from tobacco, a sensible diet and control of weight.

Arterial thrombosis

Thrombosis and fibrinolysis are physiological responses which are altered when an artery is operated upon and in many arterial and systemic diseases. The final phase of the coagulation cascade is the conversion of fibrinogen to fibrin clot in the presence of calcium ions, thrombin, platelets and other factors. Liquefaction of clot, or fibrinolysis, is the digestion of fibrin by plasmin.

Treatments to prevent and reverse arterial thrombosis are routinely prescribed by vascular surgeons. Following severe haemorrhage, the blood can lose its capacity to clot because of a consumptive coagulopathy known as disseminated intravascular coagulation (DIC). Blood is taken for coagulation studies and any heparin effect is reversed with protamine. Transfusions of fresh frozen plasma, cryoprecipitates, platelets and fresh whole blood are commenced. Trasylol (aprotinin), in a loading intravenous dose of 500 000 u or more, can be a helpful addition to the armamentarium of treatments for this worrying complication.

Thrombotic disorders

Certain uncommon disorders have been identified in patients at increased risk of thrombosis; clinical findings include a family history, thrombosis at an early age and recurrent thrombotic episodes. Arteriograms show poor run-off vessels and bypasses seldom remain patent. Diagnosis is by specific assay and treatment is by prolonged anticoagulation. A thrombotic tendency arises from deficiencies of protein C, protein S and antithrombin III, and from the presence of lupus anticoagulant in the blood. In systemic disorders such as Crohn's disease, ischaemia can be caused by the release of powerful vasoconstrictor peptides such as endothelin; the vasoconstrictor effect can be abolished by resection of the affected bowel.

Anti-thrombotic treatment

Aspirin prolongs the bleeding time by interfering with platelet function, and is the initial treatment of transient cerebral ischaemia, in a daily dose of 70–100 mg. It is effective in preventing further symptoms of transient ischaemic attacks (TIAs) and is also used postoperatively following carotid endarterectomy to cover healing of the endarterectomized flow surface, and after prosthetic femoropopliteal bypass. Some dyspeptic patients find that their indigestion is worse, and prefer an enteric-coated preparation. Aspirin has profound effects on the coagulation system and is best discontinued preoperatively to allow platelet function to recover.

Anticoagulants

Heparin was discovered in 1916 by Jay McLean, medical student at Johns Hopkins University, and was introduced into clinical practice in 1940 when Murray of Toronto used it to prevent arterial thrombosis during replacement of a popliteal aneurysm by a vein graft. Today, a systemic dose of 5000 u is routinely administered intravenously before arteries are incised or dilated. The effect wears off after an hour and reversal with protamine is not required.

Other indications for its use include an acute arterial embolus to an extremity, prior to embolectomy. An intravenous dose of 10 000 u is administered when the diagnosis is made to limit the propagation of thrombus. Heparin is also used to prevent arterial thrombosis as a continuous intravenous infusion, either in a full (40 000 u/24 h or partial dose (24 000u/24 h). The dose is monitored by measuring the activated partial thromboplastin time (APTT). The partial dose is useful post-reconstruction since a full dose can cause anastomotic bleeding.

Warfarin is an oral anticoagulant which is used routinely to prevent further emboli and to reduce the mortality in patients who have undergone balloon catheter embolectomy. Treatment should be continued for a year, by which time the risk is reduced of further emboli from, for example, a mural thrombus associated with a myocardial infarct. Patients taking anticoagulants are at increased risk of bleeding, so that care is needed if an intervention is contemplated. It is reasonable to do a femoral arteriogram or an operation involving the extremities after discontinuing warfarin for 2–3 days. For intra-abdominal operations, warfarin should be stopped for a week and normal coagulation verified by an international normalized ratio (INR) blood test.

Acute ischaemia

Arteries and veins differ markedly in their response to cessation of flow and consequent intraluminal thrombus formation. In arteries, this process is irreversible unless the thrombus is extracted mechanically or dissolved by thrombolysis. Veins, on the other hand, undergo spontaneous recanalization with restoration of the lumen, although the valves are destroyed.

The commonest cause of acute arterial ischaemia is *thrombosis within a pre-existing atheromatous stenosis*. The artery most frequently affected is the superficial femoral artery in the thigh. There is a sudden worsening in the perfusion of the limb, with the onset of claudication if walking was previously unrestricted, or critical ischaemia superimposed on claudication. The diagnosis is made clinically and confirmed by an arteriogram. Treatment is carried out by advancing the tip of an arteriogram catheter into the thrombus, and by constant or bolus infusion of a fibrinolytic agent such as streptokinase, recombinant tissue plasminogen activator (rtPA), or urokinase. This clears the thrombus and reveals the underlying stenosis which is dilated with a balloon catheter.

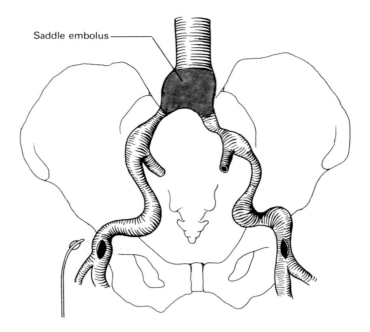

Figure 38.3 Saddle embolus at the aortic bifurcation prior to balloon catheter embolectomy

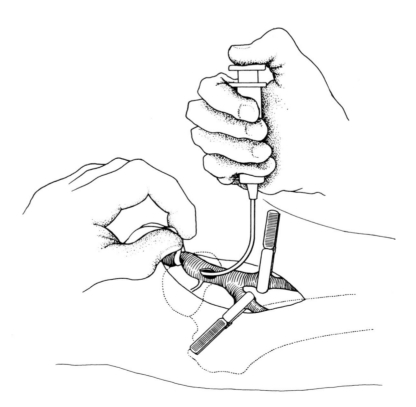

Figure 38.4 Balloon catheter placed through the embolus and inflated in the aorta prior to withdrawal

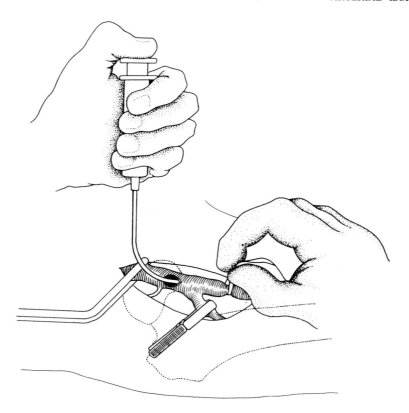

Figure 38.5 Balloon catheter placed distally via the superficial femoral and popliteal arteries to the calf, and inflated prior to withdrawal

Centrally-originating emboli arise from the auricular appendage of the left atrium in atrial fibrillation, and from left ventricular mural thrombus a few days after a severe myocardial infarction. Vegetations on the aortic and mitral valves were a common cause before bacterial endocarditis became effectively treated by antibiotics and valve replacement. The femoral artery is exposed in the groin, often under local anaesthesia, and the embolus and propagated thrombus are extracted by a Fogarty-type balloon catheter (Figures 38.3–38.5). The thrombus is sent for culture and histology, since occasionally a bronchogenic carcinoma embolizes. Postoperatively, anticoagulation with warfarin is routine. It should be noted that an embolectomy balloon is elastic, unlike an angioplasty balloon, which is made of rigid plastic and distends to a fixed diameter and no more.

Aortic dissection presents uncommonly as acute leg ischaemia. There is usually a history of retrosternal and back pain, and the patient is hypertensive. The mechanism of ischaemia is that the true aortic lumen is obstructed by the dissected false lumen (Figure 38.6). In most instances there is adequate residual perfusion, and resolution follows treatment of the underlying problem.

Arterial injuries arise from road accidents, stabbings and broken glass (Figure 38.7). Teenagers and

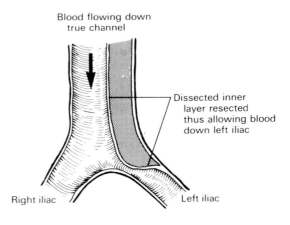

Blood flowing down true channel

Dissected inner layer resected thus allowing blood down left iliac

Right iliac

Left iliac

Figure 38.6 Mode of obstruction of an iliac artery by an aortic dissection

young adults are mainly affected. In closed injuries, the arterial intima is disrupted and the outer layers are usually intact. This leads to thrombosis which extends to collaterals on either side (Figure 38.8). Haemorrhage from an associated fracture may additionally compress the vessels (Figure 38.9). The results of direct arterial repair and vein bypass are good except where there are severe injuries elsewhere,

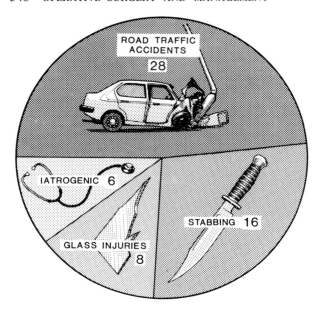

Figure 38.7 Main causes of 58 arterial injuries in Bristol

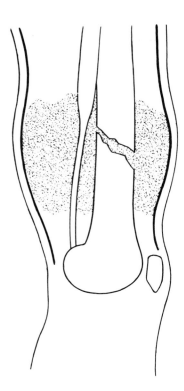

Figure 38.9 Arterial injury resulting from a fractured femur. The mechanism of injury is the bow-string impact of a spike of bone. The injured vessels are compressed by subfascial haematoma from the fracture

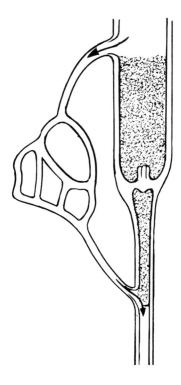

Figure 38.8 Closed arterial injury with thrombosis following disruption of the arterial intima. Note the narrowed distal vessel and reduced distal perfusion via collaterals

a crush injury involving small arteries, or there is a delay in the diagnosis which leads to tissue damage and the compartment syndrome. In this condition, oedema following reperfusion leads to increased pressure within closed fascial compartments of the calf, which is swollen and tense and leads to reduced perfusion of the extremity. Treatment is to relieve the intra-compartment pressure by fasciotomy via medial and lateral incisions so that the swollen muscles bulge into the wounds.

Iatrogenic injury occasionally follows diagnostic and therapeutic percutaneous arterial cannulation. It presents as distal ischaemia, an expanding haematoma and hypotension from retroperitoneal blood loss. The punctured artery is repaired with fine polypropylene sutures under local anaesthesia.

Chronic ischaemia

Chronic arterial ischaemia is virtually always caused by occlusive atherosclerosis and affects the lower limb, carotid, renal, mesenteric and the coronary arteries, which are considered elsewhere. End-organ ischaemia arises by two mechanisms – reduced arterial perfusion and atheroembolism.

Reduced perfusion presents at two levels – a detectable but asymptomatic resting underperfusion with ischaemic pain when flow is augmented. Examples include calf claudication and mesenteric angina. Severely reduced perfusion causes ischaemic pain at rest, which typically affects the distal forefoot and toes.

Atheroembolism occurs when cholesterol fragments and fibrin-platelet thrombi become detached from an atheromatous plaque, and is a mechanism of TIAs. Cholesterol chips and fibrin-platelet clusters can be seen fundoscopically in the retina in *amaurosis fugax* – transient monocular blindness.

In the *blue-toe syndrome*, a toe is discoloured and is disproportionately ischaemic in comparison with the remainder of the foot and leg, where the pressures are relatively good and pulses can sometimes be felt. Embolism from an atheromatous plaque is the explanation (Figure 38.10); the treatment is to remove the embolic source by endarterectomy or exclusion and bypass.

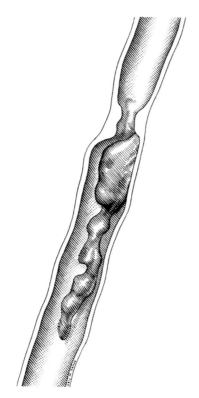

Figure 38.10 Atheromatous stenosis with a tail of thrombus seen on arteriogram which caused distal emboli

Intermittent claudication

Claudication is the most common symptom of chronic arterial ischaemia. It affects some 3% of mainly tobacco-smoking men over 50 years of age and is a cramp-like pain in the muscles of the calf which is caused by walking and is completely relieved by resting for 1–2 min. The onset of pain is more rapid if there is an uphill gradient, an adverse wind, a weight to carry or steps to climb. The cause is usually an atherosclerotic occlusion of the superficial femoral artery in the thigh. On examination, the leg looks healthy and the femoral artery pulsates normally in the groin. However, the popliteal and pedal pulses are

missing. The popliteal pulse is notoriously difficult to palpate and it is worth noting *en passant* that if it is easily felt, a popliteal aneurysm, a rare cause of claudication, should be suspected.

Where claudication is due to aorto-iliac disease, palpation reveals that the femoral artery pulsates weakly, often with a murmur on auscultation which is enhanced by exercise. If completely obstructed, it can be felt as a solid non-pulsatile cord. The muscles affected in proximal disease are the *glutei*, presenting as buttock claudication, or the *vasti* muscles of the thigh, which cause the entire leg to feel tired and heavy. Calf claudication is rare in patients younger than 40 years of age, and if it is encountered obstruction of the popliteal artery by cystic adventitial disease and external compression by an abnormal gastrocnemius band should be considered.

The *haemodynamic basis* for claudication is established by demonstration that the resting Doppler ankle systolic pressure is reduced when compared with the arm or the normal contralateral leg, and falls further after hyperaemia is induced by exercise, pneumatic cuff occlusion, or local vasodilator injection. Indicative figures for treatment of claudication in superficial femoral artery disease are a resting ankle pressure of half the arm pressure – an ankle brachial pressure index (ABPI) of 0.5 – and a fall to 0.3 after exercise. In proximal disease of the iliac arteries, with a weak femoral pulse, the threshold for treatment is higher, with a resting ABPI of 0.7 or 0.8 and a post-exercise fall to 0.6. These values are restored towards normal after successful treatment (Figure 38.11) by balloon angioplasty and bypass.

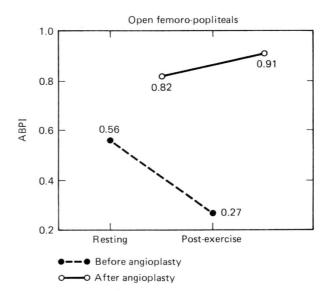

Figure 38.11 Resting and post-exercise ankle pressure index before and after femoro-popliteal angioplasty. Note the rise in the resting index and the abolition of the post-exercise fall following successful dilatation

Differential diagnosis of claudication

The main differential diagnosis of exercise-related leg pain is with lumbar osteoarthritis and other neuro-orthopaedic conditions. A past history of low back pain should be sought as well as pain of sciatic distribution and sensory symptoms such as tingling and paraesthesia. Some patients with *neurogenic* claudication can bicycle for longer than they can walk. The main back conditions to be considered are nerve-root compression, spinal stenosis and ischaemia of the cauda equina.

Other non-vascular conditions to be considered are calf cramps and restless legs at night, painful arthritis of the hips and knees, post-phlebitic swollen painful legs and lymphoedema with cellulitis. If gout is suspected, the uric acid should be checked. Diabetes can be associated with paraesthesia, numbness and severe leg pain, as well as infections and ulcers of the feet. Finally, reflux sympathetic dystrophy should be considered. It is an exaggerated response of an extremity to injury (see below).

Critical ischaemia

Patients with chronic critical ischaemia have such severe *pain* in the foot that they require analgesia. The pain is made worse by lying flat in bed, so they hang the leg down or sleep sitting in a chair. The foot is cold and is red when dependent and white upon elevation, with venous guttering and sluggish capillary return. There may be indolent ulcers or dry gangrene of the toes, bony pressure points and heel. Faint, damped Doppler signals can usually be detected in at least one of the tibial or peroneal arteries at the ankle, especially if the leg is dependent. Resting systolic ankle pressures are in the order of 30–60 mmHg. There is no advantage in exercising the patient as flow is already fully augmented. Most require a vein bypass to the popliteal or calf arteries.

Transient cerebral ischaemia

'A mild attack of apoplexy may be called death's retaining fee.' (Giles Menage, 1613–1692)

There are two main varieties of TIA. Many are of cortical origin and present as a mini-stroke, with numbness and weakness of a hand and leg on the contralateral side to the affected cerebral hemisphere. There may be a loss of speech and facial weakness, with the symptoms lasting for a minute or two, and followed by complete recovery. Other TIAs present as transient monocular blindness, known as amaurosis fugax, in which there is a curtain-like loss of vision, due to retinal artery emboli of cholesterol fragments (Figure 38.12) and platelet-fibrin clusters. A carotid source is sought on the ipsilateral side, as a murmur

on auscultation with a stethoscope. This sign, if positive, confirms the diagnosis. However, a murmur is not always heard. The investigation of choice is a *duplex ultrasound scan*, in which atheromatous narrowing at the origin of the internal carotid artery is imaged by ultrasound, and a high-speed jet of blood through the stenosis is detected by the Doppler part of the instrument. Carotid arteriography and cranial computed tomography (CT) and magnetic resonance (MR) scans to show cerebral infarcts will often help to clarify whether or not difficult cases should undergo carotid endarterectomy. Aspirin, in a low daily dose of 70–100 mg, is effective in eliminating TIAs but less so in preventing stroke. Meanwhile, the blood pressure is checked and any hypertension is treated.

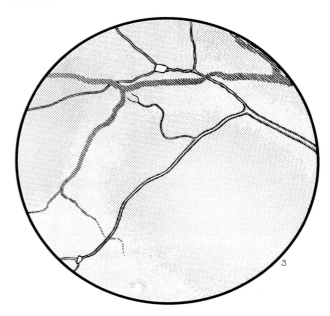

Figure 38.12 Diagram of retinal photograph showing cholesterol fragments lodged in the retinal arteries in a patient with amaurosis fugax

An occasional patient presents with a history of a mild stroke, followed by full recovery within a few days, and investigations show a complete occlusion of the symptomatic internal carotid artery, beyond the reach of surgical cure. In these circumstances, it is likely that the stroke was caused by thrombosis within a pre-existing carotid stenosis.

Renal ischaemia

Renal artery stenosis is associated with hypertension and loss of renal function (Figure 38.13). It is caused by atherosclerosis in the middle-aged and elderly, and by fibrous dysplasia in children and young adults. However, not every renal artery stenosis causes hypertension and decreased renal function, and careful evaluation is needed before correction is contemplated. The modalities available are medical treatment, surgical bypass or endarterectomy, and balloon dilatation.

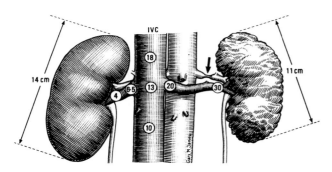

D.W.–42 YRS. LEFT RENAL ARTERY STENOSIS
(PLASMA RENIN ACTIVITY – ng/ml/hr)

Figure 38.13 A left renal artery stenosis in a hypertensive patient showing a shrunken left kidney producing an excessive output of renin

Mesenteric ischaemia

Intestinal ischaemia is rare, difficult to diagnose, and is always dangerous for the patient. *Acute intestinal ischaemia*, or abdominal apoplexy, is caused by sudden occlusion of the superior mesenteric artery (SMA) by an embolus of central origin. The symptoms are of severe generalized abdominal pain, in an elderly patient, which may be of vague and insidious origin. Physical signs are deceptively sparse, and plain abdominal X-rays have a non-specific ground-glass appearance. A raised white cell count is a helpful trigger to early laparotomy. At operation, the infarcted small bowel is blue and flaccid, with a cord-like, pulseless SMA. The situation is irremediable and the abdomen is closed, opiates administered for pain relief, and the relatives prepared for the inevitable outcome.

In the occasional middle-aged patient, irreversible ischaemia is confined to the ileocaecal region, and a local excision and exteriorization of the bowel ends is feasible. It is sometimes possible to restore arterial perfusion by balloon catheter embolectomy via an arteriotomy high in the SMA at the confluence of the root of the mesentery and the transverse mesocolon, adjacent to the take-off of the middle colic artery. This approach has the advantage of allowing a direct reconstruction if the embolectomy fails. Overall, visceral infarction has a greater than 90% mortality.

Chronic intestinal ischaemia presents with a triad of clinical features of food fear leading to weight loss, and atheroma elsewhere. The pathophysiology is as follows: atheromatous occlusions at the origins of the

coeliac axis and SMA lead to a reliance on collateral blood vessels, particularly the marginal artery of Drummond, which is seen on arteriography. Although the vascularity of the jejunum and ileum remain adequate while fasting, it is insufficient for the metabolic demands of even small meals. This leads to the dull ache of intestinal angina, which starts about half an hour after eating. Large meals cause more pain, which leads to food avoidance, weight loss and emaciation. These mainly male patients have been unable to stop smoking, and may have previously had a coronary or lower limb arterial bypass for chronic ischaemia.

The diagnosis is confirmed by duplex SMA flows before and after a test meal. A lateral aortogram shows short flush occlusions of the SMA and coeliac axis and excellent relief is produced by vein or prosthetic revascularization. The aorta may be small and calcified, or have undergone prosthetic replacement, with few soft areas onto which to sew the proximal anastomosis. The absence of body fat makes for easy access to the SMA and hepatic artery (Figure 38.14). Confidence in pain-free eating leads to regained body weight.

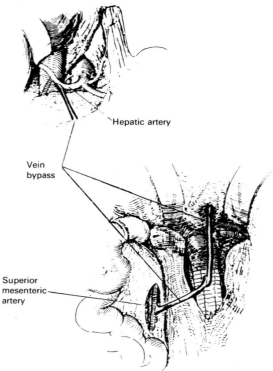

Hepatic artery

Vein bypass

Superior mesenteric artery

Figure 38.14 Vein bypass from a previously implanted aortic prosthesis to the superior mesenteric and hepatic arteries

Rare causes of mesenteric ischaemia include microcirculatory or 'non-occlusive' disease in which a segment of bowel is affected. The main arteries pulsate normally, and there is small vessel vasospasm on the arteriogram. The bowel becomes thickened and a stricture may develop. The cause is presumed to be a small vessel arteritis. Various treatments have been tried, including vasodilators, anticoagulants and steroids. Abdominal pain may be such that the affected segment of bowel has to be excised.

Colonic ischaemia in aortic surgery

A small proportion of patients, perhaps 1–2%, develop severe left colon ischaemia after aortic surgery. It is manifest as bloody diarrhoea with painful abdominal distension and the necrotic colon may have to be removed in a Hartmann's procedure. Lesser forms of mucosal ischaemia are seen if patients are colonoscoped in the days after a patent inferior mesenteric artery (IMA) has been ligated as part of an aorto-bifemoral Dacron bypass. The risk is minimized if it is possible to preserve flow in one or both internal iliac arteries by aortic or femoral end-to-side anastomoses.

Giant cell arteritis

Giant cell arteritis is an uncommon systemic vascular disease which affects the temporal, carotid, subclavian and brachial arteries. It is a granulomatous arteritis of unknown origin, with destruction of the internal elastic lamina and giant cells seen in a biopsy. The usual presentation in Europe is as temporal arteritis in patients over 50 years of age, possibly with polymyalgia rheumatica, and a markedly elevated ESR of more than 50 mm in the first hour. Diagnosis is by temporal artery biopsy. Treatment is by high-dose steroids, tapered as the ESR falls, and maintained long term in a low dose to prevent recurrence. Takayasu's arteritis is a form of giant cell arteritis which occurs in young Oriental females.

Radiation arteritis

Radiotherapy for malignant disease of the breast and cervix can cause radiation fibrosis of the axillary and iliac arteries. The damage becomes apparent many years later, as extremity ischaemia with absent distal pulses. Reconstruction is by remote bypass well away from the irradiated area.

Diseases of small arteries

These conditions cause ischaemia of the fingers and toes in the presence of palpable pulses at the wrist and ankle. They include vasospastic diseases, vibration white finger, reflex sympathetic dystrophy, frostbite, some emboli, arteritis, ergotism and acrocyanosis. Hyperhidrosis, though not a vascular disease, is included because it shares treatment by sympathectomy with other conditions in this section.

Primary vasospasm

This condition was first described by Maurice Raynaud in 1888. The fingers of both hands turn white and numb following exposure to cold. As rewarming occurs, sometimes after several hours, the fingers become blue, then bright red with throbbing pain as the circulation returns.

By definition, no underlying cause is found. Treatment is mainly directed towards preventing the cold-challenge by wearing warm clothes, including battery-heated gloves in severe cases. Systemic vasodilator therapy with nifedipine can help. However, most patients with benign, primary Raynaud's disease are young women, in 85% of whom the condition stabilizes or improves.

Secondary vasospasm

This affects mainly middle-aged women and is caused by connective tissue diseases such as scleroderma (systemic sclerosis), systemic lupus erythematosus and rheumatoid arthritis. Abnormal blood tests include raised ESR/viscosity, and the presence of anti-nuclear antibodies, lupus erythematosus (LE) cells and rheumatoid factor. Obstruction of blood flow by clumping of red cells in polycythaemia and in patients with cold agglutinins are other causes. Unilateral vasospasm is uncommon and, if encountered, a cervical rib (*vide infra*) should be sought. Treatment is directed in the underlying condition along with supportive measures for primary vasospasm.

The immediate effect of sympathectomy is to produce a warm, dry extremity. However, the benefit only lasts for a few months before vasospasm recurs. In view of this, its use is confined to helping to heal painful fingertip ulceration (Figure 38.15) in selected severe cases which are resistant to intra-arterial infusion of vasodilators such as reserpine, guanethidine and prostaglandins.

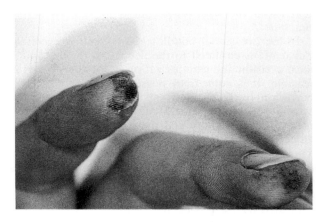

Figure 38.15 Fingertip ischaemic ulceration in severe vasospasm, prior to sympathectomy

Vibration white finger

This is an industrial disease caused by hand-held powered tools. It affects caulkers, riveters and grinders in the boilermaking, shipbuilding and repair industries, and forestry workers using chainsaws. The typical patient is male, aged 35–55 years, with a history of 10 years or so of exposure to vibrating tools for several hours each working day. The fingers tingle and become numb, and he is unable to perform the fine movements of tying shoelaces and doing up shirt buttons. There is a variable vasospastic component, and multiple digital artery occlusions on an arteriogram. The referral is often directed towards compensation, by solicitors instructed by the man's trade union. If a boilermaker, an ENT opinion may similarly be sought for industrial deafness. The diagnosis is confirmed, and its severity graded, by the Taylor–Pelmear scale. The condition is not reversible, and use of vibrating tools should be abandoned and alternative work sought.

Reflex sympathetic dystrophy

This is a persistent pain syndrome in an extremity following injury. It is otherwise known as algodystrophy, causalgia and Sudeck's atrophy, and results in failure of rehabilitation following an injury, which may have been quite minor. The extremity is painful and sensitive to touch, and disuse atrophy and osteoporosis develop. Treatment in the initial stages is based on education, reassurance and rehabilitation. In chronic cases, pain relief may be achieved by regional intravenous guanethidine and by sympathectomy. The condition may have a benign course, leading to resolution, or it may be severe, last for years with chronic pain and disability.

Frostbite

This is freezing of tissues from exposure to cold. Ice crystals form, with vasoconstriction, increased blood viscosity and sludging. Treatment is by thawing, though this should not be done until the risk of further exposure to cold has been overcome. Rapid rewarming is by immersion in warm water (38–42°C), and is painful. Vesicles form, and a line of demarcation gradually develops. This process may be helped by sympathectomy, or vasodilators including prostaglandins. The evidence tends to favour sympathectomy for the late sequelae of cold sensitivity and pain.

Emboli

Emboli to digital arteries may not be easily recognized, particularly since the main pulses are palpable. They may present in a lower extremity as the blue-toe syndrome, or in the fingers from thrombi in the subclavian artery in the thoracic outlet syndrome.

Today, bacterial endocarditis is seldom the underlying cause. Treatment is directed towards the underlying cause.

Small vessel arteritis

This encompasses a heterogeneous group of rare inflammatory vascular conditions, many of which cause secondary vasospasm, as described earlier. Others affecting the extremities include Buerger's disease (thromboangiitis obliterans) and diabetic microangiopathy.

Ergotism

This is a cause of severe ischaemia of the extremities which is occasionally encountered in patients who overtreat themselves for migraine. A careful history reveals the diagnosis, and the intense pharmacological vasospasm once known as St. Anthony's Fire is rapidly relieved when the ergot preparation is discontinued.

Acrocyanosis

This is a cyanotic discoloration of the hands and fingers of unknown cause. It is a benign condition and is mainly a cosmetic problem. No treatment is necessary. Livedo reticularis is a similar mottled discoloration of the extremities.

Hyperhidrosis

This is uncontrolled and excessive sweating of the hands and axillae of mainly 15–25 year olds. It causes social embarrassment from wetness of the hands and axillae. The rest of the body is often involved. Sometimes work is affected in those who handle paper, including bank clerks, and in waitresses because of patches of wetness in the armpits of their uniforms. The first line of treatment is to apply an antiperspirant overnight as a solution or roll-on of aluminium chloride hexahydrate. Conservative measures do not always work, and some seek bilateral upper thoracic sympathectomies which provide immediate and permanent relief. However, the operation, even when done endoscopically, is not without complications, including the small risk of a Horner's syndrome, and compensatory hyderhidrosis elsewhere, and a full discussion beforehand is advisable.

Reconstruction for aorto-iliac disease

Aorto-iliac arterial reconstruction is the treatment of choice for atherosclerotic occlusions of the infrarenal aorta, the common and external iliac arteries, the common femoral artery and the origin of the profunda femoris artery. The aim of reconstruction is to improve the perfusion of the profunda femoris and, if patent, the superficial femoral artery.

The clinical diagnosis of proximal disease is made by palpating a weakly pulsating or non-pulsatile femoral artery in the groin. The ankle pressures are checked, and treadmill testing is done in claudicants to confirm the haemodynamic basis for the symptoms. The general fitness of the patient for any intervention is assessed, and an arteriogram is done.

The following treatment options are considered, in increasing order of invasiveness and risk: balloon angioplasty; common femoral endarterectomy and profundaplasty; Dacron tube bypasses including femoro-femoral crossover, axillo-bifemoral bypass, and aorto-bifemoral bypass.

Balloon angioplasty

This treatment is the best option for iliac and aortic stenoses, since it is safe, effective, repeatable and requires no more than an overnight stay in hospital. For aortic stenosis, twin balloons are placed, one from each groin (Figure 38.16). It is not suitable for complete occlusions, which require an operation, and for stenoses within 5 cm of the puncture site in the common femoral artery, because of the need to insert a sheath, through which the balloon catheter is passed.

Occlusion of the common femoral artery

This, and isolated stenosis at the origin of the profunda femoris artery, are best dealt with surgically. The common and profunda femoris arteries are dissected through a groin incision, and a longitudinal arteriotomy is made. The occlusion is cleared by an endarterectomy, and the arteriotomy is closed directly or with a vein or prosthetic patch, using continuous 5/0 prolene sutures.

Unilateral iliac artery occlusion

This is treated, where possible, by a femoro-femoral crossover using an 8 mm Dacron tube (Figure 38.17). If the donor iliac artery has a stenosis with a pressure gradient (Figure 38.18) it is treated by balloon angioplasty prior to bypass.

Bilateral iliac occlusions

This, and aortic occlusion, are best treated by an aorto-bifemoral Dacron bifurcation prosthesis. This option is selected for occlusive atheroma which is too extensive for the lesser procedures, which have a lower mortality (1%) than aortic surgery (3%). An axillo-bifemoral bypass using 8 mm Dacron tubes is an alternative which avoids the need to enter the abdomen (Figure 38.19). It is considered for the occasionally unfit patient, with critical ischaemia, and for the 'unfavourable' abdomen. In the long term,

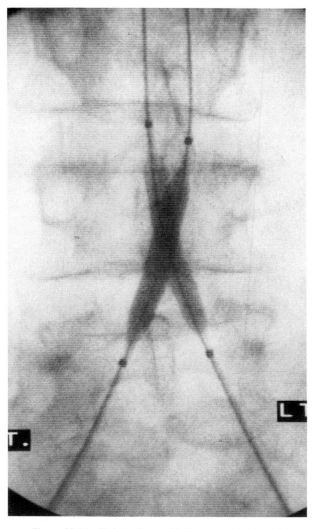

Figure 38.16 Twin balloons dilating an aortic stenosis

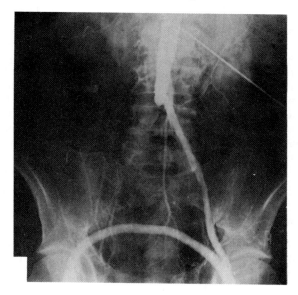

Figure 38.17 Arteriogram of a femoro-femoral crossover graft

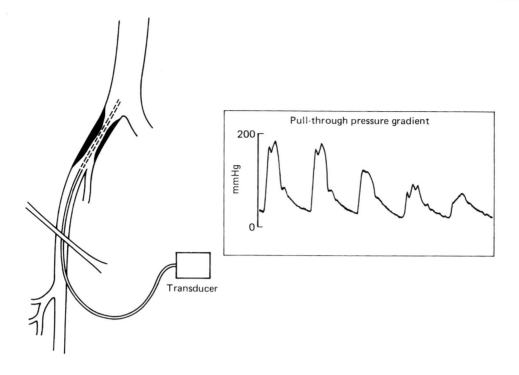

Figure 38.18   Confirmation of the haemodynamic effect of an iliac artery stenosis by showing a pull-through pressure gradient at arteriography. The effect is enhanced if papaverine is injected

orthotopic aortic reconstruction is more durable, with less need for secondary procedures to restore patency following late thrombosis of a limb of the prosthesis. Patients undergoing aortic surgery generally have poor cardiac reserve, with reduced left ventricular function. Their intravascular capacity is brittle, so that volume changes of 100–200 ml can tip the balance either way. Intraoperative haemorrhage, or sudden aortic declamping, can lead to hypotension and underperfusion of the renal and coronary arteries. Excess fluid replacement, on the other hand, causes congestive failure and pulmonary oedema. Dopamine has a useful inotropic effect and is frequently used intraoperatively.

Aorto-bifemoral Dacron bypass

Patients being prepared for aortic surgery often have other medical conditions, including hypertension, a past history of myocardial infarction, diabetes mellitus, polycythaemia and respiratory disease secondary to tobacco inhalation. Careful preoperative evaluation is required, and operation should not be undertaken within 6 months of a myocardial infarction. The possibility of predonation for autologous blood transfusion should be considered.

After arterial, venous and thoracic epidural lines have been inserted, and a urethral catheter placed, the common femoral arteries are exposed in the groins. If the superficial femoral artery is occluded, as is commonly the case, the profunda femoris arteries are dissected to beyond the circumflex femoral branches. This is likely to involve ligation of profunda veins. Attention is then turned to the aorta, which is exposed through a midline or supra-umbilical transverse incision. The viscera are carefully checked, along with the position of the nasogastric tube. Asymptomatic stones in a thin-walled gallbladder can be disregarded. Access is facilitated by a post-held ring or fish-bone retractor of Bookwalter or Omni-tract type. The posterior peritoneum is incised (Figure 38.20) and the aorta encircled between the inferior mesenteric artery origin and the left renal vein (Figure 38.21) Retroperitoneal tunnels are created by finger dissection to both groins. A Dacron bifurcation graft is selected of a size, usually 16 × 8 mm, which corresponds to the aortic diameter. A woven graft is a safe choice for the uninitiated, since it does not require preclotting. Some surgeons prefer knitted grafts, which are softer to handle, though preclotting is required. Grafts which are coated with collagen or gelatin are much more expensive for an arguably marginal advantage.

A graft is preclotted by immersion in 30 ml of the patient's blood until clotting occurs. This prevents the escape of blood through the interstices during implantation. However, the latticework of Dacron fibres allows for later fibrous ingrowth and incorporation of the prosthesis. An intravenous dose of 5000 u

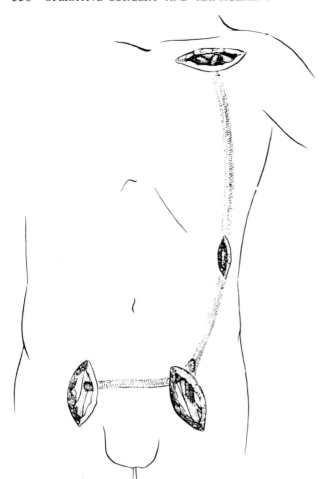

Figure 38.19 An axillo-bifemoral bypass

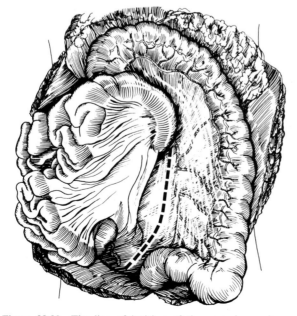

Figure 38.20 The line of incision of the posterior peritoneum between the inferior mesenteric vessels and the duodenum

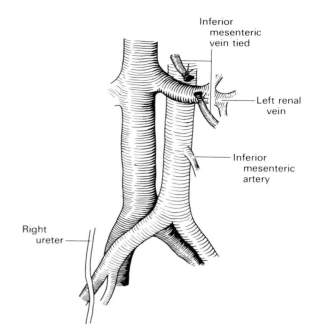

Figure 38.21 The aorta is exposed from the inferior mesenteric artery to the left renal vein. The inferior mesenteric vein has been ligated to aid access

heparin is administered and the aorta is clamped just below the renal arteries. If the aorta is occluded (Figure 38.22) it is transected and the prosthesis is sewn end-to-end with 3/0 prolene continuous sutures. Care is taken to ensure that the suture line is of adequate tension throughout. The aortic clamp is released to check for haemostasis, the distal limbs are tunnelled to the groins, and implanted by end-to-side anastomoses of 5/0 prolene. If the occlusions are mainly iliac, and the aorta is open, the proximal anastomosis may be made by the end-to-side technique (Figure 38.23). Haemostasis is checked, and the incisions are closed in layers. Antibiotic prophylaxis is provided by intravenous cefuroxime 750 mg at the induction of anaesthesia, with a further dose after 2 h. Overnight graft patency is checked by palpating the groin pulses. The patient sits out of bed on the first postoperative day, the epidural is tailed-off in 3–4 days and discharge from hospital is at a week.

Complications of aortic surgery

The general complications of aortic bypass are those of major abdominal surgery in patients with atherosclerosis, and include a myocardial infarction, and failure of the cardiac, respiratory and renal systems. The first postoperative night is frequently spent in the intensive treatment unit where there is careful monitoring and incipient system failures can be treated early.

Early surgical complications include intra-abdominal haemorrhage, which should be suspected and corrected in the early postoperative hours if there is a continuing transfusion requirement and a fall in the hourly urinary output. Graft thrombosis is uncommon; the cause tends to be poor run-off from a femoral anastomosis; operative revision is required to establish lasting patency.

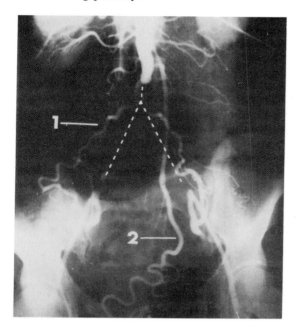

Figure 38.22 A translumbar aortogram showing total aortic occlusion. Large iliolumbar (1) and inferior mesenteric (2) collaterals

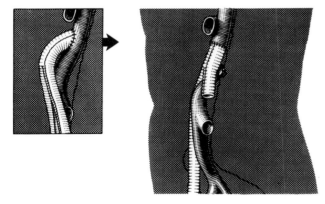

Figure 38.23 End-to-side (*above*) and end-to-end (*below*) Dacron-to-aorta anastomoses

Lymph fistula

This is a tiresome copious discharge of clear watery fluid from a groin incision, starting on the 3rd to 5th postoperative day. The loss of fluid from the wound may reach 200–300 ml/24 h and requires frequent changes of dressings; the output is sometimes contained by an adhesive plastic bag. The fluid is initially sterile, but before long a low-grade infection develops and antibiotics are needed. In most cases the wound heals within a month, although occasionally a chronically discharging sinus develops. The incidence of this complication is about 2%. In some cases, the wound is re-explored and the sartorius muscle is detached from its proximal attachment to the anterior superior iliac spine, and swung medially to cover the Dacron-to-artery anastomosis. This effectively stops the leak, although a lymphocele in the thigh may take a little time to settle.

Dacron/femoral artery false aneurysm

The development of an expansile pulsating mass in the groin signals a false aneurysm, which arises from a weakened femoral artery adjacent to the suture line (Figure 38.24). It occurs often several years after the bypass, and is treated by inserting a short segment of Dacron tube to extend the original bypass to more healthy femoral artery beyond the original anastomosis.

Late graft occlusion

About 10% of graft limbs become occluded within 5 years, usually from progression of atherosclerosis in the run-off vessels. The perfusion of the affected leg can be restored by a femoro-femoral crossover Dacron bypass from the remaining patent limb to the distal profunda femoris artery.

Graft infection

The incidence of graft infection is about 1%. Most infections are of unknown cause and occur several years after the original operation.

A *groin wound sinus* develops after breakdown of a painful red swelling with the classical features of infection. Treatment is initially by culture-specific intravenous antibiotics, assisted by irrigation of the wound with antiseptics to encourage granulation. In many instances, healing occurs with this conservative approach. However, if bleeding should occur, conservative treatment is no longer an option, and the femoral arteries are ligated and the Dacron limb is excised. At operation, the suture lines lie slackly because the arterial wall has become weakened by infection. A remote bypass is usually required to revascularize the extremity.

An *aortoenteric fistula* presents as anaemia from gastrointestinal blood loss, and presents as haematemesis and melaena. Investigations, including endoscopy, arteriography, and CT scanning with intravenous contrast, may well not slow the site of the fistula, which is between the Dacron-to-aorta anastomosis and the fourth part of the duodenum. Bleeding tends to be incremental rather than catastrophic, and several episodes may occur before the diagnosis is made.

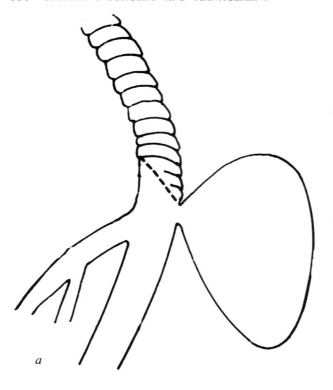

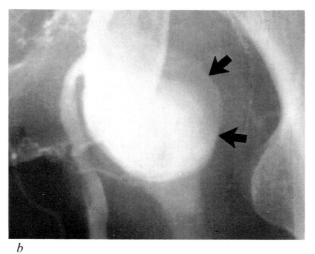

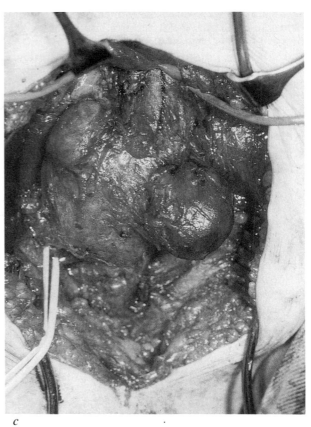

Figure 38.24 Dacron-to-femoral artery anastomotic aneurysm in the groin. *a*, Diagram showing that the false aneurysm arises from a defect in the wall of the femoral artery adjacent to the suture line. *b*, Arteriogram with the aneurysm arrowed. *c*, Operative photograph showing the aneurysm and a loop around the profunda femoris artery. The Dacron graft is visible at the top

At operation, the fistula is disconnected and the duodenal defect is closed with two layers of Vicryl. The arterial defect can be closed directly with 3–4 interrupted prolene sutures and the repair covered by omentum. Alternatively, where there is severe infection and frank pus, the Dacron graft is excised, the aortic stump oversewn, and an extra anatomical axillo-femoral bypass is done. This more radical procedure has the advantage of removing the infected Dacron at the site of the fistula. Problems with this approach include the high operative mortality, which is partly due to the complexity and long time it takes to do the operation, and to the risk of disruption of the aortic stump. The axillo-femoral bypass may

thrombose or become cross-contaminated. It is because graft infections are so difficult to treat that so much care is taken to prevent them in the first place.

Reconstruction distal to the groin

Balloon angioplasty

Where feasible, this is the treatment of choice. It works well for stenoses, and for many complete occlusions of the superficial femoral and proximal popliteal arteries of up to 10 cm in length (Figure 38.25). Some cannot be negotiated because they are

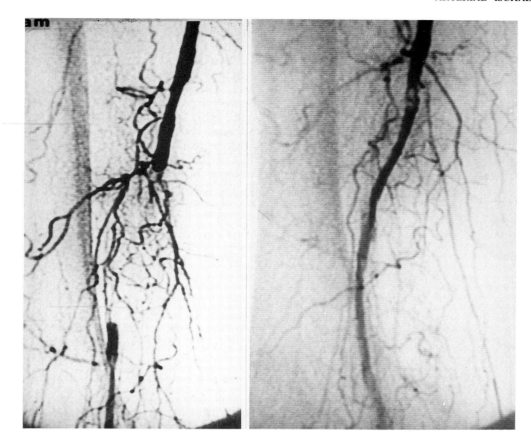

Figure 38.25 Arteriogram before (*left*) and after (*right*) recanalization and dilatation of a short, mid-superficial femoral artery occlusion with a balloon catheter

too long, involve the origin of the superficial femoral artery (SFA), have an adjacent tributary which diverts the recanalizing wire, and are so hard that they cannot be penetrated. As with bypass, long-term patency is better with 2–3 vessel run-off than with 0–1 patent calf vessels. In the past 10 years this method has proved to be safe, effective, repeatable and durable. In consequence, it has been used to treat milder forms of claudication and less fit patients than was the case when bypass was the only available intervention. Selection for angioplasty depends on the patency of the proximal SFA so that the guide wire and sheath are positioned to provide access for the balloon catheter. The duplex ultrasound scanner will show patency of this vital segment of SFA, without the need for a preliminary arteriogram.

Femoro-popliteal vein bypass

This has been the mainstay of distal reconstruction since the first report from Paris by Kunlin and Leriche in 1949. The bypass material they used was reversed long saphenous vein, which remains the gold standard to this day (Figure 38.26). In the past 10 years, equivalent results have been obtained with the non-reversed vein left largely *in situ*, with destruction

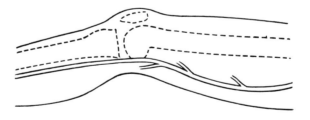

Figure 38.26 The long saphenous vein positioned well posteriorly on the medial side of the thigh

of the valves and ligation of the tributaries (Figure 38.27). If the vein is unavailable or unsuitable, reversed veins can be used without valve avulsions, including the contralateral long saphenous vein, short saphenous and arm veins. The position and size of the veins are measured preoperatively with the duplex scanner. Only after these possibilities have been exhausted are the alternatives used. Vascular operating theatres generally keep lengths of 6 mm diameter polytetrafluoroethylene (PTFE) to cover this contingency.

Apart from the conduit, the preoperative evaluation includes assessment of the run-in, run-off and of

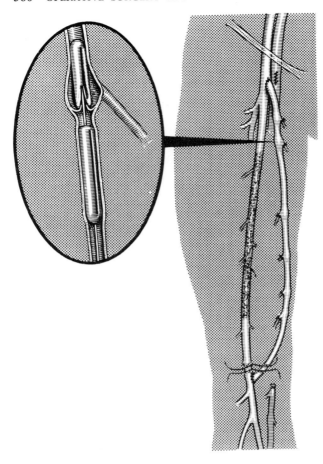

Figure 38.27 A femoro-popliteal bypass using *in situ* long saphenous vein. Insert shows avulsion of valves using Hall's valvulotome

the general fitness of the patient. In advanced ischaemia, there has to be the expectation that a healed, weight-bearing extremity can be achieved. The operation takes 2–3 h and is done under light general or regional anaesthesia. The common femoral and popliteal arteries are exposed via anterior and medial incisions. The long saphenous vein is carefully dissected *not quite* flush to the vein, to prevent avulsions of tributaries which would require suture ligation and a threat to the lumen. The sapheno-femoral junction is divided with a Satinsky clamp on the femoral vein, which is sutured with 5/0 prolene. Heparin, 5000 u intravenously, is administered, and the proximal saphenous vein anastomosed end-to-side to the common femoral artery. A 2 mm and 2.5 mm Hall's valvulotome is passed several times to avulse the venous valves so that a good jet of blood is produced. A good vein has the flow capacity of 400 ml/min. The knee is fully extended and vein length is judged so that it lies slackly; the distal anastomosis is made end-to-side to the popliteal artery with 6/0 prolene. Flow in the graft is slow to begin with, perhaps 100–150 ml/min, depending on the run-off. Injection of papaverine into the graft dilates the distal vessels and the

Doppler flow may reach double the resting value, with sustained diastolic flow. An operative arteriogram provides welcome reassurance, although experience is needed with timing of the injection and the position of the limb so that a well-filled image of the distal vein, the anastomosis and the run-off are obtained. Up to a quarter of vein grafts are at risk of occlusion in the first year. The main causes are an undivided vein-valve cusp, external pressure from a muscle or tendon at the distal end, an unligated vein tributary causing an arteriovenous fistula, a stiff, narrowed post-phlebitic segment of distal vein, anastomotic narrowing and unrecognized run-off vessel disease. Many of these problems can be discovered if a postoperative graft arteriogram is done at a week, and correction undertaken before the patient leaves hospital (Figures 38.28 and 38.29). Regular graft surveillance is advisable, and a policy of intervention yields better secondary patency rates than efforts to reopen occluded grafts by thrombolysis or balloon catheter embolectomy. After a month, once the phase of technical problems has passed 90% of these bypasses remain patent and the main risk to the patient is from associated coronary artery disease.

Alternatives to vein

As mentioned earlier, the long saphenous vein is not always available; it may be varicose, phlebitic, have multiple small branches, or have been already used as a bypass. With the help of vein from other sites, the use of autologous vein should reach 90%. Which alternatives are worth while for the remaining cases? The main contenders are 6 mm diameter lengths of PTFE, umbilical vein graft and, to a lesser extent, knitted Dacron. Each has an external support – an adherent polypropylene coil for the synthetics and a polyester mesh for the biological. All are inferior to autologous vein, and the development of an ideal arterial substitute has not advanced since these materials became available some 20 years ago.

The factors affecting patency are: the level of the *distal anastomosis* – above-knee popliteal, below-knee popliteal and infrapopliteal; the *indication* – claudication, critical ischaemia; and the number of patent *run-off vessels.* The results are best with an above-knee bypass for claudication, and few surgeons achieve prolonged patency for prosthetic bypass to a single calf vessel. As far as complications are concerned, the risk of wound infection is less because the short incisions are confined to the sites of anastomoses. However, there is a 4% risk of graft infection for PTFE compared with 1% for autologous vein.

PTFE

This is currently the most widely used alternative to vein. In a randomized trial, the cumulative primary patency rate at 2 years for bypass to the below-knee popliteal artery was 54% compared with 76% for

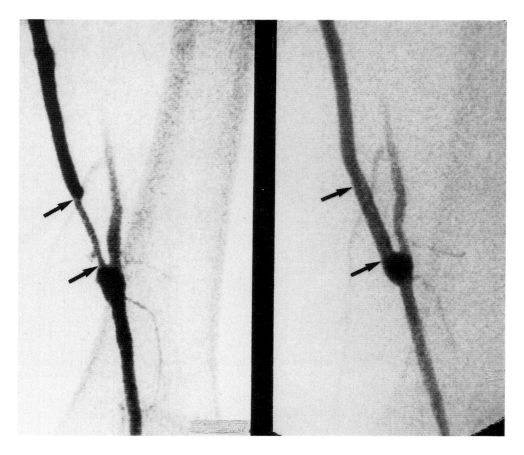

Figure 38.28 Arteriogram at a week (*left*) after femoro-popliteal bypass, showing narrowing of the vein adjacent to the distal anastomosis. Replacement by a healthy vein segment led to a normal arteriogram at 3 months (*right*)

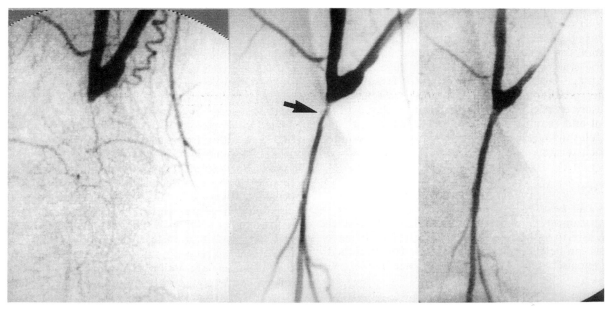

Figure 38.29 Postoperative occlusion of distal popliteal artery after femoro-popliteal bypass (*left*); popliteal artery cleared by selective intra-arterial infusion of streptokinase (*centre*) with disclosure of post-anastomotic narrowing (arrow). Good result following balloon dilatation (*left*)

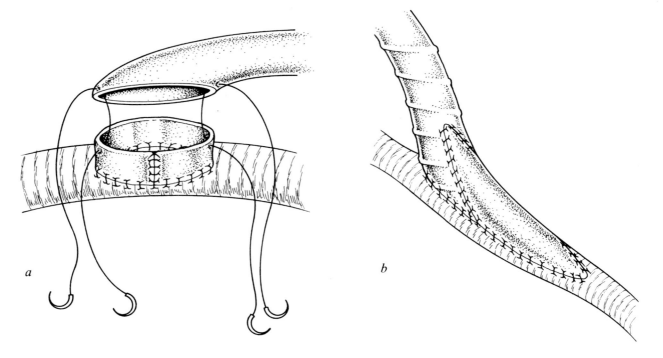

Figure 38.30 Techniques to improve the distal anastomoses of PTFE bypass. *a*, The Miller cuff. A strip of vein is sewn to the artery, to which the PTFE bypass is anastomosed. *b*, The Taylor patch. A gusset of vein is incorporated into the PTFE-to-artery anastomosis (After Bell, Jamieson and Ruckley, 1992)

autogenous saphenous vein. Incorporation of a vein cuff or patch at the distal anastomosis improves both the short- and long-term results (Figure 38.30).

UMBILICAL VEIN

Human umbilical cord vein, tanned with glutaraldehyde to stabilize the tissues and prevent immunological rejection, covered in Dacron mesh and stored in ethanol, is a useful alternative to autogenous vein. In several studies, it has been shown to have a patency advantage over PTFE. However, it is subject to biodegradation after 5 years, with the graft becoming diffusely dilated along its length. It is stored in alcohol and requires rinsing in saline before use, and the full thickness of the graft has to be incorporated in each suture.

DACRON

This can be used for above-knee anastomoses with good run-off, supported by antiplatelet treatment with aspirin and dipyrimadole. The proximal anastomosis can be at femoral or iliac level. These grafts do not remain patent if they cross the knee joint.

Ischaemic rest pain, ulceration and gangrene

Balloon angioplasty and femoro-popliteal bypass are the main interventions for lower limb ischaemia of all grades of severity. The techniques which follow are used primarily for ischaemic rest pain, ulceration and gangrene.

Thrombolysis is used for acute-on-chronic ischaemia where there has been sudden worsening within a few days, and no opacification beyond the thigh on an arteriogram. The technique is not applicable if the ischaemia is so severe that there is numbness and paralysis of the foot muscles. Treatment is by embedding and progressively advancing along the superficial femoral and popliteal arteries a catheter through which streptokinase is infused. If thrombolysis reveals patent run-off vessels, then any underlying atheromatous stenosis or thrombosed popliteal aneurysm is dilated or bypassed and the foot is saved (Figure 38.31). Failure to open the distal vessels usually results in an amputation (see Chapter 39).

In *femoro-distal bypass*, the distal anastomosis is to one of the calf vessels because the popliteal is occluded. Every effort is made to identify the least diseased calf vessel, which is hopefully in continuity with an intact pedal arch. This is done by arteriogram and Doppler. In severe ischaemia, the distal vessels may not opacify well on a preoperative arteriogram, even if digital subtraction techniques are used. Better images can be obtained from an operative pre-reconstruction arteriogram, during which the resistance to pressure on the plunger of the syringe can be felt. Alternatively, patency is established by insonating the arteries at the ankle with the leg dependent using a

arteries, there is only a fine margin of technical error in placing the sutures, and magnification with loupes will give the best chance of success. There is no good evidence that postoperative treatment with heparin, warfarin or antiplatelet agents enhances patency rates. Even so, minimizing the risk of thrombosis seems prudent if the bypass appears to be vulnerable. The results at a year are that two-thirds are patent and most of the occlusions have had an amputation.

Carotid endarterectomy

Carotid endarterectomy is done to prevent stroke in patients with focal premonitory symptoms of cerebral ischaemia in whom investigations reveal severe carotid stenosis. Recent randomized multicentre trials in Europe and North America have shown that the protection which endarterectomy provides amounts to an eight-fold reduction in disabling and fatal strokes compared with medical treatment. Even so, operation is not without risk, and 3.8% of the surgical group with more than 70% carotid stenosis in the European trial died or had a disabling stroke in the perioperative period. This risk is compared with the stroke risk with medical treatment – 17% within 3 years in the European trial – in discussion with patients and their families before the decision to operate is taken.

The focal premonitory symptoms are TIAs causing numbness and weakness of the hand which lasts for a minute or two; the leg, face and speech are also affected. TIAs can be multiple and frequent and are presumed to arise from lodgement in the contralateral cerebral hemisphere of a cluster of fibrin-platelet microemboli, which then dissolve by fibrinolysis leading to resolution of the symptoms. This explanation is consistent with the effectiveness of aspirin in abolishing the symptoms. Occasionally TIAs last for hours, or more than a day, as a 'mini-stroke'. The risk of stroke is even higher with 'crescendo TIAs' and 'stroke-in-evolution'. Provided that permanent neurological damage has not yet occurred, these clinical presentations can all be investigated for carotid stenosis.

In the eye ipsilateral to the lesion, the retinal artery can become thrombosed, causing irreversible blindness. The more usual presentation is of *amaurosis fugax*, or transient monocular blindness. This is a curtainlike loss of the upper part of the field of vision, which is fully restored after a minute or two. Fundoscopic examination reveals cholesterol or fibrin-platelet emboli in the retinal arteries.

For both ocular and cortical TIAs, the carotid bifurcation is auscultated in the neck for the localized systolic murmur which indicates a carotid stenosis. Confirmation comes from duplex ultrasound scanning, which reveals the extent and severity of the stenosis, the nature of the plaque, whether of inactive fibrous type or of embologenic heterogeneous type,

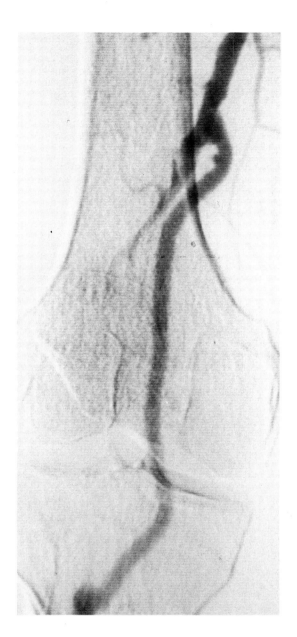

Figure 38.31 Postoperative arteriogram showing a patent vein bypass of a thrombosed popliteal aneurysm

hand-held Doppler probe. Finally, the technique of pulse-generated run-off may be employed, in which a pneumatic cuff is sharply inflated at the knee, and the artificial pulse which is created is listened for with the Doppler at the ankle. In the absence of adequate run-off, a bypass will fail and the best that can be offered is a chemical lumbar sympathectomy or an amputation.

The operation proceeds along the lines of a femoropopliteal bypass, except that the distal vessel exposure is of a tibial or the peroneal artery. The flow through the bypass is low, and seldom stabilizes at more than 80–120 ml/min. Because of these low flows into small

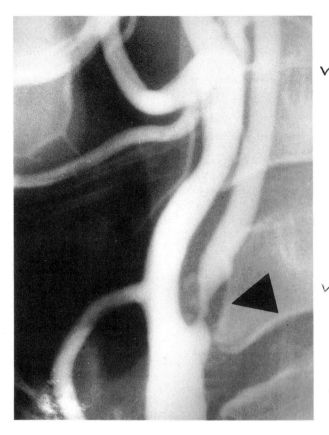

Figure 38.32 Arteriogram showing a severe, localized stenosis at the origin of the internal carotid artery (arrowed)

and the level of the carotid bifurcation in relation to the angle of the jaw. If further clarification is required, an arteriogram is done (Figure 38.32). Sometimes the clinical features are of a small stroke perhaps several days earlier, with a good if incomplete recovery. In these circumstances, a head CT scan should be done for a cerebral infarct. If found, endarterectomy should be postponed for 6 weeks to allow time for the infarct to stabilize.

The operation is done under general anaesthesia. An incision is made behind the angle of the jaw in the line of the anterior border of sternomastoid. Transverse cervical sensory nerves are inevitably sacrificed, leading to postoperative numbness anterior to the incision. The carotid arteries are partly covered by the internal jugular vein and its facial vein tributary, which is ligated. As the carotids are carefully encircled the vagus, descendens hypoglossi and hypoglossal nerves are seen. The internal carotid artery is dissected until it becomes soft beyond the atheroma, usually at the level of the posterior belly of the digastric muscle. During the dissection, the heart rate may slow to 30–40 beats/min because of excessive vagal stimulation; an injection of 1% lignocaine into the carotid sinus will restore the heart rate. After 5000 u heparin has been administered, a longitudinal arteriotomy is made in the common and internal carotids, and a short plastic tapered Javid shunt inserted to preserve blood flow to the brain. The stenosis is cleared by an endarterectomy, taking care to minimize any shelf of atheroma in the common carotid, and feathering the atheroma distally. The arteriotomy is closed with 6/0 prolene (Figure 38.33) and flow is checked with a sterile Doppler probe or flowmeter. If the arteries are small, or the atheroma extensive, a

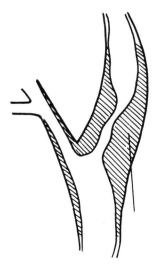
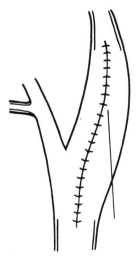

Figure 38.33 A carotid endarterectomy with direct closure of the arteriotomy

prosthetic patch is inserted. Particular care is taken with haemostasis, since most patients are on aspirin and postoperative oozing can cause a wound haematoma for which a suction drain offers scant protection. The postoperative stay is usually short and with anticipated discharge home within 48 h.

Operations for the arm and hand

Brachial embolectomy

Emboli from the heart can cause ischaemic symptoms of recent sudden onset. On examination the hand is cold and the pulses are absent. Heparin is administered and the brachial artery is exposed at the elbow under local anaesthesia. The embolus is cleared proximally, and the smallest (no. 2 or 3) embolectomy catheter is passed distally in the radial and ulnar arteries. The arteriotomy is closed with 6/0 prolene, using a vein patch if the arteries are small. Heparin is continued postoperatively followed by warfarin.

Arterial injuries

Closed injuries can arise in children from compression of the brachial artery by a supracondylar fracture. The pulse is restored when the fracture is reduced. Avulsion of the axillary artery and brachial plexus is an occasional high-speed injury in motorcyclists. Repairs can be undertaken, but the result is determined by the nerve injury and is generally a flail arm. The axillary artery can also be damaged in a shoulder dislocation and in fractures of the neck and shaft of the humerus. An arteriogram is done prior to repair by vein bypass.

The brachial artery is vulnerable to thrombosis after cannulation for radiological procedures; prompt local repair is required. The risk of thrombosis is less if the axillary artery is used, but this route brings the risk of haemorrhage from the puncture site within the adjacent fascial sheath of the brachial plexus, and the risk of arm paralysis if the haematoma is not decompressed without delay and haemostasis secured. These injuries are rare now that the femoral artery is the preferred portal of entry for cardiac catheterization.

Atherosclerotic occlusion

Atherosclerotic occlusion of the left subclavian artery is not infrequently encountered. The blood pressure in the left arm is reduced, and perfusion is provided by retrograde flow in the left vertebral artery, causing a so-called 'subclavian steal'. Symptoms are uncommon, whether of hind-brain ischaemia or arm claudication, so that arterial reconstruction is not normally required.

Upper thoracic sympathectomy

The indications for upper thoracic sympathectomy are hyperhidrosis and severe fingertip ischaemia with ulceration, arising from vasospasm and digital artery occlusion. The endoscopic transaxillary approach is preferred to the surgical transaxillary and supraclavicular approaches. There is a small risk of a Horner's syndrome, about which the patient should be warned preoperatively.

General anaesthesia is induced and a double lumen endotracheal tube is inserted. The procedure is frequently done bilaterally; in turn, ventilation of the lung on the operated side is discontinued, and a Verrer's needle inserted into the pleural space, and 1.5 litres of carbon dioxide insufflated to assist in collapsing the lung. A telescope is inserted through the 3rd rib interspace in the axilla, through which the sympathetic chain is seen, crossing the necks of the ribs. Through another portal of entry, a dissector is used to penetrate the parietal pleura and to mobilize the second and third thoracic ganglia. The chain is divided above the second ganglion with scissors, and the ganglia are destroyed by diathermy. The lung is reinflated and the procedure repeated on the other side. The patient awakes with warm dry hands. A chest X-ray is done in the recovery room to check for a pneumothorax. A chest drain is seldom required, and discharge home can be anticipated within 48 h.

Thoracic outlet syndrome

The thoracic outlet syndromes are caused by abnormal compression or irritation of the subclavian artery, vein or brachial plexus as they cross the first rib (Figure 38.34) or a cervical rib. The symptoms depend on the structure that is predominantly affected.

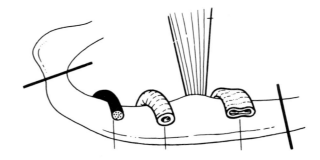

Figure 38.34 The subclavian artery, vein and T8 root of the brachial plexus as they cross the first rib. The lines of excision of the rib are marked

The subclavian artery can become compressed if a cervical rib is present. The extra rib is attached to the scalene tubercle and the artery is wedged next to the scalenus anterior muscle, causing a stenosis, below which there is a post-stenotic dilatation in which thrombus can develop and embolize to the fingers. Treatment is by removing the cervical and first ribs (Figure 38.35).

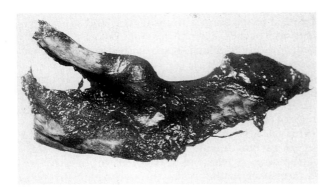

Figure 38.35 Cervical and first ribs excised via a transaxillary approach

The subclavian vein may become thrombosed by scissor-like compression between the first rib and the clavicle. The clinical features are of a swollen arm and the diagnosis is confirmed by a venogram. The swelling resolves rapidly with elevation of the arm and heparin anticoagulation, and no further treatment is necessary.

The C8/T1 root of the brachial plexus can be irritated by the first rib, leading to pain, numbness and weakness of ulnar distribution. The diagnosis is confirmed by a careful neurological examination, X-rays of the thoracic outlet, and nerve conduction studies. Treatment is initiated by analgesics, physiotherapy and correction of posture. In a few patients with severe, focal symptoms, removal of the first rib can offer the best chance of relief. However, in 10% of patients undergoing operation, the symptoms are unrelieved and may be worse.

Transaxillary excision of the first rib

The patient lies in a lateral position and the arm is held up by an assistant. A transverse incision is placed low in the axilla between latissimus dorsi and pectoralis major. The incision is deepened to the chest wall, and an axillary tunnel is extended to the first rib, taking care to preserve the intercostobrachial nerve. The first rib, and a cervical rib if present, are cleared using a periosteal elevator. Scalenus anterior is divided and the ribs mobilized posteriorly to beyond the T1 root, and anteriorly to the costochondral junction. It is then excised with right-angled rib shears, and any residual spicules of bone are carefully removed. All fibromuscular bands around the vessels and nerve are carefully removed, haemostasis checked and the wound closed with a drain if the pleura has inadvertently been entered. A chest X-ray is done in the recovery room. Three to five postoperative days in hospital are required.

Further reading

Aldoori, M. I., Baird, R. N., Al-Sam, S. Z., Cole S. E. A., Mera S. and Davies, J. D. (1987) Duplex scanning and plaque histology in cerebral ischaemia. *Eur. J. Vasc. Surg.*, **1**, 159–164

Baird, R. N. and Abbott, W. M. (1976) Pulsatile blood flow in arterial grafts. *Lancet*, **2**, 948–950

Barros D'Sa, A. A. B., Bell, P. R. F., Darke, S. G. and Harris, P. L. (eds) (1991) *Vascular Surgery: Current Questions*, Butterworth-Heinemann, Oxford

Bell, P. R. F., Jamieson, C. W. and Ruckley, C. V. (eds) (1992) *Surgical Management of Vascular Disease*, W. B. Saunders, Philadelphia

Browse, N. L. and Ross-Russel, A. O. (1984) Carotid endarterectomy and the Javid shunt. The early results of 215 consecutive operations for transient ischaemic attacks. *Br. J. Surg.*, **71**, 53–56

Clarke, A. M., Poskitt, K. R., Baird, R. N. and Horrocks, M. (1989) Anastomotic aneurysms of the femoral artery: aetiology and treatment. *Br. J. Surg.*, **76**, 1014–1016

Cole, S. E. A., Baird, R. N., Horrocks, M. and Jeans, W. D. (1987) The role of balloon angioplasty in lower limb ischaemia. *Eur. J. Vasc. Surg.*, **1**, 61–65

De Bakey, M. E., Cooley, D. A., Crawford, E. S. and Morris, G. C. (1957) Clinical application of a new flexible knitted dacron arterial substitute. *Arch. Surg.*, **74**, 944

Eastcott, H. H. G., Pickering, G. W. and Rob, C. (1954) Reconstruction of internal carotid artery in a patient with intermittent attacks of hemiplegia. *Lancet*, **2**, 994–995

European Carotid Surgery Trialists' Collaborative Group (1991) MRC European carotid surgery trial: interim results for symptomatic patients with severe (70–90%) or mild (0–20%) carotid stenosis. *Lancet*, **337**, 1235–1243

Fogarty, T. J., Cranley, J. J., Krause, R. J., Strasser, E. S. and Hafner, C. D. (1963) A method of extraction of arterial emboli and thrombi. *Surg. Gynaecol. Obst.*, **116**, 241–244

Greenhalgh, R. M. (ed.) (1989) *Vascular Surgical Techniques*, W. B. Saunders, Philadelphia

Leriche, R. and Kunlin, J. (1949) Possibilité de greffe veineuse de grande dimension (15 á 47 cm) dans les thromboses arterielles étendues. *Lyon Chir.*, **44**, 13–18

NASCET Collaborators (1991) North American symptomatic carotid endarterectomy trial – first results. *N. Engl. J. Med.*, **325**, 445–453

Rutherford, R. B. (ed.) (1989) *Vascular Surgery*, 3rd edn, W. B. Saunders, Philadelphia

Thomas, W. E. G. and Baird, R. N. (1983) Arterial injuries in two Bristol hospitals from 1974 to 1980. *Injury*, **15**, 30–34

Veith, F. J., Gupta, S. K., Ascer, E. *et al.* (1986) Six-year prospective multicentre randomised comparison of autologous saphenous vein and expanded polytetrafluoroethylene grafts in infra-inguinal arterial reconstruction. *J. Vasc. Surg.*, **3**, 104

Young, J. R., Graor, R. A., Olin, J. W. and Bartholomew, J. R. (eds) (1991) *Peripheral Vascular Diseases*, Mosby-Year Book, St. Louis

39

Arterial aneurysms

R. N. Baird

Introduction

An aneurysm is a permanent localized dilatation of an artery. Aneurysms have been feared since Galen's time because of the risk of rupture. In 1785, John Hunter successfully ligated an enlarging popliteal aneurysm; vein bypasses were first done in 1906 by Goyannes in Madrid and in 1912 by J. Hogarth Pringle in Glasgow. The first successful replacement of an aortic aneurysm was achieved in Paris by Dubost and colleagues in 1951, by extraperitoneal excision and replacement with an aortic homograft (Dubost *et al.*, 1951). In the following 10 years, the procedure was simplified using a synthetic Dacron tube implanted within the opened aneurysm sac which was left in place. This standardized operation gave good long-term results and has become deservedly popular in the past 30 years. Today, specialist units report elective operative mortalities of about 4%. These results owe much to better identification of predictive factors associated with poor outcomes, and to finely tuned surgical, anaesthetic and intensive care. Despite these advances, the operative mortality of repair following rupture remains at 30%, from blood loss causing pulmonary, cardiac and renal failure. These intractably bad results, and the unpredictability of rupture, have encouraged preventive operations so that most aneurysms are now dealt with electively.

Surgical anatomy

The aorta below the renal arteries is most commonly involved. Larger aneurysms may extend to the iliac arteries. Aortic tributaries at this level include paired lumbar arteries, median sacral and inferior mesenteric arteries. The infrarenal neck of the aneurysm is close to the inferior vena cava, left renal vein and lumbar veins, and is covered by the fourth part of the duodenum. A plexus of autonomic nerves covers the aortic bifurcation. The iliac arteries are crossed by the ureters and are closely adherent to, and sometimes inseparable from, the iliac veins.

Popliteal aneurysms occur in males over 50 years of age. The popliteal artery behind the knee is dilated from its normal diameter of 1 cm to 2–4 cm, and is closely adherent to the popliteal veins. They are uncommon, there being 10 aortic for every popliteal aneurysm, and are frequently bilateral. Aneurysms occurring rarely at other sites involve the carotid, hepatic, splenic, renal and femoral arteries.

Pathology

Abdominal aneurysms exist in up to 3% of the elderly male population and are primarily aortic, fusiform and atherosclerotic, unlike those in centuries past that were mainly syphilitic. The pathogenesis is unknown, apart from one or two tantalizing clues. Collagen and elastin are the main strength-giving components of the arterial wall, and they can be degraded by collagenase and elastase, both of which are found in increased concentrations in aneurysm patients. Congenital aneurysms in patients with connective tissue abnormalities such as Marfan's and Ehlers–Danlos syndromes have weakened or absent collagen cross-links. In some animals in whom spontaneous aneurysms occur, namely *Blotchy* mice and pigs, there is a deficiency of an enzyme, lysyl oxidase, which is essential for elastin cross-linking. The enzyme contains copper and the animals have deficient copper metabolism. In humans, there is abnormal copper metabolism in the rare Menkes syndrome, in which tortuous, dilated arteries and reduced arterial wall elastin have been found. Tilson (1982) has found decreased hepatic copper levels in 13 patients with abdominal aneurysms compared with a similar number of patients with atherosclerotic occlusive disease.

In 7% of abdominal aneurysms, there is a dense peri-aortic fibrotic reaction, indistinguishable from retroperitoneal fibrosis. The aorta, ureters and vena cava may be involved. They have been labelled 'inflammatory' because of the histology, high ESR and response to steroid therapy.

Mycotic aneurysms were first described by Osler over 100 years ago, arising from infective emboli from bacterial endocarditis. Septic foci weaken the arterial wall, causing a *bacterial arteritis*, with a leucocytosis and blood cultures yielding salmonella, streptococci and other gut organisms, sometimes in an immunocompromised patient. In a false aneurysm, or communicating haematoma, the pulsating mass of blood has escaped beyond the arterial wall, and is restrained by interstitial tissues. The femoral artery is most commonly involved, following the insertion of an arterial catheter.

Diffuse dilatation of the arteries is known as

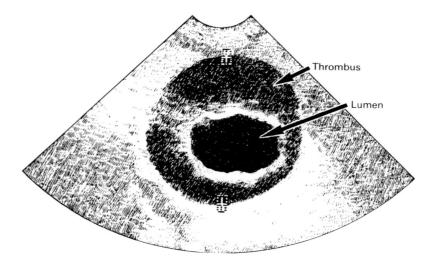

Figure 39.1 Diagram of ultrasound scan of an abdominal aneurysm showing cursors measuring its anteroposterior diameter, as well as the lumen and mural thrombus

arteriomegaly or arterial ectasia. It is widespread, and the risk of rupture is less than for a localized aneurysm.

Aortic aneurysm

Clinical features

Most abdominal aneurysms do not give rise to symptoms, and are discovered by the patient as a central pulsating abdominal tumour. Others come to light on abdominal palpation during a routine medical checkup or during examination for a non-specific abdominal or back pain. The aneurysm may be seen on an abdominal radiograph as calcification in the wall of the sac. The pulsating mass may visibly displace the anterior abdominal wall in a thin patient.

On palpation, the aneurysm may be tender and the convex left border is easily felt; the right border and the upper edge are often delineated with less certainty.

Confirmation comes from abdominal ultrasound which clearly shows the dilated aortic wall, lumen and mural thrombus (Figure 39.1), and gives accurate anteroposterior diameters. The upper limit of the aneurysm often overhangs the renal arteries and this important relationship is not shown well by ultrasound. The origin of the superior mesenteric artery is a reliable landmark, and if the aortic diameter at this level is normal, the aneurysm can be assumed for practical purposes to be infrarenal. The lower extent of the aneurysm can usually be imaged, whether at the aortic bifurcation or extending into the iliac arteries. The differential diagnoses are with a tortuous but normal-sized aorta and a retroperitoneal, pre-aortic mass, such as a lymphoma, and each can be identified by ultrasound.

Aneurysms less than 4 cm in diameter

The risk of rupture of small aneurysms, less than twice the size of a normal abdominal aorta (2 cm), is so low that operative replacement is seldom justified. Enlargement is monitored by repeating the scan in 1 year's time or if symptoms develop. Serial studies show that the average growth rate of a small aneurysm is 0.5 cm/year.

Aneurysms greater than 6 cm in diameter

Large aneurysms are potentially lethal and a Dacron replacement should be inserted unless there are good reasons for not doing so.

Aneurysms of intermediate size (4–6 cm)

An aneurysm of intermediate size should be dealt with in an otherwise fit, thin, motivated patient provided that a straightforward operative replacement is forecast and an experienced surgical team is available.

Selection for operation

Broadly speaking, a patient with an aneurysm is likely to do well if he or she feels healthy, walks unaided and can respond sensibly to an explanation of the benefits and risks of operation.

Many patients have coexisting disease. This in itself does not disqualify them from having the aneurysm repaired. Hypertension, angina, diabetes and a previous myocardial infarct are often acceptable risks, provided that hypertension and diabetes are moderate, whether requiring drugs or not, angina is mild and stable, and any myocardial infarct has occurred more than 6 months earlier. Good surgical results can

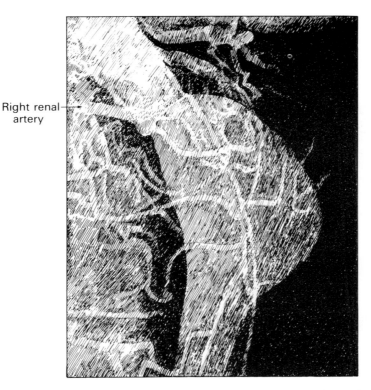

Right renal artery

Figure 39.2 Diagram of lateral view of an arteriogram of an aortic aneurysm showing the right renal artery arising from aorta of normal diameter above the aneurysm

also be obtained in combined dilating and occlusive arterial disease. In these circumstances an arteriogram is recommended to outline distal vessels.

An aneurysm is suspected of extending above the renal arteries if the pulsatile mass extends high into the epigastrium on abdominal palpation, if abdominal ultrasound shows a dilated suprarenal aorta, and if a dilated thoracic aorta is shown on a chest radiograph. Arteriograms will show the upper limit of the aneurysm (Figure 39.2) and CT scanning will clearly show its extent. Pre-aortic structures such as a horseshoe kidney and inflammatory aneurysms are well shown by CT scanning.

Adverse factors include preoperative breathlessness at rest, whether of pulmonary or left ventricular origin, right heart failure, a recent myocardial infarct (within 6 months) and a host of system failures, degenerative and neoplastic diseases. Operations for aortic aneurysm should only be undertaken in those with a worthwhile future ahead of them who have reserves of physical and mental strength to recover from a complex major procedure.

Efforts should be made to improve coexisting disease; the obese should lose weight; smokers should abstain; hypertension should be controlled.

Preoperative assessment

A detailed history-taking and examination are undertaken several days preoperatively to assess fitness for operation. Routine investigations include urinalysis, haemoglobin, platelets, urea and electrolytes, chest radiograph and electrocardiogram.

Further investigations are done selectively: arterial gases and pulmonary function tests if there is a risk of ventilatory failure; creatinine clearance, intravenous urography and angiography if poor renal function is suspected; and prothrombin time, platelet function and clotting screen where indicated.

The assessment is used to identify predictive factors of serious or fatal postoperative complications. Indices of cardiac risk such as those devised by Goldman *et al.* (1977) have been used to quantify the effects of predictive factors on outcomes following operations.

Contained rupture

The accuracy of diagnosis of tender aneurysms is improved by ultrasound and CT, which may show a contained rupture (Figure 39.3). Extravasated blood from a rent in the wall of the aneurysm is contained *for a time* by tamponade of surrounding tissues. If this finding is encountered, preparations are made for operation, as further bleeding will occur, usually without warning.

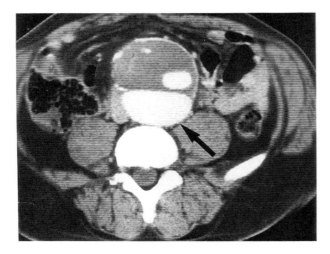

Figure 39.3 CT scan of an abdominal aortic aneurysm with intravenous contrast enhancement, showing a large, thin-walled, thrombus-filled sac with a small eccentric lumen. The arrow indicates a posterior contained rupture extending beyond the partly calcified aneurysmal wall

Preparation for operation

Six units of *whole* blood are made available. There is no place for the use of packed cells to replace intraoperative blood loss in arterial surgery.

ECG electrodes are attached. Peripheral and central venous lines, an arterial line, a thoracic epidural and a urinary catheter are inserted. In high-risk cases a Swan–Ganz catheter is used. The patient is placed on a warming blanket.

Perioperative antibiotics are administered intravenously in three doses of a cephalosporin 8-hourly, starting at the induction of anaesthesia.

Ruptured aneurysms

Abdominal aneurysms rupture intraperitoneally, retroperitoneally and rarely into the vena cava or duodenum. The first operative priority is to apply an arterial clamp safely to normal aorta between the neck of the aneurysm and the renal arteries. Following this, the blood pressure picks up immediately and improves the perfusion of the heart, kidneys and brain.

Without operation, virtually all patients with ruptured aneurysms die. Hypovolaemic shock causing damage to the heart, kidneys and lungs is the most common cause of death. Since surgery offers the only

hope for survival, it should seldom be withheld. Octogenarians, those who have required resuscitation for hypovolaemic cardiac arrest, patients with physical and mental disability, and the grossly obese, should only undergo operation if there is a reasonable expectation of a favourable outcome.

Once the diagnosis has been made, a large-bore intravenous line is inserted, blood taken for a 10-unit cross-match, and the patient transferred directly to the operating theatre. The fall in blood pressure can *only* be corrected by controlling and clamping the aorta above the site of rupture. Because of this, the highest standard of professionalism is required by all concerned to get the patient onto the operating table as quickly as possible. A midline abdominal incision is made immediately and the aorta controlled while an endotracheal tube is inserted. Once the aortic clamp is safely applied, the patient is resuscitated and the operation proceeds expeditiously but with less urgency once the emergency has passed. If the neck of the aneurysm is inaccessible, the aorta can be clamped at the oesophageal hiatus, via the lesser omentum above the stomach. Alternatively, the aneurysm is entered and plugged with a thumb (Figure 39.4), following which a clamp is applied or a large spigoted Foley catheter is inserted, and the balloon inflated.

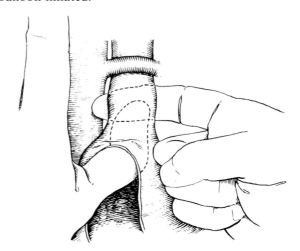

Figure 39.4 Ruptured aortic aneurysm. With the left thumb in the aorta, mobilization is achieved by encircling the normal aorta with the right index finger, following which a clamp may be applied by the operator or the assistant

Whatever technique is used, the first priority is to achieve haemostasis. Once cardiovascular stability is restored, the clamps are positioned to ensure blood flow to the kidneys.

If an aortocaval fistula is present, venous bleeding occurs when the aneurysmal sac is opened. The fistula is usually small and is controlled by direct pressure while being sutured from within the wall of the aneurysm sac. Care is taken to avoid squeezing atheroma and thrombus through the fistula into the vena cava as a pulmonary embolism can result.

Rupture of an aneurysm into the duodenum presents as gastrointestinal bleeding. At operation the fistula is disconnected, the duodenum closed, the aneurysm replaced by a Dacron graft and omentum interposed to prevent recurrence.

Elective operation

Aortic aneurysm

Incision

A transverse upper abdominal incision provides excellent access, can be readily extended towards the left chest for high aneurysms, heals well and has minimal risk of an incisional hernia. A long midline incision is a satisfactory alternative.

Findings

The gallbladder is checked for gallstones. The duodenum is inspected and the oesophageal hiatus and stomach are palpated. The colon is examined throughout its length. If carcinoma of the stomach or colon is discovered, the neoplasm should be resected and the aneurysm left unoperated. Duodenal scarring, hiatus hernia and diverticular disease are frequently encountered. They are carefully noted and do not preclude aneurysm repair. The small bowel is reflected to reveal the aneurysm. The size is measured with a ruler to compare with the preoperative investigations and any localized weakness is noted.

Procedure

The posterior parietal peritoneum is incised vertically to provide direct access to the aneurysm between the fourth part of the duodenum and the inferior mesenteric vein. The incision is continued upwards to reveal the left renal vein. The neck of the aneurysm is initially cleared on the left side and in front. Attention is then turned to the right side of the infrarenal aorta. A quadrilateral space is developed by gentle blunt dissection between the aorta and the cava with the renal vein above and the aneurysm below (Figure 39.5). Finally, the posterior aspect of the aorta is cleared *in direct vision* to ensure that the lumbar vessels are avoided.

The peritoneum is then incised downwards, skirting to the right of the inferior mesenteric artery to avoid its left colic branches, as far as the common iliac arteries. They are often normal or slightly dilated, and are exposed sufficiently to be controlled. The femoral pulses are palpated in the groins to ensure that intraluminal thrombus has not been dislodged distally by the dissection.

A tubular Dacron prosthesis is selected and preclotted. Its diameter is usually between 16 and

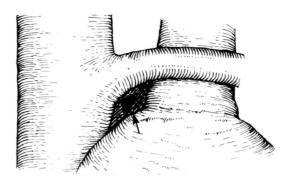

Figure 39.5 Diagram showing dissection of the neck of the aneurysm. A space (arrowed) is developed between the right side of the aorta and the vena cava, with the left renal vein above and the aneurysm below

20 mm, although a full range of sizes from 12 to 25 mm should be available. A prosthesis of *knitted* manufacture is soft, easy to sew and becomes well incorporated after implantation. There is an initial blood loss from the porosity of the material until the interstices are sealed with fibrin and platelets. Grafts of *woven* manufacture are virtually impervious to blood loss and in consequence are preferred where there are anxieties about preclotting and blood loss.

Heparin, 5000 u, is administered by central venous line and the aorta and iliac arteries are clamped and the aneurysm opened. Intraluminal thrombus is removed (Figure 39.6) and back-bleeding from any of the lumbar, median sacral and inferior mesenteric arteries is controlled by suture ligation. Dilute heparin/saline solution (10–20 ml) is instilled into the clamped iliac arteries to minimize the risk of thrombosis in the absence of flow.

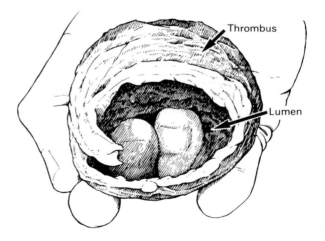

Figure 39.6 Intramural thrombus removed from within the aneurysmal sac

The graft is anastomosed to the intrarenal aorta using a 2/0 or 3/0 continuous prolene suture. The aortic clamp is released to check that the suture line is intact (Figure 39.7). The graft is reflected upwards to check the posterior part of the anastomosis (Figure 39.8) while it is readily accessible. The upper anastomosis may prove difficult. Rarely, it may be necessary to divide the left renal vein in order to expose the upper end of the resected aorta. Should this prove necessary, renal function will almost certainly be retained as the collateral venous drainage of the kidney is excellent.

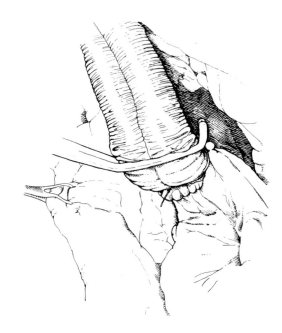

Figure 39.8 The posterior part of the top anastomosis being checked so that any additional suture can be inserted under direct vision

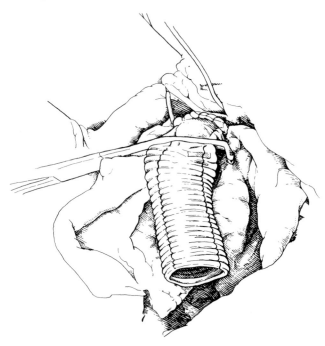

Figure 39.7 Checking the front of the top anastomosis. Note the opened aneurysmal sac left in place

The distal graft is trimmed to size and anastomosed to the aortic bifurcation with continuous 3/0 prolene (Figure 39.9). Prior to completion of the suture line the clamps are momentarily released to clear any thrombus or loose atheroma before flow is restored.

Declamping is done slowly, in patient cooperation with the anaesthetist, to minimize the hypotension that accompanies a reduction in afterload. When the clamps are finally released and normal arterial pressure restored, haemostasis is checked and the Dacron graft is covered by the aneurysm sac (Figure 39.10) and the posterior peritoneum closed. The femoral pulses are palpated once more to ensure that the arterial supply of the legs has been restored to normal.

At this stage, further consideration is given to dealing with any other problems concurrently, e.g. gallstones, inguinal hernia, etc.

The position of the nasogastric tube is checked and

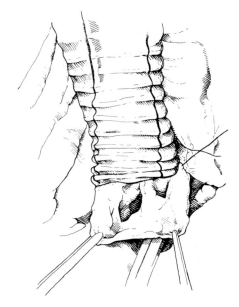

Figure 39.9 The lower anastomosis partly completed at the aortic bifurcation

the foot pulses checked by palpation, Doppler or pulse volume recordings and the abdomen closed with a continuous strong nylon suture.

Aorto-iliac aneurysm

Large aortic aneurysms frequently extend to the common iliac arteries. They are similarly amenable to operative repair, but require a bifurcation graft

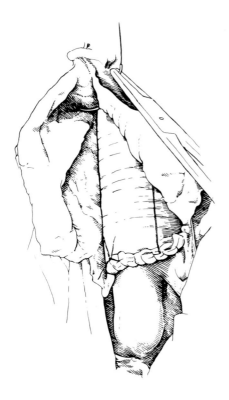

Figure 39.10 Closure of the empty aneurysmal sac over the Dacron prosthesis on completion of the anastomoses

(Figure 39.11) instead of a simple tube. In these circumstances, the limbs of the bifurcation graft are anastomosed to the common iliac, external iliac or common femoral artery depending on the extent of the aneurysm. The ratio of tube to bifurcation graft is 3:2.

Suprarenal aorta

Control of the aorta at the level of the diaphragm is occasionally required for the repair of aortic rupture or injury and for high aneurysms. It is achieved by compression of the aorta on the lumbar spine, by clamping in the hiatus via the lesser sac, or by intraluminal occlusion using a Foley balloon catheter. The occlusion time should be as short as possible (<30 min) to minimize ischaemic damage to the kidneys.

These techniques afford limited access for repairs at renal artery level. Aneurysms of the upper segment of the abdominal aorta are best approached postero-laterally by Crawford's technique, after incising the peritoneum lateral to the left colon and developing a plane behind the colon, spleen, pancreas and left kidney. The aorta is opened longitudinally well behind the left renal artery orifice and a woven Dacron tube sewn into the aorta above the neck of the aneurysmal sac. Oval opening(s) are made in the graft to accommodate the origins of the coeliac axis,

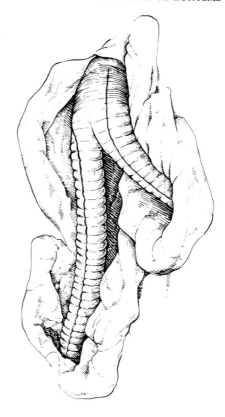

Figure 39.11 A bifurcation prosthesis for an aneurysm involving the aorta and both iliac arteries

superior mesenteric and renal arteries and anastomoses are completed with circumferentially running sutures. Finally, the distal aortic anastomosis is performed.

Horseshoe kidney

A horseshoe kidney is uncommonly encountered. In the straightforward case, the renal arteries are normal, the isthmus does not have an independent blood supply and there are no accessory renal arteries. Access to the neck of the aneurysm is obtained by reflecting the left kidney and isthmus upwards and to the right, and a Dacron replacement is undertaken. If there is a complicated anomaly, the feasibility of aneurysm replacement depends on the numbers and locations of accessory renal arteries, and in some cases with multiple vessels, reconstruction may not be possible.

Inflammatory aneurysm

Another uncommon operative finding is an aneurysm encased in marble white retroperitoneal fibrous tissue, the so-called inflammatory aneurysm. This fibrous tissue has to be cut into to free the duodenum, and to find the limits of the sac. Thereafter grafting proceeds as described earlier. The retroperitoneal reaction resolves postoperatively and the ureter and the vena cava need not be freed. Occasionally, the reaction is so dense and extensive that it is safer to leave the aneurysm unresected.

Postoperative care

In fit, elective cases, awakening from anaesthesia is straightforward and the patient is observed in the recovery area of the operating theatre for 3–4 h before the arterial line is removed and the patient is returned to the ward. During this time, hypertension may need treatment with incremental doses of intravenous labetalol or hydralazine, or by a top-up of epidural analgesia.

Less fit elective cases are booked into the intensive care unit so that arterial line monitoring is continued overnight. During this time, the legs become rewarmed. Pulses, Doppler ankle pressures and pulse volume recordings are checked. As the patient rewarms and vasodilates, the need for a gentle top-up transfusion of 1–2 units of blood should be considered. Hypovolaemia is manifest as a fall-off in hourly urinary output, arterial and central venous pressures. If a sluggish urinary output persists after volume replacement and there is no intra-abdominal blood loss, an intravenous dose of Lasix (frusemide) usually brings an ample reward.

All ruptured cases should be treated in the intensive care unit postoperatively because of the morbidity and mortality of the operation in these circumstances. They are at risk of multisystem failure and the respiratory system is particularly vulnerable from pre-existing disease and the adverse effects of pulmonary oedema resulting from intraoperative transfusion of large fluid volumes. Frequent blood gas estimations are made and treatment includes oxygen therapy, nebulizers and physiotherapy. Endotracheal intubation and ventilation with positive end-expiratory pressure are used to relieve the severest hypoxaemia.

Complications

Early complications

The main early complications are those of all arterial surgery, namely bleeding, thrombosis and embolism.

Reactive *haemorrhage* from a suture line is suspected if there is a continuing transfusion requirement within hours of operation, and leads to hypotensive collapse if untreated. At re-exploration, the anastomoses are inspected and additional sutures placed. Sometimes an active bleeding point is not identified.

Graft or *distal artery thrombosis* is suspected if

the limb(s) fail to rewarm postoperatively. Loss of femoral artery pulsation in the groin will prompt a return to the operating theatre for clearance with a balloon catheter.

Embolism is an intraoperative complication in which atherothrombotic material (see Figure 39.6) is propagated distally when the aneurysm is being dissected free of surrounding structures. The toes become acutely painful, discoloured and ischaemic despite good pedal pulses. The condition is known by the picturesque name of 'trash-foot'. The buttocks are also affected. The embolic material rests beyond the reach of a balloon catheter. Heparin and dextran may help, and the toes recover from all but the most extensive emboli.

Lymph fistula is a tiresome occasional sequel of any groin incision in which the femoral arteries are exposed. The groin incision becomes red, swollen and discharges copious volumes of clear lymph towards the end of the 1st postoperative week. Cultures may yield staphylococci and other organisms. Treatment usually consists of antibiotics, rest and elevation of the limb. The fistula may take up to 6 weeks to dry up completely. Throughout this period there is anxiety lest the Dacron prosthesis should become infected. A more aggressive approach is to cover the femoral artery and Dacron with the sartorius muscle by transposing it medially, freeing its proximal attachment from the anterior superior iliac spine and tacking it lightly to the inguinal ligament over the prosthesis. The fistula usually dries up when this is done.

Rare complications include graft infection and colon ischaemia following ligation of the inferior mesenteric artery. General postoperative complications affect the cardiac, respiratory and renal systems. As ever, prevention is infinitely better than cure. For example, the risk of respiratory complications is minimized by stopping smoking and preoperative physiotherapy, avoiding intraoperative pulmonary oedema caused by fluid overload and relieving postoperative pain by thoracic epidural to encourage deep breathing and coughing.

Aneurysm patients usually have diseased coronary arteries which can become thrombosed causing myocardial ischaemia or infarction. Excess intraoperative blood loss and inadequate replacement increase the chance of this happening.

Late complications

The main late complications are myocardial infarction, false aneurysm and secondary aorto-enteric fistula.

Myocardial infarction is the commonest cause of death after aneurysm operations. Its prevalence dominates the survival curves to such an extent that some specialized centres, notably Hertzer's group at the Cleveland Clinic (Diehl *et al.*, 1983), advocate preliminary coronary artery bypass in selected patients before the aneurysm is dealt with.

Anastomotic false aneurysms arise years later from suture line weakening of the wall of the host artery. Silk used in the anastomoses was at one time a contributory factor. False aneurysms are noted most commonly in the groins, but also occur at more deeply sited anastomoses. Good results are obtainable from local repair (see Chapter 38).

Aorto-enteric fistulas occur rarely after aneurysm repair. An intra-abdominal suture line forms the link between the arterial and gastrointestinal systems, resulting in haematemesis. Delays in recognizing the diagnosis are frequent. The most common fistula is between the upper aortic anastomosis and the fourth part of the duodenum. At operation, the aorta and graft are controlled, the fistula disconnected, the enteral aspect closed and separated by omentum from the aorta. Thereafter, opinions are divided on how the aortic deficit should be handled. Conservative surgeons simply close the defect in the Dacron–aorta anastomosis. A more radical approach is to remove the entire Dacron graft on the grounds that it must be infected, ligate the aorta and restore blood flow to the legs by an axillo-bifemoral bypass. However, the aortic stump may become disrupted later, creating a difficult situation.

Popliteal aneurysm

Clinical features

Popliteal aneurysms are uncommon, and few vascular surgeons see more than two or three a year. They mainly present as limb ischaemia resulting from thrombosis or embolism from the aneurysm. Occasionally, rupture occurs, with a tender, expanding mass (Figure 39.12); more usually, a pulsatile lump in the popliteal fossa is an incidental finding. Bilaterality is frequent, as is an associated aortic aneurysm, so clinical examination has to be thorough. The initial assessment is by duplex ultrasound to measure the external diameter, and to distinguish an aneurysm from a Baker's cyst. The foot pulses are checked before and after exercise, to rule out occlusive atheroma and distal embolism. An arteriogram will often be helpful (Figure 39.13); on other occasions the aneurysm is poorly seen because of thrombus within the wall (Figure 39.14).

Selection for operation

Popliteal aneurysms which are leaking and large, and those causing ischaemia, are treated by femoro-popliteal vein bypass as described in the preceding chapter, provided that there is adequate run-off and the patient is fit for operation.

Advice on small asymptomatic aneurysms is not easily provided, since their rate of growth and risks of thrombosis/embolism are unknown. The outcomes following prophylactic bypass and a 'watch' policy are similar; the occasional bad surgical outcome is matched by the occasional ischaemic extremity in the conservative group that is irrecoverable by thrombolysis.

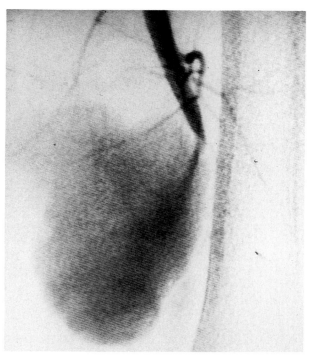

Figure 39.12 Digital subtraction angiogram showing a jet of contrast escaping from a ruptured popliteal aneurysm

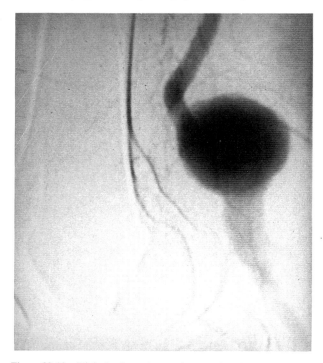

Figure 39.13 Digital subtraction angiogram showing a 4 cm diameter popliteal aneurysm

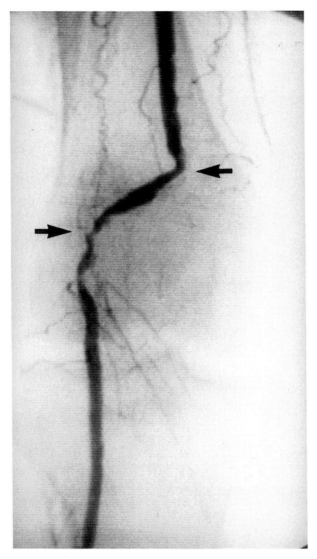

Figure 39.14 Digital subtraction angiogram of a popliteal aneurysm with so much thrombus within the sac that the diagnosis cannot be made from the arteriogram. Kinking of the residual lumen (arrowed) marks the extent of the aneurysm, which is clearly visible on ultrasound, CT and MR images

References

Diehl, J. T., Cali, R. F., Hertzer, N. R. *et al.* (1983) Complications of abdominal aortic reconstruction. An analysis of perioperative risk factors in 557 patients. *Ann. Surg.*, **197**, 49–56

Dubost, C., Allary, M. and Oeconomos, N. (1951) A propos du traitement des aneurysmes de l'aorte. *Mem. Acad. Chir.* (Paris), **77**, 381–384

Goldman, L., Caldera, D. L., Nussbaum, S. R. *et al.* (1977) Multifactorial index of cardiac risk in non-cardiac surgical patients. *N. Engl. J. Med.*, **297**, 846–850

Tilson, M. D. (1982) Decreased hepatic copper levels. A possible chemical marker for the pathogenesis of aortic aneurysms in man. *Arch. Surg.*, **105**, 338–344

Further reading

Baird, R. N. (1989) Mycotic aortic aneurysms. *Eur. J. Vasc. Surg.*, **3**, 95–96

Brown, S. L., Blackstrom, B. and Busuttil, R. W. (1985) A new serum proteolytic enzyme in aneurysm pathogenesis. *J. Vasc. Surg.*, **2**, 393–399

Crawford, E. S. and Cohen, E. S. (1982) Aortic aneurysm: a multifocal disease. *Arch. Surg.*, **117**, 1393–1400

Delin, A., Ohlsén, H. and Swedenborg J. (1985) Growth rate of abdominal aortic aneurysms as measured by computed tomography. *Br. J. Surg.*, **72**, 530–532

Fielding, J. W. L., Black, J., Ashton, F. *et al.* (1981) Diagnosis and management of 528 abdominal aortic aneurysms. *Br. Med. J.*, **283**, 355–359

Fowkes, F. G. R., Macintyre, C. C. A. and Ruckley, C. V. (1989) Increasing incidence of aortic aneurysms in England and Wales. *Br. Med. J.*, **298**, 33–35

Johansson, G., Nydahl, S., Olofsson, P. and Swedenborg, J. (1990) Survival in patients with abdominal aneurysms. Comparison between operative and non-operative management. *Eur. J. Vasc. Surg.*, **4**, 497–502

Malins, A. F., Goodman, N. W., Cooper, G. W. *et al.* (1984) Ventilatory effects of pre- and postoperative diamorphine. A comparison of extradural with intramuscular administration. *Anaesthesia*, **39**, 118–125

Sethia, B. and Darke, S. G. (1983) Abdominal aortic aneurysm with retroperitoneal fibrosis and ureteric entrapment. *Br. J. Surg.*, **70**, 434–436

40

Congenital heart disease

J. D. Wisheart

Introduction

History

The surgical treatment of congenital abnormalities of the heart and great vessels began in 1937, when Robert Gross, in Boston, successfully ligated a patent ductus arteriosus. Just after World War II, Alfred Blalock described the systemic-to-pulmonary artery shunt, known by his name, to relieve the effects of Fallot's tetralogy; this was the first palliative procedure for an intracardiac anomaly. Further such palliative procedures were developed, and in addition the relief of such simple abnormalities as valvular pulmonary stenosis using closed techniques was described by Holmes-Sellors and Brock, in London. Definitive correction of intracardiac abnormalities awaited the development of cardiopulmonary bypass by Gibbon in 1954, and of whole body hypothermia by Bigelow in Toronto and Drew in London which permitted periods of total circulatory arrest.

During the past 20 years there have been four major advances in the management of congenital heart disease. The first of these is the widening recognition that many abnormalities should be corrected in the first year of life. Refinement of techniques of bypass and hypothermia enabled correction of intracardiac abnormalities to be carried out in infancy relatively safely from 1970 onwards (Barratt-Boyes et al., 1971). The previous two-stage policy of early palliation and correction later was challenged by the development of one-stage surgical correction in infancy, which gained increasing acceptance through the 1970s. In the 1980s the more positive view has become established that the child's best interests are served by correction in infancy where possible. Thus, in the UK the percentage of open operations which were carried out in the first year of life rose from 13% in 1977 to 30% in 1988 (UK Cardiac Surgical Register).

The second important development was the introduction of ultrasound and Doppler imaging of the heart. This non-invasive method provides dynamic and detailed information about the heart and may be repeated as often as is wished without risk to the patient. Many operations are now performed on the basis of ultrasound imaging alone without cardiac catheterization.

Thirdly, the introduction of prostaglandins a decade ago has transformed the prospects for babies born with conditions in which pulmonary or descending aortic blood flow depends on continuing patency of the ductus arteriosus. Prostaglandins prevent the duct closing and thus permit infants needing aortopulmonary shunts or coarctation repair to be operated relatively electively and in good condition.

Finally, the introduction of non-surgical interventions and therapies has rendered certain operative procedures virtually obsolete. Thus balloon valvuloplasty means that pulmonary valvotomy is now rarely carried out surgically, balloon dilatation of recurrent coarctation is effective so that very few operations are now performed for recurrent coarctation, and non-surgical occlusion of a patent ductus arteriosus is now being carried out in selected patients.

The foundations of paediatric cardiac surgery are:

1. Precise preoperative diagnosis.
2. Reliable and refined techniques of cardiopulmonary bypass.
3. Accurate methods of surgical repair.
4. Rational methods of intensive postoperative care.

Preparation for surgery

Once the complete diagnosis has been established by ultrasound and/or cardiac catheterization, the decision to operate may be considered and taken. The next step is to advise the parents, setting out fully the potential benefits and risks of the operation in both the long and short term. Admission should be at least 2 days before the operation to enable all necessary investigations and preparations to be made. Prophylactic antibiotics are used for 48 h, beginning with the induction of anaesthesia.

Surgical techniques

Approach to the heart

In extracardiac operations right or left thoracotomy is commonly used and this approach is fully described elsewhere. For intracardiac repair access is virtually always by median sternotomy (see Chapter 58).

The midline incision extends from just below the suprasternal notch to the xiphisternum; it is deepened to expose the sternum and linea alba. The sternum is divided vertically using heavy scissors or a mechanical saw and the two halves separated using a spreader. After the thymus has been divided and cleared from the pericardium superiorly, and the anterior fibres of the diaphragm cleared inferiorly, the pericardium may be opened by a vertical midline incision. The cut edges of the pericardium are sutured to the skin.

Cannulation

The heart is inspected and a 3 mm tape is passed around the aorta using a plane within the aortic sheath. In preparation for cannulation a double purse-string of 4/0 or 5/0 prolene is placed in the ascending aorta just proximal to the innominate artery. Further single purse-strings of 3/0 or 4/0 prolene are placed in the right atrial appendage and on the lateral wall of the right atrium near the inferior vena cava, for venous cannulation. Before cannulation the presence of a left superior vena cava and a patent ductus arteriosus are excluded. Arterial and venous cannulas are selected, which are of a suitable size to accommodate the perfusion flows. After total body heparinization (3 mg/kg) the aortic cannula is inserted, and is connected to the bypass machine following careful displacement of all air bubbles. The venous cannulas are then inserted through the right atrium and passed into the cavae; when they are connected, cardiopulmonary bypass may begin. Most forms of bypass in children utilize some degree of cooling, and while the temperature is being reduced 3 mm tapes are placed around the cavae and 'snugged' so that all venous return, other than coronary venous blood, is removed from the heart. Some surgeons use a vent sucker in the left ventricle, which helps provide a bloodless field, decompresses the left side of the heart and is a useful means for expelling air at the end of the operation.

Management of the operation

To carry out an accurate repair it is helpful to have a still heart and a bloodless field, which is usually achieved by cross-clamping the aorta; it is therefore also necessary to take steps to protect the myocardium from potential ischaemic damage. Thus, immediately after cross-clamping the aorta cardioplegic solution at 4°C is injected into the aortic root. This solution contains potassium (K^+) at a concentration of 16 mmol/litre which leads to the immediate cessation of both mechanical and electrical activity by the heart. Its low temperature, combined with topical cooling with cold isotonic crystalloid solution also at 4°C, lowers the myocardial temperature which should be maintained below 20°C while the aorta is cross-clamped. These measures minimize the damage which may be done to the myocardium during the period of ischaemia, by reducing oxygen requirement. A more sophisticated technique for myocardial protection uses blood as the vehicle to deliver the cardioplegia to the myocardium. Thus, ideal circumstances for precise and accurate operating may be combined with a high degree of myocardial protection.

Management in infancy

The organization of the operation described above had been found unsuitable in infants, partly because the trauma of the surgical approach and cannulation often led to hypotension or cardiac arrest and, secondly, because long periods of bypass were poorly tolerated. These difficulties were largely overcome by a technique popularized by Sir Brian Barratt-Boyes in 1969; the effects of circulatory embarrassment before bypass are reduced by initial surface cooling, and the period of bypass is shortened by the use of profound hypothermia and circulatory arrest. Thus bypass is only used to complete the cooling, to achieve rewarming and for whatever time is required to achieve stability of cardiac performance. This technique is fully described in Chapter 58.

Withdrawal of bypass and closure

Once the repair is complete and the cardiotomies closed, full rewarming of the patient is achieved. Cardiac action will be restored but it is unlikely that blood will be ejected into the aorta as the cavae are still snared and the systemic ventricle vented. Care must be taken to ensure that all air has been removed from the heart and aortic root, and to do this two important rituals should be carried out. First, a freely bleeding hole is placed at the highest point of the ascending aorta. Secondly, the anaesthetist should inflate the lungs while the surgeon elevates the apex of the heart, permitting blood and air to be expelled through the site of insertion of the ventricular vent. The caval snares are now released and the ritual repeated. Ejection may occur when the heart is replaced and will increase as the vent suction is reduced. The aortic hole should continue to bleed for 5–10 min after ejection has started.

After closure of the aortic hole the bypass flow is gradually reduced and then stopped as the heart maintains the circulation. The volume of blood transfused from the pump will be determined by the left or right atrial pressure, which is commonly 12–15 mmHg at this stage, and by the systolic arterial pressure which should be maintained at not less than 70–80 mmHg immediately after bypass. Once the circulation is stable the perfusion cannulas should be removed; the effects of heparin may then be reversed by giving protamine.

Prior to closing the chest, surgical haemostasis must be achieved throughout the wound from the heart to the skin edge. When it is required, catheters may be placed to monitor left atrial and pulmonary artery pressures in addition to the right atrial pressure.

Drains are placed in the pericardium, the retrosternal space and in a pleural cavity if it has been opened. Temporary pacing wires are sutured to the surface of both the right atrium and the right ventricle. The pericardium is usually left open. The sternum is approximated with wire or heavy non-absorbable sutures, and the superficial layers are closed accurately with slowly absorbable sutures. Finally, the skin is closed with a subcuticular technique.

Postoperative care

The postoperative intensive care of infants and small children is a team discipline, involving anaesthetic, cardiology and nursing staff, in addition to the surgical team who have the central and coordinating responsibility. Inasmuch as it is not taken for granted that any physiological system will function properly after bypass, the structure of intensive care is designed to monitor and support, if necessary, each individual system, but chiefly the cardiovascular and respiratory systems. Great attention to detail is required in observing these small children whose condition may change very rapidly, and in the accurate ordering of all treatment and dosages.

Reception in intensive care

When the patient arrives from theatre the nursing staff are informed of the surgical procedure and the various drains, pacing wires and monitoring cannulas are identified. In the case of infants or small children the environmental temperature must be high to minimize heat loss and it may be convenient to use a cot with an overhead heater. The monitoring lines are immediately connected (Figure 40.1) so that the lines are maintained patent by continuous flushing with heparinized Hartmann's solution, or half-normal saline in very small children. Artificial ventilation is advisable until stability is assured, or more commonly for longer. A nasotracheal tube is more suitable than an endotracheal tube for long-term ventilation in children. Care of the airway must be rigorously maintained by regular instillation of saline (0.2–1 ml) followed by suction, to avoid obstruction of the nasotracheal tube by inspissated secretions – a real danger in a small-calibre airway. A chest radiograph is immediately carried out and blood specimens sent for haemoglobin, packed cell volume, platelets, urea, electrolytes and sugar estimation, and for a coagulation screen.

Management in the first 24 hours

It is wise to note initially the weight (kg), the body surface area (m^2) and the estimated circulating volume (70–80 ml/kg) for the child. All blood loss is usually replaced volume-for-volume (with plasma if the packed cell volume exceeds 34). If additional blood is required to maintain the cardiac output in the presence of a normal or a low left atrial pressure it is convenient to order this in increments of approximately 2–5% of the estimated circulating volume; 0.5–1 ml of 13.4% calcium chloride should be given with each 100 ml of blood.

Total clear fluid intake is restricted and for the day

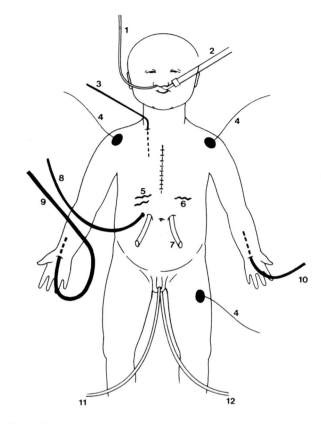

Figure 40.1 Postoperative monitoring. 1, Nasogastric tube. 2, Nasotracheal tube for ventilation. 3, Central venous cannula. 4, Electrodes for ECG. 5, Atrial pacing wires. 6, Ventricular pacing wire. 7, Pericardial and mediastinal drains. 8, Left atrial catheter, 9, Radial artery catheter. 10, Peripheral intravenous catheter in back of hand. 11, Urinary catheter. 12, Rectal temperature probe

of operation is $20\,ml/m^2$ per hour; this should be increased by 25% if the patient is nursed under an overhead heater.

Supplementary potassium may be needed on the day of operation and if so it should be given sparingly, prescribing a dose based on the formula 10 mmol of potassium per m^2 per 24 h; potassium should only be given if urine has been passed and if the serum potassium is in the low normal or below the normal range. Intravenous potassium may only be given diluted and infused over a half to one hour. Minimum urine output should be 0.5 ml/kg per hour. It is important to discuss the operation and progress of the child with the parents as early as possible.

Early complications

1. BLEEDING

Excessive bleeding may require replacement to such an extent that the complications of massive transfusion may ensue. Re-exploration to secure surgical haemostasis should be carried out if the blood loss exceeds 10% of the estimated blood volume in the first hour or 20% in the first 4 h, and so forth (Figure

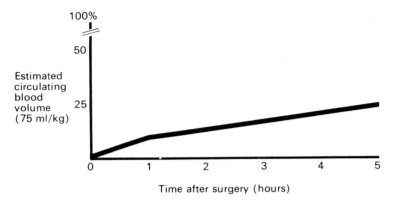

Figure 40.2 Postoperative blood loss. The level of accumulated blood loss after the operation which indicates the need for reoperation. Blood loss is expressed as a percentage of the estimated circulating volume

40.2). These rules should still apply if clotting is abnormal and the appropriate coagulation factors should be given during the surgical procedure.

2. TAMPONADE

Tamponade is the collection of blood and clot around the heart, limiting diastolic ventricular filling and leading to a fall in cardiac output and usually a rise in atrial pressure. This condition may be rapidly fatal but is completely treatable if the diagnosis is made and immediate re-exploration carried out – in the bed if need be.

3. LOW CARDIAC OUTPUT

If the cardiac output is low and both hypovolaemia and tamponade are excluded, then an inotropic drug should be used by continuous intravenous infusion; dopamine is widely used and may be combined with a vasodilator such as sodium nitroprusside or glyceryl trinitrate. Alternatives include dobutamine and adrenalin.

4. DYSRHYTHMIAS

A variety of atrial and ventricular dysrhythmias and disorders of rate may occur. It is essential to exclude possible underlying causes such as hypokalaemia, hypoxia, metabolic or respiratory acidosis, digoxin toxicity or beta-adrenergic infusion, hypovolaemia or tamponade. If none of these factors is present, then empirical therapeutic measures should be instituted.

5. PULMONARY HYPERTENSIVE CRISES

In infants and small children with elevated pulmonary vascular resistance (PVR) prior to surgery, the level of PVR in the early postoperative period is labile. When PVR rises acutely the pulmonary artery and right ventricular pressures rise, and the right ventricular stroke volume falls, leading to a reduction in cardiac output and systemic arterial pressure and a threat to the life of the child. In patients who are thought to be at risk for these events, a monitoring line should be placed in the pulmonary artery and preventive measures should be taken, including excellent oxygenation, hypocarbia, heavy sedation, muscle relaxation and arteriolar dilatation using phenoxybenzamine. Before performing airway toilet in the postoperative period, the child should be preoxygenated.

Later postoperative management

As the patient progresses, the framework of care described above may be relaxed progressively. Spontaneous breathing may be restored, using intermittent mandatory ventilation and continuous positive airway pressure for a time if needed; oral intake may be resumed, the monitoring arrangements withdrawn and the drains removed. A stable chronic therapeutic regimen designed to counter heart failure should be established if required.

Patent ductus arteriosus

Physiology and natural history

Isolated patency of the ductus arteriosus is the second most common congenital cardiac anomaly, accounting for 12% of the total. The ductus connects the aorta – usually just distal to the origin of the left subclavian artery – to the pulmonary artery just to the left of its bifurcation (Figure 40.3a). Blood passes from the aorta to the pulmonary artery. Spontaneous closure of the ductus is usual in the first few days of life, but if still patent it rarely closes later than the 3rd month. In infancy, left ventricular failure may develop, but usually a patent ductus is discovered as an incidental finding in an otherwise asymptomatic

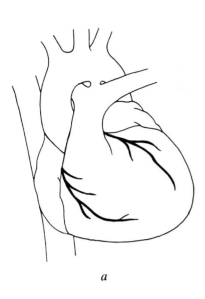

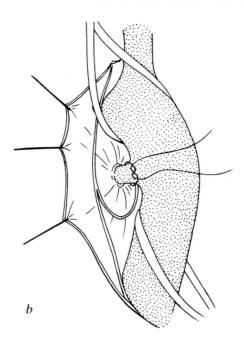

Figure 40.3 Ligation of patent ductus arteriosus. *a*, The PDA in relation to both the aorta and the pulmonary artery. *b*, The ductus is ready for ligation, and its relation to the vagus nerve and to its recurrent laryngeal branch is shown

child. In 5–7% of cases pulmonary vascular resistance will eventually rise sufficiently to cause reversal of the shunt, while in those who survive to middle age aneurysmal dilatation or calcification of the duct may occur. Bacterial endarteritis may complicate 1% of cases.

Anatomy

The ductus is thin walled and conical in shape with its wider part at the aortic end; a fold of pericardium overlies the pulmonary end. It is closely related to the vagus nerve and its recurrent laryngeal branch. Where there are anomalies of the aortic arch, the ductal anatomy may vary considerably.

Diagnosis and indications for operation

When a patent ductus arteriosus presents in childhood with a classical clinical picture, the diagnosis may be evident and in the past cardiac catheterization has not been deemed necessary for confirmation. With the advent of ultrasound and Doppler imaging it would be customary always to confirm the diagnosis by this method. In these circumstances cardiac catheterization would only be required in the presence of an unusual clinical feature or associated abnormality not made clear by the ultrasound imaging, if the level of pulmonary vascular resistance needs to be measured or if the patent ductus arteriosus presents in adult life. A demonstrably patent ductus arteriosus

should be closed operatively and this would usually be performed in infancy or the early years of life. In the presence of elevated pulmonary vascular resistance with pulmonary hypertension and shunt reversal, surgery is contraindicated. Techniques of non-surgical closure of a patent ductus as an extension of cardiac catheterization are being developed and applied to a limited degree.

Operative surgery

Operative technique

The object of surgery is to divide or ligate the duct, which may be approached using a left lateral thoracotomy at the level of the fourth intercostal space. With the lung retracted forwards and downwards the aortic arch, left subclavian artery and descending aorta, together with the phrenic and vagus nerves, may be seen and a thrill may be felt over the ductus. A vertical incision is made into the aortic sheath extending from the left subclavian artery to well below the level of the ductus. The aortic sheath is reflected forwards, using both sharp and blunt dissection, and is maintained in position by stay sutures which also serve to keep the left lung out of the immediate operative field. The posterior part of the aortic sheath is dissected and tapes passed around the aorta. The anatomy of the arch and ductus may now be confirmed (Figure 40.3b). Further dissection in the same plane will safely reflect forwards the vagus and recurrent laryngeal nerves, and will also permit all aspects

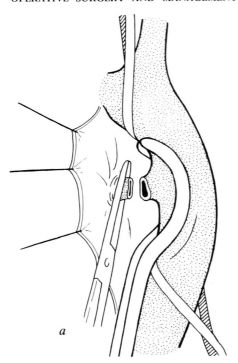

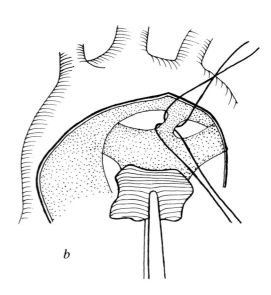

Figure 40.4 *a*, Division of patent ductus arteriosus. The ductus is divided and the cut ends will now be sutured. *b*, Closure of ductus from anterior approach. After dissecting along the pulmonary artery, the ductus is demonstrated and ready for ligation, prior to going on to cardiopulmonary bypass

of the ductus to be demonstrated. A right-angled dissecting instrument may now be passed behind the ductus; if this is difficult the aorta may be lifted forwards using the tapes, and the dissection behind the ductus completed under direct vision. The effect of 'test-clamping' the duct should be observed; the arterial pressure will normally rise a little and the heart rate remain stable. In the presence of known pulmonary vascular disease the pulmonary artery pressure should be measured before and after clamping; if it fails to fall the operation should be abandoned. Two ligatures of no. 1 linen or 2 mm braided silk are passed around the ductus and the aortic end ligated first (Figure 40.3b). Secure ligation is made safe by temporary reduction of the aortic pressure which is easily achieved by cross-clamping the aorta proximal to the ductus for the 20 s needed to apply the first two throws to the knot. A second ligature is applied to the pulmonary end of the ductus.

Other techniques

1. DIVISION OF THE DUCTUS

This is most easily carried out by applying a side-biting clamp to the aorta at the origin of the ductus and a straight clamp to its pulmonary end. The cut ends may be secured by running sutures of 4/0 or 5/0 prolene (Figure 40.4a).

2. CLOSURE OF A DUCTUS ASSOCIATED WITH INTRACARDIAC ANOMALIES

In these circumstances the ductus should be closed at the time of total correction. Control of the ductus should be obtained prior to instituting cardiopulmonary bypass in order to avoid loss of perfusion to the lungs. The anterior approach to the heart permits the pulmonary artery end of the ductus to be identified and ligated (Figure 40.4b); alternatively the ductus may be closed from within the pulmonary artery after cardiopulmonary bypass has been established.

3. CLOSURE OF A CALCIFIED OR ANEURYSMAL DUCTUS

No direct approach is appropriate in these circumstances. The safest technique is to use cardiopulmonary bypass and to open the descending aorta between clamps, so that the orifice of the duct may be closed by a patch under direct vision.

4. CLOSURE OF THE NEONATAL DUCT

Duct patency is likely to persist in those born prematurely and may also do so during the neonatal period of a full-term baby. This may lead to heart failure, respiratory distress syndrome and ventilator dependence. If medical attempts to close the duct using

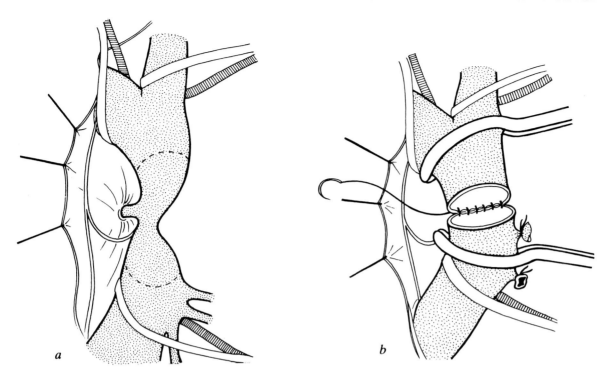

Figure 40.5 Coarctation of the aorta: direct anastomosis, *a*, shows the coarctation, its relation to the vagus nerve and its recurrent laryngeal branch, the ligamentum arteriosum and the intercostal arteries. The proposed lines of resection are indicated. *b*, The aorta has been clamped, the intercostal arteries divided and the coarctation resected. Direct end-to-end anastomosis, using a simple continuous stitch, is being performed

indomethacin fail, surgical closure by ligation or clip should be performed, usually with excellent results.

Results

Operative mortality in children is less than 0.5% but may be slightly higher in infants, adults or in the presence of pulmonary hypertension. The long-term results are usually excellent in terms of symptoms and cardiac performance. Recanalization is extremely rare.

Coarctation of the aorta

Physiology and natural history

A coarctation is a localized severe narrowing, usually at the level of the aortic isthmus just distal to the origin of the left subclavian artery (Figure 40.5a). It accounts for 6% of congenital cardiac anomalies.

There may be a pressure gradient of 40–60 mmHg across the coarctation. The resulting proximal hypertension causes left ventricular hypertrophy with ischaemia and fibrosis of the myocardium which eventually leads to left ventricular failure. Aneurysms may develop on the intracranial and intercostal arteries or the aorta. Distally the circulation is maintained

by many collaterals and the resulting flow has either dampened or absent pulsations which are thought to stimulate the renal mechanisms contributing to the hypertension.

In infancy, an isolated coarctation may lead to left ventricular failure and threaten life. Coarctation presenting in childhood is free of symptoms, but life is threatened later by the mechanisms already described which lead to an average life expectation of about 40 years.

Anatomy and classification

The luminal narrowing of a coarctation is caused by the narrowing of the aortic wall as seen on external inspection of the vessel, and an internal shelf or diaphragm, which together may limit the opening to 1 or 2 mm in diameter. Coarctations are usually divided into two groups: first, those which are approximately at the same level as the ligamentum arteriosum, called 'juxtaductal', and which are seen in children and adults; secondly, those which are proximal to the ductus, called 'preductal', which are seen in infants. In the latter group there is a long hypoplastic segment between the origin of the left subclavian artery and the patent ductus arteriosus; at the lower end of this hypoplastic segment there is a critical narrowing or coarctation. The patent ductus arteriosus is continu-

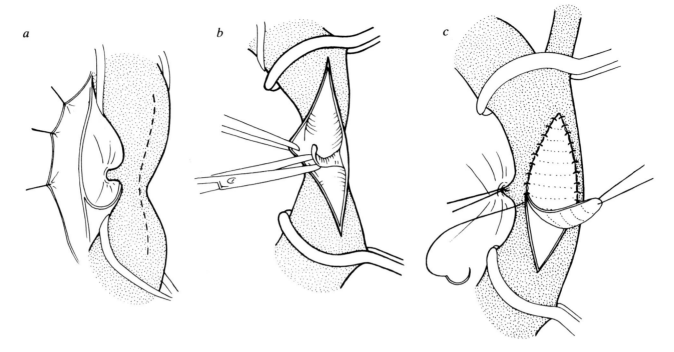

Figure 40.6 Coarctation of the aorta: aortoplasty. *a*, The proposed line of incision across the coarctation. *b*. After opening the aorta, the 'diaphragm' is excised. *c*, The aortotomy is closed using a gusset of woven Dacron

ous with the descending aorta and transmits blood from the pulmonary artery to the lower half of the body; spontaneous closure of the duct would compromise the circulation to the lower half of the body.

Abnormalities of the aortic or mitral valve may also be associated with a coarctation.

Diagnosis and indications for operation

The diagnosis in children is a clinical one based on the classic findings of elevation of the blood pressure, absent or weak and delayed femoral pulses, with evidence of periscapular collaterals. It is usually sufficient to confirm the diagnosis by ultrasound and Doppler imaging. If there is doubt about any of these findings, cardiac catheterization should be performed to measure the pressure gradient, to demonstrate by aortography the anatomy of both the coarctation and the collaterals and to clarify any associated abnormalities.

Surgical treatment is required for virtually all patients with coarctation. In the asymptomatic child, elective operation may be planned any time after the first year of life and should certainly be carried out prior to going to school, and if the diagnosis is made later the operation should not be delayed. In infancy, persistent left ventricular failure due to the coarctation alone or in association with other anomalies requires urgent surgical treatment.

Operative surgery

In 1945 both Gross and Crafoord, independently, treated patients with coarctation by resection and end-to-end anastomosis. This technique remains the most widely used in children and adults, although some surgeons prefer the plastic method first described by Vosschulte. The special problems presented by infants may be met by the subclavian artery flap method, first described by Waldhausen, and popularized in the UK by Hamilton, although many surgeons use the technique of resection of coarctation and direct end-to-end anastomoses in all age groups.

Operative techniques

The coarctation is approached through a long, left lateral thoracotomy, usually at the upper border of the 5th rib. Division of the muscles of the chest wall is time consuming and tedious as each enlarged collateral vessel must be individually ligated. Carefully controlled hypotension using trimetaphan or sodium nitroprusside is helpful. A long vertical incision is made in the aortic sheath extending from the left subclavian artery to below the coarctation. Carefully preserving the plane of the dissection, the anterior flap is reflected forwards together with the vagus and its recurrent laryngeal branch. The dissection of the aorta proximal to the coarctation may be completed and tapes passed around the left subclavian artery and the arch of the aorta distal to the left common carotid artery (Figure 40.5a). Enlarged mediastinal branches of the aorta may cause troublesome bleeding if not carefully identified and secured. Distal to the coarctation, dilated, tortuous and thin-walled intercostal arteries pass from the aorta to the chest wall; occasionally one or two pairs of these will need to be controlled or divided.

Vascular clamps are placed on the aorta above and below the coarctation and before incising the narrowed segment it should be confirmed that it is not still being filled through an uncontrolled or unidentified branch. It should be shown by formal manometry that there is a satisfactory pressure in the aorta distal to the clamp. This pressure should be not less than 45–55 mmHg.

1. END-TO-END ANASTOMOSES

The lines of resection are determined prior to application of the clamps and the coarctation should be excised (Figure 40.5a); in infants the whole of the hypoplastic segment, the coarctation and the insertion of the ductus into the aorta should be excised. After suitable mobilization of the proximal and distal aorta the two ends may be brought together using 3/0, 4/0 or 5/0 prolene and the posterior part of the anastomosis may be constructed with a simple running stitch (Figure 40.5b). The anterior part may be completed by a further continuous suture or by interrupted sutures in smaller children. The anaesthetist should be warned prior to removing the clamps so that the hypotensive agent may be stopped and blood may be available in the event of severe haemorrhage from the suture line.

2. AORTOPLASTY

This method avoids a circumferential aortic suture line by reconstructing the aorta with a gusset inserted across the narrow segment. After clamping the arch of the aorta and the left subclavian artery, a vertical incision is made in the aorta beginning near the origin of the left subclavian artery and extending down across the coarctation and into the descending aorta (Figure 40.6a). The diaphragm within the aorta at the level of the coarctation is excised (Figure 40.6b). A large oval patch of woven crimped Dacron is cut from an arterial tube graft and sewn into the resulting defect using continuous runs of prolene sutures (Figure 40.6c).

3. TUBE GRAFT

If it is not possible to bring the ends together easily, then the gap should be bridged using a circumferential graft of woven crimped Dacron of the appropriate size (Figure 40.7). The use of a circumferential graft is appropriate in fully grown children or adults, but in small children should be avoided at all costs.

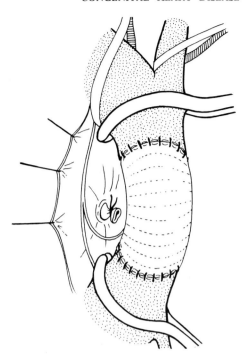

Figure 40.7 Coarctation of the aorta: tube graft. The graft is shown after its insertion has been completed. It bridges the gap between the two ends of the aorta

4. SUBCLAVIAN FLAP OPERATION

A circumferential suture line in infants commonly leads to recurrent obstruction at this site due to failure of growth of the anastomosis. This is avoided by a plastic operation using a gusset of living autologous tissue, namely the left subclavian artery which is divided proximal to its first branch. A vertical incision across the coarctation is extended into the left subclavian artery, which is thus changed from a tube to a flap (Figure 40.8a). This flap is turned down and sewn into the defect across the coarctation using a fine prolene continuous suture (Figure 40.8b).

5. USE OF LEFT ATRIOFEMORAL BYPASS

If the pressure in the descending aorta remains less than 45–50 mmHg after clamping and after the position of the clamps and medication have been suitably adjusted, then it must be concluded that the collateral circulation to the lower half of the body and in particular to the spinal cord is inadequate. It is then necessary to preserve the distal circulation by using left atrial femoral bypass, a Gott shunt or simply a Dacron tube shunt between the proximal and distal aorta.

Results

The operative mortality for uncomplicated coarctation in childhood or the teenage years is less than

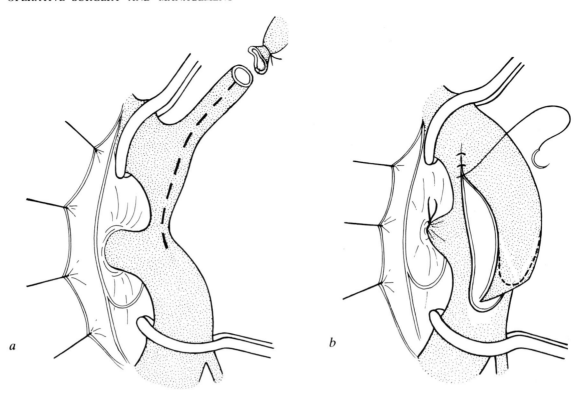

Figure 40.8 Coarctation of the aorta: subclavian flap operation. An infantile or preductal coarctation is shown. *a,* The distal subclavian artery has been ligated and the aorta clamped: the proposed incision across the coarctation and into the left subclavian artery is shown. *b,* The 'flap' of subclavian artery is being sutured into the aortic defect

2%, but in adults may be slightly higher due to technical problems arising from the degenerative changes in the aortic wall. The chief cause of operative death in these patients is severe haemorrhage. In infants where the coarctation is associated with other major anomalies, the mortality for the operation, which may include other palliative procedures, may be as high as 10–15%. Important complications include haemorrhage from the aorta or chest wall, recurrent laryngeal nerve palsy, chylothorax, or rarely renal failure or paraplegia. Local infection, either blood-borne within the aorta or outside the aorta, may have serious consequences, particularly if prosthetic material has been used in the repair. A syndrome of crampy abdominal pain mimicking an acute abdomen is described and attributed to mesenteric arteritis due to the presence of a pulsatile flow for the first time. This is usually associated with a high blood pressure immediately after operation. In the early postoperative period, if systolic pressure is greater than 170 mmHg or diastolic greater than 110 mmHg the blood pressure should be reduced by pharmacological means. The blood pressure does not fall immediately after the operation and it may not reach its final level until 6–12 weeks later.

Recurrence of coarctation is a well-documented late complication which is more likely in those of young age at operation. In the past, avoidance of this complication was based on operating at an older age of childhood rather than a younger age. However, recurrence is probably now confined to those operated in the first 2 months of life. Until recently, recurrence was treated by a second operation but it now seems to be well managed by balloon dilatation.

Congenital aortic stenosis

Physiology and natural history

Aortic stenosis accounts for about 6% of all congenital heart disorders. The obstruction causes elevation of left ventricular pressure with resulting left ventricular hypertrophy, ischaemia and fibrosis. This may be sufficiently severe to threaten life either in infancy or childhood.

Anatomy and classification

The obstruction may be valvar, subvalvar or supravalvar. In valvar aortic stenosis there may be two or three cusps, rarely one or four; the cusps themselves may be thin and pliable or thick and rigid. The commissures are usually fused and the annulus itself may be small. When the obstruction is subvalvar it is either a discrete diaphragm of fibrous tissue a few millimetres below the aortic valve or it may be caused by hypertrophic obstructive cardiomyopathy. Supravalvar obstruction is rare and is caused by a narrowing of the aorta at or just above the sinus ridge.

Diagnosis and indications for operation

The diagnosis will normally be made by ultrasound and Doppler imaging which will permit both the severity and site of stenosis to be identified. Cardiac catheterization will not normally be required in infancy or childhood. Gradients of 60–80 mmHg in the presence of symptoms and ECG changes in children are indications for surgical relief of the obstruction. In infants, smaller gradients may indicate important obstruction. The objects of surgery are to relieve the

obstruction and thereby to protect the left ventricular myocardium from the damage that would follow persistent obstruction.

Operative surgery

Operative techniques

1. VALVAR

With cardiopulmonary bypass, moderate hypothermia and a short period of ischaemic arrest, the aortic valve may be exposed by an oblique incision in the aorta (Figure 40.9a). The fused commissures should be carefully and accurately incised but no closer to the annulus than 2 mm, in case aortic incompetence should occur (Figure 40.9b). When this has been done the subvalvar region should be inspected. The aortic

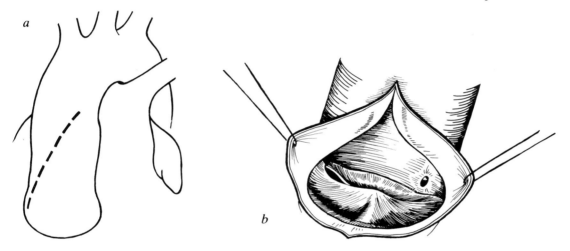

Figure 40.9 Valvar aortic stenosis. A bicuspid, stenotic valve is shown. *a*, Incision for an oblique aortotomy. *b*, The left coronary ostium is seen posteriorly

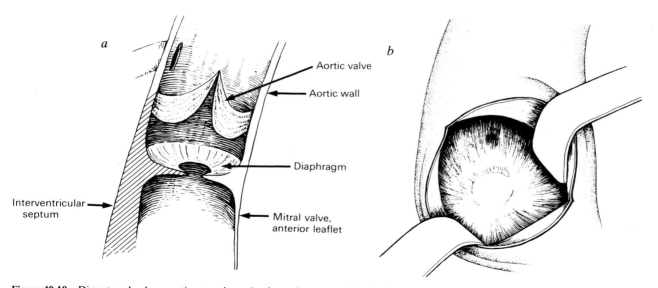

Figure 40.10 Discrete subvalvar aortic stenosis. *a*, A schematic cross-section showing the obstructive diaphragm a few millimetres below the aortic valve. *b*, The diaphragm as seen through the aortotomy with the valve cusps retracted

incision may be repaired by continuous stitches of 3/0 or 4/0 prolene.

2. SUBVALVAR

Access to the obstruction is through the aorta and aortic valve, as described above. The subvalvar region is exposed by careful retraction of the valve leaflets and annulus, avoiding pressure on the upper part of the interventricular septum, lest the conducting tissue should be temporarily injured. If a discrete diaphragm is present it may carefully be excised by a mixture of some sharp, but predominantly blunt dissection, carefully avoiding any injury to the interventricular septum, mitral valve or the aortic valve (Figure 40.10).

3. SUPRAVALVAR

These rare anomalies require major reconstruction of the proximal aorta which may also involve the annulus or the ostia of the coronary arteries.

Results

Aortic valvotomy is best regarded as a palliative operation, carried out in order to preserve life and to protect the left ventricular myocardium. Although immediate relief of stenosis is usually good, the obstruction may recur after an interval or the operation may be complicated by aortic incompetence. For either of these two reasons further surgery may be required in a high percentage of cases. When surgery is required early in infancy results are much less good and the operative mortality remains high.

Pulmonary stenosis

Physiology and natural history

Pulmonary stenosis accounts for 9% of all congenital cardiac abnormalities. There is a pressure gradient between the body of the right ventricle and the pulmonary artery resulting in hypertrophy of the right ventricle. Tiredness and shortness of breath are common and cyanosis may occur when a patent foramen ovale is also present. In severe cases, right ventricular failure, ventricular dysrhythmias, syncope or premature death may occur.

Anatomy and classification

The obstruction may be valvar, infundibular or supravalvar. In valvar stenosis the commissures, which are partly adherent to the wall of the pulmonary artery, are fused. In infundibular stenosis, hypertrophy and fusion of muscle bands impinge on the outflow tract of the right ventricle. This is a dynamic obstruction which is severe in systole.

Diagnosis and indications for operation

The diagnosis will normally be confirmed by ultrasound and Doppler imaging which will both give a measure of the pressure gradient and an indication of the level of the obstruction. Any associated abnormalities are demonstrated. The stenosis may be classified as mild if the gradient is less than 50, moderate if it is between 50 and 100, and severe if it is greater than 100 mmHg. Mild pulmonary stenosis rarely requires operation, but severe obstruction should be surgically relieved. Moderate stenosis should be relieved if it is associated with symptoms and evidence of advanced hypertrophy of the right ventricle. Occasionally, a neonate presents with life-threatening pulmonary stenosis.

Operative surgery

Relief of pulmonary valvar stenosis was devised by Holmes Sellors and Brock at about the same time, in 1947, using an instrument passed through the wall of the right ventricle to dilate the pulmonary valve. Semi-open methods using inflow occlusion and moderate hypothermia have also been used. Since cardiopulmonary bypass has become safe, open methods have nearly always been used. However, in recent years balloon valvuloplasty has proved to be an effective and safe way of relieving valvar stenosis and has largely replaced surgical pulmonary valvotomy.

Operative techniques

1. VALVAR STENOSIS

First, the presence of a patent foramen ovale should be excluded by exploration through a small incision in the right atrium; if present it should be closed. The valve is approached by a longitudinal incision in the pulmonary artery (Figure 40.11a). The commissures are freed from the wall of the pulmonary artery using fine scissors, enabling complete commissurotomies to be performed (Figure 40.11b). The arteriotomy is repaired with a continuous suture of 4/0 or 5/0 prolene.

If the valve cusps are thickened, partial or complete excision may be needed to relieve the obstruction. The resulting pulmonary incompetence is said to be well tolerated, whereas it is known that important residual obstruction is not.

In a moribund neonate there may be a place for performing a closed valvotomy using dilating instruments passed through the wall of the right ventricle.

2. INFUNDIBULAR STENOSIS

The infundibulum is exposed by a transverse ventriculotomy across the right ventricular outflow tract, carefully sited to avoid the coronary arteries.

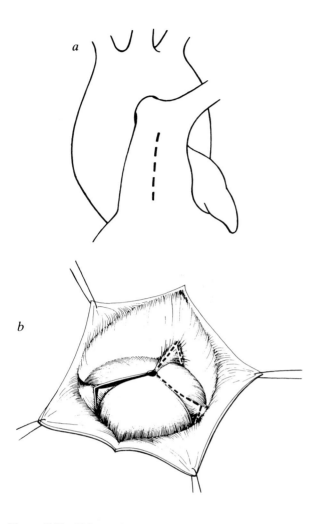

Figure 40.11 Valvar pulmonary stenosis. A tricuspid pulmonary valve with fused commissures and a small central orifice. The broken lines indicate where the commissures are freed from the arterial wall and then divided. One commissure is already divided (*b*). *a*, Line of incision in pulmonary artery

Obstructing bands of infundibular muscle, often covered with thickened endocardium, are incised or excised taking care to avoid perforating the interventricular septum or damaging the subvalvar structures of the tricuspid valve.

If the obstruction takes the form of a 'tunnel' below the pulmonary valve it may be necessary to enlarge the infundibulum using a gusset of autologous pericardium or woven Dacron.

3. SUPRAVALVAR STENOSIS

Supravalvar stenosis is not common in isolation but may occur with other abnormalities, such as Fallot's tetralogy. It is best dealt with by enlarging the narrowed area with a gusset, preferably of autologous pericardium, using a fine suture of 4/0 or 5/0 prolene.

Results

The operative mortality in children should not be more than 2%, although it may be higher in infants. An excellent result is nearly always achieved.

Atrial septal defects

Physiology and natural history

Atrial septal defects account for 10% of congenital cardiac anomalies. There is a communication between the two atria, resulting in a left-to-right shunt. Isolated simple atrial septal defects rarely threaten life in infancy or childhood, but symptoms may develop in adult life and average survival is to the fifth decade.

Anatomy and classification

There are three types of atrial septal defect (ASD):

1. Secundum atrial septal defect.
2. Primum atrial septal defect (partial atrioventricular septal defect).
3. Sinus venosus defect.

The *secundum ASD* is the most common and usually lies in the fossa ovalis, but may extend to the inferior vena caval orifice, the lateral atrial wall or the upper part of the atrial septum; it is commonly 2–3 cm in diameter. It never extends as far posteriorly or inferiorly as the coronary sinus or the tricuspid valve. A 'patent foramen ovale' is the name given to a probe-patent communication between the atria and it should be included in the group. However, it exists in 10–20% of normal people and is only of significance when associated with other lesions, particularly pulmonary stenosis.

The *primum ASD* lies in the posteroinferior part of the septum and is immediately adjacent to the tricuspid and mitral valve orifices, and also, therefore, to the conducting tissue as it passes from the atrioventricular node to the interventricular septum. The size of the defect varies and when there is virtually no interatrial septum, the condition is known as 'common atrium'. In addition to the ASD there is a cleft in the anterior leaflet of the mitral valve causing mitral incompetence. The primum ASD is due to failure of development of the septum primum and is an incomplete form of a more complex anomaly which includes both atrial and ventricular septal defects, as well as defects of the endocardial cushions which cause abnormalities in both mitral and tricuspid valves.

The *sinus venosus defect* lies high in the atrial septum and the right upper pulmonary vein may empty into the superior vena.

Diagnosis and indications for operation

Children with a secundum ASD or a sinus venosus

defect are usually free of symptoms. The diagnosis may be made by ultrasound imaging and will not usually need to be confirmed by catheterization. If the pulmonary to systemic flow ratio is believed to be greater than 2:1 the ASD should be closed, generally before school age. When adults present with an ASD it should be closed in order to reduce the effects of atrial fibrillation and to prevent further progression of pulmonary vascular disease.

Children with a primum ASD frequently have shortness of breath and increased tiredness. The diagnosis is suggested by the clinical findings of an ASD plus mitral incompetence together with the characteristic electrocardiogram. It should be confirmed by ultrasound imaging, and cardiac catheterization should usually be carried out not only to demonstrate the classical 'goose neck deformity' on the left ventricular angiogram but also the severity of the mitral incompetence and the level of pulmonary vascular resistance. These defects should always be repaired.

Operative surgery

Operative techniques

1. SECUNDUM ASD

This is an operation of low risk (less than 1%) in which there is a particular danger of air embolism. Any possibility of ejection by the left ventricle must be prevented while the heart is open; thus either the heart should be fibrillated or the aorta should be cross-clamped with either ischaemic or chemical cardiac arrest, while the defect is being closed.

Prior to bypass the heart is inspected and anomalies of the right pulmonary veins are sought. The atrium should be opened by an incision at the base of the appendage which extends towards the inferior vena cava (Figure 40.12a). The ASD is identified and the adjacent parts of the septum and fossa ovalis are inspected for additional defects or fenestrations. The defect is closed, usually by a continuous suture (Figure 40.12b). Care must be taken not to distort the orifice of the inferior vena cava. Occasionally very large defects require a patch of pericardium or Dacron for satisfactory closure.

So that all air may be removed, the heart should be fibrillated as the aortic clamp is removed. This permits full precautions to be taken before the heart may eject.

2. PRIMUM ASD

The object of this operation is to repair the mitral valve, close the ASD with a patch without causing heart block and to prevent the occurrence of air embolism.

Following the application of the aortic cross-clamp and administration of cardioplegia, the right atrium is opened. The abnormal anatomy is inspected and the

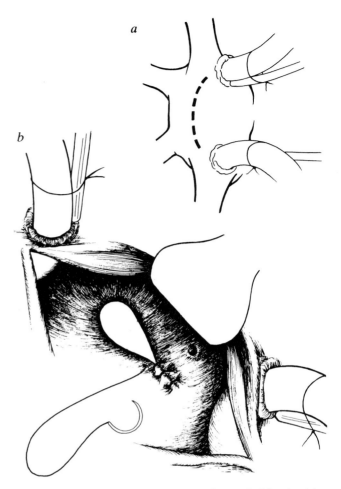

Figure 40.12 Secundum atrial septal defect. *a*, Incision in right atrium to expose the defect. *b*, A secundum ASD being closed by a continuous suture

diagnosis confirmed (Figure 40.13a); care is taken to exclude a ventricular septal defect lying below the atrioventricular valves. The mitral valve is repaired first by approximating the edges of the cleft with interrupted sutures of 4/0 or 5/0 prolene (Figure 40.13b).

The ASD is always closed with a patch, using either autologous pericardium or thin Dacron. It is of prime importance to avoid damaging the conduction tissue while inserting the patch. The atrioventricular node lies between the coronary sinus and the tricuspid valve (Figure 40.13a), while the bundle of His lies close to the tricuspid valve as it passes superiorly to enter the interventricular septum. A still heart and a bloodless field are the necessary conditions for precise suturing and avoidance of heart block, and these may be achieved by either of two techniques. The patch may be sutured to the attachment of the anterior leaflet of the mitral valve, the left side of atrial septum inferiorly and onto the edge of the defect to the right of the coronary sinus (Figure 40.13c). Alternatively,

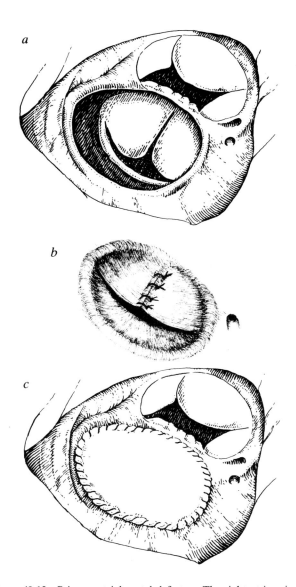

Figure 40.13 Primum atrial septal defect. *a*, The right atrium is open and the tricuspid valve is seen anteriorly. The septal defect is immediately adjacent to the tricuspid valve and the mitral valve, which with its cleft anterior cusp may be seen through the defect. The position of the atrioventricular node is indicated, lying between the coronary sinus and the tricuspid valve. *b*, The cleft is closed with interrupted sutures. *c*, The septal defect is closed with a patch sutured to the attachment of the anterior leaflet of the mitral valve

the patch may be sutured to the attachment of the tricuspid valve until the suture line is inferior to the atrioventricular node and the coronary sinus; it is then carried around the floor of the right atrium so that the coronary sinus drains to the left atrium. Either way the patch may be securely inserted and the conducting pathways preserved.

3. SINUS VENOSUS DEFECT

The sinus venosus defect is closed with a patch,

ensuring that pulmonary venous blood drains to the left atrium.

Results

The mortality for repair of secundum ASD is less than 1% and there should be close to normal cardiac function ensuring both a satisfactory length and quality of life thereafter. The mortality for repair of primum ASD is slightly higher and is between 2% and 5%. In these cases the future is determined chiefly by whether or not heart block has been avoided, and also by the severity of the mitral valve lesion. Thus a very small percentage may require permanent pacemaking, or replacement of the mitral valve later in life.

Ventricular septal defects

Physiology and natural history

Ventricular septal defects are the most common congenital cardiac anomaly, accounting for 25% of the total. Blood passes from the left to the right ventricle in volumes determined by the size of the defect and the relative resistances in the pulmonary and systemic vascular beds; this results in a high pulmonary blood flow. The natural history of the condition is complex; spontaneous closure may occur in some, but in others life may be threatened early in infancy by left ventricular failure; after infancy the development of progressive obliterative, pulmonary vascular disease may lead to a rising pulmonary vascular resistance. This will initially cause a reduction and may eventually lead to a reversal of the shunt flow (Eisenmenger syndrome). These structural changes may become advanced before teenage years in 15–25% of patients. Aortic incompetence, infundibular pulmonary stenosis and bacterial endocarditis may also occur, resulting in an expectation of life of 25–30 years if the ventricular septal defect is not closed.

Anatomy and classification

The ventricular septum may be divided into three portions – inlet, outlet (or infundibular) and trabecular (or muscular) as shown in Figure 40.14a. Each part is contiguous with part of the membranous septum. Defects may be classified as perimembranous, infundibular or muscular (Figure 40.14b). The perimembranous defect is due to a deficiency of muscle around the membranous septum and the central fibrous body forms part of the rim of the defect. The defect may extend into the trabecular, the outflow or the inflow portions of the septum, and thus perimembranous defects may be subdivided on this basis. The perimembranous defects are always contiguous with the annulus of the tricuspid valve, and the

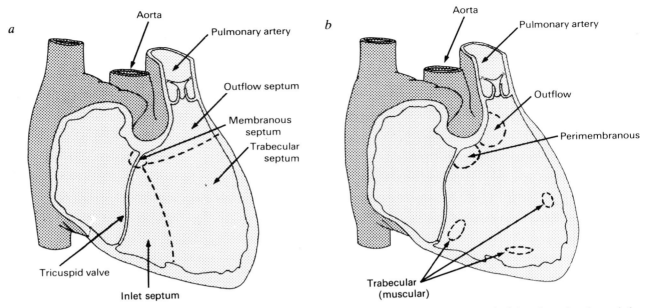

Figure 40.14 Ventricular septal defects: classification. *a*, The three parts of the ventricular septum – the inlet, the trabecular and the outflow portions, each of which impinges on the membranous septum. *b*, The sites of different types of defect, perimembranous outflow and trabecular (After Anderson, R. H. and Becker, A. E. (1983) In Stark, J. and deLeval, M. (eds) *Surgery for Congenital Heart Defects*, Grune and Stratton, London)

bundle of His always passes along the inferior margin of the defect before dividing into the right and left bundles to descend in the muscular septum. The infundibular defect lies above the crista supraventricularis and below the aortic and pulmonary valves. It is not related to the conducting tissue. Muscular defects may be single or multiple and are situated in any part of the trabecular septum.

Diagnosis and indications for operation

The diagnosis may be demonstrated by ultrasound imaging, but usually cardiac catheterization and left ventricular angiography should be carried out. This will enable pulmonary blood flow to be measured and the level of pulmonary vascular resistance to be calculated.

Surgical closure is not required if the pulmonary blood flow does not exceed twice the systemic flow and the pulmonary vascular resistance is low. If the pulmonary flow is higher than this, the defect should be closed, usually between the ages of 1 and 3 years. Earlier surgical treatment will be required if left ventricular failure in infancy does not respond to medical treatment, or if the baby fails to thrive. If very high pulmonary blood flow or elevated pulmonary artery pressure, or both, are noted early in life, they suggest the possibility of the early development of pulmonary vascular disease and the defect should often be closed before the baby's first birthday and not later than 18–24 months of age. If the patient is cyanosed due to shunt reversal, closure of the defect is contraindicated.

Operative surgery

In 1952 Muller and Dammann described how the effects of a ventricular septal defect (VSD) could be palliated by constriction of the pulmonary artery; thus by increasing the resistance to flow through the pulmonary artery the shunt flow is reduced, as is the volume load on the left ventricle. The development of pulmonary vascular disease is at least partly prevented by the reduction in pulmonary blood flow. With cardiopulmonary bypass, techniques of closure of the defect became established and satisfactory in older children; pulmonary artery banding was reserved for infants. In the past two decades cardiopulmonary bypass has become sufficiently safe in infants so that primary intracardiac correction is now the treatment of choice in infants needing surgical treatment for an isolated VSD. Pulmonary artery banding is reserved for infants in whom the VSD is associated with other complex malformations.

Operative technique for closure of VSD

The perimembranous VSD is usually approached through the right atrium and tricuspid valve, but occasionally access through the right ventricle may be used.

1. TRANSATRIAL APPROACH

This approach has the advantage of avoiding an incision in the right ventricular muscle. The right atrium is opened by an incision passing from the base

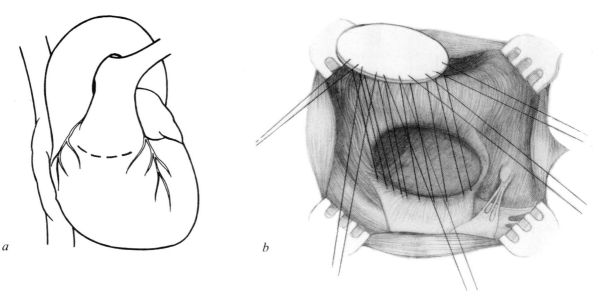

Figure 40.15 Ventricular septal defect. *a*, The site of incision when the VSD is approached through a right ventriculotomy. *b*, Closure. A view of a membranous defect from the right ventricular aspect. Sutures have been passed through the attachment of the cusp of the tricuspid valve, and then through the patch

of the atrial appendage towards the inferior vena cava, thus exposing the tricuspid valve. The septal leaflet of the valve is retracted posteriorly and to the right, permitting the VSD to be visualized. A series of double-armed sutures of 4/0 Mersilene, buttressed with small pledgets of Teflon felt, are placed in the margin of the defect. Beginning inferiorly, where the bundle of His is close to the defect, the stitches are carefully placed through the attachment of the septal leaflet of the tricuspid valve. Proceeding clockwise, care must be taken to avoid the aortic valve which is close to the defect; proceeding anticlockwise from the tricuspid valve, once the papillary muscle of the conus has been passed, stitches may be placed deeply into the muscular margins of the defect. Each stitch is passed through a knitted Dacron patch which is slid into position and the sutures carefully tied. Alternatively a continuous suture may be used incorporating the same precautions.

2. TRANSVENTRICULAR APPROACH

If access through the right atrium is unsatisfactory, the transventricular approach is used. The right ventricle is opened with a transverse incision at the level of the VSD, after carefully noting that no major branches of the coronary arteries will be injured (Figure 40.15a). The edges of the ventriculotomy are gently retracted, the crista supraventricularis and tricuspid valve are immediately noted and the VSD may then be identified behind and below the crista and above the tricuspid valve (Figure 40.15b). The papillary muscle of the conus lies posterior to the tricuspid valve. Looking through the defect, the cusps of the aortic valve may be seen. Sutures are placed as

described previously and the defect closed with a patch. The ventriculotomy is closed with two layers of simple continuous sutures of 4/0 prolene; each bite includes the whole thickness of the right ventricular wall.

3. CLOSURE OF OTHER TYPES OF VSD

Infundibular defects should be repaired either through the right ventricle or through the aortic or pulmonary valves and in either case a patch should be used. As the conducting tissue is not at risk, a simple continuous suture may be used. In the past, muscular defects were approached through the body of the right ventricle but the coarse trabecular pattern of the right side of the septum makes identification difficult and closure uncertain. It is now widely accepted that these should be approached using a 'fish-mouth' incision at the apex of the left ventricle. By this route both single and multiple defects may be identified and closed securely.

Results

The operative mortality in children ranges from 2% to 5% and is now only a little higher in infants. In nearly all, the symptomatic result is excellent but, where it was present preoperatively, pulmonary vascular disease is likely to persist. An excellent result may be defined as secure closure of the defect, a symptom-free life and a pulmonary artery pressure at or near normal levels; if this is to be obtained, operation should be carried out at not later than 2–4 years of age and in many cases before 2 years. Late complications include a residual or recurrent VSD,

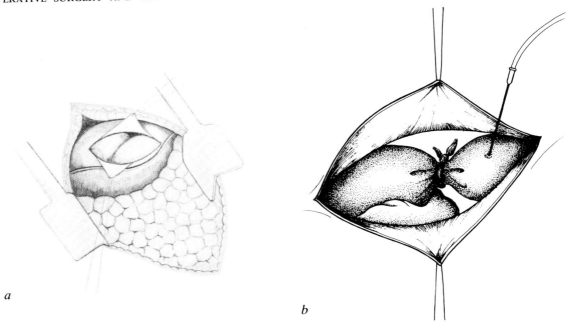

a

b

Figure 40.16 Ventricular septal defect: palliation by banding the pulmonary artery. *a*, The pericardium has been opened in front of the left phrenic nerve, exposing the left atrial appendage and the pulmonary artery. *b*, The pulmonary artery is constricted and the pressure is being measured beyond the band

complete heart block, persistence of important pulmonary vascular disease and bacterial endocarditis.

Operative technique for palliative surgery: pulmonary artery banding

This procedure is carried out through a left lateral thoracotomy at the upper border of the 4th rib. The pericardium is opened in front of the phrenic nerve and the great vessels are identified (Figure 40.16a). A right-angled dissecting instrument may be placed in the transverse sinus behind the pulmonary artery and passed forwards in a plane already established deep to the aortic sheath: 3 mm nylon tape is used to constrict the artery. Particular care is required when there is also transposition of the great arteries, as the coronary arteries arise higher than usual and are very close to the level of the band. Two methods may be used to secure the constricting band to the correct degree of tightness. Mustard and his colleagues have derived a formula relating the circumference of the band to the baby's weight; this rather arbitrary approach worked well in their hands but has not been widely applied. More commonly the band is progressively tightened until the pulmonary artery pressure beyond the constriction is reduced to 30 or 40 mmHg. If the arterial pressure, heart rate and systemic oxygenation remain stable and satisfactory, then the band should be secured; if not, it must be loosened and secured at the tightest level consistent with stable haemodynamics and acceptable oxygenation (Figure 40.16b).

The band itself must be secured to the pulmonary artery with at least three interrupted sutures to prevent its distal migration to the bifurcation, which would cause catastrophic obstruction to pulmonary blood flow. The pericardium is closed with interrupted sutures.

RESULTS

The mortality in children over 6 months with a simple VSD is substantially less than 5%, but in more complex conditions or infants under 6 months it rises to 10% or more. Ideally the band will control the haemodynamic state until the child is ready for total correction, which will include reconstruction of the pulmonary artery. Occasionally the VSD will close spontaneously, when reconstruction of the pulmonary artery alone will be required. Alternatively the constriction may be inadequate, in which case earlier intervention will be needed. Reconstruction of the pulmonary artery is most effectively done by excision of the constricted segment and end-to-end anastomoses.

Fallot's tetralogy

Physiology and natural history

Fallot's tetralogy is the most common cyanotic cardiac anomaly, accounting for 12% of the total. Classically it is described as having four abnormal features: a ventricular septal defect, pulmonary stenosis, the aorta straddles the ventricular septum, and right ventricular hypertrophy.

The abnormal circulation is determined by the VSD and pulmonary stenosis. In the face of severe stenosis the right ventricle ejects part of each stroke volume to the lungs and part through the VSD to the aorta. Thus the pulmonary blood flow is reduced and that small volume of oxygenated blood is mixed with the desaturated blood passing through the VSD resulting in arterial desaturation and cyanosis. When the myocardium contracts with greater velocity, the infundibular component of the pulmonary stenosis will be more severe, causing an acute episode of even more severe hypoxia.

Life may be threatened by hypoxia in infancy or early childhood in a substantial proportion of cases.

The remainder divide into two groups: the majority, whose condition deteriorates steadily leading to death in the teenage years, and a small minority with milder forms of the anomaly, who survive into adult life. In addition to hypoxia these children suffer from polycythaemia, cerebral thromboses and abscesses.

Anatomy and classification

The VSD is usually perimembranous in position and large, approximating to the size of the aortic valve annulus. The pulmonary stenosis is complex and is the key to the surgery of this anomaly. Invariably there is severe infundibular obstruction due to hypertrophy, thickening and fusion of the muscle bands in this area. This aspect of the obstruction is progressive, although the infundibulum is also structurally hypoplastic from birth. At valvar level there is commonly, but not always, obstruction due to fusion or thickening of the cusps. The annulus of the valve is nearly always hypoplastic, often less than half the size of the aortic annulus, and contributes importantly to the obstruction. Finally, a discrete supravalvar obstruction may occur as a stenosis of the main, right or left pulmonary arteries. The main pulmonary artery is frequently small, its size being related to the size of the valve ring. Anomalies of coronary arteries are reported in as many as 9% of cases and are of surgical importance if the anomalous vessel crosses the right ventricular outflow tract.

Diagnosis and indications for operation

Although the diagnosis may be made by ultrasound and Doppler imaging, cardiac catheterization will normally be carried out, demonstrating both the anatomy of the VSD and right ventricular outflow tract in addition to the detailed anatomy of the main right and left pulmonary arteries. Surgery is required when hypoxia is severe, whether episodic in early life or more progressive later.

Operative surgery

The history of the surgery of this condition virtually encompasses the history of cardiac surgery. Prior to cardiopulmonary bypass Blalock and Taussig realized that the life-threatening hypoxia could be relieved by increasing pulmonary blood flow. In 1945 they introduced the systemic-to-pulmonary artery shunt using the subclavian artery – the first palliative operation. In 1962 Waterston described the ascending aorta to right pulmonary artery anastomosis as an alternative in infancy to the Blalock–Taussig shunt which was technically difficult and often thrombosed in that age group. This operation has been widely used with good early palliation, but recently it has been shown to cause severe deformation of the right pulmonary artery due to kinking at the anastomosis. This results in unilateral perfusion of the right lung through the shunt and severe technical problems at eventual total correction. Brock sought to palliate this condition by increasing pulmonary blood flow by relieving the pulmonary stenosis. His technique was a closed procedure using a dilator, bougies and a punch to resect infundibular muscle. In his hands excellent results were achieved, but most surgeons found it a difficult and dangerous operation.

The two-stage philosophy of palliation and later correction for Fallot's tetralogy has been questioned by those who advance the policy of primary correction in those infants in whom surgical intervention is necessary. There is a strong tendency to correct Fallot's tetralogy at an earlier and earlier age and many surgeons report excellent results with correction in infancy. It is increasingly rare for palliation to be carried out beyond the first year of life unless there are specific anatomical reasons for doing so.

Operative technique for total correction

When cardiopulmonary bypass is begun, any systemic-to-pulmonary artery shunt is ligated or divided. A patent foramen ovale is closed or excluded through a small incision in the right atrium. The site for right ventriculotomy is selected and a vertical incision is made avoiding the coronary arteries, and their important branches (Figure 40.17a). The intraventricular anatomy is carefully inspected and the abnormal muscle bands of the outflow tract are identified and divided or, where appropriate, muscle is excised (Figure 40.17b). Care must be taken to avoid perforation of the free wall of the right ventricle or the interventricular septum, or damage to the papillary muscles of the tricuspid valve or to the aortic valve. Once adequate infundibular resection has been completed the VSD may be seen and repaired in the manner described elsewhere (Figure 40.18). The pulmonary valve may be inspected from below, or if necessary from above, using a separate pulmonary arteriotomy. Commissurotomy or excision of thick cusps should be performed.

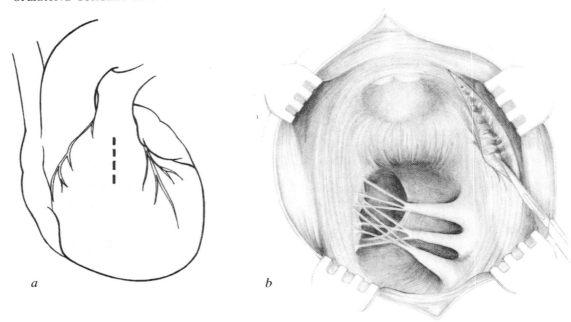

Figure 40.17 Fallot's tetralogy. *a*, Site of vertical incision in right ventricle. *b*, Infundibular resection. Through an incision in the right ventricle, there may be seen the pulmonary valve, the hypertrophied infundibular muscle and crista supraventricularis and the VSD. Resection of infundibular muscle is being carried out

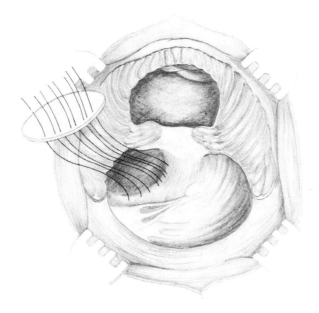

Figure 40.18 Fallot's tetralogy: patch closure of ventricular septal defect. Extensive infundibular resection has been completed. The septal defect is being closed using a patch, as previously described

The next stage of the correction remains the most difficult. There may be important residual pulmonary stenosis due to hypoplasia of the infundibulum and the valve ring. In the past if the surgeon did not expect this to be a problem then the right ventricle was closed, usually with a small outflow tract patch,

bypass withdrawn and the pressures measured in the right and left ventricles. If the right ventricular pressure exceeded 0.65–0.70 of the left ventricular pressure in the absence of a high pulmonary vascular resistance, and the right exceeded the left atrial pressure, then important residual pulmonary stenosis was said to be demonstrated and reconstruction of the right ventricular outflow tract and pulmonary artery with a transannular patch was needed.

Today, a more precise indicator of the need for this additional procedure is the size of the pulmonary annulus, as measured with bougies before closing the right ventricle. Kirklin has published tables relating annulus size to age or surface area and which indicate the probability of needing further measures to relieve pulmonary stenosis. If these are not needed the ventriculotomy is closed incorporating a small Dacron gusset simply as a technique to avoid further restriction of the outflow tract. If the annulus size indicates that further measures are needed, then reconstruction of the right ventricular outflow tract is carried out by extending the vertical incision across the pulmonary valve ring into the main pulmonary artery as far as the bifurcation (Figure 40.19). A large gusset of Dacron or pericardium is sutured into this defect to enlarge the outflow tract, the pulmonary annulus and the pulmonary artery. The pulmonary incompetence resulting from this is believed to be well tolerated in the long term.

RESULTS

The operative mortality for total correction in childhood is below 10% in most centres and in some reports has been below 5%. The most common mode of operative death is low cardiac output. Late mortality is low and a great majority of patients display excellent physical and educational development and capabilities.

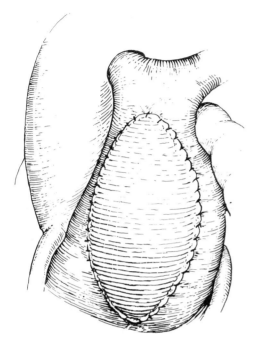

Figure 40.19 Fallot's tetralogy: reconstruction of right ventricular outflow tract. The vertical incision in the right ventricle has been extended across the annulus of the pulmonary valve, and into the pulmonary artery. The outflow pathway from the right ventricle is enlarged by closing the defect with a patch or gusset

Operative techniques for palliative surgery

1. BLALOCK–TAUSSIG SHUNT

This, the first palliative operation, remains the most important and widely used for patients aged 1–2 years or less with severe continuing or episodic cyanosis due to Fallot's tetralogy. If it is not the policy of the unit to carry out total correction at this stage, or if the individual patient is judged not to be suitable for correction, then a Blalock–Taussig shunt should be performed. The subclavian artery is selected on the side of the innominate artery. (It is most important not to insert an arterial pressure monitoring cannula in the distribution of the artery to be divided.) The chest is opened at the upper border of the 4th or 5th rib and the lungs retracted gently downwards. The pulmonary artery is identified and freed as far proximally as possible, and distally beyond the origin of the first upper lobe branch. On the right it may be necessary to divide the azygos vein. The subclavian artery is dissected carefully from its origin to beyond its first branches where it will be divided. On the right

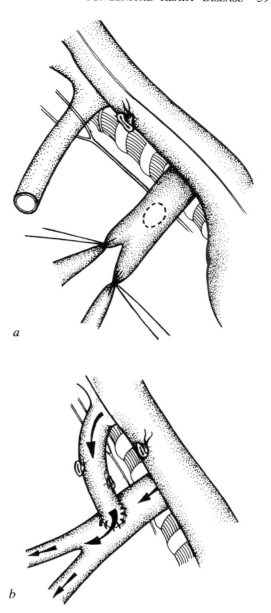

Figure 40.20 Fallot's tetralogy: palliation with right Blalock–Taussig shunt. *a*, The right subclavian artery is divided and its relationship to the vagus nerve and its recurrent laryngeal branch is shown. The right pulmonary artery is controlled distally by snares and the site of arteriotomy for the anastomosis is shown. *b*, The subclavian artery is withdrawn through the loop formed by the vagus nerve and its branch, and is anastomosed to the pulmonary artery

it should be freed from, and withdrawn through, the loop formed by the vagus nerve and its recurrent laryngeal branch, permitting its origin to be fully mobilized (Figure 40.20a). The mediastinal tissues may carefully be dissected and divided to form a bed for the artery as it passes to the pulmonary artery which is now clamped proximally and snared distally. A longitudinal arteriotomy may be made and the anastomosis should be constructed with interrupted sutures for at least half its circumference using 6/0 prolene (Figure 40.20b). When the clamps are released a thrill will be a palpable over the anastomosis. If it is necessary to use the subclavian artery arising directly from the aorta, the danger of kinking at its origin may be avoided by using a plastic technique described by Castaneda.

The modified Blalock–Taussig operation is a subclavian artery-to-pulmonary artery shunt using a 5 mm diameter Goretex graft. The subclavian artery remains in continuity and the graft is anastomosed end to side to each artery. In addition to the obvious advantage of maintaining the integrity of the subclavian artery, there is a high incidence of graft patency even in neonates, and therefore many regard this method as the technique of choice. The approach to the right and left Blalock–Taussig shunts (whether classic or modified) at the time of total correction is shown in Figure 40.21.

2. WATERSTON SHUNT

This operation is used rarely outside the neonatal period or early infancy. A right thoracotomy is performed and the pulmonary artery dissected as for a Blalock–Taussig shunt, taking care to preserve the phrenic nerve. The superior vena cava is mobilized, retracted forwards and the pericardium entered. The right convex border of the ascending aorta is seen and preparations are made to perform a side-to-side anastomosis between the posterior part of the ascending aorta and the anterior part of the right pulmonary artery, in such a way that the pulmonary artery is not deformed. A side-biting clamp is applied to isolate a segment of the aorta and cross-clamp the pulmonary artery in one bite. Corresponding incisions are made in the aorta and in the pulmonary artery so that the communication will not exceed 3 mm in a neonate, or 4 mm in an infant, and the anastomosis constructed with continuous runs of 6/0 prolene (Figure 40.22).

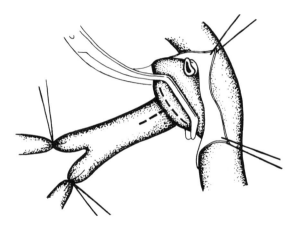

Figure 40.22 Fallot's tetralogy: palliation with Waterston's shunt. The pericardium is opened, exposing the ascending aorta. Both the ascending aorta and right pulmonary artery are controlled by a side-biting clamp, while the distal pulmonary artery is controlled by snares. The sites of incision in the aorta and the right pulmonary artery are shown

Results

The mortality of palliative surgery beyond 6 months of age is little more than 2%. Below that age it may be 10–15%. With the Blalock–Taussig operation, an inadequate or thrombosed shunt may occur, while excessive flow causing left ventricular failure is rare. With the Waterston shunt, excess flow is common and its most important late complication is deformity, possibly with obstruction, of the right pulmonary artery.

Transposition of the great arteries

Physiology and natural history

Although only accounting for 5% of all congenital

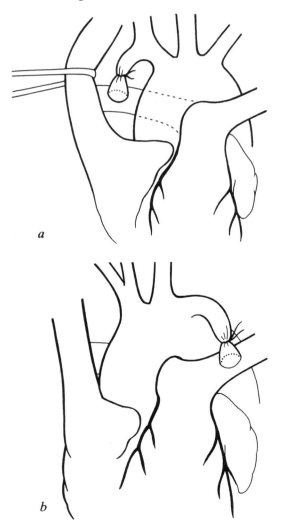

Figure 40.21 Fallot's tetralogy: ligation of Blalock–Taussig shunt at operation for total correction. Right-sided (*a*) and left-sided (*b*) anastomosis

cardiac anomalies, transposition of the great arteries is the most common condition presenting with cyanosis at birth. In transposition, the aorta arises anteriorly from the right ventricle and the pulmonary artery posteriorly from the left ventricle. Thus there are two circulations in parallel – while the systemic circulation is desaturated the pulmonary is fully saturated and survival can only occur because limited mixing occurs across an ASD. Untreated, 80–90% of babies born with this condition will not survive until their first birthday, death being chiefly due to hypoxia.

Anatomy and classification

An ASD alone is present in 70% of cases and in the remaining 30% an ASD, or VSD and pulmonary stenosis are found. Rarely, more complex associations of anomalies are present.

Diagnosis and indications for operation

A firm diagnosis in the neonatal period may be made by ultrasound and Doppler imaging which will also permit associated abnormalities to be identified. If the ASD could be enlarged, permitting increased mixing and improved systemic oxygenation, then the immediate threat to life would be averted. Attempts to achieve this by operative means carried a high mortality and have been superseded by the balloon atrial septostomy devised by Rashkind, which may now be carried out under ultrasound control and is virtually free of hazard. This procedure permits survival to the second year of life in the great majority of babies. For definitive surgery the choice must now be made as to whether this should be done by atrial redirection of venous return, which would normally be performed between 6 and 12 months of age, or by anatomical correction or switching of the great arteries which would need to be carried out in the first few weeks of life.

Operative surgery

Blalock and Hanlon described the technique of closed operative atrial septostomy in 1960. Although it carried a high mortality it remained the only palliation for this condition, until Rashkind introduced his balloon septostomy in 1966. It is now only rarely used, as many surgeons will proceed to an open corrective operation if the balloon atrial septostomy fails.

When surgeons first addressed the problem of 'correction' of simple transposition of the great arteries it was believed that 'anatomical correction' by switching the great arteries would be technically impossible due to the proximal origin of the coronary arteries. Therefore the alternative concept of redirecting flow at atrial level was formulated; pulmonary venous blood is directed to the tricuspid valve, the right

ventricle and aorta, and systemic venous blood to the mitral valve, the left ventricle and the pulmonary artery. In the late 1950s and the 1960s various techniques to achieve this goal were described, the most notable being that of Senning which used the patient's own atrial tissue and that of Mustard using autologous pericardium or Dacron as the new interatrial septum or 'baffle'. Following Mustard's description of his operation in 1964 it gained popularity and was increasingly widely applied in the early 1970s when intracardiac surgery in infants became more safe. Quaegebeur et al. (1977) described a modified Senning operation which remains widely practised. Thus definitive surgery for transposition of the great arteries based on atrial redirection of venous return uses either the Mustard or the modified Senning technique both of which achieve physiological but not anatomical correction.

In 1968, Rastelli devised an ingenious approach to anatomical correction for children with transposition of the great arteries, a ventricular septal defect and pulmonary stenosis. He suggested that the ventricular septal defect should be closed in such a way that the left ventricle drained through it to the aorta, the pulmonary valve being closed off. The right ventricle was then connected to the pulmonary artery by an external valved conduit and the atrial septal defect closed.

In 1975, Jatene performed the first successful anatomical correction of transposition of the great arteries by arterial switch, with reimplantation of the coronary arteries into the new aorta (Jatene et al., 1976). Figure 40.26 (page 602) shows one method of performing this operation, which may only be done when the left ventricular pressure is high, indicating that the left ventricle will be able to support the systemic circulation immediately after the operation. Thus the operation has a role in the correction of transposition of the great arteries combined with VSD, but has also been shown to be capable of being safely and effectively carried out in the neonatal period. This is the second option for definitive treatment of simple transposition in the neonatal period.

Operative technique for definitive surgery

1. THE MUSTARD OPERATION

The new interatrial septum or baffle may be made from autologous pericardium or Dacron and is carefully prepared to the shape preferred by the surgeon – rectangular, dumbell shaped or trouser shaped. It is convenient to cannulate the superior vena cava directly and the inferior vena cava as close to the inferior caval atrial junction as possible. After opening the right atrium its anatomy is carefully inspected and the remains of the intra-atrial septum excised (Figure 40.23). The baffle is inserted using a 5/0 prolene continuous suture. One edge is sutured around the pulmonary veins with a U-shaped suture

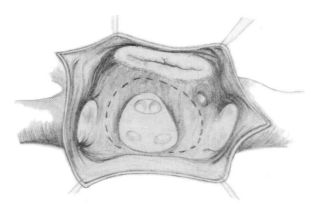

Figure 40.23 Transposition of the great arteries: the Mustard operation. The left atrium and pulmonary veins may be seen through the ASD. The dotted line indicates the line of resection of the atrial septum

line which is open towards the right. The other edge is sutured to the remnant of the atrial septum and continued in either direction around the caval orifices (Figure 40.24) to meet the first suture line. Thus systemic venous blood will flow deep to the baffle (as the surgeon sees it) to the mitral valve, while pulmonary venous blood will flow forward over the baffle to the tricuspid valve.

2. THE SENNING OPERATION

This operation is most easily performed using a single venous cannula, profound hypothermia and circulatory arrest. The right atrium is opened with a vertical incision 4 mm anterior to the crista terminalis (Figure

40.25a). The atrial septum is mobilized as a flap based on its right lateral attachment (Figure 40.25b); this flap is then attached to the left lateral wall of the left atrium in front of the pulmonary veins and behind the mitral valve, completing the suture line in the roof and floor of the left atrium (Figure 40.25c). The ASD is closed with a patch or by direct suture as appropriate. The exit for pulmonary venous blood is created by opening the left atrium at its junction with the right pulmonary veins (Figure 40.25d); this opening may be enlarged by extending the incision onto a pulmonary vein. The systemic venous pathway is now constructed by using that part of the right atrial wall which lay posterior to the original incision and suturing it to the remnant of the atrial septum and around the caval orifices (Figure 40.25d); thus caval blood passes to the mitral valve. The pulmonary venous pathway is constructed using that part of the right atrial wall which is anterior to the original incision, and its edge is sutured over the superior vena cava and inferior vena cava and around the edge of the incision in the right pulmonary veins, thus allowing pulmonary venous blood to pass forward to the tricuspid valve (Figure 40.25e). When performing the final suture line it is important to avoid damage to the sinuatrial node and to avoid constricting the suture line which passes over the cavae; the suture line around the pulmonary veins is completed using interrupted sutures.

3. THE ARTERIAL SWITCH OPERATION

The operation is performed with hypothermia and periods of circulatory arrest and/or bypass with the aorta cross-clamped. After extensive dissection of the

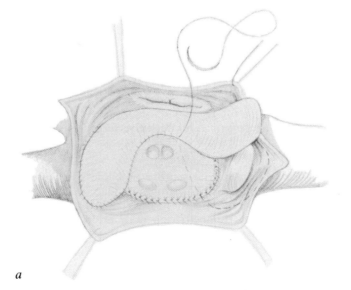

a

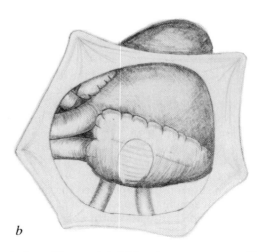

b

Figure 40.24 Transposition of the great arteries: the Mustard operation. *a,* The cut edges of the resected atrial septum are oversewn with interrupted sutures. The new baffle is partly inserted; the SVC pathway is complete and the IVC pathway is being constructed. *b,* The pulmonary venous pathway has been enlarged by making a transverse incision from the atriotomy, backwards between the right pulmonary veins. The defect is closed with a patch or gusset of Dacron or pericardium

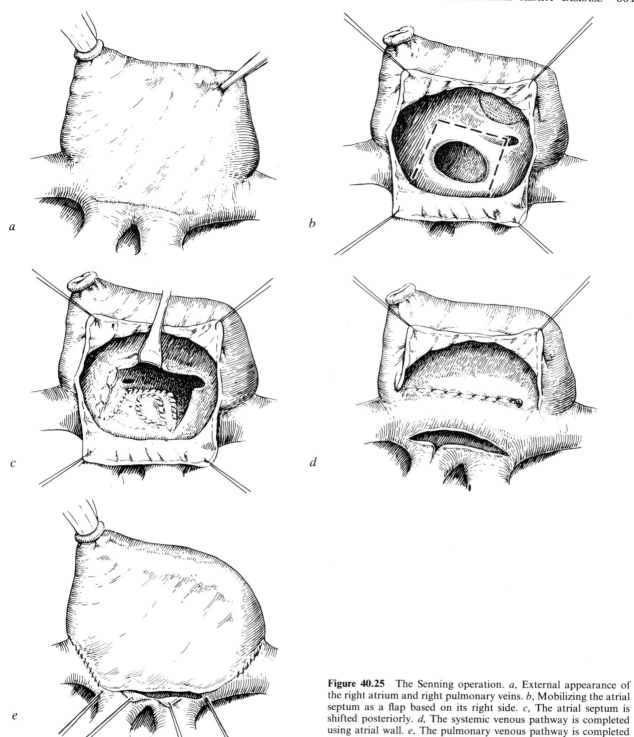

Figure 40.25 The Senning operation. *a*, External appearance of the right atrium and right pulmonary veins. *b*, Mobilizing the atrial septum as a flap based on its right side. *c*, The atrial septum is shifted posteriorly. *d*, The systemic venous pathway is completed using atrial wall. *e*, The pulmonary venous pathway is completed using the anterior part of the right atrial wall

great vessels and division of the ductus arteriosus, the arteries are transected at the same level. The coronary arteries are excised with a generous segment of aortic wall, mobilized and sutured into holes cut in the pulmonary artery sinuses. The distal aorta is now sutured to the proximal pulmonary artery to form the new aorta. The heart may now be perfused. Any intra-cardiac repair is performed at this stage. Finally the new pulmonary artery is constructed using the distal pulmonary artery and the proximal aorta; a patch of pericardium is commonly used on the posterior aspect of the new pulmonary artery (Figure 40.26).

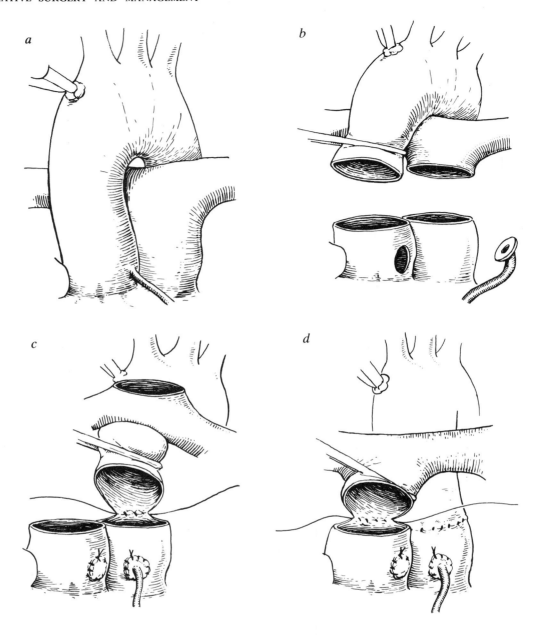

Figure 40.26 The arterial switch operations or anatomical correction for transposition of the great arteries. *a*, The abnormal anatomy with anterior aorta. *b*, Both vessels transected and coronary ostia excised with a cuff of aorta. *c*, Aorta repositioned behind the bifurcation of the pulmonary artery. The coronary arteries are reimplanted into the new aorta, and the original defect closed with a patch. *d*, The nearly finished work

Results

The operative mortality for either of the atrial operations is less than 5% regardless of age. The great majority of children have an excellent result, enjoying normal physical growth and ordinary education. Because it is a physiological and not an anatomical correction it may be regarded as a definitive, not a corrective procedure. It may be for this reason that three possible late complications may occur. First, there may be a high incidence of dysrhythmias, most commonly junctional rhythm, following the extensive atrial incisions and suturing; it is possible that this may lead to late sudden death in a very small number of patients. Secondly, narrowing of the newly constructed pathways may occur, leading to obstruction of the superior vena cava or pulmonary venous pathway; the latter is invariably fatal without further surgery to revise the pathway. Those who use the Senning operation believe that pathway obstruction will be much less common than following the Mustard procedure; much longer follow-up is necessary, however, before this hope can be confirmed. Finally, the fundamental assumption that the right ventricle and tricuspid valve can support systemic pressures indefinitely remains unproved. However, 15–20-year follow-up after the Senning operation indicates that over 90% of those with simple transposition remain free of systemic ventricular failure and it is hoped that currently performed Mustard and Senning operations will yield even better results.

Operative mortality for the arterial switch operation ranges from below 5% to over 20% in different reports. Abnormal rhythms are uncommon and ventricular function is good late after the operation. Much longer follow-up is needed before the late results can be assessed in detail.

Operative techniques for palliative surgery

The Blalock–Hanlon closed operative septectomy is carried out through a right anterolateral thoracotomy and the pericardium entered immediately in front of the phrenic nerve. Snares should be placed on the right pulmonary artery and veins. A side-biting clamp is placed on the septum, including some wall of the right and left atria and the orifices of both right pulmonary veins. Two incisions are made parallel to the septum, one anterior and the other posterior. The septum is grasped and drawn to the right as the side-clamp is partly released. A section of septum is now excised, leaving an interatrial septal defect of substantial size.

RESULTS

This operation is rarely performed now, but the operative mortality was as high as 45% in the late 1960s.

Less common anomalies

Total anomalous pulmonary venous drainage

In this condition the pulmonary veins are usually confluent and drain to the right atrium via the left innominate vein, the coronary sinus or the inferior vena cava, and not to the left atrium. Blood reaches the left side of the heart through an ASD. There may also be obstruction at some point on the pulmonary venous pathway. This condition nearly always threatens life in early infancy and corrective surgery is designed to anastomose the common pulmonary venous chamber to the left atrium. The operative mortality is between 20% and 30%. There are a small number of reports, notably from Mee in Melbourne, indicating that dramatically improved results can be obtained. The late results are encouraging.

Persisting truncus arteriosus

In persisting truncus arteriosus one great vessel only

leaves the heart and a VSD is always present. The pulmonary arteries arise directly from this vessel and, therefore, blood flow to the lungs is high and is at a high pressure. Life is threatened by left ventricular failure and pulmonary vascular disease in infancy. Palliative measures have been disappointing and anatomical correction with a valved conduit from the right ventricle to the pulmonary artery, together with closure of the VSD, is currently the treatment of choice.

Tricuspid atresia

In tricuspid atresia there is no communication from the right atrium to the right ventricle and blood passes to the left atrium through an ASD. If the great vessels are normally related there is usually severe pulmonary oligaemia, as the only sources of pulmonary blood flow are a patent ductus arteriosus and bronchial collaterals. If there is also transposition of the great arteries a large VSD is usual, with high pulmonary flows and pressures, which may lead to heart failure and pulmonary vascular disease. Palliative measures are often required in infancy and are designed either to increase or reduce the pulmonary blood flow, as indicated. The best approach to physiological correction is to perform an operation later in childhood based on the Fontan principle; in this procedure either the right atrium or the cavae are anastomosed directly to the pulmonary artery with minimal use of foreign material. The success of this operation depends on the presence of a very low pulmonary vascular resistance, and in carefully selected patients it can have a relatively low operative mortality and good functional and late outcome.

Ebstein's anomaly

In Ebstein's anomaly there is an abnormal tricuspid valve which is displaced into the right ventricle; the part of the right ventricle which lies between the actual and usual sites of the tricuspid valve is thin walled and aneurysmal; there is usually an ASD. Hypoxia, dysrhythmias and right-sided heart failure may develop during childhood or early adult life. Correction involves repair or replacement of the tricuspid valve, exclusion of the abnormal part of the right ventricle and closure of ASD. The conducting system is at risk. The operative risk is between 10% and 25%.

Atrioventricular septal defect

Atrioventricular septal defect (AVSD) is a composite defect which in its complete form involves both the atrial and ventricular septa, and the mitral and tricuspid valves. The incomplete form has been described in the section 'Atrial septal defects'. The complete form is the most common cardiac abnormality found in children with Down's syndrome, and leads to heart failure, rapid development of pulmonary vascular disease and premature death. Repair is technically complex, involving closure of the ventricular and atrial septal defects with separate patches, and repair of the atrioventricular valves, all the while avoiding the conducting tisue. Postoperative management may be made difficult by labile pulmonary vascular resistance, residual mitral regurgitation and impaired conducting tissue. The operative mortality is 20–25% and it is becoming clear that this high risk can only be reduced significantly by operating earlier, possibly in the first 6 months of life, thereby preventing the development of pulmonary vascular disease and myocardial damage.

Aortic arch abnormalities

In double aortic arch the trachea and oesophagus lie between the right and left arches and are compressed, causing stridor which usually presents in infancy. The diagnosis is based on a barium swallow which shows an indentation due to the abnormal aortic anatomy. Aortography may confirm the precise aortic anatomy and the condition is treated by division of the lesser of the two arches through a left thoracotomy.

In interruption of the aortic arch there is always a VSD and a patent ductus arteriosus which fills the descending aorta. Left ventricular failure presents in infancy and is always life threatening. Palliative approaches have yielded little success and it is now generally accepted that this abnormality should be corrected early in infancy. It is nearly always possible to restore aortic continuity and at the same procedure to close the VSD or other associated abnormality. The best results with this difficult condition have only been achieved when this approach has been used.

References

Barratt-Boyes, B. G., Simpson, M. and Neutze, J. M. (1971) Intracardiac surgery in neonates and infants using deep hypothermia with surface cooling and limited cardiopulmonary bypass. *Circulation*, 43–44, Suppl., 1–25

Jatene, A. D., Fontes, V. F., Pallista, P. P. *et al.* (1976) Anatomic correction of transposition of the great vessels. *J. Thorac. Cardiovasc. Surg.*, **72**, 364–370

Quaegebeur, J. M., Rohmer, J., Brom A. G. *et al.* (1977) Revival of the Senning operation in the treatment of transposition of the great arteries. *Thorax*, **32**, 517–524

Further reading

Blackstone, E. H., Kirklin, J. W., Bradrey, E. L. *et al.* (1976) Optimal age and results in repair of large ventricular septal defects. *J. Thorac. Cardiovasc. Surg.*, **72**, 661–679

Brawn, W. J. and Mee, R. B. B. (1988) Early results for anatomic correction of transposition of the great arteries and for double outlet right ventricle with subpulmonary ventricular septal defect. *J. Thorac. Cardiovasc. Surg.*, **95**, 230–238

Chiariello, L., Agosti, J., Ulad, P. *et al.* (1976) Congenital aortic stenosis. *J. Thorac. Cardiovasc. Surg.*, **72**, 182–193

Danielson, G. K., Exarhos, N. D., Weidman, W. H. *et al.* (1971) Pulmonic stenosis with intact ventricular septum. *J. Thorac. Cardiovasc. Surg.*, **61**, 228–234

Hamilton, D. I., DiEusanio, G., Sandrasagra, F. A. *et al.* (1978) Early and late results of aortoplasty with a left subclavian flap for coarctation of the aorta in infancy. *J. Thorac. Cardiovasc. Surg.*, **75**, 699–704

Kirklin, J. W., Blackstone, E. H., Bargeron, L. M., Jr *et al.* (1986) The repair of atrioventricular septal defects in infancy. *Int. J. Cardiol.*, **13**, 333–351

Kirklin, J. W. and Karp, R. B. (1970) *The Tetralogy of Fallot*, W. B. Saunders, Philadelphia

Lincoln, J. C. R., Deverall, P. B., Stark, J. *et al.* (1969) Vascular anomalies compressing the oesophagus and trachea. *Thorax*, **24**, 295–306

McMullan, M. H., McGoon, D. C., Wallace, R. B. *et al.* (1973) Surgical treatment of partial atrioventricular canal. *Arch. Surg.*, **107**, 705–710

Panagopoulos, P. G., Tatooles, C. J., Aberdeen, E. *et al.* (1971) Patent ductus arteriosus in infants and children. *Thorax*, **26**, 137–144

Stark, J. and deLeval, M. (1983) *Surgery for Congenital Heart Defects*, Grune and Stratton, London

Stark, J., deLeval, M. R., Waterston, D. J. *et al.* (1974) Corrective surgery of transposition of the great arteries in the first year of life. *J. Thorac. Cardiovasc. Surg.*, **67**, 673–681

Tawes, R. L., Aberdeen, E., Waterston, D. J. *et al.* (1969) Coarctation of the aorta in infants and children. *Circulation*, **39–40**, Suppl. 1, 1–173 to 1–184

Turina, M. I., Siebenmann, R., Segesser, L. *et al.* (1989) Late functional deterioration after atrial correction for transposition of the great arteries. *Circulation*, **80**, Suppl. 1, 1–162 to 1–167

41

Acquired heart disease

G. Keen

Surgery of the pericardium

Pericardial aspiration

Aspiration of the pericardium is required for either diagnostic purposes, when a small amount of fluid is removed for examination, or for the relief of large pericardial effusions which may be causing circulatory embarrassment or pericardial tamponade. These effusions may be pus or blood, or may be inflammatory or transudatory effusions.

Pericardial aspiration should not be undertaken lightly, for patients requiring this are usually very ill, and cardiac arrest may be precipitated even by experienced operators. This procedure should be carried out under sterile conditions and adjacent to facilities for immediate resuscitation and exploratory thoracotomy. This last remark applies particularly to patients undergoing pericardial aspiration for the relief of pericardial tamponade caused by stabbing, for these dangerously ill patients readily undergo cardiac arrest during this procedure.

injected down to the pericardium. The patient is monitored with electrocardiography during this procedure and this is watched very carefully for evidence of arrhythmias. Some advocate that the aspiration needle be used as an exploring electrode, contact with the heart producing an altered electrical complex, although the value of this refinement is doubtful. The aspiration needle should be strong, and at least 12 cm in length, attached to a three-way tap and a 20 ml syringe. A plastic cannula is an alternative. From the site of insertion into the skin it is passed upwards and backwards at an angle of 45° to a point midway between the patient's shoulder blades (Figure 41.2). While being inserted, continuous negative suction is applied at the syringe, and when pericardial fluid is withdrawn further insertion is terminated. The scratchy sensation of the heart moving against the end of the needle is unforgettable and when this is felt the needle must be withdrawn a little.

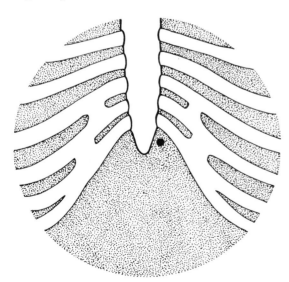

Figure 41.1 Site for pericardial aspiration

The patient is sat up at an angle of 45°. The site of insertion of the needle is between the left border of the xiphisternum and the right border of the 6th left costal cartilage (Figure 41.1). A local anaesthetic is introduced into the subcutaneous tissues and skin and

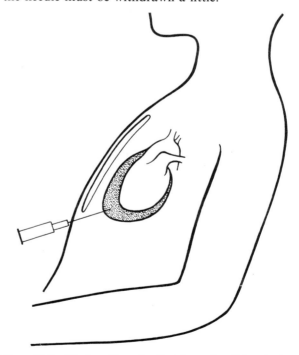

Figure 41.2. Ideal position of patient for pericardial aspiration

Treatment of chronic pericardial effusions

Such effusions may be inflammatory or malignant or may occur as an event during renal failure. Although repeated pericardiocentesis may provide temporary relief from the effusion, it is justified in some circumstances to advise surgical decompression. This may be achieved by removal of a large pericardial window. The pericardium is approached by anterior left thoracotomy through the 5th intercostal space. As large a portion as possible of pericardium anterior to the phrenic nerve is then excised, taking care to ensure haemostasis at the cut edges, which may, in inflammatory situations, be exceedingly vascular. It is, however, preferable to resect the pericardium as completely as is possible in these patients, for this is a more definitive procedure than the creation of a simple window and it is more likely to have long-term benefits for the patient.

Chronic constrictive pericarditis

Constrictive pericarditis is the terminal stage of a chronic inflammatory process which produces a fibrous, thickened and often calcified restrictive coat around the heart. This constricting layer prevents diastolic relaxation of the heart which in turn gives rise to the physical signs and symptoms of constrictive pericarditis. The cause of this condition was at one time considered to be tuberculous but more frequently it is the end result of a pyogenic or viral infection, of previous trauma, or it may be a rare late complication of haemorrhagic pericarditis. The diagnosis is made clinically, radiologically and at cardiac catheterization. Rheumatoid arthritis may be complicated by pericarditis and constriction.

Surgical treatment

The aim of surgery is to remove as completely as possible the fibrous layer and both serous layers of the pericardium. Although the thickened and calcified layer may envelop the entire heart, the deleterious effect of constrictive pericarditis is largely on ventricular relaxation. The object of surgery is to release both ventricles and as a secondary procedure to turn attention to removal of the pericardium covering the atria. The pericardium over the atria, although part of the process, rarely obstructs emptying of the atria, although some cases have been reported in which constricting bands are said to have caused narrowing at the atrioventricular ring. Again, some patients have been shown to have constricting rings of pericardium around the superior and inferior vena caval entrances into the heart, which may require attention.

Surgical approach (see Chapters 50 and 58)

The approach for the removal of the constricted and adherent pericardium may be either median sternotomy, left thoracotomy or bilateral anterior thoracotomy. Median sternotomy has the advantage that the right atrium and ventricle and the venae cavae may be safely cleared of pericardium together with the lateral aspect of the left ventricle and the inferior surface of the heart. Nevertheless, using this exposure it is frequently extremely difficult and sometimes dangerous to gain good access to the posterior aspect of the left ventricle and of the left atrioventricular groove. Since it is most important to decompress the left ventricle completely, it is considered by many that extended left thoracotomy is the exposure of choice in this condition. The incision is made through the bed of the 5th left rib. This exposure gives an excellent view of the whole of the lateral and inferior border of the heart and enables safe clearing of the left ventricle, left atrium, inferior surface of the heart and of the right ventricle to be achieved. However, the unilateral left anterior thoracic approach, although adequate for limited decortications, is considered by some to be inadequate for the more radical pericardiectomy preferred by most surgeons. Furthermore, inadequate exposure does not allow complete removal of the pericardium and does not permit the operator to handle effectively any emergency such as major haemorrhage from the right atrium or right ventricle. The extent of pericardial resection can be determined only at operation and poor results can invariably be attributed to insufficient removal of pericardium. Should left thoracotomy be chosen as the approach, and if it is then discovered that further access is required, the incision may be extended across and transecting the sternum, entering the right 4th intercostal space.

The author favours median sternotomy, with the patient in the supine position on the operating table and with the arms by the side. Should left thoracotomy be chosen, the patient should be placed in the supine position but with the arms at right angles to the side and supported by appropriate operating table fittings. The incision will then extend from the left midaxillar line to the left border of the sternum and enter the 4th intercostal space following subperiosteal stripping of the upper border of the 5th rib. Should further access be necessary, the sternum is transected with a Gigli saw, the internal mammary vessels on either side of the sternum are doubly ligated and divided and the incision then extended into the right 4th intercostal space. Median sternotomy gives the patient a far more comfortable postoperative course than does bilateral thoracotomy. It is clear that there is no ideal operative approach for this condition.

When the surgical field is exposed, it is important to select a portion of the pericardium, to begin the dissection, which is less tightly attached to the underlying heart. The important hazards of this operation are damage to the coronary arteries and the opening of a cardiac chamber. Although the heart can be repaired, perhaps with difficulty, damage to a major coronary artery is extremely serious. With the development of a plane of cleavage, scissors, knife and blunt dissection will gradually extend the dissection away from the incision. Dissection proceeds initially over the left ventricle, and after the development of a long incision in the enveloping pericardium which is

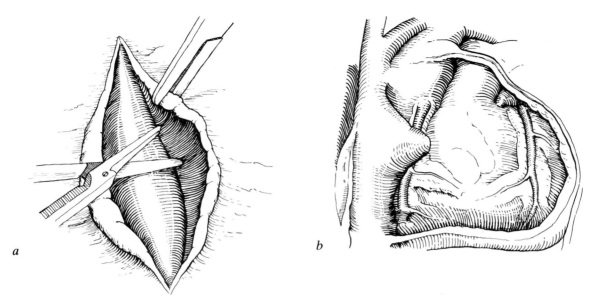

Figure 41.3 Constrictive pericarditis. Blunt dissection of the pericardium from the right and left ventricles

then undermined (Figure 41.3a), the ventricle bulges out in an unrestrained fashion, allowing immediate improvement in the patient's cardiac output. The thickened pericardium may contain layers of organizing and crumbling purulent contents, and in many instances the pericardium is heavily calcified and up to 1 cm thick. The use of bone shears is frequently necessary to complete the procedure. As much pericardium as possible is cleared from the left ventricle, followed by the right ventricle, the left atrioventricular groove and the right atrium. Should an opening into or even through the myocardium occur, it is controlled by sutures supported by Teflon felt pledgets. Should the atria be opened prior to release of the ventricles, the persistent high intra-atrial pressures will precipitate serious bleeding, difficult to control other than by a swab applied and held in place until ventricular release of the pericardial constriction allows some fall in venous pressure. Care is taken to avoid damage to the phrenic nerves, which may be difficult to identify in the inflammatory process.

The base of the heart is cleared backwards across the diaphragm for as far as it is accessible. Following removal of the thickened pericardial layer, the surface of the myocardium should be carefully examined, for there may be a considerable amount of thickened, semi-opaque serous membrane which remains to constrict the action of the heart, and this membrane must then be attended to. The myocardium is more readily seen through this membrane and a point is chosen, where no coronary vessels are seen, to begin the dissection. With patient gauze and knife dissection this layer may eventually be removed piecemeal, completing relief of the condition. Following pericardiectomy, there will be considerable oozing from the

denuded myocardial surface but this readily ceases with prolonged gauze pressure (Figure 41.3b).

The use of cardiopulmonary bypass during pericardiectomy has some advocates. This undoubtedly complicates an otherwise usually straightforward procedure, and the heparinization required will increase the operative and postoperative haemorrhage. At the present time the majority of surgeons prefer to undertake this operation without the assistance of cardiopulmonary bypass.

Acquired disease of the mitral valve

Mitral stenosis

Assessment

It is remarkable that the symptoms frequently bear little relation to the degree of mitral stenosis. Some patients with extremely severe stenosis may continue to work almost entirely without symptoms, whereas others with moderate stenosis may be extremely dyspnoeic on effort. Although in many patients the physical signs and symptoms may correlate with the degree of severity, other more objective methods of assessing mitral stenosis are required.

The most important of these are the mitral valve gradient and the pulmonary wedge or left atrial pressure measured at cardiac catheterization, both at rest and on exercise. At this investigation measurement of the pulmonary vascular resistance and an assessment of the tricuspid valve and of the aortic valve are also important. Echocardiography is routinely conducted to ensure that the patient's symptoms are not due to an atrial myxoma, and will offer reliable evidence of the degree of stenosis, the rigidity and thickness of the valve cusps and of the presence of calcification, and at the same time full echocardiographic assessment of other valves and of ventricular function can be undertaken. Unfortunately, intra-atrial thrombi are not readily detectable using echocardiography, although myxomas are readily diagnosed by this means. Left ventricular cine-angiocardiography ensures the detection of mitral regurgitation. In those with few or no symptoms, but in whom very high left atrial pressures are recorded, operation should be advised despite apparent well-being, for they may develop serious or fatal pulmonary oedema in response to stress, exercise, pregnancy or on alteration from sinus rhythm to atrial fibrillation.

Treatment

Following the earliest successful closed mitral valvotomy undertaken by Souttar in 1925, the operation was largely abandoned until 1949, when Bailey, Harken and Brock demonstrated independently the value of closed digital commissurotomy (Harken et al., 1948; Bailey, 1949; Baker et al., 1950). This operation has since been undertaken successfully in hundreds of thousands of patients with rheumatic mitral stenosis. Modifications of the technique of valvotomy, such as the use of small intracardiac knives and later the introduction of mechanical dilators, produced a more successful mitral commissurotomy, developing the standard operation for the next 25 years. With the development of open heart surgery and the current extremely low risk associated with its use, it seems clear that open commissurotomy using cardiopulmonary bypass has in most cardiac surgical centres emerged as the operation of choice and has superseded closed valvotomy almost entirely. This seems surprising when one considers the long-term relief from symptoms obtained by countless patients who have undergone closed mitral valvotomy in the past. Many long series of patients treated by closed valvotomy have been studied and these demonstrate that a large proportion are free of, or are greatly relieved of, symptoms for as long as 25 years, and that when further operation is required the subsequent open valvotomy or open mitral valve replacement is done with comparative ease and safety.

There is no doubt that in the past many patients were submitted to closed mitral commissurotomy when the valve was clearly unsuitable for this operation due to calcification, mitral regurgitation or extreme rigidity. In the presence of a rigid valve, even a full-length commissurotomy will not result in reduction of left atrial pressure, for a high left atrial pressure is required to open the rigid cusps. Nevertheless, with careful clinical examination, cardiac catheterization and angiocardiography, together with echocardiography, it should be possible to separate those whose purely stenotic, mobile and fibrous valves will be suitable for closed valvotomy from those whose rigid or calcified valves will require replacement using cardiopulmonary bypass. There is, however, the important risk of intraoperative embolism to be considered, for in many patients with chronic rheumatic heart disease and atrial fibrillation, intra-atrial thrombosis and the organization of these clots within the atrial appendage commonly occur. There is no doubt that the risk of intraoperative dislodgement of such thrombi is greater during closed surgery than it is during open heart surgery. It is unfortunately the case that there are younger patients, in sinus rhythm, who may harbour thrombi within the atrial appendage which may be dislodged during closed valvotomy.

Having excluded those with a rigid or calcified valve, those with associated important aortic or tricuspid valve disease, and others in whom intra-atrial thrombosis is likely, there remain a considerable number of patients with pure stenosis of a fibrous, mobile valve who are suitable for closed valvotomy. It is this group of patients in whom there is a predictably extremely low operative mortality and low morbidity and in whom relief of symptoms will be extremely prolonged, in many cases for 10–15 years. One danger of open commissurotomy is that inspection of the valve may persuade the surgeon that the valve is unworthy of salvage and it may consequently be removed and replaced by a prosthetic valve, perhaps unnecessarily. There seems little doubt that very many valves which have been successfully opened by closed procedures would, if viewed at open heart surgery, have been removed and replaced by a prosthetic valve, due to their unpromising appearance.

Nevertheless, the assessment of patients for closed mitral valvotomy and the undertaking of this operation are becoming less frequent each year and it is likely that future generations of cardiac surgeons will be unfamiliar with this procedure and resort universally to open operations on the mitral valve under all circumstances and will consider closed mitral valvotomy to be obsolete. Open valvotomy offers certain advantages over closed valvotomy. There is little doubt that closed valvotomy will not relieve the obstruction caused by fusion of the subvalvar mechanism and it is in this group of patients, perhaps 20% of those with mitral stenosis, that open valvotomy is so successful. Under vision, separation of the chordae tendineae which are fused to the underlying papillary muscles, debridement of calcium and selected annuloplasty are now possible. At the present time, therefore, it is fair to say that the previously widely undertaken operation of closed mitral valvotomy is rapidly giving way to open valvotomy. It is necessary to appreciate that the majority of patients with rheumatic mitral stenosis live in developing countries, and there is little doubt that closed valvotomy will be the operation of choice in those regions for very many years to come. It is inevitable that open heart surgery will not be universally available in poor countries for at least another generation.

Mitral valvotomy in pregnancy

From time to time, a previously asymptomatic patient develops pulmonary oedema in the last trimester of pregnancy, and mitral stenosis is shown to be responsible. There is little dispute that for reasons of safety, for both the mother and the unborn child, closed mitral valvotomy is the operation of choice, although closed balloon valvotomy may be successful here.

Closed mitral valvotomy

With improved selection of patients, the great majority of closed mitral valvotomies are carried out without complication. Nevertheless, there is the occasional patient prepared for closed valvotomy who is found at operation to be unsuitable, due to excessive valve calcification, intra-atrial thrombosis or the presence of previously undetected mitral regurgitation, or unsuspected atrial myxoma. Rarely, there may be an accident at the time of closed surgery, producing a serious tear of the left atrial wall or overwhelming mitral regurgitation. For these reasons, it is an advantage to have immediate pump stand-by so that the operation can be converted from a closed procedure to cardiopulmonary bypass without delay.

PREOPERATIVE PREPARATION

It is safe to discontinue digoxin 24 h prior to surgery, for many patients on this drug tend otherwise to experience significant postoperative bradycardia with consequent problems of management. Should the patient be in severe heart failure, it may be necessary to continue diuretic therapy up to the time of operation.

It is generally agreed that all patients with atrial fibrillation who are to be submitted to mitral valvotomy should be adequately treated by an anticoagulant such as warfarin for some months prior to surgery. This will frequently prevent further deposition of left atrial thrombus and enable soft thrombus, which is already within the atrial appendage and the atrium, to organize and adhere to the left atrial wall. Unfortunately, despite therapeutically maintained levels of anticoagulant therapy, there have been frequent instances of cerebral or peripheral embolism occurring during mitral valvotomy, and it is the unpredictability of this complication that prompts surgeons away from closed valvotomy and to consider open mitral valvotomy using cardiopulmonary bypass to be the lesser risk. It is wise to maintain therapeutic levels of warfarin through the operation and to continue indefinitely postoperatively, for if anticoagulant therapy is discontinued several days prior to surgery in order to diminish operative bleeding, further thrombi might form

within the left atrial appendage with possible disastrous results.

THE OPERATION

The patient is placed on the operating table lying on the right side, rotated backwards at about 30°. The incision is a left anterolateral thoracotomy extending from 5 cm from the midline, passing underneath the left breast and extending just distal to and below the angle of the left scapula. The chest is opened through the 5th left intercostal space. The pericardium is opened vertically posterior to the phrenic nerve and this incision extends from the diaphragm up to the pulmonary artery. Stay sutures are inserted into the edges of the pericardium to expose the left side of the heart and the pulmonary veins.

It is useful to measure the left atrial pressure and the pulmonary artery pressure at operation and to record these before and following valvotomy.

It is necessary that the left atrial appendage is handled as little as possible during the preliminary manoeuvres, for it is within this part of the left atrial chamber that soft, mobile thrombus may be loosely adherent. It is usual to place a purse-string of 000 prolene at the base of the appendage to aid control of the operation and finally to obliterate the appendage when it is tied. When this purse-string suture is inserted, care should be taken that only the epicardium is picked up with the needle, for penetration of the atrium at this stage may cause severe bleeding should the left atrial pressure be very high, which is usually the case. A plastic tube is slid on to the purse-string to act as a snare. The tip of the appendage is gently grasped with forceps and is opened with scissors. The appendage is then lightly grasped with the finger and thumb and forceps are placed on the edge of this incision, allowing the escape of 100 ml or so of blood, enabling loose thrombus to be washed out. The right lubricated index finger is then introduced into the left atrial appendage and the left atrium. It may be necessary to tighten the purse-string but usually the finger will fit snugly through the incision and obstruct the left atrial appendage adequately, ensuring that bleeding does not occur.

The finger is then passed to the mitral valve, where the pathology and function are assessed. Should the preoperative assessment prove to be correct, the valve will feel mobile and there will be a tightly stenotic orifice which will not admit the tip of the finger, the edges of the stenosis being fibrous and rolled. The valve should be palpated for calcium, its extent determined, and the atrium just proximal to the valve carefully assessed for mitral regurgitation, which is often difficult. Even in the presence of marked mitral regurgitation a jet may not be palpable, whereas mild regurgitation through a fine jet may readily be noted. If during the introduction of the finger large amounts of thrombus are palpated, it is wise to withdraw, ligate the purse-string and to abandon the closed procedure at this stage. The risk of producing massive systemic or cerebral embolism is so real that the operation should be conducted either at the time or later using cardiopulmonary bypass under safe conditions. Similarly, should more than a trivial amount of mitral regurgitation be encountered, the closed operation should be abandoned, for mitral valve replacement will be the operation of choice.

Should unsuspected calcification be detected in the valve, a decision needs to be made at the time whether or not mitral valvotomy should be undertaken by the closed procedure. This operation carries the risk that fragments of calcium may be carried into the systemic circulation with possible serious consequences. Furthermore, calcification of the valve implies that the valve is probably more rigid than expected and that closed valvotomy will produce an indifferent and only short-term result. Nevertheless, numerous patients with calcific mitral stenosis have undergone successful mitral valvotomy with excellent long-term results. Despite this experience it is probably wiser to convert the operation from a closed procedure to an open operation, should valve calcification be more than trivial.

Hopefully, the selection of the patient has avoided a calcified valve, a regurgitant valve, or the presence of much interatrial thrombus, and the operation can now be completed.

The original operation of mitral commissurotomy was that of opening of the adherent commissures using the finger, and was undertaken in many patients seemingly successfully for some years. Nevertheless, it is now clear that very few patients are suitable for finger commissurotomy, for the valve is usually too thickened and fused for this to be successful. In earlier days the use of small knives, which were attached to the index finger and introduced into the heart to cut the commissures, was fashionable, and certainly many patients benefited from such an operation. Nevertheless, many more patients were given important mitral regurgitation due to either an inadvertent cut into a cusp or division of the chordae tendineae below the valve. Finger commissurotomy and the use of intracardiac knives are now considered to be both dangerous and ineffective in the majority of patients. It is now the invariable practice of all surgeons to use a dilator within the mitral valve, the usual instrument being the Tubbs dilator.

A tiny stab is made at the apex of the left ventricle in the small muscular area placed between the fat surrounding the anterior descending branch of the left coronary artery and the marginal artery, using a fine artery forceps. This is enlarged with heavier artery forceps or a sound, following which the closed dilator is passed into the left ventricle. It is passed up to the mitral stenotic orifice from below, passing through into the left atrium to meet the tip of the right index finger (Figure 41.4). It is important that the instrument be passed completely into the heart, for opening of the Tubbs dilator with part of its opening mechanism within the left ventricular wall may cause tearing of this wall and serious haemorrhage. At this stage it is wise to take an extra precaution to ensure that, should a piece of calcium or clot be dislodged, these will not enter the cerebral circulation. The anaesthetist is therefore asked to compress both common carotid arteries for a 30 s period while the valvotomy is being undertaken. This compression ensures stasis of the arterial circulation to the head for this period, and it is hoped that pieces of calcium or thrombus will be swept around the aortic arch into the descending aorta. The dilator is then opened, and whether this is undertaken gradually, as several movements, or as one swifter movement is a matter for debate. It is the author's practice to use one swift movement with the dilator set at 4 cm, and it is remarkable that mitral valvotomy almost invariably occurs in the line of the fused commissures. The dilator is then withdrawn from the valve but remains in the ventricle while the valve and

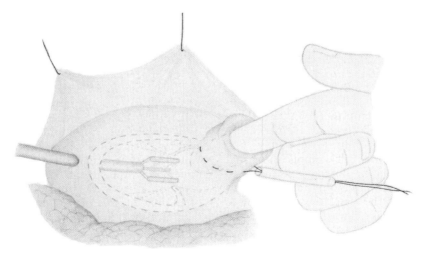

Figure 41.4 Closed mitral valvotomy. The Tubbs dilator is passed through the apex of the left ventricle towards the tip of the finger introduced through the left atrial appendage

subvalvar apparatus are palpated to estimate the degree of residual stenosis and to determine whether or not regurgitation of the valve has been produced. It is sometimes necessary to reintroduce the dilator into the valve for further commissurotomy.

Closed valvotomy is an operation which should not be overdone, for if the valve is split completely to the ring and both commissures are totally separated, interference with the support of the leaflets to the valve ring and cardiac skeleton may follow with consequent severe mitral regurgitation. Following satisfactory valvotomy, the closed dilator is withdrawn from the left ventricle and the resultant wound is covered with a small swab for several minutes. This usually seals spontaneously, but it is wise to reinforce its closure with two sutures of 3/0 Mersilene. The finger is withdrawn from the left atrial appendage and as this is done the purse-string is tied, which obliterates the left atrial appendage.

During the early years of this operation there was great controversy over the management of the atrial appendage. Many believed that the appendage should be carefully sutured and left for use at second and subsequent valvotomies, but there is no doubt that this diverticulum is an ideal site for further thrombus formation and possible embolic complications from this. It is now the practice of all surgeons to either amputate and suture the appendage or to ligate it, which obliterates this potentially dangerous backwater.

Following valvotomy the left atrial and pulmonary artery pressures are again measured and in the majority of patients a dramatic fall in left atrial pressure will have been obtained. The pericardium is irrigated and loosely closed with interrupted sutures. It is important that the pericardium be closed to avoid herniation of the heart postoperatively. The chest is closed with an intrapleural drain.

OPERATIVE COMPLICATIONS

Apart from the complications which may beset any surgical or cardiac surgical operation, the particular complications of closed mitral valvotomy are traumatic mitral incompetence and systemic embolism.

1. *Traumatic mitral incompetence.* In a patient with pure mitral stenosis, the left ventricle is a small atrophic chamber. Should even moderate mitral incompetence be produced during valvotomy the sudden increase in work required by this ventricle may overwhelm it, resulting in acute left ventricular failure with pulmonary oedema and congestive cardiac failure. This complication is seen from time to time and if mild to moderate is readily controlled by medical treatment using digoxin, diuretics and bed rest. Given time the left ventricle will hypertrophy and cope adequately with this amount of mitral regurgitation.

Severe degrees of traumatic mitral incompetence

may produce almost instant pulmonary oedema and require emergency mitral valve replacement with the use of cardiopulmonary bypass if the patient is to survive. This serious situation is very uncommon and has not been encountered in a personal experience of over 1000 closed mitral valvotomies.

Between these two extremes is the occasional patient in whom more than moderately severe mitral regurgitation is produced and who remains in severe congestive failure with pulmonary oedema postoperatively and who will require mitral valve replacement using cardiopulmonary bypass within a few days of the first operation. The author has had this experience in one patient only.

2. *Systemic embolism.* This may take the form of cerebral embolism of thrombus or of calcium, or of peripheral arterial embolism into a limb or mesenteric vessels. Invariably the thrombus which lodges peripherally originates from within the left atrium or the left atrial appendage. Occasionally small fragments of calcium produce showers of fine emboli within the brain with neurological effects which may be transient or permanent.

Following completion of closed mitral valvotomy, and after the patient is turned onto his or her back, all peripheral pulses are palpated and a comparison made with the records of pulses which were present or absent preoperatively. The limbs are watched carefully over the subsequent few hours to note coldness, pallor, loss of sensation or loss of movement. A common embolic complication is that of saddle embolism of the aortic bifurcation which is readily diagnosed by the complete absence of femoral pulses and of distal pulses in the lower limbs, pallor and perhaps mottling of the legs, together with coldness, loss of sensation and paralysis. The treatment of this condition is removal of the offending obstructing emboli by the use of Fogarty balloon catheters passed retrograde up both femoral arteries.

Mesenteric vascular occlusion is a consequence of left atrial thrombi travelling to the mesenteric vessels. The diagnosis and treatment of this condition are considered elsewhere (see Chapter 16).

POSTOPERATIVE MANAGEMENT

Those patients with poorly compliant lungs associated with either pulmonary oedema or marked pulmonary hypertension are best managed for 24 h postoperatively using intermittent positive-pressure ventilation via an endotracheal tube. This is certainly safer than immediate extubation, allowing patients to breathe as best they can, for many will become tired and have difficulty in ventilating their stiff lungs with consequent anoxia and hypercapnia. In the early days of mitral valve surgery many of the so-called 'unexplained' immediate postoperative deaths were doubtless due to hypoventilation, anoxia and retention of carbon dioxide.

Digoxin is restarted on the 1st postoperative day and diuretics with potassium supplement are given as necessary.

There is no indication for a second or subsequent mitral valvotomy being undertaken as a closed procedure.

A recent innovation has been that of closed mitral valvotomy using a dilating balloon. A catheter is introduced percutaneously into the femoral vein and passed into the right atrium, puncturing the septum whence it is introduced into the mitral valve. The attached balloon can then be forcibly dilated with fluid, producing an apparently successful mitral valvotomy.

Early reports indicate that for first-time valvotomy in patients with a non-calcified pliable valve, this has been very successful, but my own experience leads me to believe that this is an extremely dangerous procedure when undertaken in heavily calcified or fibrotic valves in elderly people. I have personal experience of total disruption of the subchordal mechanism by this very powerful hydraulic procedure. Although the use of this technique is in its early stages it is fair to say that many younger patients having first-time mitral valvotomy may be treated by this method, but extreme caution should be exercised when it is used on older patients with calcified, rigid or slightly incompetent valves and in these patients preference should be given to open operation.

Open mitral valvotomy (see Chapter 58)

This operation is undertaken using full cardiopulmonary bypass, with aortic cross-clamping and cardioplegia. Access to the mitral valve may be gained through a left thoracotomy, right thoracotomy or median sternotomy. Access via left thoracotomy is ideal when, during an attempt at closed valvotomy, it is necessary to institute cardiopulmonary bypass. Venous return may be obtained by inserting a cannula into the right ventricle or into the right atrial appendage, with arterial return into the descending aorta or left femoral artery. This approach is also useful should a left atrial myxoma be discovered during an exploration for apparent mitral stenosis.

Approach to the mitral valve via a right thoracotomy was popular at one time in patients who had previously had surgery undertaken through the left chest and in whom pleural adhesions were to be anticipated, but this approach is now obsolete.

The mitral valve is now almost invariably approached by a median sternotomy. This exposure allows surgery to be undertaken on the mitral valve, the aortic valve and the tricuspid valve and furthermore allows adequate manipulation of the left ventricle for the purpose of expelling air, a procedure which remains incomplete when surgery is undertaken through a right thoracotomy. To explore the mitral valve after median sternotomy a long incision is made in the left atrium extending from the right upper lobe pulmonary vein well down and parallel to the interatrial groove and towards the inferior vena cava (Figure 41.5). This gives excellent access to the mitral valve when using appropriate retractors. On rare occasions when the left atrium is tiny, adequate exposure may be undertaken by incising the right atrium in the horizontal plane and extending this incision back across the septum towards the tricuspid valve, also in the horizontal plane – the exposure of Dubost. Although this approach allows good visualization of the mitral valve under some circumstances, it has the disadvantage that the septal incision or its repair may interfere with atrioventricular conduction and cause permanent heart block, and furthermore the very thin portion of the septum surrounded by the annulus ovale may be difficult to resuture. The atrial cavity is carefully examined for thrombi. From time to time an extremely large thrombus occupying much of the chamber and extending into the pulmonary veins is present, and it is important that this thrombus is removed as completely as possible. Usually there is a plane of cleavage between the organized thrombus and the atrial wall, and when this is entered, and with care, the thrombus may be removed, very often in one piece.

When the thrombus is completely removed, the atrium and ventricle are irrigated with saline solution to ensure that fragments do not remain. At this stage it is wise to obliterate the orifice of the left atrial appendage using a fine continuous suture to ensure that postoperative thrombosis does not originate within the appendage, with the danger of subsequent embolization. Great care must be taken when placing this suture, for too deep an insertion may damage the circumflex coronary artery or vein in the atrioventricular groove. The insertion of a suture into the anterior and posterior leaflets of the valve is a valuable aid to the demonstration of the stenosis of the valve and of its subvalvar pathology (Figure 41.6). Horizontal traction is applied to these sutures, following which careful incision of the fused commissure can be undertaken safely. The fused commissure usually presents as a wrinkled furrow considerably thicker than the adjacent valve cusps.

The introduction of a right-angled clamp beneath the fused commissures and between the chordae aids in separation and accurate division of the commissure. The commissure is cut a few mm at a time and after each cut the valve cusps and the chordae are carefully separated to avoid damage with consequent regurgitation. In many instances the valve can be widely opened by cutting both commissures and it may be noted that there is little if any chordal fusion, enabling a competent, mobile, almost full-sized valve

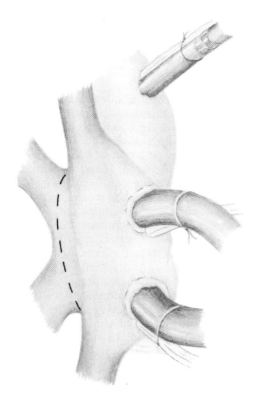

Figure 41.5 Open mitral valvotomy. The line of incision into the left atrium is parallel and posterior to the right atrium, care being taken to avoid incision too far laterally into the pulmonary veins

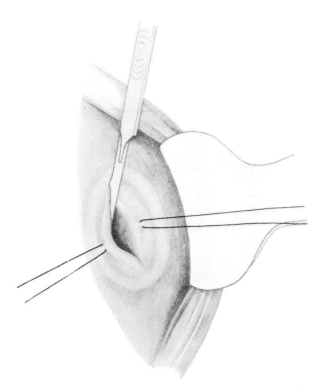

Figure 41.6 Open mitral valvotomy. The cusps of the mitral valve are retracted with stay sutures and this facilitates exposure for accurate commissurotomy

to be obtained. Unfortunately, in some instances the valve will be thickened with early calcification and with considerable subchordal fusion. Whereas it was until recently the common practice to replace such a valve, there is now a distinct leaning towards conservation of the mitral valve if at all possible, for it is clear that the patient's own mitral valve, perhaps imperfect, is far more serviceable than any prosthesis so far designed. In these patients, careful commissurotomy and removal of calcium with forceps will demonstrate the subchordal problem, and splitting of the chordae with a sharp knife or scissors may enable the valve to be separated into a good anterior and posterior leaflet, each with good chordal support mechanism (Figure 41.7). It may be that during this procedure one or two chordae are divided, but in these the valve may still be satisfactorily repaired by the placement of a few sutures in the edge of the unsupported part of the valve. At the end of this procedure it is most important to evacuate thrombus, calcium and air from the heart before ejection into the aorta begins and the bypass is discontinued.

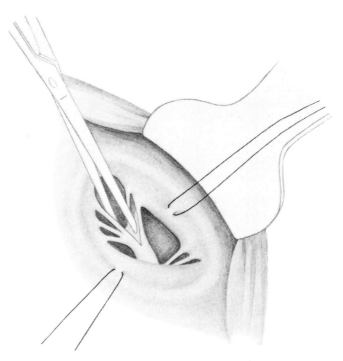

Figure 41.7 Open mitral valvotomy. Following commissurotomy the fused chordae and papillary muscles may be carefully split

PREVENTION OF AIR EMBOLISM DURING MITRAL VALVE SURGERY

In any operation which widely opens the left heart, such as aortic or mitral valve replacement, considerable amounts of air may be trapped in the pulmonary veins and the chambers of the left side of the heart, and unless great care is taken this air will be ejected through the aortic valve when the heart takes over following the termination of cardiopulmonary bypass. It is important to anticipate this problem by the use of good left ventricular venting tubes and with a supra-aortic needle vent, both of which are aspirated prior to terminating the bypass and prior to release of aortic cross-clamps. Cerebral air embolism, which was at one time a serious complication of cardiac surgery, has now been almost completely eliminated by careful attention to these details.

Acquired mitral regurgitation

Principal causes

1. Rheumatic fever.
2. Subacute bacterial endocarditis.
3. Prolapse of the cusps, especially the posterior, with herniation into the left atrium, the so-called 'floppy valve syndrome'.
4. Ruptured chordae associated with myxomatous degeneration of the central valve.
5. Mitral regurgitation following myocardial infarction due to either rupture of a papillary muscle, or due to so-called 'papillary muscle dysfunction'.
6. Following mitral valvotomy, either closed or open.
7. Mitral regurgitation associated with closed chest injuries.
8. Congenital clefts. Although these are not acquired, they may present in adult life and appear to cause acquired mitral regurgitation and will be considered in this chapter (McGoon operation).

Mitral valve repair

Until recently, the operation of choice for mitral regurgitation was replacement of the valve with a mechanical or biological prosthesis. However, the long-term complications of mitral valve replacement, together with the long-term complications of anticoagulant therapy, have made surgeons increasingly willing to explore the possibility of conserving the patient's own mitral valve. Apart from these complications there seems little doubt that left ventricular function is better preserved in the presence of papillary muscle and chordal support. There is no doubt that with increasing experience most surgeons are able to preserve more and more valves and when associated with an appropriate annuloplasty or ring insertion, many seriously regurgitant valves may be rendered quite competent.

Operation is undertaken via median sternotomy using full cardiopulmonary bypass. The left atrium is opened posteriorly to the right atrium by a vertical incision and, following exposure of the valve and appropriate retraction, the valve can be carefully examined concerning competence, leaflet perforation, chordal rupture and elongation and the condition of the papillary muscles. Other than in those valves

totally destroyed by very heavy calcification or rupture of all of the chordae of the posterior and anterior leaflets, an attempt should be made to conserve the valve and reconstruction is possible by several manoeuvres.

The original operation introduced by McGoon (1960) consisted of repair of the posterior prolapsed leaflet of the mitral valve which was due to rupture of some of the posterior chordae. This was undertaken by excising the flail segment of the valve, together with an associated wedge of left atrial wall, together with the ruptured chordae, following which the two edges of the cut valve could be reconstructed with fine sutures, rendering the valve competent.

The success of the modern operation is attributed entirely to the work of Carpentier of Paris, who had devised a number of elegant procedures on the mitral valve, such as leaflet or partial leaflet transplantation, chordal transplantation, chordal repair, chordal shortening and an appropriate annuloplasty (Carpentier et al., 1980). In his hands, very few valves need be sacrificed and his short- and long-term results for the preservation of the mitral valve in the presence of regurgitation are unsurpassed (Figure 41.8). For a fuller description of his various techniques, the reader is referred to more specialized works.

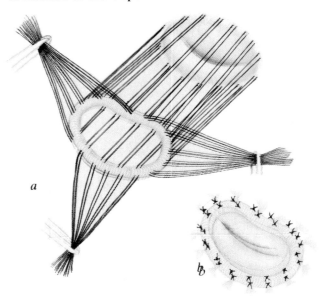

Figure 41.8 Carpentier ring used for narrowing the mitral annulus when the valve leaflets and the subvalvar mechanism are otherwise intact

Following valvuloplasty, some sort of mitral annuloplasty is necessary and this has in the past been undertaken by the insertion of a circumferential purse-string suture after the De Vega method for tricuspid annuloplasty, but this is not as successful as the insertion of the mitral Carpentier ring. The size of ring to be chosen is determined by the use of sizing obturators and it is recommended that the sizing obturator which covers the anterior cusp of the mitral valve should conform to the size of the ring to be selected. The ring will then be reduced in size to that of the anterior cusp of the mitral valve which will then readily obstruct the mitral orifice during systole, preventing mitral regurgitation.

Mitral valve replacement

Should it prove impossible to preserve the valve the cusps should be excised together with their associated chordae tendineae and tips of the papillary muscles. Care should be taken to leave a 2 mm ring of mitral valve at the ring, for complete removal of the mitral valve, especially anteriorly where the ring is not very well in evidence, may result in sutures cutting out of the thin muscle (Figure 41.9). Although the tips of the papillary muscles must be removed, care should be taken when the valve is elevated to expose the papillary muscles that the left ventricular wall is not tented inwards, with consequent damage to or rupture of the ventricular wall during excision of the papillary muscle (Figures 41.10 and 41.11). It is now the practice of many surgeons to fix the valve using a continuous suture of 2/0 polypropylene, although in those situations where the valve ring seems inadequate it is probably safer to use interrupted sutures, supported where necessary with Teflon felt buttresses (Figure 41.12).

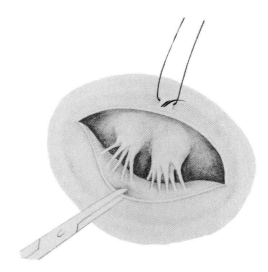

Figure 41.10 Mitral valve replacement. Following detachment of the anterior cusp of the mitral valve from the ring, the papillary muscles are seen

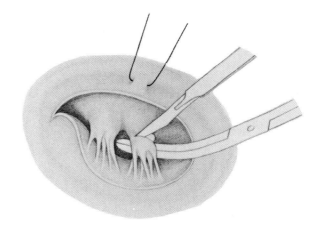

Figure 41.11 Mitral valve replacement. The papillary muscle is divided just proximal to the insertion of the chordae

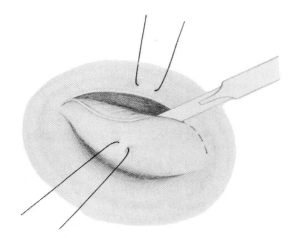

Figure 41.9 Mitral valve replacement. Traction on stay sutures facilitates accurate resection of the anterior cusp of the mitral valve

Following suture of a prosthetic valve into position it is important that it is made incompetent, otherwise the beating left ventricle may eject air into the aorta before an opportunity has occurred to evacuate this air. This is achieved by passing a fine Foley balloon catheter across the valve from the atrium into the ventricle and inflating the balloon. This will prevent the ball or disc closing and will enable free ventricular air to be ejected back into the atrium. This catheter is

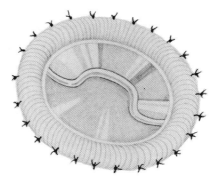

Figure 41.12 Mitral valve replacement. The mitral valve prosthesis (Bjork–Shiley) is sutured into the mitral ring using interrupted non-absorbable sutures

removed only after the atrium has been closed around it and air has been completely evacuated from all cardiac chambers (Figure 41.13).

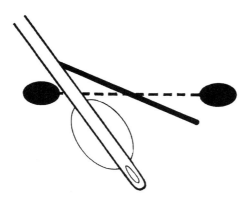

Figure 41.13 Mitral valve replacement. The use of a Foley balloon catheter (as shown) is advised during mitral valve replacement. By rendering the valve incompetent, air contained in the ventricle is displaced back into the atrium, whence it may be removed during atrial suture

Acute infections of the mitral valve

This serious illness presents as acute or subacute bacterial endocarditis of the mitral valve. The responsible organism is frequently *Streptococcus viridans* which usually originates in dental sepsis. This organism may produce subacute infection of the valve, but acute bacterial endocarditis is more likely to be caused by an organism such as *Staphylococcus aureus*. While the patient may slowly develop congestive cardiac failure, allowing an intensive 4–6-week course of the appropriate intravenous antibiotics prior to valve replacement, there are occasions when mitral regurgitation is so severe that the patient will clearly not survive to enable this long antibiotic therapy to be undertaken. In these, emergency mitral valve replacement is necessary to save life, in the face of the real risk of implanting a prosthetic valve into an infected mitral valve ring, although infection of the prosthesis is very rare in these circumstances.

Assessment of tricuspid valve

At the beginning of any open operation on the mitral valve, prior to starting bypass, digital examination of the tricuspid valve is essential. This will demonstrate the presence of previously unsuspected tricuspid valve stenosis or regurgitation, the latter being either functional or organic. Should this valve be haemodynamically seriously abnormal, attention to it is mandatory, or else, following an otherwise successful mitral valve operation, the patient may develop a serious or fatal low output state.

Management of open mitral valve operations in the presence of significant aortic regurgitation

Aortic regurgitation of either mild or moderate degree is present in many patients with mitral valve disease. In itself the aortic regurgitation may not be haemodynamically significant but during cardiopulmonary bypass the leak back through the valve into the non-beating left ventricle may cause problems.

The torrent of blood regurgitating into the left ventricle will create difficulties of visualization during the mitral valve operation, and this was a serious problem when it was customary to operate on the beating heart at normal temperatures. However, now that open mitral valve surgery is undertaken with aortic cross-clamping and the use of cold cardioplegia, the leaking aortic valve no longer presents a problem during perfusion. However, for the efficient production of a cold paralysed heart it is necessary for the aortic valve cusps to be fairly competent in order that the coronary arteries may be perfused with the injected cold solution. Should the valve be incompetent the solution will run back into the left ventricle and not perfuse the coronary arteries. This state of affairs is obvious as the aortic root will not become tense during the injection and furthermore the heart will not cool. In these circumstances it is therefore necessary to open the root of the aorta and to inspect the aortic valve. If the valve is found to be only mildly diseased, cold cardioplegia may be proceeded with by injection of the cold solution individually down both coronary arteries. If, however, the aortic valve is clearly far more diseased than was previously considered, it will be necessary to excise the aortic valve and replace it in addition to any contemplated mitral valve surgery.

Acquired disease of the tricuspid valve

The tricuspid valve may be affected by stenosis or incompetence, usually part of the rheumatic process which affects the mitral valve and perhaps the aortic valve. A significant degree of tricuspid stenosis may affect perhaps 5% of patients with mitral valve disease, but tricuspid regurgitation is more commonly seen. Tricuspid regurgitation may be organic with fibrous retraction, shortening and thickening of the leaflets by the rheumatic process or it may be functional and follow dilatation of the tricuspid valve ring associated with right ventricular dilatation consequent on pulmonary hypertension. It is unfortunately the case that serious tricuspid stenosis or regurgitation may pass unnoticed during cardiac catheterization and even clinical examination, and for this reason it is always necessary to palpate the tricuspid valve prior to cardiopulmonary bypass during open mitral valve surgery. Tricuspid stenosis is rarely amenable to separation of the commissures, for in these patients the cusps are thickened and shortened,

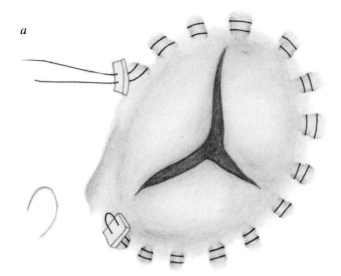

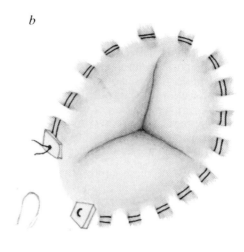

Figure 41.14 De Vega annuloplasty suture to narrow the triscupid orifice

and any such operation to relieve stenosis usually results in regurgitation. It is necessary under these circumstances to perform, in addition, some form of annuloplasty.

Tricuspid regurgitation

Tricuspid regurgitation is rarely amenable to any form of surgery to the cusps alone. Fortunately, the tricuspid ring is suitable for annuloplasty either by De Vega annuloplasty or by the ring annuloplasty of Carpentier. The annuloplasty introduced by De Vega is an excellent method of narrowing the tricuspid valve orifice in patients with tricuspid regurgitation, whether this be functional or pathological. The annuloplasty occupies about three-quarters of the circumference of the tricuspid ring, avoiding the area adjacent to the coronary sinus where lies the atrioventricular conducting bundle. A suture is introduced into the tricuspid valve ring and passed as a purse-string three-quarters of the way around the ring where it emerges (Figure 41.14a). It is then inserted into a Teflon felt buttress and retraces its steps to the original point of insertion of the suture where it is again buttressed. This suture which is of heavy prolene or heavy Ethiflex is gradually tightened over a 20 mm diameter sound and, when it sits snugly over this, it is tied. The valve will then be seen to be competent (Figure 41.14b).

The Carpentier ring annuloplasty is undertaken in much the same way as with the mitral valve. However, bearing in mind the dangerous area adjacent to the atrioventricular conducting bundle, this ring is incomplete and takes up the slack in three-quarters of the ring only. This is a most successful method of annuloplasty.

Tricuspid valve replacement

It is unfortunately the case that although many patients have undergone successful tricuspid valve replacement, it is in this situation that valve dysfunction and early thrombosis of the prosthetic valve, despite adequate anticoagulation, are common.

Acquired aortic valve disease

Aortic valve disease is common and there seems to be no shortage of patients who require surgery for aortic stenosis or regurgitation.

Aortic stenosis

Although aortic stenosis should be detected in childhood, it is more commonly detected in adult life with the development of calcific aortic stenosis. It is likely that the majority of patients with calcific aortic stenosis have calcified a congenitally stenotic or abnormal valve. The valve is frequently bicuspid or, if tricuspid, one cusp is larger than the others or there may be rudimentary commissures. Such an abnormal valve produces turbulence of flow through and around it and over the years the deposition of platelets and fibrin add to the rigidity of the valve which becomes thickened, fibrosed and later calcified. Rheumatic fever is a common cause of aortic stenosis with thickening and fibrous fusion of the commissures and is frequently associated with rheumatic disease of the mitral valve.

Aortic regurgitation

The causes of aortic regurgitation are:

1. Calcific aortic stenosis and incompetence.
2. Rheumatic aortic incompetence.
3. Subacute bacterial endocarditis.
4. Syphilis of the root of the aorta and aortic valve.
5. Dissection of the root of the aorta.
6. Marfan's syndrome.
7. A complication of rheumatoid arthritis and ankylosing spondylitis.
8. Traumatic aortic incompetence.

In some of these conditions, such as syphilis, dissection and Marfan's syndrome, the aortic valve is not primarily at fault. It is the associated pathology of the root of the aorta which causes dilatation and disruption at the aortic ring which produces regurgitation.

Aortic regurgitation may be associated with an ascending aortic aneurysm which often involves the aortic ring and the origin of the coronary arteries, together with the ascending aorta as far as, if not distal to, the innominate artery. Such aneurysms are frequently seen in association with Marfan's syndrome and syphilitic aortitis, and of course dissection has its own peculiar pathology.

Assessment

Many patients with aortic stenotic and regurgitant murmurs may have no symptoms and it is necessary to assess these patients clinically and haemodynamically before suitable advice may be given.

Radiological examination will disclose the size of the heart, and of the aorta, valve calcification and the vascularity of the lung fields, together with an assessment of degrees of pulmonary venous congestion denoting heart failure.

Electrocardiography is an important investigation in aortic valve disease. Left ventricular hypertrophy is commonly seen and the various criteria for determining hypertrophy are well documented. Associated evidence of ischaemic heart disease will indicate the need for coronary arteriography.

Cardiac catheterization will establish the level of the gradient across the aortic valve, the left atrial pressure, pressures in the left ventricle and the pulmonary vascular resistance, and when these are considered a fair understanding of the patient's haemodynamic state will be possible. Angiocardiography will assess incompetence at the aortic and mitral valves and left ventricular function. Echocardiography will help in the assessment of left ventricular function and also estimate the orifice size and function of the aortic valve. In most adults who are to be considered as candidates for aortic valve surgery, coronary arteriography is considered necessary. Certainly in those patients with associated angina pectoris, such an investigation is mandatory. It is sad to replace an aortic valve in a patient who dies and is discovered at autopsy to have previously unsuspected and important coronary artery disease.

The decision to operate is more readily made in those with symptoms, for it is known that patients with aortic valve disease who are experiencing anginal pain, syncopal attacks, or have evidence of left ventricular failure, have an exceedingly poor life expectation, variously estimated at between 1 and 3 years.

Subacute bacterial endocarditis may be a slow process and may respond to a prolonged course of intravenous antibiotics prior to valve replacement. However, as with endocarditis of the mitral valve cardiac failure may be so severe that emergency aortic valve replacement in the presence of a possibly inadequately sterilized aortic valve is sometimes necessary, and it is inevitable that the risk of reinfection of the prosthetic aortic valve must be taken.

Surgical treatment of acquired aortic valve disease

Closed valvotomy by means of dilators introduced through the left ventricle is obsolete.

Aortic valve surgery is now invariably an open procedure conducted using cardiopulmonary bypass, and presents the need for some form of myocardial protection, because exposure of the aortic valve requires cross-clamping of the aorta with consequent deprivation of natural coronary artery perfusion.

Methods of left ventricular protection and support during aortic valve surgery (see Chapter 58)

Surgical approach to the aortic valve

The aortic valve is invariably approached via median sternotomy and using full cardiopulmonary bypass and cold cardioplegia. The ascending aorta is mobilized and cross-clamped. The aortic incision is either a vertical hockey stick-shaped incision or a transverse incision in the aorta 1 cm above the right coronary orifice. The valve, if fibrous, is readily excised but in the presence of calcific aortic stenosis care is required when removing the cusps and calcium from the aortic root. Particular attention should be paid anteriorly at the commissure between the non-coronary and right coronary cusps, for it is at this site that the atrioventricular conducting bundle enters the ventricular septum and it is here that it may be damaged with the production of complete heart block. When the aortic ring is ready to receive the valve, the appropriate valve size is estimated by the introduction of graded obturators which are supplied with the particular valve to be used. Interrupted sutures of Ethibond are used and where the valve ring is weak or not very much in evidence support using Teflon felt buttresses is advised (Figure 41.15).

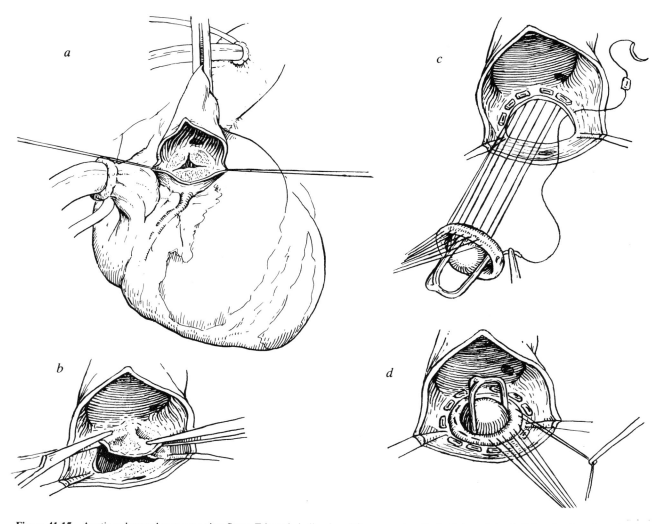

Figure 41.15 Aortic valve replacement using Starr–Edwards ball valve. After removing the leaflets and decalcifying the ring, the valve in this case is inserted using mattress sutures buttressed with Teflon felt supports

Aneurysms of the ascending aorta (Figures 41.16–41.18)

Aneurysms of the ascending aorta occur in the following conditions:

1. Atherosclerosis.
2. Tertiary syphilis.
3. Marfan's syndrome.
4. Acute dissection.
5. Traumatic aneurysms.

Aneurysms may be localized to the ascending aorta, may extend into the aortic arch and involve the descending aorta, but most frequently involve the ascending aorta only. These aneurysms will increase in size and either erode surrounding structures and eventually rupture or in addition, in many instances, so dilate the aortic ring that aortic regurgitation follows.

Aneurysms of the ascending aorta with competent aortic valve

Indications for surgery

Once such an aneurysm is more than 6 cm in diameter, the likelihood of progressive increase in size and ultimate rupture is real and surgical excision should be considered.

The operation is conducted using cardiopulmonary bypass using a single right atrial cannula with return to the femoral artery, enabling the ascending aorta to be excised without interference by aortic perfusion cannulae. When on bypass and sufficiently cooled, the aorta is cross-clamped just proximal to the brachiocephalic artery and opened just above the coronary arteries to just proximal to the distal clamp. An interposing graft of woven Dacron is sutured in place using continuous 3/0 prolene sutures and, prior to release of clamps, precautions are taken to ensure that air is completely aspirated from the prosthetic ascending aorta. The opened aneurysm is not removed and anastomoses are therefore carried out inside the sound aorta.

When the aneurysm extends so proximally that aortic regurgitation is present, it is necessary to use a composite prosthesis into which the coronary arteries are implanted. Such a prosthesis consists of a tube graft of woven Dacron to which is sutured the prosthetic valve of choice.

Most surgeons avoid the use of biological valves which are known to deteriorate in perhaps 10–12 years. However, in the very elderly, perhaps over 70 years of age, a biological valve should be considered, for the patient is then able to avoid prolonged anticoagulation with Warfarin and the problem of late degeneration of the biological valve is less likely to cause concern.

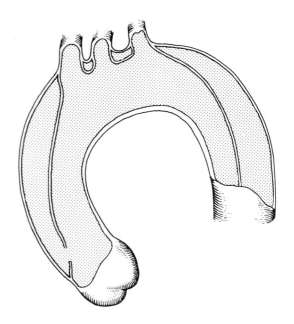

Figure 41.17 Dissecting aneurysm of the ascending aorta. The aneurysm has been opened and its anterior aspect removed demonstrating separation of the layers both proximally and distally, and in this situation the orifices of the coronary arteries are frequently involved. It is necessary to oversew the divided proximal and distal aorta with continuous sutures supported by Teflon felt prior to insertion of a composite graft

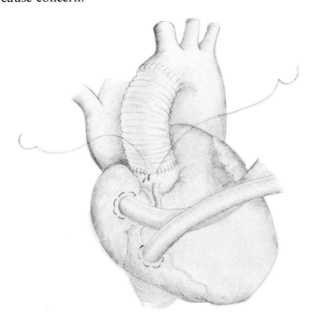

Figure 41.16 Ascending aortic aneurysm complicating aortic regurgitation. The aortic valve prosthesis has been implanted in the usual way. A woven Dacron graft is used to replace the ascending aortic aneurysm, but as is usual with simple aneurysms in this situation it has been possible to spare the proximal portion of the ascending aorta bearing the coronary arteries

Technique of composite aortic root replacement

Cardiopulmonary bypass is instituted using a right atrial cannula with return to the femoral artery. As in simple saccular aneurysm of the ascending aorta, proximal cross-clamping is undertaken near the brachiocephalic artery. It is not necessary to excise the aneurysm which is laid open. The aortic valve is removed and the prepared composite valve containing graft is sutured to the aortic ring with multiple

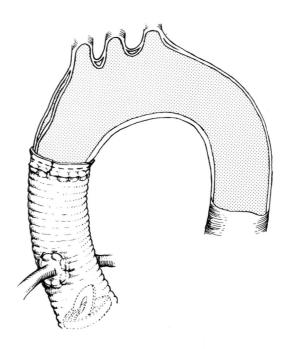

Figure 41.18 Dissecting aneurysm of the ascending aorta. A composite graft of woven Dacron with which is incorporated an aortic prosthesis is sutured directly to the aortic root below the coronary ostia. The coronary ostia are then sutured directly to small holes cut into the woven Dacron graft

interrupted mattressed and pledgeted Ethibond sutures. When this has been lowered into place and tied, holes about 1 cm in diameter are cut into the graft in an appropriate position above the prosthetic valve and adjacent to the coronary ostia in the aneurysm, and these ostia are sutured to the holes in the composite graft with continuous fine prolene sutures. Following this, the upper end of the graft is sutured to the transected aorta just proximal to the brachiocephalic artery using continuous 3/0 sutures, and after ensuring evacuation of air from the prosthesis, the cross-clamp is removed.

In the treatment of chronic aneurysm of the ascending aorta, it may be necessary to undertake coronary artery bypass grafting at the same time and it is therefore important that all such patients have preoperative coronary arteriography.

The particular problem of acute dissection of the ascending aorta

This condition presents acutely and although the majority of patients die from aortic rupture very soon after the event, many patients are diagnosed and admitted to hospital. The characteristic symptoms of acute anterior and posterior chest pain, with collapse of the patient, is now well recognized by receiving hospitals and when associated with the radiological evidence of a widened mediastinum, a presumptive and correct diagnosis is often made. Whereas acute dissection of the descending aorta is often amenable to conservative management, acute dissection of the ascending aorta is almost invariably fatal without surgery and therefore most patients should be considered for operation.

DIAGNOSIS

The clinical diagnosis is complemented by CT scan and in many patients aortography will be helpful. The CT scan, however, is usually diagnostic and the surgeon is given the information which he really requires, which is whether or not the acute dissection involves the ascending aorta, the descending aorta, the aortic arch, or all three parts of the aorta.

Aortography can be combined with coronary arteriography, but aortography in these patients may cause delay and be dangerous and most surgeons have experience of such patients rupturing their aneurysm during cardiac catheterization. This remains a vexed question, but most surgeons will now accept a clinical diagnosis supported by CT scan confirmation to enable them to embark on surgical treatment.

Acute dissection occurs in aortas affected by cystic medial necrosis and the tear usually occurs 2–3 cm above the aortic valve, usually anterolaterally and on the right side. The tear extends proximally and distally and the proximal tear may extend into the aortic ring detaching it and causing acute aortic regurgitation. This proximal tear may also extend into the pericardium causing fatal cardiac tamponade. The distal tear will extend along the head vessels, into the aortic arch and into the descending aorta, and the usual consequence of untreated dissection is external rupture into the mediastinum with immediate fatal consequences.

The surgical problem presented by acute aortic dissection is far more difficult for the surgeon than is the surgery of simple aneurysms. Whereas the aorta of atherosclerotic and syphilitic aneurysms and the aneurysms of Marfan's disease usually holds sutures well, the aortic wall in acute dissection has been likened to the consistency of wet blotting paper; cardiac surgeons engaged in this work will agree with this description.

Sutures readily tear out of the host aorta, making it mandatory for graft anastomosis to be undertaken in so far as is possible to normal aorta, and if this aorta is not normal then an aorta well supported with Teflon felt buttresses. In acute dissection it is often possible and desirable to spare the aortic valve and the coronary arteries, provided that aortic regurgitation is not a feature and that the coronary arteries are sufficiently away from the aortic tear to enable a prosthesis to be sutured safely above the coronary ostia. Very frequently the coronary ostia are spared, but the aortic valve is regurgitant due to detachment of one of the commissures, usually the commissure between the non-coronary and left coronary cusps. In these cases, if the valve is otherwise normal, the commissure can be resuspended into the aorta, or into the aortic prosthesis, with several pledgeted buttressed prolene sutures. The surgical mortality of acute aortic dissection surgery is rather lower when a composite aortic graft and coronary implantation are avoidable.

The problem of the distal anastomosis is often very trying, for no matter how distal the aorta is trimmed it is often a ragged double-barrelled mess of soggy 'blotting paper'. In these cases, it may not be possible to suture the distal end of the prosthesis as the aortic tear may extend into the aortic arch, and it is therefore necessary to take the graft as distal as is necessary, and without the use of cross-clamps. In this situation, the best approach is using a combination of profound hypothermia and circulatory arrest.

While on bypass, the patient is cooled to a temperature of 18°C. When this temperature has been reached, the patient is tilted head down to avoid air embolism to the brain and the aortic arch is opened by transection without the use of a clamp. At the same time, the extracorporeal circulation is either completely stopped or reduced to a trickle, to avoid obscuring the operative field with blood. This is a surprisingly good exposure, enabling the aorta to be trimmed as far as is necessary distally, which may include resection of the proximal brachiocephalic artery, and when good tissue is found distally, the aortic prosthesis may then be sutured more satisfactorily with continuous 3/0 prolene sutures. It may be necessary to reimplant the brachiocephalic artery into the graft. Air is then carefully evacuated from the prosthesis, the extracorporeal circulation is put back to a normal level, the patient rewarmed and happily will come off bypass without event.

The use of collagenized Dacron grafts and various surgical 'glues' has dramatically reduced intraoperative bleeding from suture lines and has made the surgery of acute dissection much safer.

Aneurysmal resection and simple graft replacement of the ascending aorta carries an acceptably low mortality of about 5%, but the insertion of a composite graft with coronary replacement increases this mortality to between 10% and 15% in average surgical units. The additional problem of ascending aortic or root replacement in acute dissection of the aorta is accompanied by a surgical mortality of between 10% and 20% in average hands, although in most centres with very wide experience this may be considerably reduced.

Replacement of the ascending aorta using an intraluminal shunt

The recent introduction of an intraluminal device which may be tied into the ascending aorta has obviated the need in many cases to undertake formal removal and replacement of the ascending aorta with a Dacron tube. The intraluminal device is inserted into the ascending aorta and its upper and lower ends are tied in place with a circumferential ligature. The use of the intraluminal shunt is precluded in those patients in whom concomitant aortic valve replacement and reimplantation of the coronary arteries are necessary.

Combined aortic and mitral valve replacement

This operation is frequently undertaken. It is important to replace the mitral valve first, for if the aortic valve is dealt with initially the consequent rigidity and fixation of the aortic root create difficulties in mobilizing the mitral valve and its replacement.

Hypertrophic obstructive cardiomyopathy

This condition has gained increasing attention in recent years. It is a muscular obstruction of the left ventricular outflow tract, characterized by marked hypertrophy in the left ventricle, particularly in the interventricular septum. During systole the hypertrophic outflow tract muscle almost completely obstructs left ventricular ejection. Fortunately, the majority of these patients respond to medical treatment, usually with beta-blocking drugs. In some patients, however, despite medical treatment, symptoms remain severe and haemodynamic and angiographic evidence of severe outflow obstruction remains. In these, resecting some of the obstructing left ventricular muscle via

a supravalvar aortotomy (Figure 41.19) or a combined supravalvar and transventricular approach has achieved relief of symptoms and has been associated with a diminution or almost complete obliteration of the measured haemodynamic gradient. Although surgical management of this condition may relieve the obstruction, it in no way influences the underlying pathology, and operative treatment is best reserved for patients with severe symptoms who have not responded to medical treatment.

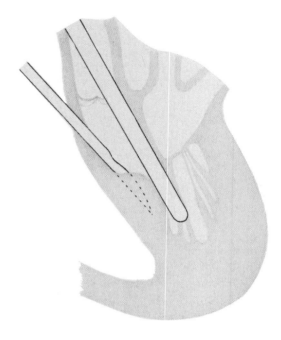

Figure 41.19 Hypertrophic obstructive cardiomyopathy. Resection of subvalvar muscle mass is safer when the spatula introduced via the ascending aorta protects other structures

Artificial heart valves

The ideal replacement heart valve has the following characteristics:

1. Central laminar flow.
2. Absence of turbulence.
3. Resistance to thrombus formation or the attraction of platelet and fibrin aggregates.
4. Resistance to wear or deterioration in function.

Artificial valves are of two basic types, the prosthetic valve and the biological valve.

Prosthetic valves

These are of three main varieties – the caged ball valve, the horizontal tilting disc valve, and the bileaflet valve.

The valves are manufactured from a non-ferrous metallic frame which is covered by artificial fabrics incorporating a sewing ring and containing a ball or

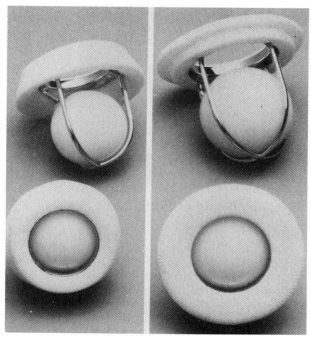

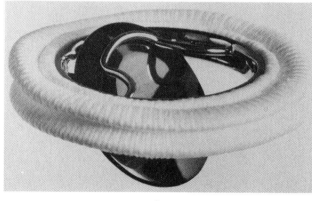

a

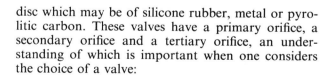

b

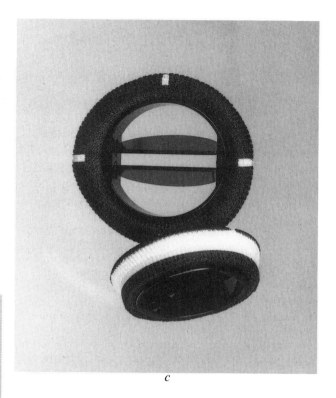

c

Figure 41.20 *a*, Starr–Edwards valves. Left, Aortic. Right, Mitral. *b*, Bjork–Shiley mitral valve. *c*, Carbomedic bileaflet valve

disc which may be of silicone rubber, metal or pyro-litic carbon. These valves have a primary orifice, a secondary orifice and a tertiary orifice, an under-standing of which is important when one considers the choice of a valve:

1. The primary orifice is the diameter of the annulus which is retained following excision of the diseased valve.
2. The secondary orifice is the diameter of the blood passage through the valve itself and this will depend largely on the thickness of the sewing ring.
3. The tertiary orifice is the effective orifice through which blood may flow following ejection through the valve and this will depend on the size of the ball in the cage or on the angle of tilt of the pivoting disc.

Furthermore, the size of the aorta or ventricle distal to the valve will determine whether or not the disc or the caged ball obstructs blood flow during systolic ejection. The valves in common use are the Starr–Edwards caged ball valve, the variations of which have stood the test of time, several types of tilting disc valve, notably the Bjork–Shiley tilting disc valve, the Lillehei–Kaster valve, and the St. Jude and Carbomedic bileaflet valves (Figure 41.20).

Whether or not a caged ball valve is used in preference to a disc valve or a bileaflet valve is often a matter of personal preference. It should be said, however, that the presence of a large caged ball valve within the left ventricle in mitral valve replacement may well interfere with left ventricular function, and erosion of the left ventricular muscle by the struts of such a valve has been recorded. For these reasons

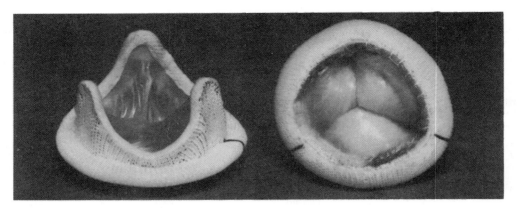

Figure 41.21 Mounted porcine xenograft for mitral position (Carpentier–Edwards)

many surgeons who use prosthetic valves in this situation prefer the use of a disc valve, which has very little protrusion into the left ventricle. On the other hand, the presence of a caged ball valve in the ascending aorta does not interfere with the function of the valve, although it may rarely obstruct a very narrow aorta. When the valves are compared there is little doubt that the secondary orifice of the pivoting disc valves, such as the Bjork–Shiley, Lillehei–Kaster or bileaflet valves, is considerably larger than the secondary orifice in the Starr–Edwards valve of similar primary orifice diameter. This is an important factor when one considers mitral valve replacement, for it is essential that this valve opens at a very low pressure and that blood passes through as wide an orifice as possible, and with little turbulence.

Biological valves

The valves now in use are homograft human aortic valves, valves prepared from calf pericardium, valves prepared from dura mater, valves prepared from fascia lata, and mounted porcine xenograft valves. With the exception of the cadaver human aortic valve and the porcine xenograft valve, those others mentioned are used very rarely and, following the disappointing experience with human fascia lata valves in the mitral and aortic positions, there is uncertainty concerning the prolonged life expectancy of dura mater valves. The great attraction of the human aortic valve or of the pig valve is its conformity with the principles of the ideal valve. It opens centrally with laminar flow and does not attract thrombus, platelets or fibrinogen and therefore requires, apart from the first few weeks postoperatively, no long-term control with anticoagulants.

Unmounted homograft aortic valves have been used with very great success by a handful of experienced surgeons in selected centres, but few are trained in this particular technique. The mounted porcine xenograft of either the Hancock or Carpentier type (Figure 41.21) is very much easier to insert than are unmounted human aortic homografts. These valves are factory prepared, already sutured to flexible metal and fabric stents stored in buffered glutaraldehyde, and are inserted in much the same way as are prosthetic valves.

Biological vs prosthetic valve replacement

The introduction of the biological valve (aortic homograft, bovine pericardial, mounted porcine xenograft) was particularly welcome to cardiac surgeons for, being far less prone to thromboembolic problems, they do not require the patient to be anticoagulated, with the attendant risks of this treatment. It was therefore not surprising that following the introduction of factory-mounted biological valves these were inserted into numerous patients. Unfortunately, after the passage of a few years it became clear that biological valves had their own disadvantages, particularly that of variable durability. It became clear that the insertion of biological valves into children (in whom chronic anticoagulation therapy is very difficult for both doctor and child) was frequently accompanied by early degeneration and calcification of the valve which was usually severe enough to require replacement with a prosthetic valve. Adults are not immune from the complication of calcification and furthermore with the passage of time more reports are emerging of these valves thickening, becoming stenotic or the cusps rupturing and producing regurgitation. It is claimed that the degeneration of biological valves is usually a very slow process, associated with gradual deterioration of the patient, enabling doctors to diagnose and treat valve failure in good time and before the patient becomes very ill. This, unfortunately, is not always the case for some patients who appear to be well, then deteriorate and die very quickly and are subsequently shown to have extensively calcified and stenotic biological valves. Furthermore, rupture of a cusp of a biological valve may occur suddenly with early deterioration and death of the patient.

There is no doubt that the factory-made prosthetic valve is extremely durable and the modern valve rarely, if ever, suffers from ball variance or from valve failure, although a large batch of prosthetic valves recently exhibited strut failure and fracture with release of the disc into the circulation with fatal consequences for many patients. Despite this, however, it is safe to say that the factory-produced prosthetic valve is far more durable than the biological valve and the insertion without complication of such a valve into a patient is likely to provide the patient with a well-functioning valve for very many years and possibly the remainder of his or her lifetime. It must be emphasized, however, that the long-term anticoagulation required for the safe maintenance of the prosthetic valve is accompanied by significant mortality and morbidity caused by anticoagulant related haemorrhage (see below).

The biological valve is particularly suited for the elderly in whom the criterion of long-term durability is not a primary consideration, for it is particularly in these patients that it is desirable, if at all possible, to avoid anticoagulation. It is the view of some cardiologists that the biological valve should be favoured when operating on women of childbearing age in order to avoid anticoagulants, some of which may be teratogenic.

There is no ideal valve for all patients and it is largely consideration of the individual patient and the experience of the individual surgeon which will determine the choice of valve. Bearing in mind the problems which may arise with either biological or prosthetic valves, it is certain that cardiac valve replacement should not be undertaken lightly and if it is at all possible to preserve the mitral valve this should be attempted.

Complications of artificial valve replacement

Both prosthetic and biological valves are subject to similar postoperative complications.

1. Thromboembolic events

There is no doubt that all prosthetic heart valves are liable to attract thrombi, platelets and fibrin with consequent risk of obstruction of the valve by clot and the embolization of this clot to peripheral vessels or to the central nervous system. For this reason, and with few exceptions, patients bearing a prosthetic valve must inevitably be treated with anticoagulants for life. Other drugs, such as aspirin and dipyridamole (Persantin), are used in an attempt to avoid the use of anticoagulants, but at the time of writing their use is not well established. Biological valves are far less likely to produce thromboembolic complications and consequently anticoagulants are used for the 1st month postoperatively to allow endothelization of the fabric and of the sutures and are then discontinued.

In the rare event of almost total thrombosis of a prosthetic valve, very urgent treatment is required, for the patient is in immediate danger of dying. At one time the first line of approach was to operate on the patient as soon as possible with a view to valve replacement, but in a patient who has had previous surgery, pericardial adhesions may cause considerable delay before cardiopulmonary bypass may be instituted.

A more recent approach to this problem is the immediate use of large doses of intravenous streptokinase which almost invariably dramatically improve the patient by rapid dissolution of much of the thrombus with consequent reopening of the mitral orifice. This relief, however, may be at a price, for the author has experience of this relief being associated with either femoral embolism or cerebral embolism. However, the treatment may be so satisfactory as to require no further treatment, but in many instances it is but a delaying manoeuvre to enable a fitter patient to come to operation to replace the thrombosed valve.

At reoperation it may be enough to clear the valve completely of clot, but usually the fibrous clot with the associated new thrombus is so thick and adherent that replacement of the valve, probably using a tissue valve, is advisable.

2. Anticoagulant-related morbidity and mortality

It is inescapable that of any group of patients who are on lifelong anticoagulant therapy, a small but significant number will suffer haemorrhage which may be cerebral, retroperitoneal or gastrointestinal. Although some of these, particularly those with gastrointestinal or retroperitoneal haemorrhage, will cause no permanent problems, those patients suffering cerebral haemorrhage will usually die. It is also the case that it is not necessarily those patients whose anticoagulant control has gone wildly wrong who will experience such a disaster, for many patients with cerebral bleeding are shown to have their anticoagulant control at therapeutic levels. This problem has, of course, prompted many surgeons away from the use of prosthetic valves and towards the universal use of tissue valves, which in many cases do not require anticoagulant therapy.

3. Infection

All artificial valves, whether prosthetic or biological, are liable to septic complications. This disaster usually becomes apparent some weeks after the patient leaves hospital and is associated with a regular fever and evidence of septicaemia. Although in many instances the infection may be cured by the vigorous use of intravenous antibiotics over a prolonged period, it may be necessary to replace such a valve on account of septicaemia, valve failure, or for both these reasons.

4. *Paravalvar leak*

This complication follows detachment of the sewing ring from the patient's own valve ring, and usually occurs very shortly after operation. It may be associated with infection or be due to the cutting out of a suture from a weak area or a region from which calcium has been inadequately removed. This complication may produce cardiac failure and resuture or replacement of the valve will be necessary. More frequently, heart failure is not severe but the regurgitant jet may result in haemolytic anaemia and mild jaundice. If this is not severe the patient may be maintained by the use of iron, but frequently valve resuture or valve replacement is required.

5. *Fatigue and wear of the valve*

The earlier models of prosthetic valves were liable to many complications such as ball variance which resulted in splitting and sometimes escape of the silicone ball from the cage, rupture of struts, wearing and fragmentation of the cloth covering the struts, and fracture or escape of the disc from low profile valves. Although these complications are still from time to time reported they are now fortunately rare. Such wear may be suspected in a patient who has remained well for some years postoperatively and who develops signs of cardiac failure. In these circumstances, early cardiac catheterization or echocardiography should be undertaken to establish the function of the prosthetic valve and, if shown to be faulty, replacement may be a matter of urgency.

6. *Degeneration of biological valves*

Biological valves such as homografts, xenografts, or those valves designed from fascia lata, dura mater or pericardium, have an excellent appearance and function well when inserted. Unfortunately, some have not stood the test of time and particularly unfortunate was experience with fascia lata valves when used in the mitral position. In a large number of patients the cusps of this valve underwent thickening and retraction with consequent severe regurgitation. Other biological valves have undergone late calcification or rupture of the cusps. In some instances, late degeneration has been attributed to the method of sterilization of the valve, whether by freeze drying, irradiation or the preservation in unsuitable buffer media or unsuitable antibiotics. It is now the practice to use almost fresh human homograft aortic valves, and in those centres where this has been practised the incidence of breakdown of homograft aortic valves is now very low. The mounted porcine xenograft valve is preserved in buffered glutaraldehyde and seems to stand up extremely well, although after several years of use occasional case reports are now emerging of calcification, stenosis, or rupture of the cusps. Degeneration in biological valves will result in either stenosis or more usually regurgitation at the valve which is readily diagnosed both clinically and by cardiac catheterization. When such degeneration has been demonstrated there is no alternative but to replace the valve.

Cardiac tumours

Metastatic tumours of the heart may be detected either clinically or at autopsy, but with few exceptions surgery plays no part in their management. Likewise primary malignant tumours of the heart are rarely amenable to surgical excision.

The common tumour of the heart is the benign atrial myxoma that arises from the annulus ovale and protrudes into the left atrium, where it may fill the cavity and then project through the mitral valve. This tumour may arise from a similar site in the right atrium, but those on the left side are 10 times more frequently seen.

These tumours may cause obstructive, embolic or systemic disturbances and their diagnosis is sometimes long delayed, being frequently mistaken for mitral stenosis or heart failure. When suspected, the diagnosis is confirmed by echocardiography and angiocardiography.

Treatment

The treatment of this condition is urgent surgical removal, for increasing delay increases the likelihood of tragic embolism.

Operation

These tumours are invariably removed using cardiopulmonary bypass. The left atrium is approached as for mitral valve surgery, i.e. via median sternotomy. However, on those rare occasions when a left atrial myxoma is diagnosed during left thoracotomy, under the mistaken diagnosis of mitral stenosis, the operation may be converted into an open heart procedure through the left chest, as described on page 612, and removal of the myxoma undertaken at that time.

The serious hazard of this operation is the danger of fragmentation of the myxoma with consequent peripheral and cerebral emboli. It is therefore advised that, while the tumour is being handled, the heart is arrested by cold cardioplegia and cross-clamping the aorta during this procedure, lest an uncontrolled heartbeat eject fragments of tumour into the aorta. When the left or right atrium is involved, the tumour is noted to be friable and gelatinous, with a mixture of solid and cystic elements. It should be removed whole if possible and the use of a large spoon is helpful in this situation. The tumour will be seen to originate from a pedicle on the annulus ovale. It is advised that a disc of the atrial septum bearing this pedicle be removed and that the resultant atrial septal defect be sutured. Failure to remove completely the pedicle of the tumour has been regarded as contributory to recurrence of this tumour. The atrium and ventricle are carefully washed out to remove remaining loose fragments. The atrium is repaired, air evacuated from the heart and aorta, and bypass terminated, allowing the heart to take over the circulation.

Surgical treatment of ischaemic heart disease

After many false starts spanning the past 50 years, the surgical treatment of ischaemic heart disease at last seems rational and is based more on objective assessment rather than on the previous purely subjective complaints of the patient. Advances in treatment have been stimulated by the development of selective coronary arteriography, good cine-angiocardiography, and well-developed techniques of echocardiography, which enable an accurate diagnosis to be made of both structure and function. Furthermore, postoperative objective studies have been undertaken in many who have undergone surgical treatment for either angina pectoris or the complications of myocardial infarction, making available an enormous amount of data assessing the value of this treatment. Although there is little doubt that operations for the relief of ischaemic heart disease have been undertaken in many doubtful situations and on many occasions, the passage of time will enable a more rational assessment and it is hoped that in due course a better understanding of the indications and anticipated results of such treatment will be available. Ischaemic heart disease presents to the surgeon in the following ways:

1. Angina pectoris.
2. The complications of myocardial infarction, which are left ventricular aneurysm, ventricular septal defect or mitral regurgitation.

Treatment of angina pectoris

Although the diagnosis of angina pectoris may readily be made by good history taking, it is well established that many patients with the typical clinical features of angina pectoris prove on investigation to have a perfectly normal coronary arterial tree. It may be that in some of these patients the condition of coronary arterial spasm does exist, but it is also likely that in some their symptoms are due to other conditions such as hiatus hernia, pancreatitis or gallbladder disease. There remains a group of patients in whom full investigation will detect no such abnormality.

It is clear that the aorto-coronary bypass procedure can restore generous blood flow to ischaemic myocardium but it cannot revitalize dead muscle or make scar tissue contract. The operation was originally offered to patients with severe but stable angina,

refractory to medical treatment and in most patients the results are truly dramatic – 85% relieved of angina with an operative mortality of less than 2%. Exercise tolerance is usually improved, but there is no good evidence that, in the majority, survival is prolonged beyond that associated with good medical management. However, there are reliable data suggesting that patients with triple vessel disease who receive complete revascularization and those with left main coronary disease who have successful operations, will gain an increased life expectation.

Indications for operation

The patient with disabling angina pectoris unresponsive to a good clinical trial with nitrites and beta-blocking drugs should be considered for surgery, prior to which selective coronary arteriography is, of course, mandatory. It is important to consider the degree to which the angina affects the patient's lifestyle. Clearly, the pain experienced by an elderly patient and regarded as tolerable will, in a younger person, possibly interfere with his or her work and lifestyle to such a degree that surgical relief is indicated.

Coronary arteriography will demonstrate the number and location of blocks and it seems that obstructions of less than 50% of the diameter of the coronary artery are haemodynamically insignificant. In most patients with angina pectoris the operation is not urgent other than the conditions of pre-infarction or unstable angina and critical stenosis of the left main coronary artery. In the latter condition, angina is often severe and the patient is liable to massive and fatal infarction at any time.

Surgical treatment

Operations of historical interest, such as cardio-omentopexy, scarification of the pericardium, the Beck operations of arterialization of the coronary sinus, and the Vineberg operation of implantation of the freely bleeding internal mammary artery into the myocardium are no longer practised and are not described. The overall poor results of these operations, coupled with the unwarranted enthusiasm of many surgeons, prejudiced many cardiologists against operative intervention for coronary artery disease and delayed the emergence – in some centres for many years – of the modern and effective operation of coronary artery bypass grafting, using reversed lengths of autogenous saphenous vein.

Coronary artery bypass grafting

This operation was introduced by Favaloro in 1969. Lengths of the patient's own long saphenous vein are reversed and implanted proximally into the ascending aorta and distally beyond the blocked segment of the coronary artery. The operation is undertaken using

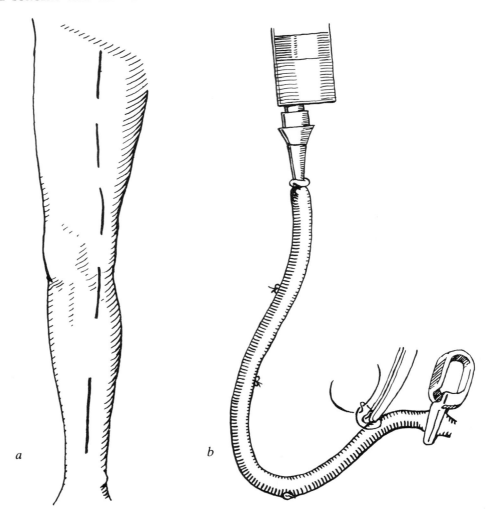

a   *b*

Figure 41.22 *a*, Exposure of the long saphenous vein for coronary artery bypass grafting is best undertaken through a series of short longitudinal incisions. *b*, Injection of reversed length of internal saphenous vein to exclude leaks

cardiopulmonary bypass and, almost invariably, cold cardioplegia, although the use of ventricular fibrillation and intermittent aortic cross-clamping has many advocates.

OBTAINING THE SAPHENOUS VEIN FOR GRAFTING

The vein may be taken from either the thigh or the leg. Whether the vein from the thigh or leg is to be preferred is a matter of controversy, but since many patients require multiple grafts it is often necessary to use the full length of the saphenous vein. The vein may be obtained either through one long incision or through multiple short incisions (Figure 41.22a). The vein is then tested for leaks by distending it with the patient's own heparinized blood or Ringer's solution. Distension of the vein in addition to identifying further leaks will reveal any twists or narrow segments when one of the side-branches has been ligated too close to the main vessels (Figure 41.22b). The vein

is carefully cleaned of adventitia and segments with aneurysmal dilatations are discarded.

ISOLATING THE CORONARY ARTERY (Figure 41.23)

The site of block of the artery has been previously determined at coronary arteriography, and may be frequently palpated as a hard mass along the line of the coronary vessel. Having identified the coronary artery, a linear incision is made into the vessel using a fine pointed scalpel, extended to about 0.75 cm in length with fine pointed Potts scissors (Figure 41.23a).

The vein to be grafted is bevelled to 45° using scissors, and care is taken to ensure that the vein is inserted in a reverse direction so that the venous valves open during flow from the aorta into the coronary artery. The vein is sutured to the open coronary artery using continuous 6/0 prolene (Figure 41.23b,c). Fine prolene is particularly suited for this

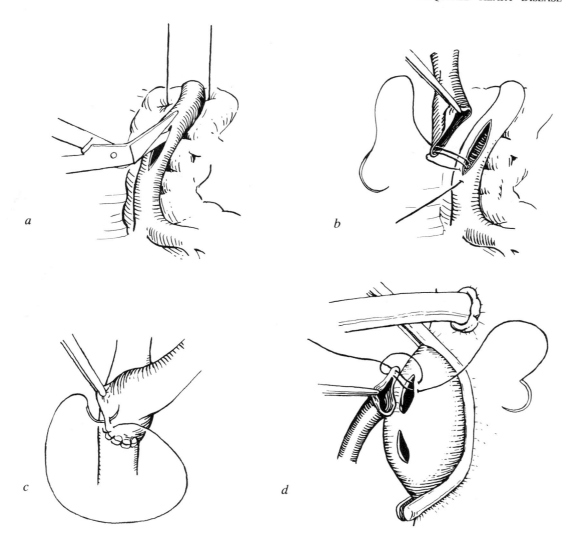

Figure 41.23 Technique of anastomosis of saphenous vein to coronary artery and of saphenous vein to ascending aorta. *a,* Following isolation of the chosen coronary artery an initial small incision is made with a pointed scalpel, following which a 6 mm incision is made with fine vascular scissors. *b,c,* Anastomosis is undertaken using continuous 6/0 or 7/0 prolene as an everting suture. *d,* Anastomosis of saphenous vein to ascending aorta using a side occlusion clamp. The anastomosis is undertaken with continuous 5/0 or 6/0 prolene as an everting suture

operation, for loops of sutures need not be drawn tight until the whole suture line is placed, and with a little traction the suture line is watertight without kinking or damage by the suture. Care must be taken to avoid purse-stringing the anastomosis. Before completing the anastomosis, fine plastic or silver probes are passed to confirm patency.

Access to the right coronary artery is best obtained by retraction of the right atrium and its cannulas to the right, and at the same time retraction of the right ventricle to the left and cephalad. Access to the marginal branches of the circumflex artery is readily obtained by elevation of the apex of the heart to the right and towards the patient's right shoulder.

The site for anastomosis is best decided prior to

operation by carefully studying the coronary arteriogram. It is usually sufficient to place one graft on the anterior descending artery, although further grafts to one or more of its diagonal branches may also be required. It is usually not possible to implant a graft into the circumflex artery for this lies deep in the atrioventricular groove, usually deep to the corresponding vein. It is usual to place one or more grafts to the lateral or obtuse marginal branches of this vessel. The right coronary artery may require disobliteration of a long atheromatous core, following which grafting may be undertaken to the main right artery or the posterior descending branch.

Following the distal anastomoses the veins are anastomosed to the ascending aorta. The ascending aorta is grasped with a vascular side-clamp and either a 5 mm hole is punched or a 5 mm slit is made with a sharp scalpel, both of which leave a clean-cut orifice on which to sew the vein. It is possible to insert two veins into the same segment of aorta which is isolated by the side-clamp. Care is taken to perform the upper anastomosis at a site where kinking is avoided. Right coronary grafts usually lie best when joined to the right side of the ascending aorta, whereas anterior descending and circumflex grafts lie best on the left side of the ascending aorta. Left-sided grafts to the anterior descending, diagonal or marginal arteries may sometimes lie more comfortably when taken in the transverse sinus behind the ascending aorta and pulmonary artery and anastomosed to the right side of the ascending aorta. A continuous suture technique is very appropriate for the proximal end of the graft using 5/0 prolene. While the upper anastomoses are undertaken, the aortic cross-clamp is released, following which the heart will rewarm and either commence spontaneous beating or require electrical defibrillation. It is the practice of some surgeons to undertake the aortic anastomoses prior to cardiopulmonary bypass and to undertake the distal anastomoses following the commencement of bypass (Figure 41.23d).

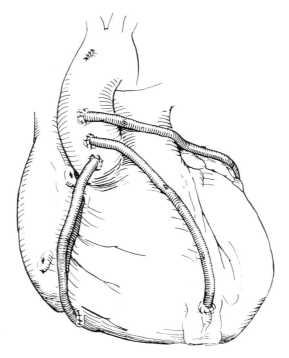

Figure 41.24 Coronary artery saphenous vein bypass grafts. Three separate grafts have been inserted into the left anterior descending coronary artery, the obtuse marginal branch of the left circumflex artery, and the right coronary artery as it turns round the base of the heart towards the posterior descending coronary artery

Having completed the grafts, it is possible to measure the flow using electromanometric devices. It is generally considered that a flow of at least 50 ml/ min will ensure a patent graft, although far higher flows are frequently recorded (Figure 41.24).

Although it has in the past been popular to provide as many as four or five separate vein bypass grafts implanted in the aorta and the recipient coronary arteries, the more recent tendency is to use perhaps only two anastomoses at the aortic end and to tailor the distal vein into sequential anastomoses, with perhaps a side-to-side anastomosis between the obtuse marginal artery and the vein continuing around the base of the heart to terminate in an end-to-side anastomosis in the posterior descending branch of the right coronary artery. By various ingenious permutations, as many as six saphenocoronary anastomoses may be undertaken with perhaps two or three segments of vein.

RESULTS

In good hands at least 80% of such bypass grafts remain patent 5 years following operation, but success relates directly to the experience of the operating surgeon.

Coronary artery bypass grafting using the left and right internal mammary arteries (Figure 41.25)

With the considerable experience available following the widespread use of the internal mammary artery during the Vineberg operation of intramyocardial insertion of a freely bleeding internal mammary artery, many surgeons were familiar with the technique of isolating the internal mammary artery from the chest wall. It was but a small step for surgeons to anastomose the distal end of the internal mammary artery to the coronary arteries using very fine suture material.

The internal mammary artery is isolated from the chest wall in a pedicle consisting of extrapleural tissues containing the internal mammary artery and vein, ligating or clipping the intercostal branches and tributaries. Although it is usually possible to bypass a block in the anterior descending coronary artery or the diagonal vessels only, more experienced surgeons are able, using both internal mammary arteries, to bypass two or more blocked coronary vessels and have in addition used this vessel for sequential grafting of up to four coronary arteries.

The advantage of the internal mammary is not only that of availability but it has been shown that over periods as long as 10 years the internal mammary–coronary artery anastomosis remains patent more frequently than do similar anastomoses undertaken using reversed lengths of internal saphenous vein. The native internal mammary artery grows and is able to deliver a far greater flow as time goes on and it is likely that more surgeons will in future utilize the internal mammary artery for at least some of the grafting undertaken at surgery (Green, 1984). More recently, the right gastro-epiploic artery has been used as a conduit in coronary bypass surgery.

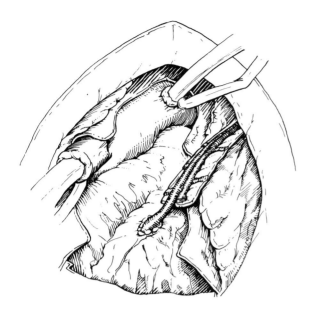

Figure 41.25 Coronary artery bypass grafting using the internal mammary artery. Mobilized pedicle of the internal mammary artery, internal mammary vein and associated chest wall tissues are brought down, following which the end of the internal mammary artery is carefully bevelled and anastomosed to the opened left anterior descending coronary artery using continuous 7/0 prolene sutures

Endarterectomy (Figure 41.26)

It is frequently the case that a coronary artery, usually the right, is almost completely blocked by a large length of atheroma. It is usually possible to remove a long sausage-like piece of this atheromatous deposit following incision into the artery, following which saphenous vein grafting may be undertaken. The atheroma may be removed either with fine dissecting instruments or by the use of carbon dioxide gas injectors.

Percutaneous transluminal coronary angioplasty

This recently introduced procedure (Grüntzig *et al.*, 1979) is a technique whereby coronary artery atheromatous obstructions may be dilated via a balloon introduced into the coronary artery at cardiac catheterization and is undertaken by either the physicians or radiologists skilled in this technique.

A fine guidewire is introduced via the femoral artery and is passed up the aorta and introduced into the orifices of the left or right coronary artery. A fine catheter is threaded over this guidewire and is passed through the coronary artery block using the image intensifier. With the injection of dye into the coronary artery the block can be readily identified and the balloon placed in an ideal situation, following which

it is forcibly dilated by the injection of a small amount of saline.

In many instances the dilatation of the atheromatous plaque is dramatic, converting a serious or almost complete obstruction of a coronary artery into a less obstructed vessel. It is rarely, if ever, possible to restore the lumen completely to normal but initial reports, extending over a period of several years, indicate that the relief of angina may be maintained for a prolonged period and at the same time further coronary arteriography may demonstrate the relief of obstruction to be well maintained over a period of several years. Several vessels may be dilated at the same sitting. Although ideally suited for the dilatation of coronary blocks, this technique may usefully be applied to those patients who have had previous surgery and in whom the current angina is caused by stenosis at the anastomosis between the saphenous vein and coronary artery.

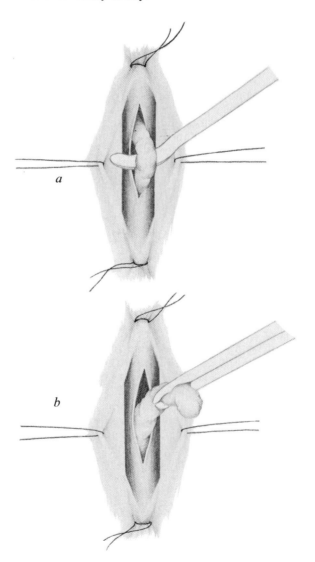

Figure 41.26 Coronary endarterectomy

It is not yet possible to assess the influence of percutaneous transluminal coronary angioplasty on the volume of surgical operations undertaken for coronary artery disease. At the present time dilatation is reserved for one or two vessels only, although in very skilled hands three or four vessels are being dilated at one sitting. So far, the influence on the volume of surgery is minimal. However, as it emerges that this is a fairly safe and successful technique, it is clear that this treatment will in due course be available in all major cardiac centres. It is likely that this technique will be reserved for patients with one- or two-vessel disease and that fewer operations for one- or two-vessel disease will be undertaken by surgeons, the operation of aorto-coronary bypass being reserved for patients requiring four or more grafts.

Whether patients in the future are treated by surgeons, or by physicians, will in no way make either of them less busy for the foreseeable future, for there are clearly far more patients requiring relief of coronary artery obstruction than there are facilities, surgeons or physicians available to treat them.

COMPLICATIONS

The important complication is dissection of an important coronary artery with the production of early myocardial infarction. Should dissection of the vessel occur during percutaneous transluminal coronary angioplasty it is imperative that the patient is transferred to the operating theatre immediately for formal aorto-coronary venous bypass operation. For this reason the medical operation of percutaneous transluminal coronary angioplasty is undertaken only in hospitals where cardiac surgeons are immediately available with a vacant operating theatre to deal with this complication.

Recurrence of angina following coronary artery bypass grafting

Although this may be due to progression of disease, the most likely cause is obstruction of the vein grafts, which may in turn be due either to complete thrombosis of the vein or more likely to obstruction at the anastomosis. This latter complication when occurring early is probably associated with a technical fault, for despite the many variables involved, it seems that a good initial anastomosis in the presence of good 'run-off' offers the patient the best chance of late patency of the graft. Recurrence of angina requires further coronary arteriography and, if indicated, further bypass grafting.

Surgical treatment of complications of myocardial infarction

Infarction followed by necrosis and fibrosis may damage the ventricular septum, its free wall or the papillary muscles. Damage and perforation of the septum will result in a post-infarction ventricular septal defect which is an acute condition resulting in very severe congestive heart failure. Necrosis of the free wall of the left ventricle may result in fatal perforation into the pericardium but may frequently produce a left ventricular aneurysm. Although the aneurysm may appear much larger than the ventricle itself, it must be remembered that the original lesion which produced the aneurysm consisted of no more than perhaps 20% of the ventricular wall. Damage to the papillary muscle by either rupture or dysfunction will result in mitral valve regurgitation.

Post-infarction ventricular septal defect

This is a serious condition. Although the patient may be in very severe heart failure, it is frequently surgically unwise to attempt closure of the defect earlier than 1 week following the myocardial infarction. The edges of the defect are otherwise oedematous and necrotic and it is unlikely that they will hold sutures. If the patient's condition allows a waiting period of 2 weeks following the myocardial infarction, the edges of the acquired ventricular septal defect will usually become thickened and fibrous. The defect may occur anywhere in the septum and when the anterior descending coronary artery has been obstructed the defect is often anterior and low in the septum and may be difficult to find from the right ventricular aspect where it may be overlain by large trabeculae and papillary muscles. The defect should be closed using a Dacron patch held in place by interrupted non-absorbent sutures, or with a sandwich of two patches of Teflon outside the heart.

Left ventricular aneurysm

Although aneurysms may appear on the left border of the heart, they are best approached via median sternotomy using cardiopulmonary bypass. The patients are often in a poor condition and, following the rapid establishment of cardiopulmonary bypass, dissection of the pericardium from the aneurysm may then proceed. It is unwise to attempt dissection earlier for this may produce troublesome arrhythmias and furthermore there is the real danger of perforating the very thin aneurysm before cardiopulmonary bypass is established, or of dislodging thrombi into the circulation.

When on full bypass a left ventricular vent is inserted through the aneurysm. Aspiration of this vent collapses the aneurysm which appears as a saucer in the left ventricle and the extent of the aneurysm is then clearly defined.

During excision of the aneurysm it is important to leave in place a rim of fibrous tissue to enable sutures to hold well. The interior of the heart is carefully examined and frequently large amounts of adherent thrombus will be found which require removal. At the same time the septum is examined for a previously

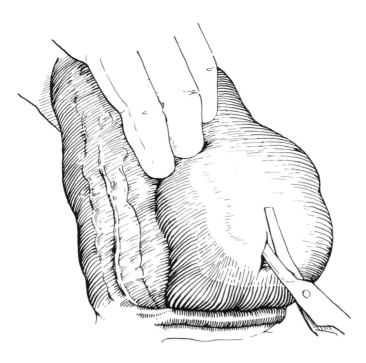

Figure 41.27 Opening into left ventricular aneurysm. This aneurysm is on the base of the heart in the territory supplied by the right coronary artery and the heart has been elevated and turned backwards to expose the aneurysm

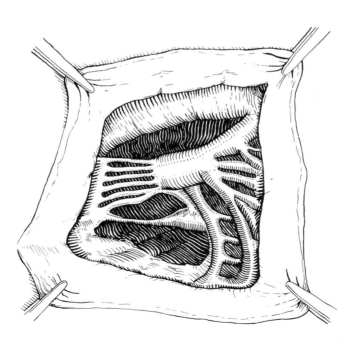

Figure 41.28 The left ventricular aneurysm has been opened and much of it excised apart from a 1 cm rim of fibrous tissue around its edge for secure suturing. The interior of the heart and the papillary muscles of the left ventricle are shown

undetected ventricular septal defect. While the aneurysm is being excised it is usual to cross-clamp the aorta to ensure that any detached thrombi in the left ventricle are not carried into the general circulation and to protect the heart by the use of cold cardioplegia. Following removal of the wall of the aneurysm and removal of clots from the ventricle, the aortic clamp may then be opened, allowing continuous coronary perfusion and normal heart action (Figures 41.27 and 41.28).

Closure of the ventricle

This is achieved using continuous and interrupted sutures of heavy prolene, taken in two layers. Support of these sutures with Teflon felt buttresses is usually necessary (Figure 41.29).

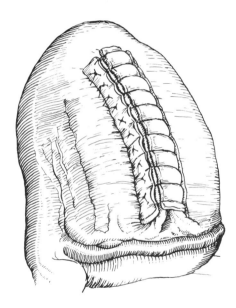

Figure 41.29 Closure of left ventricular aneurysm using heavy prolene sutures buttressed with Teflon felt supports; these sutures may be interrupted or continuous

Mitral regurgitation

Mitral regurgitation following myocardial infarction may be due to so-called 'papillary muscle dysfunction' or to rupture of a necrotic papillary muscle. In any event, these patients are extremely seriously ill and although their only hope is mitral valve replacement, using cardiopulmonary bypass, the results of this treatment are poor, reflecting the gravity of the condition which is treated.

Treatment of patients with very poorly functioning left ventricle

Although cardiac surgery for ischaemic heart disease may safely be undertaken in patients with an ejection fraction as low as 20%, or in some hands even lower, it is realistic to suppose that such surgery is probably inadvisable. Patients with very poor left ventricles usually do not complain of angina so much as shortness of breath due to left ventricular failure, and it is in these patients that other treatment is advised.

The most straightforward treatment is that of cardiac transplantation and there are now more centres where this may be made available to the patient. However, a newly developed operation of cardiomyoplasty is undergoing clinical investigation and the results are variable. The basis of this operation is in the physiological observation that skeletal muscle which is slowly contracting may be trained by the use of a pacemaker to contract more rapidly.

Cardiomyoplasty

The pedicled latissimus dorsi is wrapped around the heart. It is then made to function by the use of a specially implanted pacemaker causing contraction at about 70 beats/min. This in experimental animals and in some patients has been shown to be very efficacious in raising the ejection fraction to as high as 50% of normal, with great improvement in all parameters and in the clinical condition. Should this procedure prove to be successful in the long term, and reliable, it may well supplant cardiac transplantation, but it is far too early to make other than a very general philosophical statement.

Pulmonary embolism

Treatment of massive pulmonary embolism

Whereas the treatment of massive pulmonary embolism was until recently a choice between operation or treatment with anticoagulants, the subject has been further complicated by the introduction of powerful thrombolytic enzymes used intravenously, of which streptokinase is the most favoured. The protagonists of anticoagulant and thrombolytic therapy appear convinced that few patients now need surgical removal of pulmonary emboli and that the great majority of these patients will survive with this conservative management.

On the other hand, the view of many physicians and surgeons is that the simplicity of removal of these large obstructing emboli and the urgency of this operation must inevitably be the preferred treatment in the collapsed and possibly dying patient. These apparently opposing views are not irreconcilable.

Although the direct removal of massive pulmonary emboli from the pulmonary artery was first attempted by Trendelenburg in 1908, few successes were reported until the advent of cardiopulmonary bypass.

Pulmonary embolectomy

Indications

The criteria for surgical intervention will vary and in some centres little time is lost in operating on patients who in other centres would be treated conservatively for a further period. It is, of course, important that the diagnosis be established, for all of the following conditions have been mistakenly treated as massive pulmonary embolism and submitted to surgery:

1. Myocardial infarction, or myocarditis.
2. Postoperative septic shock.
3. Postoperative low output state.
4. Mesenteric vascular occlusion.
5. Acute pericarditis.
6. Acute pancreatitis.

The diagnosis is best established by pulmonary arteriography, together with lung scanning, but these facilities may not always be available. It is not always the case that these patients present with so-called 'typical' physical findings and patients may suffer with major pulmonary embolism, having a normal jugular venous pressure. Electrocardiography is frequently of very great assistance, a recent change of axis from left to right being significant. No reliance whatsoever should be placed on the appearances at chest radiography, for many patients dying with massive pulmonary embolism have an apparently normal plain chest radiograph. The timing of operation is important, for published figures indicate that the chance of survival is poor for patients who have their operation following resuscitation from an episode of cardiac arrest.

Arbitrary definitions and levels of 'shock', hypotension, oliguria or even anuria are referred to in the literature when the indications for surgical intervention are discussed. If the patient is allowed to deteriorate before surgery is recommended, this reflects the conservative approach of many clinicians. On the other hand, operative intervention on a diagnosis alone in a reasonably fit patient will clearly produce excellent operative results, albeit at the expense of some unnecessary surgery. These disparate views are reflected in the excellent results of this operation in some hands and the poor experience of others. It is clear that to await a prolonged period of severe hypotension, oliguria or anuria is to court disaster. Once considered, operation should be undertaken as soon as possible, and in an institution where those familiar with cardiothoracic surgery are present or available the timing of such an operation should be fairly well defined and the operative results acceptable.

Methods

Pulmonary embolectomy may be undertaken in one of two ways:

1. Using cardiopulmonary bypass.
2. Using inflow occlusion without cardiopulmonary bypass.

1. USING CARDIOPULMONARY BYPASS

General anaesthesia should be induced very carefully, for the patient's circulation may be maintained only by intense peripheral vasoconstriction. If this compensatory effect is abolished by the hasty administration of intravenous anaesthetics and relaxants, further hypotension and cardiac arrest may occur.

Full cardiopulmonary bypass is instituted following median sternotomy (Figure 41.30). The main pulmonary artery is opened vertically above the valve and the clot is removed with forceps and suction. Desjardin's common bile duct forceps are very useful, for their angles make it possible to explore the distal branches of both the right and left pulmonary arteries in order to secure clots. The right and left pleural cavities may be opened to enable the lungs to be gently massaged in order to extrude further thrombi in a retrograde direction, and at this stage forced ventilation of the lungs by the anaesthetist is useful to this end. When all clots have been removed the interior of the right ventricle and right atrium should be inspected and if necessary explored, for large coiled-up thrombi are often impacted in these chambers. The pulmonary artery is closed with a fine continuous suture and the patient gradually weaned from bypass.

Following this procedure it is considered by some surgeons that attention should now be turned to the inferior vena cava to undertake a procedure that will hopefully prevent further peripheral and pelvic thrombi from reaching the heart (see Chapter 45).

2. USING INFLOW OCCLUSION

Whereas pulmonary embolectomy using cardiopulmonary bypass is ideal, many patients present with major pulmonary embolism in hospitals where cardiac surgeons and cardiac surgery are not available. Although cardiac surgeons have from time to time travelled together with their equipment to undertake embolectomy in such hospitals, it is clear that this is unlikely to become a routine procedure. It is also clear that it is usually not possible to transfer such patients to cardiac surgical centres. It is, however, possible for cardiac surgeons or general surgeons to undertake pulmonary embolectomy in hospitals lacking the equipment for cardiopulmonary bypass and using the simplest of equipment.

Median sternotomy is undertaken using a Gigli saw, which is usually available in most general hospitals. The pericardium is opened vertically, and following a period of oxygenation of the patient with 100% oxygen for several minutes, the superior and inferior venae cavae are occluded using shod intestinal clamps (Figure 41.31). The heart is allowed to beat for a

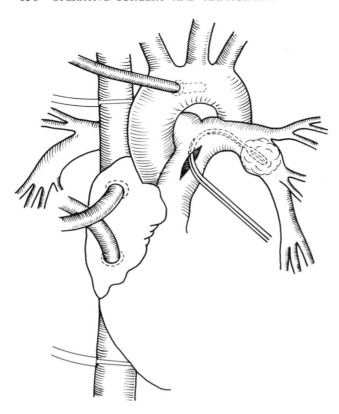

Figure 41.30 Pulmonary embolectomy using cardiopulmonary bypass. Desjardins' fully curved bile duct forceps are very useful for grasping distal thrombi

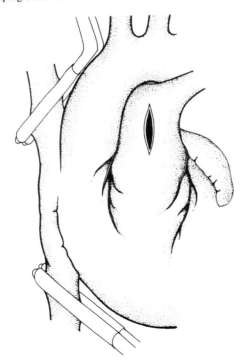

Figure 41.31 Pulmonary embolectomy without cardiopulmonary bypass. Inflow occlusion by caval clamping is well tolerated for several short periods

further 10–15 s to empty it of blood and the pulmonary artery, which is usually bulging and tense with clot, is incised vertically for 3 cm just above the pulmonary valve. This incision will be rewarded by the expulsion of a certain amount of blood together with masses of old and organizing thrombus. As much as possible is removed from the distal pulmonary arteries using Desjardins' clamps and the heart is massaged in order to milk further thrombus from the right ventricle. At the moment of caval occlusion the clock is watched carefully, and after a period of 2 min the superior vena caval clamp is removed, allowing the heart to fill with blood and to eject from the incision in the pulmonary artery. At that moment the pulmonary artery incision is occluded with a Satinsky or similar clamp, and the inferior vena caval clamp is then removed. To facilitate the reapplication of the Satinsky clamp, stay sutures of 4/0 Mersilene are placed in the pulmonary artery prior to its incision. The circulation is thus restarted and it is likely that the administration of inotropic drugs such as adrenaline, isoprenaline or dopamine will be required. Following a further period of 5 min of resumed circulation with both cavae unclamped, the Satinsky clamp is again removed, allowing a further 2 min period of exploration of the pulmonary artery.

In most patients one or two periods of pulmonary artery exploration will enable the majority of thrombus to be removed and following the final application of the Satinsky clamp the pulmonary artery is repaired using the previously placed stay sutures as a continuous running stitch.

Although undertaking pulmonary embolectomy by caval occlusion is less satisfactory than it is with the use of cardiopulmonary bypass, it remains the only hope for the majority of patients requiring pulmonary embolectomy, for it is unrealistic to advocate cardiopulmonary bypass when in the majority of instances it is not available.

Acknowledgement

The editor wishes to thank W. B. Saunders Company of Philadelphia and Dr Denton Cooley of the Texas Heart Institute for permission to copy and modify the following illustrations in this chapter: Figures 41.3, 41.15, 41.22, 41.23, 41.26, 41.27–41.29.

References

Carpentier, A. *et al.* (1980) Reconstructive surgery of mitral valve incompetence: ten year appraisal *J. Thorac. Cardiovasc. Surg.*, **79**, 338

Favaloro, R. G. (1969) Saphenous vein graft in the surgical treatment of coronary artery disease: operative technique. *J. Thorac. Cardiovasc. Surg.*, **58**, 178

Green, G. E. (1984) Internal mammary–coronary anastomosis for myocardial ischaemia. In *Gibbon's Surgery of the Chest*, 4th edn (eds D. C. Sabiston and F. C. Spencer), Saunders, Philadelphia, pp. 1451–1458

Grüntzig, A. R., Senning, A. and Siegenthaler, W. E. (1979) Non-operative dilatation of coronary artery stenosis. *N. Engl. J. Med.*, **301**, 61–68

Harken, D.E., Ellis, L.B. *et al.* (1948) The surgical treatment of mitral stenosis. *N. Engl. J. Med.*, **239**, 804

McGoon, D.C. (1960) Repair of a mitral insufficiency due to ruptured chordae tendineae. *J. Thorac. Cardiovasc. Surg.*, **39**, 357

Further reading

Amoury, R. A., Bowman, F. O., Jr *et al.* (1966) Endocarditis associated with intracardiac prostheses. *J. Thorac. Cardiovasc. Surg.*, **51**, 36

Bailey, C. P. (1949) The surgical treatment of mitral stenosis (mitral commissurotomy). *Dis. Chest*, **15**, 377

Bailey, C. P., May, A. *et al.* (1957) Survival after coronary endarterectomy in man. *J. Am. Med. Ass.*, **164**, 641

Baker, C., Brock, R. C. *et al.* (1950) Valvulotomy for mitral stenosis. *Br. Med. J.*, **1**, 1283

Barratt-Boyes, B. G., Roche, A. H. G. *et al.* (1969) Aortic valve replacement – a long-term follow-up of an initial series of 101 patients. *Circulation*, **40**, 763

Beck, C. S. (1948) Revascularization of the heart. *Ann. Surg.*, **128**, 854

Berger, S. and Salzman, E. W. (1974) Thromboembolic complications of prosthetic devices. In *Progress in Haemostasis and Thrombosis*, Vol. II (ed. T. Spaet), Grune and Stratton, New York, p. 273

Bradley, M. N., Bennett, A. L., III, *et al.* (1964) Successful unilateral pulmonary embolectomy without cardiopulmonary bypass. *N. Engl. J. Med.*, **271**, 713

Braun, L. O., Kincaid, O. W. and McGoon, D. C. (1973) Prognosis of aortic valve replacement in relation to preoperative heart size. *J. Thorac. Cardiovasc. Surg.*, **65**, 381

Braunwald, E., Lambrew, C. T. *et al.* (1964) Idiopathic hypertrophic sub-aortic stenosis. *Circulation*, **30**, Suppl. 4, 1

Cooley, D. A., Leachman, R. D. *et al.* (1973) Diffuse muscular sub-aortic stenosis: surgical treatment. *Am. J. Cardiol.*, **31**, 1

Cooley, D. A., Ott, D. A. and Reul, G. J. Jr (1987) The aortic arch. In *Operative Surgery and Management*, 2nd edn (ed. G. Keen), Wright, Bristol

Cutler, E. C. and Levine, S. A. (1923) Cardiotomy and valvulotomy for mitral stenosis. *Boston Med. Surg. J.*, **188**, 1023

Hammermeister, K. E. (1983) *Coronary Bypass Surgery*, Praeger, New York

Holman, E. and Willett, F. (1955) Results of radical pericardiectomy for constrictive pericarditis. *J. Am. Med. Ass.*, **157**, 789

Miller, G. A. H., Sutton, G. C. *et al.* (1971) Comparison of streptokinase and heparin in treatment of isolated acute massive pulmonary embolism. *Br. Med. J.*, **2**, 681–684

Moor, G. F. and Sabiston, D. C., Jr (1970) Embolectomy for chronic pulmonary embolism and hypertension. Case report and review of the problem. *Circulation*, **41**, 701

Muller, W. H., Jr, Dammann, J. F., Jr *et al.* (1960) Surgical correction of cardiovascular deformities in Marfan's syndrome. *Ann. Surg.*, **152**, 506

Mullin, M. J., Engelman, R. M. *et al.* (1974) Experience with open mitral commissurotomy in 100 consecutive patients. *Surgery*, **76**, 974

Pluth, J. R. and McGoon, D. C. (1974) Current status of heart valve replacement. *Mod. Concepts Cardiovasc. Dis.*, **43**, 65

Robinson, M. J. and Ruedy, J. (1962) Sequela of bacterial endocarditis. *Am. J. Med.*, **32**, 922

Roe, B. B., Edmunds, H., Jr *et al.* (1971) Open mitral commissurotomy. *Ann. Thorac. Surg.*, **12**, 483

Ross, D. N. *et al.* (1979) Allograft and autograft valves used for aortic valve replacement. In *Tissue Heart Valves* (ed. M. Ionescue), Butterworths, London

Sabiston, D. C., Jr and Wolfe, W. G. (1968) Experimental and clinical observations on the natural history of pulmonary embolism. *Ann. Surg.*, **168**, 1

Sauvage, L. R., Wood, S. J., Eyer, K. M. *et al.* (1963) Experimental coronary artery surgery: preliminary observations of bypass venous grafts, longitudinal arteriotomies and end-to-end anastomoses. *J. Thorac. Cardiovasc. Surg.*, **46**, 825

Selzer, A. and Cohen, K. E. (1972) Natural history of mitral stenosis: a review. *Circulation*, **45**, 878

Sharp, E. H. (1962) Pulmonary embolectomy: successful removal of a massive pulmonary embolus with the support of cardiopulmonary bypass. A case report. *Ann. Surg.*, **156**, 1

Sones, F. and Shirey, E. K. (1962) Cine coronary angiography. *Mod. Conc. Cardiovasc. Dis.*, **31**, 735

Souttar, H. S. (1955) Correspondence to Blades B. Intrathoracic surgery (lungs, heart and great vessels: surgical management of diseases of the oesophagus), 1905–55. *Int. Abstr. Surg.*, **100**, 413

Speller, D. C. E and Mitchell, R. G. (1973) Coagulase-negative staphylococci causing endocarditis after cardiac surgery. *J. Clin. Pathol.*, **26**, 517

Starr, A. and Edwards, M. L. (1961) Mitral replacement: clinical experience with a ball valve prosthesis. *Ann. Surg.*, **154**, 726

Starr, A., Grunkemeier, G. L. and Lambert, L. E. (1977) Aortic valve replacement. A ten-year follow up of non cloth covered vs cloth covered caged ball prostheses. *Circulation*, **56** (Suppl. 2), 133

Stinson, E. B., Griepp, R. B. *et al.* (1974) Clinical experience with a porcine aortic valve xenograft for mitral valve replacement. *Ann. Thorac. Surg.*, **18**, 391

Stinson, E. B., Griepp, R. B. and Oyer, P. E. (1977) Long term experience with porcine valve xenografts. *J. Thorac. Cardiovasc. Surg.*, **73**, 54

Trendelenburg, F. (1908) Ueber die operative Behandlung der Embolie der Lungenarterie. *Arch. Klin. Chir.*, **86**, 686

Vineberg, A. M. (1946) Development of an anastomosis between the coronary vessels and a transplanted internal mammary artery. *Can. Med. Assoc. J.*, **55**, 117

Wallace, R. B., Londe, S. P. *et al.* (1974) Aortic valve replacement with preserved aortic valve homografts. *J. Thorac. Cardiovasc. Surg.*, **67**, 44

Zacharias, A., Grones, L. K. *et al.* (1975) Rupture of the posterior wall of the left ventricle following mitral valve replacement. *J. Thorac. Cardiovasc. Surg.*, **69**, 259

42

The aortic arch

D. A. Cooley, D. A. Ott and G. J. Reul, Jr

Managing aneurysms of the transverse aortic arch remains a challenge for surgeons. Because the great vessels arising from the aortic arch provide the cerebral blood flow, manipulation of these vessels during operation may result in severe neurological complications. Clamping the arteries without the proper support may result in permanent neurological damage from cerebral ischaemia. Manipulation of the arteries may release atherosclerotic debris, or air may be introduced causing cerebral embolization. Proximal and distal clamping of the transverse aorta without support results not only in cerebral ischaemia but also in ischaemia to most vital structures, that is, the spinal cord, abdominal viscera, the kidneys and, proximally, ischaemia to the heart. Without careful placement of clamps or sutures, damage to other anatomical structures such as the recurrent laryngeal nerve, the venous drainage or the oesophagus may occur.

Most pathological conditions of the transverse arch and its branches have generalized involvement of the proximal and distal arteries and aorta, so that haemostasis and adequate restoration of flow are difficult. This, along with supportive measures during repair, may result in excessive bleeding. Furthermore, there are other operative risk factors in most patients such as old age, generalized arteriosclerosis, coronary arteriosclerosis, hypertension with early renal failure and/or chronic obstructive pulmonary disease.

Aneurysms of the aortic arch can, however, be treated successfully. This chapter describes our operative approach.

Surgical anatomy

The thoracic aorta is divided into the ascending, transverse arch, and descending aorta. The transverse aortic arch is that portion of the thoracic aorta that extends from the origin of the innominate artery or whichever is the first major great vessel to the last great vessel. In most cases, the last great vessel is the left subclavian artery. The distal portion of the aortic arch is also demarcated inferiorly by the ductus arteriosus or its remnant the ligamentum arteriosum. At the most distal portion of the transverse arch, the recurrent laryngeal nerve crosses over the ligamentum arteriosum. The reflexion of the pericardium extends to the level of the origin of the innominate artery. The innominate vein overlies the uppermost portion of the aortic arch and the origin of the innominate artery. The trachea and oesophagus are immediately posterior to the ascending aorta and arch (Figure 42.1).

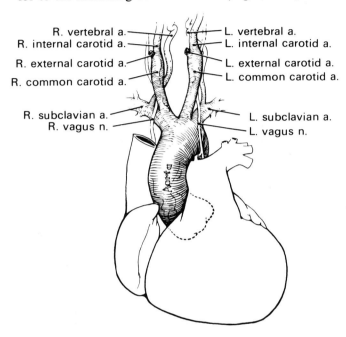

Figure 42.1 Anatomy of the aortic arch and great vessels. The transverse aortic arch is that part of the aorta which lies in between the first and last great vessel

Pathology

The major pathological lesions discussed here are aneurysms and occlusive lesions of the arch and/or its branches. Traumatic lesions may occur either by deceleration injuries with blunt trauma or by penetrating and perforating injuries caused by various missiles or sharp instruments. The approach to traumatic lesions of this area is similar to the approach for the other pathological lesions. Several reviews have been written on this subject (Reul et al., 1973; 1974; Reul, 1976; Schaff and Brawley, 1977).

The pathology of aneurysms and occlusive lesions of the arch and great vessels is of particular significance and in some instances quite different from aneurysms and occlusive lesions in other areas of the vasculature.

Table 42.1 Types of arch aneurysm

Anatomical classification
  Saccular
  Fusiform
  Dissecting
  Pseudo-aneurysm

Aetiological classification
  Congenital
    Marfan's syndrome
    Ehlers–Danlos syndrome
    Poststenotic from congenital lesions

Degenerative
  Arteriosclerosis
  Cystic medial necrosis
  Fibromuscular intimal hyperplasia

Inflammatory
  Syphilis
  Mycotic
  Postoperative infection

Mechanical
  Dissecting
  Iatrogenic – catheterization, cannulation, etc.

Aneurysmal and occlusive lesions

Aneurysms

A clinically applicable classification of arch aneurysms on an anatomical basis is difficult, since there has been confusion with regard to terminology (Table 42.1). Fusiform aneurysms involve the entire circumference of the aorta and usually have a more ovoid configuration. In a sacciform aneurysm, the defect in the aortic wall is confined to a portion of the circumference, whereas the remainder of the aortic wall is uninvolved.

Other considerations in management of the aneurysm are whether it is dissecting, i.e. a double lumen is present, or whether the aneurysm is false, i.e. it does not comprise all layers of the aorta. Most dissecting aneurysms are fusiform; however, some may be saccular. False aneurysms, on the other hand, are frequently saccular and rather extensive. Arteriosclerotic aneurysms are usually fusiform, whereas most syphilitic aneurysms are saccular.

Another useful classification is based on the cause of aneurysms of the transverse aortic arch: congenital, degenerative, inflammatory or mechanical. Most commonly, congenital aneurysms found in the thoracic aorta are associated with Marfan's syndrome. Rarely are such aneurysms caused by Ehlers–Danlos syndrome. In addition, some aneurysms of the aortic arch may result from poststenotic dilatation caused by obstructing congenital lesions or pseudo-coarctation of the aorta. These aneurysms may occur in severe cases of supravalvular aortic stenosis or congenital aortic stenosis or in cases of coarctation of the

thoracic aorta. Such aneurysms are rare, since the aorta most commonly becomes dilated or tortuous under these circumstances.

In developed countries degenerative aneurysms of the thoracic aorta are most common and are seen in older patients, whereas in underdeveloped countries inflammatory aneurysms are more common and are seen in younger patients. In the USA, the most common cause of degenerative aneurysm is arteriosclerosis. In most instances, other portions of the thoracic or abdominal aorta are involved, the most common site being the infrarenal abdominal aorta. When the arch is involved, arteriosclerosis is most frequently associated with uncontrolled hypertension and other risk factors associated with generalized arteriosclerosis. There may also be occlusive lesions of the great vessels and their branches. Fortunately, in most instances when the aortic arch is involved with arteriosclerosis, there is merely a dilatation, and other aneurysms of the aorta take precedence. There usually is a large amount of arteriosclerotic debris and clot inside the aneurysms, which may result in cerebral embolization.

Another type of degenerative process that may result in aneurysm formation is cystic medial necrosis. The media and, in most cases, the elastic lamina of the aorta degenerate and are replaced by necrotic cystic material. Medial necrosis may also occur without cyst formation. This type of degenerative process may be associated with dissection and formation of a saccular or fusiform dissecting aneurysm. The pathological findings are similar to those of Marfan's syndrome.

In the great vessels fibromuscular intimal hyperplasia may also result in aneurysm formation. This is probably due to poststenotic dilatation that results from the stenotic lesions.

Of the inflammatory lesions that cause aneurysm formation, syphilis is the most common. Although syphilitic lesions of the aortic arch have become rare in this country, they are common in other countries. The syphilitic aorta is somewhat different grossly from the arteriosclerotic aorta; the syphilitic aorta is thickened from chronic inflammation, and there may be several layers of calcium and gummatous deposits. Debris, which is present in large amounts in these aneurysms, acts as a potential source for embolization. Because the entire aorta is involved, proximal and distal anastomoses can be difficult to make. The origin of the great vessels may also be involved with occlusive lesions.

Mycotic aneurysms are also inflammatory lesions. True mycotic aneurysms of the aortic arch are quite rare. Marasmic implantations are spared in this area, probably because of the high rate of blood flow. Rarely, following arch replacement or great vessel surgery, a postoperative infection may occur, resulting in an infected graft or in pseudo-aneurysm formation. Usually the surrounding structures are also involved, i.e. lungs, heart and oesophagus. Because of the vital structures involved, aneurysms of the aortic arch are extremely difficult to treat.

Dissecting aneurysms have mechanical causes. These are perhaps the most difficult aneurysms to manage surgically. The lesions may be quite complex, involving the entire aorta and extending into the great vessels. If the aneurysm is acute, the consistency of the aorta is altered by oedema and inflammation. The presence of a double lumen also weakens the aortic wall, making suturing difficult. Dissection may extend into the aortic root and cause dehiscence of the aortic valve, necessitating aortic valve replacement and/or coronary artery reimplantation.

The most common causes of dissecting aneurysm of the aortic arch are medial degeneration and necrosis of the thoracic aorta, resulting in a mechanical tearing of the intima and a large false lumen or haematoma confined by a partial layer of media and adventitia. There may or may not be a re-entry site. Degeneration from arteriosclerosis has been the commonest cause of dissection in our series. The arteriosclerosis is associated with hypertension. Syphilitic lesions rarely cause dissection. Post-traumatic deceleration injuries of the thoracic aorta may cause retrograde or antegrade dissection into the aortic arch.

Iatrogenic manipulations such as cardiac catheterization or cannulation for cardiopulmonary bypass may also cause aortic arch dissection. Because they are acute, they may be difficult problems to manage.

Dissecting aneurysms of the aortic arch may originate with an intimal tear of the ascending aorta. The aneurysm may dissect into the entire distal aorta involving the arch, the descending thoracic aorta and abdominal aorta. In most instances these aneurysms can be managed by replacing the ascending thoracic aorta and obliterating the distal lumen just proximal to the arch.

The most difficult dissections to handle are the acute dissections that occur when a descending thoracic aortic aneurysm ruptures retrograde into the arch, ascending aorta and coronary arteries (Reul et al., 1975).

Dissecting aneurysms involving the ascending aorta and aortic arch require resection only when they cannot be controlled by proximal or distal aortic surgery – that is, false lumen obliteration by resecting the ascending aneurysm portion. If the major great vessels are involved as indicated by loss of pulse or neurological deficit, then limited surgical intervention by bypass to the involved vessel may be done along with repair of the distal or proximal thoracic aorta. If the arch portion is dilated and is aneurysmal with a large haematoma or a thin outer layer, that is, if potential rupture is apparent, then arch replacement should be done.

In chronic dissecting aneurysms of the aortic arch, occasionally a large dilatation, causing respiratory obstruction or a potential danger of rupture, may be an indication for surgical intervention (Grande et al., 1984).

Occlusive lesions

Occlusive lesions of the great vessels of the aortic arch are most commonly caused by arteriosclerosis. The arteriosclerotic plaques are localized usually to the sites of origin of the great vessels. Frequently other branches of the great vessels are involved such as the subclavian artery, vertebral artery and internal or external carotid arteries.

Syphilis rarely may cause areas of obstruction of the great vessels and is usually associated with generalized aortic disease (Duncan and Cooley, 1983c).

A unique type of obliterative process of the great vessels, described by Takayasu (1908), causes hypoplasia of the great vessels that may obliterate the lumen in advanced cases (Figure 42.2). Takayasu's arteritis most commonly occurs in young girls of Oriental descent (Shimizu and Sano, 1951). The pathological conditions causing occlusive lesions of the aortic arch have been described as the 'aortic arch syndrome' (Duncan and Cooley, 1983a–c).

Clinical picture

Aneurysms of the aortic arch, like aneurysms in other areas of the aorta, are frequently asymptomatic. For symptoms to occur, the aneurysm must be large. Actual erosion into the sternum may occur with chronic aneurysms, particularly the syphilitic type. Pain from pressure of the aneurysm on the sternum or surrounding structures is probably the most common presenting symptom (Kampmeier, 1938). Symptoms of hoarseness or chronic 'brassy' cough may occur as a result of stretching or damage to the left recurrent laryngeal nerve, which passes over the ligamentum arteriosum. Respiratory symptoms associated with chronic respiratory distress and in some cases acute respiratory distress have been described (Lefrak et al., 1972). The trachea may be compressed if the aneurysm expands posteriorly. Haemoptysis is a distressing sign, since this may indicate erosion of the aneurysm into the pulmonary parenchyma or bronchi. In most instances when frank haemoptysis appears in association with an arch aneurysm, rupture is imminent.

Some patients feel the sensation of a large mass in their neck. This may be associated with dysphagia, when the aneurysm compresses the oesophagus during swallowing.

When dissecting aneurysms of the aortic arch are associated with aneurysms of the ascending or descending aorta, symptoms are pain, cough, dyspnoea, loss of pulse, or neurological signs.

Patients with occlusive lesions of the great vessels most often have cerebrovascular symptoms. Stroke, transient ischaemic attacks or localized neurological signs, or any combination of these, may occur, depending on the blocked vessel. In some instances, a transient ischaemic attack occurs not from the vascular obstructive lesion, but from embolization of debris

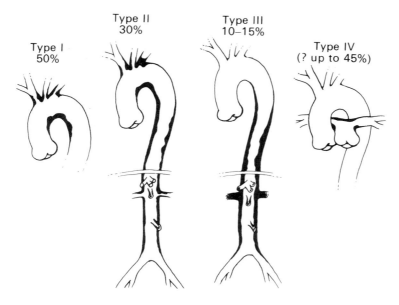

Figure 42.2 A simplified classification of Takayasu's syndrome, with the incidence of the various types

from an ulcerative plaque. Most arteriosclerotic plaques of the great vessels are not ulcerated, although ulcerative plaques are commonly found in the internal carotid artery at the common carotid artery bifurcation.

When the origin of the subclavian artery is occluded the 'subclavian steal syndrome' may result. This happens because the ipsilateral vertebral artery supplies blood to the upper extremity in a retrograde manner by way of intracranial collateral arteries, in particular the basilar system and posterior circulation. This is most frequently an angiographic finding rather than a true clinical syndrome, because in most cases cerebrovascular symptoms associated with exercise of the ipsilateral extremity occur infrequently. On the other hand, in some instances vertebrobasilar insufficiency may be associated with these lesions, and corrective surgery can abolish the symptoms. True claudication of the hand may also occur, depending on the collateral circulation and the level of obstruction. Gangrene of the upper extremity, which is only rarely associated with occlusive lesions of the aortic arch, may be related to distal embolization of necrotic debris from an aortic arch aneurysm or to ulcerative plaques of the great vessels.

Diagnosis

Although both aneurysmal and occlusive lesions may be suspected by careful observation of the patient's signs and symptoms, diagnosis is usually made by using X-rays, computed tomography or arteriography. Plain chest radiographs may show a large superior mediastinal mass in patients with transverse arch aneurysm and, in most cases, there is deviation

of the trachea to the right, although deviation of the trachea to the left may also occur. Pulsation of the sternal notch or sternum may be present with large aneurysms.

Computed tomography gives a definitive diagnosis of thoracic aneurysms and is especially useful in delineating dissection. Computed tomography will also show clot-filled aneurysms, bony erosions, peri-aortic masses and dissected intima (Doust, 1984). Computed tomography demonstrates both the lumen and mural thrombus, whereas angiography demonstrates the patent channel and the patent branches.

Angiography gives a definitive diagnosis of aneurysms of the transverse arch and aids in determining the type of approach, the extent of repair and the type of support for surgery. Good arteriograms will determine the presence and the extent of the dissection. The origin of the arch vessels can also be evaluated for obstruction. Occasionally, the patent channel may appear normal on angiography because of extensive mural thrombus. Further study may be essential to demonstrate the coronary arteries to rule out occlusive disease or to demonstrate the aortic root and aortic valve function.

There is some danger in aortography. In dissecting aneurysms, the dissection may be extended or perforated by the catheter. A small test dose injection should be done to determine whether the catheter is in the true lumen or in the false lumen so that rupture or further dissection can be avoided. Immediate surgery is indicated when sudden rupture or cardiac tamponade occurs during angiography.

In occlusive lesions, a plain chest radiograph may show calcium in the aortic arch or in its branches. Bruits may be present on auscultation in the neck at the level of stenosis or obstruction. Distal pulses may be decreased, and an occluded artery may take on a cord-like pulseless character.

Occlusive lesions can be shown angiographically, by using a variety of techniques that visualize the aortic arch and the take-off of the major branches. In addition, since more distal lesions or intracranial lesions may cause the same symptoms, views of the bifurcation of the common carotid artery and intra-cerebral circulation in both anterior–posterior and lateral positions should be taken. In many cases, occlusive lesions of the great vessels are only demon-strated when complete cerebral vascular studies are done to rule out other causes of extracranial cerebral vascular disease of a more distal nature, such as occlusive lesions of the internal carotid or vertebral arteries. If proper arch studies have not been done prior to surgery for distal lesions, occlusive lesions of the arch vessels may be suspected if there is poor antegrade blood flow after the clamp on the common carotid artery is released.

Operative management

Indications

The indications for operation upon aneurysms of the transverse arch depend on many factors, including the presence or absence of painful symptoms, com-pression of the respiratory passages (trachea and bronchi), age of the patient, severity of concomitant respiratory or renal complications, and other con-siderations. The mere presence of an aneurysm in this location does not justify immediate or routine surgi-cal intervention. Because of an inherent risk in such extensive surgery, surgery is justified when the lesion reaches a diameter of 6–8 cm and when the lesion is already impinging upon vital structures and inducing respiratory or other symptoms. We have classified aneurysms of the transverse aorta by extent and involvement of the ascending or descending aorta, or both (Figure 42.3).

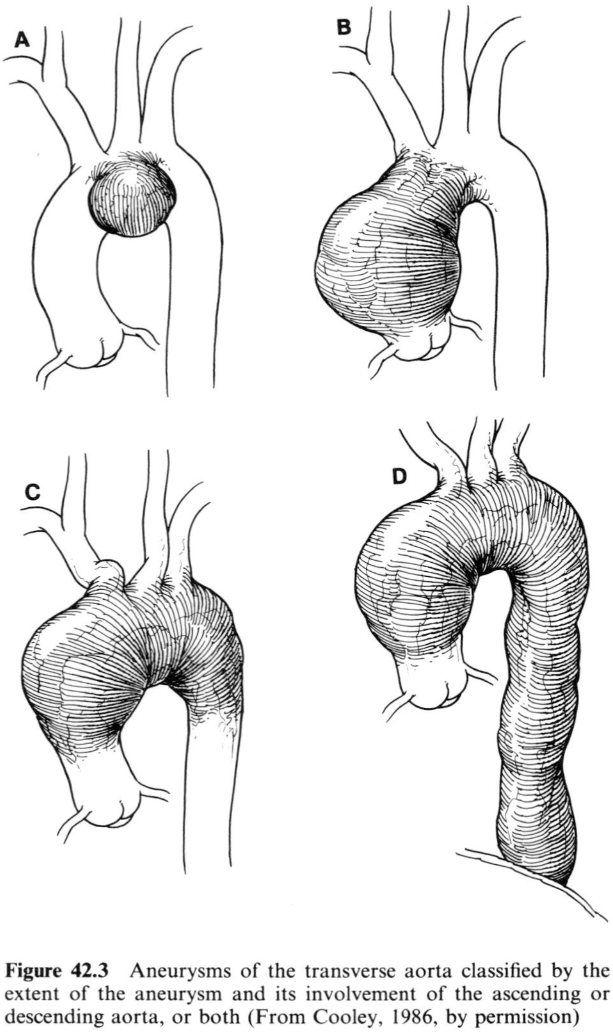

Figure 42.3 Aneurysms of the transverse aorta classified by the extent of the aneurysm and its involvement of the ascending or descending aorta, or both (From Cooley, 1986, by permission)

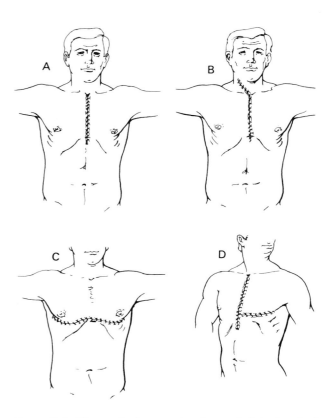

Figure 42.4 The standard approaches for surgical treatment of aneurysms of the aortic arch. A, Small- or moderate-sized aneur-ysms that do not extend far distally into the thoracic aorta can be treated by median sternotomy. B, If a bypass must be done to the great vessels, a neck extension to the right or left can be done. C, For large aneurysms of the ascending aorta, arch, and descending thoracic aorta, a bilateral anterior thoracotomy provides suf-ficient exposure. D, In some instances when a median sternotomy has already been accomplished, a sideward extension through the 3rd or 4th interspace must be done to obtain control when the descending thoracic aorta is involved with aneurysm

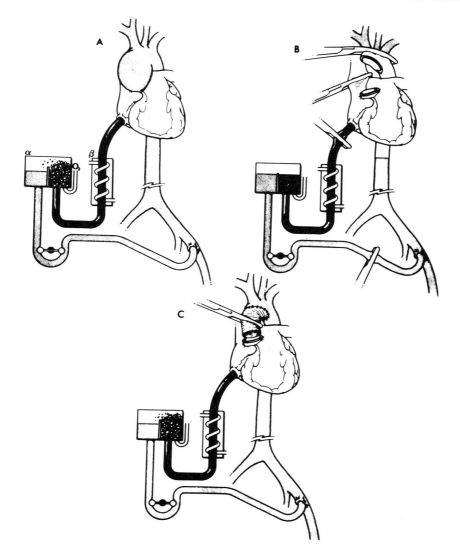

Figure 42.5 Techniques of circulatory arrest during moderate hypothermia (20°C) with partial exsanguination

Surgical approach

There are several surgical approaches to the aortic arch and its branches (Figure 42.4). We prefer to use the simplest approach, one that causes the least disability. For aneurysms of the aortic arch that do not extend far distally into the descending thoracic aorta and are not massive, we perform a median sternotomy with occasional extension into the neck (to the right or left). For a large aortic arch aneurysm, a bilateral transverse thoracotomy through the 3rd interspace is done to expose the entire ascending aortic arch and descending thoracic aorta and origin of the great vessels. This approach allows for treatment of large dissecting aneurysms in which the distal thoracic aorta must be repaired to obliterate the distal lumen or to control the saccular dilatation distally.

Occasionally, extension of the median sternotomy to the left 3rd or 4th intercostal space is necessary to further control the distal thoracic aorta, especially in emergency situations.

Type of support

Perhaps the most important determinant to a good result in surgery of the aortic arch is the type of circulatory support used during the operative procedure. Multiple techniques have been described for supporting cardiopulmonary, cerebral and renal function during operative repair of aortic arch aneurysms. Circulatory support may be divided into three basic types: (1) conventional cardiopulmonary bypass (Gwathmey *et al.*, 1958; Muller *et al.*, 1960; Hu *et al.*,

1964; Larmi and Pentti, 1974; Panday *et al.*, 1974), (2) cardiopulmonary bypass with cerebral extracorporeal perfusion (Cooley *et al.*, 1957; DeBakey *et al.*, 1957; Pearce *et al.*, 1969; Philips and Miyamoto, 1974) and (3) hypothermia with circulatory arrest (Barnard and Schrire, 1963; Nicks, 1972; Griepp *et al.*, 1975; Ott *et al.*, 1978; Livesay *et al.*, 1982, 1983; Speir *et al.*, 1982; Kay *et al.*, 1986; Cooley, 1986). The first two techniques have been used in the past, but the third technique is now preferred.

HYPOTHERMIA WITH CIRCULATORY ARREST

We have found the best technique for maintaining circulatory support to be moderate total body hypothermia by core cooling followed by total circulatory arrest (Figure 42.5). In this technique, the femoral artery and in some instances the ascending aorta are cannulated, and core cooling is accomplished to a temperature of approximately 20–24°C. When short periods of circulatory arrest (less than 30 min) are anticipated, a core temperature of 20°C is sufficient. Usually, the temperature falls below the level at which cold perfusion is discontinued, and may be 2–4°C lower after the circulation is arrested. Topical cortical cooling is achieved by applying ice bags to the head and neck. When the temperature has been reduced to the desired level, arterial perfusion is discontinued at the same time that the venous outlet line is occluded. When possible, the aortic arch vessels are cross-clamped to prevent air entrapment in those vessels, but this manoeuvre is not essential. The aneurysm is opened, and internal inspection of the aortic arch ensues. A plan of reconstruction is decided, and rapid restoration of the internal vessels by endoaneurysmorrhaphy is done (Cooley, 1984). Recently, in some cases, we have continued a very low flow perfusion, approximately $10 \text{ cm}^3/\text{kg}$ body weight, during this period to ensure some circulation to the lower half of the body and to prevent air entrapment. Once the distal anastomosis restores circulation, the aortic graft is clamped, allowing perfusion to the arch vessels. Air is evacuated from the arterial system, and retrograde perfusion of the femoral artery to the cerebral circulation is restored. The proximal anastomosis to the ascending aorta or the aortic annulus is then completed during the period of rewarming. Cardiac preservation may be enhanced during this period by further hypothermia or by introduction of cardioplegic solution if aortic valve replacement is necessary.

In our opinion, moderate body hypothermia with total circulatory arrest is the best supportive technique for arch replacement. This simple method of cerebral protection is associated with a lower rate of complications.

Operative technique for arch aneurysms

The operative technique depends on the type of

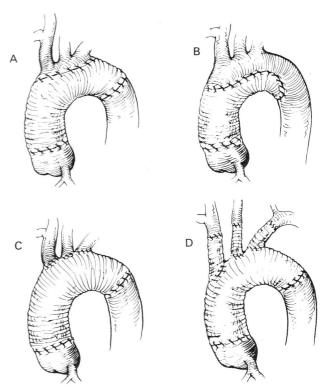

Figure 42.6 Different types of arch repair. A, The arch has been replaced with a Dacron graft and the great vessels placed to the Dacron graft as one unit. B, The inferior portion of the arch aneurysm has been resected, and a single anastomosis is used for the entire distal aorta with its great vessels. C, Separate reimplantation of each artery is done to the graft that has replaced the transverse arch. D, Interposition grafts are done from the transverse arch graft to the great vessels individually. Grafts have been fabricated that avoid the proximal anastomosis of graft to graft. This technique is reserved for cases where the arch vessels are severely involved with aneurysmal or occlusive disease in conjunction with an aortic arch aneurysm

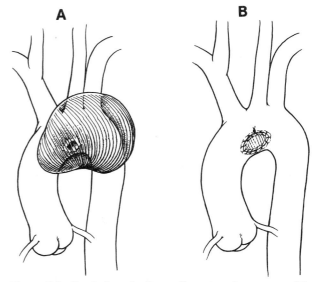

Figure 42.7 Surgical repair of a sacciform, type A aneurysm of the transverse aorta (A). This type of lesion may be repaired during moderate induced hypothermia (24°C) and a brief period of circulatory arrest (B) (From Cooley 1986, by permission)

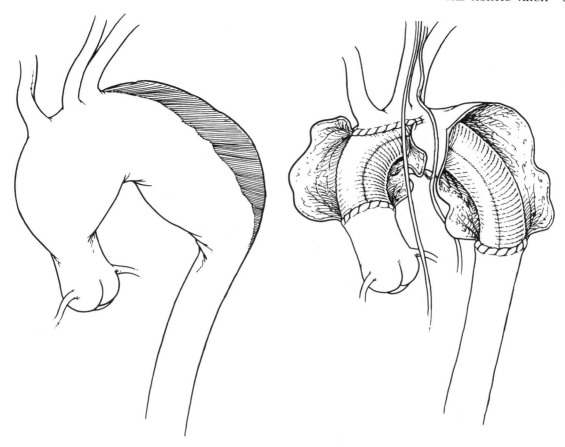

Figure 42.8 Repair of a large fusiform aneurysm of the ascending thoracic aorta, aortic arch and proximal descending aorta. A 24 mm Dacron graft is used with a distal anastomosis end-to-end, arch vessels as a unit side-to-side, and proximal end-to-end anastomosis in that sequence (From Cooley, 1986, by permission)

circulatory support used during occlusion of the great vessels in repair of aortic arch aneurysms. Our preferred method has already been stated, as have other methods of reconstruction of the aortic arch. Whenever possible, the simplest approach should be used, to allow the arch vessels to be retained on the distal aortic segment. In this manner, one anastomosis accomplishes repair of the entire aneurysm (Figure 42.6). This approach can be used in instances when the great vessels are not occluded by plaque (Figure 42.7).

In some instances, if the vessels are occluded by plaque, endarterectomy may be done to one or two or all of the great vessels. The proximal anastomosis can be achieved by anastomosis to an area usually above the annulus, because, in most instances of pure arch aneurysm, the aortic valve is not involved (Figure 42.8). When, however, the aortic valve is involved, replacement rather than resuspension is done. Reimplantation of the coronary arteries can be accomplished by a variety of techniques (Kidd *et al.*, 1976). Saphenous vein grafts may be placed to the right or left coronary system, or the right coronary artery and left coronary artery may be reimplanted.

We prefer to use a tightly woven Dacron graft (Meadox*) that is large enough to fit snugly into the inner lumen of the aorta. Size must be appropriate for both the proximal and distal aorta. When a single distal anastomosis is performed for all arch vessels, a 26 or 30 mm graft is most frequently used. A multifilament-coated Dacron suture is used for the anastomosis. Because of problems with haemostasis in these patients, we prefer a single running suture for the entire anastomosis (Figure 42.9).

Dissecting aneurysms originating in the ascending aorta (type A) should be managed by the open technique, using induced hypothermia and circulatory arrest (Cooley and Livesay, 1981; Speir *et al.*, 1982; Livesay *et al.*, 1983). In the acute dissection, cross-clamping of the aorta is contraindicated, since it lacerates the internal lumen and, thus, prevents an adequate repair. Open distal anastomosis is essential for an adequate repair of an acute dissection and also facilitates repair in a chronic lesion. Usually the distal anastomosis may be done proximal to the origin of

* Meadox Medicals Inc., P.O. Box 530, Oakland, New Jersey 07436, USA.

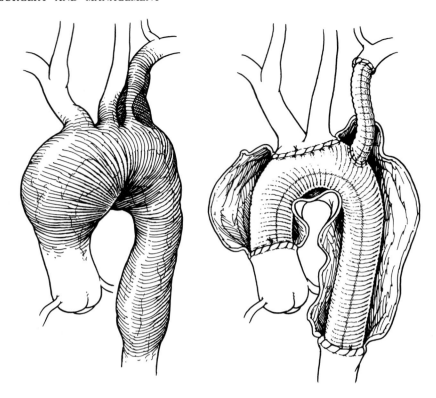

Figure 42.9 Surgical repair for a type D aneurysm of the transverse arch with involvement of the left subclavian artery. This drawing illustrates the current technique of endoaneurysmorrhaphy, which has replaced the older concept of total excision proposed by us in the early 1950s (From Cooley, 1986, by permission)

the arch vessels. The graft should be telescoped into the true lumen of the aorta to ensure that major blood flow is directed centrally. Extension of the dissection into the descending aorta is common; however, if the site of origin of the dissecting process is repaired, the distal dissection usually becomes quiescent. Surgical removal of residual dissection is technically almost impossible and may lead to complications due to compromise of blood supply to the spinal cord or kidneys. Thus, the concept of treatment for dissections is to repair the site of origin and to prevent acute rupture into the pericardial sac with tamponade. Also, restoration of aortic competence is necessary. When commissures are detached from the aortic wall by the dissecting process, then reattachment and reconstruction of the valve are essential. In severe valve disruptions, the valve may require replacement with a prosthesis.

Operative technique for occlusive lesions

The operative technique for occlusive lesions differs from that of arch replacement because flow does not have to be interrupted through the entire transverse arch. The basic techniques of reimplantation, endarterectomy and bypass have been used in the past.

Reimplantation of a great vessel, after resection of the diseased portion, may be done; however, reimplantation is technically difficult because, in most instances, the aortic arch is arteriosclerotic, making anastomosis difficult. In addition, not enough length of the distal vessel can be obtained following resection of the diseased segment.

Another technique is that of endarterectomy of the diseased artery. The artery is opened over the area of blockage and the intimal plaque carefully removed. This can be done only in selected cases, when the arterial occlusive lesion is short and isolated and when there is no severe distal or proximal disease. Therefore, endarterectomy is most often performed in younger patients who do not have diffuse arteriosclerosis. We have also used it in several instances of isolated innominate artery stenosis.

Perhaps the most useful and simple technique is that of bypass of the diseased vessel using either an extrathoracic or intrathoracic approach (Figure 42.10). The approach chosen depends on the accompanying lesions and the general condition of the patient, along with the distal and proximal anatomical disease. Any combination of techniques is possible; the choice is left to the imagination of the vascular surgeon. In general, we prefer to use a

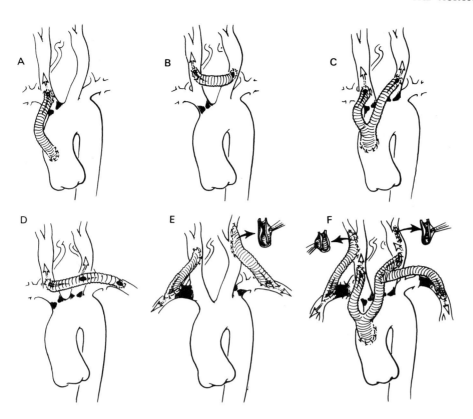

Figure 42.10   The various types of extrathoracic and intrathoracic bypass graft techniques for the treatment of occlusive lesions of the great vessels. A, Ascending aorta to innominate artery bypass is done through a transthoracic approach. B, The same lesion can be treated by left carotid to right carotid bypass. This avoids the intrathoracic approach. C, An inverted Y bifurcation graft is shown from the ascending aorta to the innominate artery and left carotid. D, With the similar obstruction as C, an extrathoracic approach can be used by placing a Dacron graft from the left subclavian artery to both carotid arteries. E, Carotid subclavian bypass is shown for treatment of either carotid or subclavian occlusive disease. On the left carotid, carotid endarterectomy is done and the Dacron graft acts as a long patch graft over the endarterectomized segment and is placed to the subclavian artery. F, Bilateral carotid endarterectomies have been done as staged lesions and the bypass grafts placed as shown. The extrathoracic or intrathoracic approach to these lesions should be individualized for each case

double velour Dacron graft (Meadox) for these bypasses. The graft is usually 7 or 8 mm in diameter. A multifilament-coated Dacron suture is utilized for both anastomoses. Bifurcation grafts or specially designed grafts may be used for multiple distal anastomoses from one proximal anastomosis on the aorta. An inverted 12 × 7 mm double velour bifurcation graft may be used to bypass two vessels from the ascending thoracic aorta. In the case where endarterectomy is done in conjunction with the bypass procedure, such as a carotid endarterectomy with carotid subclavian bypass, the distal portion of the bypass graft may function as a large patch graft over the endarterectomized segment; the proximal portion is placed to the subclavian artery.

In aortic arch syndrome, most often bypasses must be done from the ascending aorta because of the multiple vessel involvement and the length of the stenotic lesions. In some instances distal vessels are completely occluded. In such cases, bypass may be done to one or two non-major distal arteries, such as the vertebral artery or external carotid artery, to increase the collateral circulation (Figure 42.11). Frequently, the ascending aorta is likewise involved, and the proximal anastomoses may be quite difficult.

Conclusion

Because of problems related to air embolization, bleeding and the need of continued cerebral perfusion, aneurysms of the aortic arch were felt to be beyond the realm of surgical therapy as recently as 25 years ago. Overall surgical mortality for these otherwise fatal aneurysms has been as high as 43%, but the recent institution of techniques using moderate hypothermia and circulatory arrest has decreased our operative mortality for resection of arch aneurysms to 10%. The haemorrhagic, neurological, renal and pulmonary complications have likewise been reduced dramatically by adoption of the technique of moderate body hypothermia followed by total circulatory arrest.

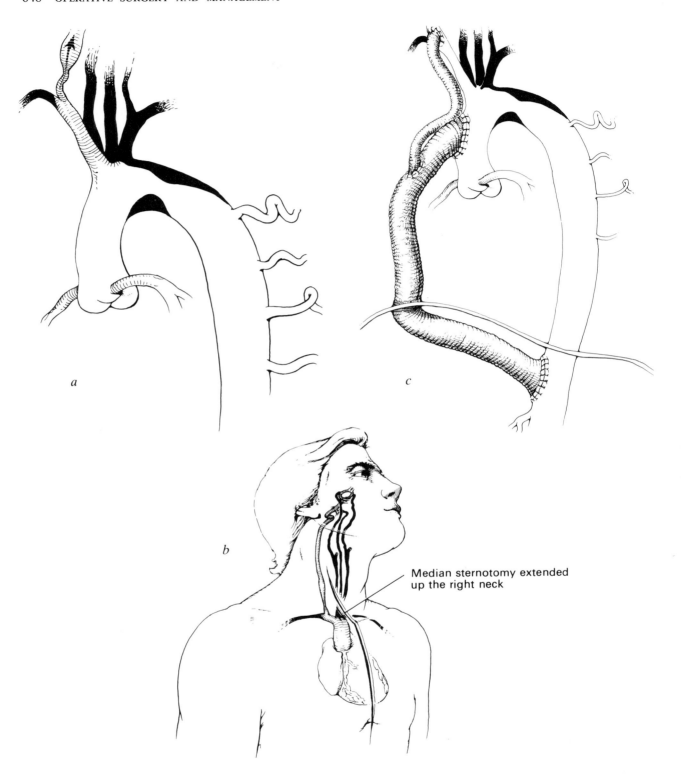

Median sternotomy extended
up the right neck

Figure 42.11 A complicated case of Takayasu's disease. *a*, Complete occlusion of the great vessels. The only artery supplying the cerebral circulation is a tortuous and dilated right vertebral artery arising from a right innominate artery. In addition, there is a coarctation of the aorta. *b*, The surgical approach to this lesion. A median sternotomy with extension to the right neck was done. The large tortuous vertebral artery can be seen to be the only artery supplying the brain. *c*, Treatment of the coarctation was done by anterior approach through a median sternotomy. A Dacron graft was placed from the ascending aorta to the abdominal aorta just below the diaphragm. The bypass graft was then placed from the aortic graft to the vertebral graft. The remaining arteries were characteristically small and hypoplastic and could not be bypassed. This procedure offers an alternative for treating a difficult case of Takayasu's syndrome

Results in surgical repair of occlusive lesions of the great vessels of the aortic arch have been good. The ultimate result is determined by the many previously stated factors; however, with the techniques of endarterectomy, bypass or reimplantation, the mortality rate is less than 1% and related to the extent of the disease process and general condition of the patient. It is obvious that for a simple carotid–subclavian bypass, the mortality rate is virtually negligible. In more complex cases, such as the aortic arch syndrome where multiple bypasses are done, from diseased proximal segments to diseased distal segments, the mortality is somewhat higher. The incidence of transient neurological problems is less than 5% and permanent neurological problems less than 2% in our experience. Long-term patency rates approach 90%, and 85% of the patients experience relief of symptoms without recurrence. Since the lesions are so varied, an individual approach to each patient with regard to prognosis and choice of operation must be exercised.

References

Barnard, C. N. and Schrire, V. (1963) The surgical treatment of acquired aneurysm of the thoracic aorta. *Thorax*, **18**, 101–115

Cooley, D. A. (1984) Endoaneurysmorrhaphy revisited. *Texas Heart Inst. J.*, **11**, 8–9

Cooley, D. A. (1986) *Surgical Treatment of Aortic Aneurysms*, W. B. Saunders, Philadelphia, pp. 73–79

Cooley, D. A., DeBakey, M. E. and Morris, G. C. (1957) Controlled circulation in surgical treatment of aortic aneurysm. *Ann. Surg.*, **146**, 473–486

Cooley, D. A. and Livesay, J. J. (1981) Technique of 'open' distal anastomosis for ascending and transverse arch resection. *Cardiovasc. Dis., Bull. Texas Heart Inst.*, **8**, 421–426

DeBakey, M. E., Crawford, E. S., Cooley, D. A. *et al.* (1957) Successful resection of fusiform aneurysm of aortic arch with replacement by homograft. *Surg. Gynecol. Obstet.*, **105**, 657–664

Doust, B. D. (1984) Computed tomography and ultrasound in evaluation of aortic aneurysms. In *Vascular Surgery*, (ed. R. B. Rutherford), W. B. Saunders, Philadelphia, pp. 786–797

Duncan, J. M. and Cooley, D. A. (1983a) Surgical considerations in aortitis with special emphasis on Takayasu's arteritis. *Texas Heart Inst. J.*, **10**, 233–247

Duncan, J. M. and Cooley, D. A. (1983b) Surgical considerations in aortitis. II. Mycotic aneurysms. *Texas Heart Inst. J.*, **10**, 329–335

Duncan, J. M. and Cooley, D. A. (1983c) Surgical considerations in aortitis. III. Syphilitic and other forms of aortitis. *Texas Heart Inst. J.*, **10**, 337–341

Grande, A. M., Eren, E. E., Hallman, G. L. *et al.* (1984) Rupture of the thoracic aorta: emergency treatment and management of chronic aneurysms. *Texas Heart Inst. J.*, **11**, 244–249

Griepp R. B., Stinson, E. B., Hollingsworth, J. F. *et al.* (1975) Prosthetic replacement of the aortic arch. *J. Thorac. Cardiovasc. Surg.*, **70**, 1051–1063

Gwathmey, O., Pierpont, H. C. and Blades, B. (1958) Clinical experiences with the surgical treatment of acquired aortic vascular disease. *Surg. Gynecol. Obstet.*, **107**, 205–213

Hu, Y. U., Shank, T. Y. and Wy, Y. K. (1964) Surgical treatment of aneurysm of the thoracic aorta. *Chin. Med. J.*, **83**, 740

Kampmeier, R. H. (1938) Saccular aneurysm of the thoracic aorta: a clinical study of 633 cases. *Ann. Intern. Med.*, **12**, 624–651

Kay, G. L., Cooley, D. A., Livesay, J. J. *et al.* (1986) Surgical repair of aneurysms involving the distal aortic arch. *J. Thorac. Cardiovasc. Surg.*, **18**, 397–404

Kidd, J. N., Reul, G. J., Jr, Cooley, D. A. *et al.* (1976) Surgical treatment of aneurysms of the ascending aorta. *Circulation* **54**(6), Suppl. III, 118–122

Larmi, T. K. I. and Pentti, K. (1974) Resection of the transverse aortic arch. *J. Thorac. Cardiovasc. Surg.*, **68**, 70–75

Lefrak, E. A., Stevens, P. M. and Howell, J. F. (1972) Respiratory insufficiency due to tracheal compression by an aneurysm of the ascending, transverse, and descending thoracic aorta: successful surgical management in a 76-year-old man. *J. Thorac. Cardiovasc. Surg.*, **63**(6), 956–961

Livesay, J. J., Cooley, D. A., Duncan, J. M. *et al.* (1982) Open aortic anastomosis: improved results in the treatment of aneurysms of the aortic arch. *Circulation*, **66** (Suppl. 1), 122–127

Livesay, J. J., Cooley, D. A., Reul, G. J., Jr *et al.* (1983) Resection of aortic arch aneurysms: a comparison of hypothermic techniques in 60 patients. *Ann. Thorac. Surg.*, **36**, 19–28

Livesay, J. J., Cooley, D. A., Ventemiglia, R. A. *et al.* (1985) Surgical experience in descending thoracic aneurysmectomy with and without adjuncts to avoid ischemia. *Ann. Thorac. Surg.*, **39**, 37–46

Muller, W. H., Warren, W. D. and Blanton, F. S. (1960) A method for resection of aortic arch aneurysms. *Ann. Surg.*, **151**, 225–230

Nicks, R. (1972) Aortic arch aneurysm: resection and replacement: protection of the nervous system. *Thorax*, **27**, 239–245

Ott, D. A., Frazier, O. H. and Cooley, D. A. (1978) Resection of the aortic arch using deep hypothermia and temporary circulatory arrest. *Circulation*, **58**(3), Suppl. 1, 1227–1231

Panday, S. R., Parulkar, G. B., Chauker, A. P. *et al.* (1974) Simplified technique for aortic arch replacement: first stage right subclavian to left carotid bypass. *Ann. Thorac. Surg.*, **18**, 186–190

Pearce, C. W., Weichert, R. F. and del Real, R. E. (1969) Aneurysms of aortic arch: simplified technique for excision and prosthetic replacement. *J. Thorac. Cardiovasc. Surg.*, **58**, 886–890

Philips, P. A. and Miyamoto, A. M. (1974) Use of hypothermia and cardiopulmonary bypass in resection of aortic arch aneurysms. *Ann. Thorac. Surg.*, **17**, 398–404

Reul, G. J., Jr. (1976) Vascular injury and arteriovenous fistula. In *Practice of Surgery: Cardiovascular Surgery* (ed. D. C. Sabiston), Harper and Row. Maryland, pp. 15–16

Reul, G. J., Jr, Beall, A. C., Jr, Jordan, G. L., Jr *et al.* (1973) The early operative management of injuries to the great vessels. *Surgery*, **74**, 862–873

Reul, G. J., Jr, Cooley, D. A., Hallman, G. L. *et al.* (1975) Dissecting aneurysm of the descending aorta: improved surgical results in 91 patients. *Arch. Surg.* **110**, 632–640

Reul, G. J., Jr, Rubio, P. A. and Beall, A. C., Jr (1974) The surgical management of acute injury to the thoracic aorta. *J. Thorac. Cardiovasc. Surg.*, **67**, 272–281

Schaff, H. V. and Brawley, R. K. (1977) Operative management of penetrating vascular injuries of the thoracic outlet. *Surgery*, **82**(2), 182–191

Shimizu, K. and Sano, J. (1951) Pulseless disease. *J. Neuropathol. Clin. Neurol.*, **1**, 37

Speir, A. M., Grey, D. P. and Cooley, D. A. (1982) Resection of the aortic arch with moderate hypothermia and temporary circulatory arrest. *Texas Heart Inst. J.*, **9**, 311–320

Takayasu, M. (1908) Case of queer changes in central blood vessels of retina. *Acta Soc. Ophthalmol. Jap.*, **12**, 554

43

The descending thoracic aorta – spinal cord protection

G. Keen

Operations on the descending thoracic aorta are indicated for acute traumatic rupture, acute dissections and for chronic aneurysms, but a common indication is for the resection and anastomosis of coarctation of the aorta. The surgical management of coarctation of the aorta is dealt with in Chapter 40, but much of this present chapter is appropriate to the management of coarctation in certain circumstances.

Operations on the descending thoracic aorta are complicated by the need to cross-clamp the aorta high up and at the same time prevent left ventricular strain and to protect the kidneys, spinal cord and abdominal viscera from the effects of ischaemia. In experimental animals, aortic cross-clamping at this level without bypass results in a marked rise in left ventricular, left atrial and pulmonary artery pressure, and if aortic occlusion is maintained for longer than about 20 min at normal temperatures the risk of paraplegia becomes very great (Kahn, 1970; Taber, 1970; Keen, 1972).

In the first reported successful repair of traumatic rupture of the aorta (Passaro and Pace, 1959), the surgeon cross-clamped the aorta of a 30-year-old man without bypass for a 17-min period, during which he sutured a 3 mm tear at the isthmus. He noted that the heart became grossly distended and the electrocardiograph pattern bizarre, with conduction defects and T-wave inversion, and that the proximal blood pressure rose to 200 mmHg. Although the patient survived, this experience was sufficiently worrying to persuade the surgeon to recommend hypothermia on future occasions. Others have stated that patients in whom restorative surgery is undertaken rapidly have no need of bypass support, but the development of paraplegia in some cases following this technique suggests that is no safer, and perhaps more liable to medicolegal problems than is the use of some form of bypass (Crawford et al., 1970). Moreover, it takes no account of possible renal damage, especially in the elderly.

Paraplegia and aortic surgery (see Chapter 44)

In 1972, Brewer and colleagues studied a collected series of 12 532 cases of repair of coarctation of the aorta which were complicated by 51 instances of severe neurological damage, usually paraplegia, an incidence of 0.41% or about 1 in 240 cases. In addition, they discovered a total of eight patients with this condition who developed paraplegia without surgical operations. They carefully reviewed this complication from the standpoint of the blood supply of the spinal cord and it is this blood supply and its variations which may determine whether or not a patient having descending aortic surgery is likely to be at risk of neurological damage.

In 1987, Keen enquired into the clinical practice and paraplegia rate associated with operations for coarctation of the aorta undertaken by surgeons in the UK. Paraplegia occurred in 16 patients in a total of 5492 operations, an incidence of 0.3% or once in every 343 operations. There were, in addition, a further 3 patients who suffered temporary paraplegia with full recovery within 10 days. Additionally, several patients in this series developed unusual gaits after operation, which may have been due to a mild cauda equina lesion. This enquiry established the need for accurate electromanometric measurement of proximal and distal to coarctation aortic pressures and the need to establish left atriofemoral bypass should distal pressures fall below 50 mmHg, especially in secondary operations for this condition. Keen advocated that serious consideration should be given to developing spinal cord monitoring using somatosensory evoked potentials, which had been shown by others to be of clinical value (Laschinger et al., 1982; Keen, 1987, 1990).

Anatomy (Figures 43.1 and 43.2)

The traditional concept of the blood supply to the spinal cord is that the anterior spinal artery forms a single continuous channel which flows uninterrupted from the cervical to the lumbar region. There are, however, many variations. The first accurate description of the circulation of the spinal cord was reported by Adamkiewicz (1882) and Kadyi (1886, 1889). They showed that the anterior spinal artery is not a continuous vessel and that not every intercostal vessel in the thoracic region will have a radicular branch to supply the anterior spinal artery.

The anterior spinal artery is divided into end arteries at several levels making possible a functional division of the blood supply to the cord. The upper division, which is the upper cervical and thoracic regions, is supplied by branches of the vertebral

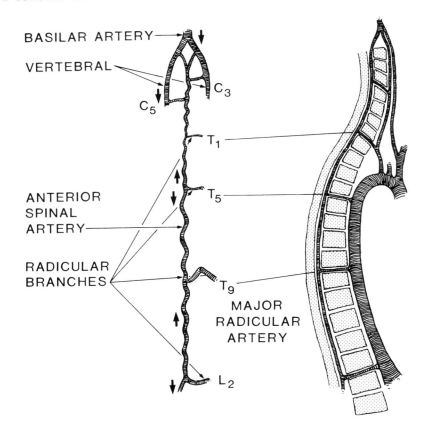

Figure 43.1 Segmental blood supply of the anterior spinal arteries via the radicular branches of the intercostal and other aortic vessels, together with a supply from the vertebral arteries. The anterior spinal artery is shown as a continuous vessel, but common variations make the continuity of the anterior spinal artery precarious and undependable

arteries which form the anterior spinal artery and by a number of spinal arteries which vary in location, the most constant branch accompanying a radicular branch of C4 and which receives its blood supply from the superior intercostal vessels. The middle division from the middle of the lower thoracic region of the cord has the poorest segmental blood supply and is usually dependent on one radicular artery which commonly arises from T7, T8 or T9.

The lower or lumbar division is supplied almost exclusively by the unpaired great radicular artery of Adamkiewicz and this artery shows considerable variation. When it arises from a lower thoracic intercostal vessel, the branch to the middle division may be absent and when the great radicular artery arises in the lumbar region the blood supply to the lower, thoracic cord is poor in the absence of T7–T9 radicular branches. Under normal circumstances, there is little exchange between the territories of the various radicular arteries, and variations in number and origin of important radicular arteries may result in an inability of the anterior spinal artery to function as a collateral. In effect, occlusion of intercostal vessels may be harmless in one patient and dangerous in another.

Although these anatomical variations are of particular importance in the management of coarctation of the aorta, they are of course most relevant when undertaking surgery for traumatic and degenerative conditions of the aorta. It is important that the surgeon determines whether the collateral circulation is adequate in the distal aorta after cross-clamping, and it is clear that the only safe measure is that of recording intra-aortic pressures in the descending aorta during surgery. Although the majority of patients with coarctation of the aorta will maintain a high distal pressure after cross-clamping (i.e. above 50 mmHg mean), all, or nearly all, patients with surgery for acquired conditions, and who have no collateral circulation, will produce no distal aortic pressure following cross-clamping. It is clear that those patients with coarctation of the aorta, who after cross-clamping produced little or no distal pressure, and all patients having surgery for acquired diseases, will need some form of bypass.

Laschinger *et al.* (1983) undertook an investigation of the experimental and clinical assessment of the adequacy of partial bypass in the maintenance of spinal cord blood flow during operations on the thoracic aorta using spinal cord impulse conduction (somatosensory evoked potentials). This group found

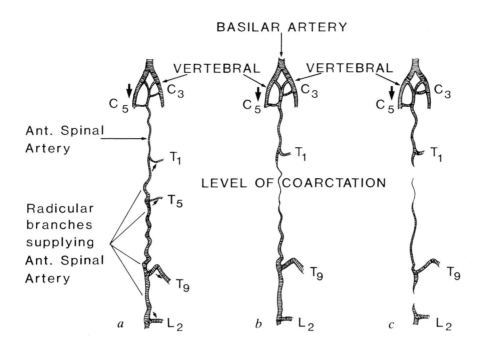

Figure 43.2 Variations in the supply to the anterior spinal artery. In (*a*) the spinal artery is supplied by many good radicular vessels, but in (*b*) there is clearly limitation of anterior spinal artery flow between T1 and T9. In (*c*), owing to the poor radicular supply from the intercostal vessels, there is discontinuity in the anterior spinal artery between T1 and T9 and again between T9 and L2, and it is in such cases that the spinal cord is endangered during operations on the descending thoracic aorta. The large radicular artery at the level of about T9 (the artery of Adamkiewiez) is a very constant and reliably large branch to the lumbar cord

no significant changes in spinal cord blood flow or somatosensory evoked potentials in any animal with a distal aortic pressure greater than or equal to 70 mmHg. With a pressure of 40 mmHg, normal flow and somatosensory evoked potentials were maintained in five of the six experimental animals. Loss of somatosensory evoked potentials, with simultaneous loss of spinal cord blood flow at the level of T6, occurred in one dog. Restoration of distal aortic pressure to 70 mmHg in all animals resulted in immediate return of somatosensory evoked potentials and loss of somatosensory evoked potentials routinely occurred in animals with a distal aortic pressure less than 40 mmHg. They concluded that maintenance of a distal aortic pressure greater than 60–70 mmHg will uniformly preserve spinal cord blood flow in the absence of critical intercostal exclusion. Should distal aortic pressure be inadequate, early reversible changes in the somatosensory evoked potentials will alert the surgeon and failure to institute measures to reverse these changes may result in paraplegia.

In those centres where extensive experience of descending aortic surgery has been obtained, some surgeons advocate descending aortic surgery without the use of left heart bypass or some form of shunting. It must be borne in mind that this small and select group of surgeons operates with extreme rapidity,

thus avoiding prolonged periods of spinal cord ischaemia. For the majority of surgeons, however, who have less experience but who from time to time necessarily undertake these operations, such surgery without bypass is probably more prone to paraplegia than otherwise.

Left atriofemoral bypass

Left atriofemoral bypass (Cooley *et al.*, 1957; Gerbode *et al.*, 1957) is employed in many cases in which surgery of the descending thoracic aorta is undertaken. This technique allows satisfactory operating conditions, preventing proximal hypertension and left ventricular strain during aortic cross-clamping and also ensuring adequate renal and spinal cord perfusion. Heparinization and its reversal by protamine pose no undue problems, but should intra-abdominal or intracerebral bleeding be taking place, heparinization might aggravate this. The patient is positioned on the operating table in the right lateral position – that is, with the left chest uppermost – with the pelvis rotated 45° backwards and the left hip joint fully extended, the chest being thus exposed for full thoracotomy and access provided to the femoral vessels. The left femoral artery is first prepared for cannulation and the chest is opened widely through the 4th intercostal space. Before mobilization of the aorta the pericardium is opened posteriorly to the phrenic nerve and the left atrial appendage snared by a purse-string. These precautions allow for immediate left atriofemoral bypass should haemorrhage occur during dissection of the acute aortic rupture. A large-bore cannula is introduced into the left atrium, whence blood is drained by gravity into an open reservoir and thence returned via a roller pump to the femoral artery. Heparinization is required in a dosage of 1 mg/kg body weight and is subsequently reversed with protamine in similar dosage. A distal flow rate of 40 ml/kg body weight per minute ensures adequate decompression of the proximal aorta with adequate perfusion of the kidneys and spinal cord. During perfusion, the radial arterial pressure should be maintained at 80 mmHg and urine should be passed. A modification of left atriofemoral bypass has been described in which a pulsatile pump containing porcine valves and tubing coated with a non-thrombogenic compound are used, thus avoiding the use of heparin (Connolly *et al.*, 1971).

Moderate hypothermia

Moderate hypothermia at 30°C, which has now been superseded by bypass procedures, was used when surface cooling had an important place in cardiac and vascular surgery. Although several successful cases of suture of ruptured aortas and resection of thoracic aneurysms have been reported, the period of safe aortic occlusion in these conditions is so unreliable and variable and the risk of ventricular fibrillation during the surface cooling of badly injured people is so high that the use of this technique is no longer advised (Neville *et al.*, 1968).

Femoral venous-to-arterial oxygenation

Femoral venous-to-arterial oxygenation was described in 1968 in the treatment of 19 patients who underwent resection of aneurysms of the descending aorta or the repair of ruptured aortas (Neville *et al.*, 1968). A large-bore catheter is inserted into the inferior vena cava via the femoral vein, whence blood is drained into a disposable bubble oxygenator and returned to the femoral artery. This allows a measured perfusion of the lower part of the body during aortic cross-clamping and decompresses the upper aortic segment. It has the additional advantage of removing cannulas and tubing from the operative field and avoids cannulation of the left atrium. Although the use of this method does not seem to be widespread, it offers an attractive alternative to left atriofemoral bypass.

Arterial shunts

In 1970, Molloy reported the successful repair of ruptured thoracic aorta in three patients with the use of a left ventriculo-aortic shunt (Figure 43.3). A plastic cannula was used, one end of which was inserted into the left ventricle at its apex and the other into the descending thoracic aorta below the site of trauma. The only complication reported was clotting of blood in the cannula on one occasion. The advantages of this method are the avoidance of heparinization on the one hand and the avoidance of elaborate bypass procedures on the other. It is extremely simple and it may well be that it will ultimately be favoured as the procedure of choice in the repair of traumatic rupture of the descending aorta. However, great care must be taken to ensure that the cannula does not pass back into the left atrium, or flow will cease.

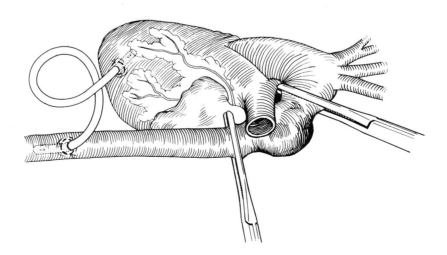

Figure 43.3 Left ventriculo-aortic shunt using heparinized bonded shunt. This is a most useful procedure when dealing with traumatic rupture of the descending aorta (Molloy)

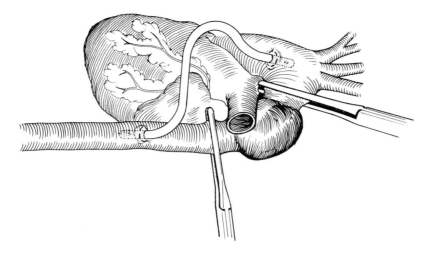

Figure 43.4 Aorto-aortic shunt using heparinized bonded shunt. The shunt is inserted into the ascending aorta and into the femoral artery or the descending aorta, and is a most useful method of dealing with large aneurysms of the descending thoracic aorta.

Another author (Kahn, 1970) described the use of a similar type of temporary plastic shunt inserted at one end into the ascending aorta and at the other into the descending aorta in operations to repair traumatic rupture of the aorta (Figure 43.4), but reported the occurrence of paraplegia in one patient which may have been due to too small a diameter of shunt. A further report (Gott, 1971) described the use of a shunt from the left subclavian artery to the left femoral artery using a plastic tube lined with a non-thrombogenic substance.

At the present time some surgeons are veering away from complicated extracorporeal systems, utilizing left ventriculo-aortic bypass, or subclavian-aortic bypass, with the Gott plastic shunt which is internally heparin-bonded and non-thrombogenic (Keen, 1972).

Acute dissection of the aorta

Acute dissection of the aorta is a specific clinical and pathological entity. The underlying aetiology is degeneration of the elements of the media which may be localized or diffuse, so-called 'cystic medial necrosis'. The cause of the initial tear in the intima and the media is not understood, although severe hypertension is often associated with this disease. The tear usually occurs in the ascending aorta 2–3 cm above the aortic valve or in the region of the ligamentum arteriosum or in the abdominal aorta. More rarely, the tear originates in the transverse arch of the aorta. The layers of the aorta are then dissected by the forceful torrent of blood, usually at the junction of the middle and outer thirds of the media, which may progress to involve part or all of the circumference of the aorta and may extend for a short or a long distance along the aorta. Dissection of the entire

aorta may occur quickly or in stages and the intramural channel may rupture back into the lumen at another level or may rupture externally causing fatal haemorrhage into the pleural or abdominal cavity or into the pericardium causing fatal tamponade. In chronic cases the dissection channel may heal and may become endothelialized and many instances are recorded where such healed dissections are found at routine autopsy in elderly patients who have died of unrelated disease. Dissection may extend along the larger branches of the aorta, interfering with the blood supply to the kidneys, limbs or brain. The intercostal and lumbar arteries are frequently torn or separated by splitting of the aortic wall and paraplegia is a common consequence of such injury. A localized and rapidly increasing dilatation may occur, particularly in the descending aorta.

Classification

DeBakey and his colleagues in 1965 introduced a classification of dissections of the aorta.

Type I DeBakey (Stanford type A) (Figure 43.5)

The dissection which has arisen in the ascending aorta has extended distally and throughout the remaining aorta including the arch, descending aorta and major terminal branches, and is often associated with aortic regurgitation.

Type II DeBakey (Stanford type A)

The disease is limited to the ascending aorta and originates from a transverse tear in the intima which usually begins just above the aortic valve and is also associated in many cases with acute aortic regurgitation.

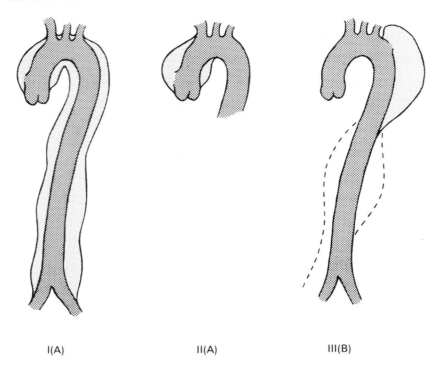

I(A)   II(A)   III(B)

Figure 43.5 Classification of aortic dissections: types I, II, III DeBakey; types A and B Stanford

Type III DeBakey (Stanford type B)

The dissection arises in the descending thoracic aorta usually at or just distal to the origin of the left subclavian artery extending distally for a varying distance.

Since this description there has been a variety of other classifications, including the Stanford classification, but from the point of view of the surgeon the type II affects the ascending aorta and type III affects the descending aorta. These are entirely separate conditions and require an entirely different surgical approach.

Acute dissection of the ascending aorta (type II DeBakey)

This subject, together with its effect on competence of the aortic valve, is dealt with in Chapters 41 and 42.

Acute dissection of the descending aorta (type III DeBakey)

The clinical picture is usually characteristic and the diagnosis is readily made by aortography. Recently, the use of the CT scan has shown that dissections can be accurately diagnosed and furthermore accurately localized, avoiding in many instances the need for aortography.

Treatment

The surgical management of acute dissection of the aorta was rationalized by DeBakey *et al.* (1955) and although the surgical mortality at that time was high it has progressively declined and in those units where this disease is managed surgically and frequently the results are now very good indeed, achieving an acceptably low mortality for what is an otherwise highly lethal disease. In 1965, Wheat introduced the concept of the medical management of acute dissections of the distal aorta (Wheat *et al.*, 1965). He maintained that progression of a dissection was the consequence of the extremely high blood pressure and was associated with a very high pulse pressure. He also maintained that if the mean blood pressure could be reduced and if the bounding pulse pressure could also be reduced, the progress of dissection would be arrested and healing would be expected in many patients who would, therefore, survive without what was at that time a very risky operation.

The selection of cases for such conservative management should be very carefully supervised by a team consisting both of surgeons and physicians, for the complications of dissection such as aortic rupture with haemopericardium, haemothorax, together with the dangers of obstruction, occlusion or separation of one or more aortic branches, causing myocardial infarction, stroke, paraplegia, intestinal, renal or distal limb ischaemia, are very real and their development or impending development might indicate the need for emergency operation. The advocates of a universal surgical attack on this disease criticize the conservative approach, for it is their view that should one of these complications develop rapidly it is by that time probably too late to save the patient, and since these complications are so common the risk should be avoided. On the other hand, Wheat and his associates point out that a large number of patients who are treated conservatively do survive without operation, and since the patient group under discussion is often elderly and otherwise unfit, conservative management should be considered in all patients with acute dissections of the descending thoracic aorta.

It is, however, necessary to say that acute dissections arising in and involving the descending thoracic aorta, which are associated with progressive extension, occlusion of vital arteries, significant aortic dilatation or leak, should be treated by immediate surgery, and that patients with any form of aortic dissection, either acute or chronic, complicating Marfan's syndrome are candidates for surgical treatment because of the high incidence of recurrent dissection and rupture. However, in elderly patients in whom there is clinical and radiological evidence of a localized dissection of the *descending thoracic aorta without any of these complications*, it is reasonable to conduct a trial of hypotensive therapy. It is essential that when such conservative management is undertaken, the patient is treated in the intensive care unit. An indwelling radial artery cannula is inserted in order to monitor the arterial pressure and the patient is treated actively with beta-blockers, and after-load reducers such as sodium nitroprusside. The intention is to maintain the mean pressure at a low enough level hopefully to prevent further extension of the tear but at the same time to maintain an adequate pressure for the patient to perfuse his or her own vital organs.

It is now clear that although a great number of these patients will be managed safely only by operative intervention, at the same time a large number of patients will respond satisfactorily and do leave hospital with a healed or healing dissection following the careful use of conservative treatment.

Operative management (Figure 43.6)

Dissections of the descending aorta are approached through an extended left posterolateral thoracotomy. It is necessary to exclude the descending aorta containing the intimal tear if possible, and an appropriate size Dacron graft is inserted to restore aortic continuity. Certainly at the distal end of aortic resection and to some extent at the proximal end, the aorta will be separated into layers which will require initial circumferential resuturing prior to the insertion of a Dacron graft (Figure 43.6b). The native aorta, especially distally, is extremely friable and often requires Teflon felt support to prevent sutures cutting through. Although many experienced surgeons advocate the undertaking of this operation using aortic cross-clamping without using any adjuncts to avoid distal ischaemia or to provide proximal decompression, it is the view of others that some form of

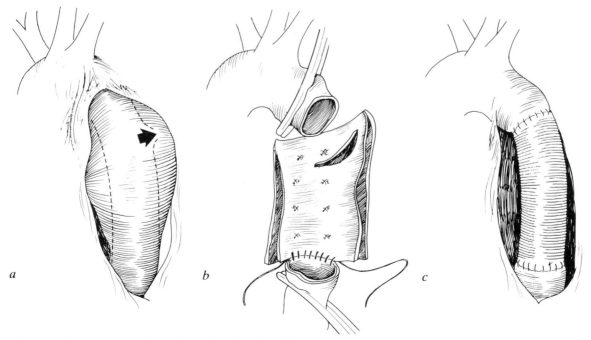

Figure 43.6 Operative management of acute dissection of the descending thoracic aorta. The segment bearing the tear (*a*) is isolated (*b*) and replaced with a Dacron graft (*c*). Intercostal vessels are sutured and the separated distal and proximal aortic layers are sutured into one layer prior to graft replacement

support such as left atriofemoral bypass, femoral vein to femoral artery bypass, or the use of heparin-bonded shunts, should be used to avoid the complications of distal ischaemia or proximal cardiac overload. In view of the friability of tissues and severe haemorrhage associated with heparinization, many experienced surgeons undertake this operation using aortic cross-clamping without any form of bypass and very good results are recorded in their reports. It must, however, be pointed out that these selected groups of experienced surgeons are technically able to insert the aortic Dacron graft very rapidly, thus avoiding neurological and other complications. Unhappily the great majority of acute dissections of the descending aorta are treated in units lacking the experience of these large series of patients and in these cases the period of aortic cross-clamping will usually be prolonged. It is then recommended that some form of circulatory support such as left atriofemoral bypass or the use of heparin-bonded shunts should be used to avoid complications of distal ischaemia or proximal cardiac overload.

Intraluminal prosthesis
(Figures 43.7 and 43.8) (Sariel *et al.*, 1978)

A modification of aortic replacement is the recent introduction of the intraluminal prosthesis. This consists of a low-porosity woven Dacron tube with expanded polypropylene ends which are grooved to accept a peri-aortic tape and these ends are covered with Dacron velour. These prostheses are manufactured in varying lengths and diameters (Figure 43.7). The prosthesis may be introduced into the ascending or descending aorta in patients with localized dissections or traumatic tears. When used in the ascending aorta, full cardiopulmonary bypass with aortic cross-clamping and cold cardioplegia are required. When used in the descending thoracic aorta, aortic cross-clamping and some form of left heart bypass are considered mandatory by most surgeons. When controlled, the aorta is opened longitudinally and the intraluminal prosthesis placed within the true lumen across the pathological or traumatic tear following which the peri-aortic tapes are tied above and below thus securing the prosthesis. The aortic wall is then sutured over the prosthesis anteriorly (Figure 43.8).

Although this prosthesis has been recently introduced, there are now several encouraging reports and if in the long term this prosthesis appears to have no disadvantages, it will offer a real advantage in the reduction of aortic cross-clamp time and in the amount of blood loss, as long and often leaky anastomotic suture lines are avoided.

The concept of the intraluminal prosthesis is not new, having been introduced by Carrel (1912) and Blakemore *et al.* (1942). In 1951, Hufnagel introduced such a prosthesis carrying a ball valve into the des-

cending thoracic aorta and this was used extensively in patients during the early 1950s. Although this valve was frequently obstructed by clots, there were few difficulties associated with the tube itself.

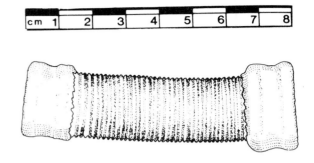

Figure 43.7 Intraluminal prosthesis

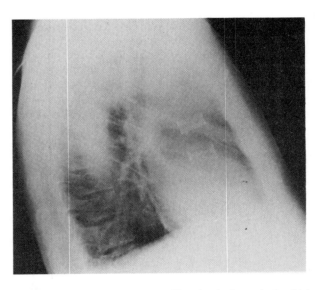

Figure 43.8 Lateral chest X-ray of intraluminal prosthesis which has been inserted in the ascending aorta to repair acute dissection of the aorta.

Acknowledgement

Figures 43.1 and 43.2 have been copied with kind permission of C. V. Mosby from the article by Brewer *et al.* (1972).

References

Adamkiewicz, A. (1882) Die Blutgefasse des Menschlichen Ruckenmarkes. I. Teil. Die Gefasse der Ruckenmarksubstanz. II. Teil. Die Gefasse der Ruckenmarkoberflache. *Sitz. Akad. Wiss. Wein. Math. Natur. Klass.*, **84**, 469; **85**, 101

Blakemore, A. H., Lord, J. W., Jr and Stefko, P. L. (1942) The severed primary artery in the war wounded. *Surgery*, **12**, 488–508

Brewer, L. A., Fosburg, R. G., Mulder, G. A. *et al.* (1972) Spinal cord complications following surgery for coarctation of the aorta. A study of 66 cases. *J. Thorac. Cardiovasc. Surg.*, **64**(3), 368–381

Carrel, A. (1912) Results of the permanent ventilation of the thoracic aorta. *Surg. Gynecol. Obstet.*, **15**, 245–248

Connolly, J. E., Wakabayashi, A., German, J. C. *et al.* (1971) Clinical experience with pulsatile left heart bypass without anticoagulation for thoracic aneurysms. *J. Thorac. Cardiovasc. Surg.*, **62**, 568–576

Cooley, D. A., DeBakey, M. E. and Morris, G. C. (1957) Controlled extra-corporeal circulation in surgical treatment of aortic aneurysm. *Ann. Surg.*, **146**, 473–486

Crawford, E. S., Fenstermacher, J. M., Richardson, W. *et al.* (1970) Reappraisal of adjuncts to avoid ischaemia in the treatment of thoracic aortic aneurysms. *Surgery*, **67**, 182–196

DeBakey, M. E., Cooley, D. A. and Creech, O., Jr (1955) Surgical considerations of dissecting aneurysms of the aorta. *Ann. Surg.*, **142**, 586

DeBakey, M. E., Henly Walter, S., Cooley, D. A. *et al.* (1965) Surgical management of dissecting aneurysms of the aorta. *J. Thorac. Cardiovasc. Surg.*, **49**, 130–147

Gerbode, F., Braimbridge, M., Osborn, J. J. *et al.* (1957) Traumatic thoracic aneurysms: treatment by resection and grafting with the use of an extra-corporeal bypass. *Surgery*, **42**, 975–985

Gott, V. L. (1971) Discussion of paper by Connolly *et al.* (1971), *op. cit.*

Hufnagel, C. A. (1951) Aortic plastic valvular prosthesis. *Bull. Georgetown Univ. Med. Center*, **4**, 128–129

Kadyi, H. (1886) Uber die Blutgefasse des Menschlichen Ruckenmarkes. *Anat. Ann.*, **1**, 304 (1889, Lemberg: Gubrynowicz and Schmidt)

Kahn, D. R. (1970) Discussion of paper by Crawford *et al.* (1970), *op. cit.*

Keen, G. (1972) Closed injuries of the thoracic aorta. *Ann. R. Coll. Surg. Engl.*, **51**, 137–156

Keen, G. (1987) Spinal cord damage and operations for coarctation of the aorta; aetiology, practice and prospects. *Thorax*, **42**, 11–18

Keen, G. (1990) Spinal cord damage associated with surgery of the descending aorta. In *Current Surgical Practice*, Vol. 5 (eds J. Hadfield, M. Hobsley and T. Treasure), Edward Arnold, London

Laschinger, J. C., Cunningham, J. N. and Catinella, F. P. (1982) Detection and prevention of interoperative spinal cord ischaemia after cross clamping of the thoracic aorta. Use of somatosensory evoked potentials. *Surgery*, **92**, 1109–1114

Laschinger, J. C., Cunningham, J. N., Jr, Nathan, I. M. *et al.* (1983) Experimental and clinical assessment of the adequacy of partial bypass in maintenance of spinal cord blood flow during operations on the thoracic aorta. *Ann. Thorac. Surg.*, **36**, 417–426

Molloy, P. J. (1970) Repair of the ruptured thoracic aorta using left ventriculo-aortic support. *Thorax*, **25**, 213–222

Neville, W. E., Cox, W. D., Leininger, B. *et al.* (1968) Resection of the descending thoracic aorta with femoral vein to femoral artery oxygenation perfusion. *J. Thorac. Cardiovasc. Surg.*, **56**, 39–42

Passaro, E. and Pace, W. G. (1959) Traumatic rupture of the aorta. *Surgery*, **46**, 787–791

Sariel, G. G., Ablaza, M. D., Suresh, C. *et al.* (1978) Use of a ringed intra-luminal graft in the surgical treatment of dissecting aneurysms of the thoracic aorta. *J. Thorac. Cardiovasc. Surg.*, **76**, 390–396

Taber, R. E. (1970) Discussion of paper by Crawford *et al.* (1970), *op. cit.*

Wheat, M. W., Palmer, R. F., Bartley, T. B. *et al.* (1965) Treatment of dissecting aneurysms of the aorta without surgery. *J. Thorac. Cardiovasc. Surg.*, **50**, 364–371

44

The descending thoracic aorta and thoraco-abdominal aneurysm

M. Horrocks

Introduction

Operations on the descending thoracic aorta and thoraco-abdominal segment of the aorta are principally for acute traumatic rupture, acute dissection, coarctation of aorta and chronic atherosclerotic aneurysms. The surgical management of coarctation of aorta and traumatic rupture of the thoracic aorta are dealt with elsewhere and many of the principles described there apply in the management of chronic thoraco-abdominal aneurysms. Operations on the descending thoracic aorta are complicated by the need to cross-clamp the aorta high in the chest and at the same time prevent left ventricular strain and to minimize the effects of ischaemia on the kidneys, spinal cord, abdominal viscera and the legs (see Chapter 43).

Current anaesthetic techniques allow cross-clamping of the thoracic aorta with minimal rise in blood pressure, allowing adequate time of thoracic aortic cross-clamping to enable aneurysm repair to be undertaken, and without the need for bypass (but see Chapter 43 for counter-arguments).

Aneurysms that extend into both the thoracic and abdominal cavities are traditionally classified as thoraco-abdominal aneurysms, principally because both cavities have to be entered for the necessary exposure. In all cases disease is very extensive and most patients are elderly, have generalized arterial disease and are also at risk from myocardial and cerebrovascular ischaemia. Treatment consists of graft replacement of the affected vessel with restoration of circulation, to all the branches of the aorta involved, as well as the aorta itself. These aneurysms, although fairly rare, now comprise a significant proportion of the workload of major vascular referral centres. It is estimated that one thoraco-abdominal aneurysm will be found for every 50 infrarenal aortic aneurysms.

Aetiology

The vast majority of thoraco-abdominal aneurysms are atherosclerotic, but some are due to dissection, cystic medial necrosis, infection or trauma. Some, particularly in the younger age group, are due to connective tissue disorders such as Marfan's syndrome. No matter what the aetiology, all present as an enlarged pulsatile mass in the chest or upper abdomen causing compression, erosion or spontaneous rupture. Rupture is catastrophic and may involve fistulation into the airway, bowel, chest or abdominal cavity.

Most aneurysms are fusiform in shape, with the exception of mycotic aneurysms which tend to be saccular. These are often located in the aortic arch or in the abdominal aorta behind the origin of the visceral vessels. On exploration of such aneurysms there is often only a small area of weakness in the aortic wall which gives rise to this saccular aneurysm.

Most thoraco-abdominal aneurysms require complete prosthetic replacement of the aneurysm with reimplantation of the major branch arteries. Those aneurysms which involved the arch of the aorta will frequently require aortic valve replacement and require cardiopulmonary bypass.

Predisposing factors

The presence of diffuse atherosclerosis is a frequent finding with thoraco-abdominal aneurysms, but may well not be the prime factor. The mechanism of aneurysm formation in the presence of atherosclerosis is not well understood, but clearly other factors are involved as the majority of patients with atherosclerosis do not develop aneurysm formation. The age of patients presenting with extensive aneurysm disease is on average 10 years older than those presenting with occlusive disease, and patients with thoraco-abdominal aneurysms are no exception.

Factors in aneurysm formation

1. Hydraulic stress

The frequent occurrence of aneurysmal dilatation of the aortic bifurcation has led to the suggestion that the reflected blood pressure wave down the aorta gives rise to stress on the infrarenal abdominal aorta. The majority of thoraco-abdominal aneurysms involve the infrarenal abdominal aorta and one theory suggests that the relative narrowing and obliquity of the level of the renal arteries gives rise to reflected waves which can produce the thoracic component in a thoraco-abdominal aneurysm. The presence of occlusive disease in the iliac vessels will further increase the reflected wave force, adding to the hydraulic stress factors on the aortic wall.

2. Structure

The relative scarcity of medial vasa vasorum and the relatively few number of lamellae units in the human aorta compared with other animals has led to the theory of a combination of relative ischaemia and poor physical properties predisposing to aortic aneurysm formation. The observation by Sumner who noted a 50% decrease in collagen and elastin in the wall of aortic aneurysms, lends some support to this theory. The role of collagenolysis has also been alluded to in the aetiology of rupture in aortic aneurysms. It is well recognized that the aneurysm wall contains significant collagenous activity which is not present in occlusive aneurysmal disease. Furthermore the level of collagenolysis is related to the rate of expansion of abdominal aneurysms. Similarly the level of elastase is raised in patients with aneurysmal disease, although the correlation with size is less clear. Copper metabolism has also been implicated as a factor in aneurysm formation; copper is known to be an essential code factor in lyasizeoxidase which catalyses to cross-linking of collagen and elastin. Although copper levels have been found to be slightly lower in aneurysm patients compared with controls, this may be clinically significant.

3. Vibration forces

It has been suggested that vibration forces within the aortic wall, either distal to the left subclavian or distal to the renal arteries, can be implicated in collagen disruption and early aneurysm formation. Once a small aneurysm has developed, tension on the wall increases according to Laplace's law, where wall tension is proportional to intraluminal pressure and wall radius. Although this law does not strictly apply to pulsatile flow in a tube, it is self-evident that as wall thickness grows with tension and an aneurysm expands then wall thickness must increase, resulting in further increased tension and ultimate rupture.

4. Genetic factors

The frequent discovery of aortic aneurysms in males and also a strong family history suggests an X-linked or autosomal inheritance. Currently this remains under investigation, but clearly some pattern of genetic inheritance seems likely.

Historically, syphilis was the most common cause of thoracic aneurysms involving the ascending aorta and occasionally the descending and upper abdominal aorta. Fortunately, syphilic aneurysms are now very rare.

5. Cystic medial necrosis

This was first described by Gazelle in 1928. Histologically there is necrosis and loss of the elastic laminae, with the appearance of cystic spaces filled with a hyaline material. This can occur throughout the arterial tree, but is most striking in the ascending aorta and more rarely in the descending aorta. It usually occurs in young men and is often associated with Marfan's syndrome which may not have other stigmata of the syndrome. This pathological condition predisposes to acute aortic dissection.

6. Clinical presentation

Symptoms of thoraco-abdominal aneurysms relate to pressure on adjacent structures. Most thoraco-abdominal aneurysms will present either as a chance radiological finding or because of erosion into the spine causing chronic back pain. Occasionally patients may present with pulmonary complications such as pneumonia due to bronchial compression or even with haemoptysis from aortobronchial fistulae. Many of these patients will present with the abdominal component of the thoraco-abdominal aneurysm alone, in the form of a pulsatile swelling, back pain, a pulsatile mass or embolization into the legs, or leakage.

7. Natural history

The natural history of thoraco-abdominal aneurysms is now reasonably well understood and it seems that only half of the patients presenting with thoraco-abdominal aneurysms will survive 5 years. Factors which predispose to rupture are the large size of the aneurysm, the presence of symptoms and the associated severe cardiovascular disease. Presler and MacNamara showed that 60% of large atherosclerotic aneurysms rupture within 3 years and only 20% survive 5 years if untreated. This study showed that survival following operation was both better in the long and short term. DeBakey demonstrated an approximately 60%, 5-year survival of untreated thoraco-abdominal aneurysms.

Diagnosis

Although symptoms of pneumonia, respiratory obstruction, thoracic pulsation or persistent cough or a hoarse voice may suggest the diagnosis, confirmation is necessary radiologically. The thoracic aorta is readily seen on a standard posterior anterior chest X-ray. A lateral chest X-ray may further help in diagnosis, which is best confirmed by contrast enhanced CT or MRI; arteriography is rarely necessary. Where the upper limit of an abdominal aortic aneurysm is uncertain a CT scan may also be unhelpful, and longitudinal MRI or aortography with a lateral view will help to separate the origin of the renal arteries and the upper end of the aneurysm. In the presence of an obvious thoraco-abdominal aneurysm, arteriography is of little value other than to help to delineate the anatomy of the visceral and renal arteries.

For details of the anatomy of the spinal cord blood supply see Chapter 43.

Types of thoraco-abdominal aneurysms

True thoraco-abdominal aneurysms have been classified into the following four distinct groups. Type 1 aneurysms involve the descending thoracic aorta and extend down into the proximal abdominal aorta but do not extend much below the renal vessels but require a thoraco-abdominal approach for repair. Type 2 aneurysms involve the whole thoracic aorta and the entire abdominal aorta from the left subclavian artery down to the aortic bifurcation. These are the most extensive aneurysms and carry the greatest risk. Type 3 aneurysms involve the lower part of the descending thoracic aorta and the entire abdominal aorta. Type 4 aneurysms start at the diaphragm and extend down to the aortic bifurcation.

Preoperative preparation

In view of the high morbidity and mortality in this patient group it is essential to exclude those patients who are unlikely to survive surgery. All should undergo routine preoperative blood testing, including full blood count, clotting screen, urine and serum electrolytes, chest X-ray, ECG, etc., to assess general fitness. In order to assess more carefully their respiratory function, a routine respiratory function test should be performed and blood gas estimations obtained. If fit, exercise ECG is advisable and if there is any doubt about fitness then more sophisticated cardiac function tests should be performed including ultrasound scan and, if indicated, cardiac catheterization. Renal functions should be formally assessed by a serum creatinine and a 24-hour creatinine clearance, as patients with pre-existing renal disease and in particular those with established renal failure have a poor surgical prognosis.

Careful assessment should be made of the peripheral circulation, including the presence of palpable pulses, resting ankle pressures and pre- and postexercise ankle–brachial ratio; pulse volume recordings are a useful peroperative measure, as repeated measurements can be made before, during and after the operation; these give an excellent indication of adequate reperfusion following release of aortic clamps.

Operative technique

The best surgical approach is through a left thoraco-abdominal incision. The patient is placed on the operating table with the buttocks flat on the table but the left chest rotated forward approximately 60° with the left arm placed across the face on an arm rest. The whole chest, abdomen and groin are prepared with an antiseptic solution, such as chlorhexidine in spirit, and it is preferable to use sterile drapes and adhesive plastic skin barrier as this maintains the drapes correctly.

The incision extends upwards from the pubis to the umbilicus and then obliquely to the left costal margin and then through the preselected intercostal space. If the aneurysm is type 1 or type 2, the fourth or fifth intercostal space will be entered and type 4 aneurysms can be exposed quite easily through the eighth or ninth intercostal space. The commonest mistake in this situation is to make this incision too low which does not allow adequate exposure of the upper end of the aneurysm. Occasionally it is necessary to open both the eighth or ninth and the third or fourth intercostal space to provide adequate exposure for a very extensive thoraco-abdominal aneurysm. Exposure of the aorta is then achieved by incision of the pleura on the posterolateral aspect of the aorta at the upper end of the aneursym, and a tape passed round to obtain control. The peri- and infra-diaphragmatic region of the aorta should then be exposed through an extraperitoneal approach in a so-called bloodless plane; this plane is easy to dissect up to the lateral border of the aorta where quite major veins can be encountered. A frequently unrecognized problem here is a posterior renal vein and more rarely a left-sided inferior vena cava crossing either in front of or behind the aorta at the level of the renal veins. This may necessitate division and subsequent reanastamosis of the left renal vein, but it is usually possible to repair the aneurysm without having to divide the left inferior vena cava. The left kidney and spleen are carefully mobilized and moved across to the right side to allow for this exposure. It is a good idea to mobilize the spleen carefully prior to traction, otherwise the splenic capsule may tear, requiring splenectomy. It is unwise in these extensive operations involving significant blood loss to leave a spleen with a capsular tear. Having mobilized the left colon, the whole of the thoraco-abdominal aneurysm is exposed from top to bottom and the proximal left external and internal iliac vessels are identified. If they are not adherent, tape can be passed behind to obtain control. The right proximal external and internal iliac arteries are best approached through a separate right-sided peritoneal incision and controlled with a tape. In order to expose the thoraco-abdominal portion of the aneurysm it is essential to divide the diaphragm; this is best done with cutting diathermy and the diaphragm should be marked with regular sutures to aid closure. In those aneurysms of type 3 or 4 it is often unnecessary to divide the diaphragm completely, but division allows adequate exposure and helps to preserve diaphragmatic function.

Prior to any further manipulation of renal vessels,

frusemide and mannitol may be given intravenously to help preserve renal function by inducing a diuretic state. Ilosone may also be given, some 15–20 min before clamping, and this may prolong the warm ischaemic time. Heparin is not normally recommended because of the extensive blood loss, but if Aprotinen is given routinely then a small dose of heparin may help prevent intravascular coagulation. Throughout dissection there should be close cooperation with the anaesthetist, with constant exchange of information about progress; it is important that the timing of cross-clamping of the aorta is coordinated so that pharmacological manipulation of the blood pressure can be achieved by the anaesthetist with no sudden rise or fall in the upper body blood pressure. When everything is ready for cross-clamping, then speed is of the essence to reduce the warm ischaemic time of the distal organs; careful blood replacement ensures that the patient remains cardiovascularly stable. Distal clamps can then be applied to the internal and external iliac arteries and the aneurysm is opened through a posterior incision just to the left of the midline.

Grafting technique

The technique of inserting the graft depends on the type of aneurysm encountered. With types 1, 2 or 3 aneurysms it is necessary to replace the whole of the aneurysm by a tube Dacron graft. Straightforward end-to-end anastomosis of the upper end is usual, although the use of an intraluminal graft with a rigid polypropylene cuff at the top end can speed up this part of the procedure (see Chapter 43); the intraluminal graft is sutured with four anchoring stitches and then secured by two tied tapes around the grooves of the collars, which will reduce the time of the upper anastomosis significantly. The principal disadvantage is that a considerable length of thoracic aorta above the neck of the aneurysm needs to mobilized and exposed, with the concomitant risk of damaging vital intercostal arteries. In the case of type 4 aneurysms, a long tongue of the anterior wall of the supradiaphragmatic region of the aorta may be left with the origins of the coeliac axis, superior mesenteric and renal arteries in place. This necessitates a long oblique anastomosis, but on completion of the anastomosis the blood supply to kidneys, gut and coeliac axis can be released, thus reducing the overall ischaemic time. This particular technique is very useful with juxta-renal and low thoraco-abdominal aneurysms and is associated with a low morbidity and mortality. The risk of paraplegia is proportional to the length of time of thoracic cross-clamping and so any procedure to reduce this important time interval is helpful. The additional use of intravenous thiopentone 20 mg/kg given prior to aortic clamping may also help in reducing spinal cord ischaemia. Other techniques, including reimplantation of intercostal arteries and drainage of cerebrospinal fluid during cross-clamping

(which keeps the pressure below 10 mmHg), have all been advocated to try to reduce the incidence of paraplegia, but without convincing success.

The number of patches required for reimplantation of all the visceral arteries will depend on the anatomical configuration of these arteries and the space between them. It is common to be able to reimplant the coeliac axis and the superior mesenteric on one patch, and the renal arteries are extremely variable and may have to be implanted separately or in conjunction with the other arteries. Although preoperative angiography may reveal the presence of peripheral renal arteries, it is always wise to explore carefully as sometimes an unexpected upper or lower peripheral renal artery may be seen and reimplanted at the same time.

Frequently, considerable back-bleeding may be encountered from the visceral arteries.

Following successful revascularization of the abdominal visceral arteries, offloading of the heart follows and the patient becomes more stable. The distal end of the graft is then sewn to the distal abdominal aortic bifurcation, or in the presence of iliac disease a bifurcated graft will be needed to the distal common iliacs. Following completion of the distal anastomosis, run-off should be restored into the internal iliac arteries after careful back-bleeding. The external iliac arteries can then be selectively declamped according to the patient's general condition.

Occasionally the ostia of the renal arteries are tightly stenosed which may not have been apparent in the preoperative investigations. Endarterectomy can be achieved within the aneurysm sac, but frequently this is difficult and the end-point uncertain; it is often easier to expose the renal arteries and reimplant them directly into the aortic graft. Following completion of the operation, restoration of circulation to the legs can be checked by clinical examination and by Doppler ankle pressures or pulse volume recording measures. The re-establishment of renal flow is usually followed by early production of urine and if any doubt exists then an intravenous injection of patent blue, producing blue urine, confirms that urine has been produced following the revascularization. All peripheral vessels are checked for the presence of pulsation and it is clear to all when the liver, spleen and bowel have restoration of normal circulation. Careful haemostasis must be achieved and it is wise to check clotting at this time and to correct any abnormality; if there has been extensive blood loss, fresh platelets and fresh frozen plasma may be necessary even if haematological assessments suggest that clotting is within normal limits. Once haemostasis has been achieved, the chest should be closed with two large chest drains placed through separate stab incisions in the left chest and the abdomen closed in the usual way with a suction drain under the left diaphragm.

In those patients where the principal aneurysm is thoracic with a minimal abdominal component, the reverse tongue can be used where the artery wall containing the coeliac access, superior mesenteric and either the right or both renal arteries is cut out separately as a tongue of normal aorta and the graft is sewn down behind it. This enables rapid restoration of blood supply to the visceral organs and reduces the warm ischaemic time.

Note on prevention of paraplegia

Paraplegia remains the most unfortunate and sinister of complications following apparently successful repair of thoraco-abdominal aneurysm, and perhaps has attracted the greatest controvesy. The use of a variety of heparin-bonded shunts, in particular femorofemoral and atriofemoral bypass shunts, has not reduced the incidence of paraplegia and they are associated with considerable technical problems. The routine use of spinal fluid drainage can theoretically improve spinal cord perfusion and may well increase the safe clamp time. However, in a recent prospective randomized study involving 200 patients, no benefit accrued from the routine use of spinal fluid drainage.

The incidence of paraplegia increases with the complexity and extent of the aneurysm, and even the implantation of arteries thought to coincide with the artery of Adamkiewicz seems to show no benefit in terms of paraplegia.

The technique of spinal cord drainage after induction of anaesthesia

A size 18 spinal needle is introduced intrathecally, usually between the fourth and fifth lumbar vertebrae, and a Silastic catheter implanted. A total of 100–150 ml of spinal fluid may be withdrawn and the needle subsequently removed, leaving the intrathecal catheter in place. This catheter is then connected to a pressure transducer for monitoring and spinal fluid is withdrawn when the pressure exceeds 10 mmHg; by this technique quite large volumes of cerebrospinal fluid can be withdrawn and this may be maintained into the postoperative period. On rare occasions paraplegia may occur several days following operation when the aetiology is less clear. It is thought that this may represent a reperfusion injury and steroids may be helpful to reduce the incidence of this complication. Other factors which may decrease reperfusion injury include cooling and the use of thiopentone sodium, both of which have been shown experimentally to prolong the warm ischaemic time.

During the extensive dissection involved in thoraco-abdominal aneurysm repair, the patient's core temperature may well drop down to 33–34°C, even before thoracic aortic cross-clamping. This may be achieved by a relatively cool operating theatre and avoidance of a heating blanket. After completion of revascularization and restoration of flow to visceral organs, the patient may then be warmed by a combination of increasing the room temperature, switching on the warming blanket and giving warmed blood and crystalloid. Although individually all these methods may be of marginal benefit, the complication of paraplegia is so catastrophic that all techniques would appear to be justified.

Complications and results

The team approach to repair of thoraco-abdominal aneurysm, with attention to all the many details which help to improve the outcome, should provide an acceptable morbidity and mortality.

Results with an overall mortality as low as 2% have been recorded, with paraplegia and paraparesis occurring in 6%. The incidence of paraplegia may be as low as 1.5% when all types of aneurysm are taken into account. Renal failure appears to be a relatively rare complication and is usually associated with pre-existing renal artery disease, often undiagnosed preoperatively. In these patients, care must be taken to ensure that the reimplanted renal arteries are patent with adequate perfusion and any renal artery stenosis should be corrected. Transient elevation of creatinine and urea postoperatively is quite common but rarely requires dialysis and the prognosis seems to be excellent.

Major complications include myocardial infarction and pulmonary problems which may require prolonged ventilation. Overall this group of patients represents a considerable surgical challenge, but with a meticulous approach and good teamwork excellent results can be achieved with reasonable long-term survival.

45

The peripheral veins

K. Burnand

Disorders of the peripheral veins of the lower limb are common, whereas disorders of the veins of the upper limbs are rare (Browse *et al.*, 1988). Varicose veins are perhaps the price the human race pays for adopting the erect posture. The calf pump mechanism and to a lesser extent the thigh and foot pumps encourage venous return against the force of gravity. Failure of these 'peripheral hearts' leads to a persistently elevated venous pressure on standing and walking and causes the changes in the skin and subcutaneous tissues which lead to venous ulceration. Poor venous return is a factor in the development of thrombosis within the deep veins of the calf and thigh in the postoperative period and is an important and largely preventable cause of morbidity and mortality.

Surgical anatomy of the veins of the lower limb

The venous drainage of the superficial tissues of the leg is by three main routes: the long and short saphenous veins and the communicating or 'perforating' veins and the deep veins (Figure 45.1). Valves direct blood flow proximally and through communicating veins into the deep veins. The deep tissues of the calf drain into the paired venae commitantes of the three main lower leg arteries which coalesce to form the popliteal vein. This receives soleal and gastrocnemius tributaries before it ascends through the thigh as the superficial femoral vein. Venous blood is directed proximally by numerous valves and propelled against the force of gravity by the powerful contractions of the calf muscles squeezing the soleal sinusoids. The long and short saphenous veins have relatively thick muscular coats, but the walls of their tributaries are thin and dilate to form 'varicose veins' or 'varices'.

Varicose veins

Varicose veins are defined by the World Health Organization as tortuous and dilated veins. Primary varicose veins are often familial, while secondary varices are often the result of post-thrombotic deep vein damage. Rare causes of secondary varicose veins include the Klippel–Trenauney syndrome, and acquired or congenital arteriovenous fistulae. Most primary varicose veins are associated with incompetence of the valves within the long or short saphenous veins. Much less common are vulval and pudendal varices. Dilated venules (venous flares, venous stars or telangiectases) are quite common, but these dilated cutaneous venules are not varicose veins and are only of cosmetic importance.

The aetiology of varicose veins is disputed. It may be a primary disorder of the valves (Ludbrook, 1963) or an inherited disorder of collagen and connective tissue (Svejcar *et al.*, 1963) which allows the vein wall to dilate and the valves to become secondarily incompetent. Apparently rare among rural Africans, varicose veins are quite common in industrialized Western society (Borschberg, 1976). A smooth muscle abnormality has been demonstrated (Rose, 1986), but it is not known if this is cause or effect. Catabolism of connective tissue in patients with primary varicose veins is greater than in normal controls (Buddecke, 1975) and this seems to be related to increased local lysosomal enzyme activity (Niebes and Laszt, 1971) and to increased serum levels of these enzymes (Niebes and Berson, 1973). Venous dilatation secondary to wall weakness prevents the valve cusps from meeting and reflux then increases the dilatation. The valves themselves are not damaged by this process. A familial tendency is well recognized (Gunderson and Hauge, 1969) and the incidence is increased by occupations which involve prolonged standing (Lake *et al.*, 1942).

Primary varices often appear initially during the first pregnancy and disappear after childbirth, only to reappear and persist with each subsequent pregnancy (McCausland, 1943; King, 1950). Raised oestrogen levels cause a generalized smooth muscle relaxation, there is an increase in circulating blood volume and the bulk of the gravid uterus may obstruct venous return.

Symptoms and complications

The commonest symptom is aching, particularly after prolonged standing, and night cramps are quite common. Venous eczema and lipodermatosclerosis suggest the possibility of deep vein damage or incompetence of the calf communicating veins and indicate the potential for future venous ulceration. Varices may bleed and this can be catastrophic unless the patient or a companion elevates the limb and compresses the bleeding point. Superficial thrombophlebitis is a common complication of varicose veins and may propagate to the deep veins.

Many patients, especially women, complain of the disfigurement of varicose veins and the ache that

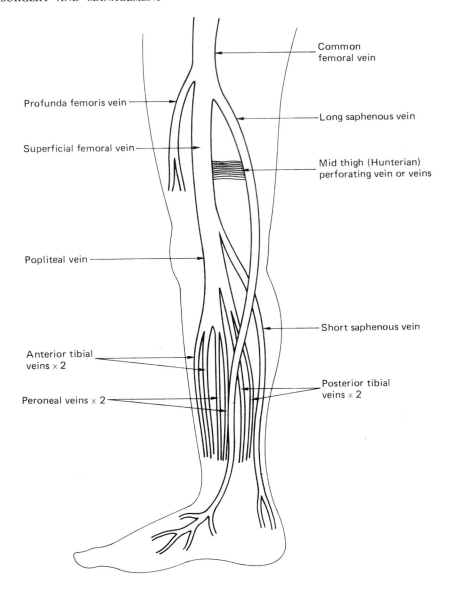

Figure 45.1 Major venous pathways of the lower limb

accompanies unsightly veins is often ephemeral. Varicose vein pain is never felt at night, is worse at the end of the day and felt in or over the major varicosities. If the pain is 'atypical', another cause must be sought such as oestoarteritis of the hip and knee, intermittent claudication, lumbar disc pain and peripheral neuritis.

Examination of the patient

All patients with varicose veins must have a general physical examination, the urine should be tested and the blood pressure taken. The abdomen should be examined to exclude a pelvic tumour or other abnormality. The legs, including the peripheral pulses, are examined with the patient lying on a couch, but the veins are only properly assessed with the patient standing.

The examination is carried out in a warm cubicle in a good light with the patient properly undressed. The patient should stand on a stool and the surgeon should sit opposite on a low chair for maximum ease of examination. The limbs must be carefully inspected from the front and the back for the presence and distribution of the varicosities. The dilated tributaries should be carefully charted on printed outlines of the lower limbs. The presence of lipodermatosclerosis, venous ankle flare, atrophie blanche and 'blow outs' should be noted.

A hand is run over the course of the saphenous veins as some varicosities are more easily appreciated on palpation than inspection. One or two fingers (the index and middle) should be placed over the sapheno-femoral junction (2 cm below and lateral to the pubic tubicle) and the patient is then asked to cough. The presence of a thrill is indicative of long saphenous incompetence. A finger is used to percuss over any dilated varicosities on the medial side of the leg. The presence of a percussion wave detected by the fingers over the saphenofemoral junction also indicates long saphenous incompetence. The process can be reversed by tapping over the saphenofemoral junction and placing the detecting fingers over the dilated varices. Groin varices and suprapubic veins should be sought as these indicate the presence of an iliac vein stenosis or occlusion. Pulsating varices are found when an arteriovenous fistula is present. The popliteal fossa is palpated with the knees slightly flexed to determine if a dilated short saphenous trunk is present. This is indicative of short saphenous incompetence, which is confirmed by tourniquet tests (see below) and special investigations.

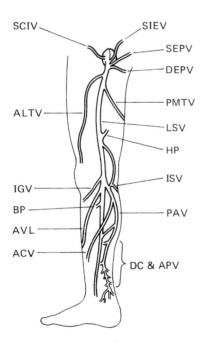

Figure 45.2 Long saphenous vein and its tributaries. SCIV, Superficial circumflex iliac vein. SIEV, Superficial inferior epigastric vein. SEPV, Superficial external pudendal vein. DEPV, Deep external pudendal vein. ALTV Anterolateral thigh vein. PMTV, Posteromedial thigh vein. LSV, Long saphenous vein. HP, Hunterian perforator. IGV, Infragenicular vein. ISV, Intersaphenous vein. BP, Boyd's perforator. AVL, Anterior vein of leg. PAV, Posterior arch vein (of Leonardo da Vinci). ACV, Anterior crural vein. DC and APV, Direct calf and ankle perforating (communicating) veins

Surgical anatomy

The long saphenous vein and its tributaries are shown in Figure 45.2. Four main tributaries enter the long saphenous vein near its termination; these are the superficial and deep external pudendal veins, the superficial

epigastric and circumflex iliac veins. Lower down, two large tributaries enter the long saphenous vein (the anterolateral and posteromedial thigh veins). Below the knee the anterolateral vein and the posterior arch vein of Leonardo join the long saphenous, and the important medial calf direct (perforating) communicating veins link the posterior arch vein with the posterior tibial vein. The main long saphenous stem rarely becomes dilated in the lower leg. There is often a small medial tributary which communicates with the short saphenous vein which can lead to confusion in diagnosis. The long saphenous vein is accompanied by the saphenous nerve which is closely applied to the vein in the lower one third of the leg where it may be damaged by the passage of a stripper (Cox and Wellwood, 1974). At the ankle the long saphenous vein lies in front of the media malleolus.

The tributaries of the long saphenous vein often have a variable termination. The long saphenous vein itself may be duplicated (Figure 45.3) and may sometimes join the common femoral vein deep to the external pudendal artery (Figure 45.4). Occasionally a high bifurcation of the common femoral artery results in the profunda femoris artery lying medial to the femoral vein. The long saphenous vein may have two terminations into the common femoral vein at the groin (Figure 45.3).

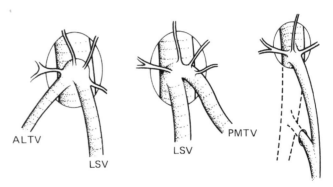

Figure 45.3 A bifid or duplicated long saphenous termination. ALTV, Anterolateral thigh vein. PMTV, Posteromedial thigh vein. LSV, Long saphenous vein

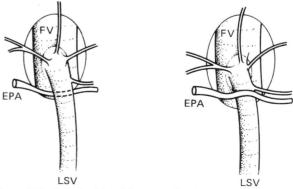

Figure 45.4 Relationship of the external pudendal artery (EPA) to the termination of the long saphenous vein (LSV). FV, Femoral vein

Special tests

Tourniquet test

A rubber tourniquet is placed tightly around the upper thigh after the superficial veins have been emptied by elevation. The patient is then asked to stand quickly and the limb is observed to discover whether the varices remain empty or refill. Good tourniquet control implies that the major problem is saphenofemoral incompetence and this is confirmed by rapid refilling of the varices when the tourniquet is released after about 30 s. If the tourniquet does not control the varices, it is reapplied below the knee. Control at this point indicates short saphenous incompetence, while a further failure of control implies incompetence of the calf communicating veins.

Doppler tests

Retrograde flow, detected by a zero-crossing Doppler probes placed over the dilated veins during a Valsalva manoeuvre or when the tourniquet is released, confirms long saphenous reflux. Biphasic flow may also be heard over the long saphenous termination during calf squeezing and release. Duplex Doppler is an even more accurate method of visualizing the deep to superficial communications and detecting reflux in both superficial and deep veins, but its use is rarely necessary in uncomplicated long saphenous incompetence (Hoare et al., 1974) (Figure 45.5).

Venography and varicography

Varicography and ascending phlebography should be reserved for the investigation of limbs which prove difficult to assess by the techniques described above (Browse et al., 1988). These tests are especially useful in patients with recurrent varicose veins or when post-thrombotic changes are suspected (Figures 45.6 and 45.7).

Management

On completion of the history and examination most patients can be categorized and scheduled for surgery or sclerotherapy. A few patients require further investigations and those with post-thrombotic limbs are probably best treated by elastic support stockings which may be prescribed in pregnancy or when patients are very old or unfit. In principle, patients with long or short saphenous incompetence are best treated by surgical ligation of the saphenofemoral or saphenopopliteal junctions. Stripping of the trunk vein appears to reduce the incidence of recurrence (Munn et al., 1981). The value of ligating the calf communicating veins has been questioned (Sethia and Darke, 1984), but this observation does appear to reduce the incidence of recurrent varicose veins and ulceration in patients with normal deep veins. Sclerotherapy appears to be equally efficacious in treating calf communicating vein incompetence (Hobbs, 1974). Sclerotherapy is ideal treatment for simple tributary incompetence and is very useful in removing

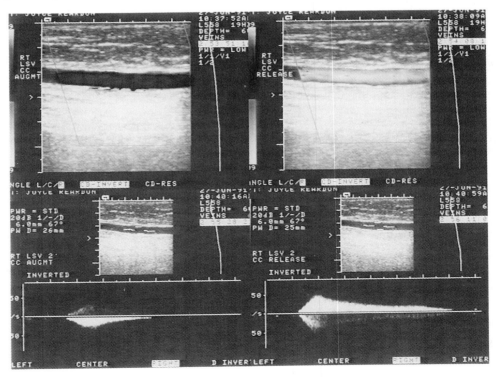

Figure 45.5 A colour duplex scan showing reflux down the long saphenous vein

minor residual veins or recurrent varicose veins after saphenous surgery.

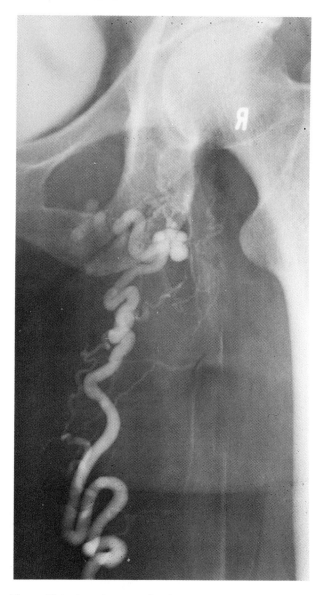

Figure 45.6 A varicogram showing a groin recurrence after a previous high saphenous ligation

High saphenous ligation and long saphenous stripping

Patients are re-examined in the ward before operation and the tributaries are carefully marked on the skin surface with an indelible pen. The more accurately the tributaries are marked, the easier they are to find and avulse at the time of surgery. Marks are placed over the termination of the saphenous veins and circles are placed over the sites of suspected communicating vein incompetence. General anaesthesia is normally used in the UK, although local anaesthesia is widely used elsewhere (Nabatoff, 1970). It is difficult to provide suitable anaesthesia for stripping unless a spinal or epidural is used. The patient is positioned with the legs widely abducted on a padded board (Figure 45.8) and the operating table is tilted to elevate the feet as far as possible without the patient slipping off the table! Chlorhexidine in spirit or povidone-iodine is used to prepare the skin. The former allows the skin markings to be seen more easily.

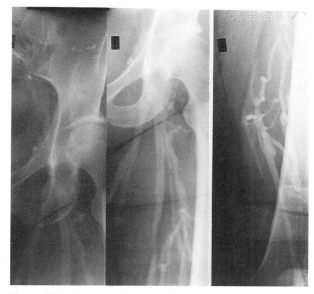

Figure 45.7 An ascending venogram showing post-thrombotic changes

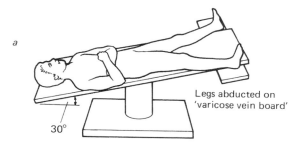

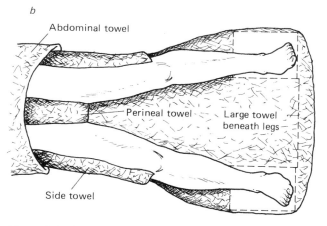

Figure 45.8 Position on the table (*a*) and towelling up (*b*) of the patient for a high saphenous ligation and long saphenous stripping

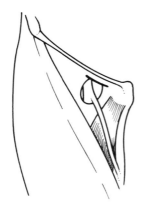

Figure 45.9 Incision for high saphenous ligation

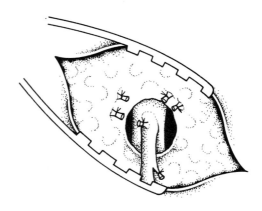

Figure 45.12 Division of the tributaries entering the long saphenous and femoral veins near the saphenofemoral junction

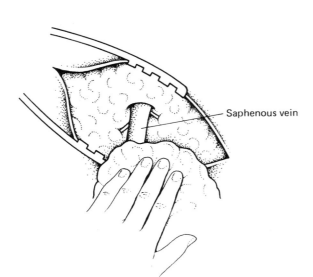

Saphenous vein

Figure 45.10 Exposure of the long saphenous vein in the subcutaneous fat

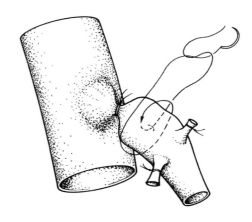

Figure 45.13 Double flush ligation of the long saphenous vein at its termination using a transfixion suture

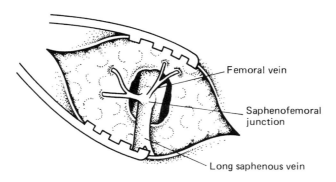

Femoral vein

Saphenofemoral junction

Long saphenous vein

Figure 45.11 Insertion of a self-retaining retractor to display the termination of the long saphenous vein

1. A skin crease incision is made centred on a point 2.5 cm below and lateral to the pubic tubercle (Figure 45.9). The length of the incision varies with the size of the patient (thin, short, fat, long), but must allow adequate exposure of the saphenofemoral junction.

2. The subcutaneous fat is split by placing a swab on either side of the incision and gently but firmly parting the fingers. The long saphenous vein is exposed as it passes across the centre of the wound (Figure 45.10). If this manoeuvre does not display the trunk of the vein blunt dissection, opening the points of the scissors in the plane of the vein, separates the fat and exposes its upper surface.

3. Once the vein has been identified it is traced upwards by bluntly dissecting the fat off the adventitia with scissors or a small artery forcep. A self-retaining retractor such as a Travers, Cockett's or West is inserted to hold the fat apart (Figure 45.11).

4. As the vein is dissected upwards a number of tributaries are found entering the main trunk (see Figure 45.2); small veins may be ligated. These small

veins need to be divided between small artery forceps and ligated with catgut or an absorbable soluble suture such as polyglycolic acid or they may be ligated in continuity and divided (Figure 45.12).

5. The main trunk of the saphenous vein should not be divided until its termination in the femoral vein has been confirmed. This avoids accidental division of a superficial femoral vein or artery which can be mistaken for a saphenous vein in a thin individual. This is a disastrous mistake!

6. As the long saphenous vein nears its termination it dips down through the cribriform fascia. The superficial external pudendal artery usually passes just beneath the saphenous vein as it dips down (see Figure 45.4), but it may pass in front and can be divided with impunity.

7. A white 'line' of fascial condensation marks the saphenofemoral junction. The femoral vein should be dissected free from its surrounding fascia for approximately 1 cm above and below the saphenofemoral junction. The deep external pudendal vein commonly terminates either at the sapheno-junction or in the common femoral vein and must be carefully ligated and divided.

8. At this point, and not before, the long saphenous vein can be divided between ligatures. The upper ligature should be flush with the saphenofemoral junction. Double ligatures of catgut or polyglycolic acid may be used at the top end or a transfixion suture may be preferred to prevent the knot from slipping (Figure 45.13). Non-absorbable sutures should not be used as they can lead to sinus formation if a groin infection occurs. A short length of long saphenous vein is left beyond the ligature with its attached tributary. This helps to prevent the ligature from rolling off the end of the vein.

Stripping the long saphenous vein

A Miles flexible internal stripper or one of its modifications is used (Figure 45.14). Some prefer a plastic disposable stripper (Figure 45.15) (Corbett and Harris, 1991). Plastic strippers are expensive and it is more difficult to direct their tips down the vein. Metal strippers must be carefully maintained and rough handling renders them difficult to use if kinks have been made in the flexible wire.

In most patients the varicose calf tributaries of the long saphenous vein join the main trunk just below the knee and the long saphenous vein itself is not usually varicose below this level. It is therefore quite sufficient to strip down to the upper one-third of the lower leg. This avoids the risk of damaging the attached saphenous nerve which is closely applied to the saphenous trunk in the lower leg (Cox and Wellwood, 1974).

1. The upper end of the long saphenous vein is held taut by traction on an artery forceps which occludes the lumen. A ligature is placed around the vein a centimetre or two below the artery forceps and held

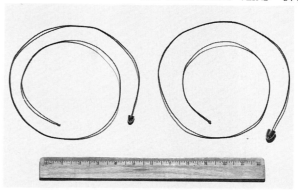

Figure 45.14 A flexible metal stripper

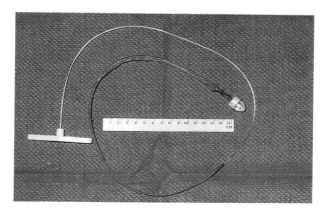

Figure 45.15 A plastic disposable stripper with the long saphenous vein on it

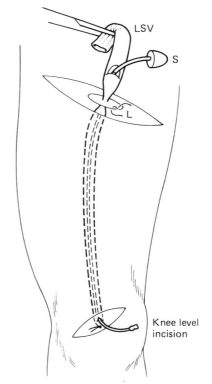

Figure 45.16 Passage of the stripper down the long saphenous vein (LSV). S, Stripper. L, Ligature

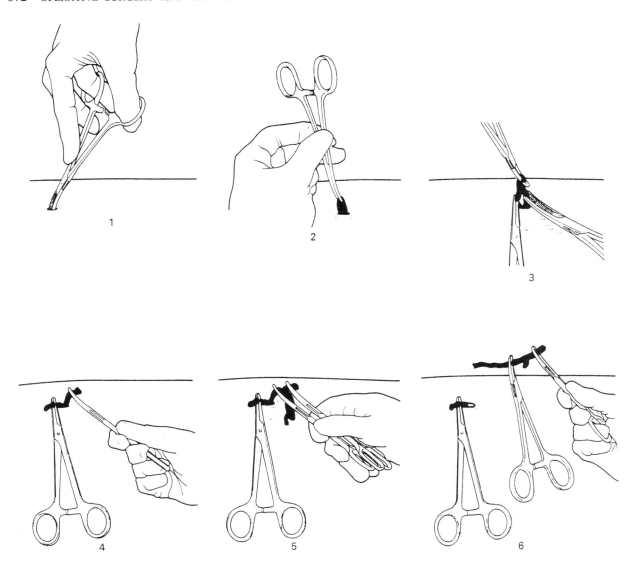

Figure 45.17 Technique for avulsing varices. (After Browse, Burnand and Lea Thomas, 1988)

taut to prevent blood from escaping when a small transverse venotomy is made to insert the tip of the stripper.

2. The ligature is tied down once the tip of the stripper has passed down the vein to prevent further blood loss (Figure 45.16). The passage of the stripper is aided by pulling up on the proximal artery forceps to straighten and tauten the vein and allow the tip to be forced through any residual or valve remnants. The point may be negotiated down the vein by gentle rotatory movements of the free upper end of the stripper which encourages the tip to enter different passages as it descends. An undesirable 'course' should be remedied by withdrawal and repassage of the stripper.

3. When the stripper has been passed down the vein and identified under the skin in the upper one-third of the leg it should be located through a small incision made directly over its tip. The vein containing the stripper is identified, divided and ligated, allowing the stripper to be brought out onto the surface. The vein is fixed onto the stripper with a ligature before a handle is attached and the vein is stripped out by continuous downward traction on the handle causing the vein to concertina up on the top 'olive'.

Avulsions of tributaries

After the long saphenous has been stripped its varicose tributaries are avulsed through a number of small incisions placed at strategic sites along their course.

1. Tiny 2 mm stab incisions are made using a pointed no. 11 scapel blade. These incisions which are

made in Langer's lines are usually placed about 5–10 cm apart.

2. The vein is seen as a white worm in surrounding yellow fat. It is picked up by mosquito forceps and dissected free from the surrounding fat and overlying skin. It is then pulled onto the surface by gentle traction and a loop is developed (Figure 45.17).

3. The loop is freed and divided between mosquito forceps. Both ends of the vein are then teased and pulled out of the subcutaneous fat by a process of firm persistent traction on the artery forceps, combined with subcutaneous blunt dissection by opening the points of the mosquito forceps pushed in alongside the vein (Figure 45.17).

4. Curved hooks have been designed to hook up the vein and free it from the fat by passing them alongside the vein beneath the skin (Chester and Taylor, 1990).

5. White veins avulse well, blue veins tend to tear. As the vein is pulled out of the stab incision, other mosquito forceps are applied to obtain better traction and prevent the vein from disintegrating. Gentle rotatory movements of the attached forceps, combined with blunt dissection under the skin by the mosquito forceps, help in this process. Three to 10 cm of vein can be avulsed through each incision.

6. When the vein eventually tears, haemorrhage is controlled by firm external pressure using a swab. Ligation is rarely necessary but can be used at the distal end of a tributary to prevent continuing haemorrhage.

7. Some surgeons carry out avulsions and stripping in an exsanguinated limb using a tourniquet to provide a bloodless field. This is released before the wounds are closed (Royle, 1984).

Wound closure and bandaging

Subcuticular 3/0 prolene or polydiaxanone sulphate (PDS) is used for closing the groin incision except in the obese, in whom interrupted 2/0, 3/0 or 4/0 nylon sutures should be used. Very small avulsion incisions can be closed with Steri-strips, with a single 4/0 prolene or nylon stitch or even left open if not bleeding. Small incisions are covered by tiny pieces of gauze held in place by plastic spray. Mepore dressings are more comfortable for larger incisions such as the groin.

The leg is bandaged with 10 or 15 cm Elastocrepe or Tensopress bandages and the patient returns to the recovery room with the foot of the bed elevated. Most patients prefer to have both legs operated on at the same time, choosing some additional temporary discomfort to more prolonged treatment.

Postoperative care

Active movement is encouraged. The patient should walk the following morning after the addition of a second pair of bandages over the first set. Most patients leave the hospital by lunchtime on the first postoperative day, with instructions to walk as much as possible, not to stand still or sit with their legs down, to lie on a bed when not walking or sit with the leg elevated on a stool. Patients need to reattend hospital if pain develops in the limb, especially if this becomes severe or if the toes become numb.

Bandages are worn until the sutures are removed after 5–7 days. One set of bandages is reapplied when the patient stands and these are worn for two or three weeks until the bruising has settled and the patient feels comfortable. Elastic stockings are an expensive alternative to bandages. Pain is controlled by suitable oral analgesia (soluble aspirin, paracetamol, codeine phosphate or a nonsteroidal anti-inflammatory) and walking is encouraged. Patients should return to work after a week to 10 days, although some take three or four weeks off.

Complications of high saphenous ligation and stripping

1. Groin haemorrhage occasionally results from a slipped saphenofemoral ligature. Haemorrhage can be controlled by pressure on the femoral vein above and below the junction, and the sucker allows the termination of the long saphenous vein to be identified and controlled by the application of an artery forcep. Double ligation or transfixion ligation usually avoids this problem. If it occurs, the junction may be closed by a continuous 5/0 running prolene suture.

2. Partial damage to the common femoral vein can usually be repaired without serious side effects. A wider incision allows the vein to be controlled above and below the saphenofemoral junction by finger compression. Bulldog clamps can then be applied and the tear closed with a continuous 5/0 or 6/0 prolene suture.

3. Division of the femoral artery or an abnormal profunda femoris artery can occur. Haemorrhage can be controlled by finger pressure. The artery is exposed and controlled. Heparin is given, clamps are applied and repair is effected with an arterial suture of 5/0 or 6/0 prolene, with or without a vein patch as necessary.

4. Wound sepsis is rare, provided that haematoma formation is avoided.

5. Saphenous neuritis is uncommon if the long saphenous vein is not stripped to the ankle.

6. Other nerves such as the lateral popliteal may occasionally be damaged during the avulsion of varices. Awareness of this possibility and reasonable care should prevent this complication.

7. Deep vein thrombosis and pulmonary embolism are very uncommon.

8. Haematoma and bruising in the track of the stripped long saphenous vein always occurs to some extent but rarely cause major problems. If the bandages are loosened in the early stages, haematoma formation is inevitably more severe.

9. Lymphatoma or lymph fistula in the groin

wound may occur, especially during re-exploration (see below), and can prove troublesome. They may occasionally require exploration for drainage and to ligate the lymphatics.

Surgery of the short saphenous vein

SURGICAL ANATOMY

The short saphenous vein passes upwards from behind the lateral malleolus along the middle of the back of the calf to the popliteal fossa, where it usually joins the popliteal vein (Figure 45.18). It often perforates the deep fascia in the lower third of the calf and lies beneath the fascia until its termination (Figure 45.19). It is commonly connected to the deep veins by a communicating vein which passes between the twin bellies of gastrocnemius. A number of tributaries join the short saphenous vein in the popliteal fossa. Important tributaries include the persisting posterior axial vein which runs down the middle of the posterior surface of the calf and another which joins the long saphenous vein. In the lower third of the leg the short saphenous vein is closely accompanied by the sural nerve which must be identified and preserved.

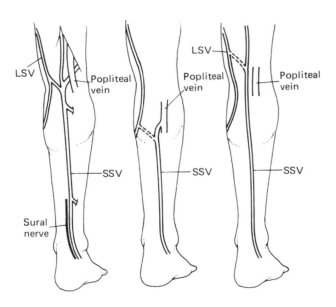

Figure 45.18 Termination of the short saphenous vein (SSV) in the popliteal fossa. LSV, Long saphenous vein

ANATOMICAL VARIATIONS

The short saphenous vein has a very variable termination (Figure 45.20). The most common 'anomaly' is a high termination (33%) (Kosinski, 1926). It may end in the centre of the thigh (persistent post-axial vein or vein of Jacomini) either in the profunda system of veins or by joining the long saphenous vein (Figures 45.18 and 45.20). A low termination occurs in about

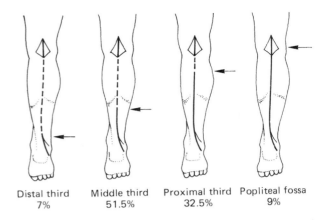

| Distal third 7% | Middle third 51.5% | Proximal third 32.5% | Popliteal fossa 9% |

Figure 45.19 Points at which the short saphenous vein pierces the deep fascia

9%; the vein either terminates in the long saphenous vein or joins the gastrocnemius veins below knee level (Figure 45.20). The saphenopopliteal junction may then be missed if a conventional popliteal skin crease approach is used (see below). Preoperative varicography (Lea Thomas and Bowles, 1985) (phlebography without tourniquets with injections made directly into the major varicose veins) or duplex scanning (Hoare and Royle, 1984) can prevent such mistakes.

SHORT SAPHENOUS LIGATION AND STRIPPING

Incompetence of the short saphenous vein may occur in isolation or may accompany long saphenous incompetence. Both can be dealt with under the same anaesthetic, with the short saphenous vein approached first. The examination of the patient and preoperative preparation are similar to that described for the long saphenous vein.

1. The anaesthetist must intubate and ventilate the patient. The patient is then placed face downwards with the chest and abdomen resting on pillows. The legs are widely abducted on a padded board.

2. The short saphenous vein is located at the ankle through a short transverse incision placed just behind the lateral malleolus (Figure 45.21). The sural nerve usually lies posteriorly (Figure 45.18) and is pushed away from the short saphenous before the vein is ligated distally. A second suture is passed around the vein proximally and held up to prevent backbleeding.

3. A transverse venotomy allows the stripper to be inserted and pushed up to the popliteal fossa. The termination of the short saphenous vein is usually close to the point where the stripper can no longer be palpated.

4. The popliteal fossa is explored through a 7–10 cm long skin crease incision (Figure 45.21) sited on the basis of the preoperative investigations or made at the point where the stripper can no longer be palpated.

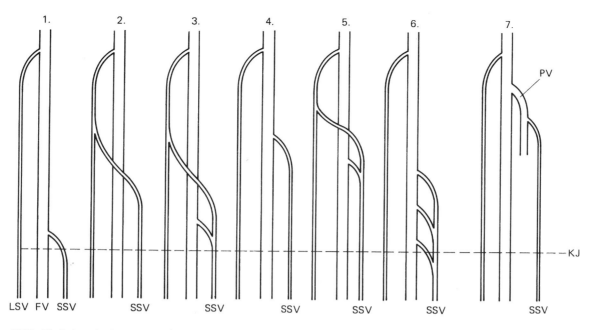

Figure 45.20 Variations in the termination of the short saphenous vein (SSV). KJ, Level of knee joint. LSV, Long saphenous vein. FV, femoral vein. PV, Deep femoral vein

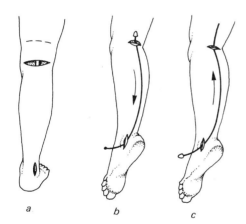

Figure 45.21 Stripping the short saphenous vein

confirmed, as this avoids inadvertent damage to the popliteal vein. Blunt dissection with division of the tributaries enables the saphenopopliteal junction to be defined.

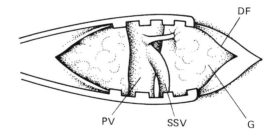

Figure 45.22 Dissection of the saphenopopliteal junction. PV, Popliteal vein. SSV, Short saphenous vein. DF, Deep fascia. G, Gastrocnemius muscle

5. Superficial veins are ligated and divided and the deep fascia is opened in the line of the incision. The sural nerve is identified and the short saphenous vein is found passing up in the subcutaneous fat. The vein is easily located because it contains the semi-rigid stripper (Figure 45.21).

6. The short saphenous trunk is traced to its termination at a T-junction with the popliteal vein. This dissection is aided by insertion of a self-retaining retractor or using a couple of Langenbeck's retractors held by an assistant (Figure 45.22). The dissection is easier if the knee is flexed as this relaxes the deep fascia and the muscles of the popliteal fossa. The vein must not be divided until its termination has been

7. The short saphenous vein is flush ligated in continuity, divided and stripped. The deep fascia and skin are closed after any haematoma has been expressed. The bandaging and postoperative care is the same as for operation on the long saphenous vein.

COMPLICATIONS

These include haematoma formation, wound infection and sural nerve damage. The most serious problem is damage to the popliteal vein which can be avoided if the anatomy is carefully confirmed before any veins are ligated or divided. Recurrent popliteal fossa varicosities develop if ligation of the sapheno-popliteal junction is imprecise. This is usually because the vein has been ligated some distance from its termination, leaving the distal tributaries still draining into its upper end.

Surgery of the incompetent calf communicating veins (perforating veins)

SURGICAL ANATOMY

The calf communicating (perforating) veins are those veins which penetrate the deep fascia to join surface veins with the deep veins of the calf. A number of unimportant indirect perforating veins enter the muscles in the upper half of the leg before joining the deep veins. Three or four important direct perforating veins are present on the medial side of the lower calf (Cockett and Elgan Jones, 1953) (see Figure 45.2). These arise from the posterior arch vein and join the posterior tibial vein. There are one or two direct perforating veins on the lateral side of the leg which connect the short saphenous to the peroneal veins (see Figure 45.19). Each perforating vein contains a valve which directs blood from the superficial to the deep veins (Thompson, 1979).

Communicating veins exist in Hunter's canal, in the upper thigh and in the upper calf, Boyd's perforating vein and the gastrocnemius perforating (see Figure 45.2) veins. These communicate with varicosities but are not usually a cause of venous ulceration.

Incompetence of the valves of the communicating veins may be associated with primary varicose veins and with long or short saphenous incompetence. Communicating vein incompetence missed at operation is often responsible for recurrent varicosities. Secondary incompetence of the perforating veins is usually the result of a previous thrombosis in the calf veins extending into the communicating veins. Post-thrombotic deep vein incompetenceis nearly always associated with perforating vein damage and results eventually in lipodermatosclerosis and ulceration (Burnand et al., 1976). The middle and lower medial calf communicating veins are the commonest to become incompetent: the lateral peroneal perforator rarely becomes incompetent, as does the lowest medial perforator which lies behind the medial malleolus.

INDICATIONS AND CONTRAINDICATIONS

The indications and contraindications for the treatment of varicose veins secondary to communicating vein incompetence are identical to those which apply to long or short saphenous incompetence. Injection sclerotherapy may be selected if there is no associated long or short saphenous incompetence. Post-thrombotic incompetence of the communicating veins is considered with the management of the post-thrombotic syndrome..

EXAMINATION

The presence of an ankle flare, lipodermatosclerosis or large dilated veins (blowouts) over the recognized sites of calf communicating veins suggests that the valves in the these veins have become incompetent. Failure of the tourniquet to control calf varicosities and a failure of the surface veins to empty during walking with a below knee tourniquet applied to the limb (Perthes, 1895) (Perthes' walking test) makes the diagnosis of perforator incompetence extremely likely. Other clinical tests such as the application of multiple tourniquets, the palpation of fascial defects and the sliding finger test to control 'leak points' are of dubious value, with a localization accuracy of around 60% (O'Donnell et al., 1977; Lamont et al., 1986). Bipedal ascending phlebography and duplex scanning avoid false positives but may miss some incompetent veins. Thermography, hand-held Doppler and fluorescein testing have all been discredited. Accurate localization cannot be ensured by any of these tests and if their ligation is considered to be important a full exposure of the medial sub-fascial space must be carried out (e.g. to prevent venous reulceration). A local exploration based on preoperative localization by duplex scanning or phlebography is often appropriate for perforating incompetence that is not associated with any skin changes. Clinical examination is an unreliable method of locating the sites of incompetent perforating veins.

INCOMPETENT MEDICAL CALF COMMUNICATING VEINS (PERFORATORS)

Patient preparation and anaesthesia are as before and a head-down tilt reduces bleeding. These veins are best approached through a long vertical subfascial incision described by Linton (1938) (Figure 45.23). The posterior stocking seam incision of Dodd (1964) is an alternative if lipodermatosclerosis spares the posterior surface of the leg. The extrafascial approach of Cockett (1955) is not recommended, as excessive undermining which may be necessary invariably leads to skin edge necrosis.

1. The incision is placed one finger's breadth behind the posterior border of the tibia and extends from the medial malleolus to nearly halfway up the leg where the calf muscles begin to swell (Figure 45.23). The subcutaneous fat and deep fascia are divided in the same line as the incision. Any subcutaneous veins that are encountered are ligated and divided.

2. The anterior flap with its attached deep fascia is elevated and any communicating veins which cross this plane close to the posterior border of the tibia are identified. The veins with their accompanying arteries are then ligated with 2/0 chromic catgut and divided.

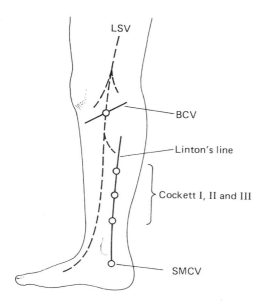

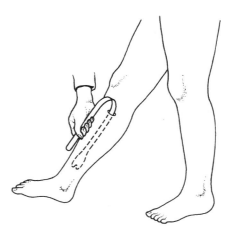

Figure 45.25 Use of the Edwards phlebotome

Figure 45.23 The Linton/Cockett incision. LSV, Long saphenous vein. BCV, Boyd's communicating vein. SMCV, Submalleolar communicating vein

By gently stripping the muscles away from the deep fascia of the posterior flap, other communicating veins are identified, ligated and divided (Figure 45.24).

3. The deep fascia does not need to be closed but can be approximated with 2/0 continuous catgut. The skin is closed with interrupted 2/0 prolene or nylon sutures or alternatively with a subcuticular PDS and Steristrips. An incompetent long saphenous vein can easily be found under the upper end of this incision and stripped out at the same time.

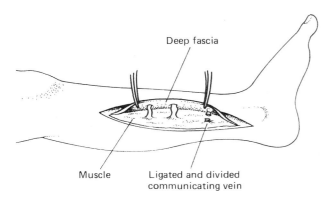

Figure 45.24 Exposure of the medial incompetent communicating veins through the subfascial approach

ALTERNATIVES

Edwards (1976) designed a phlebotome to be pushed down beneath the deep fascia to 'shear' off the communicating veins as they leave the muscle (Figure 45.25). This causes considerable haemorrhage but avoids the long incision in poor-quality tissues.

INCOMPETENT LATERAL COMMUNICATING VEINS

These are approached by local cut-downs and ligated as they cross the deep fascia.

A HIGH MEDIAL CALF PERFORATOR (BOYD'S PERFORATOR)

This is approached through a longitudinal or oblique incision placed directly over the site of the vein.

GASTROCNEMIUS PERFORATING VEINS

The gastrocnemius perforating veins are located by varicography or duplex scanning. They are isolated, ligated and divided as they leave the muscle belly.

HUNTERIAN PERFORATING VEINS

If the long saphenous veins have been ligated rather than stripped, Hunterian perforating veins are rarely a problem. Recurrent varicose veins not infrequently arise from a Hunterian perforator which joins a residual long saphenous trunk (see below). These veins are approached through a longitudinal incision which often has to be fairly long to allow accurate ligation at the junction with the femoral vein.

TENSOR FASCIA LATA PERFORATOR

This rare communicating vein joins the muscular veins of the thigh to the primitive lateral vein which is present in patients with Klippel–Trenauney syndrome. Treatment is by local exploration, ligation and division.

POSTOPERATIVE CARE AND COMPLICATIONS

The long medial incision of Linton or Cockett is often slow to heal. If the incision is made through indurated subcutaneous tissues, the wound edges may necrose, especially if they are undermined. Skin edge necrosis can complicate between 5% and 10% of operations. The aftercare is similar to that described above.

Injection sclerotherapy

Sclerotherapy produces obliteration by injecting a detergent which strips off the endothelium. Application of compression reduces thrombosis and encourages cross-luminal adherence. Injections should be made into a collapsed vein, followed immediately by the application of prolonged pressure. The final result should be a thin fibrous cord. Failure to apply adequate prolonged pressure leads to thrombosis which is lumpy and painful and may become recanalized.

INDICATIONS

Injection sclerotherapy is indicated in the treatment of isolated below-knee varicosities in limbs without evidence of long or short saphenous incompetence. Patients may sometimes request injection sclerotherapy rather than operation because they wish to avoid being admitted to hospital. They should be advised that, in the presence of major saphenous incompetence, recurrence is inevitable (Hobbs, 1968).

CONTRAINDICATIONS

1. Major long or short saphenous incompetence.
2. Varicosities in the upper thigh, especially if this is fat, as compression is difficult to apply, and where thrombosis may extend into the femoral vein.
3. Veins of the foot, where there is a risk of mistakenly injecting into arteries.
4. A history of allergy, especially if this is to a previous injection of sclerosant.
5. Any condition which increases the risk of thrombosis, e.g. pregnancy or the contraceptive pill.

TECHNIQUE

The patient stands on a stool and the veins are carefully marked with a felt tip pen. 3% sodium tetradecyl sulphate is the most commonly used sclerosant (Fegan, 1967). The patient then lies down and injections are made along the course of the venous tributaries at 5–10 cm intervals (Hobbs, 1968, 1974). These are best placed at junctions. The vein is transfixed; the plunger of the syringe is withdrawn and the needle pulled back through the vein. When blood enters the barrel of the syringe, 0.5 ml of sclerosant is injected. Up to 10 injections can be made at a single sitting. A small cottonwool ball held on by a Micropore tape is placed over the puncture site by an assistant. After the last injection has been given, the leg is elevated and a Tensopress covered with a tubular bandage is applied.

The patient is instructed to walk 5 km (3 miles) a day) (Fegan, 1967), advised to avoid prolonged standing and asked to report back if the bandages become too loose, too tight or uncomfortable. The patient is seen after 3 weeks. The bandages can be removed a few days before reattending the clinic and the patient may have a bath. The legs are inspected. Lumpy thrombi can be evacuated through small cutaneous punctures made with a large needle. Remaining varicosities are injected and cottonwool pad pressure and bandages are reapplied for a further 3 weeks. Alternatively, the second limb can be injected at this time.

COMPLICATIONS

1. A painful thrombus results if the vein is distended during the injection or inadequately compressed after the injection. If the thrombus is not evacuated, a brown stain of the skin can result. This stain gradually fades but may take one to two years to do so.
2. Extravasation of sclerosant can cause skin ulceration. This should be avoided by always confirming the presence of back-bleeding before making the injection.
3. Sensitivity reactions may occur, and anaphylactic shock and death have been reported. Adrenaline, hydrorcortisone and antihistamines must be immediately available.
4. Deep vein thrombosis and pulmonary embolism are avoided by never injecting more than a small volume of sclerosant at any one sitting and by brisk walking immediately after the injections.
5. Accidental arterial injection has occurred and caused peripheral gangrene which required amputation (MacGowan, 1985). Injections into the lower calf perforators or foot are especially dangerous, as it is easy to inject mistakenly into arteries at these sites. Always draw back blood into the syringe and confirm that it is of venous colour and non-pulsatile. Do not inject if you have any doubt! If an intra-arterial injection is made inadvertently it should be stopped immediately. Intra-arterial injection is suspected because it causes severe pain. The patient should be placed on heparin and given dextran. A prostaglandin infusion and lumbar sympathectomy may be of value in avoiding tissue loss.

Venous flares

These are only of cosmetic importance and can be masked by cosmetic camouflage creams. Injection sclerotherapy and laser ablation have also been used with variable success.

Recurrent varicose veins

Recurrent varicosities may develop even after careful and accurate surgery or because of imprecise or inaccurate surgery. Careful clinical examination is essential and varicography, duplex examination and ascending phlebography may be required to define the anatomy of recurrence accurately.

Groin and thigh recurrence

Groin recurrences occur when the long saphenous vein has been ligated but not stripped or when one or more of its proximal tributaries has been left unligated. Under certain circumstances new vessels arise at the upper end of the saphenous vein reconnecting it to the femoral vein (Sheppard, 1978). Some suggest that the deep fascia should be closed to obliterate the fossa ovale. The presence of a groin recurrence can usually be confirmed by varicography (Figure 45.26), but if this is not adequate and there are large thigh varicosities which have developed after a previous high saphenous ligation, groin exploration should be considered.

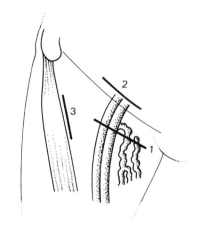

Figure 45.26 Possible approaches to a groin recurrence. 1, Li's approach. 2, Luke's approach. 3, Lateral approach (rarely used)

The old incision is opened and extended laterally over the femoral vein and artery (Li's approach) (Li, 1975). The anterior surface of the femoral artery is exposed and the femoral vein lying on its medial side is then displayed (Figure 45.27). As the anterior surface of the femoral vein is defined working across from the lateral side, the long saphenous trunk can be seen entering it anteriorly. This is dissected free and ligated in continuity by passing a catgut tie around it, using a right angle forceps. The distal end can then be clamped, ligated and divided. If a residual long saphenous vein is found passing down into the thigh, this may be dissected out and a stripper passed down it to the knee.

Re-exploration of the groin is never easy. There is often a considerable amount of fibrous tissue present and a direct approach risks massive bleeding from multiple thin-walled veins that pass between the end of the long saphenous vein and the femoral vein. The lateral approach reduces some of the risk of haemorrhage and avoids inadvertent injury to the femoral artery and vein which are displayed and carefully protected. Lymphatic damage is quite common and there is a higher risk of lymphocele and leg swelling after re-exploration of the groin.

Popliteal recurrence

These may arise from the divided end of the short saphenous or from gastrocnemius communicating veins. Varicography may be helpful. It may be best to explore the popliteal fossa through a long vertical incision or a lazy S incision (Figure 45.28). The popliteal vein is defined at the upper end of the popliteal fossa and mobilized until it disappears below the gastrocnemius muscles. All the tributaries that enter its superficial surface are ligated and divided. Care is taken to avoid damaging the popliteal artery and the popliteal and cutaneous nerves.

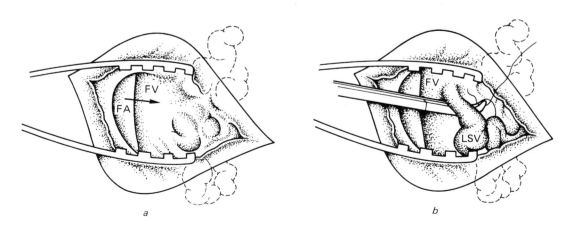

Figure 45.27 Li's approach to a groin recurrence. FA, Femoral artery. FV, Femoral vein. LSV, Long saphenous vein

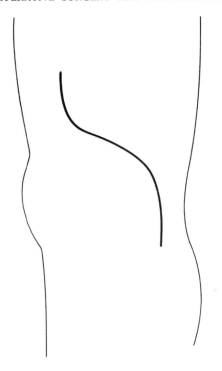

Figure 45.28 Lazy S approach to a popliteal recurrence

Other recurrences

Incompetent Hunterian perforating veins should be ligated after careful localization by saphenography or duplex scanning. Many other recurrent varicosities are best treated by sclerotherapy.

Deep vein thrombosis

This can be defined as thrombosis within the stem veins beneath the deep fascia of the lower limb and includes thrombosis extending into the pelvic veins and inferior vena cava. The thrombosis commonly starts in the soleal sinuses and extends up the leg as propagated thrombus (Nicolaides *et al.*, 1971). Some thrombi do start in the femoral veins and thrombosis can start in the profunda and internal iliac veins. Venous thrombosis is rare in the upper limb except when the veins have been cannulated. Axillary vein thrombosis usually results from some form of unusual exercise (effort thrombosis) (Tilney *et al.*, 1970).

Lower leg deep vein thrombosis may sometimes indicate the presence of an occult cancer (Sproull, 1938). In younger patients it may be associated with a deficiency of fibrinolytic activity (Nilsson *et al.*, 1961) or antithrombin III (Egberg, 1965), although these conditions are rare. It may complicate superficial thrombophlebitis in varicose veins which extends through the saphenous opening or through other communicating veins.

Deep vein thrombosis often develops as a complication of bed rest and major illness such as a myocardial infarction or trauma, whether surgical or accidental. Pregnancy and the puerperium are predisposing conditions, but the incidence should decline as measures to combat its onset become more effective (Berquist, 1983). It should occur in less than 10% of patients with the introduction of effective prophylaxis. The incidence of post-partum thrombosis has been reduced by prescription of anti-embolism stockings and a policy of early mobilization. Head and neck, upper limb and breast surgery have a very low incidence of thrombosis. Hip operations and lower limb fractures carry a high risk of thrombosis (50–70%) if no prophylaxis is given. Clinical pulmonary embolism occurs in about 1% of general surgical patients and is fatal in about 0.4%. Hip surgery has a much higher incidence, 2% or even 3% in some series. Thrombosis is confined to the calf in 85% and only a minority propagate into or arise in the femoral or iliac veins (excluding thromboses associated with hip surgery). Iliofemoral venous thrombosis is more common in the left leg, probably as a result of left iliac vein compression by the right common iliac artery (Cockett and Lea Thomas, 1965).

Prevention of postoperative deep vein thrombosis

The risk of developing postoperative deep vein thrombosis is increased by the following factors (Berquist, 1983; Browse *et al.*, 1988):

1. A past history of deep vein thrombosis.
2. Malignancy.
3. The contraceptive pill.
4. Major abdominal or thoracic surgery.
5. Hip and lower limb fracture or surgery, particularly hip replacement.
6. Obesity.
7. Polycythaemia, thrombocythaemia, hyperfibrinogenaemia and raised blood viscosity.

Methods of prophylaxis

1. EARLY AMBULATION

2. MECHANICAL METHODS

'Anti-embolism' stockings. These graduated low-compression stockings reduce the incidence of postoperative deep vein thrombosis from 30% in control limbs to just over 10% in treated limbs (Holford and Bliss, 1976). This is thought to be the result of increasing the velocity of the blood flow in the deep vein. They have almost no side effects, although ischaemia of the lower limb has been reported.

Intermittent calf compression. This can achieved by inflatable plastic leggings (Sabri *et al.*, 1971; Hills *et al.*, 1972) or by electrical calf muscle stimulation

(Browse and Negus, 1970). Both techniques reduce the incidence of deep vein thrombosis but are now less commonly used than stockings.

3. PHARMACOLOGICAL METHODS

Full anticoagulation with warfarin effectively prevents postoperative deep vein thrombosis (Sevitt and Gallagher, 1959), but is often contraindicated when major surgery is contemplated.

Subcutaneous heparin. Five thousand units of heparin are given subcutaneously with the premedication and continued in a dose of 5000 u twice a day until the patient is fully mobile or ready to leave hospital. This regimen has reduced the incidence of postoperative deep vein thrombosis and pulmonary embolism (*Lancet*, 1975). Haematoma formation is quite common and severe postoperative bleeding occurs occasionally (Briton *et al.*, 1977). This method should not be used when a significant raw area is present, e.g after prostatectomy or abdominoperineal resection of the rectum.

Heparin fragments. Smaller fragments of heparin have been developed in the hope that they would produce better anticoagulation with fewer side effects. Given once a day, rather than twice, they appear to be more effective in preventing thrombosis after orthopaedic surgery (Leyvraz *et al.*, 1991), but have not been shown to have fewer side effects and cost considerably more.

Intravenous low molecular weight dextran. This is given in a dose of 500 ml during the operation and continued for 2 days postoperatively in a dose of 500 ml per day. This is effective in preventing pulmonary embolism but does not reduce the incidence of deep vein thrombosis (Kline *et al.*, 1975). Circulatory overload can occur and dextran should be avoided in patients with any impairment of renal function. Acute anaphylaxis is an extremely rare but serious complication.

Ultra-low dose heparin. A very low dose of 1 u of heparin/kg/h has shown to be effective in early trials (Negus *et al.*, 1980), but these results need confirmation.

Diagnosis of suspected deep vein thrombosis

Calf tenderness and ankle oedema are important physical signs. Extensive deep vein thrombosis may have pitting oedema of the ankle as the only physical sign. An increase in calf temperature may be present, but Homans' sign is of little value (Browse *et al.*, 1988). An unexplained low-grade pyrexia may indicate occult deep vein thrombosis, but major pulmonary embolism can occur without pyrexia or other physical signs.

Massive occlusive iliofemoral deep vein thrombosis is usually obvious. Both the thigh and calf are swollen and the skin is pale (phlegmasia alba dolens) or cyanosed (phlegmasia caerulea dolens). Occasionally venous gangrene may develop. Massive thrombotic occlusion of the inferior vena cava is rare and often associated with terminal carcinomatosis.

Methods of diagnosis

1. ASCENDING PHLEBOGRAPHY

This is the most accurate means of diagnosis. Contrast medium is injected into a dorsal foot vein, monitored by an image intensifier and recorded on serial films using a rapid cassette changer. Non-irritant, non-ionic contrast media have improved the comfort and safety of phlebography. The risk of contrast-induced thrombosis is now negligible (Lea Thomas and Briggs, 1984). The thrombus is seen as a filling defect (Figure 45.29).

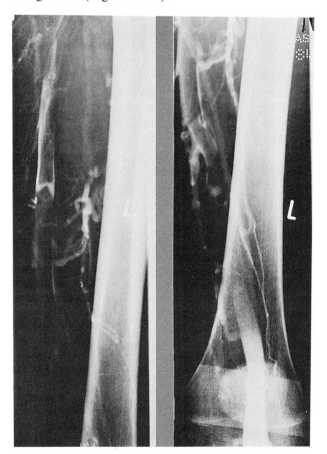

Figure 45.29 A phlebogram showing a filling defect in the deep veins caused by thrombus

2. DOPPLER ULTRASOUND

Ultrasound can detect major venous obstruction by loss of the flow signal over the femoral vein on calf squeezing (Evans and Cockett, 1969). It is a simple but unreliable test which is especially inaccurate in picking up calf or non-occlusive thrombi in the femoral veins.

3. ^{125}I-FIBRINOGEN TEST

This depends on the incorporation of isotopically labelled human serum fibrogen into developing thrombus. Any increase in radioactivity is detected with a scintillation counter. It is very accurate in the calf and lower thigh (Flanc *et al.*, 1968; Negus *et al.*, 1968). It is, however, expensive and time consuming and is much less accurate after the thrombus has formed. Its main use is as a screening test for new methods of prophylaxis. The isotope is being withdrawn because of worries over its safety.

4. OTHER ISOTOPICALLY LABELLED COMPOUNDS

These include streptokinase, plasminogen, plasminogen activators and indium-labelled platelets (Browse *et al.*, 1988). None of these has found a routine place in clinical practice.

5. INFRARED THERMOGRAPHY

A developing thrombus shows up as a 'hot spot'. Small transportable thermographic cassettes are now available, but the accuracy of this test for screening symptomless patients is poor.

6. PLETHYSMOGRAPHY

This detects obstruction to venous outflow. It can be measured using a strain gauge, air-filled cuffs or indirectly by changes in electrical conductivity (impedance plethysmography). It is reliable only in detecting obstructing thrombi in or proximal to the popliteal vein.

7. DUPLEX DOPPLER SCANNING

This uses the imaging capacity of the duplex scanner to visualize the deep veins of the calf, thigh and pelvis. Thrombus is suspected when the lumen of the vein cannot be obliterated by pressure from the probe head or when filling defects are seen within the vein (Figure 45.30). False positives and negatives occur in post-thrombotic limbs and calf thrombus is poorly visualized (70% accuracy) (Lensing *et al.*, 1989; Mitchell *et al.*, 1991). It is, however, a very good method of detecting popliteal and femoral thrombus, with an accuracy approaching 100%.

8. D DIMER

This antibody detects the presence of cross-linked fibrin degradation products in the blood and is a useful negative screening test (Gaffrey, 1983). Few patients with low levels of D dimer have a venous thrombosis of any consequence. A diagnosis suspected from high titres must be confirmed by phlebography or duplex scanning.

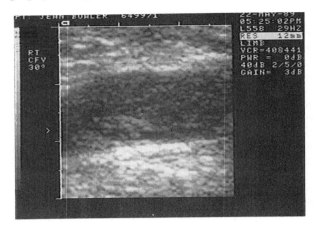

Figure 45.30   A duplex scan showing venous thrombus

Conservative management of established deep vein thrombosis

Anticoagulation remains the most important measure in the treatment of deep vein thrombosis. Pulmonary embolism must always be treated by full anticoagulation and the source of the emboli should be confirmed by phlebography

Anticoagulants

Intravenous heparin in a dose of approximately 40 000 u/24h is given as a continuous infusion using a mechanical pump. Daily kaolin cephalin clotting times (KCCTs) or accelerated partial thromboplastin times are measured to ensure adequate heparin anticoagulation and to ascertain if resistance is developing as a result of heparin antibody formation. The KCCT is arbitrarily defined as a level of anticoagulation between two and three times longer than normal controls.

A loading dose of warfarin is given (usually 10 or 15 mg on two or three consecutive days) after 24 or 48 h of heparin which is continued until adequate warfarin anticoagulation has been achieved (usually after 2–3 days.) A patient with pulmonary embolism should be treated for five or six days with heparin before converting to warfarin. The warfarin dosage is adjusted according to serial prothrombin times, and continued for 3–6 months to prevent recurrent thrombosis or embolism (Lagerstedt *et al.*, 1985). Recurrent pulmonary embolism is an indication for permanent anticoagulation.

Fibrinolytic agents

Urokinase, streptokinase and tissue plasminogen activator may be of value in the treatment of massive pulmonary embolism. These agents are best administered through a catheter placed in the pulmonary artery (Miller and Sutton, 1970). They may have a place in the treatment of peripheral venous thrombosis, but this has not clearly been established. Fresh thrombus can be lysed, but there is little evidence that this reduces the incidence of post-thrombotic limb syndrome (Kakkar and Lawrence, 1985) and successful thrombolysis may encourage pulmonary embolism. Local infusion of the fibrinolytic agent through an indwelling catheter achieves the best results. Urokinase and tissue plasminogen activator are expensive, but have the advantage that they are less antigenic than streptokinase. Steroid cover is required for streptokinase and a second course cannot be given. Fibrinolytic treatment is contraindicated if there has been recent surgery or the patient has been injured. This excludes most patients with postoperative deep vein thrombosis from treatment. Fibrinolytic therapy is always followed by a course of anticoagulants.

Surgical treatment of deep vein thrombosis

Deep vein thrombosis can be treated by thrombectomy or by a 'locking-in' procedure to prevent further embolism. The latter includes venous ligation, the application of clips and the insertion of intracaval filters (Browse et al., 1988).

Successful treatment depends on an accurate knowledge of the site, extent and degree of fixity of the thrombus. Precise diagnosis depends on phlebography or duplex ultrasound to assess the amount of thrombus present within the deep veins, whether it is large, loose and liable to embolize, or whether it is minor, old, occlusive and unlikely to cause further problems.

Surgical thrombectomy is only indicated for recently formed non-adherent thrombus in the iliac or femoral veins (Burnand and Baker, 1992), especially if there is gross venous obstruction causing phlegmasia caerulea dolens or venous gangrene. It may be used when anticoagulants are contraindicated, although in these circumstances 'locking-in' procedures are more popular. Insertion of an inferior vena caval filter is the most commonly performed procedure to 'lock-in' thrombus, as it can be safely performed without general anaesthesia and probably causes the fewest side effects. 'Clipping' of the inferior vena cava is an alternative procedure. The operation of femoral vein ligation is now rarely performed, as the risk of causing a severe post-thrombotic limb is too great. This probably does not occur if the ligature is carefully placed below the junction of the profunda femoris and common femoral veins (Young et al., 1974).

Venous thrombectomy

INDICATIONS

1. Recent iliofemoral thrombosis shown by phlebo-

graphy (usually in patients presenting with pulmonary embolism).
2. Phlegmasia caerulea dolens where peripheral ischaemia is threatening the viability of the limb.
3. When anticoagulation cannot be used and the size and lack of fixity of the thrombus poses a threat to life.

CONTRAINDICATIONS

Old adherent thrombus is difficult to remove and rapid re-thrombosis is common. Patients must be fit for general anaesthesia.

THE OPERATION

Full anticoagulation with heparin should be continued to the time of operation and 2 u of blood should be cross-matched. A general anaesthetic must be used, as positive pressure ventilation is required while the thrombus is extracted. An image intensifier is desirable and the patient should be placed on a radiolucent operating table. The patient is placed flat with the legs apart and with a small amount of head-down tilt (Burnand and Baker, 1992).

1. A longitudinal groin incision is made over the femoral vein starting just medial to the mid-inguinal point and continuing into the upper thigh for 5–10 cm to allow adequate exposure of the femoral vein (Figure 45.31).

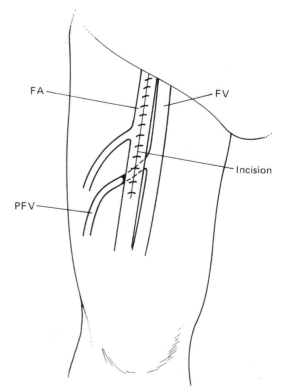

Figure 45.31 Exposure of the femoral vein in the upper thigh. FA, Femoral artery. FV, Femoral vein. PFV, Profunda femoris vein

2. The superficial femoral vein is found on the medial side of the artery, and dissected proximally to the level of the inguinal ligament. The profunda femoris and other smaller tributaries are dissected and controlled by fine slings (Figure 45.31).

3. A segment of femoral vein is isolated between soft bulldog clamps and a transverse or longitudinal venotomy made close to the profunda termination.

4. A no. 7 or 8 Fogarty balloon catheter is passed proximally through the venotomy into the inferior vena cava.

5. The balloon is inflated and a second catheter is inserted and passed up to the level of the first catheter (Figure 45.32); the slings are pulled taut to prevent continuous bleeding. The balloon of the second catheter is then inflated and withdrawn. This process is repeated until no more thrombus is extracted. The vein is flushed with heparin saline solution (1000 u of heparin in 200 ml of normal saline). This process should remove the venous thrombus, while the initial blocking catheter prevents embolization into the lungs from thrombus that is dislodged by the passage of the second catheter.

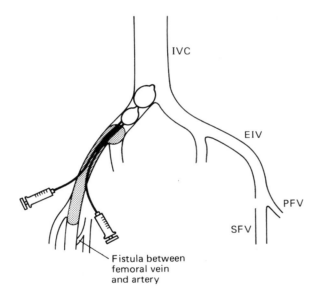

Figure 45.32 The technique for venous thrombectomy. IVC, Inferior vena cava. EIV, External iliac vein. PFV, Profunda femoral vein. SFV, Superficial femoral vein

6. When no more thombus is obtained, contrast can be instilled up the vein to check that the vein is patent and to confirm that all the thrombus has been removed. The blocking catheter is then carefully withdrawn.

7. When the thrombus is confined to the iliac segment the operation is complete and the venotomy can be closed. Recently Ecklof and others (Plate *et al.*, 1984) suggested that the formation of a temporary arteriovenous fistula made at the site of the venotomy on completion of the thrombectomy reduces the risk of re-thrombosis (Dodd, 1964; Egberg, 1965).

The fistula is closed after 6 weeks, when a prolene ligature left around the communication is found, freed and tied.

8. An attempt may be made to pass the catheter down the limb if distal thrombosis has been demonstrated. Difficulty may be encountered in negotiating the catheter past competent distal valves.

9. If this attempt fails, thrombus may be extracted from the distal veins by tightly compressing the limb with an Esmarch bandage applied from the foot to the thigh. The distal bulldog is then released to evacuate loose thrombus from the calf and thigh veins.

10. It is provident to 'lock-in' residual thrombus by ligating the superficial vein below the profunda termination. This reduces the risk of subsequent embolism.

11. The venotomy is then closed with a continuous 6/0 prolene suture.

12. The incision is closed in layers with suction drainage. Anticoagulation is continued for at least 3 months.

COMPLICATIONS

Haemorrhage in a fully anticoagulated patient is a risk but is fortunately rare. Superficial wound infection can occur at a later stage. The most common complication is re-thrombosis despite prolonged and adequate anticoagulation. The use of an arteriovenous fistula and careful radiographic control usually reduces this risk. Further pulmonary embolism is quite common and may necessitate placement of a caval filter.

Superficial femoral vein ligation

INDICATIONS

1. Recurrent pulmonary embolism arising from the lower leg in spite of adequate anticoagulation.
2. Following incomplete superficial venous thrombectomy.
3. Deep vein thrombosis in the lower leg when anticoagulation is contraindicated, e.g. active peptic ulceration.

THE OPERATION

The patient's position and preparation is the same as for venous thrombectomy. A similar vertical incision is made. The superficial femoral and profunda femoris veins are dissected free and snares placed around them. A 2/0 silk or prolene ligature is passed around the superficial femoral vein just below the orifice of the profunda vein and tied down. The incision is closed with Redivac drainage.

COMPLICATIONS

Further distal thrombosis can occur, causing a

painful swollen limb with a high risk of post-thrombotic complications developing at a later stage. Rethrombosis is always a risk. Anticoagulation must be continued.

Inferior vena caval interruption

INDICATIONS

1. Thrombosis in the iliofemoral segment associated with recurrent pulmonary embolism.
2. Incomplete distal thrombectomy.
3. Recurrent pulmonary embolism; source not demonstrated by phlebography.
4. Anticoagulants contraindicated.

METHODS

A number of plastic clips have been described. The most commonly used are those of DeWeese and Miles (DeWeese and Hunter, 1958; Miles et al., 1964).

1. The vena cava is approached through a transverse muscle-cutting incision on the right side of the abdomen just above the level of the umbilicus. A vertical incision can also be used.

2. The peritoneum can be opened and the hepatic flexure of the right colon and duodenum mobilized medially to expose the vena cava below the level of the renal veins (Figure 45.33). Alternatively, it is possible to stay extraperitoneally and approach the vena cava by reflecting the peritoneum to the left.

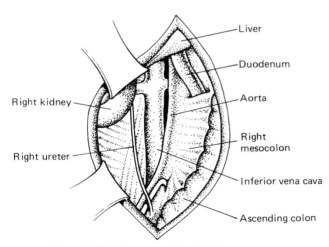

Figure 45.33 Exposure of the inferior vena cava

3. The exposed vena cava is dissected free and encircled with a snare. The clip is passed around the vein and its free ends ligated to divide the main channel into four smaller channels (Figure 45.34). The wound is closed in layers with suction drainage. Plication with sutures is an alternative method, but this is less satisfactory and more difficult.

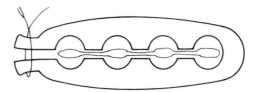

Figure 45.34 A Miles/DeWeese clip

COMPLICATIONS

The vena cava may thrombose below the clip and emboli may arise from its proximal extent. These complications are reduced by continuing anticoagulation.

Insertion of a vena caval filter

There are a number of filters that can be inserted into the vena cava under radiographic control. The Mobbin-Uddin umbrella (Mobbin-Uddin et al., 1967) has been superseded by the Greenfield Kimway filter (Croonfield et al., 1981) because of better configuration and the barbed feet reduce the risk of migration. Gunther, Helical and Bird's-nest filters are alternatives that can be inserted percutaneously (Roehim et al., 1984). The Greenfield filter has now been adapted for percutaneous insertion.

The Greenfield filter should, if possible, be inserted through the internal jugular vein. A radiographer and image intensifier must be available with the patient placed supine on an X-ray table with a screen to allow draping over the head.

1. Local anaesthetic is infiltrated into the skin above the clavicle. Intravenous Diazemuls or diazepam can be given to allay anxiety.

2. The internal jugular vein is exposed through a transverse supraclavicular incision centred over the sternomastoid muscle. The sternomastoid is split upwards between the sternal and clavicular heads and the internal jugular vein exposed lying just beneath the deep fascia.

3. The vein is dissected free and two snares are passed around it. These are pulled up to isolate a 1 cm segment of vein (Figure 45.35).

4. A vertical venotomy is made in the isolated segment, the edges of which are held apart by 5/0 prolene stay sutures. A medium-sized (20–24 Clutton's) sound is then passed down the lumen to dilate the vein and gauge the direction of the vessel as it passes beneath the clavicle.

5. The catheter containing the loaded filter is inserted through the venotomy which is held open by the stay sutures. A guidewire which passes down the centre of the filter can be used to direct the catheter through the right atrium, but this is usually unnecessary as X-ray screening shows the catheter crossing the right atrium and entering the inferior vena cava (Figure 45.35).

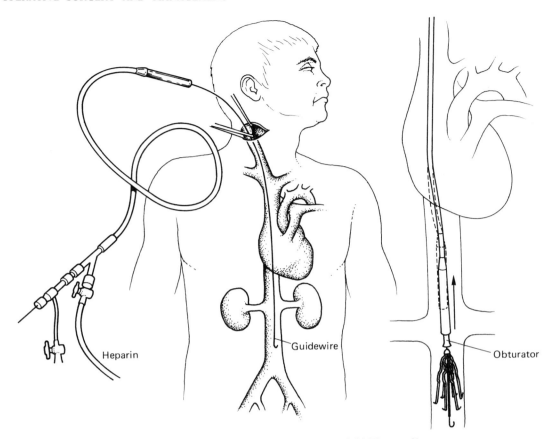

Figure 45.35 Insertion of a Greenfield Kimway filter

6. When the catheter is thought to lie between the iliac bifurcation and the renal veins, radiographic contrast medium is injected to confirm the exact position and the filter extruded by unscrewing the safety lock and pushing the plunger.

7. The catheter is then withdrawn and the venotomy closed with 6/0 prolene before the platysma and skin are approximated.

COMPLICATIONS

1. Cardiac irregularity during insertion.
2. Poor siting of the filter (in the iliac veins or above the renal veins).
3. Retroperitoneal haematoma from the sharp 'feet' perforating the inferior vena cava.
4. Thrombosis of the filter.
5. Continued embolism arising from the proximal end of the filter.

Venous ulcers

Venous leg ulcers are common, with a prevalence of approximately 0.2% (Callam et al., 1985). They are caused by a sustained rise in the venous pressure during walking as the result of a defective calf pump mechanism. This may be the result of post-thrombotic damage to the deep veins, incompetence of the perforating (calf communicating) veins or saphenous incompetence (Browse et al., 1988) (although primary saphenous incompetence without associated incompetence of other communicating veins is a rare cause of ulceration).

Venous ulcers tend to develop in the medial gaiter area of the leg between the malleoli and the fleshy muscles of the calf. They are usually surrounded by lipodermatosclerosis (pigmentation, induration and inflammation) of the calf skin and subcutaneous fat. They have a gently sloping edge and a base of slough or granulation tissue. Varicose calf veins are often present and there may be localized venous dilatations ('blowouts') in the area around the ulcer. Lateral ulcers may occur and are usually related to incompetence of the short saphenous and peroneal perforating veins. Circumferential ulcers are not uncommon. An ankle flare of dilated venous capillaries situated below the malleolus is indicative of a high venous pressure and the likelihood of incompetent communicating veins.

Other causes for the ulceration must be considered and ischaemia, neuropathy, vasculitis and skin tumours must be excluded.

Management

Patients should initially be managed by compression bandaging and this allows about 80% of all venous ulcers to heal within 6–12 months (Blair *et al.*, 1988). Failure to achieve healing or a progressive increase in ulcer size should lead to changes in the treatment.

Skin grafting

The possibilities are split-skin grafting with or without ulcer excision, pinch grafts, postage stamp grafts, mesh grafts, cross-leg grafts (Ryan, 1983, 1990) and autografts of synthetically grown keratinocytes (Leigh *et al.*, 1987). Most patients are best treated by excising the ulcer to obtain a granulating base before the immediate application of a one to one and a half times meshed split-skin graft. Additional skin should always be taken and banked. All ulcers can eventually be healed by this technique, provided that patients and surgeons persist! Unfortunately many ulcers recur.

Once the ulcer has healed

The patient should be investigated to ascertain the type and extent of the venous abnormality (Browse *et al.*, 1988). Phlebography gives anatomical information on the deep veins and physiological information on the communicating veins. Duplex scanning and descending venography document deep venous reflux (Baker *et al.*, 1993) and foot vein pressure measurement or plethysmography (Norgren, 1973) allows calf pump function to be assessed. If the deep veins appear 'normal' on phlebography, it is worth obliterating all sites of superficial venous incompetence (long and short saphenous systems and incompetent calf communicating veins). There is little evidence that this type of surgery is of any lasting benefit if the deep veins are severely disrupted, and patients should be prescribed elastic stockings for the rest of their life. Recurrent ulceration, despite the conscientious wearing of stockings should raise the possibility of valvular reconstruction (Kistner, 1985), transplantation (Taheri *et al.*, 1982a) or venous bypass (Palma and Esperon, 1960; Dale and Harris, 1966; Dale *et al.*, 1984), although an attempt will usually have been made to operate on the superficial veins first.

Surgery of the deep veins

There are no really good controlled clinical trials which have demonstrated the benefit of this type of surgery in preventing recurrent ulceration. The types of procedure that have been attempted include:

1. Femorocaval bypass (Dale *et al.*, 1984) using an externally supported polytetrafluorethylene (PTFE) prosthesis with a temporary adjuvant arteriovenous fistula (Figure 45.36). This provides good venous outflow but does not prevent reflux.

2. A Palma–Esperon femorofemoral crossover bypass (Palma and Esperon, 1960), using the contralateral saphenous vein with a temporary arteriovenous fistula to provide outflow from a limb with an iliac occlusion (Figure 45.37).

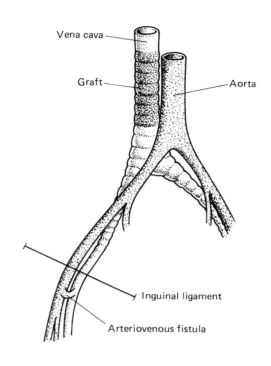

Figure 45.36   Replacement of the inferior vena cava by PTFE with an arteriovenous fistula to enhance patency

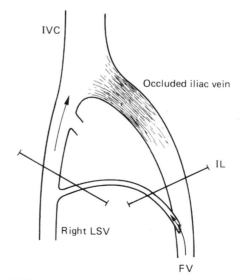

Figure 45.37   A Palma–Esperon bypass. IVC, Inferior vena cava. LSV, Long saphenous vein. FV, Femoral vein. IL, Inguinal ligament

3. A popliteofemoral bypass (Husni, 1970; May, 1985) anastomosing the ipsilateral long saphenous vein to the popliteal vein (Figure 45.38). This procedure has a high occlusion rate and no real advantage over the natural state of affairs, when incompetent communicating veins bypass the deep veins via the saphenous systems.

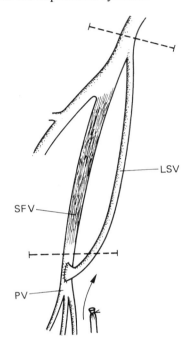

Figure 45.38 A popliteal-to-femoral saphenous vein bypass. LSV, Long saphenous vein. PV, Popliteal vein. SFV, Superficial femoral vein

4. Femoral-to-profunda or femoral-to-saphenous transposition (Kistner and Sparkhul, 1979) (Figure 45.39). This has been shown to be unsatisfactory in the long term because the previously competent valves became incompetent (Queral *et al.*, 1980).
5. Axillary vein valve transplant (Taheri *et al.*, 1982b). An axillary vein valve is resected and inserted between the superficial femoral vein in the lower thigh to prevent reflux (Figure 45.40). The valve may become incompetent later and the best site for the transplant is still undecided.
6. The Veno-cuff (Jessup and Lane, 1988). A perforated silicone cuff is placed around an incompetent valve and tightened to render the cusps competent by external compression (Figure 45.41).
7. Valvuloplasty (Kistner, 1975). A number of plicating sutures are inserted into the valve cusp to 'reef' it up and to prevent the free margin from inverting which may account for reflux (Figure 45.42).
8. Gracilis sling valvuloplasty (Psthakis and Psthakis, 1985). There are a number of variations in the technique used to sling the gracilis muscle around the femoral vein to act as an external valve.

These techniques now need to be assessed and compared with conservative management in controlled clinical trials of ulcer prophylaxis. The Palma crossover bypass and the caval bypass are of established benefit in reducing symptoms of venous claudication in patients with post-thrombotic venous claudication. Axillary vein transposition and the 'veno-cuff' require critical assessment.

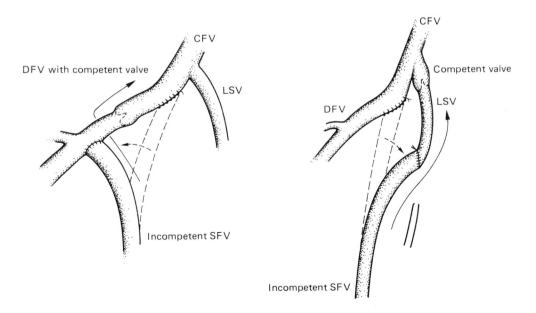

Figure 45.39 A femoral-to-profunda and femoral-to-saphenous transposition. DFV, Deep femoral vein. CFV, Common femoral vein. LSV, Long saphenous vein. SFV, Superficial femoral vein

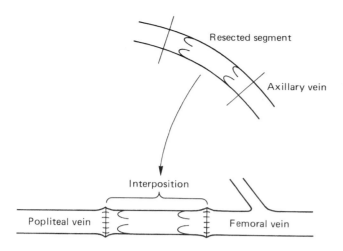

Figure 45.40 Axillary vein valve transposition

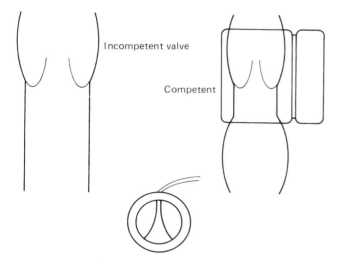

Figure 45.41 Application of the Veno-cuff

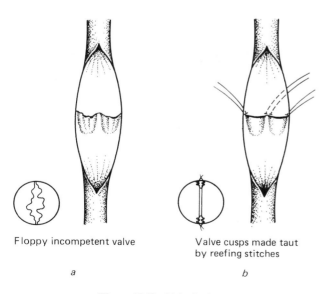

Floppy incompetent valve

a

Valve cusps made taut by reefing stitches

b

Figure 45.42 Valvuloplasty

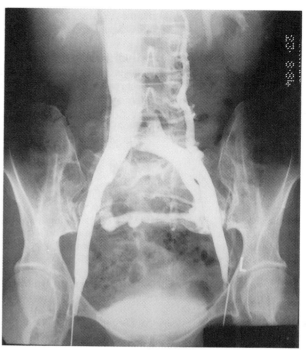

Figure 45.43 A patient with iliac vein compression syndrome

Iliac vein compression syndrome

Patients with the iliac vein compression syndrome (Figure 45.43) are best treated by a Palma crossover using the left long saphenous vein. Elevation of the artery by a plastic bridge or division of the artery anastomosing it behind the vein are not recommended.

Rare venous anomalies

1. Arteriovenous fistulae may produce large pulsatile varicose veins, and these are usually associated with a generalized enlargement of the limb (Browse *et al.*, 1988). Treatment is by surgical excision in localized cases or by radiological embolization (ligature coils or autologous thrombus).

2. The Klippel–Trenauney syndrome (Klippel and Trenauney, 1900) consists of a capillary haemangioma (portwine stain) associated with enlargement of the primitive lateral vein of Servelle and limb enlargement (Servelle, 1985). Bony abnormality and lymphoedema may be present. Varicose veins may be excised, but patency of the deep veins must be confirmed as some patients have aplastic femoral and popliteal veins. Patients with Klippel–Trenauney syndrome have a high incidence of deep vein thrombosis and pulmonary embolism after surgery (Baskerville *et al.*, 1985).

3. Cutaneous capillary haemangiomas. Flat portwine stains are treated by cosmetic creams or by

excision if small (Mulliken and Young, 1988). Laser ablation may be tried. Strawberry marks – raised capillary haemangiomas – often regress spontaneously but may be excised if large or troublesome.

4. Localized venous angiomas can be excised, but diffuse angiomas extending through the muscles of the thigh or calf cannot be removed without destroying function. Investigation by phlebography and CT scanning must precede any decision on the advisability of surgery.

References

Baker, S., Burnand, K. G., Sommerville, K. M., Lea Thomas, M. and Wilson, N. M. (1993) Comparison of venous reflux assessed by duplex scanning and descending phlebography in chronic venous disease. *Lancet*, 341, 400–403

Baskerville, P. A., Ackroyd, J. S., Thomas, M. L. and Browse, N. L. (1985) The Klippel–Trenauney syndrome: clinical and haemodynamic features and management. *Br. J. Surg.*, 72, 232

Berquist, D (1983) *Postoperative Thrombembolism*, Springer-Verlag, Berlin.

Blair, S. D., Wright, D. D. I. *et al.* (1988) Sustained compression and healing of chronic venous ulcers. *Br. Med. J.*, 297, 1159–1161

Borschberg, E. (1976) *The Prevalence of Varicose Veins of the Lower Extremity*, Karger, Basel

Briton, B. J., Finch, D. R. A. *et al.* (1977) Low dose heparin. *Lancet*, 11, 604

Browse, N. L., Burnand, K. G. and Lea Thomas, M. (1988) *Diseases of the Veins*, Edward Arnold, London

Browse, N. L. and Negus, D. (1970) Prevention of postoperative deep vein thrombosis by electrical muscle stimulation. An evaluation with I^{125} labelled fibronogen. *Br. Med. J.*, 3, 615–618

Buddecke, E. (1975) Allersveranderungen der Poroteogllykane. *Verh. dt. Ges. Pathol.*, 59, 43

Burnand, K. G. and Baker, S. R. (1992) Venous thrombectomy in the lower limb. In *Emergency Vascular Surgery* (eds R. M. Greenhalgh and L. I. F. Hollier), W. B. Saunders, London

Burnand, K. G., O'Donnell, T. F. *et al.* (1976) Relationship between postphlebitic changes in the deep veins and results of surgical treatment of venous ulcers. *Lancet*, 1, 936–938

Callam, K., Ruckley, C. V. *et al.* (1985) Chronic ulceration of the leg: the extent of the problem. *Br. Med. J.*, 290, 1855

Chester, J. F. and Taylor, R. S. (1990) Hookers and French strippers: a technique for varicose vein surgery. *Br. J. Surg.*, 77, 560–561

Cockett, F. B. (1955) The pathology and treatment of venous ulcers of the leg. *Br. J. Surg.*, 43, 260–278

Cockett, F. B. and Elgan Jones, D. (1953) The ankle blow out syndrome. A new approach to the varicose ulcer problem. *Lancet*, 1, 17–23

Cockett, F. B. and Lea Thomas, M. (1965) The iliac compression syndrome. *Br. J. Surg.*, 52, 816–821

Corbett, C. R. R. and Harris, W. J. (1991) Which vein stripper: plastic or metal disposable? *Phlebology*, 6, 149–151

Cox, S. J. and Wellwood, J. M. (1974) A saphenous nerve injury caused by stripping the long saphenous vein. *Br. Med. J.*, 1, 415

Croonfield, K., Peyton, R., Crutes, S. and Barnes, R. (1981) Greenfield vena caval filter experience: late results in 158 patients. *Arch. Surg.*, 116, 1451

Dale, W. A. and Harris, J. (1966) Cross over vein grafts for iliac and femoral venous occlusions. *Ann. Surg.*, 168, 319

Dale, W. A., Harris, J. and Terry, R. B. (1984) Polytetraflurethylene reconstruction of the inferior vena cava. *Surgery*, 95, 625

DeWeese, M. S. and Hunter, D. C. (1958) A vena caval filter for the prevention of pulmonary emboli. *Bull. Soc. Chir.*, 17, 17

Dodd, H. (1964) The diagnosis and ligation of incompetent ankle perforating veins. *Ann. R. Coll. Surg. Engl.*, 34, 186–196

Edwards, J. M. (1976) Shearing operation for incompetent perforating veins. *Br. J. Surg.*, 63, 885

Egberg, O. (1965) Inherited anti thrombin deficiency causing thrombophilia. *Thromb. Diath. Haemorrh.*, 13, 516

Evans, D. S. and Cockett, F. B. (1969) Diagnosis of deep vein thrombosis with an ultrasonic Doppler technique. *Br. Med. J.*, 2, 802–804

Fegan, W. G. (1967) *Varicose Veins: Compression Sclerotherapy*, Heinemann, London

Flanc, C., Kakkar, V. V. *et al.* (1968) The detection of venous thrombosis of the legs using ^{125}I labelled fibrinogen. *Br. J. Surg.*, 55, 742–747

Gaffney, P. J. (1983) The occurrence and clinical relevance of fibrin fragments in blood. *Ann. N.Y. Acad. Sci.*, 408, 407–423

Gunderson, J. and Hauge, M. (1969) Hereditary factors in venous insufficiency. *Angiology*, 20, 346

Hills, N. H., Pflug, J. J. *et al.* (1972) Prevention of deep vein thrombosis by intermittent pneumatic compression of the calf. *Br. Med. J.*, 1, 131–135

Hoare, M. C. *et al.* (1974) Investigations and management of varicose veins. *Ann. R. Coll. Surg. Engl.*, 55, 245–252

Hoare, M. C. and Royle, J. P. (1984) Doppler ultrasound detection of sapheno femoral and sapheno popliteal incompetence and operative venography to ensure precise sapheno popliteal ligation. *Aust. N.Z. J. Surg.*, 54, 49

Hobbs, J. T. (1968) The treatment of varicose veins: a random trial of injection–compression therapy versus surgery. *Br. J. Surg.*, 55, 777–780

Hobbs, J. T. (1974) Surgery and sclerotherapy in the treatment of varicose veins. *Arch. Surg.*, 109, 793–796

Holford, C. P. and Bliss, B. P. (1976) The effect of graduated static compression on isotopically diagnosed deep vein thrombosis of the leg. *Br. J. Surg.*, 63, 157

Husni, E. A. (1970) In situ sapheno popliteal bypass graft for incompetence of the femoral and popliteal veins. *Surg. Gynecol. Obstet.*, 130, 297

Jessup, G. and Lane, R. J. (1988) Repair of incompetent venous valves. A new technique. *J. Vasc. Surg.*, 8, 569–575

Kakkar, V. V. and Lawrence, D. (1985) Haemodynamic and clinical assessment after therapy for acute deep vein thrombosis: a prospective study. *Ann. J. Surg.*, 156, 54

King, E. S. J. (1950) The genesis of varicose veins. *Aust. N.Z. J. Surg.*, 20, 126

Kistner, R. L. (1975) Surgical repair of the incompetent femoral vein valve. *Arch. Surg.*, 110, 1336

Kistner, R. (1985) Deep venous reconstruction. *Int. Angiol.*, 4, 429

Kistner, R. L. and Sparkhul, M. D. (1979) Surgery in acute and chronic venous disease. *Surgery*, **85**, 31

Kline, A., Hughes, L. E. *et al.* (1975) Dextran 70 in prophylaxis of thromboembolic disease after surgery: a clinically orientated randomized double-blind trial. *Br. Med. J.*, **2**, 109–112

Klippel, M. and Trenauney, P. (1900) Du naevus varigueux ostero-hyper tropique. *Arch. Gen. Med. (Paris)*, **185**, 641

Kosinski, C. (1926) Observations on the superficial venous system of the lower extremity. *J. Anat.*, **60**, 131–142

Lagersted, C. I., Olsson, C. G. *et al.* (1985) Need for long term anticoagulant treatment in symptomatic calf vein thrombosis. *Lancet*, **ii**, 516–518

Lake, M., Pratt, E. H. and Wright, I. S. (1942) Atherosclerosis and varicose veins: occupational activities and other factors. *J. Am. Med. Ass.*, **119**, 696

Lamont, P., Bavin, D. *et al.* (1986) Accuracy of clinical versus doppler examination for detecting incompetent perforating veins. *Br. J. Surg.*, **73**, 493

Lancet (1975) An international multicentre trial into the prevention of fatal pulmonary embolism by low doses of heparin. *Lancet*, **11**, 45–51

Lea Thomas, M. and Bowles, J. N. (1985) Incompetent perforating veins: comparison of varicography and ascending phlebography. *Radiology*, **154**, 619

Lea Thomas, M. and Briggs, G. M. (1984) Low osmolarity contrast media for phlebography. *Int. Angiol.*, **3**, 73

Leigh, I. M., Purkis, P. E. and Navsaria, H. A. (1987) Treatment of chronic venous ulcers with sheets of cultural allogenic keratinocytes. *Br. J. Dermatol.*, **117**, 591–597

Lensing, A. W., Pradoni, P., Brandjes, D. *et al.* (1989) Detection of deep vein thrombosis by realtime B mode ultrasonography. *N. Engl. J. Med.*, **320**, 342–345

Leyvraz, P. F., Bachmann, F., Hoek, J. *et al.* (1991) Prevention of deep vein thrombosis after hip replacement: randomised comparison between unfractionated heparin and low molecular weight heparin. *Br. Med. J.*, **303**, 543–548

Li, A. K. C. (1975) A technique for re-exploration of the sapheno-femoral junction for recurrent varicose veins. *Br. J. Surg.*, **62**, 745

Linton, R. R. (1938) The post-thrombotic syndrome of the lower extremity: its aetiology and surgical management. *Ann. Surg.*, **107**, 582–593

Ludbrook, J. (1963) Valvular defect in primary varicose veins: cause or effect. *Lancet*, **2**, 1289

McCausland, A. M. (1943) Influence of hormones upon varicose veins. *West J. Surg.*, **51**, 199

MacGowan, W. A. L. (1985) Sclerotherapy: prevention of accidents. A review. *J. Roy. Soc. Med.*, **78**, 136

May, R. (1985) The femoral bypass. *Int. Angiol.*, **4**, 435

Miles, R. M., Chappell, F. and Renner, O. (1964) A partially occluding vena cava clip for the prevention of pulmonary embolism. *Ann. J. Surg.*, **30**, 40

Miller, G. A. H. and Sutton, G. C. (1970) Acute massive pulmonary embolism. Clinical and haemodynamic findings in 23 patients studied by cardiac catheterization and pulmonary arteriography. *Br. Heart J.*, **32**, 518–523

Mitchell, D. C., Grasty, M. S., Stebbings, W. S. L. *et al.* (1991) Comparison of Duplex ultrasonography and venography in the diagnosis of deep vein thrombosis. *Br. J. Surg.*, **78**, 611–613

Mobbin-Uddin, K., Smith, P. E. and Martinel, L. D. (1967) A vena caval filter for the prevention of pulmonary embolism. *Surg. Forum*, **18**, 209

Munn, S. R., Morton, J. B., Macbeth, W. A. G. and McLeish, A. R. (1981) To strip or not to strip the long saphenous vein? A varicose veins trial. *Br. J. Surg.*, **68**, 426

Nabatoff, R. A. (1970) Three thousand stripping operations for varicose veins on a semi ambulatory basis. *Surg. Gynecol. Obstet.*, **130**, 497

Negus, D., Freidgood, A. *et al.* (1980) Ultra-low dose intravenous heparin in the prevention of post-operative deep vein thrombosis. *Lancet*, **i**, 891–894

Negus, D., Pinto, D. *et al.* (1968) The reliability of the ^{125}I fibrinogen uptake method in the diagnosis of occult deep vein thrombosis. *Br. J. Surg.*, **55**, 858

Nicolaides, A. N., Kakkar, V. V. and Field, E. S. (1971). The origin of deep veins thrombosis: a venographic study. *Br. J. Radiol.*, **44**, 653

Niebes, P. and Berson, I. (1973) Determination of enzymes and degradation production of mucopolysaccharide metabolism in the serum of healthy and varicose subjects. *Bibl. Anat.* **11**, 499

Niebes, P. and Laszt, L. (1971) Influence in vitro d'une série de flavonoides sur des enzymes du métabolisme des muocopolysaccharides des veines saphenes humaines et bovines. *Angiologia*, **8**, 279–302

Nilsson, I. M., Krook, H. *et al.* (1961) Severe thrombotic disease in a young man with bone marrow skeletal changes and a high content of an inhibitor in the fibrinolytic system. *Acta Med. Scand.*, **169**, 323

Norgren, L. (1973) Functional evaluation of chronic venous insufficiency by foot volumetry. *Acta Chir. Scand.*, Suppl. 444

O'Donnell, T. F., Burnand, K. G. *et al.* (1977) Doppler examination versus clinical and phlebographic detection of the localisation of incompetent perforating veins: a prospective study. *Arch. Surg.*, **112**, 31

Palma, E. C. and Esperon, R. (1960) Vein transplants and grafts in surgical treatment of the post-phlebitic syndrome. *J. Cardiovasc. Surg.*, **1**, 94

Perthes, G. (1895) Uber die Operation der Unterschenkel varices nach Trendelenburg. *Dtsch. Med. Wochenschr.*, **21**, 253

Plate, G., Einaksson, E., Ohlin, P. *et al.* (1984) Thrombectomy with temporary arteriovenous fistula. The treatment of choice in acute ilio femoral venous thrombosis. *J. Vasc. Surg.*, **1**, 867

Psthakis, N. D. and Psthakis, D. N. (1985) Rationale of the substitute valve operation by technique II in the treatment of chronic venous insufficiency. *Int. Angiol.*, **4**, 397

Queral, L. A., Whitehouse, W. M., Flinn, W. R. *et al.* (1980) Surgical correction of chronic deep venous insufficiency by valvular transposition. *Surgery*, **87**, 688

Roehm, J. F. O., Glaurturco, C., Barth, M. H. and Wright, K. C. (1984) Percutaneous trans catheter filter for inferior vena cava – a new device for treatment of patients with pulmonary embolism. *Radiology*, **150**, 255

Rose, S. S. (1986) Some thoughts on the aetiology of varicose veins. *J. Cardiovasc. Surg.*, **27**, 534–543

Royle, J. P. (1990) Treatment of varicose veins. In *Vascular Surgical Techniques* (ed. R. M. Greenhalgh), Butterworths, London 1990

Ryan, T. J. (1983) *The Management of Leg Ulcers*, Oxford Medical Publications, Oxford

Ryan, T. J. (1990) *The Management of Leg Ulcers*, 2nd edn, Oxford Medical Publications, Oxford

Sabri, S., Roberts V. C. *et al.* (1971) Prevention of early post-operative deep vein thrombosis by intermittent compression of the leg during surgery. *Br. Med. J.*, **4**, 394–396

Servelle, M. (1985) Klippel–Trenauney's syndrome. *Ann. Surg.*, **201**, 365

Sethia, K. K. and Darke, S. G. (1984) Long saphenous incompetence as a cause of venous ulceration. *Br. J. Surg.*, **71**, 754

Sevitt, S. and Gallagher, N. G. (1959) Prevention of venous thrombosis and pulmonary embolism in injured patients. *Lancet*, **2**, 981

Sheppard, M. (1978) A procedure for the prevention of recurrent sapheno femoral incompetence. *Aust. N.Z. J. Surg.*, **48**, 322

Sproull, E. E. (1938) Carcinoma and venous thrombosis: the frequency of association of carcinoma in the body or tail of the pancreas with multiple venous thrombosis. *Am. J. Cancer*, **34**, 566.

Svejcar, J., Prerovsky, I., Linhart, J. *et al.* (1963) Content of collagen, elastin and hexosamine in primary varicose veins. *Clin. Sci.*, **24**, 325–330

Taheri, S. A., Lazar, L. and Elias, S. M. (1982a) Surgical treatment of post-phlebitic syndrome. *Br. J. Surg.*, **69** (Suppl.), 54

Taheri, S. A., Lazar, L. *et al.* (1982b) Vein valve transplant. *Surgery*, **91**, 28

Thompson, H. (1979) The surgical anatomy of the superficial and perforating veins of the lower limb. *Ann. R. Coll. Surg. Engl.*, **61**, 198–205

Tilney, N. L., Griffith, H. J. G. and Edwards, E. A. (1970) Natural history of major venous thrombosis of the upper extremity. *Arch. Surg.*, **101**, 792

Young, A. E., Lea Thomas, M. and Browse, N. L. (1974) Comparison between sequelae of surgical and clinical treatment of venous thromboembolism. *Br. Med. J.*, **4**, 127

46

Portal hypertension

J. Terblanche

The clinical syndrome of portal hypertension exists when there is raised pressure within the portal venous system. The most common cause is cirrhosis or other liver disease causing obstruction to portal flow. Extrahepatic venous obstruction is less common and involves either the portal vein or the hepatic veins and vena cava. The obstruction leads to the development of a collateral venous circulation which bypasses the liver. A small proportion of the total collateral circulation passes through the submucosal veins of the lower oesophagus, but these are of vital importance because bleeding is usually caused by rupture of these varices. Patients may develop specific gastric lesions with bleeding, and occasionally bleed from rectal varices. Unusual causes of portal hypertension require consideration, as the optimal treatment may be different. Rare patients with portal hypertension have troublesome ascites or portasystemic encephalopathy requiring surgical management.

Aetiology

Most patients with portal hypertension have intrahepatic pathology, usually cirrhosis. The most common cause in Western society is alcoholic cirrhosis. Prognosis is poor, with few patients surviving longer than 5 years unless they abstain from alcohol abuse. Viral hepatitis (other than hepatitis A) is a common cause of cirrhosis world wide. Cirrhosis can also be caused by drugs, biliary disease and other liver insults, as well as certain inherited conditions. Liver damage is followed by fibrosis and nodule formation which causes obstruction to flow through the liver. The most common cause of portal hypertension world wide is schistosomiasis, although it is unusual in the West. The prognosis is usually good with correct treatment but in some areas combined schistosomiasis and hepatitis B cirrhosis make prognosis less satisfactory. Non-cirrhotic portal fibrosis, which occurs in India and the East, has a good prognosis. The geographical variation in the prevalence and the causes of portal hypertension is important in assessing the results from various centres.

Patients with portal hypertension due to primary extrahepatic portal vein obstruction have an excellent prognosis, but when portal vein thrombosis occurs secondary to underlying liver cirrhosis, the prognosis is usually poor. The Budd–Chiari syndrome with hepatic vein and/or vena caval obstruction has a variable outcome, but early surgical management should be considered.

Variceal bleeding is the most important complication of portal hypertension. Most variceal bleeding occurs from the submucosal veins in the lower 5 cm of the oesophagus. Bleeding results from disruption of the varices, usually due to increased pressure within the lumen and thinning of the overlying supportive structures as the varices increase in size. Although the size and endoscopic appearance of the varices are important, they are usually not accurate predictive factors for subsequent variceal bleeding.

Indications for surgical management

Oesophageal varices

The majority of patients with portal hypertension and gastrointestinal haemorrhage are bleeding from oesophageal varices. Almost invariably the site of bleeding is the lower 5 cm of the oesophagus. The mortality of an acute variceal bleed in a patient with cirrhosis is as high as 50%. This can be lowered by specific treatment in a specialized centre.

Patients with good liver reserve have a better chance of surviving an acute variceal bleed than those with poor liver reserve. Bleeding with shock leads to further deterioration in liver function, which may precipitate more variceal bleeding and a vicious cycle ending in death. Patients with portal hypertension and oesophageal variceal bleeding frequently die because of an acute variceal bleed. The risk of death is highest at the time of the acute bleed and diminishes rapidly over the next few months to return to the pre-bleed level (Burroughs et al., 1989).

After a variceal bleed 70% of patients will have a further bleed and other specific long-term therapy is indicated. Patients who have never bled from their varices only have a 30% chance of ever bleeding and should therefore be treated expectantly.

Gastric lesions in portal hypertension

The main lesions are gastric varices and portal hypertensive gastropathy.

Gastric varices usually present in association with oesophageal varices and are frequently a direct continuation of the oesophageal varices. Bleeding usually occurs from the oesophageal rather than the gastric varices. The gastric varices usually disappear when the oesophageal varices are adequately treated with sclerotherapy or surgery. Occasionally gastric variceal bleeding presents after successful sclerotherapy or oesophageal transection. Treatment is a problem because sclerotherapy is technically difficult in the stomach. Although sclerotherapy is often attempted, if gastric variceal bleeding persists, the patient may require either a portasystemic shunt or an extensive devascularization operation.

Localized splenic vein thrombosis produces segmental portal hypertension in the left upper quadrant with associated isolated gastric varices without oesophageal varices. Although rare, the condition is cured by gastric devascularization with splenectomy.

The dilated submucosal vessels produced in the stomach by portal hypertension are termed portal hypertensive gastropathy. The whole gastric mucosa is involved, but the upper stomach is often more severely affected. It is not surprising that these lesions may bleed and that treatment is difficult. Propranolol may be effective and a portacaval shunt provides definitive treatment in the rare patients with recurrent bleeding from portal hypertensive gastropathy.

Anorectal varices and other gastrointestinal varices

Varices may present at the stoma in patients with portal hypertension and an ileostomy or a colostomy. Local measures usually suffice, but occasionally portasystemic shunting is required.

Isolated varices in the submucosa of the duodenum or the remainder of the small or large bowel are very rare, but may rupture and cause significant bleeding. Because the majority of patients with portal hypertension bleed from oesophageal varices, the condition is usually not considered and difficult to diagnose. Angiography may be required. Treatment is difficult. When recurrent bleeds occur, portasystemic shunting is curative.

Anorectal varices are a specific condition and must be differentiated from haemorrhoids. Bleeding from the anorectal area in portal hypertension is invariably due to anorectal varices. Diagnosis is by anorectoscopy. If the bleeding is massive, bleeding oesophageal varices have to be excluded. Treatment is controversial. The site of bleeding must be identified by local examination. The site is invariably within the upper anal mucosa. The varix including the bleeding site should be underrun with a continuous suture (Hosking and Johnson, 1988)

Other causes of variceal bleeding

Portal vein obstruction

Primary portal vein obstruction is an important cause of portal hypertension and haemorrhage in children, but can present in adults. In this group the prognosis is usually excellent, with long-term survival regardless

of the therapy used. Sclerotherapy is the most successful form of treatment in children. We have demonstrated the success of repeated sclerotherapy in managing adult patients with primary extrahepatic portal vein obstruction. In adults, distal splenorenal shunting has been used and is an alternative management to be considered.

Budd–Chiari syndrome

Patients with acute occlusion of the hepatic veins, with or without occlusion of the vena cava, tend to have a poor prognosis without treatment. The outcome of management of the Budd–Chiari syndrome depends on the underlying cause of the hepatic vein block, as well as the acuteness of the presentation and the prior management. Although some patients survive for long periods, the majority have rapidly deteriorating liver function, particularly when the onset is acute. They require an urgent liver transplant or a shunt operation to decompress the liver. Sclerotherapy can be used to control variceal bleeding when it occurs, but this does not help the associated deteriorating liver function.

A side-to-side portacaval shunt is advocated when the inferior vena cava is patent and there is no significant pressure gradient across the retrohepatic vena cava. When the vena cava is either occluded or markedly narrowed, a meso-atrial shunt, using a reinforced PTFE graft, is the most successful treatment (Klein and Cameron, 1990)

Schistosomiasis

The prognosis is usually good with correct treatment unless there is associated underlying liver disease from another cause, such as viral hepatitis. Standard portacaval shunting has given poor results, but groups from Brazil and Egypt have reported excellent results using medical treatment for the underlying infestation combined with either an extensive oesophagogastric devascularization operation plus splenectomy or with a distal splenorenal shunt (Da Silva et al., 1986).

Non-cirrhotic portal fibrosis

Although rare in the West, this is an important cause of portal hypertension in India and the Far East. Most patients have a good prognosis with correct treatment. Portacaval shunting is contraindicated. The currently advocated therapy of choice is either sclerotherapy or a major devascularization and transection operation.

Ascites

This can be a major problem in patients with severe intrahepatic obstruction to portal venous flow due to cirrhosis. Fortunately, most patients with severe ascites can be managed by a combination of minimal salt intake and careful diuresis. Patients with resistant ascites are currently treated by repeated partial tapping of the ascites and replacement with an albumin-rich solution. Peritoneojugular shunting is seldom utilized because of side effects, but can produce dramatic results. Here in the University of Cape Town, a Le Veen or Denver catheter shunt is used. One end of the catheter is placed into the peritoneal cavity and the other end is passed subcutaneously to the neck where it is inserted into the subclavian vein. The shunt has a one-way valve system which allows peritoneal fluid to pass into the venous system. Where a portasystemic shunt is performed for ascites, a side-to-side portacaval shunt must be used. Although successful, it is rarely indicated.

Portasystemic encephalopathy

Portasystemic encephalopathy occurs spontaneously in patients with cirrhosis and portal hypertension due to the presence of collateral channels with intestinal blood bypassing the liver at first passage. The treatment is medical. The precise cause remains controversial. Portasystemic encephalopathy can be a particular problem after a large collateral is formed surgically when a portacaval shunt is constructed. The occurrence of encephalopathy cannot be predicted. When severe and incapacitating, it may be necessary to take down the shunt and treat the patient's portal hypertension and varices by some other means. This, however, is fortunately uncommon. Total colectomy to remove the source of the breakdown products produced by bacteria is no longer used.

Management of oesophageal varices

Acute variceal bleed management

Patients with massive upper gastrointestinal haemorrhage should be suspected to be bleeding from varices if they are either known to have portal hypertension or if they have clinical features of either portal hypertension or underlying hepatic dysfunction. The only way to prove that they are actually bleeding from varices is to perform an emergency endoscopy. This will exclude patients who do not have varices and diagnose the other source of bleeding. When considering invasive therapy for acute variceal bleeding, it must be remembered that between 40% and 60% of patients with a variceal bleed will stop bleeding spontaneously. This allows time for adequate resuscitation and work up, prior to performing some form of definitive management. Those patients who continue to bleed from their varices pose a difficult management problem. Therapy can be divided into immediate and subsequent emergency therapy.

Immediate management

Patients are admitted to hospital and are preferably managed in an intensive care unit (ICU). Standard resuscitation for massive haemorrhage is instituted. Such patients should be treated in a unit with special expertise because one or more forms of complex therapy may subsequently be required.

While arrangements are made for emergency fibreoptic endoscopy, pharmacological therapy is usually instituted in patients with massive or continued variceal bleeding. The aim is to control the acute bleed which will facilitate the diagnostic endoscopy and management. The most widely used therapy is a continuous intravenous infusion of vasopressin using a constant infusion pump at 0.4 u/min. This is frequently combined with nitroglycerine which reputedly reduces the side effects of vasopressin while potentiating its haemodynamic effects in the portal bed. Nitroglycerine is best administered as sublingual tablets, one tablet half-hourly for up to 6 h. The synthetic analogue of vasopressin (glypressin) or synthetic somatostatin are alternative therapies which are being evaluated. Recent studies favour somatostatin. All have the effect of lowering portal pressure and, by implication, intravariceal pressure, although this is not proven for somatostatin. Drugs with other actions including metoclopramide, which causes constriction of the lower oesophageal sphincter, are sometimes used.

Emergency fibreoptic endoscopy is mandatory to confirm that the patient has varices. Diagnosis may be difficult during active bleeding. Patients with varices fall into three broad groups: those with actively bleeding varices, those with varices that have stopped bleeding and those with varices but who are bleeding from another lesion. Clearly the latter need to have the alternative lesion treated on merit. Approximately one-third of patients fall into each of these three categories. Variceal bleeding which has stopped is diagnosed if an adherent blood clot is noted on a varix or if varices are present in a patient with upper gastrointestinal bleeding where panendoscopy discloses no other explanation for the bleeding. Both patients with active variceal bleeding and those with variceal bleeding that has stopped should have definitive emergency sclerotherapy at the time of the first emergency endoscopy. Where this is not possible, either because expertise is lacking or because it is not technically feasible due to the presence of active bleeding, some additional measure is required. If pharmacological therapy has already been started, then the only method of controlling active bleeding is by a correctly placed balloon tube for tamponade.

A correctly used four-lumen modified Sengstaken balloon tube (Minnesota tube) is highly effective in temporarily controlling bleeding. As its use is associated with complications, including aspiration, balloon tube tamponade should only be used when required to control active variceal bleeding. Once a balloon tube has been inserted, the patient requires subsequent additional therapy to prevent recurrent bleeding, which will otherwise occur in 60% of patients. Such therapy must be performed early, within 6–12 h, to prevent local complications. If bleeding continues the tube should be checked by an expert and, if correctly placed, the patient should be re-endoscoped to determine whether the bleeding is caused by another lesion or is arising from the gastric mucosa. A balloon tube is depicted later, in Figure 46.1.

Subsequent management

Once the active variceal bleeding episode has either ceased spontaneously or been temporarily controlled, there is a danger of early recurrent variceal bleeding. This rises from approximately 40%, with spontaneous cessation of haemorrhage, to over 60% in patients who require pharmacological therapy or a balloon tube for temporary control. Clearly, additional therapy is required as each recurrent acute variceal bleed is associated with a high mortality.

The mainstay of subsequent emergency therapy is sclerotherapy, although emergency shunts and emergency transection and/or devascularization operations are under evaluation. The available controlled trials and considerable uncontrolled data have demonstrated that sclerotherapy will control acute variceal bleeding in 90–95% of patients. The techniques of sclerotherapy are depicted in Figures 46.2 and 46.3 and described later.

Emergency sclerotherapy is either performed at the time of the first diagnostic endoscopy or on the next available list the following morning. Where a balloon tube has been inserted, this should be removed and sclerotherapy performed within 6–12 h to prevent complications. Balloon tube control allows time for resuscitation and to improve the patient's general condition. One or two emergency injection treatments during a single hospital admission will control active variceal bleeding in more than 90% of patients. The 5–10% of patients who have further recurrent variceal bleeds after two injection treatments pose a particularly difficult management problem. Here, we advocate temporary balloon tube tamponade followed by one of the surgical treatment options.

Some groups use either a portasystemic shunt or an oesophageal transection as the primary procedure for the majority of patients with acute variceal bleeding who do not respond to conservative measures. The surgical shunt options are depicted in Figures 46.4–46.6. Of these, only the end-to-side, side-to-side or narrow diameter PTFE portacaval shunts are widely used in acute variceal bleed management (Figure 46.4). Some use an emergency mesocaval shunt (Figure 46.5A,B) or a distal splenorenal shunt (Figure 46.6B) in some patients.

Preferred treatment here for the failures of sclerotherapy is emergency staple gun oesophageal transection (Figure 46.9A). More extensive devasculari-

zation (Figure 46.9B) or combined transection and devascularization operations (Figure 46.10) are usually reserved for long-term management.

Sclerotherapy failures are defined as those patients in whom bleeding recurs after two emergency injection treatments. In our institution, only those patients who fail to respond to emergency injection sclerotherapy are treated with either a staple gun oesophageal transection or an emergency portacaval shunt. Unfortunately, the mortality in this group is high, particularly in patients who have poor hepatic reserve.

Long-term management after a variceal bleed

Some form of specific therapy is usually advocated in patients after a variceal bleed because they have a 70% chance of a further variceal bleed with the attendant morbidity and mortality. No single therapy has proved superior and alternatives need to be weighed up for each patient.

The alternatives are conservative medical management, waiting to see whether the patient has a further bleed and then instituting emergency treatment followed by some specific management, if indicated; pharmacological therapy, usually aimed at lowering portal pressure; sclerotherapy; a portosystemic shunt; or a devascularization and transection operation. The only definitive treatment for patients with end-stage liver disease and variceal bleeding is liver transplantation. This not only cures the underlying liver disease but eradicates the portal hypertension and its complications. All patients presenting with a variceal bleed should be considered for liver transplantation, although very few will ultimately receive a transplant. Likely transplant candidates should preferably be treated with sclerotherapy because major surgery, particularly portacaval shunting, makes subsequent transplant surgery more difficult.

Long-term pharmacological therapy has attracted attention as an appealing management option. The most widely used and tested treatment is beta-blockade with propranolol. The dose of propranolol is adjusted to reduce the pulse rate by 25%. Where this is effective, it has been shown to lower portal pressure. Individual controlled trials have produced conflicting results, but statistical meta-analysis of the available controlled trials, despite its problems, has suggested a positive role for beta-blockade (Hayes *et al.*, 1990). There are many problems with current drug therapy, including patient compliance (particularly in alcoholic patients), the side effects of the drugs and the need for lifelong therapy. Pharmacological therapy is being increasingly used, but this should be restricted to major institutions.

Sclerotherapy is the most widely accepted long-term management option after a variceal bleed. The various techniques are depicted in Figures 46.2 and 46.3. Sclerotherapy should be performed at weekly intervals until the varices are eradicated. Patients are followed for life. The first repeat endoscopy should be performed at 3 months to confirm eradication of varices and thereafter at 6-monthly or yearly intervals. Whenever recurrent varices are diagnosed, an identical treatment policy of repeated injections should be undertaken at weekly intervals until eradication has been achieved. A number of groups have shown the efficacy of repeat sclerotherapy in managing patients after an oesophageal variceal bleed. Varices are eradicated in over 90% of patients. Varices usually remain eradicated for 1–2 years and then recur if the patient survives. Survival with sclerotherapy appears to be related to the number of variceal bleeds that occur and the patient's underlying liver condition. Repeated sclerotherapy usually eradicates varices and, after eradication, variceal bleeding is significantly diminished. Improvement in survival remains in question, particularly if conservatively treated patients have the best available treatment for any subsequent acute variceal bleeds. A major problem is that patients require lifelong follow-up and that varices recur and require repeated injections. Although repeat injections can be performed on an outpatient basis, sclerotherapy places an increasing strain on a specialist unit interested in portal hypertension.

For this reason a number of authorities advocate either portasystemic shunting (Figures 46.4–46.6) or a transection or devascularization procedure (Figures 46.9 and 46.10) as the primary therapy. Several trials have been published and others are under way comparing these procedures with sclerotherapy.

Sclerotherapy as primary treatment with early surgical salvage for the failures of sclerotherapy is widely accepted as the main modality of treatment today. Failure of sclerotherapy is defined as either repeated variceal bleeds, or varices that are difficult to eradicate, despite adequate sclerotherapy management.

The most favoured shunt is the distal splenorenal shunt (Figure 46.6B). There appears to be little difference in the overall results between this operation and a standard portacaval shunt (Figure 46.4A) in alcoholic cirrhotic patients. Because a standard portacaval shunt is technically simpler, some reserve the distal splenorenal shunt for non-alcoholic cirrhotic patients. An alternative shunt which is being evaluated is the narrow diameter PTFE portacaval H-graft (Figure 46.4C).

An alternative to shunting is extensive oesophagogastric devascularization with associated oesophageal transection using the staple gun (Figure 46.10B).

Prophylactic long-term management

Prophylactic therapy for patients with portal hypertension is defined as treatment to prevent the first variceal bleed. As only 30% of patients with cirrhosis and diagnosed oesophageal varices will bleed from their varices during their lifetime, any form of therapy instituted routinely in patients who have not bled

from varices is likely to be used unnecessarily in 70% of these patients. Most, therefore, treat patients expectantly and only consider specific therapies once the patient has had a variceal bleed. There is a significant mortality with the first variceal bleed and if a group of patients could be identified who are at high risk for the first bleed then selective specific therapy would be justified. According to the North Italian Endoscopic Club (1988), a combination of the endoscopic findings of large varices with overlying red markings, together with clinical and biochemical evidence of poor hepatic function, may identify such high-risk patients.

Prophylactic management options that have been tested in patients prior to a variceal bleed include pharmacological therapy, sclerotherapy, portasystemic shunts or a devascularization and transection operation.

Pharmacological therapy with beta-blockade using propranolol is controversial but may be effective. It required the statistical technique of meta-analysis of multiple trials to demonstrate a lower first bleed rate and lower mortality (Hayes et al., 1990). Multiple sclerotherapy trials have produced conflicting results. Prophylactic sclerotherapy may even precipitate bleeding with associated mortality in a patient who has never bled before. Japanese surgeons advocate prophylactic major surgical procedures for patient groups identified as being at high risk of bleeding. Any form of prophylactic therapy in patients who have not yet bled from oesophageal varices should only be undertaken in major centres investigating prophylactic treatment.

Surgical techniques in portal hypertension

Balloon tube tamponade

The Minnesota modification of the Sengstaken balloon tube is currently preferred. It has four lumens. One opens into the stomach for suction and to instil medications. One has openings into the upper oesophagus for suction of secretions to prevent aspiration. The last two lumens are connected to the balloons, one for the stomach and the other for the oesophagus (Figure 46.1).

Balloon tube tamponade is used to control active variceal bleeding, usually when the endoscopist is unable to perform emergency sclerotherapy because of poor visualization due to active haemorrhage.

A well-lubricated tube is passed via the mouth (rather than the nose) after previous test inflation of the balloons and suction deflation, ensuring that all the air has been removed. The tube is passed until the tip is well within the stomach. Passage of the tube is usually easy in a cooperative patient. When the patient is stuporous or uncooperative it is sometimes essential to insert an endotrachial tube first to protect the airway. In stuporous patients a laryngoscope and forceps may be required to assist with tube insertion. The siting of the tube in the stomach can be checked by auscultation while blowing air through the tube. The gastric balloon is inflated with 200 ml of air and drawn up tightly against the oesophagogastric junction. This provides compression of the submucosal varices at the oesophagogastric junction. The oesophageal balloon is inflated to 40 mmHg using a sphygmomanometer and a three-way tap. The gastric balloon is the important functional component of balloon tamponade. Having pulled the tube up tightly against the oesophagogastric junction, compression is maintained by strapping a split tennis ball to the tube at the patient's mouth (Figure 46.1). The tube should be left *in situ* for as short a time as possible because of the potential danger of erosion at the oesophagogastric junction.

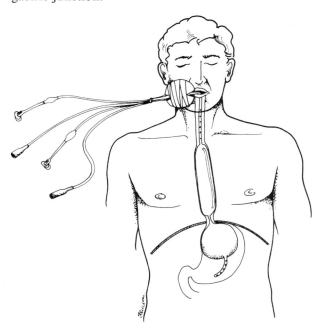

Figure 46.1 Four-lumen modified Sengstaken balloon tube (Minnesota tube). The tube is pulled up tightly against the oesophagogastric junction and held in place with a split tennis ball at the mouth

The patient must be nursed in an ICU with the airway protected by regular suction, unless the patient is intubated. Resuscitation is continued and between 6 and 12 h after insertion the patient is endoscoped in the endoscopy suite or in the ICU and sclerotherapy performed. After removing the tennis ball, the oesophageal balloon is deflated and the tube either removed or moved downwards into the stomach immediately prior to passing the fibreoptic endoscope. The tube should not be replaced after the sclerotherapy because of the danger of causing ulceration with subsequent bleeding. The major complications of balloon tube tamponade are aspiration

and local ulceration, caused particularly by excessive and prolonged pressure of the gastric balloon on the oesophagogastric junction.

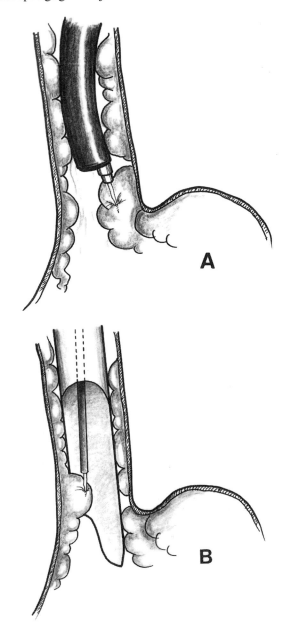

Figure 46.2 Intravariceal sclerotherapy. A, Intravascular sclerotherapy with the flexible endsocope. B, Intravascular sclerotherapy with the rigid endoscope

Injection sclerotherapy

The techniques of sclerotherapy are shown in Figures 46.2 and 46.3. The rigid endoscope (Figure 46.2B) has been supplanted by the fibreoptic scope. There are three different techniques. Direct intravariceal injection thromboses the varices, thereby controlling acute bleeding and preventing recurrences (Figure 46.2A).

Paravariceal or submucosal injections produce sub-mucosal oedema which stops early rebleeding and later causes thickening of the overlying mucosa with repeat injections. This prevents recurrent bleeding (Figure 46.3A). The third is a combination of intra-variceal and paravariceal techniques (Figure 46.3B).

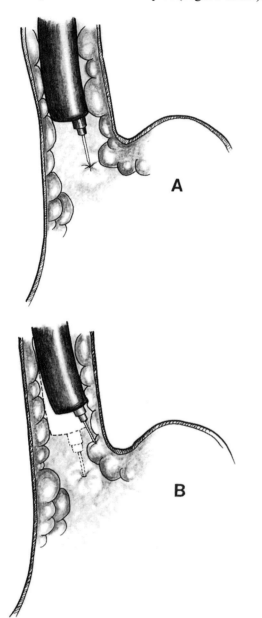

Figure 46.3 Sclerotherapy. A, Paravariceal sclerotherapy. B, Combined paravariceal and intravariceal sclerotherapy

A variety of sclerosant agents have been used. Ethanolamine oleate 5% is favoured for intravariceal injections. The alternatives are 5% sodium morr-huate, 5% sodium tetradecyl sulphate or combination sclerosant therapy. Polidocanol 1% is most widely used for paravariceal injections. Our group use com-bined intra- and paravariceal sclerotherapy for acute variceal bleeding and a predominantly intravariceal technique for long-term management using 5% etha-nolamine oleate.

Combined sclerotherapy technique

This is used for emergency sclerotherapy, preferably at the time of the first diagnostic endoscopy or after the removal of a balloon tube. The patient is lightly sedated unless stuporous, when no sedation is given. Occasionally a light general anaesthetic is required for difficult patients. With the patient either head up or on the side, and with adequate suction available, the endoscope is passed to the oesophagogastric junc-tion. If active bleeding is present this is controlled first by sclerotherapy and the remainder of the diag-nostic endoscopy performed thereafter. If bleeding has stopped, panendoscopy is performed first and sclerotherapy undertaken once other causes of bleed-ing have been excluded.

Injections are localized to the 5 cm area immedi-ately above the oesophagogastric junction. One to 2 ml of ethanolamine oleate is injected above or on either side of each varix, raising a bleb which provides partial compression of the variceal channel and a further 2–5 ml of solution is injected into the variceal channel (Figure 46.3B). After the intravariceal injec-tion the needle is withdrawn and the injection site is tamponaded with either the injector sheath or the endoscope. Any residual bleeding or oozing from the needle puncture site in the varix is controlled by further small paravariceal injections, raising blebs with 1–2 ml of ethanolamine oleate on either side of the bleeding point. Once satisfactory haemostasis has been achieved the endoscope is removed. The balloon tube should not be reinserted after sclerotherapy. The patient is monitored in an ICU. Any evidence of rebleeding requires a further diagnostic endoscopy and additional injection sclerotherapy, if necessary.

Intravariceal sclerotherapy

This technique is used for repeated injections to eradicate varices (Figure 46.2A). Sclerotherapy is per-formed on an outpatient basis with the patient under light sedation. With the patient on the side and with adequate suction available, the endoscope is passed and full panendoscopy performed. Sclerotherapy is undertaken after documenting the size and extent of the varices. The needle is inserted directly into the varix immediately above the oesophagogastric junc-tion and between 3 ml and 6 ml of ethanolamine oleate is injected into each varix; 8 ml may be needed for an individual large varix. Lesser volumes are used as obliteration occurs. On removing the needle, the puncture site is tamponaded. If oozing or bleeding persists, additional paravariceal injections are usually successful.

The procedure is usually performed in the morning and the patient is observed for 3–4 h before being allowed to proceed home, with instructions to return immediately should there be any evidence of bleeding.

Paravariceal sclerotherapy

The most widely used technique is that described by Paquet (1983). Here, multiple 0.5–1 ml injections of 1% polidocanol are placed circumferentially around the lower third of the oesophagus, commencing at the oesophagogastric junction and moving proximally in a helical fashion giving 30–50 injections and 30–50 ml of polidocanol. The technique has been successfully used for both acute bleed management and long-term control.

Complications

The incidence of complications is low, but is cumulative with time in long-term sclerotherapy. Local slough or superficial ulceration is common, but usually not troublesome unless it overlies a major varix and bleeding occurs. Stricture of the oesophagus is rare unless high concentration agents are used, particularly 3–5% polidocanol, and the stricture is easily treated by dilatation. Local injection site leak or rupture of the oesophagus are described and, although rare, are more serious complications. Sclerotherapy has proved remarkably safe, considering its widespread application (Kahn et al., 1989).

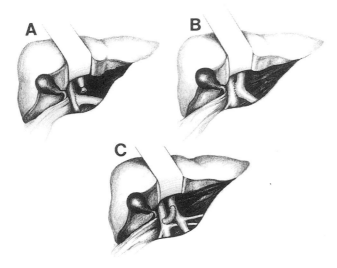

Figure 46.4 Portacaval shunts. A, End-to-side shunts. B, Side-to-side shunts. C, H-graft (From Terblanche, 1989, by permission)

Portasystemic shunts

These are broadly divided into portacaval (Figure 46.4), mesocaval (Figure 46.5) and splenorenal shunts (Figure 46.6).

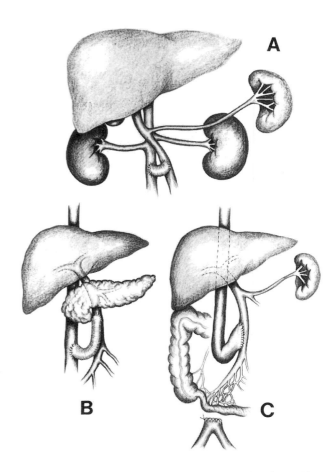

Figure 46.5 Mesocaval shunts. A, H-graft. B, C-graft. C, Clatworthy shunt (From Terblanche, 1989, by permission)

A portacaval shunt may be a totally diverting end-to-side shunt (Figure 46.4A) or a side-to-side shunt (Figure 46.4B), which is largely reserved for treating patients with ascites. The H-graft or interposition shunt between the portal vein and the vena cava (Figure 46.4C) utilizes a narrow-diameter PTFE graft. The procedure is simple as the whole circumference of the portal vein does not have to be dissected free. It is said to have the theoretical advantage of maintaining moderately raised portal pressure and liver perfusion (Sarfeh et al., 1986)

The previously popular wide-lumen prosthetic graft mesocaval shunt (Figure 46.5A), which is reputedly easier to perform than a standard portacaval shunt, has been largely abandoned because of a high graft thrombosis rate. The exception is the C-mesocaval graft (Sarr et al., 1986) (Figure 46.5B). Clatworthy's shunt, where the divided vena cava is anastomosed end-to-side to the superior mesenteric vein, was described for use in children but has been largely abandoned (Figure 46.5C).

The originally described central splenorenal shunt entailed removal of the spleen with the splenic vein being anastomosed to the renal vein as an end-to-side procedure (Figure 46.6A). This shunt is rarely used today. Probably the most popular shunt is the Warren selective distal splenorenal shunt (Figure 46.6B). This has the theoretical advantage of selectively shunting left upper quadrant venous blood. The shunt decompresses the lower oesophagus (the site of variceal bleeding) and upper stomach via the spleen, while at the same time theoretically preserving the superior mesenteric blood flow to the liver and retaining a high pressure in that system. The shunt is reported to produce a lower encephalopathy rate than standard shunts.

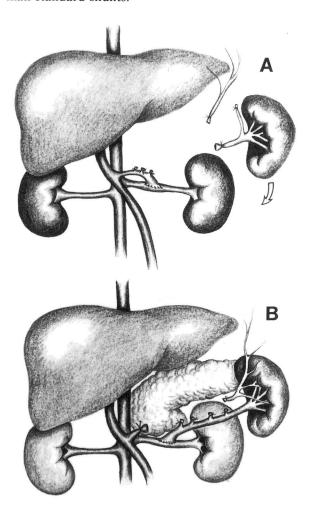

A

B

Figure 46.6 Splenorenal shunts. A, Central splenorenal shunt. B, Selective distal splenorenal shunt (From Terblanche, 1989, by permission)

Portacaval shunt

This is indicated for acute variceal bleeding and for long-term management after a bleed. The patient is supine on the operating table with the right side elevated. A right subcostal incision extended to the left provides good exposure. Careful dissection with diathermy or ligation of all vascular connections is

required. The colon is mobilized downwards from the liver and the duodenum is Kocherized and mobilized to the patient's left to expose the underlying vena cava (Figure 46.7A). The vascular retroperitoneal tissues overlying the vena cava are divided with diathermy and suture ligation to expose enough of the anteromedial wall of the cava to place a Satinsky clamp at a point suitable for the anastomosis (Figure 46.7B). The porta hepatis structures are dissected, working from posterolaterally and exposing the portal vein. It is not necessary to expose the bile duct or the hepatic artery which are retracted to the patient's left (Figure 46.7A). Careful dissection exposes the full circumference of the portal vein. Small medial tributaries may have to be divided and ligated. This is the most hazardous part of the operation. A sling is placed round the portal vein and it is pulled to the patient's right and dissected up to the bifurcation and down to the pancreas. Sufficient length is freed to perform the anastomosis. If the caudate lobe of the liver is in the way, it is retracted upwards. Portal pressure is measured with a needle and manometer and thereafter the portal vein is clamped above and below the proposed site of transection. The upper end is either oversewn or ligated. Ligatures are sometimes best placed around the individual right and left portal vein branches to ensure adequate length for the anastomosis. The vein is divided obliquely, as demonstrated in Figure 46.7B. Stay sutures are inserted (Figure 46.7C) and the anastomosis performed with a continuous running 5/0 vascular suture for the posterior wall (Figure 46.7D). Many use a continuous suture for the anterior wall, but this anastomosis can be effected with two or three separate sutures. Sutures should be carefully inserted to prevent tearing the vein wall as this will lead to subsequent bleeding. Prior to completing the anastomosis, the clamps are temporarily released and blood clots washed out of the lumen with heparinized saline. After completing the anastomosis, the Satinsky clamp on the vena cava is released to expel air. The clamp on the portal vein is removed last. Portal pressure is measured and should have diminished significantly. The completed operation is depicted in Figure 46.4C.

The abdomen is closed with continuous sutures without drainage. Patients require postoperative monitoring in an ICU. The most important late postoperative complication is unpredictable hepatic encephalopathy.

Distal splenorenal shunt (Warren shunt)

Preoperative investigations must confirm prograde flow to the liver and panangiography displays the vasculature and the relationship of the splenic vein to the renal vein. The shunt should be restricted to the long-term management of better risk patients in Child's A and B groups.

The patient is supine on the operating table and a bilateral subcostal incision, frequently with a vertical

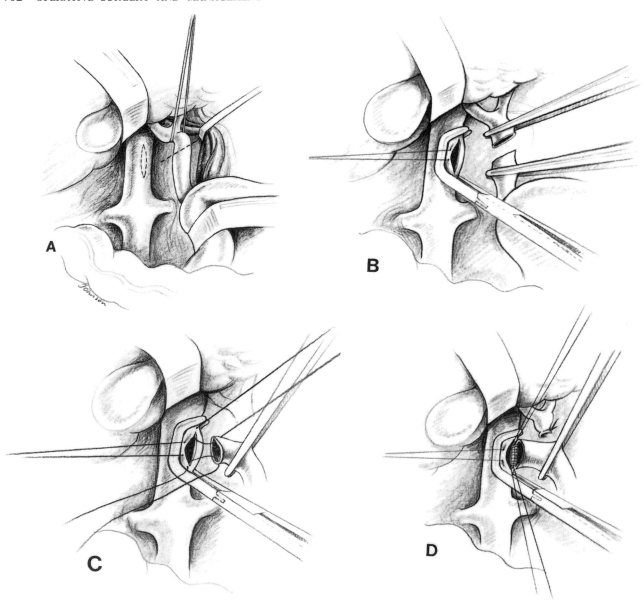

Figure 46.7 End-to-side portacaval shunt. A, Exposure of the inferior vena cava and the portal vein. B, Partial clamping of the inferior vena cava and oblique transection of the portal vein. C, Preparing for the portacaval anastomosis. D, Posterior layer of the portacaval anastomosis

midline extension, is used. Dissection is performed carefully to avoid bleeding using diathermy or ligation of all structures containing vessels. The gastrocolic omentum is divided in its full length and the splenic flexure of the colon separated from the spleen. The peritoneum overlying the inferior wall of the pancreas is incised, largely with diathermy. The splenic vein is identified by retracting the pancreas upwards, and is encircled by careful dissection near its junction with the superior mesenteric vein (Figure 46.8A). The inferior mesenteric vein is ligated. The left gastric or coronary vein is carefully isolated and

divided, if visible. If not visible at this stage, it is subsequently divided at a higher level above the stomach. A tape is placed around the splenic vein (Figure 46.8A). The splenic vein is dissected out of the pancreas, ligating and dividing the small vessels encountered. For non-alcoholic cirrhotic patients, dissection of the vein to near the tail of the pancreas is probably adequate. In alcoholic cirrhotic patients, total splenopancreatic disconnection is required with dissection of the vein to the hilum of the spleen. This is a more complex and tedious procedure.

Attention is directed to the renal vein. The retroperitoneal tissue overlying the renal vein (as identified by the preoperative angiogram) is divided between clamps. The vein is situated deeper than anticipated by the uninitiated. Its anterior wall is exposed, the adrenal vein is divided and ligated and the antero-superior margin of the left renal vein is prepared for the anastomosis by placing a Satinsky partially occluding clamp (Figure 46.8B).

The splenic vein is clamped adjacent to the superior mesenteric vein and oversewn (Figure 46.8B). An ellipse of the renal vein is removed and an end-to-side anastomosis is performed with a 5/0 vascular suture, using a continuous layer for the posterior anastomosis which is performed from within the lumen (Figure 46.8C). The anterior layer of the anastomosis can be completed with a continuous suture or with interrupted sutures. Prior to completing the anastomosis, the clamps are temporarily released and the lumen washed clear of blood clots with heparinized saline. The Satinsky clamp is removed from the renal vein first to check for bleeding and finally from the splenic vein. Isolation of the oesophagogastric and splenic compartment is completed by dividing any additional venous connections with the superior mesenteric compartment. A schematic representation of the completed procedure is presented in Figure 46.6B. Haemostasis is checked and the abdomen closed without drainage. Careful postoperative monitoring in an ICU is required.

Devascularization and transection operations

Oesophageal or gastric transection alone is largely reserved for the emergency management of acute bleeding varices (Figure 46.9). Both have the disadvantage of recurrent varices occurring in a percentage of patients, but these can be treated by subsequent sclerotherapy. Oesophageal transection was originally performed by hand, but most surgeons now use the staple gun (Figure 46.9A). The alternative is to transect the stomach a short distance below the oesophagogastric junction, either by hand or with stapling instruments. Devascularization alone was widely used in the past but it is only of use in patients with schistosomiasis (Figure 46.9B).

The extensive abdominothoracic devascularization and transection procedure described by Sugiura, or one of its modifications, is still widely used in Japan (Figure 46.10A). Most Western surgeons use a transabdominal devascularization and oesophageal transection procedure using the staple gun (Figure 46.10B).

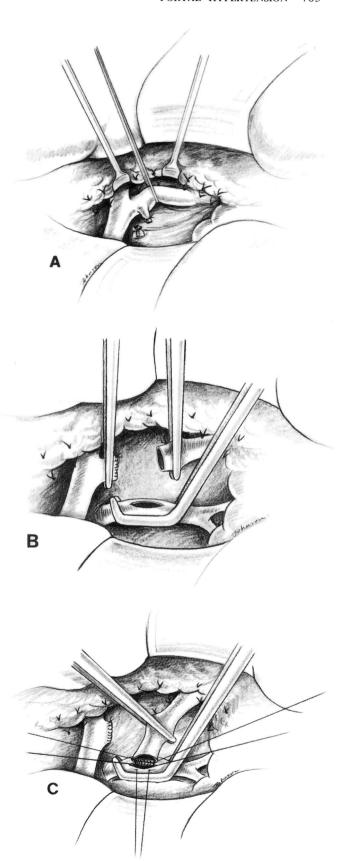

Figure 46.8 Selective distal splenorenal shunt. A, Mobilization of the splenic vein from behind the pancreas. Ligation of the inferior mesenteric vein. B, Transection of the splenic vein adjacent to the superior mesenteric vein and preparation for the splenorenal anastomosis. C, Posterior layer of the splenorenal anastomosis

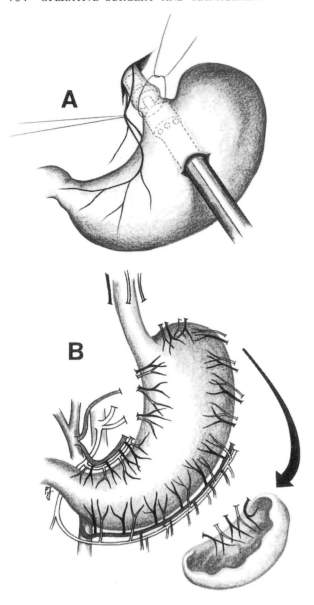

Figure 46.9 Transection or devascularization operations. A, Oesophageal transection with a staple gun. B, Gastric devascularization alone (From Terblanche, 1989, by permission)

Staple gun transection

This is a relatively simple technique but is made difficult when peri-oesophageal fibrosis occurs after previous sclerotherapy or when there are extensive major collateral veins around the lower oesophagus. It is contraindicated when the lower oesophageal wall is extensively thickened by fibrosis following sclerotherapy. This is fortunately uncommon. It is particularly indicated for acute variceal bleeding, either as a primary procedure or after failed sclerotherapy. It should not be used for long-term management because much lower recurrence rates can be achieved by combined procedures. Patients requiring balloon tube tamponade should only have this removed after the initial dissection is complete.

With the patient supine, a left subcostal incision or a left subcostal incision extended to the right is used. The lower oesophagus is carefully isolated after identifying and isolating the anterior and posterior vagus nerves with slings. This requires careful dissection with a combination of diathermy and suture ligation to prevent excessive bleeding. Once the oesophagus has been encircled with a sling some 4–5 cm are freed. A transverse gastrotomy is performed (Figure 46.9A) and the staple gun is fitted with the largest cartridge which will easily enter the oesophagus. In our experience after sclerotherapy, this is often the smallest of the three cartridges. A 0 or 00 non-absorbable strong thread, such as Ethibond, is passed around the oesophagus and tied firmly between the separated staple cartridge and the anvil. The cartridge and anvil are approximated by turning the handle of the gun and the gun fired. The procedure removes a complete circle of the oesophageal wall while at the same time staple suturing the two cut ends and transecting all of the oesophageal wall variceal connections. The gun is gently removed and the single complete ring segment of the oesophagus checked. The gastrotomy is closed with a single layer of continuous 3/0 PDS suture. The abdomen is closed without drainage.

Recurrent acute bleeding during this hospital admission is exceedingly uncommon after staple gun transection. Complications include leakage or stenosis of the anastomosis, both of which are uncommon. These complications occur less frequently when the transection is performed alone rather than when combined with an extensive devascularization procedure. Late rebleeding does occur and recurrent varices should be treated by sclerotherapy.

Combined oesophagogastric devascularization and oesophageal transection

This is indicated for the long-term prevention of oesophageal variceal bleeding after a previous bleed. A variety of procedures are described. The procedure used by the Cape Town group is presented in Figure 46.10B.

With the patient supine, a left subcostal incision extended to the right is made. Dissection and haemostasis are carefully achieved by a combination of diathermy and suture ligation. The lesser curve of the stomach is devascularized as for a highly selective vagotomy (Figure 46.10B). The dissection need not extend as low as for a standard highly selective vagotomy. The vagal nerves are not specifically identified, but the procedure is performed entirely from the front to the back of the lesser curve adhering closely to the stomach. The areas between vessels are divided with diathermy and each individual vessel is doubly ligated and divided with the vagal trunks to the body of the stomach. The dissection proceeds across the

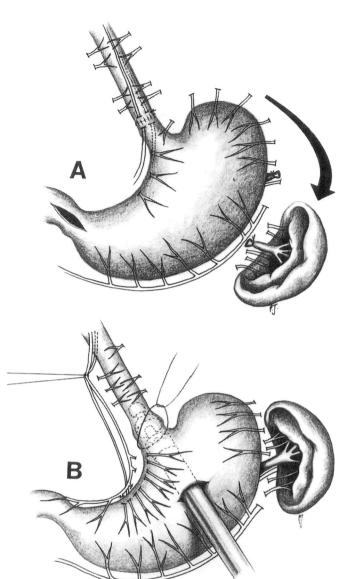

Figure 46.10 Combined transection and devascularization operations. A, Sugiura operation. B, Transabdominal oesophagogastric devascularization and staple gun oesophageal transection with preservation of the spleen (From Terblanche, 1989, by permission)

curve up the right side and then up the left side of the oesophagus. The bundle of tissue containing the anterior and posterior vagal nerves, which are encircled with tape, are pulled to the patient's right while the oesophagus, also encircled with tape, is pulled to the patient's left. Great care is taken to ensure that no major veins entering the oesophagus at a high level are missed. If any are found, they are ligated and divided. At this point the stomach and oesophagus can be lifted up to facilitate the oesophageal transection with the staple gun. The transection is performed as described above via a small gastrotomy (Figure 46.10B). After removal of the staple gun the gastrotomy is closed with a continuous 2/0 PDS suture. A loose wrap of the fundus of the stomach around the lower oesophagus, as would be used in performing a 'floppy' Nissan operation, may be performed to prevent reflux and to bolster the anastomosis. The abdomen is closed without drainage. The patient usually requires postoperative intensive care. The complications include leakage from the anastomosis, which is unusual, or very rarely a stricture of the lower oesophagus. Late rebleeding is uncommon.

References

Burroughs, A. K., Mezzanotte, G., Phillips, A. *et al.* (1989) Cirrhotics with variceal hemorrhage: the importance of the time interval between admission and the start of analysis for survival and rebleeding rates. *Hepatology*, **9**, 801–807

Da Silva, L. C., Strauss, E., Gayotto, L. C. C. *et al.* (1986) A randomized trial for the study of the elective surgical treatment of portal hypertension in mansonic schistosomiasis. *Ann. Surg.*, **204**, 148–153

Hayes, P. C., Davis, J. M., Lewis, J. A. *et al.* (1990) Meta-analysis of value of propranolol in prevention of variceal haemorrhage. *Lancet*, **336**, 153–156

Hosking, S. W. and Johnson, A. G. (1988) Bleeding ano-rectal varices – a misunderstood condition. *Surgery*, **104**, 70–73

Kahn, D., Bornman, P. C. and Terblanche, J. (1989) Incidence and management of complications after injection sclerotherapy: a 10-year prospective evaluation. *Surgery*, **105**, 160–165

Klein, A. S. and Cameron, J. L. (1990) Diagnosis and management of Budd–Chiari syndrome. *Am. J. Surg.*, **160**, 128–133

North Italian Endoscopic Club for the Study and Treatment of Esophageal Varices (1988) Prediction of the first variceal hemorrhage in patients with cirrhosis of the liver and esophageal varices. A prospective multicentre study. *N. Engl. J. Med.*, **319**, 983–989

Paquet, K-J. (1983) Endoscopic paravariceal injection sclerotherapy of the esophagus – indications, technique, complications: results of a period of 14 years. *Gastrointest. Endosc.*, **29**, 310–315

Sarfeh, I. J., Rypins, E. B. and Mason, G. R. (1986) A systematic appraisal of portacaval H-grafts diameters. Clinical and hemodynamic perspective. *Ann. Surg.*, **204**, 356–363

upper stomach immediately below the oesophagogastric junction. The spleen is left *in situ* and the short gastric vessels are divided starting at approximately the mid-point of the greater curve of the stomach. When the spleen is very large and adherent to the stomach, this can be the most difficult part of the operation. It should be possible to perform the whole procedure with minimal blood loss. The operating surgeon works alternately from above or below until the upper half of the stomach has been mobilized. At this point the stomach can be lifted up, which greatly facilitates the devascularization of the lower 5–7 cm of the oesophagus. This commences from the lesser

Sarr, M. G., Herlong, H. F. and Cameron, J. L. (1986) Long-term patency of the mesocaval C shunt. *Am. J. Surg.*, **151**, 98–103

Terblanche, J. (1989) The surgeon's role in the management of portal hypertension. *Ann. Surg.*, **209**, 381–395

Further reading

Henderson, J. M., Millikan, W. J. and Galloway, J. R. (1990) The Emory perspective of the distal splenorenal shunt in 1990. *Am. J. Surg.*, **160**, 54–59

Terblanche, J. (1990) Has sclerotherapy altered the management of patients with variceal bleeding? *Am. J. Surg.*, **160**, 37–42

Terblanche, J., Burroughs, A. K. and Hobbs, K. E. F. (1989) Controversies in the management of bleeding esophageal varices. *N. Engl. J. Med.*, **320**, 1393–1398, 1469–1475

Terblanche, J., Kahn, D. and Bornman, P. C. (1989) Long-term injection sclerotherapy treatment for esophageal varices: a 10-year prospective evaluation. *Ann. Surg.*, **210**, 725–731

47

Soft-tissue sarcomas

G. Westbury

Soft-tissue sarcomas constitute a relatively rare group of neoplasms which account for less than 0.5% of all cancers registered in England and Wales, although they are proportionately commoner in childhood, ranking third in the Manchester Children's Tumour Registry. They may occur in any anatomical region but are commonest in the lower limb.

Pathology

The histological classification is somewhat complex and is based on the resemblance of the tumour cells to the various normal components of the soft supporting tissues, e.g. *lipo*sarcoma, *fibro*sarcoma, *synovial* sarcoma and malignant *fibrous histiocyt*oma, the last being the commonest of all though its identity was recognized only in the 1960s. Malignant tumours of smooth muscle, the *leiomyo*sarcomas, arise principally in the gastrointestinal tract and uterus; they are not mentioned further as their management falls within the scope of the general abdominal surgeon and the gynaecologist. Malignant tumours of striated muscle, the *rhabdomyo*sarcomas, are extremely rare in the adult. The embryonal rhabdomyosarcomas of infancy and childhood are noteworthy in that they are uniquely responsive to systemic cytotoxic therapy, which plays a major role in their management. For the purpose of tumour staging, prognosis and management the histological *grade* is all important. This depends on an amalgam of factors including histological type, cellularity, mitotic activity and amount of necrosis. The concept of a two- or at the most three-grade classification has the virtues of simplicity and practical clinical value.

The gross appearance of most soft-tissue sarcomas is misleading as they often seem to be encapsulated. This is, however, a *pseudocapsule* since it contains tumour cells. Surgical enucleation through this false plane of cleavage will nearly always be followed by local recurrence. Fascial planes, major nerve sheaths and the adventitia of larger arteries are relatively resistant to invasion and sarcomas tend to spread along the lines of least resistance, as is exemplified most clearly within the musculofascial compartments of the limbs. Invasion of major arteries and nerves and of bone occurs relatively late. Lymph node involvement is unusual and is seen mainly in rhabdomyosarcoma and synovial sarcoma. It carries a grave prognosis. Regional node dissection is only rarely indicated.

Diagnosis

Clinical diagnosis of this rare group of tumours depends on a high index of suspicion when a soft-tissue mass is encountered in any anatomical site, especially if deep to the deep fascia or in the retroperitoneum (10% of soft-tissue sarcomas). Sarcoma must be distinguished from the many benign lesions which can produce similar signs, e.g. lipoma, ganglion, bursa, haematoma, cold abscess.

Plain radiographs of the mass are of limited value but occasionally provide incidental evidence to aid differential diagnosis, e.g. tuberculosis of bone. Computerized axial tomography (CT) usually provides excellent definition of the extent of the lesion, especially when this is within the abdominal cavity. It is the most sensitive detector of pulmonary metastases. It is of particular value for tumours of the pelvis and trunk. Arteriography usually (though not always) shows a pathological circulation and demonstrates both the volume of the mass and its relation to the major arteries. Neither CT nor arteriography precludes the need for a tissue diagnosis to exclude other pathology and, if sarcoma is confirmed, to define its histological type and grade of malignancy.

Biopsy

Fine-needle aspiration cytology and large-needle Trucut type biopsy yield a high percentage of accurate results for the very experienced interpreter and such methods, under CT control, are the investigations of choice when diagnosing and grading retroperitoneal sarcomas. Most pathologists prefer larger tissue samples. Individual soft-tissue sarcomas may show wide variation in their histological appearance from one area to another, and needle biopsy can lead to sampling error with regard to type and grade of tumour. Larger tumours usually contain areas of necrosis which may produce false-negative findings. Small samples may also lead to false-positive reports whereby benign lesions such as the pseudosarcomas (fibromatosis, fasciitis, etc.) or even simple reactive processes can be erroneously labelled as sarcomas.

Excision biopsy

This is indicated for small, superficially sited lumps. The entire lesion is available for pathological evaluation and should sarcoma be diagnosed this simple surgery will not prejudice subsequent definitive management.

Incision biopsy

This is the orthodox diagnostic procedure for the larger, deeply placed mass. The incision must always be placed with the possibility of subsequent definitive surgery in mind. It should lie over the midpoint of the mass and run in the direction of the local musculofascial planes which in the limbs is *vertical*. Transverse or eccentrically placed incisions, even though sometimes appropriate for access to certain benign conditions, usually prejudice the definitive operation which follows. The tumour surface is exposed with the minimum laying open of tissue planes. Sarcomas are often highly vascular and haemostasis should be meticulous. An adequate sample of solid-looking tumour is taken, avoiding the often gelatinous or grossly necrotic areas in the deeper zones as these may be of no diagnostic value. If in doubt, frozen section confirmation of a cellular sample is helpful; the delay involved is far preferable to the need for repeat biopsy. The deep fascia is closed. Drainage is avoided where possible, but if necessary the drain is placed so as to emerge at one end of the wound: or if of Redivac type the puncture is made close to and in the line of the incision to facilitate subsequent re-excision of all potentially contaminated tissue planes.

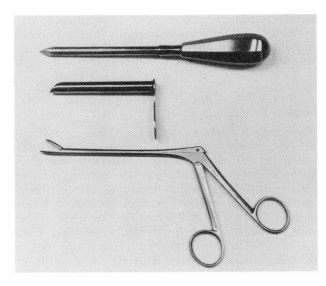

Figure 47.1 Punch biopsy set

Punch biopsy (Figure 47.1)

This is the author's usual preference as it is simple,

relatively non-traumatic, avoids embarrassing haemorrhage and the opening of tissue planes, and provides adequate material. The apparatus consists of a standard 1.0 cm trocar and cannula together with a pair of Tilley–Heinkel forceps. A stab incision just sufficient to take the cannula is made over the prominence of the mass. The trocar and cannula are inserted to the centre of the tumour and the trocar removed; bloody fluid and/or gelatinous material may be released. The forceps are then inserted through the cannula and multiple samples taken from various sites within the tumour. Frozen section control is again helpful in case of doubt. The cannula is removed, gauze pressure applied to the wound for a few moments and the skin closed with one or two sutures. A firm pressure dressing is applied.

General principles of management

The overall management of the soft-tissue sarcomas includes the eradiction of local disease at the primary site and the control of metastases. The latter aim calls for more effective systemic cytotoxic therapy than is currently available, except in the case of the embryonal rhabdomyosarcomas of infancy and childhood, and is not further discussed except to state that very occasionally selected patients whose primary disease is controlled and who have apparently solitary or few pulmonary metastases may enjoy prolonged disease-free survival following appropriate pulmonary resection. This chapter is concerned principally with the management of the primary disease, and to establish a perspective it should be borne in mind that the 5-year survival for the soft-tissue sarcomas as a group is approximately 50%, although shorter for larger, fixed tumours of high-grade malignancy than for smaller, low-grade lesions.

Eradication of the primary tumour is therefore of cardinal importance and in the case of the limbs this aim is achieved, wherever possible, without amputation. The available treatment methods of proven value are surgical excision and radiotherapy; these are often used in combination. Intra-arterial chemotherapy either by isolated, extracorporeal perfusion or by various techniques or intra-arterial infusion produces undoubted anti-tumour effects. Its place in combined management is under study but has yet to be established and is therefore not further considered here.

Surgery

The chances of local cure with surgery alone depend to a major degree on the scale of the operation undertaken. Considerations of pathology indicate that in the case of the soft-tissue sarcomas a radical operation is one which encompasses the entire musculofascial compartment in which the tumour is located.

This ideal is usually attainable only in the limbs and even then depends on whether the tumour originates within or remains confined to such a compartment. The popliteal fossa and femoral triangle, for example, have very incomplete anatomical boundaries and radical surgery is not possible. The same is true for sarcomas which arise in or involve the skin and subcutaneous tissues. The close confines and anatomical complexity of the head and neck prohibit radical operation for most sarcomas of this area and satisfactory clearance can seldom be achieved in the wide ill-defined tissue planes of the retroperitoneum. Enneking (1983) has suggested a unified classification of the types of operation for sarcoma which can be applied to any anatomical region. This is shown in modified form in Figure 47.2. Radical excision includes the entire musculofascial compartment. Wide excision implies clearance by several centimetres though less than strictly radical. Marginal excision means enucleation through the pseudocapsule with clear removal of all visible tumour. Intracapsular excision leaves gross residual tumour. Note that even amputation is not a radical cancer procedure if the plane of transection passes through the involved compartment. The validity of these concepts is confirmed by the recorded incidence of local failure following surgery as the sole method of treatment; radical limbsparing surgery, 30%; wide local excision, 40–60%; marginal excision, 95%.

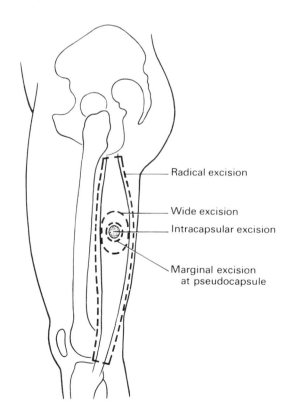

Figure 47.2 Classification of types of surgery for soft-tissue sarcoma (After Ennecking, 1983)

Radiotherapy

Although it was generally held for many years that the soft-tissue sarcomas were radio-resistant, they are in fact responsive to a variable degree to irradiation towards the upper end of the therapeutic dose range and a small percentage are totally sterilized. Radiation is therefore useful for palliation of sarcomas which are unresectable by reason of site, organ involvement (e.g. retroperitoneal sarcoma) or fixation. It is also of proven value as an adjuvant to surgery where radical dosage can, for example, reduce the local failure rate following marginal resection from 95% to in the region of 30% or less. It is therefore indicated postoperatively whenever the surgery carried out is for any reason less than radical, and for all high-grade sarcomas. The field of treatment is determined by the same pathological factors as guide the surgeon, i.e. it must cover the compartment at risk and not be restricted to the immediate vicinity of the apparent tumour. Radiotherapy is indicated as a preoperative measure for tumours which are fixed or of dubious mobility; not uncommonly the mass will shrink and become more mobile thus facilitating excision. Such shrinkage may sometimes take several months to become manifest. For this reason the decision to amputate for limb sarcoma should not be taken with undue haste and in any event never without repeat biopsy confirmation of tumour. There is no evidence that such delayed amputation, or amputation following failure of a planned combined surgical/radiation approach, carries a lower chance of survival than does immediate amputation. The prognosis for life is principally determined by the tumour stage at first presentation.

Surgery following radical dose irradiation calls for the usual added caution attached to the tendency to impaired tissue healing. Skin tension and dead space are particularly dangerous, especially in relation to the major arteries.

Surgery of specific regions

The anatomical ubiquity of the soft-tissue sarcomas precludes complete coverage of their operative surgery within a single chapter. Many operations do not conform to classic textbook descriptions because the tumour makes its own rules. The surgeon must always be prepared to extemporize and design each operation to suit the individual sarcoma. Facilities must be available for replacement of involved skin, chest or abdominal wall, major artery or, where necessary, long bone. Skin cover may require Thiersch grafts, pedicled cutaneous, muscle or myocutaneous flaps or even free flap transfer with microvascular anastomosis. The value of the greater omentum for cover at certain sites should be borne in mind. Sarcomas of the head and neck, which are uncommon, will usually require the services of a specialist surgical team. The embryonal rhabdomyosarcomas of infancy and childhood occur mainly in the head and neck area and in the pelvis; they call not only for specialized surgical skills but should also be managed within the context of a multidisciplinary paediatric oncology unit. Retroperitoneal sarcomas fall within the province of the general surgeon. Their removal, which can seldom be complete, may involve resection of solid and hollow viscera; infiltration of the small bowel mesentery or involvement of the great veins may restrict surgery to a debulking procedure. Sarcomas of the limb girdles may be removable only by forequarter or hindquarter amputation. When, however, the main neurovascular bundle is free, it is possible to perform satisfactory, individually tailored resections of, for example, scapula, the scapula with clavicle and head of humerus (Tikhoff–Linberg operation) or partial resection of the pelvis, with retention of a useful limb.

Two standard operations are illustrated in full which, together with the modifications described, provide a basis in principle for the surgery of most soft-tissue sarcomas of the limbs and trunk.

from the gluteal fold to just above the popliteal crease and includes the previous biopsy scar by a 5 cm margin on either side to clear the potentially contaminated subcutaneous fat. The incision will need to be modified if the biopsy has been incorrectly sited.

Full-thickness skin flaps are raised widely as far as the mid-adductor plane medially and the corresponding plane laterally. The deep fascia is incised along the length of these two planes. With the ensuing release of tension with the compartment, the tumour mass immediately 'loosens' and the extent of the proposed resection becomes more clearly defined.

The fascia along the lower edge of gluteus maximus is divided and upwards retraction of this muscle exposes the origins of the hamstrings from the ischial tuberosity. The hamstrings are put on the stretch by the encircling index finger and detached flush with the bone; the angled diathermy point is a convenient instrument for this step. For a proximally situated tumour whose upper pole is close to bone, more effectively clearance is achieved by dividing the tuberosity horizontally using the osteotome or power saw so that the complete muscle origin, together with its attached plate of bone, is included in the specimen.

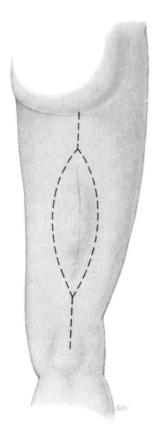

Figure 47.3 Skin incision which includes biopsy scar

Posterior thigh compartmental resection
(Figures 47.3–47.7)

The skin incision extends in the posterior midline

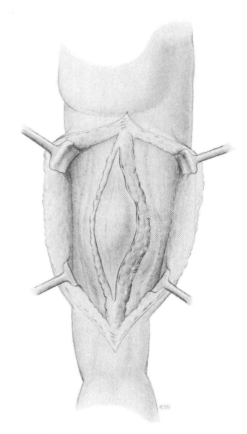

Figure 47.4 Elevation of skin flaps

The detached muscle origins are grasped with tissue forceps and lifted up so that the relatively avascular medial and lateral planes of separation of the com-

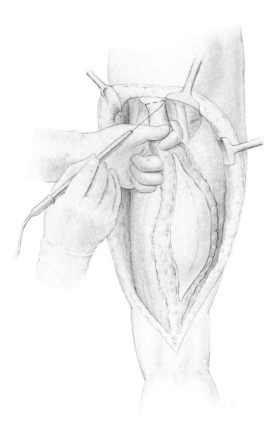

Figure 47.5 Division of origin of hamstrings

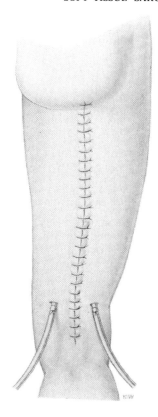

Figure 47.7 Sutured incision and suction drains

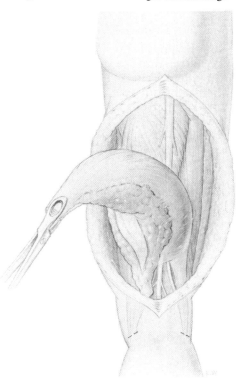

Figure 47.6 Posterior thigh compartment with contained tumour partially dissected to expose sciatic nerve. Sites for division of hamstring insertions indicated by dotted lines

partment become readily apparent and are cut by running the curved scissors along their length. If the tumour has invaded into the lateral or medial compartments, the resection must extend to include appropriate portions of the vastus or adductor muscle groups; in the latter case the superficial femoral artery may be exposed on its posterior aspect.

The proximal end of the sciatic nerve has been uncovered and its relation to the deep aspect of the tumour can now be ascertained. In the case illustrated in Figures 47.3–47.7, the tumour is totally enclosed within a musculofascial envelope and the nerve lies clear. Sometimes the nerve is found closely applied to the tumour pseudocapsule though not grossly invaded. It is entirely justified to dissect the nerve off the tumour, if necessary deep to the perineurium, because, provided that adjuvant radiotherapy is given, recurrence along the nerve occurs only exceptionally. In the unusual event of frank invasion, or for the rare primary neurogenic sarcoma of the main trunk, the entire sciatic nerve can be sacrificed and, provided that there is a good peripheral circulation, the patient retains a useful limb with a foot free from trophic ulceration.

Division of the short head of the biceps close to the linea aspera exposes the perforating branches of the profunda femoris artery and vein, several of which may require division and ligation. The specimen is now attached only by the insertions of the hamstring muscles which are finally divided at the level of the knee joint.

The skin is closed with interrupted sutures placed sufficiently close to secure an airtight wound for effective suction drainage via two large-bore tubes which are laid along the length of the cavity. A firm pressure dressing is applied. Gentle active movements are encouraged from the outset and walking started as soon as the drainage tubes are removed, usually on the 4th or 5th day.

Anterior and medial thigh compartmental resections

These follow the same lines, but the femoral vessels require special consideration. As with the sciatic nerve, frank invasion of the wall of the superficial femoral artery is uncommon and it can usually be dissected off the tumour mass in the subadventitial plane (Figure 47.8). A tape is placed under the artery proximal to the tumour and used to apply gentle traction while the vessel is mobilized by serial division of its branches until it lies entirely free along its length. The tumour mass is mainly supplied by the profunda artery and this usually requires division close to its origin from the common femoral artery. Its perforating branches are again encountered close to the linea aspera. The superficial femoral vein can often be dealt with in similar fashion, but if this thin-walled structure is adherent to tumour it should be sacrificed and little ultimate disability results. If the femoral artery cannot be readily separated from the tumour the adherent segment is resected *en bloc* and continuity restored, preferably using autogenous long saphenous vein. Residual muscle, if available, is used to cover the exposed femoral artery or graft. If not, and where there is any doubt about the integrity of skin cover, especially after radical radiotherapy, serious consideration must be given to skin or myocutaneous flap replacement for the proximal segment of the limb, or a greater omental flap which will readily reach the knee.

The approach to resections in other limb segments follows the same general guidelines. Loss of the gastrocnemius/soleus complex or of the anterior or posterior compartments of the upper limb leaves remarkably little functional disability. The planning of rational surgical excision in the forearm is less straightforward because of the complexity of the muscular anatomy and the proximity of important major nerves. Any resulting disability may be considerably helped by simple splints or by operative measures, e.g. arthrodesis of the wrist or tendon transfers. The surgeon must at all times consider the crucial question: will the residual limb be of greater value to the patient than a prosthesis? The same question applies to the rare soft-tissue sarcoma of the hand where, for example, excision of the ulnar three fingers and corresponding palm will leave a more useful functional unit than any artificial limb.

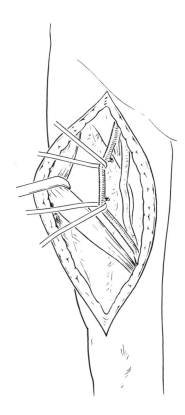

Figure 47.8 Femoral artery elevated off underlying mass in quadriceps group. Femoral vein still undissected. Sartorius retracted

Amputations for sarcoma

Amputation is indicated when, in the absence of metastases, the tumour is locally irremovable or when its removal would leave a limb of less value to the patient than a prosthesis. Palliative amputation is occasionally required for massive, fungating disease even in the presence of distant metastases.

As mentioned above, amputation must be planned with respect to the potential longitudinal spread of the tumour. This will usually mean section through the site of election proximal to the next joint, e.g. above knee for tumours of the leg. For sarcomas of the proximal arm or thigh forequarter or hindquarter, amputation will usually be necessary. Failure to observe these principles carries the risk of stump recurrence.

Full-thickness resection of chest wall
(Figures 47.9–47.13)

The case illustrated depicts the operative management of a sarcoma involving the chest wall and overlying skin. The proposed line of incision is outlined with Bonney's blue dye and clears gross tumour by a margin of 5 cm all round. The incision is deepened through the cephalad intercostal space to enter the pleural cavity and allow palpation of the deep aspect of the lesion to confirm operability. The

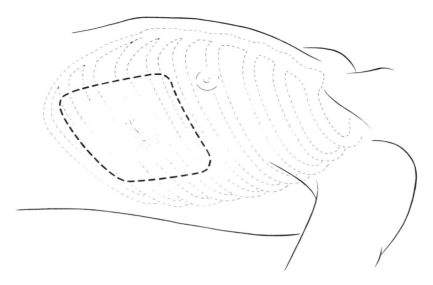

Figure 47.9 Outline of proposed skin incision

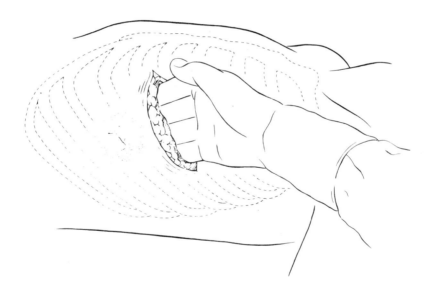

Figure 47.10 Preliminary thoracotomy to assess deep aspect of lesion

anterior and posterior incisions are then deepened with successive section of the appropriate ribs and the specimen finally freed by division of the muscles and pleura of the caudad intercostal space.

The defect is bridged by a sheet of Marlex (polypropylene) mesh cut to shape and sutured under moderate tension to the surrounding muscles using interrupted non-absorbable sutures, e.g. monofilament nylon. Added strength is provided by passing a few sutures around the cephalad and caudad ribs and through drill holes close to the cut rib ends anteriorly and posteriorly. An underwater chest drain is inserted via a separate stab incision prior to the completion of this stage.

Finally, the skin defect is restored by a cutaneous transposition flap and the resulting donor area surfaced with split skin which may be applied either at the time or 48 h later in the ward. It is not necessary to insert drains deep to the flap as this space is drained via the pleural cavity through the interstices of the Marlex. A light dressing is applied which avoids pressure on the skin flap and allows ready inspection of its viability.

Resection of abdominal wall

This proceeds as for the chest wall. Peritoneum can be sacrificed with impunity as, like the pleura, it is

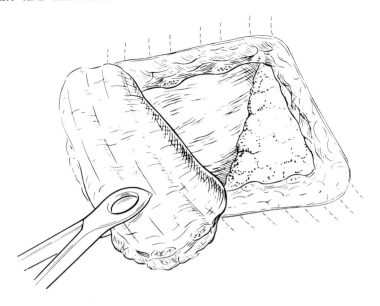

Figure 47.11 Tumour-bearing segment elevated

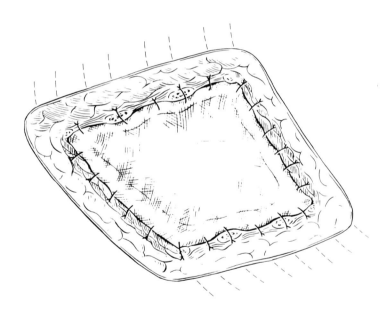

Figure 47.12 Marlex mesh sutured in place

rapidly reformed on the deep surface of the mesh. The skin may be closed by direct suture provided that there is no tension, but in case of doubt an appropriate cutaneous (or myocutaneous) flap should be used. Dead space between the skin and Marlex is obliterated by use of suction drains introduced via separate stab incisions.

Excision of retroperitoneal sarcomas

Retroperitoneal sarcomas are often large and clinically advanced at first presentation, despite a short duration of symptoms. They frequently involve multiple organs and it is this fact and not tumour size which determines the ability to achieve complete excision. In a large study of 120 retroperitoneal sarcomas (Alvarenga *et al.*, 1991), a transperitoneal approach was preferred since it provided better access to the blood vessels related to the tumour. In view of possible bowel involvement, thorough preoperative bowel preparation is advised. Survival was better after complete excision of the primary tumour, but there was still a high probability of local relapse (80%) by 5 years.

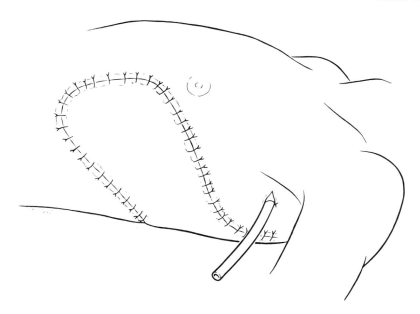

Figure 47.13 Cover by posteriorly based skin flap. Underwater chest drain inserted

If complete excision is not possible, the survival chances are so low that radical surgery is not worth while. Such surgery should be avoided in patients with high-grade tumours and/or concurrent metastases unless it is essential for palliation. Such information can often be obtained by CT scan and CT-guided needle biopsy. It should be possible to avoid surgical exploration merely to obtain accurate prognostic factors and organ involvement.

References

Alvarenga, J. C., Ball, A. B. S., Fisher, C. *et al.* (1991) Limitations of surgery in the treatment of retroperitoneal sarcoma. *Br. J. Surg.*, **78**, 912–916

Enneking, W. F. (1983) *Musculoskeletal Tumor Surgery*, Churchill Livingstone, New York

Further reading

Das Gupta, T. K. (1983) *Tumors of the Soft Tissues*, Appleton-Century-Crofts, Norwalk, Conn.

Enzinger, F. and Weiss, S. W. (1983) *Soft Tissue Tumors*, C. V. Mosby, St. Louis

Thoracic surgery

48

Tracheostomy

G. Keen

History

'The evolution of tracheostomy can be divided into five stages. The first and longest period (covering roughly 3000 years from 1500 BC to AD 1500) begins with references made to incisions into the "windpipe" in the Abers Papyrus and the Rig Veda. However, Alexander the Great, Asclepiades, Aretaeus and Galen are all recorded as having used this operation. Between 1546 with the writings of Brassarolo until 1883, the procedure was considered futile and irresponsible and few surgeons had the courage to perform it. The third period starts with Trousseau's report of 200 cases in the therapy of diphtheria in 1833. Tracheostomy became a highly dramatized operation for asphyxia and acute respiratory obstruction. In 1932 Wilson suggested its prophylactic and therapeutic use in poliomyelitis. Tracheostomy was then recommended for a large variety of assorted maladies. This started a tremendous period of enthusiasm' (Frost, 1976) (Figure 48.1).

There are now fewer indications for tracheostomy as the efficient use of endotracheal tubes, which may be left *in situ* for prolonged periods, will usually be adequate to tide most patients over their acute respiratory or airway problem. Nevertheless, should the need for tracheal intubation persist, tracheostomy may become necessary.

Opinions vary concerning the safe maximum period of orotracheal intubation. Certainly in the days of rubber tubes, tracheal damage and stricture formation were frequently recorded. Modern tubes of clear soft plastic seem less traumatic and it is safe to leave such tubes in place for up to 2 weeks before tracheostomy need be considered. In infants and children, however, modern nasotracheal tubes which are made of non-irritant plastic may safely be left in place for periods of 4–6 weeks, frequently avoiding the necessity for tracheostomy. When necessary, tracheostomy should be undertaken optimistically and confidently at a time when benefits are possible and should not be reserved for patients in a terminal state. The more frequent use of tracheostomy and widespread understanding of tracheostomy care has made this operation the safe and useful procedure it now is. Tracheostomy and tracheostomy suction, are well tolerated by the patient who needs less sedation than the patient with an orotracheal tube.

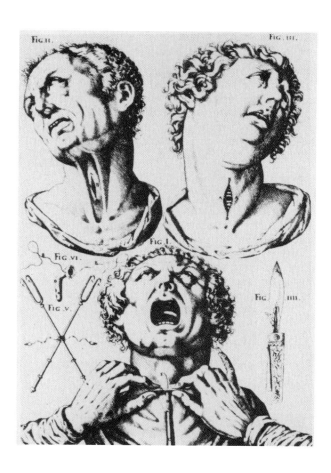

Figure 48.1 Early illustration of tracheostomy from the Tabulae Anatomicae of Julius Casserius (1627)

Indications

Tracheostomy is indicated in the following conditions. It will be resorted to only after an appropriate period of treatment using an endotracheal tube.

1. In infants and children

When treating severe respiratory or cardiac disease, prolonged ventilation, sometimes for periods of several months, may be necessary and a well-planned tracheostomy using well-designed tubes should be readily tolerated.

2. Chest trauma

The combination of an unstable chest wall and lung damage, perhaps associated with a head injury, frequently requires very long-term airway maintenance with possibly the addition of assisted ventilation. Following a reasonable period of treatment using an orotracheal tube, tracheostomy should be undertaken when it seems clear that long-term treatment is appropriate.

3. Pulmonary insufficiency

In elderly patients with poor pulmonary function complicated by infection, tracheostomy will considerably decrease the anatomical dead space and allow secretions to be removed with less difficulty. This operation should not be undertaken lightly in such patients, but from time to time has given some of these a useful and comfortable life when other forms of treatment seem ineffective.

4. Neurological problems

Patients in coma due to head injury or cerebrovascular accidents frequently require long-term maintenance of a good airway and the removal of secretions. In other patients with conditions such as bulbar palsy, poliomyelitis or the Guillain–Barré syndrome, ventilatory support may also be necessary. Tracheostomy is frequently the most comfortable and effective method of dealing with these patients.

5. Laryngeal and hypopharygeal disease

Permanent end tracheostomy for malignant disease of the larynx and hypopharynx.

The operation

This should be performed by an experienced surgeon in an operating theatre in good light with adequate surgical assistance and instruments. Although this may be self-evident, one may still encounter the lone doctor attempting tracheostomy in the ward by hand-held lights and with few instruments. That a successful tracheostomy is ever completed under these circumstances is cause for congratulation, but in no way condones such heroic attempts. The availability of adequate endotracheal tubes has almost completely eliminated the need for emergency tracheostomy and the operation should be delayed until good facilities and competent personnel are available. Should the patient be encumbered by splints, intravenous infusions, chest drainage tubes and various electrical leads, it is quite in order to undertake the operation in the bed rather than move the patient on to the operating table, and this is facilitated in those beds from which the head can be removed.

A small sandbag is placed between the shoulders, enabling the neck to be extended. The skin incision is transverse, 2.5 cm above the suprasternal notch and 5 cm in length. The platysma and pretracheal fascia are opened and the strap muscles held aside by the assistant. It may be necessary to retract or divide the thyroid isthmus. The removal of large discs of trachea or the suturing of tracheal flaps to the skin is unnecessary and furthermore may be followed by stricture formation at the site of this stoma. An adequate opening into the trachea is readily achieved by a simple longitudinal midline incision through the second, third and perhaps fourth tracheal rings, and when this is held apart an appropriate size tracheostomy tube may be readily introduced (Figures 48.2 and 48.3). One or two skin sutures on either side of the tube are adequate. The tracheostomy tube tapes should be firmly tied by the surgeon using tight knots with instructions that the tapes be left well alone for 48 h. Tying these tapes with pretty bows invites well-intentioned staff to interfere with these at the earliest opportunity, with possible dislodgement of the tube. After 48 h the tube may safely be changed.

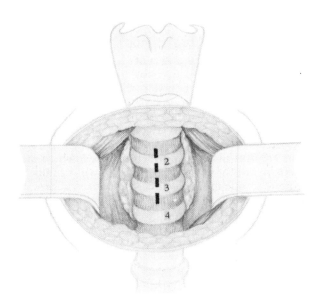

Figure 48.2 Incision through the second and third rings in tracheostomy

Care of tracheostomy

Tracheostomy, while of great benefit to the patient, creates its own acute problems:

1. Increased liability to local and pulmonary infection.
2. Decreased ability of patient to clear secretions.
3. Inadequate humidification of inspired air.

All procedures involving handling of the tracheostomy should be undertaken using sterile precautions.

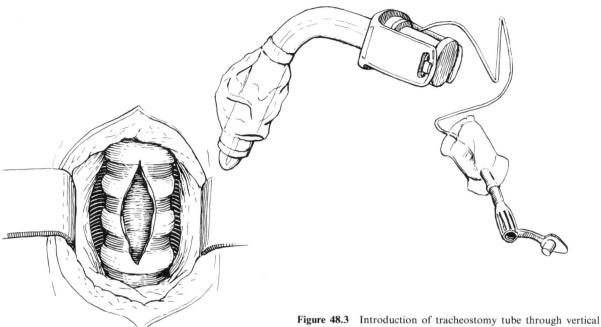

Figure 48.3 Introduction of tracheostomy tube through vertical slit in trachea. Retractors of the tracheal incision are not shown

The tracheostomy wound should be swabbed with non-irritant antiseptic solutions. Ideally nursing staff should avoid contact with other patients, for cross-infection may become a serious problem in special care units and when, from time to time, several patients become infected with organisms such as *Pseudomonas, Escherichia coli* or *Staphylococcus*, serious generalized infections may threaten the work of the department. Local infections may not only proceed to tracheal stricture formation but in the short term may cause severe and even fatal pulmonary infection. These patients are often debilitated and septicaemia readily occurs.

As with endotracheal tubes, tracheostomy bypasses the vocal cords interfering with the patient's ability to build up that head of pressure within the lungs which is necessary to expel secretions. Weak coughing is possible, which moves peripheral secretions into the central bronchi, but for their further clearance suction is necessary. Furthermore, following the introduction of an endotracheal tube or of a tracheostomy tube it is recognized that within 48 h the ciliary action of the tracheal mucosa is grossly upset.

Humidification

Humidification is essential, for the nasopharynx which normally provides warming humidification is bypassed. The drying of inspired gases is not only damaging to the tracheal mucosa but encourages thickening of secretions. To ensure adequate humidification it is important that the patient be well hydrated with both oral and intravenous fluids, for general tissue dehydration will eventually affect all mucosal surfaces. It may from time to time be useful to inject small quantities of sterile saline down the tracheostomy tube prior to routine suctioning. This certainly aids both coughing and loosening of secretions. It is important, especially in infants, that this is not overdone or considerable amounts of fluid may be absorbed.

Humidifiers, heated or unheated, saturate the inspired air with water vapour, and recently ultrasonic nebulizers, which add an extremely fine water spray into the inspired gases, have been used with great benefit.

The humidifier and connecting tubes should be frequently sterilized.

Care of the tracheostomy cuff

The tracheostomy cuff (Figure 48.4) prevents aspiration of nasopharyngeal secretions and forms an airtight fit, enabling the ventilator to build up an appropriate intrabronchial pressure. A well-designed cuff will position the distal end of the tube centrally within the trachea and it is hoped that the inflated cuff exerts minimal pressure on the tracheal mucosa and the tracheal microcirculation. The most suitable form of cuff seems to combine the characteristics of high compliance, softness and large volume, and although numerous types of cuff are in use it is likely that the large-volume floppy cuff will gain wide acceptance. Cuffs containing plastic foam have been designed and exert low pressure on the tracheal wall. Cuffs may cause complications which include difficulty of insertion of the tube or of occlusion of the end of the tube if badly fitting.

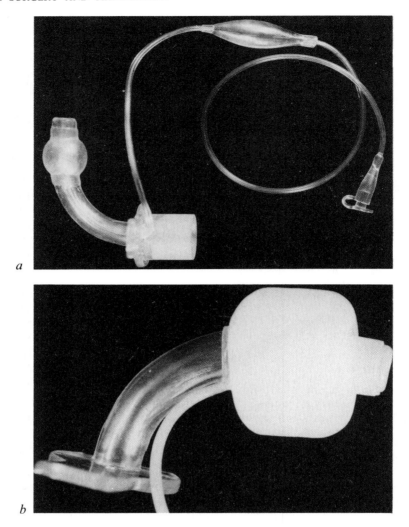

a

b

Figure 48.4 *a*, Conventional tracheostomy tube with cuff inflated with 3 ml of air. *b*, Tracheostomy tube carrying latex rubber floppy cuff inflated with 8 ml of air. Pressures measured in the cuffs under these conditions indicate that the floppy cuff pressure is about 10% of that within the standard cuff (Grillo *et al.*, 1971, from Keen, 1984)

The ideal tracheostomy tube should be smooth and of inert material, polyvinyl chloride tubing being superior to either metal or rubber. The tube should be non-kinking, the internal diameter remaining constant at body temperature. It should have the largest possible diameter together with the smallest wall thickness commensurate with strength, flexibility and non-kinking. Although there is a need for a sensitive indicator of cuff pressures this is by no means readily available. With the cuff just inflated to create an airtight seal very little extra air introduced into the cuff is needed to increase pressure on the tracheal wall to a degree which will cause local necrosis, and perhaps late stricture.

Although it might seem obvious that intermittent deflation of the cuff minimizes the risk of ischaemic damage to the tracheal mucosa, such a programme has its disadvantages. In those patients who require

ventilation, deflation of the cuff may deprive the tube of its airtight fit and prevent adequate ventilation, and allow aspiration of nasopharyngeal secretions. On the other hand, an over-inflated cuff will cause ulceration in a very short time, for the tracheal mucosa is soon damaged by pressure necrosis and it is unlikely that any of the currently advised regimens of intermittent inflation and deflation of the cuff will prevent this. It is suggested by some that where possible the cuff should be deflated for 5 min in every hour, but it is likely that the adoption of low-pressure floppy cuffs will prove of greater benefit than such arbitrary periods of cuff deflation.

Removal of tracheostomy tube

In due course the tracheostomy tube may be dispensed with. As a primary measure the cuffed tube may be exchanged for a smaller-size uncuffed tube, enabling the patient to breathe through the tube and breathe normally. A speaking tube may be used for a time, enabling the patient to cough and speak normally for a trial period, following which the tube may be removed and the wound covered. At this stage it is well worth closing the tracheostomy wound with a few stitches. This will produce a more cosmetic scar.

Complications

These may occur early in the postoperative period; late, following discharge from hospital; or at any other time.

Early complications

1. Displacement of tube

Displacement of a tube shortly after the operation of tracheostomy is an unforgivable disaster and is related entirely to inadequate fixation of the tracheostomy tube associated with careless nursing of the patient. Should this occur, it is far safer to reintubate the patient using an endotracheal tube passed through the mouth rather than to fumble in the neck of an anoxic, engorged patient. Following the introduction of such a tube, the patient may then be returned to the operating theatre for reintroduction of the tracheostomy tube and its more satisfactory fixation. Some surgeons consider that at the primary operation the tracheal edges should be sutured to the skin wound in order to facilitate reintroduction of a displaced tube, and Björk developed his flap operation to cover this eventuality. The former manoeuvre generally fails in its purpose for the sutures tend to cut out of the tracheal wall which is pulled forward under tension, and the Björk flap is considered unnecessary.

2. Herniation of cuff

In some cases an overinflated cuff may prolapse distally and occlude the end of the tracheostomy tube. This now rarely occurs with the better design of tubes, but is diagnosed when attempts at ventilation fail due to an apparent obstruction. The cuff should be deflated which will provide an instant diagnosis, following which the tube should be changed.

3. Infection

Infection of the tracheostomy site is a rare occurrence in clean experienced units, but it occurs more readily when good surgical and sterile techniques are wanting. The dangers of local necrosis, stricture formation, severe haemorrhage and fistula formation are increased in the presence of infection.

Intermediate complications

1. Haemorrhage

Haemorrhage may occur from the tracheostomy wound shortly following operation, and when control is ineffective by local packing alone it is wise to return the patient to the operating theatre for exploration, when the bleeding point may be ligated or sutured.

A most serious complication is erosion of the trachea and innominate artery, causing tracheo-innominate fistula, usually fatal. Fortunately many of these patients have several small premonitory arterial haemorrhages. These may warn the surgeon of an impending disastrous and terminal event which may, on occasions, be avoided by immediate surgery.

TRACHEO-INNOMINATE ARTERY FISTULA

Tracheo-innominate artery fistula occurs most commonly from the low placement of a tracheostomy so that the tube lies against the innominate artery at the inferior lateral margin of the stoma and erodes it directly. Less commonly, a high-pressure cuff or the tip of a tracheostomy tube may erode through the anterior wall of the trachea, into the overlying innominate artery. In the latter case the stoma is high and uninvolved in the fistula. The first type of lesion may be controlled acutely by direct pressure at the inferior margin of the stoma against the leaking innominate artery, with concomitant placement of an endotracheal tube through the stoma to seal and maintain the airway. The emergency management of the second type of lesion can only be done by the rapid insertion of an endotracheal tube through the stoma with the inflation of a high-pressure cuff against the leak to tamponade the bleeding. The point of fistulization is not available in this case to a tamponading finger.

Both these lesions must be treated surgically immediately. Anaesthesia is induced through the endotracheal tube which has already been placed. Complete division of the sternum provides maximum access to the artery and arch of the aorta if necessary. A collar incision above provides cervical access. Dissection is done proximally around the origin of the innominate artery, taking care not to injure the artery at this point, and distally beyond the point of leakage, which is just below the bifurcation of the subclavian and common carotid arteries. One may resect the perforated artery, closing both proximal and distal arterial ends with two layers of running arterial sutures.

The stumps of the artery are then carefully buried centrally under thymic tissue and laterally under strap muscles. In the case of a stomal erosion, the trachea does not require further treatment except to seal off the tracheostomy from the general incision during the course of the closure. In erosion by a cuff the injured segment of trachea is resected and an end-

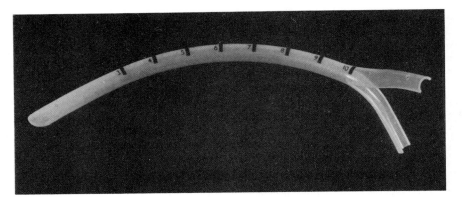

Figure 48.5 Matthews' mini-tracheostomy tube

to-end tracheal anastomosis is performed. Primary arterial grafting is avoided because of the contaminated field.

2. Tracheo-oesophageal fistula

When a tracheo-oesophageal fistula results from the erosion of an endotracheal tube cuff through the membranous wall, often by compressive action against an inlying nasogastric tube, the problem may be life endangering. Repair of such a fistula is unlikely to succeed if the patient remains on a respirator, since a cuff will be very likely to be adjacent to the suture line. These patients are therefore tided over by placement of a tube with a large-volume, low-pressure cuff seal, the removal of the nasogastric tube, cessation of oral feedings, placement of a gastrostomy tube for gastric drainage to prevent reflux, and jejunostomy tube for long-term feeding. If the patient still suffers excessive contamination of the lungs from salivary excretion, the proximal oesophagus is exteriorized in the neck as an end salivary fistula and the distal end is temporarily closed. This is rarely necessary.

CLOSURE OF TRACHEO-OESOPHAGEAL FISTULA

The approach to the fistula is very much the same as that of the anterior approach to the trachea for resection. Usually a collar incision alone is sufficient, although occasionally an upper sternal vertical incision is also needed. The level of the stoma is usually 1–3 cm above that of the fistula itself, since the fistula was due to a cuff. The dissection is carried out as previously described with intubation across the operative field. The diseased segment of trachea is elevated, excising not only it but the fistula in continuity. The oesophagus is closed vertically with two layers of interrupted sutures. A pedicled strap muscle flap is often placed over this because of the contiguity, otherwise, of this suture line with the transverse suture line of the trachea. End-to-end repair of the trachea is next accomplished as described previously.

Late complications

1. Stricture formation

Most reported series of tracheal strictures indicate that the majority are associated with the use of tracheostomy in the treatment of chest injuries. This may reflect the widespread and perhaps sometimes indiscriminate use of this operation by the less expert in ill-equipped centres, although this complication may follow tracheostomy undertaken with great skill and in a good environment. Apart from clinically manifest tracheal strictures, tracheoscopic and tomographic examination undertaken some months following tracheostomy will in many cases show some degree of tracheal narrowing. Tracheal strictures may complicate tracheostomy or the prolonged use of endotracheal tubes. The stricture may present clinically either shortly after removal of the tracheostomy tube or after a delay of some months. The stricture may be at the site of the inflatable cuff, at the site of the stoma or more distally, when it is due to damage by aspiration catheters. Stomal strictures may be associated with the removal of excessive amounts of tracheal wall at operation or the use of tracheal flaps. The most common aetiological features, however, are pressure necrosis and infection. The adoption of low-pressure cuffs and the insistence on aseptic nursing techniques, together with less destructive surgery, should go some way towards reducing the incidence of this complication.

2. Failure of spontaneous closure of tracheostomy stoma

This complication is considered in Chapter 49.

Mini-tracheostomy

Matthews (Matthews and Hopkinson, 1984) has introduced an ingenious method of undertaking

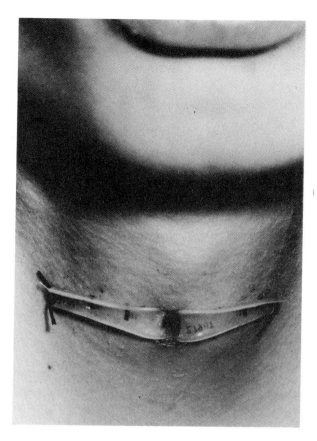

Figure 48.6 Matthews' mini-tracheostomy tube in place. The tight-fitting tube does not allow escape of air around it

tracheostomy via the cricothyroid membrane using a fine tube. This apparatus is marketed as a set by Portex Ltd of Hythe, Kent, England and consists of a 4 mm diameter tracheal cannula mounted on an introducer accompanied by a guarded scalpel which can penetrate to a maximum of 0.5 cm (Figure 48.5).

This tracheostomy cannula is readily introduced in the ward in the patient's bed under local anaesthesia and provides a route for adequate suction in those patients who are unable to cough but who nevertheless are able to breathe spontaneously. Entry into the trachea is so small that the tight-fitting tube does not allow escape of air around it and consequently the patient is able to cough forcibly and speak normally while this tube is in place (Figure 48.6).

Clearly this tube offers a very successful alternative to the prolonged use of an endotracheal tube or a tracheostomy in patients whose ventilatory ability is adequate but who suffer from the serious effects of sputum retention.

References

Frost, E. A. M. (1976) Tracing the tracheostomy. *Ann. Otol.*, **85**, 618–624

Keen, G. (1984) *Chest Injuries*, 2nd edn, John Wright, Bristol

Matthews, H. R. and Hopkinson, R. B. (1984) Treatment of sputum retention by mini tracheostomy. *Br. J. Surg.*, **71**, 147–150

49

Tracheal surgery

H. C. Grillo and D. J. Mathisen

Surgical anatomy

The trachea in the average adult measures only 11 cm from the inferior border of the cricoid cartilage to the carinal spur (Grillo, 1989). The carina serves as a definite point of reference although the trachea ends a short distance above this point, and variations in length (approximately 10–13 cm) depend roughly on the individual's height. There are between 18 and 22 cartilaginous rings in the human trachea, approximating two rings in each centimetre. The average internal diameter in the adult is 2.3 cm from side to side and 1.8 cm anteroposteriorly. This results in a roughly elliptical shape. In the infant, however, the anteroposterior diameter is greater. In older patients, with chronic obstructive lung disease, an increase in anteroposterior diameter over the lateral diameter is also seen, particularly in the lower two-thirds ('saber sheath' trachea).

Calcification may occur as the larynx and trachea age and in areas of injury. The degree of flexibility present in youth is increasingly lost with age. The trachea may move up and down quite easily in youth, sliding in the connective tissue which surrounds it, and the segmental blood supply also rises and falls with it. The trachea is tethered inferiorly by the arch of the aorta which passes over the left main bronchus. In a thin young person, over 50% of the trachea may rise into the neck with cervical extension, while in an aged, kyphotic, obese person, where the trachea is much more horizontal, the larynx may be fixed in the retrosternal notch.

The blood supply of the trachea comes principally in its upper portion from segmental branches from the inferior thyroid artery and inferiorly from the bronchial arteries (Salassa et al., 1977). Collateral circulation between these nearly end vessels is relatively poor. The vessels enter the trachea laterally, usually after dividing to provide both oesophageal and tracheal branches. Circumferential dissection of any significant length of trachea may easily disrupt this blood supply and lead to necrosis, with either perforation or restenosis of a devascularized trachea.

From a surgical standpoint it must be emphasized that the trachea is short, is an unpaired organ, is relatively non-extensible, is adjacent to the innominate artery and aorta, recurrent laryngeal nerves and oesophagus, and has an essentially segmental blood supply. These facts demand thoughtfulness and caution in surgical approaches.

Indications for operation

1. Benign strictures.
2. Benign and malignant tumours.

Tracheal resection is performed principally for the relief of obstructive lesions with concomitant reconstruction for restoration of an essentially normal airway (Grillo, 1979b; Grillo and Mathisen, 1990).

1. Benign strictures

The most common indication for such surgery has been for correction of the tracheal stenosis resulting from intubation for mechanical ventilatory support in respiratory failure (Grillo, 1979b, 1981). The most common lesions are circumferential stenoses related to injury by high-pressure sealing cuffs on both endotracheal and tracheostomy tubes or large-volume 'low-pressure' cuffs used within a high enough range of inflation to convert them to high-pressure cuffs. Next most common are stenotic lesions at the site of a tracheal stoma which has been eroded by leverage by equipment attached to the tracheostomy tube. Occasionally both lesions present in the same patient, either separated or confluent.

2. Benign and malignant tumours

Primary tumours of the trachea, both benign and malignant, are relatively rare but provide the second most common indication for reconstruction (Eschapasse, 1974; Pearson et al. 1984; Perelman and Koroleva, 1987; Grillo and Mathisen, 1990). The primary tumours most often seen are squamous cell carcinoma and adenoid-cystic carcinoma (cylindroma). After this, lesions vary widely with no predominance of a single type. Resection is less often justified for secondary tumours, but is indicated for slowly growing papillary and follicular carcinoma of the thyroid gland (Grillo et al., 1992a) and for selected cases of carinal involvement by bronchogenic carcinoma (Mathisen and Grillo, 1991). Less common indications for tracheal reconstruction include: congenital stenosis, post-traumatic stenosis, post-infectious stenosis (tuberculosis, histoplasmosis, diphtheria), idiopathic stenosis, compressive malacia and postoperative stenosis (Grillo, 1990).

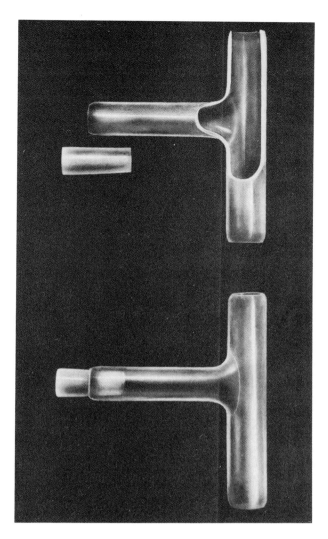

Figure 49.1. Montgomery tracheal T-tube. This silicone T-tube (E. Benson Hood Laboratories, 575 Washington St., Pembroke, Ma 02359) serves as a tracheal stent and tracheostomy tube. It is available in multiple diameters and lengths. With the side-arm plugged the patient has an inlying tubular stent (From Montgomery, 1973, by permission)

Limitations of reconstruction

Most patients with benign stenosis of the trachea can be managed by dilatation of the stenosis and the placement of an appropriate splinting tracheostomy tube or T-tube. Therefore undue risks should not be taken in the surgical resection and reconstruction. It is rare for inflammatory lesions, however, to be of such length that they cannot be resected and reconstructed at the *initial* operation. This is all the more reason why the initial operation must be well designed, well executed and not done by an occasional operator. If the trachea has been subtotally destroyed by previous surgery and reconstruction is hence not possible, the best available manoeuvre is to place a Montgomery Silastic T-tube (Montgomery,

1964) across the whole length of the damaged trachea internally (Figure 49.1). This will provide a safe, dependable airway which only needs occasional replacement. It does not create the hazards which are attendant on resecting the trachea and attempting to place a prosthesis across the gap so created. The functional effect of a replacement prosthesis is the same as that with a T-tube, but the hazards of erosion of the innominate artery or of granulation tissue obstruction at either end are considerable.

Diagnostic investigations

Once a lesion is suspected, appropriate roentgenograms of the trachea without contrast medium will suffice to delineate these lesions precisely in their disposition, length and degree of airway compromise (MacMillan *et al.*, 1971; Weber and Grillo, 1978). Equally important are definition of the functional state and involvement of the larynx and the amount of trachea which remains uninvolved by the process. The glottis must be adequate prior to any tracheal reconstruction. CT scanning has proved to be useful only in delineation of the extent of lateral spread of tumours.

Bronchoscopy is frequently reserved for the time of surgical correction, particularly if the degree of obstruction is great. The manipulations performed at bronchoscopy may well precipitate an obstructive episode in such cases. Biopsies of tumours may be done and frozen section diagnosis obtained just prior to resection. Surgery of tracheal tumours requires frozen section control of the margins of resection.

Emergency relief of obstructed airways may be obtained by dilatation of benign stenosis or coring-out of tumours via the rigid bronchoscope under general anaesthesia (Mathisen and Grillo, 1989). Bleeding is usually manageable. Laser treatment offers no advantages.

Operative technique

Anaesthesia for tracheal resection and reconstruction must be induced with care, preferably with a gentle inhalation induction to avoid obstruction (Wilson, 1987). Bronchoscopy is next performed with a rigid instrument which permits manipulation and adequate biopsy. Endotracheal tubes may usually be passed beside a tumour unless it is a rare circumferential one. Very tight stenoses may be dilated under direct vision using ventilating bronchoscopes serially in size, but with lesser degrees of obstruction an endotracheal tube is positioned above the lesion. The patients breathe spontaneously throughout the operation and ventilation is maintained at all times with judiciously placed endotracheal tubes across the operative field, as indicated later. High-frequency ventilation may be used and is especially applicable in intrathoracic cari-

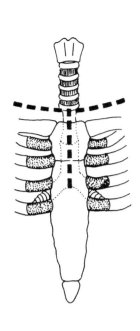

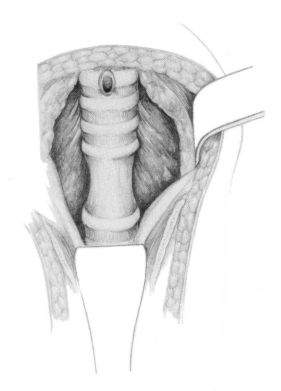

Figure 49.2 Cervical or cervicomediastinal approach for tracheal reconstruction

nal reconstruction (El-Baz *et al.*, 1982). The patient should, in general, be extubated at the conclusion of the procedure and be able to breathe independently. If ventilatory support is needed postoperatively it should be for very brief periods of time only. There is no need for cardiopulmonary bypass in any but the most complex and unusual cases, and in the most complicated cases, where extensive intrathoracic manipulation is necessary, the anticoagulants required for bypass pose lethal hazards.

Inflammatory stenoses and post-intubation stenoses are operated on through an anterior cervical or cervicomediastinal approach. Upper tracheal tumours are similarly approached. Tumours of the lower trachea or carina are best approached through a transthoracic route. Median sternotomy with exposure between superior vena cava and aorta affords difficult but adequate access for small distal tumours, but is inadvisable for complex problems. Special approaches must be designed for special problems (Grillo, 1988, 1989, 1990).

Anterior approach (Figure 49.2)

With the patient supine, the neck is hyperextended with the aid of an inflatable bag placed beneath the shoulders. The field is draped so that the entire neck from the chin down is accessible and also the pre-sternal area. A low collar incision is most frequently employed. After elevation of flaps and retraction of the strap muscles the anterior surface of the trachea is

exposed from the level of the cricoid cartilage to the carina (Figure 49.2). The thyroid isthmus is usually divided and reflected laterally. If the lesion is lower in the trachea or if the extent of resection is such that the final suture line will lie quite deeply in the upper mediastinum, it is necessary to obtain wider access to the operative field. The collar incision is extended with a vertical limb over the midline of the sternum. This is carried only 1 or 2 cm below the sternal angle. The sternum is divided to this point and a small spreading retractor is used to separate the sternum. It is not necessary to divide the sternum laterally at the lower end of the sternal incision. The bone always yields at an appropriate point. Complete sternotomy does not aid the exposure and adds nothing but further pain and potential instability. Even partial sternal division is less often needed in young patients since a large portion of the trachea rises into the neck with hyperextension.

Where operation is being performed for a post-intubation stenosis or other inflammatory lesion, dissection is kept very close to the surface of the trachea. Where the resection is being performed for tumour it is preferable to include adjacent overlying tissue with the specimen including a lobe of thyroid gland, if this overlies an area of possibly invasive tumour. If the innominate artery is adherent to an area of inflammatory stenosis the dissection must be kept very much on the tracheal surface, and no effort should be made to isolate the artery itself since this may lead to postoperative haemorrhage from a damaged arterial wall. In inflammatory stenosis the recurrent laryngeal nerves are not dissected, damage to nerves being avoided by keeping the plane of dissection against the trachea. On the other hand, in the case of a tumour, the nerve should be identified and isolated at a distance from the tumour and a decision made on whether or not the nerve must be sacrificed because of actual involvement by tumour.

When the level of the lession is identified the dissection is carried circumferentially around the trachea at a point just below the lesion in most cases. Dissection is not carried circumferentially around the trachea for any distance longitudinally since this will result in destruction of the segmental blood supply which reaches the tracheal wall laterally (Salassa *et al.*, 1977). If the lesion is very low in the trachea, the dissection is sometimes carried around the trachea more simply just above the lesion. With care and patience it is possible then to pass a tape about the trachea without injury either to the membranous posterior wall or to the oesophagus. If the dissection is kept fairly close to the level of the inflammatory lesion, any inadvertent injury to the membranous wall of trachea can be encompassed in the subsequent line of resection. With the approximate line of division now established, lateral traction sutures of heavy material (2/0 Vicryl) are placed in the midlateral line on either side, approximately 2 cm distal to the anticipated line of division. These sutures pass through the tracheal wall. An armoured flexible endotracheal tube of appropriate size is arranged in the operative field along with connecting anaesthesia tubing which is passed to the anaesthetist. The trachea is divided below the lesion and the patient is intubated directly across the operative field (Figure 49.3) or a catheter if high-frequency ventilation is elected. Conservatism governs the initial tentative division below or above an inflammatory lesion. Additional rings of trachea may be taken subsequently. In the case of a tumour the exploratory opening of the trachea is done on the side opposite the tumour base to avoid crossing tumour tissue. If this exploratory opening of limited extent is not sufficiently distant from the tumour, successive levels may be selected until an appropriate one is obtained.

The lesion is elevated after grasping the ends of the trachea with Allis forceps and the trachea is dissected away from the oesophagus. If there is neoplastic involvement of the oesophageal wall, which usually has been determined preoperatively by oesophagoscopy or barium roentgenogram, a portion of oesophageal wall may also be resected. The specimen is finally removed by transecting the trachea above the level of the lesion or, in the case of low stenotic lesions, completing the division below the lesion. In the latter case the trachea is divided just above the lesion, a tight stenosis is dilated and the endotracheal tube is passed through the lesion. Traction sutures are placed in the mid-lateral position proximal to the upper line of tracheal division. Thus, when resection

is completed circumferential dissection of the remaining trachea has extended a distance no greater than 1.5 cm either proximal or distal to the line of division. This prevents devascularization, which could lead to later sloughing of the tracheal cartilages and subsequent stenosis.

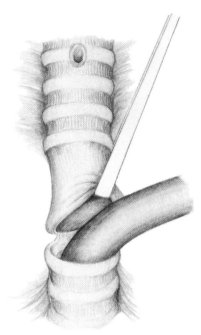

Figure 49.3 Tracheal stricture. Following division below the stricture the trachea is intubated across the operative field

If the upper end of the lesion is at the cricoid cartilage the transection must be done at this level. Great care must be taken posteriorly where the recurrent laryngeal nerves are closely applied to the posterolateral angles of the trachea, coursing up behind the cricoid plate just inside the inferior cornua of the thyroid cartilage. In such cases the lateral traction sutures must be passed through the substance of the larynx proximally. Where the lesion is circumferential, the anterior surface of posterior cricoid plate is bared and later covered by advancing a flap of membranous wall of distal trachea (see Figure 49.7).

Ease of approximation is tested after the segment has been resected. The anaesthetist places a hand behind the patient's head and flexes the neck, directing the chin towards the sternum. The surgeon and assistant on each side apply counter-traction between the upper and lower traction sutures drawing the ends of the trachea (or the larynx and the trachea) together. If the ends approximate without significant tension, anastomosis is possible with no other manoeuvre than the already described pretracheal dissection and the addition of cervical flexion. In young adults this may be all that is required even for resection of 50% of the trachea (Figure 49.4). In older patients, however, who are kyphotic, whose trachea is somewhat more horizontal, and in whom the larynx and trachea do not rise on cervical hyperextension, even very limited resection may result in an unacceptable degree of tension. Under these circumstances the next most useful manoeuvre is a suprahyoid laryngeal release (Figure 49.5) (Montgomery, 1974).

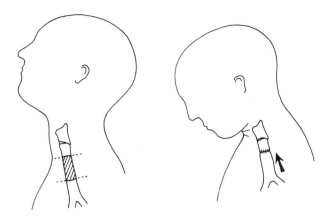

Figure 49.4 Following tracheal resection, extreme flexion of the neck ensures that approximation and suture of the trachea may be done without tension in most cases

Once it has been demonstrated that approximation may be obtained with safe degrees of tension, the anastomotic sutures are placed. Since the suture line may become relatively inaccessible after major resections, it is best to use strong suture material and to place all of the sutures in serial fashion prior to tying any of them. Although it is attractive conceptually to complete the posterior portion of the suture line and then to place the anterior sutures, it is not really optimal to accomplish this satisfactorily after extended resection. Sutures of polyglycolic acid polymer (Vicryl 4/0) are recommended. The use of such absorbable material minimizes the suture line granulomas which occur with non-absorbable material (Grillo, 1979a; Grillo et al., 1985).

The anastomotic sutures are placed so that the knots will lie outside the tracheal lumen. The first suture is placed in the midline of the membranous wall, passing through the wall approximately 3 or 4 mm from the edge, outside to inside and then to the outside again. This suture is grasped with a fine haemostat which in turn is clipped to the drapes of the field close to the midline superiorly. Additional sutures are placed individually at approximately 4 mm intervals, working out laterally from the initial posterior midline suture. Each suture is grasped and similarly clipped in sequence with fine haemostats. The sutures are placed in series, recognizing that they will later be tied starting from the most anterior suture. It is therefore necessary to be certain that each suture will lie anterior to the line of the just previously placed suture. The sutures are placed serially from the posterior midline to the mid-lateral line on either side. Two-thirds of the anastomotic sutures have now been placed. The remaining anterior third are placed and then temporarily aligned on the anterior chest wall. It is occasionally necessary to remove the endotracheal tube intermittently from the distal cut trachea while the sutures are placed, although in some patients with an appropriately sized endotracheal tube it is possible to work around the tube (Figure 49.6a). Once all the sutures have been placed the distal trachea is carefully suctioned from across the operative field and the original endotracheal tube, which had been retracted upwards to be out of the way of the operator, is readvanced into the distal trachea (Figure 49.6b). In cases of high lesions it is very helpful to suture a catheter to the tip of the proximal endotracheal tube after tracheal division to guide it back through the glottis at this point.

The patient's neck is sharply flexed and securely

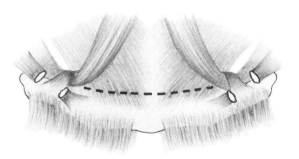
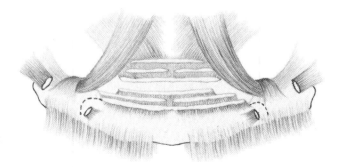

Figure 49.5 Suprahyoid laryngeal release. The suprahyoid release described by W. W. Montgomery has the advantage of providing 1–2 cm of anterior release without interfering as markedly with the function of the superior laryngeal nerves as does the thyrohyoid release. Exposure is frequently made through a separate horizontal incision. The mylohyoid, geniohyoid and genioglossus muscles are dissected from the superior border of the hyoid bone. The stylohyoid tendons are detached from their points of fixation on the hyoid. The lesser cornua of the hyoid are divided to release the chondroglossus muscles and then the body of the hyoid divided just medial to the sling of the digastric muscles on either side. The pre-epiglottic space is thus opened

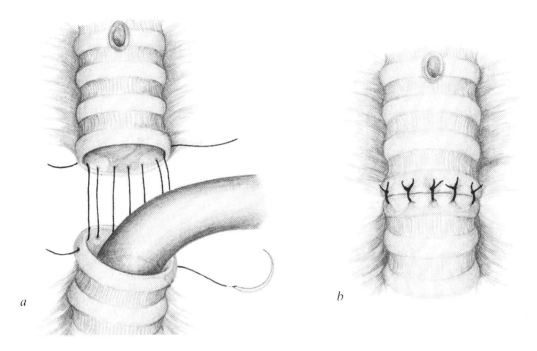

Figure 49.6 Tracheal stricture. Resuture of trachea following stricture resection

supported in this position. The surgeon and assistant draw the lateral traction sutures together, tying them so that the ends of the airway are approximated but not intussuscepted. The anastomotic sutures are thus tied without tension. The anterior sutures are tied first, continuing posteriorly until the midline is reached first from one side and then from the other. The most posterior sutures, particularly if the suture line is near the larynx, cannot be seen at this point even if gentle rotatory force is applied to the lateral traction suture. However, it is possible to feel the setting of the knots very accurately. After the anastomosis has been accomplished, the field is flooded with saline and the anastomosis is tested for airtightness.

Where the entire anterior cricoid cartilage has been removed, the distal trachea is gently bevelled backwards, taking care, however, not to create too small a segment of free cartilaginous ring. An exact fit is not required, and the anastomotic principles otherwise are precisely the same, taking care to correct visually for any discrepancy between larynx and trachea. There is no need to gather the membranous trachea together posteriorly or to create a groove in the cricoid plate, direct suture technique being possible (Figure 49.7). Where the posterior cricoid has been exposed, a previously fashioned flap of membranous tracheal wall is advanced to cover it (Pearson *et al.*, 1975; Grillo, 1980; Grillo *et al.*, 1992b).

Closure is made in the usual fashion, wiring the sternum together and approximating the strap muscles in the midline. Suction drains are placed both in the pretracheal and retrosternal spaces. Tracheostomy is hardly ever used following such a reconstruction.

The management of an existing tracheostomy is relatively complicated. Sometimes where it is clearly going to have to be resected it may be included in the line of the original incision. If this forces the incision to be placed in an ungainly spot, the cutaneous stoma may be removed independently leaving a second small incision. Sometimes a tracheostomy may be left in place and allowed to close spontaneously later. If it binds the trachea and prevents its advancement for anastomosis, the skin may require detachment from the trachea and the tracheostomy re-exteriorized through a new opening following the anastomosis, or it may be closed (Figure 49.8). If the tracheostomy ends up in the mediastinum as a result of the advancement, closure is done either by pedicling a strap muscle over it or, if there has been epithelium-to-epithelium healing prior to the reconstruction, the inversion technique may be used (Lawson and Grillo, 1970).

The operation is completed by placing one or two heavy sutures from the horizontal crease just beneath the point of the chin to the skin of the presternal area. This acts as a guardian suture to prevent sudden extensile motions in the 1st postoperative week. It is more effective and much more comfortable than splints or collars.

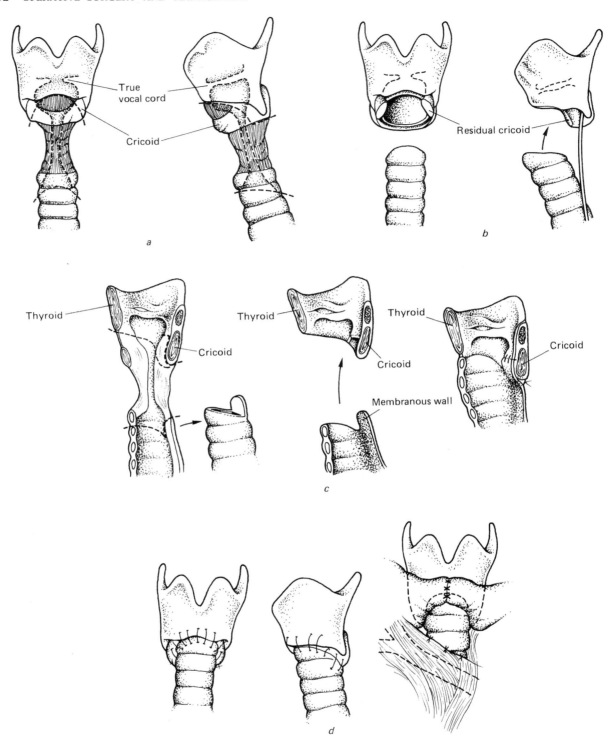

Figure 49.7   Resection and reconstruction of stenosis affecting subglottic larynx and upper trachea. *a*, Line of resection, including anterior subglottic larynx but preserving the posterior plate of cricoid. The inferior line of division is sloped. *b*, The cricoid as initially divided. If there is posterior stenosis in front of the posterior cricoid plate, this is excised along with the mucosa. Recurrent laryngeal nerves are carefully preserved by this dissection. *c*, In the case where there is posterior stenosis, the mucosa over the cricoid plate has been excised and a broad-based flap of membranous wall prepared inferiorly for surfacing of the cricoid. *d*, The completed anastomoses. Strap muscle is sutured over the innominate artery if it is close by to protect it in case a tracheostomy is needed. The thyroid isthmus or other tissue may be sutured over the anastomosis itself

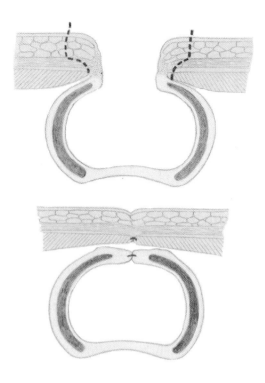

Figure 49.8 When it is necessary to close a persistent tracheostomy stoma it is essential to separate the trachea from the superficial musculocutaneous layer. If the skin has healed to the tracheal mucosa, the stoma is circumcised and a small margin of skin inverted with a subcuticular suture to provide epithelial closure. This prevents granuloma formation. In other cases, closure with adjacent strap muscle is accepted

Transthoracic approach (Figure 49.9)

Transthoracic tracheal reconstruction

The best approach has been through a high right posterolateral thoracotomy, although occasionally sections of the lower trachea and carina are approached through a trapdoor type of incision which consists of a right anterolateral thoracotomy and a median sternotomy up to the neck or, less effectively, through median sternotomy alone. After the trachea and an area of pathology, including carina in some cases, have been mobilized, additional mobilization is performed as is deemed to be necessary. This may consist of division of the inferior pulmonary ligament, dissection of the pulmonary vessels, intrapericardial release of the pulmonary vessels and carinal mobilization. Proximal and distal lateral traction sutures are placed as described earlier. If the point of division below the lesion is just above the carina, intubation is performed into the left main bronchus. The right pulmonary artery is occluded atraumatically only if physiological evidence develops of a shunt into the unventilated lung. Approximation and anastomosis are done as previously described.

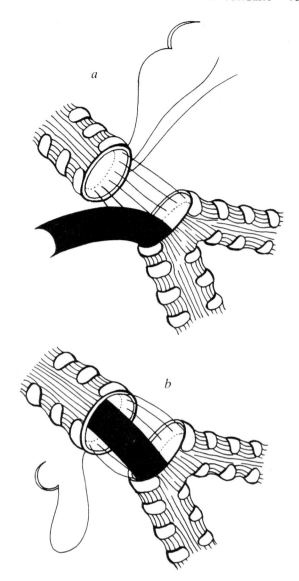

Figure 49.9 Transthoracic resection of low tracheal stricture. Posterior view (*a*) following resection and, while some sutures are placed, the left main bronchus is intubated directly across the operative field (*b*) to be later replaced by an endotracheal tube

Carinal reconstructive methods

When the carina is resected without removal of a large segment of trachea, the reconstruction is performed either by end-to-end anastomosis of trachea to right main bronchus, or to left main bronchus, with then the implantation of either the right or left main bronchus into a lateral opening in the devolved trachea, a short distance above the line of end-to-end anastomosis. Direct reconstruction of the carina itself by approximation of right and left main bronchi presents more difficulties unless the resection has been very limited. This is because the aortic arch anchors and tethers the left main bronchus, and the consequent suturing of right-to-left main bronchus means that the trachea must be devolved even further down for approximation to be accomplished. Carinal reconstruction is complex, difficult and prone to complications, even when expertly done (Barclay *et al.*, 1957; Grillo, 1982; 1988).

If greater lengths of trachea are resected, reconstruction is done by the technique of Barclay *et al.* (1957), anastomosing the left main bronchus to the side of the right bronchus intermedius, following end-to-end anastomosis of right main bronchus to trachea (Grillo, 1982).

Tracheal fistulas

1. Tracheo-oesophageal fistula

When a tracheo-oesophageal fistula results from the erosion of an endotracheal tube cuff through the membranous wall, often by compressive erosion against an inlying nasogastric tube, the problem may be life endangering. Repair of such a fistula is unlikely to succeed if the patient remains on a respirator, since a cuff will very likely be adjacent to the suture line. These patients are therefore tided over by placement of a tube with a large-volume, low-pressure cuff seal, the removal of the nasogastric tube, cessation of oral feedings, placement of a gastrostomy tube for gastric drainage to prevent reflux, and jejunostomy tube for long-term feeding. If the patient still suffers excessive contamination of the lungs from salivary secretion, the proximal oesophagus is exteriorized in the neck as an end salivary fistula and the distal end is temporarily closed. This is rarely necessary and frequently impossible. The oesophagogastric junction is never ligated.

Once the patient has been weaned a single-stage repair of the tracheo-oesophageal fistula is preferred.

Closure of tracheo-oesophageal fistula

The approach to the fistula is very much the same as that of the anterior approach to the trachea for resection. Usually a collar incision alone is sufficient, although occasionally an upper sternal vertical incision is also needed. The level of the stoma is usually 1–3 cm above that of the fistula itself since the fistula was due to a cuff. The dissection is carried out as previously described with intubation across the operative field. The diseased segment of trachea is elevated, excising not only it but the fistula in continuity. The oesophagus is closed vertically with two layers of interrupted sutures. A pedicled strap muscle flap is placed over this because of the contiguity, otherwise, of this suture line with the transverse suture line of the trachea. End-to-end repair of the trachea is next accomplished as described previously. The interposed muscle flap prevents recurrence of fistula (Grillo *et al.*, 1976).

In patients in whom circumferential damage to the trachea does not accompany the fistula, the tracheal and oesophageal openings are sutured after division of the fistula, and muscle interposed, without tracheal resection. Special care must be taken not to injure the recurrent laryngeal nerves.

2. Tracheo-innominate artery fistula

Tracheo-innominate artery fistula occurs most commonly from the low placement of a tracheostomy so that the tube lies against the innominate artery at the inferior lateral margin of the stoma and erodes it directly. Less commonly, a high-pressure cuff or the tip of a tracheostomy tube may erode through the anterior wall of the trachea, into the overlying innominate artery. In the latter case the stoma is high and uninvolved in the fistula. The first type of lesion must be controlled acutely by direct pressure at the inferior margin of the stoma against the leaking innominate artery, with concomitant placement of an endotracheal tube through the stoma to seal and maintain the airway. The emergency management of the second type of lesion can only be made by the rapid insertion of an endotracheal tube through the stoma with the inflation of a high-pressure cuff against the leak to tamponade the bleeding. The point of fistulization is not accessible in this case to a tamponading finger (Grillo, 1990).

Both of these lesions must be treated surgically immediately. Anaesthesia is induced through the endotracheal tube which has already been placed. Complete division of the sternum provides optimal access to the artery and arch of the aorta if necessary. A collar incision above provides cervical access. Dissection is done proximally around the origin of the innominate artery, taking care not to injure the artery at this point, and distally beyond the point of leakage, which is just below the bifurcation of the subclavian and common carotid arteries. The author has resected the perforated artery, closing both proximal and distal arterial ends with two layers of running arterial sutures. The stumps of the artery have been carefully buried centrally under thymic tissue and laterally under strap muscles. In the case of a stomal erosion the trachea does not require further treatment except to seal off the tracheostomy from the general incision during the course of the closure. In erosion by a cuff, the injured segment of trachea is resected and an end-to-end tracheal anastomosis is performed. Primary arterial grafting has been avoided because of the contaminated field. Thus far no neurological injuries have been seen, but some hazard exists.

References

Barclay, R. S., McSwan, N. and Welsh, T. M. (1957) Tracheal reconstruction without the use of grafts. *Thorax*, **12**, 177

El-Baz, N., Jensik, R., Faber, J. P. and Faro, R. S. (1982) One-lung high-frequency ventilation for tracheoplasty and bronchoplasty: a new technique. *Ann. Thorac. Surg.*, **34**, 564

Eschapasse, H. (1974) Les tumeurs trachéales primitives. Traitement chirurgicale. *Rev. Fr. Mal. Respr.*, **2**, 425

Grillo, H. C. (1979a) Complications of tracheal operations. In *Complications in Thoracic Surgery* (eds A. R. Cordell and R. Ellison), Little, Brown, Boston

Grillo, H. C. (1979b) Surgical treatment of postintubation tracheal injuries. *J. Thorac. Cardiovasc. Surg.*, **78**, 860

Grillo, H. C. (1980) Primary reconstruction of airway after resection of subglottic laryngeal and upper tracheal stenosis. *Ann. Thorac. Surg.*, **33**, 3

Grillo, H. C. (1981) Tracheostomy and its complications. In *Davis-Christopher Textbook of Surgery*, 12th edn (ed. D. C. Sabiston, Jr), W. B. Saunders, Philadalphia

Grillo, H. C. (1982) Carinal reconstruction. *Ann. Thorac. Surg.*, **34**, 356

Grillo, H. C. (1988) The trachea. In *Atlas of General Thoracic Surgery* (eds M. M. Ravitch and F. M. Steichen), W. B. Saunders, Philadelphia, pp. 293–331

Grillo, H. C. (1989) Tracheal anatomy and surgical approaches. In *General Thoracic Surgery*, 3rd edn (ed. T. W. Shields), Lea and Febiger, Philadelphia

Grillo, H. C. (1990) Congenital lesions, neoplasms and injuries of the trachea. In *Gibbon's Surgery of the Chest*, 5th edn (ed. D. C. Sabiston, Jr.), W. B. Saunders, Philadelphia

Grillo, H. C. and Mathisen, D. J. (1990) Primary tracheal tumors: treatment and results. *Ann. Thorac. Surg.*, **49**, 69

Grillo, H. C., Mathisen, D. J. and Wain, J. C. (1992b) Laryngotracheal resection and reconstruction for subglottic stenosis. *Ann. Thorac. Surg.*, **53**, 54

Grillo, H. C., Moncure, A. C. and McEnany, M. T. (1976) Repair of inflammatory tracheo-oesophageal fistula. *Ann. Thorac. Surg.*, **22**, 112

Grillo, H. C., Suen, H. C., Mathisen, D. J. and Wain, J. C. (1992a) Resectional management of thyroid carcinoma invading the airway. *Ann. Thorac. Surg.*, **54**, 3

Grillo, H. C., Zannini, P. and Michelassi, F. (1985) Complications of tracheal reconstruction: incidence, treatment and prevention. *J. Thorac. Cardiovasc. Surg.*, **91**, 322

Lawson, D. W. and Grillo, H. C. (1970) Closure of a persistent tracheal stoma. *Surg. Gynecol. Obstet.*, **130**, 995

MacMillan, A. S., James, A. E., Jr, Stitik, F. P. *et al.* (1971) Radiological evaluation of post tracheostomy lesions. *Thorax*, **26**, 696

Mathisen, D. J. and Grillo, H. C. (1989) Endoscopic relief of malignant airway obstruction. *Ann. Thorac. Surg.*, **48**, 469

Mathisen, D. J. and Grillo, H. C. (1991) Carinal resection for bronchogenic carcinoma. *J. Thorac. Cardiovasc. Surg.*, **102**, 16

Montgomery, W. W. (1964) Reconstruction of the cervical trachea. *Ann. Otol.*, **73**, 5

Montgomery, W. W. (1973) *Surgery of the Upper Respiratory System*, Vol. II, Lea and Febiger, Philadelphia, p. 384

Montgomery, W. W. (1974) Suprahyoid release for tracheal anastomosis. *Arch. Otolaryngol.*, **99**, 255

Pearson, F. G., Cooper, J. D., Nelems, J. M. *et al.* (1975) Primary tracheal anastomosis after resection of the cricoid cartilage with preservation of recurrent laryngeal nerves. *J. Thorac. Cardiovasc. Surg.*, **70**, 806

Pearson, F. G., Todd, T. R. J. and Cooper, J. D. (1984) Experience with primary neoplasms of the trachea. *J. Thorac. Cardiovasc. Surg.*, **88**, 511

Perelman, M. I. and Koroleva, N. (1987) Primary tumors of the trachea. In *International Trends in General. Thoracic Surgery*, Vol. 2 (eds H. C. Grillo and H. Eschapasse), W. B. Saunders, Philadephia, p. 91

Salassa, J. R., Pearson, B. and Payne, W. S. (1977) Gross and microscopic blood supply of the trachea. *Ann. Thorac. Surg.*, **23**, 100

Weber, A. L. and Grillo, H. C. (1978) Tracheal tumors: radiological, clinical and pathological evaluation. *Adv. Otol. Rhinol. Laryngol.*, **24**, 170

Wilson, R. S. (1987) Anesthesia management for tracheal reconstruction. In *International Trends in General Thoracic Surgery*, Vol. II (eds H. C. Grillo and H. Eschapasse), W. B. Saunders, Philadelphia, pp. 3–12

50

The lung, pleural cavity and mediastinum

R. Hurt

Part 1 Anatomy, bronchoscopy, mediastinoscopy, anterior mediastinotomy, surgical access, preoperative assessment and postoperative management.

Part 2 Acute and chronic empyema, chronic sinus, recurrent and chronic pneumothorax, chylothorax.

Part 3 Assessment for resection of lung carcinoma, technique of pneumonectomy, lobectomy (including 'sleeve' resection), segmental resection, management of post-resection empyema and bronchopleural fistula.

Part 4 Mediastinal tumours, myasthenia gravis and thymectomy, chronic superior vena caval obstruction.

Part 5 Pleural biopsy, pleural and chest wall tumours, malignant pleural effusion.

Part 6 Emphysematous and hydatid cysts.

Part 7 Surgical treatment of pulmonary tuberculosis.

Part 1

Surgical anatomy of the lungs

The two lungs are basically very similar, despite the fact that on the right side there are three lobes and on the left two. The lingular segment of the left upper lobe corresponds to the right middle lobe and is the first branch of the left upper lobe bronchus. Each lobe is divided into segments which function as individual units, each having its own bronchus, artery and vein. The segmental arteries run very close to the bronchi, usually on their superior or lateral aspect, whereas the segmental veins run *between* the segments, from which they receive tributaries. The segments are held together by loose connective tissue and no bronchi or arteries cross the intersegmental plane.

Nomenclature of bronchopulmonary segments

The classification adopted by the Thoracic Society of Great Britain (1950) (see also Brock, 1950; Boyden, 1955) is as follows:

Right lung

The three lobes have 10 main segments:

RIGHT UPPER LOBE

1. Apical segment.
2. Posterior segment.
3. Anterior segment.

RIGHT MIDDLE LOBE

4. Lateral segment.
5. Medial segment.

RIGHT LOWER LOBE

6. Apical segment.
7. Medial basal (cardiac) segment.
8. Anterior basal segment.
9. Lateral basal segment.
10. Posterior basal segment.

Left lung

The two lobes have nine main segments (segment 7 is omitted in the left lung):

LEFT UPPER LOBE

1. Apical segment.
2. Posterior segment.
3. Anterior segment.
4. Superior division of lingula.
5. Inferior division of lingula.

LEFT LOWER LOBE

6. Apical segment.
8. Anterior basal segment.
9. Lateral basal segment.
10. Posterior basal segment.

Anatomy of the bronchial tree

The anatomy of the bronchial tree is illustrated in Figure 50.1. Each lung has an *upper lobe*, which is divided into anterior, apical and posterior segments. On the right side, these segmental bronchi branch as a trifurcation, but on the left side there is usually an apicoposterior stem bronchus and a separate anterior segmental bronchus. It is important to appreciate that the origin of the right upper lobe bronchus is only just distal to the carina, with the result that the right main bronchus is very short.

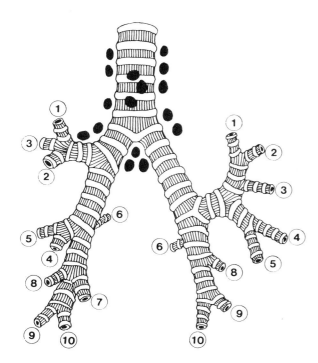

Figure 50.1 Anatomy of the bronchial tree. The position of the paratracheal, pretracheal, superior and inferior tracheobronchial lymph nodes is shown

The right *middle lobe* lies anteriorly and is a branch of the intermediate bronchus. In the left lung, however, the middle lobe is represented by the lingular segment, the first segmental bronchus of the left upper lobe which passes anteriorly and inferiorly.

The *lower lobe* on each side is composed of three basal segments, together with an apical segment lying posteriorly, which in the right lung arises immediately opposite the middle lobe. In the right lower lobe there is, in addition, a medially placed cardiac segment arising between the apical segmental bronchus and the basal divisions.

Three surgical anatomical points

There are three important surgical points to note:

1. The right main bronchus is situated more vertically than the left; therefore inhaled foreign bodies are more common on the right than on the left.
2. The origin of the right upper lobe is *very* close to the carina. Indeed at bronchoscopy the right upper lobe orifice and the carina appear to be almost the same distance from the upper jaw.
3. The middle lobe and the apical segment of the right lower lobe arise from the intermediate bronchus immediately opposite each other. This is of importance in right lower lobectomy.

Bronchial vessels

The lung has a systemic as well as a pulmonary blood supply. The bronchial arteries arise from the descend-

ing thoracic aorta or upper intercostal arteries and run along the corresponding bronchi. They become very much dilated in chronic infective disease (e.g. bronchiectasis) and also in congenital heart disease when the pulmonary arterial flow is reduced (e.g. tetralogy of Fallot). The bronchial veins drain into the systemic and pulmonary circulation.

Pulmonary arteries (Figure 50.2)

Each main pulmonary artery gives off lobar and segmental branches corresponding to the lobar and segmental branches of the bronchial tree. Although these usually follow a regular pattern there is no substitute for careful dissection and identification of these arteries, for variations are common.

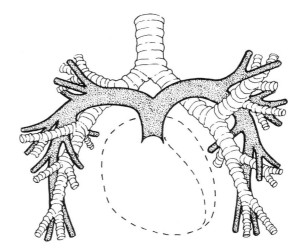

Figure 50.2 Distribution of the pulmonary arteries. Note that the pulmonary segmental arteries are closely related to the segmental bronchi

Pulmonary veins (Figure 50.3)

The segmental veins run in the planes between the segments, joining to form the lobar veins which drain into the main pulmonary veins. Of particular importance is the middle lobe vein which drains into the right upper pulmonary vein and must be preserved when upper lobectomy is performed.

Bronchoscopy

Therapeutic bronchoscopy may be required to remove secretions from the tracheobronchial tree of severely ill patients suffering from sputum retention (including postoperative sputum retention and lobar collapse) or to remove foreign bodies, which are especially liable to be inhaled by infants and young children. *Diagnostic* bronchoscopy is one of the most commonly used methods of investigation in the study of chest disease, both to establish the diagnosis and to assess operability and the type of operation to be performed.

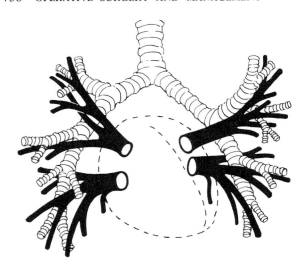

Figure 50.3 Pulmonary venous drainage

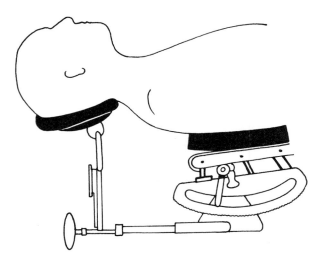

Figure 50.4 Position for bronchoscopy. Note extension of patient's head

Bronchoscopy is preferably done under general anaesthesia. In cases of sputum retention it is important that the patients wake up as rapidly as possible so that they may again be encouraged to cough – it is probably better in these cases to carry out the bronchoscopy under local anaesthesia. The modern Sanders technique of oxygen jet-injection has made it possible to maintain adequate oxygenation even during a prolonged examination, and this is especially valuable during the removal of foreign bodies in children (Sanders, 1967). No patient is too ill to be bronchoscoped and if necessary the examination may be carried out under local anaesthesia in the patient's bed.

The flexible fibreoptic bronchoscope, more commonly used by physicians, may be passed to view and biopsy upper lobe lesions. It is also of value for forceps biopsy or brush biopsy of peripheral lesions under radiographic control.

A happy compromise is first to pass the rigid bronchoscope under general anaesthesia. If this examination (even with the use of the right-angled telescope) fails to provide sufficient information, the flexible fibreoptic instrument may then be passed through the rigid bronchoscope and a further examination made.

Technique (Figures 50.4 and 50.5)

The Negus rigid bronchoscope is preferable since its lumen is slightly elliptical and for any given size of instrument there is less pressure on the teeth or gums. The more modern Storz bronchoscope, however, has very much better illumination and a wider range of accessories. Unless the patient is distressed due to sputum retention, superior vena caval obstruction or heart failure, and the examination is therefore being done in the sitting position, the patient lies supine, without pillows and with the head moderately extended.

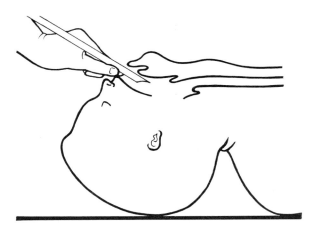

Figure 50.5 Introduction of bronchoscope. Note the protection of the upper lip, teeth and jaw by the operator's fingers. The bronchoscope must rest on the thumb to prevent any injury to the teeth or gums

Complications

1. Haemorrhage

The main complication of bronchoscopy is haemorrhage, which may occur after biopsy of an unusually vascular carcinoma or more commonly a carcinoid tumour (adenoma), for these tumours are often very vascular. It may also occur after a biopsy from the region of the middle lobe or left upper lobe bronchus, to both of which a pulmonary artery branch is closely related. Haemorrhage may be controlled by locally applied swabs soaked in 1 in 1000 adrenaline. This, together with suction, is usually adequate. The bronchoscope should be left in place until the effects of the anaesthetic have worn off and the patient is beginning to cough. The bronchoscope may then be removed and the patient laid on the side from which the haemorrhage is coming, to prevent inhalation of blood into the contralateral lung. Rarely an emergency thoracotomy may be required, in which case a Thompson blocker or Fogarty catheter should be used to occlude the bronchus and prevent inhalation of blood into the remaining lung.

2. Laryngeal oedema

Laryngeal oedema is not uncommon in infants or children, and is best treated by humidification of the inhaled air or a steam tent, together with systemic steroids. A tracheostomy is only rarely necessary.

Mediastinoscopy

This investigation, which was first carried out by Carlens in 1959, has proved to be a most valuable procedure for establishing the diagnosis of intrathoracic disease, without embarking on the more major procedure of an exploratory thoracotomy (Pearson *et al.*, 1972; Paulson, 1974; Nohl-Oser, 1976). Positive histology may often be obtained in cases of mediastinal or hilar lymph node enlargement and the diagnosis of bronchial carcinoma, Hodgkin's disease, sarcoidosis, tuberculosis, pneumoconiosis or other disease confirmed. Anterior mediastinal conditions such as thymic tumours cannot be approached by this procedure as they lie in front of the great vessels. In the presence of superior vena caval obstruction there is a special risk of haemorrhage – the operation is best avoided.

Operative technique

Mediastinoscopy is carried out under general anaesthesia.

The patient lies supine with a sandbag under the shoulders so that the neck is extended and the head turned slightly to the left. The table is tilted slightly foot downwards to reduce venous congestion. The surgeon stands on the patient's left side.

A transverse incision is made through the skin and platysma 5 cm in length just above the suprasternal notch. The pretracheal muscles are separated by blunt dissection in the midline, taking care to avoid the inferior thyroid veins which can usually be retracted laterally but may need to be divided. The pretracheal fascia, which has now been exposed, is incised transversely so that a tunnel may be made by blunt dissection with the index finger down into the mediastinum *behind* the pretracheal fascia immediately in front of the trachea (Figure 50.6). It is absolutely vital for the finger to be in the correct plane, otherwise the great vessels in the mediastium (in particular the left innominate vein) are likely to be damaged (Figure 50.7). If the dissection is in the correct plane immediately in front of the trachea, the area is avascular and, in addition, the pretracheal fascia will protect the

great vessels during the subsequent introduction of the mediastinoscope.

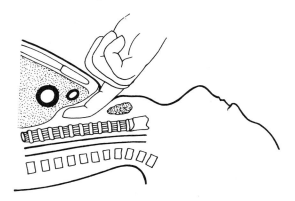

Figure 50.6 Mediastinoscopy. Creation of plane deep to the pretracheal fascia

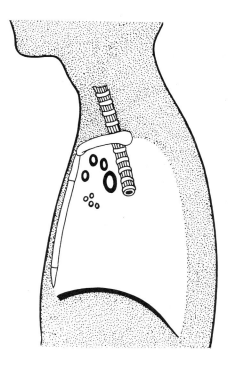

Figure 50.7 Mediastinoscopy. Major vessels are at risk in the superior mediastinum

The Carlens mediastinoscope has a slit along the whole of the right side and this facilitates the introduction of forceps and suction without obstructing the view of the operator. The surgeon moves to the head of the table and the mediastinoscope is gently introduced into the mediastinal tunnel already made by the index finger (Figure 50.8). The instrument must remain in the midline and the tracheal rings should therefore be visible. At the preliminary digital exploration enlarged glands may have been palpated.

These, together with other lymph nodes, are exposed by blunt dissection. It is often difficult to distinguish lymph nodes from veins because of the bluish colour of both structures. Further dissection will often distinguish a node from a vein, but before taking a biopsy it is always wise to carry out a preliminary diagnostic aspiration. A blind biopsy should never be taken.

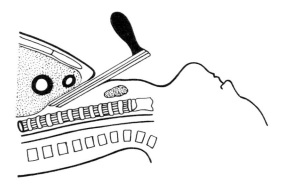

Figure 50.8 Mediastinoscopy. Introduction of the mediastinoscope anterior to the trachea and posterior to the great vessels

Complications

The most important complication is haemorrhage. This may well cease on removal of the mediastinoscope, with or without packing the area with gauze. If haemorrhage persists then a posterolateral thoracotomy must be carried out on the side from which the biopsy was taken. It is unwise to use an anterior approach through a midline sternotomy to deal with this problem. Other complications are injury to the recurrent laryngeal nerve and pneumothorax.

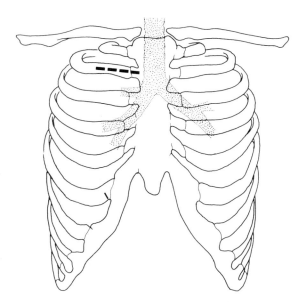

Figure 50.9 Incision for mediastinotomy

Anterior mediastinotomy

Diagnostic exploration of the mediastinum may also be carried out by anterior mediastinotomy (Evans *et al.*, 1973). Through a short horizontal incision about 10 cm long lateral to either side of the sternum, the 2nd or 3rd costal cartilage is excised subperichondrially and the incision in the rib bed extended laterally along the upper border of the rib (Figure 50.9). The internal mammary vessels are ligated and the mediastinum may be explored extrapleurally. Hilar and paratracheal lymph nodes or any anterior mediastinal mass are easily accessible for biopsy. If necessary, the pleura may be opened for inspection and biopsy of the lung or pleural cavity. If the pleura is opened, an underwater drain should be inserted through a separate stab incision. This procedure disturbs the patient very little more than a mediastinoscopy and provides very much more information.

Surgical access in thoracic operations

Preoperative assessment

The preoperative assessment of patients undergoing thoracic surgery is most important. There are no definite standards to establish whether a patient is sufficiently fit to tolerate a major lung resection or other intrathoracic procedure. Many factors must be taken into account. An obese, bronchitic, middle-aged patient may not tolerate thoracotomy, whereas a relatively thin man of 75 years may tolerate the procedure very well.

History

A history of recurrent bronchitis or bronchospasm increases the operative risk and the likelihood of the patient becoming a respiratory cripple after operation, especially pneumonectomy.

Clinical examination

The chest movements and configuration of the chest must be assessed by clinical examination. Patients with a 'barrel-shaped' chest (large anteroposterior diameter) often suffer from chronic bronchitis and emphysema, and this will be confirmed by the radiological signs of lack of lung markings and depressed diaphragms. Excessive obesity increases the operative risk.

Lung function studies (Saunders, 1975)

It is customary to undertake extensive lung function studies in patients being considered for lung resection. These tests of respiratory function will provide valuable confirmatory evidence of impaired lung function.

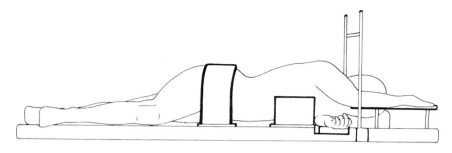

Figure 50.10 Position on operating table for right thoracotomy. Note position of chest and hip supports. The pad under the chest is hidden by the chest support

They are often very difficult to interpret, however, and do not replace the simple tests of asking the patient how short of breath he is on exercise and of walking with him up two flights of stairs.

Preoperative treatment

The preoperative preparation of patients for thoracic surgery is most important and 2–3 days' intensive treatment will often shorten the patient's stay in hospital by 2–3 weeks – it may even be life saving.

Treatment should be directed to:

1. Reduction of bronchial infection by the appropriate antibiotic, together with postural drainage if necessary.
2. Reduction of bronchospasm by antispasmodic drugs such as ephedrine or salbutamol (Ventolin), together with steroids if necessary.
3. Correction of anaemia.
4. Instruction in breathing exercises by the physiotherapist.

Techniques of thoracotomy

There are five standard approaches for entering the thorax and the anatomical position of the lesion will determine the correct incision. The five approaches are:

1. Posterolateral thoracotomy.
2. Anterolateral thoracotomy.
3. Median sternotomy.
4. Thoraco-abdominal.
5. Face-down or Overholt position (obsolete).

1. Posterolateral thoracotomy

A posterolateral thoracotomy, along the upper border of the 6th rib, is suitable for all lung resections and for many other intrathoracic procedures. Repair of a diaphragmatic hernia is best carried out through the 8th rib bed and operation for coarctation of the aorta or patent ductus arteriosus through the 4th rib bed. The patient lies in the lateral position with a pad under the chest to spread the ribs and with chest and hip supports (Figure 50.10). The knees and hips are flexed. The diathermy pad is under the buttock or strapped to the thigh.

The skin incision (Figure 50.11) begins below the nipple over the 5th or 6th rib, runs backwards 2–3 cm below the angle of the scapula and then turns upwards to a point halfway between the vertebral border of the scapula and the midline. The muscle layers are then divided with the diathermy needle in the line of the incision. The first layer consists of the latissimus dorsi and trapezius, and the second layer, the rhomboids and serratus anterior. It is often possible to retract the serratus anterior and not divide it. The scapula is then elevated using a scapular retractor and the ribs counted from above downwards to select the correct rib. The periosteum is elevated from the upper border of the 6th rib and the pleura entered through the rib bed, taking care not to damage the underlying lung. The costotransverse ligament should be divided with a rougine or grooved chisel. It is not necessary to resect a rib, though in the older patient, whose ribs are more brittle, it is probably wise to divide the back end of the rib. Any adhesions in the neighbourhood of the incision are divided and then a Finochietto type of rib spreader introduced to spread the ribs.

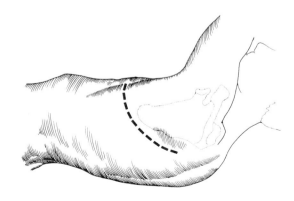

Figure 50.11 Incision for left posterolateral thoracotomy. The anterior end of the incision should be over the 5th rib

CLOSURE OF CHEST

After almost every thoracotomy an apical (air) or basal (fluid) tube is inserted – very often both. These tubes remain in place for 1–7 days, depending on the amount of drainage (see Postoperative Management, below). The tubes must be of adequate internal diameter – 7 mm is recommended – and of adequate rigidity so that they do not kink. They are placed through separate stab incisions below the thoracotomy wound, anteriorly in the axillary line so that the patient will not compress the tubes when sitting up in bed after operation. The tubes are introduced by drawing them through the chest wall from within with a strong clamp (Figure 50.12). The posterior tube is a basal tube and its end lies at the level of the dome of the diaphragm. The anterior tube is an apical tube which passes up inside the chest to the apex (Figure 50.13). A stitch should be placed around the tube through the intercostal muscle on the upper border of the thoracotomy incision to prevent it falling away from the apex when the patient sits up. Stitches are placed to fix the tubes to the skin and also to close the stab incision when the tube is removed. Both tubes are connected to underwater seals.

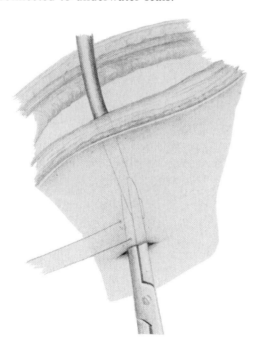

Figure 50.12   Introduction of pleural drainage tube

The chest wall is then closed. A rib approximator is useful to bring the ribs together. The rib bed is closed with a continuous non-absorbable suture (using 2/0 nylon), placed through the intercostal muscle parallel to the rib above and below the rib bed incision. It should *not* encircle the rib as this will compress the intercostal nerve and cause persistent postoperative pain. The two muscle layers are then closed separately with continuous Dexon, nylon or catgut. Finally, the skin is closed with a continuous suture.

This standard posterolateral thoracotomy may be enlarged if necessary by extending the incision anteriorly as far as the costal cartilage, and by dividing the back ends of one or more adjacent ribs.

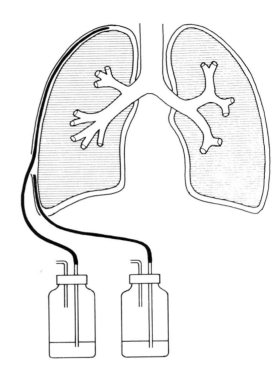

Figure 50.13   Position of basal and apical tubes following pulmonary resection. The end of the basal tube should be at the level of the dome of the diaphragm

2. Anterolateral thoracotomy

This incision is used for closed mitral valvotomy and may sometimes be appropriate for anterior mediastinal tumours. It provides poor access to the hilum of the lung. The patient lies on his or her back with a pad under the left shoulder to give a slight tilt to the right. The upper left arm is bent over the head. The incision starts at the 5th left costal cartilage (counting from the first cartilage downwards) and runs along the line of the rib in the submammary groove to end in the mid-axillary line (Figure 50.14). The pectoralis major is divided over the 5th intercostal space and retracted (with the breast in a female patient) upwards. The dissection is carried well back by splitting the serratus anterior and undercutting the skin incision to expose the ribs as far as the posterior axillary line. The perichondrium and periosteum on the lower border of the 5th rib and cartilage are elevated and the rib bed opened. The internal mammary vessels are divided between ligatures, the 5th costal cartilage divided and a rib spreader and protecting towels introduced. If further exposure is required, the sternum may be transected with a Gigli saw and the incision extended into the right chest, with division of the right internal mammary vessels. Alternatively the 4th left costal cartilage may be divided.

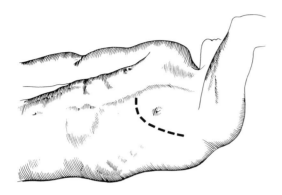

Figure 50.14 Left anterior thoracotomy

The wound is closed in layers in the same way as a posterolateral thoracotomy, with an underwater-seal drainage tube inserted through a separate stab incision low down in the chest in the line of the axilla. If the sternum has been divided the edges should be brought together with three no. 24 SWG wire sutures inserted with an awl and using a protective spoon.

Postoperative management

After operation it is important to prevent tracheo-bronchial infection and its sequelae, and in the case of segmental resection and lobectomy to encourage expansion of the remainder of the lung. Postoperative physiotherapy is vital and may be life saving. The following are most important:

1. Expectoration

This should be encouraged as much as possible, partly verbally and partly by manual support of the operated side of the chest. This encouragement is extremely effective in helping a patient to maintain a clear airway. If the sputum is thick and tenacious, inhalations are useful.

2. Analgesics

These should be given as necessary to relieve the pain of the thoracotomy incision. Sputum retention or lobar collapse may occur as a result of the excessive administration of analgesics, which reduce the cough reflex, but on the other hand the same effect may occur from the *inadequate* relief of postoperative pain.

3. Postural drainage

Postural drainage ('tipping') should be instituted for 1 hour 3 times a day, or more often if there is any tendency for sputum retention. If inhalations have been given, then the period of 'tipping' should be immediately afterwards.

4. Antibiotic cover

This should be continued for at least 10 days after operation. It may be necessary to check the bacteriology of the sputum, for sometimes the predominant organism alters after operation, in which case the type of antibiotic may have to be changed. In elderly patients, chloramphenicol is very often life saving.

5. Ambulation

The patient should be encouraged to move about in bed as much as possible, and it is a help if there is a cord attached to the foot of the bed for the patient to pull up on. Patients should be allowed out of bed as soon as their general condition permits (on the 2nd or 3rd day, if possible), even though a drainage tube is still in position.

6. Management of chest tubes

The chest tubes drain blood and air from the pleural cavity and are connected to underwater seals to which suction is applied. They are removed after a varying number of days, depending on the amount of drainage of air or fluid, and also on the radiographic appearance.

After a pneumonectomy, the management of the chest tube is different and is described on page 758.

Complications of thoracotomy

1. Sputum retention

Collapse-consolidation of a lobe or lung will occur if the patient is unable to expectorate the bronchial secretions adequately, in spite of intensive physiotherapy. Sooner or later respiratory insufficiency will occur, leading to general weakness and still further difficulty in expectoration. The treatment is bronchoscopy or, if this has to be repeated more than once daily, a mini-tracheostomy (Matthews and Hopkinson, 1984) or even intubation with an endotracheal tube.

2. Atrial fibrillation

Most patients undergoing lung resection for a tumour are over the age of 50 years and may develop atrial fibrillation after operation, especially if the pericardium has been opened. This most commonly occurs during the first 10 days, and if the heart rate is fast may produce a shock-like condition. The irregularity should be confirmed by an electrocardiogram and careful digitalization carried out as a matter of urgency. More modern antiarrhythmic drugs offer few advantages and more dangers than digoxin.

3. Bronchospasm

Bronchospasm may occur, leading to dyspnoea, tachycardia and cyanosis. Ephedrine, salbutamol (Ventolin) or hydrocortisone should be given.

4. Surgical emphysema

Surgical emphysema may occur if the drainage tubes are blocked or, when the tube is functioning, if the air leak from the raw surface of the lung is greater than the suction pump can handle. The treatment is to unblock the drainage tube, introduce a new tube or *remove* the sucker so as to allow the free escape of air.

5. Haemorrhage

Excessive haemorrhage will require exploration.

Part 2

Acute empyema (Le Roux *et al.*, 1986; Smith *et al.*, 1991)

The advent of modern chemotherapy has radically altered the natural history of empyema and many cases are now relatively late in their development. The most important factor in the diagnosis of an empyema is an awareness that it may be present. In some cases an empyema may be 'sterile' when first diagnosed, due to use of an antibiotic early in any pulmonary infection, and these patients may be best treated by decortication. In any patient over the age of 40 years, it is important to exclude an underlying carcinoma by examination of the sputum for malignant cells and by bronchoscopy.

The *choice of treatment* depends on the thickness of the pus and the patient's clinical state. Treatment may be by:

1. Aspiration and instillation of an antibiotic.
2. Drainage by rib resection or intercostal tube.
3. Decortication.

1. Aspiration and instillation of an antibiotic

Some patients may be treated successfully by this method if the pus is thin *and remains thin*. An arbitrary definition of thin pus is pus that contains less than one-third sediment after 24 h. Treatment must be carried out under radiological control and aspirations carried out every 2nd or 3rd day until no more fluid is formed. On each occasion as much fluid as possible should be removed. A large dose of the appropriate antibiotic is instilled and in addition the patient must be given systemic chemotherapy, also in high dosage so that the antibiotic reaches the pleural cavity. If this regimen is successful the fluid will become sterile after about 1 week and will become less purulent at each aspiration. The radiograph will show continued expansion of the lung and only minimal residual pleural thickening will remain. Physiotherapy must be given throughout this period to maintain equal movement of both sides of the chest. If pus is still being produced after 10 days, this method of treatment should be abandoned, and tube drainage or rib resection carried out.

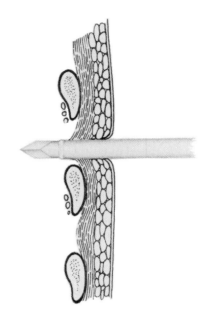

Figure 50.15 Introduction of intercostal drainage tube. It is important to stay close to the upper surface of the lower rib to avoid damage to the intercostal bundle

It is important to appreciate the limitations of this method of treatment. If the patient remains febrile, if aspirations become increasingly difficult because of frequent needle blockage by fibrin, if the organism is resistant to antibiotics, or if the radiograph shows multiple fluid levels due to loculation, then this regimen must be abandoned and rib resection and drainage instituted. The use of fibrinolytic enzymes such as streptokinase is not recommended. If significant fibrin is present, it is better to proceed to immediate rib resection and drainage in order to prevent the development of a chronic empyema.

Aspiration treatment is especially valuable in children or in the elderly.

2. Drainage

Drainage may be by intercostal tube or rib resection.

Intercostal tube (Figures 50.15 and 50.16)

Intercostal tube drainage may be necessary as an emergency procedure in the patient's bed. It is indicated:

(a) In an acutely ill patient with severe toxaemia.
(b) When an empyema is associated with a bronchopleural fistula and threatens to 'drown' the patient due to inhalation of pus into the contralateral lung.
(c) In a case of delayed diagnosis of a ruptured oesophagus, which is usually associated with severe toxaemia.
(d) In an acute lung abscess associated with an empyema.

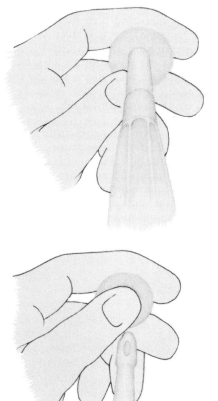

Figure 50.16 Introduction of intercostal drainage tube

TECHNIQUE OF INSERTION

If there is a bronchopleural fistula, the patient must be in a sitting position, leaning forwards over a bed-table. The site of drainage is usually the 8th or 9th intercostal space in the posterior axillary line but this must be confirmed by chest radiography, which will include a lateral view.

The site of insertion is infiltrated down to the pleura with 20 ml 0.5% lignocaine with adrenaline. The presence of pus must be confirmed either by aspiration through the needle used for the local anaesthetic or a large-bore needle if the pus is thick.

If no pus is obtained another site must be chosen. It is a mistake to aspirate too low. A large-size trocar and cannula should be used, together with the largest Malecot catheter that when stretched will go through the cannula. A small incision is made in the skin and the trocar and cannula introduced into the empyema by a steady, thrusting movement accompanied by rotation. The trocar should be kept as close as possible to the rib below to avoid damage to the intercostal vessels, and the forefinger should be in contact with the patient's chest in order to guard against uncontrolled entry of the trocar. The trocar is withdrawn and the opening in the cannula is immediately closed with the thumb to prevent the entry of air into the chest – this is *most* important (Figure 50.16). The Malecot catheter, held stretched over the introducer, is then introduced simultaneously as the thumb is moved from the opening in the cannula. The cannula is now removed from the chest, *while keeping the catheter stretched on the introducer.* Before finally removing the cannula from the tube, the catheter must be occluded between the index finger and thumb, again to prevent the entry of air into the chest. The catheter, still occluded by finger and thumb, is then connected to an underwater-seal bottle by an assistant. Alternatively, the tube may be clamped first.

The disposable Argyle catheter and introducer may be used instead of the Malecot catheter.

Aftercare. Each day the drainage is measured and a known volume of sterile water replaced. The tube must be clamped while the bottle is being changed. Physiotherapy is most important to encourage both lung expansion and the restoration of chest wall movement.

Rib resection

Rib resection drainage is indicated if the pus is thick (more than one-third sediment), if aspiration and antibiotic replacement therapy has failed, or as a later procedure following intercostal tube drainage. *It must not be delayed too long*, or the empyema will become chronic. It must also be *adequate and dependent.*

If the empyema is drained at the correct time and proper aftercare is instituted, the lung will soon re-expand and the empyema obliterate. If the drainage has been unduly delayed, it may be preferable to carry out a decortication operation.

TECHNIQUE

Two important facts must be established before the actual rib resection is undertaken.

Is there a bronchopleural fistula? A patient who has a bronchopleural fistula *must* be drained in the sitting-up position under local anaesthesia (Figure 50.17). If a rib resection is done under general anaes-

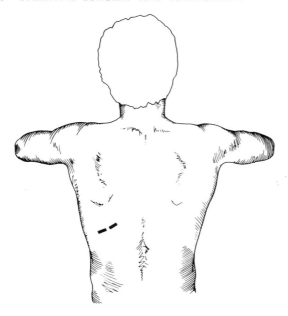

Figure 50.17 Sitting-up position and incision for rib resection and drainage of empyema

thesia in the lateral position a 'spill-over' aspiration pneumonia will occur in the contralateral lung, with a probable fatal outcome. A bronchopleural fistula may be excluded by gently turning the patient towards the opposite side – if this causes expectoration a fistula is likely. It may be confirmed by the injection of methylene blue into the empyema. If a fistula is present this will be obvious from the colour of the sputum. A radiological air/fluid level is diagnostic of bronchopleural fistula, unless a previous aspiration has been carried out or gas-forming organisms are present.

Which rib to resect? The drainage tube must be placed at the lowest point of the empyema cavity and therefore the rib to be resected must be determined before operation by radiography. Ten millilitres of Lipiodol or Dionosil (propyliodone) are injected into the empyema and posteroanterior and lateral chest radiographs are taken (*with extra penetration*) to show not only the radio-opaque dye at the bottom of the cavity but also the lowermost ribs, and in particular whether or not the 12th rib is short or long (and therefore palpable), for it is from *below upwards* that the ribs are counted at operation (Figure 50.18). The 7th–9th rib in the posterior axillary line or the 8th–10th rib in the scapular line is usually the correct site for drainage, but each case must be individually assessed by radiographic localization.

Rib resection. An oblique incision through skin and muscles is made over the appropriate rib, about 5 cm of which should be resected (Figure 50.17). If much fibrin is present a longer segment should be removed to permit adequate inspection and removal of fibrin. A longitudinal incision is made with a diathermy needle in the periosteum, which is then elevated

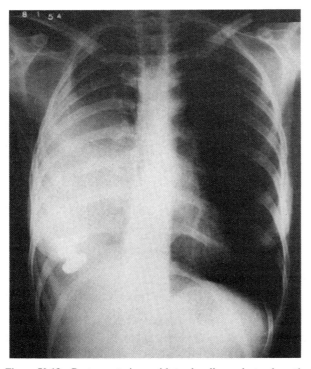
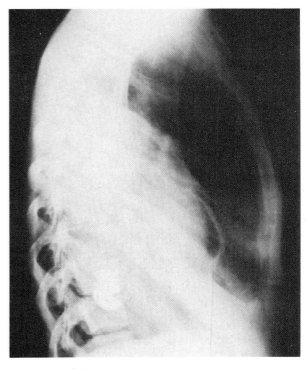

Figure 50.18 Posteroanterior and lateral radiographs to show the lowermost extent of the empyema cavity which has been demonstrated by injecting Dionosil. It is important that these radiographs are taken with extra penetration.

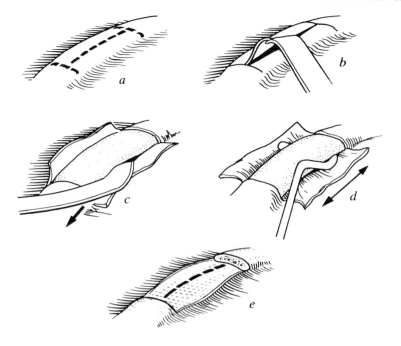

Figure 50.19 Subperiosteal resection of a segment of rib prior to drainage of empyema

towards the upper and lower borders of the rib (Figure 50.19). The periosteum is cleared from the upper and lower borders of the rib in the direction shown, to avoid damaging the obliquely placed intercostal muscles, and then from the undersurface of the rib, using a Doyen raspatory. The rib is then divided as close as possible to the edge of the elevated periosteum, to avoid leaving any rib denuded of periosteum, which might later develop osteomyelitis. A wide-bore aspirating needle should confirm that the correct rib has been removed. The rib bed is incised keeping towards its upper border to avoid damaging the intercostal vessels. A pleural biopsy should be taken if there is any suspicion of tuberculosis or carcinoma – it is probably wise to take a biopsy in all cases. The empyema cavity is opened the full length of the incision, the fluid sucked out, the cavity inspected with a sterile light, fibrin removed with sponge-holding forceps and a *wide-bore* tube (internal diameter at least 1 cm) inserted well into the cavity. The wound is closed in layers around the tube using catgut for the muscles. The tube should be fixed in place, as shown in Figure 50.20. Except in a small localized empyema, closed drainage to an underwater drainage bottle is preferable since it diminishes the number of dressings and encourages early lung expansion by re-establishing a negative intrapleural pressure (Figure 50.21).

Postoperative management

The subsequent management is most important – *inadequate postoperative care is the most common cause of a chronic empyema.* Breathing exercises are

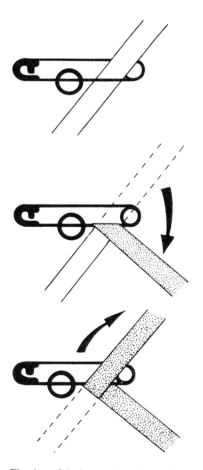

Figure 50.20 Fixation of drainage tube using adhesive strapping. Note that the adhesive surface faces outwards in the upper diagram

essential and the patient should get out of bed as soon as possible to walk round the ward. While still on closed drainage the patient should carry the bottle in a special carrier. Closed drainage may be converted to open drainage as soon as the drainage is less than 100 ml daily. Care must be taken that the tube does not become blocked by fibrin, and should this happen the tube will cease to 'swing' with respiration. Serial sinograms should be taken every week and the tube adjusted as necessary. The tube may need to be *lengthened*, even though the cavity has become smaller. The patient should be discharged from hospital as soon as possible and arrangements made for daily dressings as an outpatient and serial radiographs every 2–3 weeks.

Suction is *not* advisable. If suction is applied the lower lobe may expand prematurely so that the upper portion of the empyema becomes separated off, requiring a second rib resection higher up.

Irrigations are not necessary for they do nothing to aid recovery.

The drainage tube should *never* be removed from an empyema cavity! While there is still a cavity the tube should remain in place. It should only be removed when the sinogram shows a tube track only. *One of the commonest causes of a chronic empyema is premature removal of the drainage tube.*

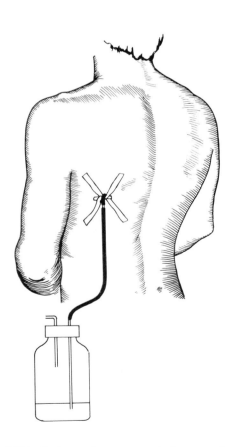

Figure 50.21 Drainage of empyema cavity into an underwater seal

3. Decortication

The operation of decortication consists of the complete removal of the fibrous walls of the empyema cavity from both the lung and the chest wall and diaphragm to allow the underlying lung to expand and fill the space previously occupied by the empyema. Originally confined to the treatment of sterile empyema, it is now being increasingly used in the treatment of cases of infected empyema following their near sterilization by intrapleural antibiotics. This is naturally a more extensive operation than a simple rib resection drainage but with the rapid expansion of the lung, the period of convalescence is reduced from many weeks to days.

The operation is a major procedure and should only be undertaken in a previously fit patient whose general condition is still reasonably good. It is not advisable in the elderly.

Operative technique

Elective hypotension may be provided by the anaesthetist, as there is always considerable oozing from the lung and chest wall during the removal of the thick layer of fibrin (Figure 50.22).

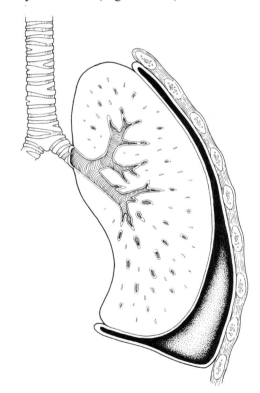

Figure 50.22 Chronic empyema cavity showing thickened, fibrous layer on its internal and external surfaces

A posterolateral thoracotomy with resection of the whole of the 5th rib will give good access. The ribs are always very close together and entry into the chest

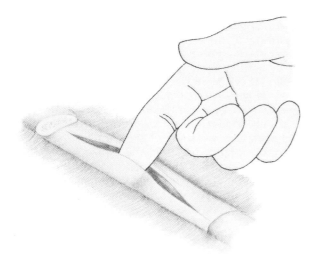

Figure 50.23 Decortication of empyema. Commencement of extrapleural strip deep to the incised periosteum

will be very difficult unless a rib is excised. Resection of 2 cm of the posterior ends of the 4th and 6th ribs will provide extra exposure if required. The rib bed is incised and the extrapleural layer entered by blunt dissection with the finger or Roberts forceps. The outer layer of the empyema is stripped off the chest wall by a combination of blunt and sharp dissection (Figure 50.23). Considerable force may be required. The mobilization of the lung is continued over the apex and down the mediastinum to the hilum (Figure 50.24). Great care must be taken not to damage the superior vena cava or azygos vein on the right side or the innominate vein or aorta on the left side, nor the vagus and phrenic nerves, though fortunately the dissection is usually easier in this area. The mobilization should be carried down to and over the diaphragm, though it may prove to be impossible to free the diaphragm completely. The inner wall of the empyema is next peeled off the surface of the lung, starting at a point where there appears to be a good plane of separation.

In practice, the empyema cavity itself may be accidentally opened before it has been mobilized from the chest wall and diaphragm or alternatively it may be necessary to open it intentionally if complete parietal mobilization proves to be too difficult. In such a case the empyema cavity should be sucked dry and all fibrin removed. A *long* linear or cruciate incision should then be made in the thickened visceral pleura until the normal lung surface can be seen underneath. The thick layer of fibrin can then be 'peeled off' the whole of the lung by a combination of sharp and blunt dissection. It is preferable to leave very adherent portions of fibrin on the lung surface rather than produce too many air leaks by their attempted removal.

Finally, and this is important and rewarding, the fissures between the lobes should be opened up. It will be surprising how much invagination of lung has

occurred and how much increased expansion of lung will be produced.

After operation there is always considerable drainage and it is therefore wise to insert *three* underwater-seal drainage tubes – one apical, one posterior basal and one anterior basal, all connected to strong suction to encourage rapid lung expansion which reduces bleeding.

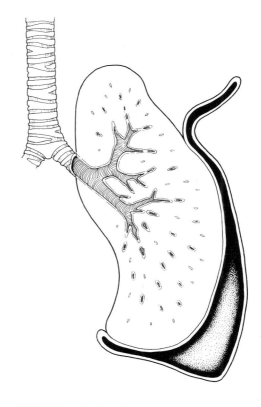

Figure 50.24 Decortication of empyema. The thick layer of fibrin on the parietal and visceral pleura is excised completely

Complications of an undrained empyema

An undrained persistent empyema may rupture into the lung and result in a bronchopleural fistula or it may rupture onto the skin surface and cause an empyema necessitas.

1. Bronchopleural fistula

This is an acute emergency. The patient will suddenly expectorate large quantities of purulent fluid, which will increase when the patient lies towards the opposite side and will cease almost immediately if laid on the affected side. If untreated the patient will develop an inhalation pneumonia into the contralateral lung or even succumb from 'drowning' if the empyema is large. It is imperative that the empyema be drained as soon as possible by intercostal tube or rib resection *under local anaesthesia in the sitting position*. Until this is done the patient *must* lie on the affected side, which will immediately prevent further expectoration.

2. Empyema necessitas

An empyema necessitas may not point immediately over the underlying empyema. The pus may track along tissue planes (including the intercostal vessels) and commonly points anteriorly. Radiographical localization must be carried out before rib resection drainage is undertaken.

Chronic empyema

An empyema which persists for more than 2 months may arbitrarily be defined as chronic, and the most common cause of this is imperfect treatment during the acute phase. The drainage may have been too late or inadequate or the drainage tube may be too small or have been removed too early. Another important cause is underlying lung disease – tuberculosis or bronchiectasis in the young or carcinoma in the middle-aged and elderly. It may also be due to a retained drainage tube or swab. A chronic empyema can usually be prevented, although the correct time for surgical drainage in the acute stage requires considerable clinical judgement and experience.

Before embarking on any further surgical treatment, underlying lung disease must be excluded by bronchoscopy, examination of pleural pus for tuberculosis or actinomycosis and histological examination of the pleura or granulation tissue for tuberculosis or carcinoma.

Treatment (if there is no underlying lung disease)

1. Redrainage

A chronic empyema will often obliterate if adequate dependent drainage is instituted, together with ardent physiotherapy and activity on the part of the patient.

2. Decortication

Simple redrainage may not produce rapid healing of the empyema and because of this a decortication (see above) is advisable if the patient is sufficiently fit for this major procedure and the underlying lung is healthy.

3. Roberts' flap operation

An alternative procedure to decortication is a Roberts' flap operation. It is indicated if it is considered that the lung would not expand sufficiently well after a decortication, perhaps because of old-standing fibrotic changes. In this operation a subperiosteal resection of the ribs overlying the empyema cavity and well beyond the margins of the cavity posteriorly

is carried out. This decostalized portion of chest wall (consisting of thickened parietal pleura, periosteum and intercostal muscle) is then made into a U-shaped flap by cutting along its anterior, upper and inferior borders. It is hinged posteriorly to preserve its blood supply (Figures 50.25 and 50.26). This flap is then turned inwards against the medial wall of the cavity, the whole of which has been freshened by thorough curettage. The two walls of the empyema are maintained in contact by a flavine gauze pack placed outside the flap. The skin, subcutaneous tissues and chest wall muscle are sutured over the pack and a further pad strapped over the skin surface. Ten days later the pack is removed, a temporary corrugated rubber drain inserted in its place, and the wound resutured. A sinus may persist for a few weeks after this operation but usually it will ultimately heal.

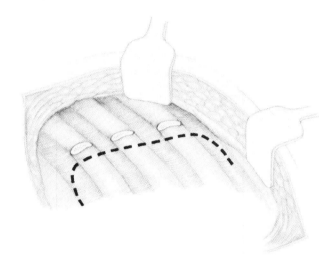

Figure 50.25 Roberts' flap operation for chronic empyema. Rib resection prior to incision into empyema cavity to produce U-shaped flap, hinged posteriorly

4. Schede operation

Schede operation is indicated if the empyema cavity is very small. The cavity is 'unroofed' by resecting subperiosteally the overlying rib or ribs, excising the thickened parietal pleura over the cavity, and packing the cavity open with dry gauze. The gauze pack is changed regularly until the residual cavity has filled with granulation tissue and is covered by epithelium.

Both the Roberts' flap and Schede operations are now rarely performed.

Chronic sinus

A chronic sinus (which implies the discharge of a small amount of pus on the skin surface) must always be examined radiographically following the injection of radio-opaque material. It may be due to an underlying empyema, often surprisingly large. It may also be due to osteomyelitis at the end of the previously resected rib, a retained nylon stitch, infected costal cartilage, a tuberculous gland under a rib, or even a retained drainage tube or swab. These causes will all be apparent on the chest radiograph or at subsequent operation.

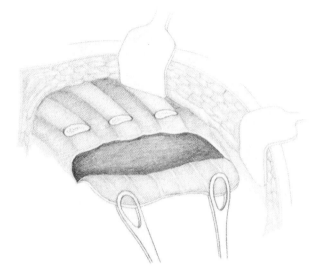

Figure 50.26 Roberts' flap operation for chronic empyema showing posterior hinged flap

Any underlying cause must be treated. An osteomyelitic portion of rib should be excised or infected cartilage removed. If the infected cartilage is part of the 6th–10th cartilage complex, all of the cartilage must be removed and the operation may be much more extensive than had been anticipated. A tuberculous gland should be removed after excision of the overlying rib. If there is no underlying cause and the empyema is small, a Schede type of operation should be carried out. If the underlying empyema is large, an adequate redrainage operation may be sufficient to obtain healing. Alternatively a decortication or a Roberts' flap operation will be required.

Recurrent and chronic pneumothorax (Smith and Rothwell, 1962; Sengupta, 1963; Killen and Gobbel, 1968)

A chronic pneumothorax implies the persistence of a small bronchopleural fistula which maintains the pneumothorax and causes minimal symptoms. This persisting pneumothorax is usually due to a leaking bleb or bulla, though there may be no apparent cause. It most commonly occurs in the 20–30-year age group due to a congenital bleb, or in the 50–60-year age group due to an emphysematous bulla. In some elderly patients there may also be gross emphysema

associated with bronchospasm. At any time, however, the fistula may become valvular, causing an increase in size of the pneumothorax or even a 'tension' pneumothorax.

Although there is wide divergence of views concerning the treatment of recurrent and chronic pneumothorax, ranging from observation alone to bilateral parietal pleurectomy (on the basis that the underlying lung pathology is a bilateral condition), the generally accepted regimen for the treatment of this condition is:

1. Intercostal tube for first and second attack.
2. Parietal pleurectomy for third or subsequent attacks and also for chronic (persisting) pneumothorax, together with ligation of bullae if present.
3. Instillation of a pleural irritant for elderly patients not fit for pleurectomy due to chronic bronchitis and emphysema.

These patients should not be treated conservatively because of the risk of tension pneumothorax or a haemothorax from a torn adhesion.

Differential diagnosis

It is most important to differentiate a pneumothorax from a large emphysematous bulla – if an intercostal tube is inserted into a bulla, a tension pneumothorax may occur. An unusual but not very rare presentation of a bronchial carcinoma may be by spontaneous pneumothorax – this underlying pathology will usually be apparent on the chest radiograph.

Treatment

1. Intercostal tube

The tube should be inserted in the 2nd intercostal space in the mid-clavicular line.

2. Parietal pleurectomy

Parietal pleurectomy should be advised in a patient who has had two or more previous pneumothoraces, who has a persisting pneumothorax, or who has radiological evidence of a bulla, provided that the patient is fit for thoracotomy. It is carried out through a small posterolateral or axillary thoracotomy in the 5th space. The plane between the parietal pleura and the endothoracic fascia can easily be developed by blunt dissection and the parietal pleura stripped from the chest wall over the upper half of the thoracic cage above the thoracotomy incision – over the apex and down over the mediastinum to the level of the hilum, anteriorly to the sternum and posteriorly to the paravertebral gutter. If any blebs, bullae or cysts are present they should be treated as described on page 770.

3. Instillation of a pleural irritant

This procedure is reserved for patients who are considered unfit for thoracotomy, usually because of age or poor respiratory function. The daily injection through the intercostal tube of 50 ml 50% glucose will almost always seal the air leak. Iodized talc may also be used to produce a chemical pleurisy, though the recurrence rate is at least 30% and probably higher. Silver nitrate produces very severe pain and is not now advised, nor is camphor in oil.

Chylothorax (Gingell, 1965; Roy et al., 1967; Ross, 1978; Milsom et al., 1985)

Anatomy of the thoracic duct

The thoracic duct ascends from the abdomen through the aortic opening in the diaphragm to the left of the vena azygos. It passes up the posterior mediastinum, to the right of the midline between the azygos vein and the aorta. At the level of the 7th thoracic vertebra the duct passes obliquely upwards to reach the left side of the mediastinum at the level of the 5th thoracic vertebra. It passes behind the oesophagus at this level and then passes upwards along the left border of the oesophagus to the neck where it enters the junction of the internal jugular and subclavian veins. Occasionally there is an extra terminal branch which enters the veins on the right side of the neck. In about 50% of individuals, two or more ducts are present at some stage in its course through the mediastinum. There are, in addition, numerous other connections between the main thoracic duct and the azygos, intercostal and lumbar veins. This collateral circulation is so extensive that the duct may be ligated at any point in its course without any untoward effect.

Aetiology

The duct may have been damaged during an operation in its vicinity, e.g. Blalock operation, operation for coarctation of the aorta or thoracoplasty (though curiously oesophageal operations are rarely complicated by a leak of chyle), or there may be evidence of malignancy or a history of hyperextension injury, which may rupture the duct just above the diaphragm. In many cases no cause can be found. Treatment must be active because 50% of cases are said to die from inanition.

Treatment

The initial treatment is repeated aspiration of the pleural cavity to dryness, in the hope of obtaining full expansion of the lung and cessation of the leak. With this regimen the leak will cease in 50% of cases within 2–3 weeks. The advice regarding diet during this time is conflicting. Some advise a low fat and protein diet in the hope of reducing chyle secretion and therefore aiding closure of the leak. This would seem logical, and it should be combined with supplementary intravenous feeding if necessary. Others advise a high fat and protein diet in order to prevent deterioration of the patient's condition from dietary insufficiency. This will, of course, *increase* chyle production, and tend to keep the leak open.

If chyle production continues unabated, closed intercostal drainage will be necessary to try to obtain complete lung expansion, and if this fails, early thoracotomy is indicated. Cream taken by mouth 4 h before operation will help to identify the damaged duct. If the cause was a recent operation, then that area should be explored and the injured duct sutured. If no previous operation has been carried out, then a thoracotomy on the side of the effusion should be undertaken. The chyle is aspirated and the pleura will be seen to be covered by a whitish exudate. The mediastinum will look swollen and be exuding chyle. This area should be opened up and an attempt made to identify the duct, which should then be sutured on either side of the tear. If this is not possible the area should be encircled with sutures tied over generous quantities of fibrin foam. If these procedures fail to cure the leak, then the duct should be ligated through a low thoracotomy just above the diaphragm. This is much easier through a right thoracotomy, for at this level the duct is to the right of the midline. If a left-sided approach is used, it may be necessary to mobilize the aorta to gain access to the duct. Iodized talc pleurodesis (see above) has also been suggested as a treatment for chylothorax.

Intractable cases may be treated by the Denver double valve peritoneal shunt (Milsom et al., 1985)

Part 3

Tumours of the lung

The most common tumour of the lung is carcinoma which arises in a main or lobar bronchus, or less often more peripherally. Other tumours, comprising about 4% of cases, may be innocent hamartoma, carcinoid adenoma of low-grade malignancy, or an adenoid cystic carcinoma (cylindroma) of relatively low-grade malignancy.

Resection is the treatment of choice for carcinoma of the lung, by standard pneumonectomy (simple extrapericardial), extended pneumonectomy (radical intrapericardial), lobectomy, or by segmental resection, provided (1) the patient is fit enough to undergo operation (see page 740), (2) there is no evidence of spread of the growth outside the chest, (3) there is no clinical or investigatory evidence of inoperability, and (4) the growth is not undifferentiated small cell carcinoma, although there is undoubtedly a small group of patients with this histological type of growth in whom resection *is* advisable (Levison 1980; Shore and Paneth, 1980; Prasad *et al.*, 1989)

Evidence of spread of growth outside the chest

Metastases may occur in the supraclavicular glands, liver, lumbar and thoracic vertebrae, pelvis, ribs, brain and long bones and these must be excluded as far as possible. Supraclavicular glands may be palpable on the same or contralateral side, and growths in the left lung not uncommonly spread to the right supraclavicular area. Secondary deposits in the liver are best diagnosed by CT scan. Radioactive liver scan reports are often equivocal and the place of ultrasound has not yet been established – it is probably more reliable than a radioactive scan. A recent onset of pain in the back must be investigated by appropriate radiographs, including lateral tomography, together with radioactive bone scan. Likewise, a recent onset of headache, muscular weakness in a limb or epileptiform fits must raise the possibility of a cerebral secondary deposit and suggest the need for brain or CT scan.

Clinical or investigatory evidence of inoperability

Superior vena caval obstruction or left recurrent laryngeal paralysis causing a hoarse voice may both be presenting symptoms, usually of upper lobe growths, and both imply inoperability. Bronchoscopic evidence of inoperability includes actual involvement by tumour of the trachea or main bronchus at its origin (not merely distortion by glands or growth *outside* the lumen) or gross widening of the carina or its involvement by growth. The significance of rigidity of a main bronchus is not easy to assess. Phrenic nerve paralysis in the presence of an upper lobe growth implies inoperability, but if the growth is in the middle or lower lobe, resection may still be possible by opening the pericardium which often seems to act as a barrier to the spread of the growth. Dysphagia must be investigated by a barium swallow – actual involvement of the oesophageal mucosa indicates inoperability. Mere displacement of the oesophagus may only signify para-oesophageal glands which may be removable at operation. The Pancoast syndrome (a small growth in the apex of the lung, which involves the 1st rib, 1st thoracic and 8th cervical nerves and stellate ganglion causing a Horner's syndrome) is usually regarded as inoperable, but Paulson (1974) has treated 26 of these cases by preoperative radiotherapy followed by resection and obtained a 10-year survival in 8. Chest wall involvement is not a contraindication, for it may be possible to resect a large area and replace it with a prosthesis of tantalum gauze or Marlex mesh. A pleural effusion, whether or not bloodstained, is likewise not a contraindication, for it is not necessarily due to the carcinoma – it may be due to an infarct or infection distal to a carcinoma. Axillary node biopsy, unless the gland is hard and clearly malignant, is generally not rewarding, for such nodes are frequently palpable in otherwise normal men.

The value of routine mediastinoscopy in the assessment of patients with bronchial carcinoma is debatable. Some authorities (Nohl-Oser, 1976) are of the opinion that the presence of positive mediastinal lymph nodes contraindicates thoracotomy but, on the other hand, these nodes are often removable at operation and many such patients are known to have been cured of their growth, especially if the involved nodes are low (Shields, 1989). The crux of the matter is 'What is the significance of a positive node obtained at mediastinoscopy?' The answer is not yet known and the problem may well be more complex than it appears. CT scan of the thorax has recently been found to be of considerable value in the assessment of mediastinal gland enlargement, although unfortunately not necessarily of involvement. Contralateral mediastinal lymph node involvement is a definite contraindication to resection.

Only about one-third of patients with bronchial carcinoma are suitable for thoracotomy, and of these about 10% per cent are found to be unresectable at operation.

TNM staging of lung carcinoma (Spiro and Goldstraw, 1984)

The revised TNM International Clinical Staging System enables tumours to be classified according to their size, lymph node involvement and presence of distant metastases.

T   *Pulmonary tumour*
TX   Malignant cells in sputum or bronchial washings. Radiograph normal.
TIS   Carcinoma *in situ.*
T1   Tumour 3 cm or less in size and no evidence on bronchoscopy of invasion of a bronchus proximal to a lobar bronchus.
T2   Tumour more than 3 cm in size; or a tumour of any size that invades visceral pleura or obstructs a bronchus; or at bronchoscopy at least 2 cm distal to the main carina.
T3   Tumour of any size with direct extension into parietal pleura, chest wall, diaphragm or mediastinum; or a tumour involving main bronchus less than 2 cm distal to carina; or any tumour associated with obstruction to a main bronchus or a pleural effusion.
T4   Tumour of any size with invasion of mediastinum; or involving heart, great vessels, trachea, oesophagus, vertebral body or carina; or presence of a malignant pleural effusion.

N   *Node involvement*
N0   No involvement of regional lymph nodes.
N1   Involvement of peribronchial or ipsilateral hilar lymph nodes.

N2 Involvement of ipsilateral mediastinal lymph nodes.

N3 Involvement of contralateral mediastinal, scalene or supraclavicular lymph nodes.

M Distant metastases

M0 No (known) distant metastases.

M1 Distant metastases present.

Choice of operation

Pneumonectomy might seem to be the only logical operation for carcinoma of the lung, but as many of these patients also have chronic bronchitis this operation is often unfortunately very disabling and many are never able to resume work, especially if they are over the age of 55 years. Because of this, lobectomy and much less often segmental resection are both carried out and have provided excellent results in terms of cure rate as well as quality of life (Bates, 1981). Lobectomy for peripheral carcinoma is as effective in curing the patient as pneumonectomy – and has a lower operative mortality (Belcher, 1959; Flavell, 1962).

Segmental resection for small peripheral carcinoma in the elderly has also provided satisfactory results (Bates, 1975). Lobectomy is sometimes combined with segmental resection of an adjacent lobe, e.g. upper lobectomy with resection of the apical segment of the lower lobe, or lower lobectomy with resection of the lingular segment of the left upper lobe or the posterior segment of the upper lobe. It is often only possible to make the final decision at operation. In many thoracic surgical centres a pneumonectomy or lobectomy is carried out with equal frequency.

Indications for lobectomy

1. Patients in whom the growth is relatively peripheral and confined to one lobe (or middle and right lower lobe). In the case of an upper lobe growth, especially on the right, it is possible to obtain almost as good a clearance of lymphatic glands as by pneumonectomy.

2. Patients who are considered unfit for pneumonectomy because of age or impaired lung function.

Indications for segmental resection

A localized peripheral tumour in an elderly patient with poor respiratory function.

Operative technique for pneumonectomy

This may be *'standard'* pneumonectomy with division of the pulmonary vessels outside the pericardium, together with removal of carinal, paratracheal, pretracheal and para-oesophageal lymph nodes if they appear to be involved, or it may be an *'extended' radical operation*, with division of the vessels inside

the pericardium, and removal of all the involved lymphatic glands described above. This 'extended' operation must of necessity be more limited on the left than the right because of the interposition of the aortic arch.

A posterolateral thoracotomy through the 5th rib bed provides the best exposure and allows the hilum to be approached both from in front and behind. The apex of the lung is mobilized and drawn downwards so that the aortic arch or azygos vein is clearly seen. The rest of the lung is mobilized so that a clear view of the hilum is obtained. If the lung is very adherent to the chest wall, an extrapleural strip should be carried out over the adherent area. Operability is decided by vision and palpation, although a final opinion may not be possible until the pericardium has been opened and a hilar dissection attempted. Mediastinal lymph node involvement must be assessed and a decision made whether to open the pericardium to divide the pulmonary artery and veins. On the right side the liver should be palpated and if necessary the diaphragm opened.

Signs of inoperability

1. Inability to separate growth from aorta or superior vena cava.

2. Inability to separate tumour from lower end of trachea.

3. Spread of growth along pulmonary veins to involve left atrium to such an extent that the vein cannot be divided, even by 'pinching up' a portion of atrial wall.

4. Spread of growth along pulmonary artery to such an extent that it cannot be divided, even on the left side proximal to the obliterated ductus arteriosus.

5. Inability to separate tumour from vertebral bodies.

6. Involvement of oesophageal mucosa

Standard pneumonectomy

In all cases (including lobectomy or segmental resection) it is theoretically advisable first to divide the vein draining the part of the lung containing the carcinoma to prevent tumour embolization during its manipulation. Thereafter it does not matter in which order the hilar structures are divided, although if there is an excessive amount of sputum or haemoptysis it is preferable at least to clamp, if not actually divide, the bronchus first.

The hilar anatomy is shown in Figures 50.27 and 50.28 which demonstrate that on the left side the main bronchus is just below and behind the pulmonary artery, the superior vein is immediately below the pulmonary artery and in front of the bronchus, and below both is the inferior vein. On the right side the pulmonary artery is immediately in front of the bronchus, with the superior vein just below and a little in front, and the inferior vein lower still.

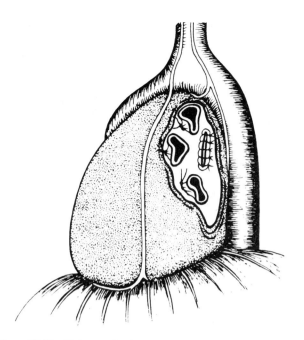

Figure 50.27 Major mediastinal structures following left pneumonectomy. The pulmonary artery is above and anterior to the left main bronchus. The superior pulmonary vein is immediately anterior to the bronchus and the inferior pulmonary vein lies below

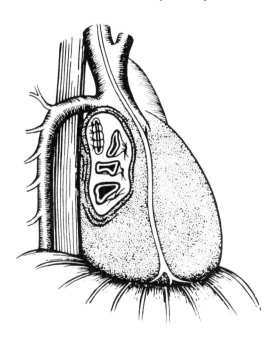

Figure 50.28 Mediastinal structures following right pneumonectomy. The pulmonary artery is anterior to the right main bronchus and the pulmonary veins lie below the pulmonary artery

The inferior or superior vein is divided first, according to the position of the tumour.

The *inferior vein* is exposed by retracting the lower lobe upwards and forwards so that the vein is approached from behind (Figure 50.29). The adven-

titia around the vein is incised, the vein isolated and then divided between two strong ligatures proximally and a clamp or another ligature distally, ensuring that an adequate cuff of vein remains. If necessary, the pericardium is opened to obtain greater length, and if still more length is required, an angled Satinsky clamp may be placed on the atrial wall, the vein divided and the atrium closed with a continuous 3/0 Mersilene stitch. The vein may be approached from in front or behind, or a combination of both. Not infrequently the tributary from the apex of the lower lobe enters the pericardium separately from the main vein to join it inside the pericardium.

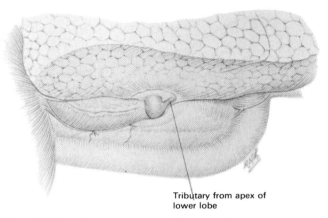

Tributary from apex of
lower lobe

Figure 50.29 Left pneumonectomy. Exposure of inferior pulmonary vein anterior to the oesophagus

Superior pulmonary vein

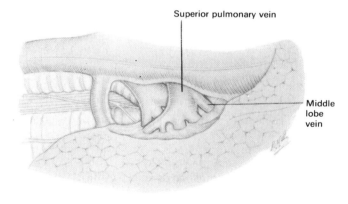

Middle
lobe
vein

Figure 50.30 Right pneumonectomy. Ligation and division of the right superior vein will expose the right main pulmonary artery and its main branches

The *superior vein* is approached from in front and the lung retracted backwards (Figure 50.30). As with the inferior vein, the pericardium is opened if necessary to obtain greater length on the vein for the ligature or to place a clamp on the atrium itself.

The *pulmonary artery* is next isolated, divided and sutured with 4/0 prolene and another ligature or clamp distally. If necessary, the pericardium may be opened and the artery divided and sutured within the pericardium. On the right side, there is a condensation of tissue between the superior vena cava and pulmonary artery which must be deliberately cut with scissors, and when it is divided a considerable extra length of pulmonary artery is obtained (Price Thomas manoeuvre). It is then very easy to encircle the artery so that it may be sutured with 0000 prolene.

Finally, the *bronchus* must be defined. The surrounding adventitious tissue containing bronchial arteries and pulmonary branches of the vagus must be divided between clamps. On the left side care must be taken to preserve the recurrent laryngeal nerve as it hooks around the obliterated ductus.

The bronchial stump is closed with interrupted figure-of-eight no. 2 SWG stainless steel wire sutures on atraumatic needles, placed so that the proximal loop is inserted under the blades of the clamp (Figure 50.33). It is important to cut the bronchial sutures short to avoid the danger of the ends of the wire suture perforating the oesophagus on the right, or the pulmonary artery on the left. Airtight closure may be confirmed by pouring saline onto the stump and requesting the anaesthetist to apply gentle pressure. It is sometimes possible to cover the bronchial stump with adjacent pleura. A pedicled intercostal muscle bundle is recommended by some surgeons.

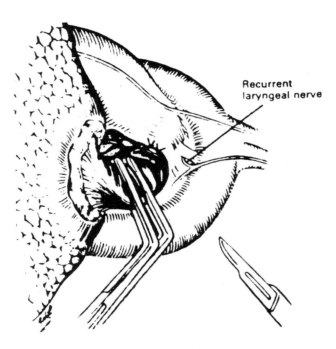

Figure 50.31 Left pneumonectomy. Following ligation of the left pulmonary artery and left upper lobe vein, the left main bronchus is dissected deep to the arch of the aorta and controlled with bronchial clamps prior to division

The bronchus must be divided flush with the carina to avoid pooling of pus in a long stump (Figures 50.31 and 50.32). If a clamp is used for bronchial closure it must be of the non-crushing variety. Alternatively, the bronchus may be divided with a knife and interrupted sutures placed in the cut open end as the division proceeds until the bronchus has been completely divided. The author's preferred technique is to use a non-crushing clamp placed on the bronchus with the handles towards the patient's head so that the membranous (posterior) wall of the bronchus is brought against the concavity of the C-shaped cartilage. Care must be taken to avoid placing the clamp too proximal or the opposite main bronchus may be narrowed or the anaesthetist's tube compressed and subsequently caught in the sutures. The bronchus is divided with a long-handled angled knife.

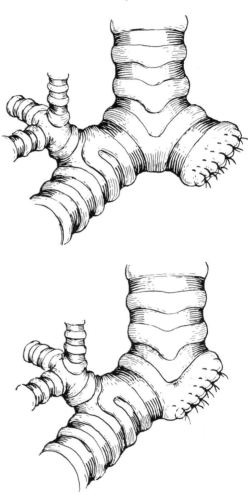

Figure 50.32 Pneumonectomy. Upper (incorrect) and lower (correct) level of division of the main bronchus.

The bronchus may also be safely closed using the 'Auto Suture' automatic stapler which inserts a double staggered row of staples through the bronchus, which can then be divided. Staples, 4.8 mm or 3.5 mm in size, are used for pneumonectomy or lobectomy, respectively. The incidence of postoperative bronchopleural fistula is considered to be less,

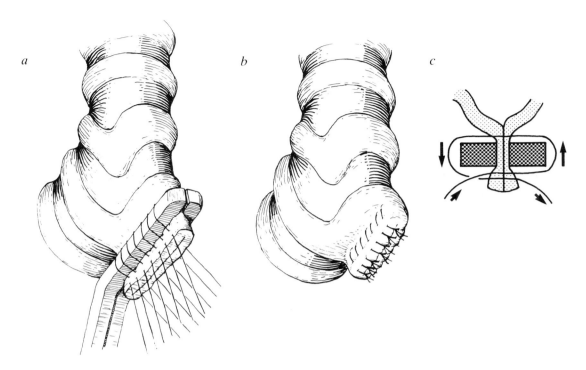

Figure 50.33 Pneumonectomy. Closure of bronchial stump using figure-of-eight interrupted wire sutures

especially if a 5/0 Mersilene continuous suture is placed along the distal end of the stapled bronchus.

Five points concerning the division of the pulmonary artery and veins

1. It is most important to ensure that the assistant relaxes on the lung retraction at the moment when the ligatures are being tied, to prevent the danger of the ligature 'cutting through'.

2. The distal ligatures may be multiple ligatures on the branches or tributaries of the vessel, rather than on the main vessel itself. Alternatively, if there is insufficient length of vessel for a distal ligature, a clamp may be used distally and the vessel divided with a knife flush with the clamp.

3. The ligature material must be reasonably thick – thin ligature may cut through the vessel.

4. The two proximal ligatures should be tied so that they overlap each other. There should be a cuff at least 1 cm long distal to the two ligatures. If this is not possible, then it is wise to apply a Satinsky clamp and after division suture the vessel with a continuous 4/0 Mersilene suture. A transfixion suture may cause problems and is not required if an adequate cuff of vessel is available.

5. The pulmonary artery and veins are all ensheathed in a layer of adventitia. It is most important to pick up this adventitia with forceps and deliberately cut it with scissors, so as to enter the correct layer. It should then be relatively and often surpris-

ingly easy, and certainly much safer, to pass a clamp around the vessel.

Extended (radical intrapericardial) pneumonectomy

If the growth is extensive with considerable mediastinal lymph node involvement, an early decision must be made whether to use the intrapericardial technique. The pericardium is opened around the whole lung root, both anteriorly and posteriorly. If possible, it is preferable to retract the phrenic nerve anteriorly and not divide it. This will avoid the paradoxical movement of the diaphragm which will occur after phrenic division and the consequent difficulty in expectoration during the postoperative period. However, the situation of the growth may make this impossible and the nerve may have to be divided.

On either side the dissection exposes the oesophagus and care must be taken not to damage it on the medial side of the main bronchus or in the region of the inferior pulmonary vein. A small portion of oesophageal muscle may be removed, provided that the mucosa is preserved. The lung is removed together with the subcarinal lymph nodes. On the right side the azygos vein is divided and the areola tissue containing the paratracheal and pretracheal lymph nodes is removed completely, exposing the side of the trachea, the superior vena cava and ascending aorta. The dissection is carried from the oesophagus behind to the internal mammary vessels in front. On the left side the vagus is divided below the recurrent laryngeal nerve unless there are so many glands in the subaortic fossa that the nerve has to be sacrificed. The lymphatic clearance is of necessity less complete on the left side.

Drainage after pneumonectomy

There is a surprising difference of opinion among thoracic surgeons concerning the advisability of draining the pleural space after pneumonectomy, and at a meeting of the Society of Cardiovascular Surgeons of Great Britain and Ireland members were equally divided in their views. It is the author's opinion that a basal intercostal tube connected to an underwater seal should always be inserted after a pneumonectomy. The tube should be clamped but be released every hour for 1 min only and the drainage noted. Suction must *never* be applied as this would lead to too much mediastinal displacement and cause hypotension by impairing venous return to the heart. The tube is removed after 24 h. If this routine is adopted, any postoperative haemorrhage will be obvious – this complication is not always easily diagnosed after pneumonectomy and patients who have not had a drain in place are known to have died without the cause being recognized. There is no risk of infection if the tube is removed after 24 h and, moreover, the need for postoperative aspiration is avoided.

If the space is not drained, the intrapleural pressure should be adjusted to a slightly negative level at the end of the operation by an intercostal catheter inserted through the third space anteriorly. This is then connected to an underwater seal and left in place until the patient has been placed on his back. It is then removed.

Operative technique for lobectomy

The final decision whether to carry out lobectomy or pneumonectomy must remain until the operation because the growth may be more extensive than anticipated. A posterolateral thoracotomy, through the 5th rib bed, is suitable for all lung resections.

In all cases of lobectomy or segmental resection, it is wise to request the anaesthetist to inflate the lung after the bronchus has been clamped and *before* it is divided, to ensure that the proposed division is not too proximal – a mistake surprisingly easy to make.

Upper lobectomy

This is a more difficult operation than lower lobectomy because of the more complex arrangement of the upper lobe arterial branches as they leave the main arterial trunk and the close proximity of the superior pulmonary vein to the main pulmonary artery to the lower lobe. This artery lies immediately posterior to the vein, damage to which will jeopardize the preservation of the lower lobe. The pulmonary

vein, which lies in front of the hilum, should be divided first, opening the pericardium if necessary.

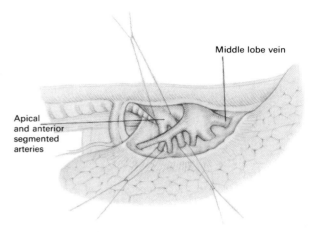

Middle lobe vein

Apical and anterior segmented arteries

Figure 50.34 Right upper lobectomy. The right upper lobe veins are ligated and divided. Note carefully that the middle lobe vein, a tributary of the right upper lobe vein, is preserved

RIGHT UPPER LOBECTOMY

The lobe is retracted posteriorly to expose the venous drainage. It is most important to preserve the middle lobe vein, which drains into the superior vein (Figure 50.34). The division of the veins to the upper lobe must therefore be distal to the middle lobe vein and this must first be identified. Division of the vein will expose the arterial branches, of which there are two or three. These are divided. The posterior segmental branch arises low down below the upper lobe bronchus and often quite close to the middle lobe artery. It may not easily be visible until the bronchus has been divided. Finally, the lobe is retracted forwards to expose the upper lobe bronchus. The margins are defined, the adventitia containing bronchial arteries divided between clamps and the upper lobe bronchus clamped. The bronchus is divided close to the main bronchus but not so close that the lumen is narrowed. This is most important to prevent postoperative lower lobe collapse. The bronchial stump is closed as described under pneumonectomy, or with simple interrupted 2/0 Ethibond sutures on a 25 mm half-circle eyeless needle. The hilar structures have now all been divided but the lobe may not yet be completely free – it may still be partially attached to the apex of the lower lobe and there may also be an incomplete fissure or no fissure between the upper and middle lobes. Attachment to the apex of the lower lobe is best managed by division of lung tissue between clamps. The apex of the lower lobe is then closed with a continuous suture over the clamp (Figure 50.35). The lobe is separated from the middle lobe by traction on the divided upper lobe bronchus and gentle blunt dissection with the index finger in the relatively avascular interlobar plane, as in segmental resection, beginning at the hilum and working towards the periphery. Inflation of the lung by the anaesthetist will help in the identification of the correct plane. Small air leaks and bleeding points are controlled by ligation. Finally, the pulmonary ligament should be divided so as to allow the lower lobe to swing upwards to fill the upper part of the chest.

If, as is usual, the fissure between the middle and lower lobes is complete, the middle lobe will be seen to be attached only by a narrow pedicle at the hilum; the lobe may therefore rotate, causing torsion, obstruction and later venous thrombosis. This can be prevented by attaching the middle lobe at 2–3 points along the periphery of the lower lobe by placing opposed artery forceps on the lung at these points and tying them together, incorporating a minute portion of lung tissue.

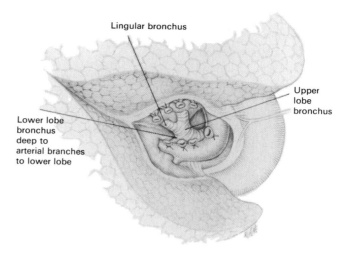

Figure 50.36 Left upper lobectomy. The left upper arterial branches have been divided and the left upper lobe bronchus is prepared for clamping and division

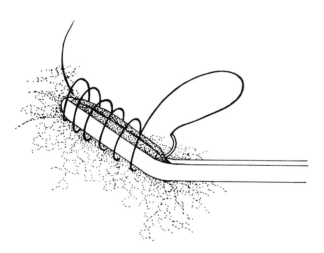

Figure 50.35 Closure of raw surface of lower lobe using a continuous suture over a clamp

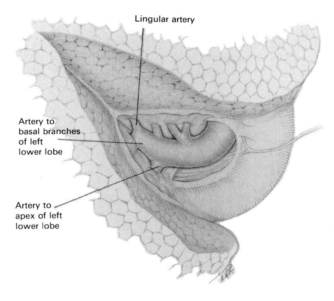

Figure 50.37 Left lower lobectomy. Note that the apical artery to the left lower lobe lies at a more proximal level than the lingular artery to the left upper lobe, necessitating individual attention to the apical lower artery and the three basal branches

LEFT UPPER LOBECTOMY

After division of the superior pulmonary vein the lobe is retracted anteriorly to expose the arterial branches, of which there are three to five (Figure 50.36). These branches are separately divided. The lingular artery may arise from a basal branch to the lower lobe and not from the main artery itself (Figure 50.37). The division must therefore not be too proximal. The artery to the lower lobe is retracted posteriorly to expose the upper lobe bronchus. The margins are defined, the adventitia containing bronchial arteries divided between clamps and the upper lobe bronchus clamped with a non-crushing clamp. The bronchus is divided close to the main bronchus but not so close that the lumen is narrowed. This is most important to prevent postoperative lower lobe collapse. The bronchial stump is closed as described under pneumonectomy, or with simple interrupted 2/0 Ethibond sutures on a 25 mm half-circle eyeless needle.

The hilar structures have now all been divided but the lobe may not be completely free – it may still be partially attached to the apex of the lower lobe. Attachment to the apex of the lower lobe is best managed by division of lung tissue between clamps. The apex of the lower lobe is then closed with a continuous suture over the clamp. Finally the pulmonary ligament should be divided to allow the lower lobe to swing upwards to fill the upper part of the chest.

Lower lobectomy

RIGHT LOWER LOBECTOMY

The inferior vein is divided first (see Operative Technique for Pneumonectomy). Care must be taken to preserve the right middle lobe artery, which arises opposite the artery to the apex of the lower lobe. The arteries to the apex of the lower lobe and the basal segments must all be divided separately. The bronchus, which lies deep to the divided arterial branches, is defined and the bronchus to the middle lobe identified – it arises opposite the apical lower lobe bronchus. It is necessary in most cases to divide the apical lower segmental bronchus and the lower lobe bronchus separately. If the middle lobe bronchus is more proximal than usual, this separate division may not be necessary.

If there is an incomplete fissure between the apex of the lower lobe and the upper lobe, the separation is as described under Upper Lobectomy.

LEFT LOWER LOBECTOMY

The inferior vein is divided first (see Operative Technique for Pneumonectomy). Care must be taken to preserve the lingular artery, which may arise from a basal branch artery or from the main artery (Figure 50.37). The arteries to the apex of the lower lobe and the basal segments must all be divided separately; it is never possible to ligate the artery to the lower lobe as a single trunk. Finally, the bronchus is defined by dividing the peribronchial tissue containing the bronchial arteries. The pulmonary artery is retracted anteriorly so that the upper lobe bronchus is identified. This identification of the upper lobe is important to prevent narrowing of the upper lobe bronchus by too proximal application of the bronchus clamp or even division of the main bronchus itself. The lower lobe bronchus is then clamped and divided close to the upper lobe, taking care not to narrow the origin of the upper lobe bronchus (Figure 50.38). The bronchial stump is closed as in upper lobectomy. A suture line flush with the upper lobe is important – a long stump is the usual cause of a bronchopleural fistula.

If there is an incomplete fissure between the apex of the lower lobe and the upper lobe, the separation is as described under upper lobectomy.

Middle lobectomy

The middle lobe is retracted posteriorly so as to expose the origin of the middle lobe vein, which is divided between ligatures close to its entry into the superior vein. The lobe is then retracted anteriorly and the oblique fissure between the middle lobe and lower lobe developed so as to expose the arterial branches to the middle and lower lobes. The middle lobe is supplied by one or two arteries which pass anteriorly from the right main pulmonary artery

opposite or just proximal to the branch to the apex of the lower lobe. The middle lobe artery is divided between ligatures, and the middle lobe bronchus can then be seen and defined. It is divided and closed as in upper and lower lobectomy. The middle lobe can now be removed by traction on the middle lobe bronchus and gentle dissection with the index finger in the plane between the middle and upper lobes. Inflation of the upper lobe by the anaesthetist will help to define the correct plane. Small air leaks and bleeding points are controlled by ligatures.

If the oblique fissure is incomplete, dissection to expose the middle lobe artery may be time-consuming or even dangerous. In such a case it may be preferable, after division of the middle lobe vein, to identify the bronchus from in front, which is situated immediately deep to the divided vein. After the bronchus has been divided the middle lobe artery or arteries will be clearly visible.

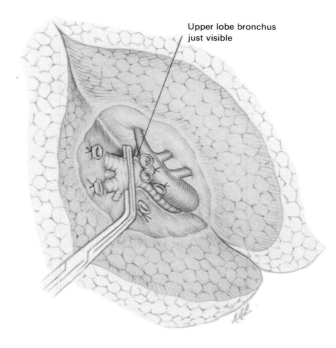

Upper lobe bronchus just visible

Figure 50.38 Left lower lobectomy. The pulmonary arterial branches to the lower lobe have been secured, preserving the lingular vessels. The left lower lobe bronchus has been clamped prior to division

Right middle and lower lobectomy

A right middle and lower lobectomy is not infrequently required for bronchial carcinoma. The technique for the venous and arterial ligation is as described for middle lobectomy and right lower lobectomy. The bronchial dissection is similar to a left lower lobectomy, i.e. the right upper lobe must be visualized before the bronchus clamp is applied so as to avoid a long bronchial stump or a narrowed right upper lobe bronchus.

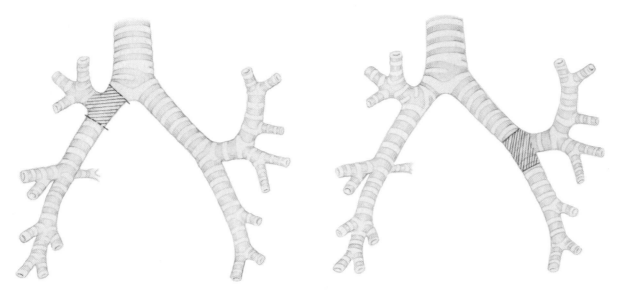

Figure 50.39 Sleeve resection of right upper lobe and left upper lobe. This is an acceptable method of dealing with malignant tumours situated at the mouth of the upper lobe in those patients with poor lung function who might not tolerate pneumonectomy

Upper lobectomy with 'sleeve' resection of the main bronchus (Johnson and Jones, 1959; Bennett and Smith, 1978; Kittle, 1989)

Upper lobectomy with 'sleeve' resection of the main bronchus is a most valuable procedure in those cases in which the growth involves the actual origin of the upper lobe bronchus at its junction with the main bronchus and where standard upper lobectomy would not provide a complete removal of the growth. In these cases a 'sleeve' of main bronchus is removed with the upper lobe and the two ends of the main bronchus are reanastomosed (Figure 50.39). This technique may be applied to the left or right upper lobe, although it is technically more difficult to perform on the left side because of the proximity of the aortic arch. The lymphatic drainage area can be removed as completely as by pneumonectomy. In older patients, or in younger patients with diminished respiratory reserve, this technique is most valuable in permitting the tumour to be removed, with preservation of the right lower and middle lobes or left lower lobe. If necessary the resection may be extended to include a 'sleeve' of the main pulmonary artery. The final decision concerning the possibility of 'sleeve' resection must be taken at thoracotomy. The technique is best reserved for squamous carcinoma or innocent tumours.

Anaesthesia into the opposite lung must be by double-lumen tube. If the tumour is localized and it is decided that this technique can be carried out, the venous and arterial dissection is performed as already described. The main bronchus is isolated and up to about 2.5 cm may be resected. The main bronchus is divided proximally and distally. The proximal end of the bronchus may be left open but the distal portion should be temporarily occluded with ribbon gauze to prevent the entry of blood. The upper lobectomy may then be completed as already described. The remaining lobe or lobes must be mobilized by division of the pulmonary ligament. The two ends of the bronchus are anastomosed with interrupted no. 3/0 Ethibond (Ethicon) on an atraumatic needle, with the knots on the outside of the bronchus. The main problem encountered is the discrepancy in size of the two portions of the bronchus. This can generally be overcome by placing the sutures closer together on the distal bronchus. If this does not suffice, the technique illustrated in Figure 50.40 may be used. Before final closure the lower lobe should be aspirated by a fine catheter. Airtight closure is easily obtained and the lower and middle lobes are then inflated by the anaesthetist. A flap of pleura should be placed between the bronchus and the pulmonary artery, to prevent the rare but well-recognized late complication of secondary haemorrhage from the pulmonary artery.

Perhaps rather surprisingly there are no special immediate postoperative problems after this operation. The main late complication is a stricture at the site of the anastomosis, but the incidence of this is not high.

Operative technique for segmental resection

Any segment of the lung may be resected, although in the case of carcinoma it is the lingula or apical segment of the lower lobe that is most commonly removed (Le Roux, 1972; Kittle, 1989).

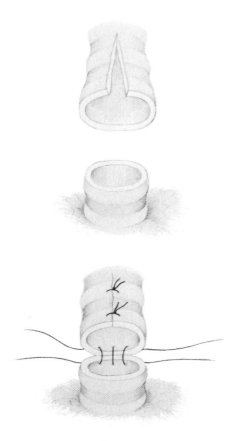

Figure 50.40 Sleeve resection. Method of tailoring the right main bronchus prior to airtight closure

General principles

Each bronchopulmonary segment has its own individual artery and bronchus. The vein runs *between* the segments in the intersegmental plane, receiving tributaries from both adjacent segments. When a segment is to be resected the appropriate segmental artery and bronchus are divided at the hilum. A clamp is then placed on the distal end of the bronchus. The segment can be separated from the adjacent lung by traction on this bronchus and gentle dissection with the index finger from the hilum outwards in the relatively avascular intersegmental plane. The correct plane is shown by the line of the intersegmental vein which must remain in place undisturbed. Its tributaries from the segment to be removed are divided. Inflation of the remainder of the lung by increased endotracheal pressure by the anaesthetist will assist in defining the correct line of separation.

There is only minimal air leak from the damaged alveoli and these soon seal off with swab pressure. Very little, if any, lung suture is required. The raw surface of the lung should not be oversewn, as any attempt to do this will only increase the air leak. The bronchial stump is closed by an 'open' technique with two or three simple stainless steel or Ethiflex sutures.

Lingulectomy

The lingular vein (situated anteriorly) is first divided. The lingular artery is next divided (for anatomy, see Left Lower Lobectomy) and finally the origin of the lingular bronchus is defined prior to its division. It is the first inferior branch of the upper lobe bronchus.

Apical lower segmentectomy

The vein is situated posteriorly. It drains into the inferior vein although sometimes it enters the pericardium separately. The artery is approached through the oblique fissure. The artery is divided and immediately underneath the segmental bronchus will be seen and this too is divided.

Other tumours of the lung

1. Hamartoma

At operation a hamartoma is freely mobile within the lung substance like a fibro-adenoma of the breast. It can always be removed by grasping the tumour between thumb and forefinger and making a small incision in the overlying lung – the tumour will then 'pop out'. The lung incision is closed by interrupted catgut sutures placed so as to obliterate the cavity. Alternatively a wedge resection can be carried out.

2. Carcinoid (adenoma)

This is a tumour of very low malignancy (Lawson *et al.*, 1976). It often presents as a well-defined red lobulated mass which protrudes into a bronchus and has a narrow pedicle. It sometimes bleeds profusely on biopsy. Local excision of the tumour by bronchotomy is the procedure of choice, provided that the tumour is small and distal bronchiectatic changes have not occurred (Hurt and Bates, 1984; McCaughan *et al.*, 1985; Stamatis *et al.*, 1990). Frequently, however, a segmental resection, lobectomy or even pneumonectomy is required.

Resection for pulmonary metastases

During the past 15 years, limited and often repeated resections of pulmonary metastases by wedge or segmental resection, or in some cases lobectomy, have been increasingly performed. The best results have been obtained if the patient is symptom free and the disease interval is greater than 1 year (Wright *et al.*, 1982; Mountain *et al.*, 1984; McIntosh and Thatcher, 1990)

Complications of lung resection

Apart from haemorrhage, bronchospasm, sputum retention, pulmonary collapse and cardiac arrhythmias, the most important complications are persistent air space, empyema and bronchopleural fistula.

1. Persistent air space

Although an important bronchopleural fistula may not be demonstrated, the majority of these patients do, in fact, have a pinhole leak which is responsible for this complication. Usually the leak will ultimately close – if not, a small thoracoplasty may be required. If infection occurs, necessitating rib resection drainage, the fistula will usually close spontaneously.

2. Empyema following lobectomy or segmental resection, uncomplicated by bronchopleural fistula

The diagnosis will be suspected by the onset of fever with radiological evidence of increased fluid. There may be discharge of pus at the site of the drainage tube. The diagnosis should be confirmed by diagnostic aspiration and the empyema should be drained.

3. Post-pneumonectomy empyema without demonstrable bronchopleural fistula (Goldstraw, 1993)

It is sometimes possible to sterilize these empyemas by daily aspiration and the instillation of antibiotics, but often rib resection drainage of the empyema will be required. Opening up and marsupialization of the space have been recommended as a method of sterilizing such a cavity. More recently, pedicled grafts of omentum have been successfully used to obliterate the residual space (Mathisen et al., 1988), or a further technique, in association with a plastic surgeon, is the use of extensive vascularized chest wall muscle flaps, using the latissimus dorsi or trapezius muscles (Miller et al., 1984; Pairolero, 1990). Finally, if these measures fail or are not used, and in the presence of persistent infection, it is worth while considering a ten-rib thoracoplasty. These major procedures should be reserved only for those patients who appear to be long-term survivors from their carcinoma.

4. Postoperative bronchopleural fistula

AFTER LOBECTOMY OR SEGMENTAL RESECTION

This complication is uncommon but must be suspected if the patient expectorates bloodstained sputum and develops an air space with a fluid level. Should this space not obliterate completely with tube drainage and suction, further operation and resuture of the bronchus or leaking lung together with removal of the fibrin peel are advised.

AFTER PNEUMONECTOMY (Goldstraw, 1993)

A bronchopleural fistula following a pneumonectomy is a very major disaster and all too often ultimately leads to the death of the patient or a permanent tube or stoma drainage of the pneumonectomy space. It may be associated from the beginning with infection in the pneumonectomy space, and it almost always occurs on the right side, usually in those cases in which the blood supply to the bronchial stump has been reduced by the removal of enlarged pretracheal or paratracheal lymph nodes. Most cases occur from 4 to 21 days after operation, but a fistula may develop months or even years after operation.

The diagnosis is made by the sudden expectoration of bloodstained sputum, exacerbated by the patient lying towards the contralateral lung and dramatically relieved by lying towards the pneumonectomy side (Figure 50.41). The development of a fistula is a surgical emergency and the patient must be instructed to lie on the pneumonectomy side (which will immediately abolish the cough and expectoration) until the chest has been emptied of fluid, either by intercostal tube or thoracoscopic suction. If the fistula is small or there is doubt concerning the diagnosis, the instillation of methylene blue dye into the pneumonectomy space will confirm the diagnosis. The sputum will immediately change colour.

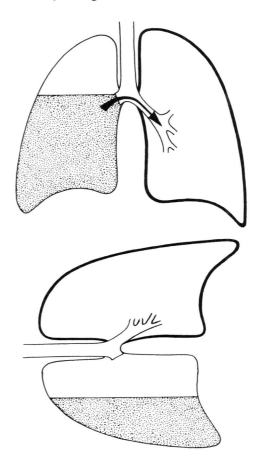

Figure 50.41 Bronchopleural fistula following pneumonectomy. Lying the patient on the operated side prevents further aspiration of bloodstained fluid

The elective treatment of the fistula depends on whether or not the pleural fluid is sterile. If the fistula has occurred 3 or more months after the pneumonectomy, bronchoscopy should be performed to determine whether or not there is recurrence of carcinoma.

If the fluid is sterile. The bronchial stump should be resutured. The operation should be carried out in the lateral position and it is unwise to rely on a cuffed endobronchial tube to prevent further spillage into the remaining lung, however expert and persuasive is the anaesthetist. The only safe procedure is to aspirate the pneumonectomy space dry through a thoracoscope with the patient in the sitting position immediately prior to induction of anaesthesia. Only by this means is the aspiration of fluid into the contralateral lung and its very serious consequences prevented with certainty.

The chest is opened, the pneumonectomy space evacuated of blood clot and fibrin, and the fistula identified – it is usually obvious. On the right side (which is almost always the side of the fistula – the author has never had a fistula on the left) a longitudinal incision is made behind the bronchial stump in the line of the oesophagus. This plane is then followed around the stump anteriorly until it is completely freed. The azygos vein is divided unless it was previously divided at the time of the pneumonectomy. The superior vena cava and the pulmonary artery stump both lie anteriorly. On the left side the dissection is much more difficult because of the very close proximity of the pulmonary artery and superior pulmonary vein, as they lie anterior to the bronchus which is deep in the mediastinum. It is preferable to open the track of the fistula first and then subsequently to mobilize the bronchial stump.

However tempting it may be, the fistula must not merely be closed by an extra two or three stitches. A recurrence of the fistula will inevitably occur. It is imperative that the whole of the previously sutured stump be re-amputated so as to provide a fresh bronchus for suture. The stump should be covered with a pedicled muscle graft.

An alternative procedure is to re-amputate and resuture the bronchial stump by a transpericardial approach, a technique which can also be used if the pneumonectomy is infected. Through a median sternotomy the pericardium is opened and the right bronchial stump approached between the ascending aorta and the superior vena cava, each of which is retracted laterally. The posterior pericardium is incised and the remainder of the right pulmonary artery divided, thus exposing the trachea and origin of the right main bronchus for division and suture. If, very rarely, the left bronchial stump is to be exposed, the remainder of the left pulmonary artery is divided under the aortic arch, thus exposing the trachea and origin of the left main bronchus (Ginsberg *et al.*, 1989).

If the fluid is infected. If the fluid is infected, then it is unwise to attempt to resuture the bronchus by a transpleural approach. Not only will this fail, but it is likely that much of the thoracotomy wound will become infected. It is better to drain the empyema by rib resection and then, about 6 months later when the infection has subsided and the patient's condition has improved, perform a lateral thoracoplasty (with preservation of the first rib) together with a modified Roberts' flap operation in which the decostalized chest wall is sutured onto the open bronchial stump (see page 750). Complete healing will usually occur within a few weeks

Alternatively the transpericardial approach described above can be used to resuture the bronchus. The residual infected pneumonectomy space can then be treated as described above by muscle flap or thoracoplasty.

If there is a recurrence of carcinoma at the bronchial stump, then resuture or lateral thoracoplasty are not advisable and the treatment can only be directed to the prevention of aspiration of infected pleural fluid into the contralateral lung. This will usually require rib resection drainage.

Part 4

Mediastinal tumours

Mediastinal tumours occur from infancy to old age in both sexes and are best classified according to their position on the chest radiograph. Neurogenic tumours occur in the posterior mediastinum, foregut duplications and lymphatic tissue tumours in the central mediastinum, while thyroid, thymic and dermoid tumours occur in the anterior mediastinum (Blades, 1941; Morrison, 1958; Wychulis *et al.*, 1971; Le Roux *et al.*, 1984; Trastek, 1987) (Figure 50.42).

Classification of mediastinal tumours

Posterior mediastinum (paravertebral gutter):
  Neurofibroma.
  Ganglioneuroma.
Anterior mediastinum (from above downwards):
  Retrosternal thyroid.
  Thymic tumour.
  Dermoid and teratoma.
  Para-pericardial cyst.
Central mediastinum:
  Foregut duplication cyst (bronchogenic or gastrogenic).
  Lymphatic tissue tumours (including sarcoid).
  Primary tuberculosis.
  Secondary bronchial carcinoma.

Any mediastinal tumour may be an aortic aneurysm or a tumour of lymphatic origin.

Diagnostic aspiration is best avoided and thoracotomy is usually required, both for diagnosis and treatment, for many of these tumours are potentially

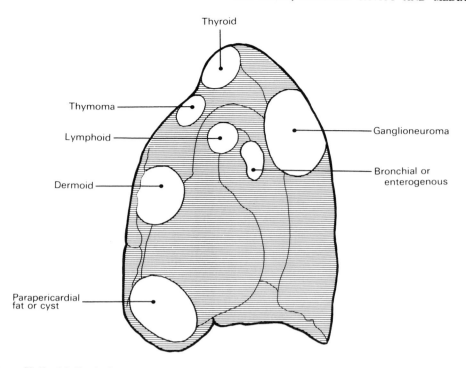

Figure 50.42 Mediastinal tumours. Those commonly seen are: anteriorly from above down, thyroid, thymus, dermoid, para-pericardial cyst; posteriorly, neurogenic tumours; centrally, bronchial or enterogenous cysts or tumours. A vascular or lymphatic swelling or tumour may occur at any site

malignant and may suddenly increase in size if a haemorrhage occurs into them.

A foregut cyst, which is often associated with a vertebral abnormality (hemivertebra), may develop a bronchial communication producing cough and sputum, together with a fluid level on the chest radiograph.

Thymic tumours, unless associated with myasthenia gravis, are usually found on routine radiographic examination, as also are dermoids, neurofibroma and ganglioneuroma, unless they are so large as to cause pressure symptoms.

Posterior mediastinal tumours

Surgical approach

A high posterolateral thoracotomy through the 4th or 5th rib bed, with division of the posterior end of the rib above if necessary, will provide an adequate exposure. If the tumour is large and closely applied to the ribs there may be difficulty in ligating the intercostal vessels. In this event it is best to secure haemostasis after the tumour has been removed. The oesophagus may be displaced by the tumour and must be identified at operation – the passage of a stomach tube may be of great help.

Complications of operation include damage to the sympathetic trunk (causing Horner's syndrome or sympathetic impairment to the upper limb) or thoracic duct (causing a chylothorax).

A neurofibroma may penetrate and enlarge an intervertebral foramen and care must be taken to avoid damage to the spinal cord when ligating the spinal branch of an intercostal artery. There may even be a prolongation into the vertebral canal ('dumbbell' tumour) causing symptoms of cord or root compression. A myelogram is necessary to ascertain the extent of the intraspinal prolongation and laminectomy may be required for its removal.

Anterior mediastinal tumours

Surgical approach

The approach may be by posterolateral thoracotomy on the side to which the tumour mainly projects or by median sternotomy if the tumour is bilateral. An anterolateral thoracotomy does not give an adequate exposure, nor is it so easy to enlarge if this proves necessary. After incision of the mediastinal pleura the tumour may be enucleated from its false sac often without division of a single blood vessel. If there has been malignant change or previous infection, the dissection may be extremely difficult and the great vessels in the mediastinum are at risk.

Central mediastinal tumours

Surgical approach

These tumours should usually be approached through

a right posterolateral thoracotomy. Division of the vena azygos will permit a full exploration of the mediastinum, the exposure of which will not be hampered by the aortic arch and its left branches. If the chest radiograph shows that the whole tumour is on the left side, or if the left lung is involved, then clearly a left thoracotomy would be necessary.

A bronchogenic cyst is usually situated high in the mediastinum, has thin walls and is relatively easily excised. A gastrogenic cyst is lined by gastric epithelium, may develop peptic ulceration and become very adherent to adjacent structures, particularly the oesophagus, aorta or bronchus.

Before embarking on a resection of a central mediastinal tumour, it is important to exclude an aneurysm of aorta, generalized disease of the lymphatic system, or secondary carcinoma.

Retrosternal thyroid

Retrosternal prolongation of a goitre may occur into the chest. It is a potentially dangerous condition because of the possibility of superior vena caval obstruction or stridor from tracheal compression. These symptoms may suddenly increase if a haemorrhage occurs into the retrosternal prolongation. The extension into the chest is usually in the plane immediately behind the sternum and *in front* of the innominate vein, though rarely it may pass behind the vein or even behind the trachea and oesophagus. The blood supply is invariably from the neck.

Operative approach

Most retrosternal prolongations of the thyroid may be removed through the neck. The thyroid is exposed by a cervical collar incision and the superior, middle and inferior thyroid vessels isolated and divided as described in Chapter 24.

The index finger is then passed down into the mediastinum and gently swept around the gland to free it from adhesions. In almost all cases the gland may be successfully delivered into the neck. It may be helpful to evacuate the contents of some of the cysts. If difficulty is encountered due to abnormal adherence, size or position of the gland, then the manubrium should be split vertically (see Chapter 58).

Myasthenia gravis

The functions of the thymus are not fully understood and there is considerable controversy concerning its exact relationship to myasthenia gravis. Initiated by Sauerbruch in 1913 and popularized by Blalock *et al.* in 1939 and Keynes in 1949, thymectomy has nevertheless now become an established procedure in the treatment of myasthenia, though its exact benefit is difficult to define since myasthenia is notorious for its spontaneous remissions. The patients who most benefit from thymectomy are young females with a short history who have a macroscopically normal thymus. The gland, though not enlarged, usually has an excess of germinal follicles.

The diagnosis of myasthenia should be confirmed pharmacologically. The combination of electromyography, single-fibre electromyography and the measurement of acetylcholine receptor bodies now allows the detection of milder cases and the exclusion of other myasthenic syndromes.

The possible presence of a tumour should be ascertained by a lateral chest radiograph and lateral tomography of the mediastinum or, if possible, CT scan. If muscle antibodies are present in the blood it is likely that there is a thymic tumour. The presence of a tumour makes a good operative result much less likely and in these cases the patient should have preliminary radiotherapy.

The surgical treatment of myasthenia gravis is still controversial because of the lack of data from controlled clinical trials and the fluctuation in the clinical course of the disease. However, thymectomy is now advised for most cases and in 1987 Simpson reported virtual recovery in 90% of cases, especially those without a thymoma and if surgery is carried out early, within 2 years of diagnosis (Simpson and Thomaides, 1987). Age and sex are not relevant factors in the results of operation. Immunosuppression with steroids or azathioprine may reduce the morbidity of the disease, but as these drugs can rarely be withdrawn completely without causing a relapse, the long-term hazards of them are serious.

Thymectomy (Keynes, 1949; Edwards and Wilson, 1972; Otto and Strugalska, 1987; Maggi *et al.*, 1989; Mulder *et al.*, 1989)

The main postoperative complication is respiratory failure from 'cholinergic crisis'. The doses of anticholinergic drugs which will produce the maximum therapeutic response must be determined by trial and error, and care must be taken to avoid overdose.

The operation is carried out through a median sternotomy. The pleura is displaced laterally by blunt dissection to reveal the yellowish-pink H-shaped thymus. The gland is grasped in light artery forceps at its two lower poles and peeled upwards, taking care not to damage either pleural cavity. The gland is gently lifted upwards until the innominate vein is exposed on its deep surface. The thymic veins which drain into the innominate vein are then divided. The upper poles of the thymus are mobilized and it is here that the thymic arteries may be seen, arising from the internal mammary artery. They are divided and the thymus removed. If either pleural cavity is opened it should be drained by an underwater-seal drainage tube inserted through the lateral chest wall.

After operation the patient is best managed in an intensive care unit, for respiratory problems are common. An immediate postoperative chest radiograph is important to exclude pneumothorax or haemothorax. Artificial ventilation through an endotracheal tube for 24 h is advisable. Thereafter assisted respiration can usually be reduced, provided that there is no respiratory infection and the patient's respiratory muscles are strong enough. A nasogastric tube will allow the crushed anticholinesterase drugs to be given into the stomach, which is the most effective route, but they should be withheld until their need is apparent, to prevent the serious complication of a cholinergic crisis. The reader is referred elsewhere for a description of the specific drug and steroid therapy suitable to this condition.

In some centres, 'maximal thymectomy' is advised, removing all mediastinal fat and possible ectopic thymus as an *en bloc* excision (Jaretski *et al.*, 1988).

Transcervical thymectomy (Donnelly *et al.*, 1984)

An alternative approach is the removal of the thymus gland via the collar incision used in thyroid surgery. Several large series of patients have been treated satisfactorily in this way. However, this is a very specialized technique and in the absence of special experience, is likely to result in the thymus being incompletely removed.

Chronic superior vena caval obstruction

Superior vena caval obstruction is usually due to advanced malignant disease and is best treated by radiotherapy. In a few cases, however, it is due to benign idiopathic mediastinal fibrosis, caseating granuloma or old-standing tuberculous glands and the obstruction may be relieved by the insertion of a conduit between the left innominate vein and the right atrial appendage. Synthetic grafts almost always thrombose due to the thrombogenicity of the graft material and the relatively slow venous flow. An autogenous venous graft is therefore advisable. A preliminary venogram, preferably by CT scan with venous enhancement, is carried out to define the caval obstruction.

A midline sternotomy is performed to confirm feasibility of venous bypass and to biopsy the obstructing lesion. The thymic remnant is excised and the pericardium opened in the midline to expose the right atrial appendage. The innominate vein is ligated as close to its entry into the superior vena cava as possible. A vascular clamp is applied to the jugulo-subclavian junction and the innominate vein divided. The graft is then anastomosed with 5/0 prolene sutures to the left innominate vein and the right atrial appendage. The graft must not be kinked as this would predispose to later thrombosis. The venous graft may be a composite spiral vein graft fashioned from the long saphenous vein (Stanford and Doty, 1986) or it may be a segment of common femoral vein. The spiral vein graft is made by opening the

segment of saphenous vein longitudinally to form a ribbon which is then wound round a stent as a spiral and made into a tube by suturing its edges together with a continuous 7/0 prolene suture. Alternatively a segment of common femoral vein is obtained by incising the deep fascia along the posterior border of the sartorius to expose the adductor canal and excising a segment of common femoral vein distal to the profunda femoris vein (the long saphenous vein must be present and normal if this technique is used) (Figure 50.43).

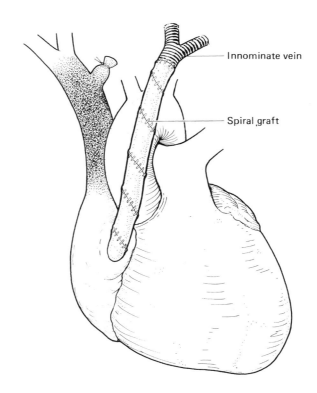

Figure 50.43 Spiral vein graft between left innominate vein and right atrial appendage

Part 5

Surgery of pleura and chest wall

Pleural biopsy

Pleural biopsy may be required for the diagnosis of pleural effusion or diffuse pleural tumours. It may be carried out by a closed 'aspirating' technique or by an open technique.

Closed technique

The site of the proposed biopsy is anaesthetized with 0.5% xylocaine (lignocaine) and then a wide-bore needle advanced into the pleural tumour. The needle is gently angulated when the end is judged to be in the tumour so as to cut off a piece of tissue. The needle is withdrawn while suction is continuously applied by means of a 20 ml syringe, and the biopsy is then expelled from the needle into fixative.

A more sophisticated method is to use an Abrams needle which has a side-hole near its end. This hole is wedged against the pleura or tumour and a small piece of tissue cut off by the sliding internal cannula (Abrams, 1958). A Tru-cut needle is also useful.

A high yield is provided by the Steel drill biopsy, in which a rapidly rotating drill 'cores out' a piece of tissue. This was originally designed for lung biopsy but is equally effective for pleural tumours (Steel and Winstanley, 1969).

Open technique

This is a more certain method of obtaining positive histology. A portion of rib is resected under local or general anaesthetic, the rib bed incised and a wedge biopsy carried out.

Tumours of the pleura

Primary tumours of the pleura are relatively rare, although secondary invasion from bronchial carcinoma or breast carcinoma is common. The primary tumour may be a fibroma or a mesothelioma.

Fibroma

A fibroma is usually found by chance on a routine chest radiograph, although it may cause a dull chest pain or hypertrophic pulmonary osteoarthropathy. It is basically an innocent tumour but should be resected together with a generous portion of adjacent chest wall (rib and intercostal muscle), for it is likely to recur and may behave as a slow-growing, low-grade malignant tumour. If an area of chest wall involving long lengths of several ribs is removed, it will be necessary to close the deficit with Marlex mesh or tantalum gauze in order to prevent respiratory embarrassment after operation. If the deficit is under cover of the scapula, however, a much larger portion of chest wall may be excised without the use of a prosthesis (Thomas and Drew, 1953; Okike et al., 1978).

Mesothelioma

A mesothelioma is usually due to exposure to asbestos, often many years previously. It may or may not be associated with a pleural effusion. If no effusion is present it commonly causes multiple pleural opacities. Treatment is generally considered to be unsatisfactory and there is evidence that resection (or even open biopsy) may hasten the growth of the tumour, which is usually much more extensive than appears on the chest radiograph. There is no evidence that radiotherapy, cytotoxic drugs or intrapleural radioactive material influence the prognosis. The duration of life after diagnosis is very variable and may be surprisingly long (Hickman and Jones, 1970; Elmes and Simpson, 1976; Butchart et al., 1976; Ginsberg, 1986).

Martini et al. (1987) classify mesothelioma into two histological types (1) a localized fibrosarcomatous tumour for which a wide excision of chest wall is advisable and which is considered to be potentially curative, and (2) a diffuse pleural epithelial tumour associated with an effusion and related to asbestos exposure, for which treatment is unsatisfactory though pleuropneumonectomy followed by irradiation may be of some benefit.

Secondary carcinoma

If secondary carcinoma from the lung or breast is associated with a recurrent pleural effusion, a pleurectomy will produce adherence of the lung to the chest wall and prevent a recurrence of the effusion and at the same time remove some of the tumour. There is a small risk of implantation of tumour cells into the chest wall. The advice of an oncologist may help the patient.

Chest wall tumours

Excision of the chest wall may be required for primary tumours such as chondrosarcoma (the commonest), chondroma (which often becomes malignant) or osteochondroma, or for secondary tumours (e.g. from the breast), provided that the primary growth is adequately controlled.

Malignant tumours, especially chondrosarcoma, have a marked tendency to recur and a wide excision must be carried out. The whole length of the ribs involved must be removed together with adjacent intercostal muscle and underlying pleura and part of the diaphragm if necessary. If the lung is involved a lobectomy may be required. It is usually possible to distinguish benign from malignant tumours by a careful study of the radiographs.

The wide excision of chest wall leads to a problem in reconstruction, in which there are two functional considerations:

1. Airtight closure.
2. Restoration of the functional integrity and rigidity of the chest wall.

If the defect is likely to be large it is important to plan the operation in conjunction with a plastic surgeon, who can prepare in advance full-thickness pedicled skin grafts to fill the chest wall deficit.

Lateral chest wall tumours

An elliptical incision is made in the line of the ribs to encircle the tumour. It is deepened to expose the chest wall. If there is doubt concerning the resectability of the tumour, only one half of the elliptical incision should be made. The periosteum of a normal rib above the tumour is incised longitudinally, stripped from its lower border and the pleura opened to ascertain the extent of the tumour and to make sure that scattered nodes are not present throughout the pleural cavity. The presence of multiple nodules would preclude resection, although an intercostal neurectomy should be carried out if the pain is severe. A frozen section is advisable to ascertain the nature of the tumour. If it is malignant the resection will need to be much wider than if innocent, although the tumour may only be malignant in part and this may not be the site of the biopsy. The periosteum is elevated from the involved ribs for a short length anteriorly and posteriorly, so that they can be divided with a costotome. The intercostal muscles and bundle are divided between clamps and longitudinal incisions are made along the adjacent normal ribs above and below so that the tumour and involved chest wall may be removed. If there is involvement of the underlying lung and diaphragm an appropriate resection must be undertaken.

If the chest wall deficit is under cover of the scapula, quite a large opening may be left unclosed. If, however, the deficit is lower down and involves more than two ribs, some type of prosthesis is required to strengthen the chest wall. The most satisfactory materials are Marlex mesh or tantalum gauze. Tantalum gauze should be turned in at its edges to avoid fraying. The edge of the prosthesis should overlap the edge of the defect by 1 cm and be fixed in place outside the chest wall with interrupted wire sutures. If the tumour has involved a wide area of skin and it is difficult to obtain complete skin closure, a pedicled skin graft may be used to cover the defect. Alternatively, muscle or musculocutaneous flaps of latissimus dorsi, pectoralis major, serratus anterior, rectus abdominis or external oblique muscle may be used (Pairolero and Arnold, 1986). The pleural cavity should always be drained by a tube inserted through a separate stab incision posteriorly in the lowest part of the chest.

Sternal tumours

Tumours of the upper end of the sternum may require the excision of the medial ends of both clavicles. If the tumour is malignant the whole sternum may need to be removed.

The restoration of rigidity of the bony cage depends on the extent of sternal excision. If a portion of manubrium can be preserved, the rest of the sternum may be excised and the deficit satisfactorily closed by bringing together the attachments of the pectoralis major from each side. If the whole of the sternum has been removed, the ribs must be stabilized by the insertion of a prosthesis of a tantalum plate or acrylic resin.

Malignant pleural effusion

Malignant pleural effusions, which are most commonly due to lung cancer, breast cancer and lymphoma, cause considerable disability, lead to repeated hospital admissions and are difficult to control. The aim of treatment is to obliterate the pleural space to prevent the continued accumulation of pleural fluid.

Tube thoracostomy, followed by the injection of a sclerosing agent, should be the first line of treatment. Under general anaesthesia the pleura is aspirated to dryness through a thoracoscope introduced in the 7th intercostal space in the mid-axillary line. An apical intercostal tube is inserted two spaces above the thoracoscope and iodized talc insufflated through the thoracoscope cannula until it discharges through the apical cannula. The thoracoscope cannula is removed, replaced with a second intercostal tube and both tubes are connected to underwater drains for 4–5 days (Cheslyn-Curtis and Treasure, 1989; Tattersall and Boyer, 1990).

In most patients a satisfactory pleurodesis will occur and no more fluid will accumulate, but if fluid does develop again either a pleurectomy (Martini *et al.*, 1975) or a Denver pleuroperitoneal shunt (Tsang *et al.*, 1990) is advisable.

Part 6

Emphysematous cysts (Connolly and Wilson, 1989)

An air-containing cyst in the lung may be a congenital bronchogenic cyst or an acquired emphysematous cyst.

A *bronchogenic cyst*, which is usually diagnosed on a routine chest radiograph, should always be removed as it is prone to become infected.

An *emphysematous cyst* should be excised if:

1. The patient is breathless.
2. There is evidence that the cyst is enlarging.
3. The cyst occupies more than one-third of the lung.
4. The patient is fit for operation – the patient must not be so incapacitated by chronic bronchitis, bronchospasm, the effects of cor pulmonale or ischaemic heart disease that the risk of operation is too high.

Careful selection of patients is most important, for the operative mortality is high in poor-risk patients with bilateral disease. Many patients fall into this group.

Surgical excision or obliteration

The method of anaesthesia is most important. The more usual technique of paralysis and manual ventilation is very likely to rupture the cyst and cause a tension pneumothorax before the chest has been opened.

Small cysts with a narrow pedicle are ligated and excised. Larger cysts are removed by incising the cyst wall at its junction with normal lung and continuing around its base (Figure 50.44). Trabeculae may need to be divided near normal lung. The cyst should then be obliterated by multiple interrupted catgut sutures placed through its wall, including its deepest part (Figure 50.45). Alternatively the cyst is excised and its base closed with the T90 'Auto Suture' stapler applied across normal lung tissue.

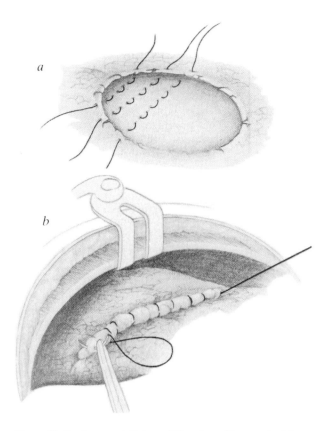

Figure 50.45 Lung cyst. Suture obliteration of lung cysts. Alternatively the base of the cyst may be stapled

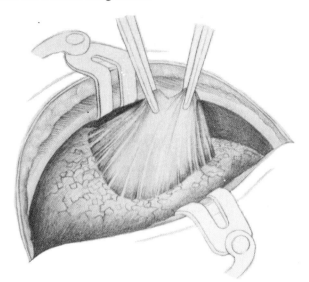

Figure 50.44 Mobilization of lung cyst prior to excision

At the conclusion of operation the anaesthetist should avoid vigorous inflation of the lungs, or new air dissections, or a contralateral spontaneous pneumothorax, may be caused.

If the whole lobe is replaced by a cyst and no functioning lung remains, a lobectomy should be carried out. However, an important aim of the operation is conservation of lung tissue – no functioning lung should be removed. Cysts should be obliterated so that the compressed lung may expand.

The chest is closed. Three tubes (apical, basal and anterior) should be inserted, as air leak is always a major problem and it is important to obtain rapid expansion of the lung. Care must be taken that the suction is sufficient to deal with the volume of air leak when the patient coughs – otherwise surgical emphysema will occur. Alternatively, one tube should be attached to an underwater seal, without suction, to allow excess air to escape readily.

Postoperatively it is important to make sure that the tubes remain patent, being removed only when all air leak has ceased.

Intracavity suction (Monaldi drainage) (Macarthur and Fountain, 1977)

This is a most valuable technique in patients with a large cyst who are severely disabled due to cor pulmonale and very poor lung function and who are unfit for thoracotomy. The cyst may be reduced in size by introducing a Malecot catheter and applying suction. A two-stage operation is required so as to ensure adherence of the two layers of pleura. At the first stage a short length of rib overlying the cavity is resected under local anaesthesia and a gauze pack soaked in 1% iodine placed against the parietal pleura. The wound is closed. Two weeks later the pack may be removed and a tube inserted into the cavity by a trocar and cannula technique. The tube is attached to suction and gradually over a period of 2–3 weeks the cavity will reduce in size. The tube may then be removed and usually the cavity remains small or actually obliterates.

A recent modification enables this operation to be carried out in one stage. A 2.5 cm length of rib overlying the cavity is excised subperiosteally and a purse-string chromic catgut suture is inserted through the parietal pleura into the visceral pleura and underlying cyst wall. The cyst is then opened through the centre of the purse-string and a large self-retaining

Foley urethral catheter inserted into the cavity. The balloon is inflated and the purse-string tightened. If a pneumothorax is inadvertently produced, a separate underwater-seal drainage is instituted (Venn *et al.*, 1988).

Obstructive emphysema

This term is used to describe two entirely separate conditions.

1. Congenital obstructive emphysema

This rare condition occurs in infants and is due to lack of cartilage support in the bronchial wall. A 'ball-valve' obstruction occurs in the affected lobe, usually the upper, which becomes increasingly distended. This causes mediastinal shift to the opposite side and severe respiratory embarrassment. Symptoms occur soon after birth. The treatment is lobectomy.

2. Obstructive emphysema due to bronchial blockage

The bronchial blockage may not be complete and a 'ball-valve' obstruction may occur due to dilatation and contraction of the bronchus with each respiration, allowing air to enter the lung but to leave less easily. The affected part of the lung gradually becomes distended and is more translucent on the chest radiograph. The cause is an inhaled foreign body or a tumour (usually innocent) blocking the bronchus. This will lead later to complete collapse of the affected lobe or lung and subsequent bronchiectasis. The treatment is that of the causative lesion. If the foreign body has caused bronchiectasis, a lobectomy may be required.

Hydatid cysts of the lung

Hydatid cysts of the lung should always be removed to prevent their subsequent rupture and the consequent spread of the parasite into the pleural cavity or the rest of the lung (Barrett and Thomas, 1952; Lichter, 1972).

Surgical technique

This will depend on whether the cyst is still unruptured in the substance of the lung or whether it has developed a bronchial communication and become infected.

1. Unruptured cyst

This is the more common situation. Posterolateral thoracotomy is performed and the lobe containing the cyst packed off from the surrounding lung and pleural cavity by large swabs soaked in 2% formal-dehyde solution. Some of the fluid in the cyst is aspirated with a fine needle to make it less tense. Ten millilitres ether or 10% formaldehyde solution may be injected into the cyst to sterilize the contents. Very great care must be taken to avoid any contamination of the pleural cavity. The 'peri-cyst' (the adventitious layer of fibrous tissue surrounding the cyst itself) is carefully incised and with gentle pressure on the lungs by the anaesthetist, the cyst itself will be extruded intact from the lung substance. The interior of the pericyst is inspected, any bleeding points or bronchial communications are closed, and the lung cavity obliterated by interrupted mattress catgut sutures. If the cyst is less than 3 cm in diameter it is best removed by a wedge resection of the lung containing the cyst.

If the cyst is very large, a lobectomy may be required.

2. Infected cyst

If the cyst has become infected a lung resection must be carried out, either a segmental resection or a lobectomy depending on the size and situation of the cyst.

Part 7

Surgical treatment of pulmonary tuberculosis
(Goldstraw, 1987; Kariuki, 1989)

The management of pulmonary tuberculosis has been revolutionized during the past 30 years by the use of modern chemotherapy. Operation may still be required, however, in patients who have developed drug resistance and are still sputum positive. This is usually due to inadequate initial treatment.

The assessment of these patients for surgery is often very difficult and controversial and note must be taken of the following:

1. The quantity of sputum, the presence of tubercle bacilli and their sensitivity to antituberculous drugs, together with the presence of other organisms and their sensitivity to antibiotics.
2. The extent of lung cavitation and infiltration and its exact location in the upper lobe or apex of the lower lobe, as shown by the posteroanterior and lateral radiographs, including tomograms.
3. Any evidence of tuberculous activity, as shown by weight loss, evening temperature, raised erythrocyte sedimentation rate (ESR) and radiological evidence of recent change. All previous radiographs should be examined if possible for evidence of previous disease.
4. The presence of bronchitis or bronchospasm.
5. The state of respiratory function, including differential lung function as shown by ventilation/perfusion studies using radio-isotope techniques.
6. The presence of bronchostenosis or endobronchitis, as shown by bronchoscopy.

Surgical procedures available

The surgical procedures available for the treatment of tuberculosis comprise resection of a part or the whole of the lung (combined with decortication if an empyema is present), thoracoplasty to obliterate an upper lobe cavity by permanently collapsing the affected lobe, and 'sleeve' resection of a bronchus for a localized bronchostenosis causing distal infection (Figure 50.46). Artificial pneumothorax and phrenic crush combined with pneumoperitoneum are no longer practised.

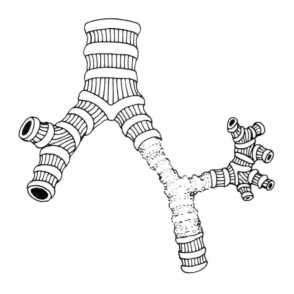

Figure 50.46 Tuberculous bronchostenosis affecting the region of the left upper lobe orifice. This is an ideal situation for left upper lobectomy with 'sleeve' resection of the main bronchus

Indications for surgery

Tuberculosis which is active must be treated medically by chemotherapy for several months before surgical treatment is considered. By this time the cavity may have closed, the sputum become negative and the disease process arrested. On the other hand the cavity may remain open and the sputum be negative or positive. If the sputum is negative, operation is only required if the cavity is large, because in many of these cases a fungal infection (Aspergilloma) will develop, leading to repeated haemoptyses, which may threaten life (British Tuberculosis Association, 1970). If the sputum is positive, then surgical treatment is advisable, probably thoracoplasty, for by this time the organisms are almost certainly drug resistant.

Indications for resection

These are now well established (Crofton and Douglas, 1969):

1. *Persistent positive sputum*, despite adequate chemotherapy.
2. *Persistent cavity* for more than 2 years (so-called 'open-negative' case). There is considerable difference of opinion concerning the treatment of this type of patient, and the present tendency is to advise resection if the cavity is thick walled, if there has been only a slow response to treatment, as shown by time taken for sputum conversion, or if the patient undertakes strenuous physical activity, or is likely to be unreliable in follow-up examination (e.g. an alcoholic).
3. *Tuberculoma*. A localized nodule greater than 2 cm in diameter. In older patients, it may not be possible to differentiate this lesion from a carcinoma unless percutaneous needle biopsy under radiological control is available.
4. *Destroyed functionless lung*. If the patient has haemoptyses or considerable sputum a pneumonectomy may be required, provided there is very definite evidence of lack of function (as shown by previous extensive disease), presence of fibrotic changes on tomography, or bronchiectatic changes on bronchography. It must be remembered that such patients may live without surgical intervention for many years and an estimate must be made of the likely progress of the patient with and without surgery. In these patients a lateral thoracoplasty (ribs 2–7) is often advisable 2 weeks after pneumonectomy, to prevent overdistension of the remaining lung.
5. *Tuberculous empyema*. If there is significant underlying lung disease, lobectomy or pneumonectomy will be required as well as the decortication.
6. *Failed thoracoplasty*. If an adequate thoracoplasty fails to close a cavity and the sputum still remains positive, a resection of the diseased part of the lung should be carried out under the thoracoplasty.

Contraindications to resection

The main contraindications to resection are inadequate cardiac reserve, respiratory insufficiency due to bronchitis and bronchospasm, tuberculous disease in the lung which is too extensive to remove without making the patient a respiratory cripple, and progressive extrapulmonary tuberculosis. In addition, active endobronchitis at the point of the proposed division of the bronchus will almost certainly lead to a bronchopleural fistula and is therefore an absolute contraindication.

Indications for thoracoplasty

This operation was devised before the advent of antituberculous chemotherapy and provided a selective permanent collapse of the upper lobe and apex of the lower lobe. The operation causes a greater loss of lung function than does resection and must be carried out as a staged procedure. For these reasons the operation is now rarely performed for tuberculosis, though it may be indicated for a post-pneumonectomy empyema (see page 764). The morbidity and mortality are less than after lung resection and because of this it is still advisable in some poor-risk patients who would not tolerate a resection.

Operative procedures

1. Lung resection

The operations available are wedge resection, segmental resection, lobectomy or pneumonectomy, together with 'sleeve' resection for a tuberculous stricture of a main bronchus. The segments most commonly excised are the apical and posterior segments of the upper lobe and the apical segment of the lower lobe (often combined with an upper lobectomy). The detailed technique is described in the section on tumours of the lung. Special points to note during resections for tuberculosis are:

(a) The avoidance of lung division across tuberculous tissue.
(b) Extrapleural separation of the lung where it is adherent to the chest wall.
(c) Increased difficulty of hilar dissection because of fibrotic changes around the blood vessels and bronchus.

It is important to obtain complete expansion of the remainder of the lung as soon as possible and in some cases a decortication of the remaining lobe will be necessary. Fortunately the portion of lung to be resected is often atelectatic and the adjacent lung will have already become overdistended. 'Sleeve resection' of the main bronchus, in combination with an upper lobectomy, is indicated if previous tuberculous endobronchitis has caused a stenosis of the main bronchus. In such a case it is necessary to excise the narrowed segment of bronchus in order to prevent the occurrence of non-tuberculous infection and subsequent bronchiectasis in the lower lobe.

2. Decortication

This may be required in cases of tuberculous empyema. The initial treatment of such an empyema must always be aspiration and streptomycin injection into the pleural cavity, at first twice weekly and then subsequently once weekly, together with systemic antituberculous chemotherapy. In some cases the empyema will absorb on this regimen, with re-expansion of the lung and obliteration of the pleural cavity.

However, most cases of tuberculous empyema require decortication, the technique of which is described on page 748. If there is underlying lung disease a lobectomy or pneumonectomy will also be required and the necessity for this must be judged

partly on a knowledge of the previous extent of the tuberculosis, as shown by previous radiographs, and partly on the findings at operation. The tuberculous disease is likely to be more extensive at the apex of the lung and the extrapleural strip must proceed with care at this point to avoid damage to the brachial plexus or subclavian artery and vein. On the mediastinal side, the dissection is less difficult and the actual hilar dissection may be surprisingly easy.

If a bronchopleural fistula has developed, shown by the expectoration of purulent fluid when the patient lies on the opposite side and confirmed by the injection of methylene blue into the pleural cavity, operation is a matter of extreme urgency in order to prevent tuberculous spread to the contralateral lung. If the patient is sufficiently fit, pleuropneumonectomy should be carried out. The empyema must first be aspirated dry through a thoracoscope in the sitting-up position and then thoracotomy performed in the face-down position or in the lateral position with an appropriate blocker or cuffed endobronchial tube to prevent a 'spill-over' into the opposite lung. If the patient is unfit for a resection, intercostal tube drainage must be instituted.

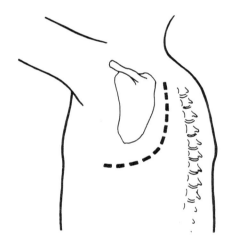

Figure 50.47 Thoracoplasty showing extended parascapular incision

3. Thoracoplasty (Thomas and Cleland, 1942) (Figure 50.47)

A thoracoplasty, together with an extrafascial apicolysis, mobilizes the chest wall and allows concentric relaxation of the affected lung. This abolishes the bronchial ball-valve mechanism which maintains the distension of the tuberculous cavity, and thus allows healing to take place. The number of ribs resected depends on the extent of the disease and it is usual to carry the resection to one rib below the lowermost area of tuberculosis, as related to the posterior end of the ribs on the posteroanterior chest radiograph. In practice, a 5–8-rib thoracoplasty is usually required.

A 6-rib thoracoplasty should never be performed, for the interior angle of the scapula 'rides' on the unresected 7th rib and causes considerable discomfort. The operation must be done in two or three stages or the patient will succumb to the effects of a large mobile portion of chest wall and resultant paradoxical respiration. The transverse processes of the vertebrae should not be removed, or a severe scoliosis will develop.

A thoracoplasty operation is nowadays rarely performed – its main indication is for the closure of a persistent apical air space following a lung resection (Hopkins *et al.*, 1985). The detailed operative technique is well described by Hewitson (1986).

References

Abrams, L. D. (1958) A pleural biopsy punch. *Lancet*, i, 30

Barrett, N. R. and Thomas, D. (1952) Pulmonary hydatid disease. *Br. J. Surg.*, **40**, 222–244

Bates, M. (1975) Segmental resection for bronchial carcinoma. *Thorax*, **30**, 235

Bates, M. (1981) Analysis of 2000 resections for bronchial carcinoma. *Ann. R. Coll. Surg.*, **63**, 164–167

Belcher, J. R. (1959) Lobectomy for bronchial carcinoma. *Lancet*, **2**, 639–642

Bennett, W. F. and Smith, R. A. (1978) A twenty-year analysis of the results of sleeve resection for primary bronchogenic carcinoma. *J. Thorac. Cardiovasc. Surg.*, **76**, 840–845

Blades, B. (1941) Intrathoracic tumours. *Am. J. Surg.*, **54**, 139–148

Blalock, A., Mason, M. F., Morgan, H. G. *et al.* (1939) Myasthenia gravis and tumours of the thymic region. *Ann. Surg.*, **110**, 544

Boyden, E. A. (1955) *Segmental Anatomy of the Lungs*, McGraw-Hill, New York

British Tuberculosis Association (1970) Aspergilloma and residual tuberculous cavities. *Tubercle*, **51**, 227–245

Brock, R. C. (1950) *The Anatomy of the Bronchial Tree*, Oxford University Press, London

Butchart, E. G., Ashcroft, T., Barnsley, W. C. *et al.* (1976) Pleuropneumonectomy in the management of diffuse malignant mesothelioma of the pleura. *Thorax*, **31**, 15–24

Carlens, E. (1959) Mediastinoscopy: a method for inspection and tissue biopsy in the superior mediastinum. *Dis. Chest*, **36**, 343–352

Cheslyn-Curtis, S. and Treasure, T. (1989) Pleural effusion in malignant disease. *Surgery*, **69**, 1645–1649, The Medicine Group, Oxford, June

Connolly, J. E. and Wilson, A. (1989) The current status of surgery for bullous emphysema. *J. Thorac. Cardiovasc. Surg.*, **97**, 351–361

Crofton, J. and Douglas, A. (1969) *Respiratory Diseases*, Blackwell Scientific Publications, Oxford, page 250

Deslauriers, J., Gaulin, P., Beaulieu, M. *et al.* (1986) Long term clinical and functional results of sleeve lobectomy for primary lung cancer. *J. Thorac. Cardiovasc. Surg.*, **92**, 871–879

Donnelly, R. J., Laquaglia, M. P., Fabri, B. *et al.* (1984) Cervical thymectomy in the treatment of myasthenia gravis. *Ann. R. Coll. Surg.*, **66**, 305–308

Doty, D. B. (1982) Bypass of superior vena cava. *J. Thorac. Cardiovasc. Surg.*, **83**, 326–338

Edwards, F. R. and Wilson, A. (1972) Thymectomy for myasthenia gravis. *Thorax*, **27**, 513–516

Elmes, P. C. and Simpson, M. J. C. (1976) The clinical aspects of mesothelioma. *Q. J. Med.*, **45**, 427–449

Evans, D. S., Hall, J. H. and Harrison, G. K. (1973) Anterior mediastinotomy. *Thorax*, **28**, 444–447

Flavell, G. (1962) Conservatism in surgical treatment of bronchial carcinoma – review of 826 personal operations. *Br. Med. J.*, **1**, 284–287

Gingell, J. C. (1965) Treatment of chylothorax by producing pleurodesis using iodised talc. *Thorax*, **20**, 261–269

Ginsberg, R. J. (1986) Diffuse malignant mesothelioma – therapeutic dilemma. *Ann. Thorac. Surg.*, **42**, 608

Ginsberg, R. J., Pearson, F. G., Cooper, J. D. *et al.* (1989) Closure of chronic postpneumonectomy bronchopleural fistula using the transternal transpericardial approach. *Ann. Thorac. Surg.*, **47**, 231–235

Goldstraw, P (1987) Surgery for pulmonary tuberculosis. *Surgery*, **45**, 1071–1082, The Medicine Group, Oxford, June

Goldstraw, P. (1993) Postpneumonectomy empyema. *J. Roy. Soc. Med.*, **86**, 559–560.

Hewitson, R. P. (1986) Thoracoplasty. In *Thoracic Surgery*, 4th edn (eds C. Rob and R. Smith), Butterworths, London

Hickman, J. A. and Jones, M. C. (1970) Treatment of neoplastic pleural effusions with local instillation of quinacrine (Mepacrine) hydrochloride. *Thorax*, **25**, 226–229

Hopkins, R. A., Ungerlieder, R. M., Staub, E. W. *et al.* (1985) The modern use of thoracoplasty. *Ann. Thorac. Surg.*, **40**, 181–187

Hurt, R. L. and Bates, M. (1984) Carcinoid tumours of the bronchus: a 33 year experience. *Thorax*, **39**, 617–623

Jaretski, A., Penn, A. S., Younger, D. S. *et al.* (1988) 'Maximal' thymectomy for mysathenia gravis. *J. Thorac. Cardiovasc. Surg.*, **95**, 747–757

Johnson, J. B. and Jones, P. H. (1959) The treatment of bronchial carcinoma by lobectomy and sleeve resection of the main bronchus. *Thorax*, **14**, 48–54

Kariuki, J. K. (1989) Surgery for pulmonary tuberculosis in the third world. *Surgery*, **75**, 1787–1790, The Medicine Group, Oxford, Dec.

Keynes, G. (1949) Results of thymectomy in myasthenia gravis. *Br. Med. J.*, **2**, 611–616

Killen, D. A. and Gobbel, W. G. (1968) *Spontaneous Pneumothorax*. Little, Brown, Boston

Kittle, C. F. (1989) Atypical resections of the lung. *Curr. Probl. Surg.*, **26**, 63–132

Lawson, R. M., Ramanathan, L., Hurley, G. *et al.* (1976) Bronchial adenoma: review of an 18-year experience at the Brompton Hospital. *Thorax*, **31**, 245–253

Le Roux, B. T. (1972) Management of bronchial carcinoma by segmental resection. *Thorax*, **27**, 70–74

Le Roux, B. T., Kallichurum, S. and Shama, D. M. (1984) Mediastinal cysts and tumours. *Curr. Probl. Surg.*, **21**, 5–76

Le Roux, B. T., Mohlala M. L., Odell J. A. *et al.* (1986) Empyema. *Curr. Probl. Surg.*, **23**, 5–38

Levison, V. (1980) What is the best treatment for early operable small cell carcinoma of the bronchus? *Thorax*, **35**, 721–724

Lichter, I. (1972) Surgery of pulmonary hydatid diseases. *Thorax*, **27**, 529–534

Macarthur, A. M. and Fountain, S. W. (1977) Intracavitary suction and drainage in the treatment of emphysematous bullae. *Thorax*, **32**, 668–672

McCaughan, B. C., Martini, N. and Bains, M. S. (1985) Bronchial carcinoids – review of 124 cases. *J. Thorac. Cardiovasc. Surg.*, **89**, 8–17

McIntosh, R. and Thatcher, N. (1990) Management of the solitary metastasis. *Thorax*, **45**, 909–911

Maggi, G., Casadio, C., Cavallo, A. *et al.* (1989) Thymectomy in myasthenia gravis. Results of 662 cases operated upon in 15 years. *Eur. J. Cardio-thorac. Surg.*, **3**, 504–511

Martini, N., Bains, M. S. and Beattie, E. J. (1975) Indications for pleurectomy in malignant effusion. *Cancer*, **35**, 734–738

Martini, N., McCormack, P. M., Bains, M. S. *et al.* (1987) Pleural mesothelioma. *Ann. Thorac. Surg.*, **43**, 113–120

Mathisen, D. J., Grillo, H. C., Vlahakes, G. J. *et al.* (1988) The omentum in the management of complicated cardiothoracic problems. *J. Thorac. Cardiovasc. Surg.*, **95**, 677–684

Matthews, H. R. and Hopkinson, R. B. (1984) Treatment of sputum retention by minitracheostomy. *Br. J. Surg.*, **71**, 147–150

Miller, J. I., Mansour, K. A., Nahai, F. *et al.* (1984) Single stage complete muscle flap closure of the postpneumonectomy empyema space: a new method and possible solution to a disturbing complication. *Ann. Thorac. Surg.*, **38**, 227–231

Milsom, J. W., Kron, I. L., Rheuban, K. S. *et al.* (1985) Chylothorax: an assessment of current surgical management. *J. Thorac. Cardiovasc. Surg.*, **89**, 221–227

Morrison, I. M. (1958) Tumours and cysts of the mediastinum. *Thorax*, **13**, 294–307

Mountain, C. F., McMurtrey, M. J. and Hermes, K. E. (1984) Surgery for pulmonary metastases: a 20 year experience. *Ann. Thorac. Surg.*, **38**, 323–330

Mulder, D. G., Graves, M. and Herrmann, C. (1989) Thymectomy for myasthenia gravis: recent observations and comparisons with past experience. *Ann. Thorac. Surg.*, **48**, 551–555

Nohl-Oser, H. C. (1976) Mediastinoscopy. *Br. J. Hosp. Med.*, **16**, 33–36

Okike, N., Bernatz, P. E. and Woolner, L. B. (1978) Localised mesothelioma of the pleura: benign and malignant variants. *J. Thorac. Cardiovasc. Surg.*, **75**, 363–372

Otto, T. and Strugalska, H. (1987) Surgical treatment for myasthenia gravis. *Thorax*, **42**, 199–204

Pairolero, P. C. and Arnold, P. G. (1986) Thoracic wall defects: surgical management of 205 consecutive patients. *Mayo Clin. Proc.*, **61**, 557–563

Pairolero, P. C., Arnold, P. G., Trastek, V. F. *et al.* (1990) Postpneumonectomy empyema. *J. Thorac. Cardiovasc. Surg.*, **99**, 958–968

Paulson, D. L. (1974) In *Surgery of the Lung* (eds R. E. Smith and W. G. Williams), Butterworths, London

Pearson, F. G., Nelems, S. M., Henderson, R. F. *et al.* (1972) The role of mediastinoscopy in the selection of treatment for bronchial carcinoma with involvement of superior mediastinal lymph nodes. *J. Thorac. Cardiovasc. Surg.*, **64**, 382–390

Prasad, U. S., Naylor, A. R., Walker, W. S. *et al.* (1989) Long term survival after pulmonary resection for small cell carcinoma of the lung. *Thorax*, **44**, 784–787

Ross, J. K. (1978) In *Operative Surgery* (eds C. Rob and R. Smith), Butterworths, London

Roy, P. H., Carr, D. T. and Spencer-Payne, W. (1967) The problem of chylothorax. *Proc. Mayo Clin.*, **42**, 457–459

Sanders, R. D. (1967) A ventilating attachment for bronchoscopy. *Del. Med. J.*, **39**, 170.

Sauerbruch, F. (1913) *Mitt. Grenzgeb. Med. Chir.*, **25**, 746

Saunders, K. B. (1975) The assessment of respiratory function. *Br. J. Hosp. Med.*, **15**, 228–238

Sengupta, A. (1963) The treatment of recurrent spontaneous pneumothorax with iodine and talc poudrage. *Br. J. Dis. Chest*, **57**, 197–199

Shields, T. W. (1989) In *General Thoracic Surgery*, 3rd edn (ed. T. W. Shields), Lea and Febiger, Philadelphia, p. 912

Shields, T. W., Humphrey, E. W. Higgins, G. A. *et al.* (1978) Long-term survivors of resection of lung carcinoma. *J. Thorac. Cardiovasc. Surg.*, **76**, 439–445

Shore, D. F. and Paneth, M. (1980) Survival after resection of small cell carcinoma of the bronchus. *Thorax*, **35**, 819–822

Simpson, J. A. and Thomaides, T. (1987) Treatment of myasthenia gravis: an audit. *Q. J. Med.*, **64**, 693–704

Smith, J. A., Mullerworth, M. H., Westlake, G. W. *et al.* (1991) Empyema thoracis: 14-year experience in a teaching center. *Ann. Thorac. Surg.*, **51**, 39–42

Smith, W. G. and Rothwell, P. P. G. (1962) Treatment of spontaneous pneumothorax. *Thorax*, **17**, 342–349

Spiro, S. G. and Goldstraw, P. (1984) The staging of lung cancer. *Thorax*, **39**, 401–407

Stamatis, G., Freitag, L. and Greschuchna, D. (1990) Limited and radical resection for tracheal and bronchopulmonary carcinoid tumour. *Eur. J. Cardio-thorac. Surg.*, **4**, 527–533

Stanford, W. and Doty, D. B. (1986) The role of venography and surgery in the management of patients with superior vena caval obstruction. *Ann. Thorac. Surg.*, **41**, 158–163

Steel, S. J. and Winstanley, D. P. (1969) Trephine biopsy of the lung and pleura. *Thorax*, **24**, 576–584

Tattersall, M. H. N. and Boyer M. J. (1990) Management of malignant pleural effusion. *Thorax*, **45**, 81–82

Thomas, C. Price and Cleland, W. P. (1942) Extrafascial apicolysis with thoracoplasty. *Br. J. Tuberculosis*, **36**, 109

Thomas, C. Price and Drew C. E. (1953) Fibroma of visceral pleura. *Thorax*, **8**, 180–189

Thoracic Society of Great Britain (1950) The nomenclature of bronchopulmonary anatomy. *Thorax*, **5**, 222–228

Tsang, V., Fernando, H. C. and Goldstraw, P. (1990) Pleuroperitoneal shunt for recurrent malignant pleural effusion. *Thorax*, **45**, 369–372

Trastek, V. F. (1987) Management of mediastinal tumours. *Ann. Thorac. Surg.*, **44**, 227–228

Venn, G. E., Williams, P. R. and Goldstraw, P. (1988) Intracavitary drainage for bullous, emphysematous lung disease: experience with the Brompton technique. *Thorax*, **43**, 998–1002

Wright, J. O., Brandt, B. and Ehrenhaft, J. L. (1982) Results of pulmonary resection for metastatic lesions, *J. Thorac. Cardiovasc. Surg.*, **83**, 94–99

Wychulis, A. R., Payne, W. S., Clagett, O. T. *et al.* (1971) Surgical treatment of mediastinal tumours: a forty year experience. *J. Thorac. Cardiovasc. Surg.*, **62**, 379–392

The nervous system

51

Intracranial neurosurgery

H. B. Griffith†

General technique

The consequences of infection or unnecessary tissue damage can be disastrous for the neurosurgical patient. Habits of handling tissue with the fingers, dabbing and wiping subcutaneous bleeding points with hand-held gauzes, and of allowing the fingers to touch the skin of the patient have no place in neurosurgery. Tissues, needles and sutures are handled only with instruments. An intelligently meticulous 'no touch' technique is mandatory. Since the hair follicles of the scalp cannot be sterilized by detergent followed by bactericide, which is the usual skin preparation, exposed skin edges must be covered and separated from the deeper parts of the exposure by on-laid strips of Lintine. Tissue exposed for several hours must be protected from bacterial fallout by tailored guttapercha sheet. Bactericidal powder applied as a light frosting is used in the extradural layers in wound closure. Subcutaneous sutures have their knot-tails cut obsessionally short and buried under the galeal layer. Talking should be kept to a minimum. Hand signals are often more appropriate and more easily understood than a preoccupied mumble. This is an additional reason for keeping the use of instruments to an easily followed sequence.

Investigation

The best way of developing an instinctive knowledge of the internal topography of the brain in relation to the surface of skull and scalp is always to look at radiographs, arteriograms, isotope scans and computed tomography (CT) scans in a standard way. For instance, a left-sided arteriogram should invariably be orientated on the screen as if the surgeon were gazing at the left side of the patient's head. Radiographs taken on a standard skull table are usually magnified by a factor of 6:5, whereas linear isotope scans are exactly the same size as the brain. In order to reinforce this three-dimensional idea of the internal architecture of the head on which the surgeon is about to operate, it is important for the surgeon in person to position the patient on the operating table headrest. If possible the surgeon should use transparent plastic drapes so that the major topographical features (nose, ears, external occipital protuberance) are visible during surgery. In this way the surgeon will

build up an unconscious awareness of the exact whereabouts of, for instance, the occipital horn, if the time comes during the operation to 'tap the ventricle'. The surgeon who hurries into the operating theatre to carry out the allegedly 'important' part of an operation on a patient, whose head has been positioned, prepared and opened by a junior, will fail to acquire this instinctive knowledge of the patient's brain.

Computed tomography scans occasionally mislead about the position of a mass inside the brain since the plane of cut may be such that a lesion situated almost in the centre of the head may appear to be just beneath the forehead (Figure 51.1).

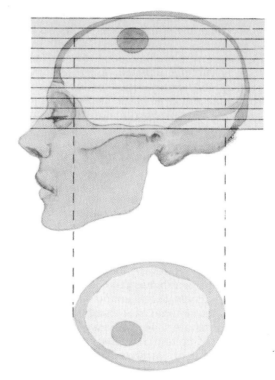

Figure 51.1 CT scan. Anatomy. To show how, for correct localization, the CT scan must be strictly interpreted according to slice levels

Magnetic resonance imaging (MRI) scanning has opened up new horizons in the diagnosis of intracranial conditions. This is especially true for vascular conditions, since flowing blood alters the MRI signal such that vessels, especially if sizeable, can be well seen. The same is also true of cerebrospinal fluid

---

†Huw Griffith died on 4 September 1993.

(CSF). In some MRI pictures the CSF in the ventricles, which is slow moving, is seen as white, and that in the third ventricle, which is moving much faster with a to-and-fro flux, is often displayed as black. In pituitary disease, especially with the smaller tumours, MRI is greatly superior to CT. Because the MRI data can be displayed in three directions at right angles without loss of discrimination, the coronal images are usually very much more detailed and informative than a reconstruction in the plane at right angles to the cut of the CT scan. In the posterior fossa too, because of the lack of bone artefact in the MRI image, structures such as acoustic neuromas, aneurysms and meningiomas are very much better seen. The same applies to imaging the foramen magnum where cerebellar tonsils which may be in the upper cervical canal can be well displayed and a correct interpretation more rapidly arrived at than with CT. There are snags of course. One is that at present the MRI scan takes a lot longer to acquire the data compared with CT scan. Where the patient is restless or disturbed, such as after a head injury, this can be the important factor which dominates the choice of imaging.

Arteriography has now largely become digital. Percutaneous puncture of the carotid in the neck is now almost unheard of, most of the cerebral circulation being outlined with modest doses of contrast introduced via a catheter inserted in the femoral artery retrogradely. By this technique, balloon occlusion of carotid fistulae and large basal aneurysms, and embolization of tumours preoperatively, can be carried out in the conscious patient.

Anaesthesia

It has been said with only a little exaggeration that neurosurgical anaesthesia consists of 'two aspirins and some oxygen'. A sizeable number of minor operations on the skull are safely performed under local anaesthesia and the history of neurosurgery early in the century is studded with examples of major procedures carried out under local anaesthesia alone. What is usually regarded as premedication for general anaesthesia, namely the injection of an opiate with atropine, is not suitable as a tranquillizing agent for neurosurgical patients. This is because opiates depress respiration, leading to the retention of carbon dioxide and the increase of intracranial pressure. The best premedication for a patient about to undergo a procedure under local anaesthesia alone is a clear and confident explanation to a patient who is able to receive the information about what is to occur. The patient should understand that the surgeon will be able to talk to him or her throughout and the patient, if not dysphasic, will be able to talk to the surgeon.

If there are any doubts about the ability of the patient to cooperate, either in understanding or in carrying out instructions, it is better to conduct the procedure under full general anaesthesia with an endotracheal tube. Since intracranial pressure is often high, an increase in cerebral blood flow by unnecessarily prolonged apnoea during induction, venous obstruction due to an awkward position of the head on the shoulders and an increase in cerebral blood flow with a use of vasodilating agents are to be avoided. A reinforced and flexible tube should be used to avoid tube obstruction and in order that the surgeon can reposition the head during operation without provoking a reaction from the patient due to relative movement between the trachea and endotracheal tube.

It is generally preferable to have the patient mechanically ventilated at an adequate gas exchange rather than to rely on the activity of a respiratory centre which may well be compromised by displacement or brain oedema. It is sometimes held that a patient breathing spontaneously will give visible evidence of interference with the respiratory mechanism during surgery in the posterior fossa, but it is far better to be assured of good operating conditions which enable the surgeon to visualize precisely the anatomy involved.

Positioning

For cranial neurosurgery there are three main positions. The *supine* position can be used for all approaches to the anterior three-fifths of the head, neck rotation being minimized by lifting one shoulder with a pad. The *lateral* position can be used for the middle three-fifths of the head, including paramedian incisions for the cerebellopontine angle of the posterior fossa. For the occipital region and the posterior fossa the best position is for the patient's body to lie in a *true lateral* posture with the head turned into the horseshoe rest, a small turn in the neck being permitted. This has the advantage that chest and abdomen are free to move and consequently require less inflation pressure from the ventilator. A modest head-up tilt deals with the problem of systemic venous pressure without the dangers of the sitting position with respect to air embolism. The prone position is now superseded, since it is inefficient on three counts: the ventilator has to lift the entire weight of the patient's trunk to ensure an adequate gas exchange, the head tends to be dependent with a tendency to venous bleeding, and access for the surgeon for lesions near the midline can be extremely awkward. The sitting position for the posterior fossa carries with it the dangers of air embolism and of uncontrollable hypotension during brisk blood loss.

Surgery of access

As the vascular supply and the cranial nerves are concentrated at the base of the brain, together with the pituitary gland, orbit and inner ear, a substantial fraction of the surgery of access to the cranium consists of an approach to the base of the brain.

Pathology near the brain convexity, whether above or below the tentorium, is approached through the skull vault. Basal pathology may also be approached via the skull vault with retraction of the inferior surface of the cerebral hemisphere. Alternatively, basal pathology can be approached more directly through the paranasal air sinuses or through the drilled petrous bone. Occasionally, such as for an acoustic neuroma, these approaches may be combined in one operation. Nevertheless, leaving aside this kind of combined approach, the account which follows will be divided into approaches via the skull vault on the one hand and via the skull base on the other.

It is important to have in one's mind a clear idea of the surface markings of the main features of the brain. In addition, the location of the main vault sutures, coronal, sagittal and lambdoid, have relation to the scalp on the one hand and to the brain on the other. The sutures can often be clearly visualized, especially the lambdoid suture, which appears as a visible ridge when the scalp is shaved. This is especially important when operating on infants where the frontal, parietal and occipital bones are still separated.

Skin incisions

These are basically of two types, namely linear and circumferential. When the approach is a limited one, such as for a burr hole or a trephine, a linear scalp incision will provide an economically large area of exposure of the scalp per unit length of incision. This is because of the shape of the skull and the elasticity of the scalp. When retractors are placed so as to distract and stretch the edges of a linear wound, a diamond-shaped exposure is obtained. When the scalp is very elastic, as in infants, a sizeable osteoplastic craniotomy can be turned via such an exposure. However, when the exposure required is large, a circumferential or scalp flap incision is more efficient. Frequently, as in exploratory head injury surgery, a burr hole to locate a haematoma can be extended into a circumferential incision when it is sited on the circumference of a future flap. Occasionally, as when tapping an otogenic and temporal lobe abscess, the requirement for future surgery may be ignored and the short burr-hole incision will be radial to the circumference of a future osteoplastic flap craniotomy for abscess removal if this subsequently proves to be necessary. Scalp lacerations can usually be extended into an S-shaped incision if a nearby compound depressed fracture needs to be dealt with (see Figure 51.14).

On each side of the head there are three main scalp nerves. These are the supraorbital (V1), auriculotemporal (V3) and greater occipital (C2). Accompanying each of these there are three main arteries (Figures 51.2 and 51.3). The supraorbital artery is a branch of the ophthalmic which, in turn, stems from the internal carotid. The external carotid artery gives rise

to the superficial temporal artery which crosses the zygoma to accompany the auriculotemporal nerve. The occipital artery branches posteriorly from the external carotid deep to the mastoid process and runs a little distance from the greater occipital nerve which is more medially situated. Scalp incisions should be placed so as to respect and preserve both innervation and arterial supply, although the latitude given to surgeons by the excellent anastomotic blood supply of the scalp makes almost any incision possible. The shape and size of the flap should respect the general rule of having a sound vascular pedicle and should preferably taper gently from base to apex. Remember that the frontalis and occipitalis muscles and the occasionally well-developed muscles attached to the ear pinna (anterior superior and posterior auriculares) are part of the scalp and are not, as are the temporalis muscles and the suboccipital muscles, attached to the skull.

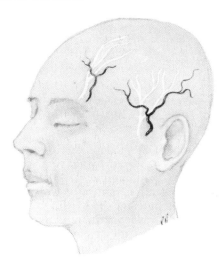

Figure 51.2 Superficial arteries and veins of the anterior and lateral scalp. Note how the anterior branch of the superficial temporal artery (external carotid circulation) can easily establish an anastomosis with the supraorbital artery (internal carotid circulation)

The major venous sinuses, namely the sagittal sinus, torcula and the transverse (lateral) and sigmoid sinuses, dominate the surgery of the skull. This is because the outer layer of these venous sinuses is composed of flimsy collagen which tears easily. It is possible to lose a large amount of blood in a short time when this occurs. The veins which bridge between the cortex and the superior sagittal venous sinus seriously hamper access to the great longitudinal fissure, and to divide them can lead to damaging venous infarction. Avoid this by utilizing, where possible, the gaps, such as at the occipital pole, which are free of such veins. The supratentorial pineal approach slips through this constant gap. There is another less complete gap in the area between frontal pole and coronal suture.

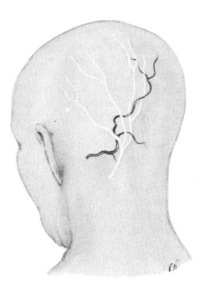

Figure 51.3 Superficial arteries and nerves of the posterior scalp. Note that the occipital artery (external carotid branch) emerges behind the mastoid process, considerably lateral to the origin of the greater occipital nerve

Surgical sequences: basic steps

Burr hole

This is the simplest method of gaining access to the brain. The hair is removed by shaving over an area measuring 10 × 12 cm minimum. After preparation and draping, the scalp is infiltrated with local anaesthetic (usually lignocaine 1% with adrenaline 1: 200 000 added as a vasoconstrictor (Figure 51.4). The pointed scalpel incises all layers including pericranium in a single cut of 3 cm length. The pericranium is swept back on either side with a curved Adson's periosteal elevator. A self-retaining retractor is inserted and opened to produce enough tension in the wound edges to stop bleeding (Figure 51.5). A small Hudson's brace with a 15 mm perforator is used. Considerable force is transmitted from the trunk via the left hand of the operating surgeon who stands (as in Figure 51.6) with the legs placed so that the forward foot is safely underneath the head of the patient. The right hand now rotates the brace at speed. It is only necessary for two fingers or the index finger and thumb to grasp the handle of the brace lightly so that the subtle changes of vibration as the perforator shaves through the outer table, diploë and inner table can be detected in sequence by a combination of feel and noise. An assistant drips saline slowly onto the rotating perforator so that it lubricates and cools the sharp cutting edge without irrigating the skin edges. When the inner table is breached over an area 2 mm across, the 16 mm tapered conical burr is used to ream out the hole. Less trunk pressure and more rotary force are used. The brace becomes difficult to turn as the burr engages in the bone. Bone

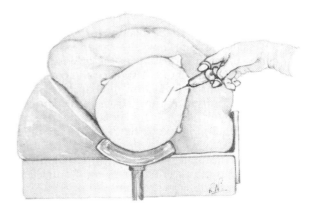

Figure 51.4 Burr-hole infiltration. A bleb of local anaesthetic raises a substantial wheal in the scalp around the intended burr incision under local anaesthetic

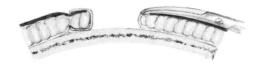

Figure 51.5 Scalp haemostasis. On the left an encompassing Raney scalp clip; on the right galeal tension by means of curved haemostatic forceps

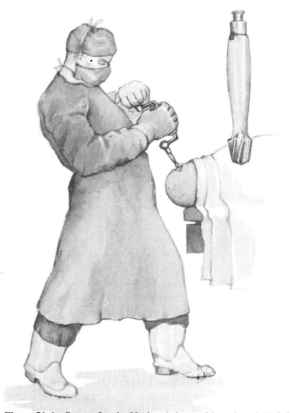

Figure 51.6 Stance for the Hudson's brace. Note that the left foot, onto which all weight is transferred, provides both a safety factor and for a more sensitive manoeuvre

left hand keeps the small exposure free of blood and CSF. As the diathermy sparks coagulate arachnoid, pia and the superficial layers of the cortex, the closed tip of the dissecting forceps is thrust through the coagulated spot to a depth of approximately 3 mm.

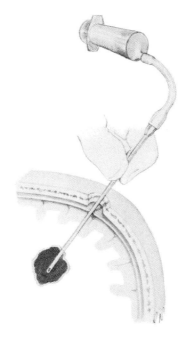

Figure 51.8   Aspiration of intracerebral abscess. Note the flexible connection to syringe to avoid needle movement

If, for example, an abscess is to be aspirated, a glioma biopsied or the ventricle visualized, a slim brain cannula or endoscope is now introduced by thumb and index finger while the heel of the hand rests on the head (Figures 51.8 and 51.9). Similarly supported, left-handed fingers grasp the butt of the cannula when the stylet is withdrawn. The syringe is inserted smoothly into the flexible rubber connector, with which all brain cannulas should be fitted. The cannula is held motionless while CSF pus or liquid haematoma or glioma fragments are aspirated. If bleeding is encountered, the cannula is not withdrawn until it stops. When the cannula is withdrawn the dura is not closed but the small dural hole is covered by a stamp of Gelfoam sponge. Scalp closure is accomplished by two interrupted inverted galeal absorbable sutures (3/0) with four through-and-through deeply biting skin sutures (2/0 or 3/0), which underrun the plentiful scalp arteries and accomplish scalp haemostasis without need for diathermization of skin edges (Figure 51.10).

A trephine disc (Figures 51.11 and 51.12)

A disc 2.5–5.0 cm in diameter must be removed when the cortical exposure needed is larger than afforded

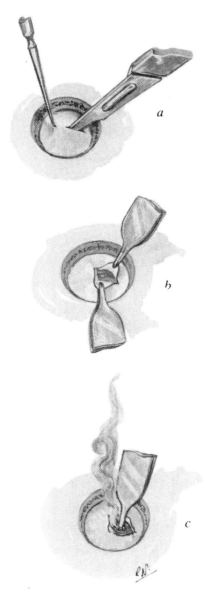

Figure 51.7   *a*, Dural opening. After burr hole or disc trephine the sharp hook tents up the dura into which a light incision is made. This is then opened by forceps or by scissors (*b*) *c*. A pial spot for ventricular cannulation or an incision is coagulated with the unipolar diathermy

flakes are now picked off the dura as the surgeon sits down comfortably. Bone dust is irrigated away from the hole. A sharp right-angled fine hook tents up the dura in the centre of the hole (Figure 51.7a) and a rounded tenotome (no. 15 blade) incises the dura with one or two deft strokes 5 mm or so in length. This short nick is pulled apart with dissecting forceps into a diamond-shaped exposure (Figure 51.7b). A pial spot on the crown of a gyrus is now coagulated lightly with the low setting of the unipolar diathermy connected to a fine non-toothed dissecting forceps held in the right hand (Figure 51.7c). A fine sucker held in the

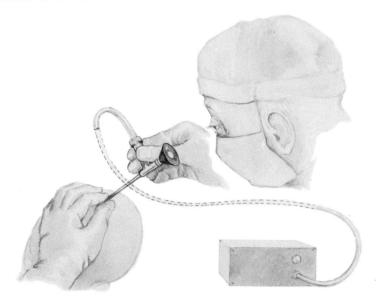

Figure 51.9 Endoneurosurgery. Note endoscope held with steadying left hand, and manipulating right hand, which should be supported

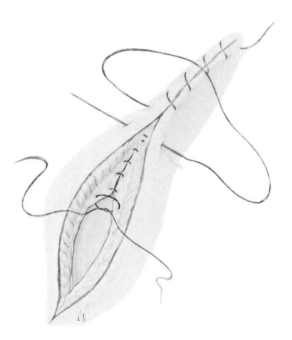

Figure 51.10 Scalp closure. The deep (galeal) sutures are tied with knots inverted, the superficial scalp being brought together by deep bites of continuous or interrupted sutures round the superficial scalp vessels

by a burr hole. For example, the aspiration of a solid intracerebral haematoma, the search for a suitable sylvian artery in superficial temporal/middle cerebral microvascular anastomosis, or the taking of a block cortical brain biopsy, usually require at least a 2.5 cm exposure. This can be obtained by the circumferential nibbling enlargement of a burr hole (as in exploration of extradural haematoma (see Figure 51.13) but the resulting skull defect then produces a visibly pulsating indent or bulge which can be upsetting for patients and relatives. A straight all-layer scalp incision about 6 cm in length is distracted by self-retaining retractors (Mollison's are convenient) into a diamond-shaped cranial exposure. In its centre a 2.5 mm twist drill guarded to a 6 mm depth produces a hole which takes the centre pin of the Scoville trephine. Taking care to avoid snagging the trephine cutting teeth on the surrounding pericranium, the trephine begins to cut a disc. An even cut is made to a depth of 3 mm or so. At this stage, the trephine is disengaged from the skull, its centre pin is removed and the trephine cuts again. As the inner table is reached, rotation is more cautious with frequent checks. This will allow the

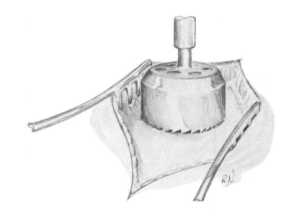

Figure 51.11 Trephine exploration

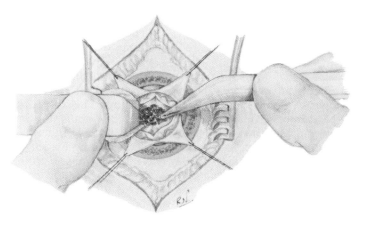

Figure 51.12 An intracerebral haematoma is being evacuated under direct vision with a retractor working opposite the sucker

surgeon to cut just through the inner table (without perforating the dura) over approximately half the circumference of the bone disc. Orientation marks to ensure correct reinsertion are now made by a small nibbling bite on inner and outer lips of the cut respectively. Bone elevators prise out the disc, taking care not to allow the disc to jump uncontrollably out of the wound with the final snap.

The dura is usually opened in a cruciate incision with scissors or director with tenotome. When a solid subcortical haematoma is to be removed, the surgeon dons a headlight, sits comfortably and, with sucker in the left hand and dissecting forceps in the right, coagulates the arachnoid and pia over a 2 cm linear incision in the crown of the gyrus. Fine brain scissors are used to divide the cortex and leptomeninges. The incision is now deepened by strokes of a narrow sucker held in the right hand while the incision is opened by a metal strip brain retractor held in the left. The brain is protected by Lintine strips overlapping the lips of the cortical incision. When the haematoma is encountered, the large sucker is used to evacuate it under direct vision, taking care not to abrade the delicate granulating walls of the cavity. For haemostasis, the emptied cavity is lightly packed with cottonwool balls soaked in 10 vol hydrogen peroxide for 4 min. During this wait, the surgeon attends to any small cortical bleeding points with the bipolar diathermy.

When haemostasis is complete, the four triangular dural flaps are drawn together with a single silk suture through their apices. Gelfoam sponge pledgets are laid over the remaining gaps in the dura. The bone disc is replaced and the pericranium and/or temporalis fascia is closed with interrupted 2/0 silk sutures so as to hold it in position. The scalp is then closed in the usual two layers without suction drainage.

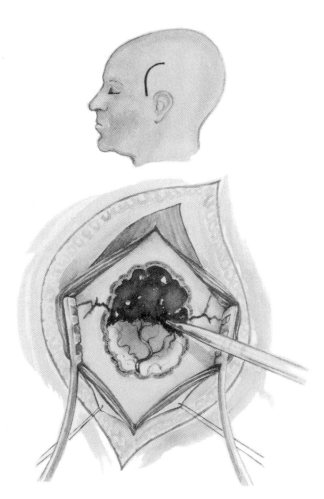

Figure 51.13 Extradural haemorrhage. Sucker evacuation of haematoma after division of temporalis muscle and enlargement of burr hole

Surgical management of extradural haemorrhage

Indications for surgery

The classic picture of a rapidly advancing extradural haemorrhage is well known. A young person, often after a relatively minor head injury, sometimes without loss of consciousness, and after a lucid interval which may vary from minutes to hours, usually first complains of increasing headache, becomes drowsy and then unconscious. Signs of increasing limb paresis may or may not be obvious. With depression of the level of consciousness, which is the most important observation, comes a progressive dilatation of the pupil on the side of the haematoma, slowing of the pulse, and increase in the systolic blood pressure so as to give a bounding pulse and, later, periodic respiration. The pupillary dilatation is due to stretching of a third (oculomotor) nerve by the medial portion of the temporal lobe, which is being squeezed through the tentorial hiatus into the posterior fossa, distorting as it does so the midbrain and producing depression of consciousness by compromise of the ascending reticular activating system. Examination of the head will usually give enough information to enable an alert surgeon to rescue a deteriorating patient. Almost invariably, and particularly in young people, a transverse lateral fracture is present low on the skull, usually in the thin and vulnerable temporal bone. Not only does the fracture lacerate the middle meningeal artery, producing a sizeable lens-shaped haematoma, often several centimetres thick, but the blood under arterial pressure leaks out under the temporalis muscle, producing the characteristic 'boggy swelling'. This feels characteristically different to the exploring finger of a surgeon from the ordinary scalp haematoma which can be indented. Skull radiographs are helpful to delineate the underlying fracture but, particularly in the restless child, indifferent skull radiographs may mislead one into the belief that a fracture is not present.

The immediate treatment is evacuation of the haematoma and hopefully a reversal of the progressive mid-brain and medullary compression, which otherwise will be rapidly fatal. The simplest manoeuvre is to make a burr hole and then enlarge this with nibbling bone forceps so that a sucker can evacuate with the solid haematoma (Figure 51.13). Dealing with the site of haemorrhage itself is not always necessary, since in many cases by the time the surgeon arrives at the haematoma the haemorrhage will have stopped. The main difficulty, however, is to site the exploring burr hole squarely over the haematoma.

The burr hole should be sited: (1) in relation to the boggy swelling; (2) in relation to the skull fracture seen on the radiograph, particularly at the place where the fracture may cross the middle meningeal artery seen on the skull radiographs; (3) in the temporal region if no boggy swelling is present and no fracture can be discerned on the skull radiograph. The side chosen is always the side of the first and larger dilating pupil.

The incision is made 3 cm long at right angles to the skull base and halfway between the bony rim of the orbit and the external auditory meatus, just above the zygoma. The scalpel cut is firmly taken down through the temporalis to the underlying bone, where an unsuspected fracture edge may be felt by the encountering blade. A periosteal elevator scrapes the temporal muscle from its underlying attachment to the bone, and the deep-bladed self-retaining retractor holds the edges of the wound apart. The perforating burr is now used, care being taken when making a burr hole adjacent to a linear fracture (Figure 51.14). Immediately the burr is lifted a tarry haematoma is apparent if the hole has been accurately sited. If dura is encountered, it should be opened if blue, since an acute subdural haematoma can mimic the clinical picture of an extradural haemorrhage. The dura, which will be tightly bulging, should be depressed gently with the periosteal elevator in the direction towards the base of the skull and swept gently round, hard against the inner table of the skull. A spurt of blood will indicate location of the adjacent haematoma and nibbling of the bone in that direction will give access to the edge of the clot. If the dura is slack then cerebral compression is not present and the situation should be reassessed. In this context the presence of fat embolism in the patient with limb fractures should not be overlooked.

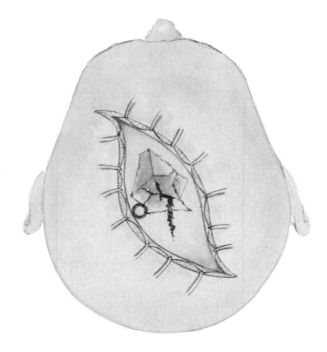

Figure 51.14 Compound depressed vault fracture. Note extension of laceration into S-shaped exposure. Burr hole placed at margin of fracture, the inner table fracture being larger than the outer table fracture

When the haematoma is encountered, further bone is nibbled away (see Figure 51.13). An extension of the burr-hole incision may be necessary to enable this to be done comfortably. The temporalis muscle is retracted to enable the direction and extent of the haematoma to be seen as it is evacuated with the sucker and periosteal elevator. Usually the clot will track down across the floor of the middle fossa towards the foramen spinosum. If a bleeding extra-dural artery can be seen it is dealt with by diathermy coagulation. The traditional matchstick plugging of the foramen spinosum is usually unnecessary. There may be multiple oozing points from the dura, and from the bone edge, the latter being dealt with by Horsley's bone wax being squeezed into the narrow diploic spaces. When the haematoma is extensive, the linear burr-hole incision may be extended into a circumferential osteoplastic flap craniotomy incision. Often, however, the application of cottonwool patties or pledgets soaked in peroxide, combined with patience, will allow the extradural space to be closed again by the steadily re-expanding brain. The dura should be inspected for rents which can be closed with interrupted fine black silk sutures.

When the bleeding has been controlled, any patties are removed, and the temporalis fascia is apposed with interrupted black silk sutures. The scalp is then closed with a layer of inverted sutures to the galea aponeurotica, and interrupted black silk or continuous nylon to the skin at 1 cm intervals. Drainage is not usually necessary, but if the ooze is persistent then a suction drainage tube can be introduced gently into the extradural space and let out through a stab wound adjacent to the main incision.

Evacuation of the haematoma is usually followed by a rapid and dramatic reversal of the deteriorating preoperative sequence. If this does not occur, then specialized help should be sought, not forgetting that a CT scan usually discloses rapidly and clearly a fresh intracranial haematoma.

Craniotomy

General principles

The need for craniotomy is dictated by two considerations. One is the size of the pathology to be dealt with. Clearly, a large tumour will usually require a sizeable exposure, not for the evacuation of the mass intact, but in order to gain access to the planes of cleavage when normal brain must be discretely and carefully separated from tumour boundary such as in the removal of a meningioma. The second reason for craniotomy is to gain access, for instance, at the skull base to an aneurysm which may itself be quite small. Here the base of the cerebral hemispheres must be retracted and although some of the space to be gained can be taken up by the removal of CSF by lumbar or ventricular puncture, the surgeon needs enough

exposure at the surface to enable him or her to deploy instruments and retractors without dangerous overcrowding. Although it is quite possible to carry out basal procedures via a 5 cm trephine, it is on the whole preferable to permit oneself the exposure which an adequately sized osteoplastic flap provides.

The siting of the craniotomy naturally will depend on the procedure. Dandy introduced the 'concealed' osteoplastic frontal craniotomy, a scalp flap designed with its incision virtually entirely hidden behind the hairline on one side overlying a modestly sized bone flap sited so as just to avoid the frontal air sinus, yet sufficiently low on the temporal bone to enable the operator to proceed along the sphenoidal ridge in the direction of the brain base. A lateral craniotomy gives access to the temporal lobe and to the tentorial hiatus at the brain base, and an occipital craniotomy, besides being the approach for occipitally placed tumours, may be used with occipital lobe retraction to give access to the pineal region. The main decision to be made when siting a craniotomy is the relation of the flap to the main venous sinuses, mainly the superior sagittal sinus, especially in its posterior portion, and the lateral and sigmoid venous sinuses (see Figure 51.16). The outer wall of the triangular lumen of a large venous sinus may be deficient, especially in the sigmoid region, and a craniotomy whose margin transgresses these structures runs a risk of torrential blood loss during the opening stages. If the medial longitudinal fissure of the brain is to be entered, then the craniotomy must go beyond the midline. Special care has then to be taken to preserve and protect the sagittal sinus. Where a bifrontal procedure has to be undertaken, such as for an anterior falx meningioma or bilateral dural repair, then a coronal scalp flap gives an excellent cosmetic result under which either a bifrontal or two separate frontal craniotomies can be turned down. A convexity meningioma may evoke a hyperostosis from the overlying skull at the site of dural attachment and this must be encompassed by the planned flap so that the attachment presents in the middle of the exposure when the skull flap is turned down.

In general it is better to allow a bone flap to remain attached by a thick pedicle of temporalis muscle as this can be conserved without impairing the operator's approach. Occasionally it is difficult to fashion and turn down a flap which does not, by its very presence, somewhat impair the operator's access to the brain base, and in these circumstances there should be no hesitation about stripping the bone from its musculofibrous attachment, to be replaced as a free bone graft at the closure.

A posterior fossa craniotomy is really a craniectomy. The thin bone of the posterior fossa is simply removed piecemeal and not replaced. There are two reasons for this. One is the technical difficulty of fashioning an osteoplastic craniotomy based on the occipital muscles without damaging the underlying cerebellum and venous sinuses, particularly at the torcula. The second is the frequent need for an adequate decompression of the posterior fossa structures after the operative procedure, since room is restricted and any swelling of the cerebellum may lead to medullary compression with dire consequences. The occipital muscle attachment regenerates a thin bony integument of the posterior fossa fairly well over the course of the next 2 or 3 months after the acute period has passed, so that lack of bone over the posterior fossa structures is neither a serious nor a cosmetic defect.

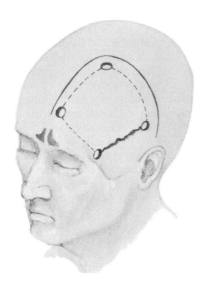

Figure 51.15 Osteoplastic craniotomy – frontotemporal. Note the scalp incision largely concealed behind the hair line

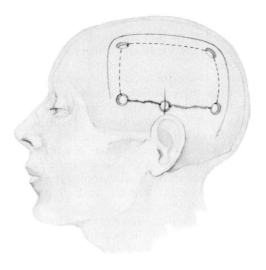

Figure 51.16 Lateral craniotomy. Note that the two posterior lowermost burr holes are placed above the transverse or lateral venous sinus

Osteoplastic craniotomy of the skull vault
(Figures 51.15 and 51.16)

After skin preparation and draping and with the patient under endotracheal general anaesthesia, the incision is made through the outer four layers of the scalp which have been infiltrated with local anaesthetic containing adrenaline. This latter procedure makes it easier to avoid incising the pericranium with the knife. The guide to complete division of the galea aponeurotica is the parting of the edge of the scalp under the slightly distracting finger pressures of operator and assistant. Scalp bleeding can always be controlled by digital pressure properly applied. Haemostats (curved artery forceps) are applied to the galea or, if preferred, removable haemostatic scalp edge clips of the Raney variety, either metal or plastic, are applied (see Figure 51.5). In infants and in the temporal region the scalp thickness may need to be augmented by folded strips of wet gauze to enable the clip to apply enough pressure to stop edge bleeding. The incision is usually completed in two sweeps of the scalpel. The scalp flap is then picked up with forceps or retractor and the areolar layer of tissue divided by sweeps of the scalpel using the broad edge rather than its point. Any bleeding vessels are now picked up with the low coagulating diathermy current directed via fine non-toothed dissecting forceps held in one hand while the sucker is used in the other. This scalp flap is then wrapped in a wet gauze and held back with stay sutures. The pericranium and temporalis, on which the flap is to be based, are now divided by the point of the cutting diathermy. The pericranium is eased back by the flat-ended periosteal rugine lubricated by a thin stream of warm saline. A four-pointed bone flap is usually adequate for most purposes if perforator and burr are to be used. The motor-driven craniotome gives a little more freedom in the shaping and extent of the exposure. Each burr hole is made with perforator, then burr, and a curved Adson's periosteal elevator is used to separate gently the somewhat adherent dura from the inner table of the skull (Figure 51.17). In older patients hyperostosis frontalis interna can promote dural shredding during the lifting of the bone flap due to great adherence of the bone to the outer dural layer.

The Gigli saw guide is now passed between the skull vault and the dura from burr hole to burr hole, except at the base of the flap which is best fractured. The Gigli saw is kept taut while its full length is used, the advancing cut being cooled by a dribble of saline (Figure 51.18). As the base of the flap, usually bridged by temporalis muscle, is thin, a few nibbles across here with a bone rongeur are sufficient to enable the skull flap to be snapped back. Carefully prising the flap will avoid a sharp bone edge penetrating the dura. Often the middle meningeal artery will have been torn as the flap is lifted and the first priority is to stop this bleeding with the bipolar diathermy. The jagged edges of the base of the flap

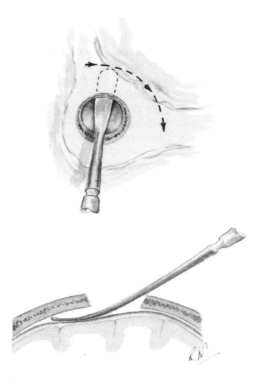

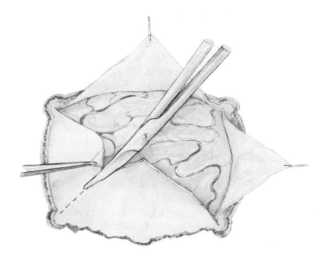

Figure 51.19 Dural opening for maximum brain exposure

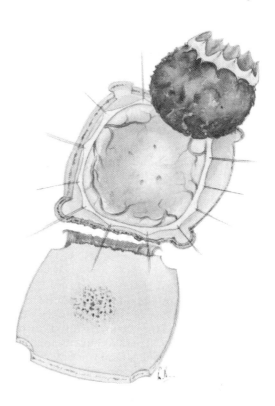

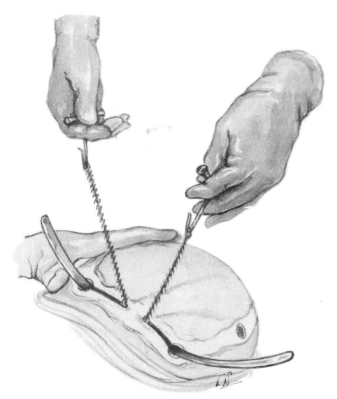

Figure 51.17 Method of dural separation from the inner scalp table

Figure 51.18 Use of the Gigli saw between burr holes, introduced by means of the De Martel saw guide

Figure 51.20 Removal of vault (or convexity) meningioma, showing hyperostosis on inner table of osteoplastic flap. Method of tumour traction utilizing dural sutures

are now trimmed with a bone rongeur and the skull flap held back by a towel clip through enveloping twisted gauze. When the craniotomy nears or encroaches upon the midline, venous bleeding from the superior longitudinal sinus or lacunae laterales is controlled by Gelfoam pledgets under stamps of gutta percha held in place by patties.

The dura is now exposed for the surgeon to make the decision as to how it should be opened (Figure 51.19). If the dura is very tight, measures must be taken to slacken it by ventricular tapping, anaesthetic hyperventilation or intravenous mannitol, since cortical herniation through even the smallest incision can produce venous bleeding that is impossible to control. The type of dural opening is dictated by the underlying pathology to be treated. For instance, a vault meningioma will usually have a dural attachment which must be removed with the tumour (Figure 51.20). A cut radial to the circumference of the tumour will bring the surgeon up to its edge. A circumferential cut around the tumour attachment is then made. The hypertrophied dural vessels are controlled with silver or tantalum dural clips. Further radial cuts in the uninvolved dura will enable the boundary of the meningioma and normal brain to be discerned so that the removal can begin. If a glioma is to be approached then there is a choice between turning a dural flap up towards the superior sagittal sinus so as to avoid damaging veins bridging cortex to sinus. Alternatively, the dura can be opened in a cruciate incision, beginning at the site most likely to reveal discernible pathology, so that the dural opening can then be restricted only to what is necessary for the biopsy or removal. When the brain base is to be approached, the dura is opened in a curved incision along but 5 mm away from the forward edge of a frontal craniotomy exposure, since there are virtually no bridging veins here. The vulnerable 'corner' of the cerebral hemisphere where convexity becomes base is protected with gutta percha strips overlaid by Lintine. The retractor which now elevates the frontal lobe for access, for example, to a pituitary neoplasm or a basal aneurysm is used to coax the brain away from the base rather than to pull it.

Closure

Hitch sutures are often employed to tie dura to pericranium at the edge of the craniotomy exposure in order to discourage the accumulation of extradural blood postoperatively. These should be placed very precisely so that no undue lateral traction on the dura ensues. If there is likely to be an appreciable period of haemostasis, as, for example, in drying up a tumour bed, then placement of these sutures is most profitably left to what would otherwise be a period of waiting. For basal approaches, however, hitch sutures are best put in before the dural opening since haemostasis will have to take place during the time that the brain is still retracted.

When all intradural bleeding points are completely controlled, leaving nothing to chance or probability, the dura is closed. Intermittent 3/0 fine silk sutures spaced at 1 cm intervals are usually sufficient. If brain swelling is thought likely then the dura is left open over the temporal lobe but closed over the convexity and the bone flap is removed. Even without brain swelling, this flap removal is sometimes best in meningiomas which are modest in size but which have provoked a marked oedematous reaction in the surrounding brain. The bone flap is replaced when the intracranial pressure normalizes, usually after 2 or 3 weeks. The flap is stripped carefully from temporalis muscle and periosteum and this layer is then sutured at 2 cm intervals with 2/0 black silk exactly in the position it would have occupied were the bone flap still in place. The elasticity of muscle and periosteum is usually sufficient to accommodate all but the most desperate of swellings.

When the dura is closed, external bleeding points on it are dealt with by very light touches with the bipolar diathermy or, if venous, by pressure on a stamp of gelatin sponge or Surgicel. When haemostasis is complete, the bone flap is fitted in position and, while an instrument wielded by an assistant holds it so, the surgeon places several 2/0 sutures through the pericranium to hold it in place. The closure is then completed with further sutures at 1.5 cm intervals. A powdery mixture of antibiotic and bone dust is compressed into each burr hole so as to prevent an unsightly dent on the forehead. The sutures are placed only in pericranium or temporalis fascia and not through muscle. Unless an air sinus has been opened, a 3 mm polythene catheter for suction drainage is now reverse introduced through the scalp about 2 cm from the craniotomy edge and allowed to lie in the subgaleal space. The scalp is closed with a galeal layer of interrupted absorbable sutures (3/0 in children) inserted so that the knots lie underneath the galea with tails cut no more than 1 mm long. These are put in at intervals of 1–1.5 cm, taking care to approximate galea only and to avoid placing the suture through potentially contaminated deep hair follicles. Alternatively, a continuous absorbable suture can be used to close this layer. The top layer is most speedily closed with a continuous 3/0 nylon suture introduced with a straight needle, but interrupted sutures or a subcuticular Dexon with Steristrip closure may also be used. If continuous sutures are employed it is unnecessary to use diathermy coagulation to control bleeding points in the vessels which lie between galea and skin.

Special manoeuvres

Aneurysm clipping

Operations to prevent rebleeding from ruptured intracranial basal aneurysms are usually undertaken in the first 3 weeks after bleeding. The common sites for these aneurysms are at the inferior aspect of the internal carotid artery just before it bifurcates into anterior and middle cerebral branches (posterior communicating site), the bi- or trifurcation of the middle cerebral artery and at the anterior communicating artery respectively. The initial approach to all these aneurysms is by retraction of the frontal lobe along the sphenoidal wing (Figure 51.21). A basic tenet of aneurysm surgery is to approach the aneurysm so that control of the vessel feeding it can be speedily undertaken were the aneurysm to rupture during dissection. Consequently, when the middle cerebral aneurysm is to be approached the sylvian fissure is opened just proximal to the aneurysm so that, before the aneurysm base is dissected, the middle cerebral artery can be prepared to take a clip in an emergency rupture. Similarly, the choice of side in the approach to the anterior communicating aneurysm is dictated by the artery which most readily fills it. This will usually give the most advantageous approach since the aneurysm will usually point away from the main feeding artery, thus presenting its neck for clipping advantageously at right angles.

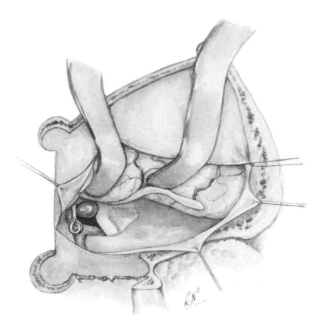

Figure 51.21 Clipping of basal aneurysm. Note that the olfactory bulb has been avulsed from the cribriform plate (unfortunately). Scoville removable spring clip applied to the neck of the aneurysm

The approach to the aneurysm is a cautious one with adjustments of the retractors and division of arachnoidal bands by sharp-pointed bayonet-shaped micro-scissors. The dissection is directed to the neck of the aneurysm and not to its vulnerable fundus, where the wall is very thin and the leak which produced the intracranial haemorrhage is sealed only by a friable fibrin plug. The expanded base of the aneurysm has to be dissected away from enveloping blood vessels so that the true neck, which may be sizeable, can be discerned. When this has been done, a temporary clipping to lower the pressure in the aneurysm or shrinkage of the neck by brief applications of the bipolar diathermy current sometimes enables an inoperable aneurysm to become operable. Removable

spring clips, of which there are many patterns, the Scoville being the most versatile, are used. When an expanded trifurcation and aneurysm of the middle cerebral are dissected, it sometimes is seen that there is no true neck and one has to be 'manufactured' by the act of clipping. When this has been done without compromise of vessels, it may be clear that some of the fundus remains proximal to the clip and further expansion of the aneurysm may yet be possible. In these circumstances the clipped aneurysm and the vessels of origin can with advantage be invested in a quick-setting acrylic resin. This can be introduced around the aneurysm and solidifies in a few minutes. Aneurysms at the posterior communicating site usually point at right angles to the surgeon and the neck is encountered first. Occasionally the arachnoid around the neck has to be divided to allow a clip to slide around it. In turn the clip may impinge on the dura of the cavernous sinus or petroclinoid ligament. Occasionally the posterior communicating artery can neither be easily seen nor dissected and is included in the clip. The anterior communicating artery dissection best takes place through an approach which removes a very small volume of gyrus rectus above the optic chiasm which is bridged by the anterior cerebral artery. Division of the arachnoid 5 mm medial to the olfactory tract, with sucking away of the subjacent brain at the level of the optic nerve, gives access to the anterior communicating region together with the terminal anterior cerebral artery. It is important to see the contralateral anterior cerebral artery and to dissect away the pericallosal arteries from the base of the aneurysm before application of the clip.

Although most aneurysm surgery is straightforward, it occasionally occurs that the clip may compromise the circulation in the distal vessels in a way which cannot be discerned from inspection even under the operating microscope. In these circumstances it has been found advantageous to carry out an operative arteriogram through a flexible catheter introduced retrogradely down the superficial temporal artery as far as the carotid bifurcation. Eight or 10 ml of radiological contrast, together with a single unscreened film under the head, usually give sufficient detail to reassure the surgeon that the clip has not embarrassed the remaining circulation. If the circulation is sparse, then the clip will have to be readjusted and a further arteriogram taken. The incision in the superficial temporal artery is closed by a continuous 10/0 nylon microsuture under high magnification.

Posterior fossa craniotomy (Figure 51.22)

There are three basic surgical approaches to posterior fossa structures. The most commonly practised posterior approach is with a craniectomy via a midline incision. Most intracerebellar tumours and cysts can be dealt with by this approach and it has the added advantage that dangerous posterior fossa herniation through the foramen magnum can be effectively decompressed. In addition, tumours which extend into the spinal canal, such as haemangioblastomas and ependymomas, can be encompassed simply by downward extension of the incision. A second approach used for surgery of tumours of the high cerebellar vermis is an occipital osteoplastic craniotomy with retraction upwards of the occipital lobe after opening the dura above the lateral sinus. The posterior fossa is opened by division of the tentorium. Another more anterior transtentorial access can be gained by a lateral craniotomy so as to lift up the temporal lobe with division of the anterior tentorium along the petrous ridge attachment. This gives good exposure of the upper cranial nerves and to aneurysms of the upper vertebral artery and of the basilar artery. The third route of entry to the posterior fossa is via its anterior wall but as this is formed by the petrous bone, this structure has to be drilled away in the translabyrinthine approach to acoustic neuromas.

Ensuring good operating conditions

Positioning for a posterior fossa craniotomy is very important. The most common position in former times was with a patient lying prone with the head flexed. The position of the operating surgeon was then somewhat awkward and with mechanical ventilation the inflation pressures required from the pump were high since each ventilatory cycle had in effect to lift the weight of the trunk. This makes for somewhat less than ideal operating conditions. The sitting position gives good operating conditions for surgeons as far as pressures are concerned, but there is a small but appreciable mortality in this position from unexpected massive air embolism even though anticipated and guarded against. In addition, hypotension due to substantial blood loss can less easily be countered in this position. The lateral position for approaches to the posterior fossa suffers from none of the disadvantages which have been mentioned. With a slight head-up tilt and the patient lying on the side operating conditions are good, the surgeon can sit comfortably in a specially designed chair for microdissection and the anaesthetist has good access to the ventral surface of the patient. The thorax and abdomen are free so that either mechanical or spontaneous ventilation can then be employed.

Many posterior fossa pathologies have secondary effects in precipitating obstructive hydrocephalus. This leads to high intracranial pressure which in turn elevates the intracranial venous pressure. As the intracranial veins are in communication with the diploic veins, the result of breaching the bone, particularly around the torcula, is brisk loss of venous blood at substantial pressure. One way of dealing with this situation is to insert a ventriculovenous

shunt some time before operation, particularly if the patient is in poor nutritional shape and is clearly not fit to face a major posterior fossa operation. However, the benefits of this somewhat complicated manoeuvre can be gained very rapidly by the insertion of a catheter into the lateral ventricle via a frontal burr hole, such as for positive contrast ventriculography. If, as usually occurs nowadays, the diagnosis has been made purely on the CT scan, a parieto-occipital burr hole inserted 3 cm from the midline just above the lambdoid suture gives access to the lateral ventricle and intracranial pressure control can rapidly be effected by draining a few millilitres of cerebrospinal fluid.

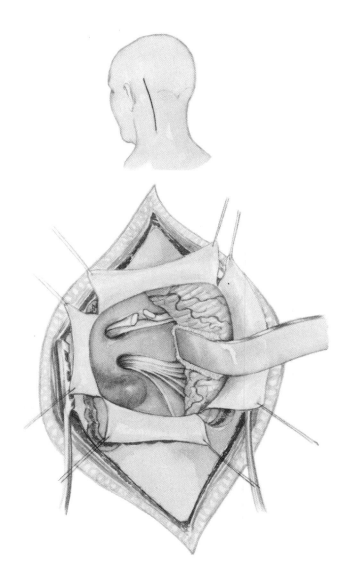

Figure 51.22 Intracranial (posterior fossa) division of vestibular nerve for Ménière's disease. Note very light retraction of cerebellum and intact jugular group of nerves

Approach

The lambdoid suture becomes visible on the shaved and prepared scalp as a slight ridge. This burr hole is marked out just above it. The midline linear incision to the posterior fossa is marked out from some 2 cm above the external occipital protuberance to a similar distance below the palpable spine of the second cervical vertebra (axis). After draping, the cut is made with one sweep of the scalpel and artery forceps are applied to the skin edges to control bleeding. Occasionally in a young person the scalp will be pliable enough for Raney scalp edge clips to be effective. With bleeding controlled, self-retaining retractors of the Mollison type now produce distracting tension to allow the muscles to be split, using the cutting diathermy and keeping strictly to the midline. If this relatively avascular midline plane is not easily apparent it is worth picking it up at the external occipital protuberance first and then following it down into the nuchal musculature. One or two veins are found crossing the midline but these can be dealt with by the coagulating diathermy. The incision is taken onto the truncated spine of the posterior arch of the atlas and below this onto the much stouter midline spine of the axis vertebra. Remember that the posterior arch of the atlas is sometimes deficient in the midline, and because of the circular venous sinus at the foramen magnum it is safer to clear the tissue from the atlanto-occipital membrane with a tenotome than with cutting diathermy.

It is important while elevating the muscles from the posterior fossa bone below the superior nuchal line to use the controlled force of a double-handed grip on the periosteal elevator. With reinsertions of the self-retaining retractor with teeth in the muscle layer, together with judicious upward cuts of the diathermy, especially at the superior nuchal line, the muscles can be elevated to display a considerable width of the occipital bone. Clearly if the structure to be approached is to one side of the midline (and this should be the side chosen uppermost when positioning the patient on the operating table) the muscles are cleared more completely on this side. Now, with an extension to the Hudson brace, a burr hole is placed to each side of the midline just below the external occipital protuberance. The Adson periosteal elevator is used to separate the dura from bone and the burr hole is enlarged by nibbling first with narrow and then with broader bone rongeurs until the foramen magnum is reached and opened to the extent of the posterior quarter of its circumference. If the cerebellar tonsils are shown, perhaps in ventriculographic or myelographic studies, to have descended below the foramen magnum, the central 3 cm of the posterior arch of the atlas are removed after elevating the periosteum from this structure. The bony removal superiorly is usually taken upwards to the inferior margin of the transverse venous sinus. This is seen as a blueness of a slightly elevated contour of the dura.

The bone, especially near the torcula, is cancellous and may bleed freely from the diploë which is plugged with bone wax.

The dura is now ready for opening but if its tension is excessive, cerebrospinal fluid should be drained via the ventricular catheter. The usual approach to a structure close to the midline is to make a Y-shaped incision in the dura, the junction of the three limbs being approximately 1 cm above the foramen magnum. It is most convenient to make the upper limbs of the incision first, making separate breaches in the dura with hook and tenotome. These are then extended with the long-handled dural scissors. The small cerebellar sinus is found in the midline. The keel of double-folded dura in which it is enclosed extends a variable distance inwards between the cerebellar hemispheres, usually no more than 0.5 cm. To encompass this, a patty is introduced on either side of the structure so as to push away the cerebellum from the advancing dural scissors with which the cut is made. The open upper end of the divided cerebellar sinus is closed either with several haemostatic dural clips of tantalum or silver or by an encircling ligature. Diathermizing it brings about excessive dural shrinkage. The lower limb of the Y is taken through the small venous sinus running circumferentially at the foramen magnum and this bleeding is likewise controlled with dural clips. The dural opening in the midline below the foramen magnum is taken to the lower margin of the cerebellar tonsils but not further unless downward extension of a tumour demands it.

Operative procedures

The dura is now drawn upwards to expose the cerebellar hemispheres and vermis and is held aside by stay sutures. If the pathology to be encountered is an intrinsic tumour of the cerebellar hemisphere, broadening of the transversely running cerebellar folia is looked for as a sign of an underlying mass. This is sought by exploration with a blunt-ended brain cannula introduced through a coagulated punctum of a pia-arachnoid, so that the increased resistance of a cyst wall or tumour margin can be felt. If an incision into the cerebellum is decided on, this is made in a direction at right angles to the folia, that is to say a cut parallel to the midline. This results in much less bleeding from the pia-arachnoid which is coagulated with successive pincer-like movements of the bipolar diathermy, the more resistant coagulated strands being divided with fine scissors. The incision is opened by either the hand-held or mechanical retractor resting on a protecting patty and deepened by light strokes of a slim metal sucker held in the right hand.

A cyst or tumour is usually encountered as a blue-grey mass looming through the white matter. With a blunt-ended brain cannula the nature of this mass is now explored and, if cystic, the fluid is aspirated. The retractors are now introduced directly into the cyst and, with headlight or operating microscope, the lining and walls are inspected for mural tumour nodules. A haemangioblastoma is usually seen as a reddish-grey nubbin of tissue often on the deep aspect of the cyst wall. There are usually prominent blood vessels running to it and these are taken with the bipolar diathermy and the nubbin removed. Astrocytoma tissue, on the other hand, is greyish-brown, relatively avascular and usually has a clear line of demarcation between it and the surrounding cerebellar white matter. The removal of solid tissue of this kind is accomplished by sweeps of the metal sucker along the line of demarcation between it and white matter with the placement of Lintine and patties so that the tumour is gradually encompassed. Depending on its extent, it can often be completely removed. The most common adult tumour to be encountered in the cerebellum is a metastasis, usually from bronchus, with tissue which is usually friable and vascular and it is removed using a similar technique. The more common childhood tumours not already mentioned are the medulloblastoma which is usually central, softer and more vascular and is best removed with a sucker. The ependymoma usually presents emerging from the foramina of the 4th ventricle and its lobules are removed piecemeal. The tumour grows out of the 4th ventricular floor and when this is the case, having removed the bulk of the tumour, it is unwise to delve too deeply into the medulla and pons, since the opportunity for irremediable damage exists and the tissue plane here is much less clear than elsewhere.

The closure is begun after haemostasis of discernible bleeding vessels with the bipolar diathermy and of an ooze by pledgets of cottonwool soaked in peroxide and introduced into the tumour bed. After 3 or 4 min these are removed gently by irrigating a flow of saline between tissue and cottonwool ball as this is then lifted gently out. When haemostasis is complete, the dura is replaced over the cerebellar hemispheres and the upper extremities of the Y are usually then closed by 3/0 black silk sutures. As the dura will usually have shrunk, a complete closure would present difficulties even if this were desirable. It is wisest to allow the incision near the midline to remain open in case of cerebellar swelling. To limit the ingress of blood and tissue exudate, strips of gelatin sponge are laid transversely across the dural exposure. Alternatively, a dural graft of artificial dural substitute or gelfilm can be sewn in. However, grafts have the possible disadvantage that they may act as an impermeable film behind which cerebrospinal fluid can leak and become trapped. It then forms a source of compression for the underlying nervous system. The muscles are closed by interrupted sutures of 1/0 silk, taking care to introduce these through the most aponeurotic part of the musculature since this will not only give the most secure closure but will avoid unnecessary muscular necrosis. Antibiotic powder is usually sprayed into the wound at this stage before the muscle closure is quite complete. After the ligamentum nuchae has been reconstituted the superficial tissues are usually drawn together in two layers. The skin is approximated either by a continuous subcuticular Dexon 2/0 suture or by a continuous over-and-over suture introduced by either straight or curved atraumatic needle.

Postoperative care

The postoperative care of patients after posterior fossa exploration begins in the anaesthetic room. It is desirable for the patient to return to a level of consciousness sufficient to obey commands and to ensure that he or she is capable of speaking, swallowing and of being able to deal with the secretions. If this is not clearly so, the patient is retained in the theatre suite recovery bay or room until these functions return. If the patient's ascent to full consciousness is delayed for no good reason connected with anaesthesia, then a postoperative clot is suspected and preparations are made to reopen the wound. The intracranial pressure can be monitored via the ventricular catheter which has been left *in situ*. If the pressure here is found to be raised, preparations are made to redrape and reopen the wound. If progress and recovery are smooth, the main precaution to take is to ensure that when the patient is first offered sips of fluid, swallowing is more likely to function properly if the 'normal' side is disposed downwards when the patient lies in the lateral position. This minimizes the risk of aspiration and pneumonia if the jugular nerves have been involved in the dissection for, for example, a sizeable acoustic neuroma. The ventricular catheter is usually removed 48 h after operation.

Cerebellopontine angle

For lateral approaches to the posterior fossa, such as into the cerebellopontine angle, a favourite incision is an inverted 'hockey stick' (with the straight limb in the midline) to 1 cm above the superior nuchal line and then sweeping laterally and downwards to the tip of the mastoid process. The muscles are detached from the posterior fossa after dividing the rather tough pericranium just above the superior nuchal line. The whole of the posterior fossa bone on one side is then exposed. The dura is uncovered by enlarging a burr hole so as to remove bone between foramen magnum inferiorly and the transverse and sigmoid sinuses superiorly and laterally. An alternative incision is to make a linear curved cut, convex laterally, which at the midpoint almost reaches the mastoid process. The cutting diathermy is used through muscle to the bone. The edges of this muscle-cutting incision are then distracted with self-retaining retractors. The bony removal is taken laterally to the mastoid air cells which may have to be opened to obtain an adequate exposure. If opened they should be sealed during the closure to prevent Eustachian CSF leakage via the mastoid air cells and middle ear cavity. It is somewhat more difficult to reach the foramen magnum by this method but for operations of short duration and limited exposure, such as division of the glossopharyngeal upper filaments for glossopharyngeal neuralgia, for division of the vestibular division of the 8th nerve for Ménière's disease or of the 5th nerve for trigeminal neuralgia, this incision suffices. The dura is opened in a curved incision 5 mm away from the transverse and sigmoid sinuses so as to uncover the minimum of cerebellum. The cerebellar hemisphere is retracted to one side to expose the inferior cranial nerves and cerebello-pontine angle (see Figure 51.22).

The removal of an acoustic neuroma by this posterior fossa approach, a procedure which is reserved for the small tumours, is achieved first of all by draining cerebrospinal fluid to allow the cerebellar hemisphere to fall away under gravity rather than be retracted. Gutta percha tissue and Lintine strips are now placed to protect the cerebellum from the mechanical retractor. The skull fixation for this is a 6.5 mm hole drilled into the skull above the lateral sinus, into which is inserted a tapered self-tapping lug from which the retractor takes origin. With the cerebellum held aside the internal auditory meatus is approached and the tumour is seen bulging into the posterior fossa cisterna. The posterior margin of the expanded meatus is now defined and the dura is divided from here backwards parallel with the superior petrosal sinus for a distance of 3 cm. This uncovers the posterior bony lip and wall of the internal auditory meatus which is now drilled away with a high-speed air drill and burrs. By this means the thinned dura lining the meatus (which forms a false capsule for the contained yellow fleshy schwannoma) can be opened with a linear cut. The cuff of dura and arachnoid which expansion of the tumour has formed as a collar at the porus is divided.

Under the operating microscope the lobules of tumour are now tilted gently away from the depths of the meatus, identifying the superior vestibular nerve from which the tumour usually arises. Superiorly and slightly anteriorly the facial nerve is to be found and the tumour is teased gently away from this. When the meatal tumour has been cleared, the arachnoid adhesions at the porus are divided by bipolar diathermy and micro-scissors and the rest of the tumour can now be debulked. It is then again teased away from the facial nerve which runs superiorly and then over the front of the tumour. The nerve here becomes expanded and thinned and greyer than expected, but great pains should be taken to identify it to avoid stretching it. No effort or time should be spared to preserve it intact. When the removal, which is usually piecemeal, is complete, the facial nerve should be traceable intact from the internal meatus to the pons. If the tumour is a large one and the nerve cannot be preserved, it should be reconstituted by laying the divided ends together on a short pledget of gelatin sponge which, with the application of fibrin, soon serves to anchor the oedematous and friable nerve. After small adjustments of the nerve ends are made to maximize close approximation, a second similar pledget of gelatin sponge is used to form a sandwich, nerve ends being the filling. Alternatively, 10/0 micro-sutures can be used to approximate ends that have been redivided.

The closure, after haemostasis is complete, is usually made with interrupted fine silk to the dura, strips of gelatin sponge over the dural incision to minimize the entry of blood from the muscle layer, which itself is closed with interrupted sutures of waxed 1/0 silk. The galeal and subcutaneous layers are closed with interrupted Dexon and the skin for a linear incision by subcuticular 2/0 Dexon.

Transphenoidal pituitary surgery

The advent of the binocular stereoscopic operating microscope has renewed interest in the transphenoidal approach to the pituitary gland which was employed in the early years of the century by Cushing and others. It was then largely given up by him in favour of the subfrontal approach. Four ways of entering the sphenoidal sinus exist. The original trans-septal approach via sublabial incision was to elevate the mucosa from either side of the nasal septum and then to resect this structure. A bivalved speculum was then opened so as to expose the midline prow of the sphenoid bone which was resected antero-inferiorly to allow entry to the sinus. The transethmoidal route exploited by Angell James approaches via a curved ethmoidal incision from the medial eyebrow downwards and medially, and then curves a short way onto the cheek. The lacrimal sac and trochlea for the superior oblique muscle are then elevated subperiosteally with the rest of the anterior orbital contents (taking care to avoid breaching the orbital periosteum) to expose the anterior ethmoidal air cells. These are punched away after a specially designed ethmoidal retractor has been introduced to hold aside the anterior orbital contents. The air cells are removed together with the upper posterior square centimetre of nasal septum where this abuts onto the prow of the sphenoid bone. The roof of the ethmoidal cells is seen above and maintained intact, as is the posterior ethmo-orbital wall. As the anterior wall with its ostium of the sphenoidal air sinus is approached, it is opened and punched away from the anterior fossa floor above so as to expose the whole of the anterior sellar wall which may of course be vastly expanded by tumour (Figure 51.23).

Although the transethmo-orbital method is a little shorter, it does have some disadvantages in that the nasal air cell system can be distorted and very occasionally intra-orbital sepsis is introduced. It has now largely been superseded by the transnasal method which relies on the fact that the piriform

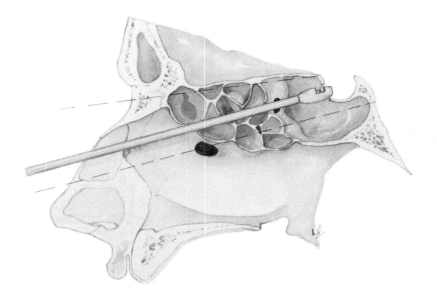

Figure 51.23 Transethmosphenoidal pituitary exposure. The bone punch nibbles out anterior wall of sella turcica

opening in the face, through which the old transeptal method of approaching the sphenoidal air sinus was carried out, is divided in the midline by the flexible cartilaginous anterior component of the nasal septum. A speculum is introduced into the right nasal cavity along the line of the middle turbinate. When opened, the septum can be deflected fully to the opposite side. The posterior nasal septum made of bone can be snapped off its attachment to the prow of the sphenoid, now giving access to the sphenoidal air sinus. This is a rapid approach, accurate, and does not need image intensification to guide the surgeon. All these advantages are likely to make this method, which we introduced in 1979, supersede the old-fashioned sub-labial transeptal approach. Consequently a transphenoidal operation for a fairly straightforward tumour of the pituitary can now be accomplished in less than three-quarters of an hour, with a hospital stay of 4 or 5 days.

The main complication of the procedure has always been the possibility of CSF leakage. However, awareness of the problem is half-way to its solution. If no CSF is seen at operation, probably sponge replacement rather than wads of muscle taken from the patient's thigh or deltoid are sufficient to prevent leakage. If CSF leakage is observed, then fascia lata has no peer as a seal applied to the dural opening. CSF occurring in the postoperative days must be treated at once by reoperation, and adjusting the graft. Cerebrospinal fluid drainage in this situation is contraindicated, since it encourages the ingress of air and sinus contents and promotes infection. The fact that the CSF leak has stopped does not mean that it is no longer a source of continued danger to the patient from infection.

The success rate of endocrine pituitary surgery in eradicating secretory tissue depends on the size of the adenoma. Secretory adenomas are usually soft, distinct in whitish colour from the surrounding yellow normal anterior pituitary gland tissue, and have no capsule. With obsessional curettage and suction, if they are small they can usually be completely removed. Larger tumours often spread into interstices in the bone, into the cavernous sinus, and into other structures such as Meckel's cave. Surgically these are not completely eradicable. Consequently cure rates are related to the size of the tumour and are greatest in Cushing's syndrome where the adenomas are smallest and central, and less efficient in the growth hormone-secreting tumours causing acromegaly, and in prolactin-secreting tumours, both larger and originating in the lateral lobes of the anterior gland.

The most important investigation, if the tumour is a bulky one and an operation is being undertaken for decompression of the optic pathways, is a serum prolactin level. This can now be provided by an expeditious laboratory in less than 2 h. Bromocriptine is such an efficient shrinker of prolactinoma that in the vast majority of cases operation is unnecessary and, when the tumour is very large, undesirable. The levels of serum prolactin should exceed 5000 iu in order to make a positive diagnosis of prolactinoma. Non-prolactinomas and craniopharyngiomas distort the pituitary portal system of the stalk, so that the inhibiting effect of prolactin-releasing hormone is lifted from some parts of the normal pituitary so that the prolactin level rises to levels which are usually less than 2000. This indicates only that some kind of pathological process is present. It is by no means diagnostic of prolactinoma.

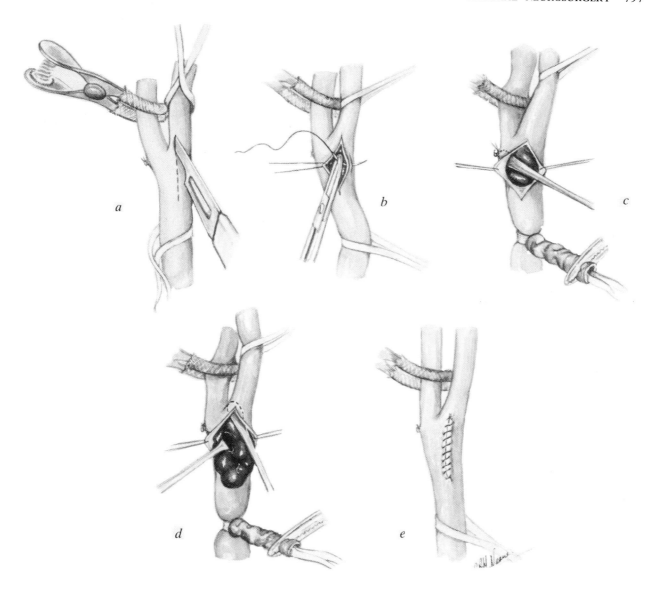

Figure 51.24 Carotid endarterectomy. This operation is undertaken at normal temperatures, carefully controlling the carotid vessels (for purpose of clarity the shunt is not shown)

Extracranial vascular surgery of the brain

Eastcott's pioneer operation for reconstitution of the internal carotid artery took place in 1954. In 1969 Yasargil first carried out an operation using a microvascular technique at which the superficial temporal artery was connected end to side with a middle cerebral branch on the cortical surface of the brain. Both operations have been progressively exploited and now are secure as part of the neurosurgical repertoire.

Carotid endarterectomy (Figure 51.24)

There is no simple explanation for the siting of atheromatous plaques at the carotid bifurcation, although flow eddies may be important. The build-up of atheroma seems to be maximal in the internal carotid at the point approximately 1 cm distal to the carotid bifurcation. Its effect is twofold. Platelet embolization from an ulcerating atheromatous plaque may give rise to stereotyped attacks of ischaemia in the territory of the ophthalmic artery and of the middle cerebral artery. Ophthalmic embolization gives rise to transient blindness sometimes called 'amaurosis fugax'. Middle cerebral embolization produces transient ischaemic attacks (defined as neurological symptoms and signs of less than 24 hours' duration) affecting the face and arm and, on the left side, speech function. Marked involvement of the leg should arouse suspicion that vertebrobasilar ischaemia is present. These transient ischaemic attacks can often be reduced or abolished by formal anticoagulant treatment or by aspirin or Persantin (dipyridamole). If the stenosis is severe then there is the danger of further thrombosis to complete occlusion. This may be silent but is more likely to produce a major infarct in the middle cerebral territory, often with propagating thrombus into the middle cerebral vessels.

Both these consequences of carotid atheroma can be effectively treated by carotid endarterectomy. Although the atheromatous plaque penetrates into the media to a varying degree, atheroma is basically an intimal process. In well-developed plaques a plane between media and plaque can be fairly easily dissected. The principle of the operation consists of removing plaque and overlying distorted intima, leaving a fairly smooth bare media with the intimal margins undisturbed in order to promote re-intimalization of the reconstituted channel.

Investigations

These patients frequently have well-developed coronary and other atherosclerosis. Part of the clinical work-up should be specially directed to the clinical assessment of these lesions and in particular to determine whether the cerebral attacks could have a basis in cardiac embolization from mural thrombus consequent on endocardial involvement in myocardial infarction. In addition the femoral arteries should be checked for patency and bruits since much selective cerebral catheterization for arteriography is nowadays transfemoral. The clinical work-up should include special attention to bruits in the neck and the patency of the superficial temporal arteries.

Selective arteriography is still *sine qua non* for carotid surgery. Pictures of the carotid bifurcation should be obtained in two directions at right angles, including if possible the skull base up to the siphon. Formal cerebral arteriograms in two directions at right angles should be taken since siphon atheroma is common and middle cerebral stenosis, best seen in an anteroposterior view, can produce transient ischaemic attacks. Both right and left bifurcations should be clearly visualized, since the contralateral internal carotid artery will bear the main burden of cerebral blood supply during occlusion of the operated side. If possible, the vertebral vessels should be visualized at the same time since these, too, can occlude silently. Pulsed Doppler images of the carotid bifurcation should be obtained and studied in conjunction with the arteriograms. These are especially valuable since they can be useful for follow-up purposes. At present, however, the clarity of the image does not permit sufficient confidence in the investigations to hinge operation on the pulsed Doppler scan alone.

Technique

During operations on the carotid arteries the necessary temporary surgical occlusion of these vessels will reduce the cerebral flow, sometimes appreciably. Nevertheless, the contralateral carotid system and the vertebral arteries are adequate to prevent cerebral ischaemic damage in the majority of patients. Various protective methods have been devised.

1. Hypothermia

Surface cooling to 30°C using a water bath or ice packs was used for many years and was found to prolong the safe ischaemic time to an acceptable level.

2. Intravascular shunts (see Chapter 38)

The introduction of intravascular shunts, which are manufactured tubes of polyvinyl chloride or Silastic rubber, has superseded hypothermia. The shunts are inserted into the common carotid proximally and internal carotid artery distal to the site of operation at the carotid bifurcation, thus maintaining the cerebral circulation.

During surgery it is necessary to monitor the electro-encephalogram, as significant deprivation of cerebral blood supply during carotid clamping is readily detected and will then declare the need for shunting. Measurement of the distal carotid pressure during clamping, so-called 'stump pressure', is also of great use and it is suggested that a distal stump pressure of less than 60 mmHg should be regarded as an indication for temporary shunting.

Although hypothermia was used for many years and intra-arterial shunting is favoured by many, the invariable need for such precautions is questioned and the author has found that provided surgery is undertaken rapidly and that continuity of blood flow is established within 20 min the patients come to no harm.

Local anaesthesia is sometimes used for endarterectomy but appears to have no particular merit. General anaesthesia cuts down the oxygen requirement of the brain by its depressing effect on metabolism. The anaesthetist can usually ensure an adequate level of systemic blood pressure for collateral circulation. In addition, inadvertent movement and what must be a somewhat stressful adventure for the patient are avoided.

The position of the patient is supine with the head turned slightly away from the side of the operation with a slight head-up tilt to disengorge the neck veins. The incision is via a collar skin crease taken approximately from the external jugular vein to somewhere near the midline. The incision is deepened through platysma and small bleeding points are picked up precisely with the bipolar diathermy. The dissection is continued towards the carotid bifurcation with the blunt-tipped dissecting scissors, when the carotid sheath can usually be seen shining through the areolar layer of connective tissue. Bifurcating veins running from the thyroid gland are ligated flush with the jugular vein and a length of 1 or 2 cm of vein is taken in case a repairing patch is needed after the endarterectomy. The carotid bifurcation is now exposed and the hypoglossal nerve and digastric posterior belly are reflected upwards. The adventitia is stripped from the lateral aspect of the bifurcation and internal carotid, the extent of the stripping being guided by palpation of the hard atheromatous plaques through the wall of the artery. This clearance is taken at least 2 cm below the carotid bifurcation. Encircling tape ligatures are now passed around the common carotid as low as possible, usually 3 cm below the bifurcation and around the main trunk of the external carotid, just above the superior thyroid artery take-off. The superior thyroid is occluded by a small bulldog clip. The internal carotid is encircled but a small curved vascular clamp is used here for occlusion.

The anaesthetist is now told that all is ready for the incision and the tapes on the common carotid and external carotid are tightened to occlusion. The clamp on the internal carotid is closed and a count started by the anaesthetist, this being for record purposes. The times are not called out as the surgeon will clearly work as rapidly as is possible with safety. An incision is made with a tenotome and no. 15 blade smoothly on the surface of the internal carotid and taken down a smooth line well into the common carotid (Figure 51.24a). Usually this will penetrate the lumen and the atheromatous plaque can be visualized. The sucker is used to empty the vessel and the plane between plaque and media is now picked up carefully and the dissection proceeds upwards and downwards to the full extent of plaque. Care is taken with the dissection to maintain the cleavage plane and, where this deepens into the media to avoid perforation, especially of the medial wall. As the dissection proceeds anteriorly it will usually be seen that a sleeve of atheroma can be disengaged from the mouth of the external carotid artery. With fine sharp-pointed scissors this sleeve is cut off flush with the intima, taking care to leave no tags or intimal fringe which could lift and form an occluding dissection between media and intima. The same principle holds for the dissection down into the common carotid but here, due to the direction of blood flow, the risk of postoperative flap occlusion is less. As the sleeve of atheroma is gently disengaged from the internal carotid, it is vitally important here to guard against later intimal lifting. Special care is necessary here. As the dissection is completed the entire atheromatous cast is lifted intact from the artery. The bed can now be inspected for tags of intima or ulcers. These are dealt with. The margin of intimal dissection in the upper internal carotid is now inspected again and any intimal lifting is dealt with either by retrimming or a through-and-through loop tacking suture inserted from without inwards and in the reverse direction again (Figure 51.24b–d).

The closure is made with a 5/0 prolene single-ended arterial needle beginning at the upper end of the arteriotomy. The sutures are placed continuously without locking approximately at 1.5–2 mm intervals. It is important to have equal bites of media on either side of the incision. The assistant maintains steady tension on the suture line, taking care to hold the suture either between finger and thumb or with a forceps protected so as to avoid damage to the suture. This closure is best done under magnification, by either loupes or operating microscope. The last three passages of the needle are not drawn tight, although the assistant maintains tension on the rest of the suture line (Figure 51.24e). The internal carotid clamp is now released and a backflow of arterial blood obtained. This briefly washes out the arteriotomy, then the arterial clamp is closed again. The remaining loops of suture are now drawn tight and the suture is securely knotted. The internal carotid clamp is now released followed by the external carotid and common carotid snares in that order. This attempts to ensure no residual fibrin or clot is delivered into the internal carotid circulation. As the clamps are removed, the suture line usually leaks. This is dealt with by laying a gutta percha strip over the suture line and packing wet saline swabs over this. Firm pressure is maintained with the fingers for 10 min by the clock, after which the leaks will usually have ceased. The gutta percha tissue is removed and antibiotic powder is lightly sprinkled into the wound. The neck closure is by buried 2/0 interrupted sutures to the platysma at 1.5 cm intervals with a continuous 3/0 Dexon subcuticular suture to the skin. If wound drainage is needed, a short length of corrugated drain emerges through the centre of the incision and clips are used for skin closure.

As anaesthesia is terminated and dressing is applied, the patient should be awake for neurological testing before return to the recovery bay or ward. Observations about manual strength and, in the case of left-sided operations, the ability to speak clearly should be continued at hourly intervals for the first 48 h after operation. Blood pressure is charted so as to guard against hypotension. Unexplained events, even those which do not at first seem to have a direct neurological cause, such as sudden severe breathlessness, should arouse suspicion of a postoperative occlusion of the artery at the arteriotomy site. Naturally hemiplegia or hemiparesis occurring under these circumstances on the appropriate side merits immediate re-exploration of the wound. Digital palpation of the internal carotid reveals thrombotic occlusion. In these circumstances the arteriotomy should be reopened and resutured again after clot removal. Secondary haemorrhage is uncommon but can occur at the period of maximum fibrinolysis at the end of the 1st week. In these circumstances the neck must be re-explored to remove the haematoma and the suture line inspected for its origin. For this reason patients must be kept under observation in hospital for over 1 week after operation. A check arteriogram is carried out to ensure patency and an adequate operation. It should not be assumed that in the absence of any neurological signs, the reconstituted artery is necessarily patent. Silent occlusion can and does occur. If, as occasionally happens, occlusion is detected only at late arteriography a decision has then to be made as to whether a superficial temporal-to-middle cerebral bypass should be performed.

External carotid/internal carotid anastomotic surgery (Figure 51.25)

The most common form of bypass surgery for complete occlusion of the internal carotid or vertebral vessels is end-to-side anastomosis of the posterior branch of the superficial temporal artery to one of the larger middle cerebral branches emerging from the sylvian fissure. The indications for this operation are still not entirely clear. Complete occlusion of the internal carotid followed by transient ischaemic attacks which persist despite anticoagulants, severe stenosis of the internal carotid artery between its origin at the common carotid bifurcation in the neck and the intracranial branching into the anterior and middle cerebral arteries or severe middle cerebral stenosis with persistent symptoms are indications for this procedure. It has also been invoked in established stroke either in the acute phase of the 1st week or in the recovery phase if this seems not to be proceeding rapidly. In addition, a prophylactic bypass may be constructed prior to aneurysm surgery (for instance, at the intracranial internal carotid bifurcation) in cases where occlusion of major branches is to be feared. The main contraindication to the operation is swelling of the underlying cerebral hemisphere as revealed by a CT scan. Lucency of cerebral tissue, often regarded as cerebral oedema in the scan, is not necessarily a contraindication. The presence of haemorrhage in the hemisphere in stroke is, however, a direct contraindication.

Arteriography preoperatively should reveal precisely the state of the neck and intracranial vessels on both sides. Four-vessel arteriography is a desideratum. Late films will often reveal a substantial intracranial anastomotic circulation via the anterior branch of the superficial temporal artery which connects with the ophthalmic artery via the supraorbital vessels. This should not be disturbed. Even in the absence of this angiographic demonstration effective collateral circulation can be demonstrated by Doppler change of phase of flow on compression of the superficial temporal artery over the zygomatic arch. For these reasons the posterior branch of the artery is used.

The operation can be carried out under local anaesthesia but general anaesthesia is preferable if there is any doubt about the patient's cooperation. The scalp is shaved over the side of the head and the continuous

wave Doppler probe is employed to map out the course of the superficial temporal artery and branches in the scalp. The point of maximum echo should be marked by Bonney's blue pricked into the skin through a sharp needle so that, after the scalp is prepared and draped, the course of the vessels can be clearly seen. The incision, after scalp infiltration with 1% lignocaine without adrenaline, is made over the posterior branch of the artery. The superficial temporal vessel is dissected under the low magnification of the operating microscope from its origin to the major branches near the vertex. This usually displays approximately 8 cm of artery, not all of which need be used. The minor side-branches of the first 5 cm of this vessel are coagulated by the bipolar diathermy and divided close to the parent vessel. A sleeve of adventitia is left on the artery.

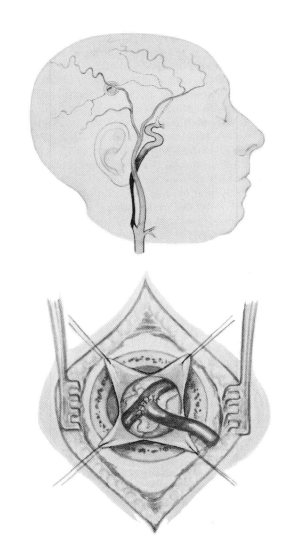

Figure 51.25 External carotid/internal carotid anastomotic surgery. The posterior branch of the superficial temporal artery is anastomosed to the middle cerebral artery or one of its branches

When a sufficient length of artery has been mobilized but not yet divided distally, the incision is deepened through temporalis and this muscle is retracted so as to expose the temporal bone lying above the sylvian fissure. A 4.5 cm trephine disc is now drilled and removed, taking great care not to breach the dura. The dura is now opened with a cruciate incision and a search is made for a suitably sized middle cerebral branch emerging from the sylvian fissure. Further extension of the bony removal may need to be taken if a large enough vessel does not immediately present itself. The vessels emerging over the upper lip are used for preference. With the high magnification of the microscope the arachnoid over the selected vessel is now cleared for approximately 1 cm and the very fine-tipped bipolar diathermy is used to coagulate perforating vessels which run down into the subjacent cortex directly from the selected vessel. After division of these coagulated vessels, a strip of gutta percha tissue is inserted so as to lie under the selected arterial segment. Specially weakened arterial spring clips are readied for occlusion. Patties and Lintine are placed so as to limit the brain exposure to the small segment of interest. Any bleeding is dealt with at this stage.

The superficial temporal artery is now divided with sufficient length to bring the end without tension to the site for anastomosis. This is usually just over 5 cm. The vascular clip is reapplied more proximally over a part of the vessel covered by adventitia. The extreme distal end of the artery is grasped firmly and the adventitia is pulled proximally for about 0.5 cm. This cuff of excess adventitia is then trimmed away. The arterial termination is then retrimmed with an oblique cut at approximately 45° to the long axis of the vessel so as to present an undamaged and unhandled media and intima for suturing.

The magnification of the operating microscope is now increased. The 1 cm segment of recipient middle cerebral branch is now isolated by application of the vascular clips at either end. A longitudinal incision in this vessel approximately 3 mm long (to correspond with the length of the obliquely cut end of the superficial temporal artery) is now made with a diamond knife or sharp scalpel. It is important to ensure that media and intima are cut together and it is often best to do this with sharp micro-scissors and with one definitive cut. Taking more than one cut usually results in fraying and disparity between media and intima. With no. 3 watchmaker's forceps in the left hand and a slightly curved micro-needle holder in the right, a 10/0 monofilament microsuture is trimmed to approximately 8 cm in length. The anastomosis begins by passing this needle from without in at one end of the arteriotomy cut, taking care to include both media and intima. The suture is now passed in the reverse direction through the much thicker-walled superficial temporal artery, selecting either the shorter

or longer end of the obliquely cut vessel as appropriate. This suture is now tied with the microvascular technique, having deposited the needle on a nearby patty. A convenient method is to zoom the microscope to a smaller magnification and increased field for tying the suture. This suture is then cut and a corresponding suture at the other extremity of the anastomosis is again placed in a similar way, after zoom up to a higher magnification.

An important point of technique is that the edges of the vessels to be sewn are not grasped by the watchmaker's forceps as this would damage seriously the delicate endothelium. The function of the forceps is to pick up the needle and to support with counterpressure the tissue through which the needle is being introduced. When the end sutures are tied the two sides of the anastomosis are constructed with interrupted sutures, an average number being 10 or 12 in a vascular reconstruction of this size. An alternative technique is to insert and tie two separate microsutures at each end of the anastomosis. The suturing is then completed with a continuous suture, each tied to the tail of the other. Care is taken during the reconstruction to avoid fibrin accumulating inside or near the cerebral vessel. A micro-sucker is used to ensure this.

The anastomosis is now wrapped in gutta percha tissue and mild pressure by saline-soaked patties is applied. The vascular clips are now removed, first from the middle cerebral branch, then from the superficial temporal artery. Unless there is uncontrollable bleeding the anastomosis is not disturbed for 10 min. When the patties are removed and the gutta percha peeled back, the suture line is usually secure and arterial pulsation can be discerned in all three segments of vessels. Unlike an end-to-end anastomosis, the test for patency is difficult without a radiographic or fluorescein angiogram which may be carried out by an injection into a specially prepared and cannulated small side-branch of the superficial temporal vessel.

The bone disc is now trimmed so as to allow appropriate access for the entering superficial temporal vessel. The dura is closed and Gelfoam pledgets placed on any gaps. The bone disc is replaced. It is held in place by sutures of 2/0 silk through the temporalis fascia, again allowing an appropriate gap for the entry of the superficial temporal artery. The scalp is closed with interrupted sutures at 1 cm intervals to the galea, with a continuous suture to the skin, taking care at the lower end of the incision to avoid traumatizing the superficial temporal vessel. Patency of the anastomosis is tested in the early days by Doppler, the vascular ultrasonic signal being fairly readily followed into the small craniectomy, where a change in the character of the signal is usually detectable. Arteriography for patency should usually be delayed since a patent anastomosis will occasionally not fill immediately.

52

Neurosurgical disorders of the spine

J. N. Rawlinson and M. G. McGee-Collett

Introduction

The musculoskeletal spinal column is the backbone of the human body, enabling an upright posture, transmitting power from the legs to allow movement, supporting the head and shoulders and providing a firm base from which the upper limbs can exert power. It is therefore a complex structure with a wide variety of tissues and many joints to give maximum flexibility. In addition, it contains and protects the spinal cord, surrounded by cerebrospinal fluid (CSF) and enclosed in its dural sheath. The segmental nerve roots leave the bony spinal canal through exit foramina between each vertebral segment. Neurosurgical disorders of the spine include disease processes arising within the spinal cord or nerve roots or their coverings, or disease processes of the surrounding musculoskeletal tissues or joints that are having a direct effect on the underlying nerve root or cord, or where there is a potential to do so.

Surgical management of spinal disorders is a rapidly changing field. Diagnosis is assisted by many new developments. Computed tomography (CT) scanning and more recently magnetic resonance imaging (MRI) have enabled very clear resolution of anatomical abnormality. Tumour markers in serum provide evidence of tumour differentiation. New methods of analysing CSF including cytology may enable histological diagnosis without open biopsy. Somatosensory evoked potentials and electromyography (EMG) also have their place.

Surgery of the spine and spinal cord has advanced dramatically with the use of the operating microscope. This enables more precise surgery to be done under better illumination through smaller access, thereby minimizing postoperative complications. In addition, the discipline of microsurgery encourages a greater understanding of the anatomy and the pathological process of the disease. The introduction of the laser and the new forms of internal fixation are further advances.

Despite all these technical advances the value of clinical diagnosis in the management of these patients cannot be underestimated. This diagnosis depends on the history, examination and special investigation in spinal disorder. A general principle is that the diagnosis is *made* on the *history*, is *confirmed* on the *examination*, and is *proven* by special *investigation*. The two main symptoms are pain and neurological dysfunction.

Pain. Although there are many causes of back pain these may be classified into three groups: pain of mechanical nature, radicular pain and pathological pain. Mechanical pain is pain confined to the back (although occasionally referred into the proximal limb) which is related to spinal posture or movement. It is therefore made better by immobility and rest.

Radicular pain is due to irritation of a nerve root causing pain in the dermatome supplied by that nerve. It is usually of a characteristic distribution. The characteristic shooting nature of the pain is valuable in diagnosis.

Pathological pain is vital to recognize since it implies a sinister process such as cord compression by tumour or infection. This is a constant gnawing back pain at rest and often therefore complained of at night. It is not related to movement.

Neurological dysfunction. Neurological symptoms are due to nerve root or spinal cord dysfunction. Nerve root disorder (radiculopathy) is either due to nerve root irritation (pain, paraesthesia) or root compression (loss of power, loss of sensation, loss of reflexes). It is common that only one nerve root is affected, producing a characteristic pattern of symptoms and signs to aid diagnosis. Disease within the spinal canal may affect the spinal cord (myelopathy). The disorder is therefore much more widespread, with characteristic upper motor neuron signs of brisk reflexes, increased tone and upgoing plantar reflexes. This pattern of symptoms and signs is of course absent in the lumbar region below L1, although the cauda equina syndrome affecting the many nerve roots in the lumbar theca produces wide-ranging disturbance.

Non-organic symptoms and signs. 'Abnormal illness behaviour' is a term to describe non-organic symptoms and signs that often become florid in chronic back disorder. These include abnormal subjective reactions such as reporting continuous pain for at least a year with no relief from any analgesia, and inconsistent objective signs such as a varying range of straight-leg raising depending on the position of the individual. These psychological manifestations of disease are surprisingly common and are not confined to psychiatrically disturbed individuals. Their presence may be so florid that the true nature of the disease process (if there is one, which is not always the case) may be masked, and the effects of surgery, however successful, may not cure the patient.

To conclude the introduction it is important to emphasize that surgical management of disorders of the spine and spinal cord is emerging as an important speciality. There is no longer a place for the occasional spinal surgeon. Many of these disorders are best treated by surgeons with a neurosurgical and/or orthopaedic training who have a particular interest or enthusiasm for spinal disorder.

This chapter will concentrate on neurosurgical disorders of the spine and spinal cord. Each condition will be discussed, emphasizing the process of clinical diagnosis with history (make it), examination (confirm it) and investigation (prove it). Management will be discussed underlying the general principles, without too much detail of specific procedures for which the reader is referred to more advanced texts of spinal surgery. The diseases are discussed in terms of disease process rather than region. A basic knowledge of anatomy and physiology is assumed.

Degenerative spinal disease

Age and use lead to degenerative disease. The intervertebral disc – 'the vertebral shock absorber' – undergoes desiccation and the space narrows. Degenerate nucleus pulposus emerges through cracks in the annulus fibrosus to prolapse into the spinal canal or lateral to the pedicle. Increased strain on the synovial joints causes osteophytosis predominantly anteriorly in the neck (from the neurocentral joints) and posterolaterally in the lumbar region (from the facet joints) (Figure 52.1).

Radiculopathy

Neurological dysfunction at the level of the nerve root (a 'lower motor neuron' lesion) is usually due to a compressive lesion, and rarely due to an intrinsic disorder of the nerve.

It is manifest clinically as pain experienced in the dermatomal distribution of the nerve root and, as the compression advances with time, nerve function will deteriorate leading to sensory disturbance and finally motor impairment. A disturbance of autonomic function may occur depending upon the magnitude of the contribution to the autonomic nervous system which a particular nerve root provides. Compressive radiculopathies occur most commonly in the lumbar region, then the cervical and rarely the thoracic region.

Cervical radiculopathy

This is usually due to a posterolateral herniation of the nucleus pulposus through a degenerating annulus fibrosus, impinging upon the nerve root in its axilla. Because of the anatomical arrangement of the cervical nerve roots a C5/6 disc protrusion (the commonest) produces a C6 radiculopathy (in the neck, the segmental nerve emerges above its corresponding vertebra – remember the C8 root!) with pain (brachialgia) and dysaesthesia in the thumb and index finger, weakness of the biceps and brachioradialis muscles and diminution of their tendon jerks. A C6/7 disc protrusion produces a C7 radiculopathy with pain (brachialgia) and sensory changes in the middle and ring fingers, weakness of the triceps and wrist flexors and extensors and reduction of the tricep jerk. Radiculopathies of the upper brachial roots are rarer and of the lower roots rarer still. Upper cervical radiculopathy is difficult to discriminate from neck pain from other causes.

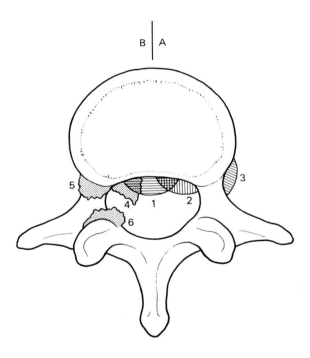

Figure 52.1 A, Disc prolapse: 1, central and 2, posterolateral (both into the spinal canal); 3, lateral. B, Osteophytes from: 4, the vertebral body and 5, neurocentral joint (both cervical spine only); 6, the facet joint

Cervical radiculopathies can also result from spondylosis with osteophyte encroachment upon the nerve root within the exit foramen. There is almost always associated neck pain, especially upon neck movement.

The standard investigation is currently water-soluble myelography (Figure 52.2) combined with CT, but MRI is improving in its spatial resolution, especially in the sagittal cuts and will, with increased availability, replace myelography. Plain X-rays (anteroposterior, lateral and oblique) readily demonstrate degenerative bony and joint changes (Figure 52.3).

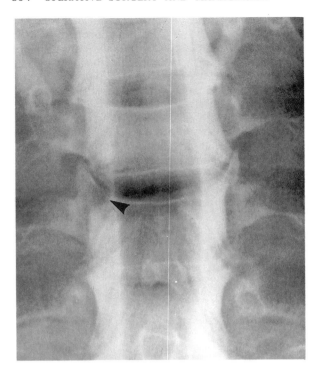

Figure 52.2 Cervical myelogram showing a lateral disc prolapse (arrowed)

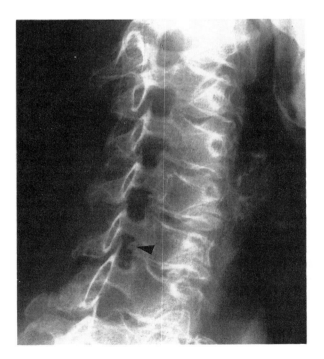

Figure 52.3 Oblique X-ray of the cervical spine to demonstrate the intervertebral foraminae, showing osteophytes from the neurocentral joint at C6/7 encroaching on the exit canal of the C7 nerve root

Nerve root compression can be treated surgically from anterior or posterior approaches. The anterior approach is accomplished by dissecting in the plane between the great vessels laterally and trachea and oesophagus medially, separating the longus colli muscles and then performing a discectomy as far laterally as possible. The posterior part of the neurocentral joint is drilled off, and disc removed, until the exit foramen is decompressed. An autologous bone graft (taken from the iliac crest) is usually placed in the prepared discectomy site to allow distraction and fusion. Cloward's instruments, or a more 'freehand' Smith Robinson technique, may be utilized for bone grafting. Relief of brachialgia should be prompt, with an ensuing improvement in neurological deficit.

The posterior approach involves removal of the small portions of two adjacent laminae and facet processes to expose the ventral and dorsal roots in their separate dural sheaths and then careful removal of the herniated disc fragment or osteophyte compressing the root usually in its axilla.

Thoracic radiculopathy

This is rare. It is usually seen in conjunction with myelopathy from neoplastic metastatic cord compression or thoracic disc herniation. Its clinical diagnosis is difficult because of the overlap of adjacent dermatomes. The characteristic pain shooting around the trunk from back to front should, however, alert the clinician to possible disc herniation, epidural abscess, neoplasm or syrinx, or rarely, tabes dorsalis.

Lumbar radiculopathy

This is probably the commonest condition seen by neurosurgeons and commonly occurs in the 30–60 age group. It is usually due to disc prolapse, but in the older patient may be due to unilateral facet joint hypertrophy.

Degeneration of the annulus fibrosus allows herniation of the nucleus pulposus posterolaterally into the vicinity of the nerve root which is compressed. It is most common within the spinal canal, but up to 6% of prolapses occur under or lateral to the pedicle outside the spinal canal (a lateral lumbar prolapse) (see Figure 52.1). A posterolateral prolapse in the canal compresses the nerve emerging at the space below. A lateral prolapse impinges on the nerve emerging at the same space. Facet joint osteophytes can compress either (Figure 52.4). The resulting neuralgia (femoralgia or sciatica) is almost always greater in magnitude than the back pain.

High disc protrusions (L1/2, L2/3) account for approximately 5% of cases and may be difficult to differentiate from renal colic. L3/4 disc protrusion compresses the L4 root as it exits the common dural sac. Pain and dysaesthesia are experienced in the thigh (femoralgia) and down to the medial malleolus. There may be weakness and wasting with fascicula-

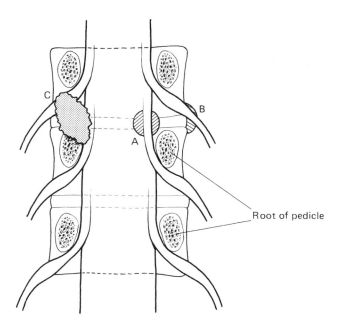

Root of pedicle

Figure 52.4 The lumbar vertebral bodies seen from behind. A, A posterolateral prolapse within the spinal canal compresses the nerve emerging at the space below. B, A lateral disc prolapse outside the pedicle impinges on the nerve emerging at the affected space. C, Facet joint hypertrophy and osteophytosis (seen here after removing the parent joint) can affect either nerve

tion of the quadriceps. The knee jerk is reduced or absent. Forced hip extension stretches the femoral nerve and its roots (including L4) over the disc herniation and exacerbates the pain.

Sciatic pain typically radiates through the buttock down the posterior aspect of the leg to the dermatomal representation of the root. L4/5 herniations are the commonest (approximately 40–45%) and cause pain and dysaesthesia travelling from the back of the thigh, outside of the lower limb, across the foot into the big toe, with weakness of ankle dorsiflexion and great toe extension. Sometimes there is a positive Trendelenburg sign (with the opposite side of the pelvis dropping when the patient stands on the affected leg) due to weakness of the gluteus medius. The angle of straight-leg raising is limited by pain. The signs are due to L5 compression.

L5/S1 disc herniation (40%) produces an S1 radiculopathy manifest by pain and dysaesthesia along the outer aspect of the root in the little toe, with weakness of plantar flexion (patients may not be able to support their weight on the toes of the affected side) and loss of the ankle and medial hamstring jerks. Straight-leg raising is reduced.

A large disc herniation may compromise the entire cauda equina, and information regarding sexual performance and sphincter function must be elicited in history-taking. Rectal tone, cremasteric and bulbo-cavernosus reflexes should be assessed.

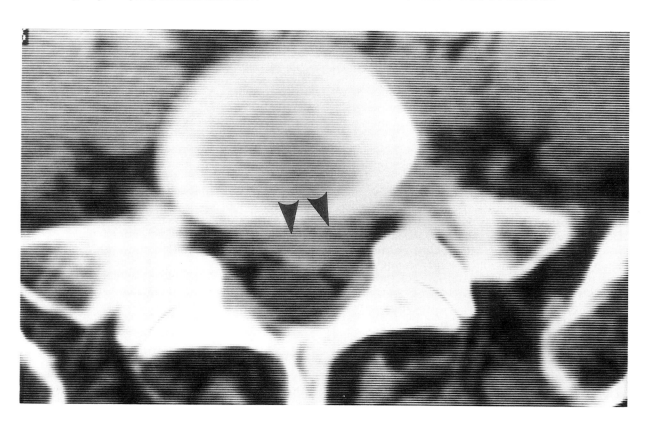

Figure 52.5 Plain CT scan showing a typical lumbar disc prolapse (arrowed)

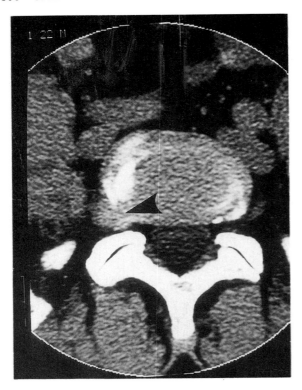

Figure 52.6 Plain CT scan showing a lateral lumbar disc prolapse (arrowed)

The standard investigation is the myelogram combining CT scanning, although plain CT on modern machines is usually adequate (Figure 52.5) and is in fact the only way to determine radiologically the presence of a far lateral herniation (Figure 52.6) which lies beyond the extent of the subarachnoid space (and therefore beyond the practical ability of myelography). Improvements in MRI will probably replace other forms of investigation. CT scanning after myelography shows facet joint hypertrophy (see Figure 52.9).

The principle of surgery is to alleviate the small number of patients who do not spontaneously recover or who deteriorate. X-ray is used to identify the correct level. A unilateral exposure of the interspace is made with removal of a small amount of the medial portion of the facet joint and the inferocaudal margin of the rostral lamina. A 'caudal bite' of the lamina below is also often necessary. A flap of ligamentum flavum is retracted or excised and the affected nerve root and the common dural sac identified within the epidural fat. At this point, magnification and lighting are of primary importance and this is achieved with the operating microscope and the use of micro-instruments and bipolar diathermy.

The root will be seen to be heaped up over the obvious disc protrusion. Sometimes a disc fragment is ruptured through the posterior longitudinal ligament and lies free within the spinal canal. With minimal root retraction the offending fragment is gently withdrawn usually lateral to the root. The hole in the annulus is then enlarged and the remaining loose pieces of degenerative nucleus pulposus cleared as completely as possible to reduce the risk of recurrent protrusion. A search is made using a blunt hook in the exit foramen and the epidural space for missed fragments of disc. The wound is closed in anatomical layers. The use of free fat grafts is common, but may only increase the amount of devitalized tissue in the wound, causing adhesions.

If the root compression is due to facet joint hypertrophy, the medial half of that joint can be removed with the high-speed drill until the exit canal is of adequate size.

In the event of far lateral protrusions, either the facet joint must be completely removed, or an approach made lateral to the facet joint where the disc fragment will be found caudal to the nerve root which is compressed against the more rostral pedicle.

Adequate patient selection and surgery should produce an 85–95% chance of immediate pain control. Neurological deficits recover more slowly depending upon their duration and magnitude. The presence of sphincter dysfunction mandates emergency treatment. It is worth while remembering that intradural neoplasms (meningiomas and schwannomas) may mimic disc lesions as may root compression by neoplastic bony involvement.

Myelopathy

Dysfunction of the spinal cord (upper motor neuron lesion) occurs when the cord is compressed anywhere in its extent between foramen magnum and its termination at L1/2. Cardinal features are weakness, spasticity and sensory disturbance. Dorsally placed lesions may selectively impair dorsal column function, producing impairment of kinaesthesia and joint position sense. The deep tendon jerks are usually increased, and the Babinski reflex is extensor, and there is loss of superficial cutaneous reflexes. There may be a sensory level above which sensation is normal, indicating the segmental level of cord compression. Anteriorly placed lesions may selectively affect the motor function below, with less effect on sensation. Myelopathy usually develops insidiously, but may occur suddenly due to cord concussion or contusion following compression, due, for example, to hyperextension of a spondylitic cervical spine or acute cervical disc protrusions.

Cervical myelopathy

This may occur from degenerative disease causing cord compression either from osteophytes located at the disc level, a prolapsed cervical disc or both. It occurs more frequently with increasing age and the presence of sensory disturbance usually excludes amyotrophic lateral sclerosis. Myelopathic cord function is evident at levels below that of the compression, due either to anterior horn cell ischaemia or osteophytic compression of the nerve root in its exit foramen. A lower motor neuron lesion may be present.

Myelography and CT demonstrate the extent of cord compression. Generally the condition is relieved by laminectomy or anterior decompression (i.e. medial corporectomy and autologous bone grafting) over the levels of decompression. The choice of approach depends on the number of levels involved and upon whether the compressing pathology is anterior or posterior to the cord.

The prime aim of surgery is to halt progression of the myelopathy and then to achieve some improvement. Myelopathy is halted in approximately 60% of cases and improvement may occur in 20–30%; but 10–20% continue to deteriorate despite adequate surgical correction.

Special situations may occur in rheumatoid arthritis where spondylotic narrowing of the spinal canal coexists with destruction of synovial joints and instability of the vertebral articulations leading to subluxation at the affected area. When decompression is performed, the vertebrae may need to be realigned with traction and metallic internal fixation systems. These are held rigid by bone grafting and splinted in Philadelphia collars or halothoracic fixation. Involvement of the atlanto-axial articulation may lead to anterior cervicomedullary cord compression by pannus replacing the dens (Figure 52.7), in addition to subluxation of C1 on C2. This difficult condition may be treated by transoral resection of the anterior compressive lesion (pannus) followed by posterior grafting and fixation.

Thoracic myelopathy

This is usually due to metastatic neoplasm, but can be due to degenerative thoracic disc protrusion. Myelopathy results in direct cord compression by the hard, often calcified, herniated disc material. MRI has replaced myelography for the radiological evaluation (Figure 52.8) but plain CT is usually necessary to assist intraoperative localization of the appropriate level. Thoracic disc herniations usually occur at the lower end of the thoracic spine, mainly T9–T12.

Laminectomy performed to gain access to a thoracic herniation has a high complication rate from further cord compression during retraction. Transpedicular removal is an alternative technique. However, the most direct attack on a thoracic disc protrusion is anterolaterally via thoracotomy. The firm disc fragment is dissected off the dura after limited bony and disc removal has afforded access and a cavity, into which the fragment may be manipulated.

Cauda equina compression

The spinal cord ends at the L1/2 interspace and

neurological deficit from compression of its distal end within the upper lumbar canal is rare but does occur due to canal stenosis from facet joint hypertrophy into the spinal canal as well as the development of osteophytes. More common is the syndrome of claudicant sciatica or pseudoclaudication. It is a clinical diagnosis, the hallmarks of which are lower limb pain and dysaesthesia, and lower limb deficit, which are precipitated by prolonged walking or standing. The spinal canal is narrowed by facet joint hypertrophy and becomes critically stenosed when the patient assumes the erect posture for walking or standing. There is believed to be an alteration of cauda equina haemodynamics, possibly due to venous stasis which produces the pain and occasional motor disturbance.

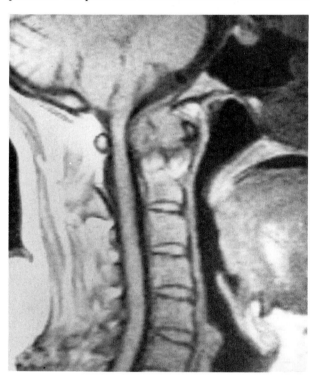

Figure 52.7 MRI scan showing destruction of the dens, and anterior compression of the lower medulla by pannus

The disease is usually worse in the lower lumbar region and so the lower roots of the cauda equina are more severely affected. The symptoms may progress to the point where the patient becomes incapacitated after standing or walking for only a few minutes. Further exercise may precipitate further deficits in the most severely affected nerve roots. Lumbar canal stenosis and pseudoclaudication occurs more frequently with advancing age.

The symptoms may readily be differentiated from vascular (intermittent) claudication by the presence of adequate distal pulses or the patient reporting that bending over (and thus opening the lumbar laminae and increasing the sagittal diameter of the spinal canal) relieves the symptoms. Physical examination is often normal.

Myelography is the most accurate investigation and demonstrates wasting of the common dural sac at the level of the facet joints. CT readily demonstrates the facet joint hypertrophy encroaching into the lumbar canal and making the cross-section 'T-shaped' rather than oval (Figure 52.9). The bony changes contribute a great deal to the radiological assessment of this condition and for this reason MRI is not yet the investigation of first choice.

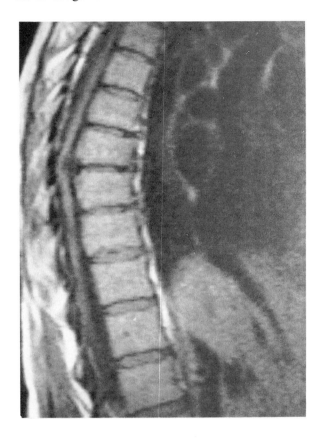

Figure 52.8 A thoracic disc prolapse well shown by an MRI scan

The treatment is decompression by wide laminectomy over the affected levels. The compromised nerve roots are decompressed by performing medial facetectomies. Because advanced degenerative changes exist prior to treatment, the new removal may compromise spinal stability and cause or exacerbate subluxation leading to further compromise of neurological function. When there is pre-existing instability the spine ought to be stabilized at the time of laminectomy. This is done by performing autologous posterolateral bone grafting and postoperative bracing in a plaster or plastic jacket. Internal fixation may be undertaken in conjunction with grafting, by pedicle screws and intersegmental rods. Generally speaking the symptoms are reversed by adequate surgical decompres-

sion. Recovery of neurological function depends on the severity and duration of the deficit.

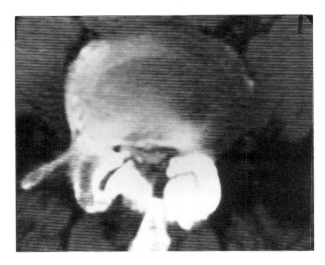

Figure 52.9 Severe lumbar facet joint hypertrophy and osteophyte formation deforming the oval shape of the spinal canal

Spinal trauma

This is common both in frequency and in the time that it occupies the mind of any clinician dealing with accident victims. However, secondary cord damage from undetected spinal instability still occurs too frequently and therefore a high degree of clinical suspicion is important.

The vertebral column encloses and protects the spinal cord and emerging nerve roots. These may be damaged directly or secondarily by trauma, and structural damage to the spinal cord is irreversible. Spinal injury is often present in victims of multiple trauma and the accompanying hypoxia and hypotension may affect the rate and degree of recovery of cord function.

Management therefore starts at the scene of the accident, and throughout the principles are to prevent further cord injury, treat existing cord damage, realign the bony vertebral column and restore stability. The role of surgery in spinal trauma is now increasing again after the trend to manage all these patients conservatively. There are now specific indications for spinal canal decompression and vertebral fixation, which include major instability, significant narrowing of the spinal canal with deteriorating nerve function, and radiculopathy. In addition there are occasional instances where vertebral stabilization is performed to facilitate nursing care even when the cord is irreversibly and completely damaged.

General pathology

The main problems requiring surgical management

include cord compression and vertebral malalignment and instability. Nerve root compression is rare. Soft-tissue injury in the neck and cord concussion also occur and cause long-term problems.

Spinal cord compression is most often due to a bone fragment, a prolapsed intervertebral disc or ligamentous buckling. Compression by extradural haematoma is very unusual, other than in patients with ankylosing spondylitis. The resulting cord damage may be partial or complete and the pattern of symptoms and signs may indicate the direction of cord compression.

The stability of the vertebral column depends on three structural pillars. The vertebral bodies with their intervening discs and the anterior and posterior longitudinal ligaments form a strong anterior pillar, and the two columns of facet joints with related intertransverse and interspinous ligaments form two posterior pillars. These three pillars surround the spinal canal. Stability is lost when more than one pillar is disrupted. This may be detected because of primary malalignment such as facet joint dislocation and vertebral body wedge fracture. However, stability may be lost with no primary malalignment and these patients are at considerable risk of secondary nerve injury if this instability is not suspected and the vertebrae are unknowingly displaced at a later stage. In an unstable spine, abnormal movement is possible between the vertebrae compromising the spinal canal. The cervical and lumbar spine are most vulnerable to instability. The rib cage provides added support in the thoracic region.

Nerve root compression can occur and is more common in the lumbar spine than cervical spine. This may either be due to bone such as a fractured facet joint, or to a prolapsed intervertebral disc.

A degenerate spine is more susceptible to injury and long-term complications.

General principles of management

Management of spinal injury starts at the scene of the accident. Emergency personnel are trained to suspect spinal injury and transport the victim of an accident to hospital in such a way that further injury is avoided. At the scene a rapid motor assessment asking for movement of the hand, arm, legs and feet is useful. The main principle, however, is that the spine should be regarded as injured and unstable until this has been excluded.

The same principle applies on reception in casualty. All cases of multiple trauma and all patients with major head injuries should be assumed to have an injury to the cervical spine. A cervical collar is applied, and the head held with sandbags and tape. If there is any suspicion of lumbar spinal injury the patient must not be moved unnecessarily, and should be turned using the 'log rolling' method. This requires at least three people and moves the patient with no movement of the spine.

Resuscitation is required in any case of multiple trauma, and this takes priority over any neurological or skeletal procedure of the spine. Hypoxia or hypotension may cause secondary cord damage in patients with partial cord lesions, and limit the degree of recovery of cord function. Hypoxia may be neurogenic with any high spinal injury where there is a mechanical inability to ventilate, and may also be due to chest injury or airway obstruction. Cord damage may also result in autonomic dysfunction where the sympathetic outflow is fractured leading to unopposed parasympathetic cardiovascular control, leading to hypotension and bradycardia. Ruptured abdominal viscera may also cause hypotension.

The role of steroids is controversial. High-dose methyl prednisolone given within 8 h of injury has a small beneficial effect in some patients. Dexamethasone has been shown to have a beneficial effect in central cord syndrome after spinal trauma.

After safe transport to hospital and resuscitation, a full assessment can begin.

Cervical injury

Occipito-atlanto axial injuries include fracture of the odontoid peg, disruption of the transverse ligament (in rheumatoid arthritis and Down's syndrome) with odontoid dislocation, and the hangman fracture of the pedicles of C2. Rarer injuries include the fracture of Jefferson (a fracture of the atlas where the posterior arch joins the lateral mass) and atlanto-occipital dislocation. At this level the spinal canal is wide, injuries affecting cord dysfunction at this level usually cause death, and so if the patient survives the spinal cord is usually unaffected. Below the axis, the typical injury is vertebral subluxation, caused by ligamentous disruption, pedicle fracture or facet joint dislocation. This may be either unilateral or bilateral. There may be an associated crush fracture of the vertebral body. It is caused by a force of flexion and compression.

Cervical disc prolapse causing cord compression is common and must be excluded by imaging any cervical spine injury where instability is detected.

Spinal injury in the neck, particularly in a degenerate cervical spine, causes a wide spectrum of soft-tissue injuries, including muscle bruising causing mechanical neck pain, dysphagia due to retropharyngeal haematoma and other non-specific symptoms of the 'whiplash' syndrome. Buckling of the ligamentum flavum can cause temporary, permanent or recurrent cord compression, particularly in children, where cord damage results due to the greater elasticity of the musculoskeletal vertebral column than the spinal cord and meninges.

Clinical diagnosis is complicated for many reasons. Conscious level may be impaired by trauma or alcohol. There may be associated brachial plexus injury with its own neurological signs, and abrasions of the neck and bruising in the supraclavicular fossa provide important clues. There may be a palpable deformity of the cervical spine and neurological examination will demonstrate quadraparesis.

A lateral cervical spine X-ray reveals most vertebral injuries if it is examined critically, and it must include the junction between the mobile cervical spine and the more rigid thoracic spine. This may require an assistant to pull on the arms to depress the shoulders. The bony contours of the anterior longitudinal ligament, the posterior longitudinal ligament and facet joints must be examined for irregularity suggesting bony malalignment (Figure 52.10). There may be opening of an interspinous space suggesting rupture of the interspinous ligaments (Figure 52.11). A retropharyngeal haematoma may be seen pushing the larynx and oesophagus forward. Abnormal narrowing or distortion of the disc space may suggest disc prolapse. An anteroposterior view may show spinal malalignment suggesting unilateral facet joint dislocation, and oblique views of the foraminae and specific views of the odontoid peg complete the plain radiological examination. The doctor responsible for the patient should supervise these X-rays and do so until satisfied that a full assessment has been performed.

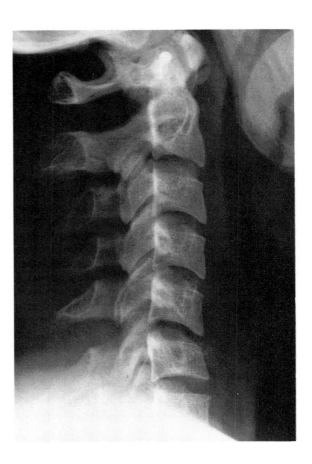

Figure 52.11 Lateral cervical spine X-ray showing widening of the interspinous space and forward angulation at C5/6

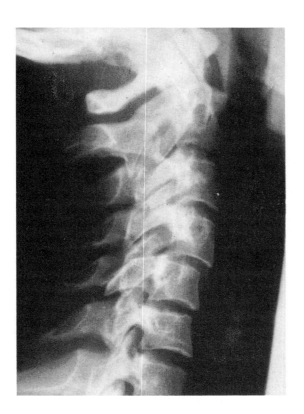

Figure 52.10 Lateral cervical spine X-ray showing a bony 'step' at C4/5, demonstrating vertebral malalignment and potential instability

If there is any doubt about stability, flexion and extension views or image intensifier screening of the cervical spine under surgical supervision will provide further information.

With any suspicion of cervical injury, CT scanning is the next investigation to demonstrate bony arrangement and also reveal any associated disc prolapse. Myelography with soluble contrast is an alternative. MRI is of limited use because it does not show bony injury and is complicated if the patient is ventilated or needing resuscitation. It is also not available in most accident units.

Successful management needs a thorough approach. It is important to avoid being distracted by a severe head injury or other injuries such that the cervical spine is overlooked. A spinal collar does play a useful role in reminding all medical personnel that the cervical spine has not been assessed. It may be removed once injury has been excluded.

Malalignment of the cervical spine must be reduced. This may be achieved by external traction with skeletal tongs which should penetrate the outer table of the skull 1 cm anterior to the coronal plane of the external auditory meatus. In this position they tend to extend the neck as traction is applied. Manipulation is performed under image intensifier control and traction maintained by weights. Care must be taken to avoid causing further ascending damage by excessive retraction. If reduction is not achieved when 50 lb (23 kg) weight is applied, then open reduction is required.

Under general anaesthetic the patient is rolled over under supervision and a repeat X-ray is taken, since the combined effect of anaesthesia and 'log rolling' may have achieved reduction. If not, the laminae are exposed and the dislocated facet joint reduced. Bone may be removed with a high-speed drill. Image intensifier control is important. After open reduction, fusion may be performed. At the same time an anterior cervical decompression may be needed to remove prolapsed disc material or bone fragments and this also may be followed by a fusion.

If reduction has been achieved without operation, the cervical spine must be immobilized and this is achieved by external splintage fixing the patient's head via a halo screwed into the outer table of the skull to a brace securely fitted to the patient's trunk. Some fixation devices do not need skull screws (Figure 52.12). This is maintained for 8–12 weeks and removed following X-ray evidence of satisfactory alignment and fusion.

In the absence of malalignment, instability or compromise to the spinal canal, symptoms due to cervical spine injury are treated conservatively with a combination of a cervical collar for comfort, analgesia, and physiotherapy and mobilization once the pain has settled. Persistent symptoms require further investigation to exclude instability of late onset and disc prolapse. Symptoms may be prolonged, particularly if litigation is ongoing.

Thoracic injuries T1–T10

Injury to this region is less common and more severe and often associated with multiple trauma. Axial loading (in the axis of the trunk) is the usual mechanism, the compression causing a burst fracture. Adjacent vertebrae can telescope together. Dislocation is rare. Bony malalignment is common, but the spinal column is still stable due to the splinting effect of the rib cage.

Cord damage is primary and most usually due to compression by bony fragments, disc material or a distorted spinal column. The thoracic spinal canal is narrow and the blood supply to this segment of the cord is most vulnerable. If cord damage occurs it is usually complete and increasing neurological deficit is unusual.

After a period of spinal shock the patient presents with a spastic paraparesis. A partial lesion is usually anterior, causing motor spinal loss with preservation of the sensation in the posterior columns.

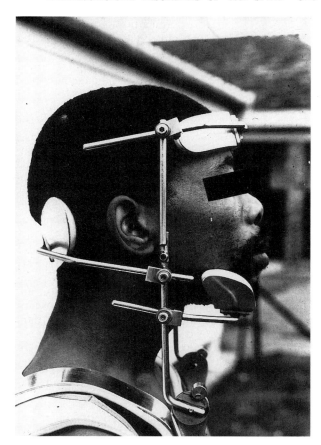

Figure 52.12 A young man with an unstable fracture at C6/7 which has been held in an external brace that does not use a skull halo. The chin piece is removed to facilitate eating (Courtesy of the Head of Department, Spinal Injury Unit, Conradie Hospital, Cape Town, South Africa)

Plain films must be over-penetrated to show the bony arrangement. The area is difficult to image because of the rib cage and mediastinal structures, but CT scanning after contrast is most helpful, and MRI, once the patient is resuscitated, may emerge as a most useful investigation.

Resuscitation is the priority in this group of spinal injuries. Other injuries may require more pressing treatment, in particular tension pneumothorax, hypoxia and hypotension. Management may include blood transfusion, oxygen, intubation, ventilation and chest drainage. Abdominal and thoracic visceral injuries may require laparotomy or thoracotomy.

Bony injury is usually stable and is best treated by bed rest for 3–6 weeks followed by mobilization with or without a moulded jacket.

Primary injury to the spinal cord is unlikely to recover, particularly if it is complete and has been present for more than 48 h. In this group, surgical decompression and stabilization does not help. However, a partial cord lesion or major dislocation that could lead to deformity are indications for surgery. A partial cord lesion is usually due to anterior compression and therefore a transthoracic approach will achieve decompression and the posterior bony structures are preserved. Total dislocation can be treated by open reduction and infusion and this will help nursing care even though the cord damage may have resulted in paraplegia.

Thoracolumbar injury

This area is vulnerable since the spinal column loses the support of the rib cage and is once again mobile. Again, multiple injury is common and hypotension and hypoxia need emergency treatment. Damage to the thoracic aorta and the radicular artery of Adamkiewicz may cause cord ischaemia, particularly of the conus.

Compression fracture of the vertebral body causes wedging and collapse and this is commonly associated with bony encroachment into the spinal canal, particularly at T12 or L1. Fracture dislocation and subluxation may also occur. Fractured transverse processes are common and associated with flank bruising, but do not cause neurological disturbance. Below L1 the dural sac contains nerve roots which are more able to withstand compression due to their greater mobility.

Examination may reveal abrasions or bruising, for example due to a seat belt. There may be a palpable step in the lumbar spine, suggesting malalignment. Leg weakness and retention of urine must be identified. Rectal examination is useful, provided that the patient is rolled with care. Injury to the conus can cause isolated difficulty with micturition and loss of perineal sensation with normal power in the legs.

Anteroposterior and lateral plain X-rays (Figure 52.13) of the lumbar spine and CT scan (Figure 52.14) with or without intrathecal contrast will show bony damage and any encroachment of the spinal canal, and will usually provide sufficient information to decide management.

If the lumbar spine is aligned with no compromise of the spinal canal, then conservative treatment with bed rest and analgesia is all that is required. A roll towel beneath the patient will restore lumbar lordosis and the patient can be mobilized with or without a moulded jacket. The duration of bed rest depends on the present state of instability. An unstable spine should be immobilized for 3 months.

Indications for surgical treatment include significant cauda equina compression (with deteriorating function), and spinal instability. Below L1 any compression of the dural sac affects nerve roots which are potentially able to recover after structural damage. The usual site of dural compression is anterior and in this area of the spinal canal it is possible to approach this following a laminectomy and removal of one or both pedicles. Access is then gained to the spinal canal anterior to the dural sac and any compressing material (bone or lumbar disc) may be removed. If this transpedicular approach is used it will of course render the spinal column unstable (the anterior 'pillar' already being fractured) and fusion is therefore required. This may be achieved using a transpedicular screw or sublaminar wires attaching the two laminae above and two laminae below the operated level to a moulded rectangular metal bar. Autogenous bone graft should be added to provide a permanent fusion.

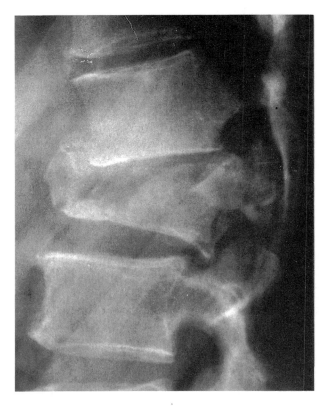

Figure 52.13 Lateral X-ray of the lumbar spine showing an anterior wedge fracture crushing the vertebral body. Posterior displacement of bone is likely in this case (see also Figure 52.14)

Penetrating cord injury

This is very rare in this country and is usually caused by bullets, stab wounds, shrapnel or other blast damage. Complications include cord damage, CSF leakage and infection. Primary impairment of cord function depends upon the path of the missile.

Cord compression occurring by a lodged bullet or dislodged bone fragments requires surgery. In the absence of cord compression, surgery is rarely indicated other than for superficial wound debridement. Persistent CSF leakage will require repair. Bullets or metal fragments are much less likely to cause infection than bone fragments, so a deep-seated foreign body causing no other complication is best left alone.

Long-term care of spinal injury

Spinal injury causing paraplegia or quadriplegia is

common in young people after accidents, and will have a devastating effect on the patient and his or her family. The long-term management requires a multi-disciplinary approach and is best performed in a specialist centre.

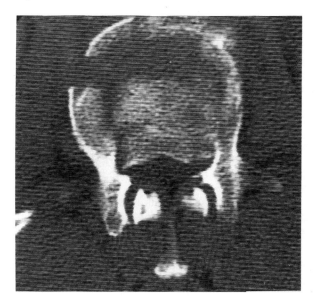

Figure 52.14 CT scan of the fracture in Figure 52.13 showing marked encroachment of the spinal canal by a peg of bone that has been ejected back from the fractured vertebral body

Bladder and bowel function is disturbed in any complete cord lesion. Good management of the paralysed bladder is most important. Prolonged distension of the bladder will limit its recovery. Initial urine drainage is achieved with a catheter. Faecal impaction must be avoided, as this in itself can cause further difficulty with micturition.

Urinary infection must be prevented and treated effectively when it occurs. Complications include pyelonephritis with compromise of renal function and renal stones, particularly in recumbent patients. Patients are taught manual expression, self-catheterization and other 'tricks' to provoke bladder contraction.

It is now possible to implant sacral nerve root stimulators surgically for patients with upper motor urine problems. These stimulators can be programmed to provide a particular pattern of frequency to nerve roots that will achieve micturition, defaecation and useful erection (see page 822).

Specialist nursing and physiotherapy are needed to prevent pressure sores and joint contractures developing which may cause problems in long-term mobilization.

This is a human tragedy which can be alleviated by good care. Early mobilization is very good for a patient's morale. Complete lesions in young people cause major social, physical and sexual consequences, all of which need very careful counselling.

Spinal tumours

As elsewhere in the body, tumours affecting the spinal column may be benign or malignant, and the malignancy may be either primary or metastatic. While this is a useful pathological classification, spinal tumours are more practically divided according to site, into those which are extradural and those which are intradural. Intradural tumours are further divided into extramedullary (outside the spinal cord) and intramedullary (intrinsic to the spinal cord). The distinction between extra- and intradural tumours is reflected in the different presentation, the risk of bony instability with extradural tumours and the difference in the surgical procedure. The principles of treatment for all these tumours is to establish a histological diagnosis, to preserve neural function and maintain vertebral stability. Recent advances include the invaluable introduction of the operative microscope, enabling more accurate surgery for intradural tumours, and the change in the management of extradural tumours where the vogue of posterior decompression by laminectomy has been replaced by a more carefully selected surgical management in terms of approach and appropriateness of surgical intervention.

Extradural tumours

The majority of these are metastases. Primary tumours are rare in the spinal column. The most common primary sites are breast, bronchus, prostate, thyroid, kidney and haemopoietic tissues. Blood-borne transmission of malignant cells via the rich venous plexus enables seeding of the vertebral bodies and pedicles. Nerve dysfunction by compression is secondary. Spinal instability is therefore a major component of these tumours. Multiple lesions are common.

Benign tumours such as neurofibromas also occur in the extradural space.

Extradural tumours present with back pain or neurological deficit. The character of the back pain is 'pathological', and is characterized by severe boring pain, unrelated to activity, which is often noted at night when the patient is recumbent. The major differential diagnosis is mechanical back pain. Patients are usually in the middle or older age group (an age group that commonly suffers mechanical low back pain) and there may be a history of malignant disease. Neurological deficit depends on the site of dural compression and is most commonly a spastic paraplegia due to thoracic or thoracolumbar disease. It may be of acute or gradual onset and can occur in the absence of pathological back pain. Examination includes detecting signs of motor and sphincter disturbance, and a sensory level may indicate the level of disease. Myelopathy may be partial or complete.

Investigation of neurological deficit is urgent. Extradural tumours may be identified on plain antero-posterior and lateral films of the affected spinal region, and are characterized by asymmetry with loss of pedicles and anterior vertebral collapse. There may be a soft-tissue shadow. In an emergency, myelography with or without CT scanning is the next investigation and it will show the typical features of extradural compression (Figure 52.15). The upper and lower limits of the lesion must be visualized if surgery is to be contemplated. If there is any suspicion about multiple deposits, a full myelogram is advisable to identify other lesions. If there is time, these may also be identified by isotope bone scan. A general examination including chest and rectal examination must be performed to identify primary disease.

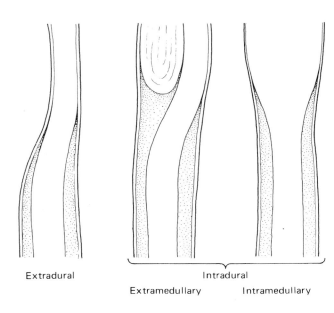

Extradural

Intradural

Extramedullary   Intramedullary

Figure 52.15 The different myelographic patterns of cord compression due to extradural, intradural extramedullary and intradural intramedullary tumours

General investigations would include a chest X-ray, acid phosphatase and other search for primary disease as time permits.

Decisions of management must be made on the basis of a histological diagnosis which may be available from known past malignancy. The aim of treatment is to prevent neurological deficit and preserve spinal stability and if a deficit is present its reversibility depends on its completeness, duration and speed of onset. A complete paraplegia of sudden onset and more than 12 h duration will not recover. It is clearly inappropriate to subject a patient to a painful operation if this will not lead to any improvement of nerve function or alteration in the course of disease. In this respect, surgery is more likely to be considered with metastases which may respond to chemotherapy, radiotherapy or hormonal manipulation than those which will not.

Histological diagnosis can initially be achieved by a CT-guided needle biopsy if early surgical decompression is not indicated. Otherwise it can be achieved at operation by frozen section. Radical surgery is best indicated where there is a long history, a mild neurological deficit and a responsive tumour.

Decompressive laminectomy is adequate in the thoracic spine and lumbar spine where there is a posteriorly placed tumour with no anterior instability. The limits of the lesion must be identified, and decompression is achieved when there is restoration of dural pulsation. More radical surgery is indicated for extensive anterior disease, particularly if there is vertebral body collapse and loss of the anterior column of stability. These tumours may be approached anteriorly to preserve the facet joint columns, or via a transpedicular approach with external spinal stabilization to restore the stability that has been lost by decompression.

Recovery of these patients needs attention involving physiotherapy, occupational therapy, home conversion and further treatment of tumour.

Intradural tumours

These are less common, but if undetected may cause profound irreversible neurological deficit. Diagnosis depends on clinical suspicion, particularly of an unusual back presentation in a young person. The lack of bony involvement and rarity of these tumours delay their detection.

Most intradural tumours are extramedullary, and benign meningiomas or neurofibromas predominate. Intramedullary (intrinsic cord) tumours are of varying behaviour, the most common being ependymoma and low-grade astrocytoma. Some tumours may seed by CSF fluid transmission, and these include medulloblastoma, high-grade ependymoma and pineal tumours, and deposits may occur typically in the lumbar region. These may be multiple and associated with malignant meningitis. Intradural tumours may occur as part of systemic syndromes such as von Recklinghausen's disease and von Hippel–Lindau disease.

These patients are often young and present with a gradual onset of progressive neurological deficit. Pain is unusual. Diagnosis on the basis of examination may be complicated if there are multiple deposits.

Detection of these lesions is complicated and specialized. There is usually time to investigate fully a patient prior to surgical treatment. A long-standing residual tumour may lead to secondary bony changes such as vertebral body scalloping or enlarging an intervertebral foramen (typical of neurofibroma), and CT myelography will identify the intradural pattern of contrast displacement demonstrating either intramedullary or extramedullary features (Figure 52.15). CT scanning after myelography gives further information. The spinal cord is well visualized by MRI scan. Differential diagnosis include syringomyelia, multiple sclerosis or spinal arteriovenous malformations (AVMs). If there is a past history of brain tumour, CSF cytology can now identify exfoliated brain tumour cells.

Surgery for these tumours requires a binocular operating microscope and microsurgical instrumentation. The spinal cord is exposed by laminectomy and the tumour removed with minimal manipulation or displacement of adjacent normal spinal cord. A cord that has been compressed and distorted by tumour is more susceptible to damage at the time of surgery. Extramedullary tumours are usually removed with ease, but intramedullary tumours require dissection from surrounding normal nerve tissue. A subtotal resection is preferable to complete removal causing neurological deficit, as these tumours usually respond to radiotherapy, which should include the entire neuroaxis if the tumour is one that can recur by CSF seeding. The CO_2 laser and ultrasonic aspirator are occasionally invaluable for surgery of intramedullary tumours. Cysts may occur adjacent to tumours. Cytology will identify any malignant disease. If the cyst fluid has the same colour and protein content as CSF it is usually benign.

Spinal infection

Infection of the spine, with the serious risk of neurological disorder, is difficult to manage well. Treatment is often inadequate and too late, because diagnosis is often missed in the early stages. This is because the disease process is relatively unusual and therefore unfamilar to most clinicians, and the symptoms may be relatively non-specific. In consequence, a high awareness is required about the conditions discussed below. Spinal tuberculosis is rare in this country, but very common in the Third World and therefore may present in immigrants.

The characteristic of the pain of spinal infection is that it is the second major cause of 'pathological pain', that being pain in the spine of a constant nature, unrelated to spinal movement and often worse at night. Infection of the spinal column occurs via haematogenous spread in most instances via the vertebral venous plexus (Batson's plexus). The patient may have a predisposition to infection (e.g. diabetes) and there is often a history of urinary tract infection, recent pelvic or bowel surgery or cutaneous sepsis.

Osteomyelitis

Haematogenous spread settles in the vertebral bodies. The most common organisms are *Staphylococcus aureus* and Gram-negative organisms (particularly in association with previous urinary tract infections and instrumentation). The intervertebral discs may rarely be the seat of infection causing discitis, and this may follow disc surgery.

The typical patient presents with severe back pain of pathological nature, lumbar spasm and limited range of spinal movement. Neurological deficit is unusual unless the disease has progressed to cause vertebral collapse or epidural abscess. The patient may or may not be toxic, and febrile.

Serological tests such as the erythrocyte sedimentation rate (ESR), protein and white cell count are raised and often diagnostic. In addition they monitor the course of the disease and its response to treatment. Plain X-rays may show evidence of discitis. Radioisotope bone scanning will reveal the causative lesion and CT scanning of the area will show any soft-tissue involvement. Diagnosis is confirmed by blood culture and CT-guided needle aspiration.

Effective treatment is with large doses of antibiotics and bed rest. If there is any suspicion of instability the patient is mobilized in a supportive jacket. Surgery is indicated when a causative organism has not been isolated or there is evidence of myelopathy.

Epidural abscess

In this case haematogenous spread of infection settles in the epidural space, most typically in the thoracolumbar junction with the pus posterior to the dura. If it is associated with osteomyelitis, then it may lie more anteriorly.

Presentation is similar to spinal osteomyelitis except that neurological deficit caused either by cord compression or ischaemia occurs much earlier, and sensory loss is usually less than motor loss. It is this group that requires early diagnosis for effective treatment, since once neurological deficit is severe and total it is unlikely to recover.

In addition to the serological investigations, the diagnosis can be made by lumbar puncture, when no CSF is obtained (dry tap). This is caused by pus compressing the dura such that no CSF is available. Occasionally pus will be seen on withdrawing the needle which is further confirmation. Myelography is often unsuccessful when a dry tap has occurred. CT scan will show evidence of soft-tissue swelling, and an isotope bone scan will show a 'hot area'. However, a toxic patient with severe pathological back pain, a tender spot in the lower spine and increasing neurological deficit is a surgical emergency which requires early surgical decompression.

It is vital to decompress the cord and obtain early diagnosis. Limited bone removal is required, since the pus may sometimes be washed out with catheter irrigation. Occasionally the epidural material is more solid and extensive laminectomy is required. Antibiotics must be given in a high dose and may be given topically via catheters that are left in the epidural space.

Tuberculosis

This is unusual in this country, but very common in

countries such as India and Pakistan, where it is commonly seen in children. The age of onset increases as social and economic conditions improve. It most often affects L1, and a typical picture is an intervertebral disc affected with spread to the adjacent vertebral bodies on either side. In addition, there may be a soft-tissue paraspinal abscess. Vertebral collapse is common in advanced disease, causing kyphosis which may compress the cord at the apex (Pott's disease).

This condition is rare in Europe and will only be diagnosed by a high degree of suspicion. Symptoms of systemic tuberculosis such as weight loss and malaise are common, the patient presenting with low back pain and local tenderness over the spine. It is unusual to have a neurological deficit. However, once collapse has occurred the kyphos may lead to a severe spastic paraparesis.

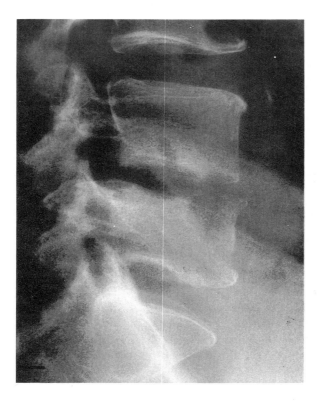

Figure 52.16 Lateral lumbar X-ray showing narrowing of the L4/5 disc space, 'softening' of the bony outlines and spread of the infection to the adjacent vertebral bodies

Serological tests will show evidence of infection. A chest X-ray may show primary disease (chest or abdominal films may show a paravertebral soft-tissue swelling suggesting a psoas abscess). Plain films of the spine, particularly a lateral view, may show the typical appearance of a disc and adjacent vertebral body involvement (Figure 52.16). If there is evidence of myelopathy, myelography combining MRI scanning or CT scanning will delineate the extent of the disease

and cord involvement. An isotope bone scan also shows affected areas of the cord. Diagnosis is confirmed by microbiological tests which are usually obtained by needle biopsy under CT guidance.

Once the diagnosis is confirmed and in the presence of spinal cord compression, the most effective treatment is surgical decompression and spinal fusion. In the absence of neurological deficit, chemotherapy alone is usually sufficient.

Congenital spinal disease

These conditions result from failure of formation, differentiation, fusion, and segmentation of the embryological components of the spinal column. These include the neural tube, mesodermal segments (forming the musculoskeletal tissues) and the overlying ectoderm (forming the skin) and the underlying endoderm (forming the intestine). The resulting multi-tissue abnormalities are collectively described as spinal dysraphism (Figure 52.17). Other congenital disorders often occur. Associated hydrocephalus is common.

Spina bifida occulta

This is the commonest congenital anomaly, occurring in approximately 1% of the population. It consists of a bony defect in the posterior neural arch of the vertebra (Figure 52.18). It may occur anywhere from C1 to the sacrum and usually affects only a single level. It should be regarded as an incidental finding, but may make the spine more prone to degenerative disease and mechanical back pain.

Spina bifida aperta

This open defect may either cause meningocele or the more common myelomeningocele.

Meningocele

The neuro-axis is essentially normal, but spinal bifida allows herniation of a CSF-filled diverticulum of meninges contiguous with the common dural sac. These are usually posterior and covered with normal skin. They may appear anywhere from the cervical to the sacral region. Neurological status is usually normal, but other anomalies of the CNS may coexist. Their repair is a cosmetic concern and must be done by a neurosurgeon after adequate radiological investigations (plain X-ray, ultrasound, myelogram and CT or MRI).

Myelomeningocele

This is the commonest dysraphic condition of clinical importance. It results from persistence of the posterior neuropore. A tangle of neural tissue (the placode),

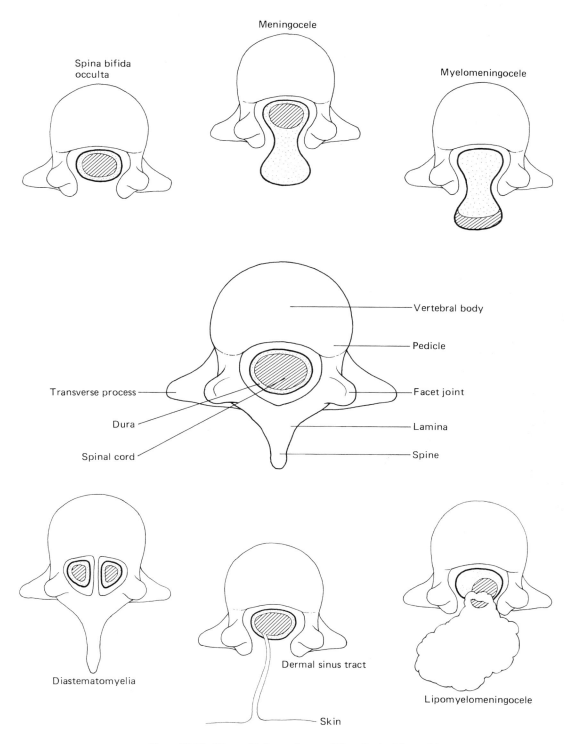

Figure 52.17   The multi-tissue abnormalities of spinal dysraphism

meninges and abnormal epithelium appear on the body surface anywhere from the cervical region to the sacrum. The commonest site is the thoracolumbar junction. The higher the lesion, the worse is the neurological deficit and the greater the incidence of hydrocephalus. This occurs in 75% of cases, the majority within the first 3–4 months. The Chiari malformation affects the CNS coincidentally with the myelomeningocele.

The best prognosis occurs with small sacral lesions. These are associated with the likelihood of normal ambulation, possible sphincter control, normal intelligence and less than 10% chance of hydrocephalus requiring shunting.

'Emergency' management involves covering the lesion with a moist sterile dressing. Antibiotics are not indicated. The immediate danger is ascending meningitis via the universally present open central canal in the placode, and the infection rate escalates after 36 h. Immediate referral to a neurosurgical service is indicated. The warm, fed normoglycaemic infant is then examined to ascertain the extent of spontaneous movement in the lower limbs, anal tone (seen as dimpling when the baby cries), urinary stream, the presence of talipes and the anterior fontanelle tension. A general paediatric examination assesses the cardiac status because of the incidence of associated defects, and plain X-rays of the spine and ultrasound and CT of brain are obtained. Imaging of the urinary tract may be required.

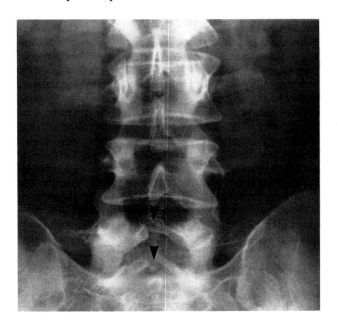

Figure 52.18 Spina bifida occulta discovered on the control film for an intravenous pyelogram, affecting the laminae of the L5 and S1 vertebrae (arrowed)

Although the parents may not comprehend the magnitude of the clinical situation, a careful attempt is made to inform them. The incidence is decreasing, although unexpected cases still occur when the diagnosis is made at birth. Surgery is now considered inappropriate if the future quality of life would be intolerable – a judgement made considering the level of the lesion, the completeness of the nerve defect, the presence of hydrocephalus, serious infection and other congenital abnormalities. The decision to withhold active treatment is very complex and needs expert and patient counselling of parents who are already distressed. The final decision must be theirs.

In almost all other cases surgery will be indicated to close the myelomeningocele and restore the normal anatomical layers covering the defect with fascia and skin. This does not produce improved function, but should prevent deterioration and ascending infection. Untreated infants do not always succumb and may present after having survived and deteriorated. Hydrocephalus is present in the majority of cases and CSF diversional shunting is undertaken when CSF samples are proven to be clear of infection after the myelomeningocele closure. Follow-up must be close, with involvement of paediatricians, therapists, urologists, orthopaedic surgeons and neurosurgeons. Wheelchairs and special educational needs also strain the already stressed family. Fifty per cent of survivors achieve some schooling, although most are handicapped.

Myelocele

This is a cystic expansion of the spinal cord through a spina bifida. The wall of the cyst consists of neural tissue and meninges and skin in disordered fashion. MRI is indicated to seek other anomalies such as syringomyelia and/or tethered cord.

Lipomyelomeningocele

This presents clinically as an asymmetrical fatty mass which distorts the buttock, often with skin dimpling. There is usually impairment of sphincter function and sometimes talipes. A myelogram and CT, or MRI, shows a low conus ending within the fatty mass, through which the nerve roots pass (Figure 52.19). Surgical intervention is directed towards untethering the conus, preserving the lowest nerve roots and reconstituting the common dural sac before further neurological deficits develop. Lipomyelomeningocele demands an exacting approach.

Diastematomyelia

In this condition there is a cleft in the spinal cord producing two hemi-cords around a septum which passes from the vertebral body sagittally through the cleft to the lamina. Its aetiology is unknown, but probably relates to duplication or persistence of the neuroenteric canal. The septum is either fibrous or bony and lies between two discrete dural tubes and their contained hemicords. The hemicords usually reunite immediately caudal to the septum which thus acts to tether the cord during active spinal movement. The lesion usually is present at the thoracolumbar junction and hemivertebrae, a tethered conus and syringomyelia may coexist.

A cutaneous marker such as a hairy patch or naevus is often present. The lesion may be obvious at birth or may be detected when symptoms such as pain or progressive (and often asymmetrical) neurological

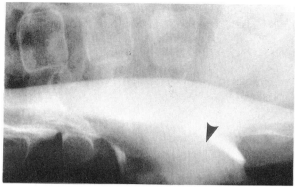

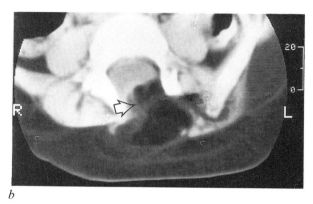

Figure 52.19 A myelogram (*a*) followed by CT scan (*b*) showing the spinal cord tethered in a spina bifida (solid arrow), and closely associated with the intradural component of a lipoma (open arrow)

disturbance of the lower limb supervene in childhood or adolescence.

Diagnosis is proven by CT myelography or MRI (Figure 52.20).

The lesion must be treated as soon as it is detected, to prevent further deterioration. Other lesions, especially a tethered conus, must be sought prior to treatment. Surgery entails laminectomy and meticulous removal of the often vascularized septum flush with the posterior aspect of the vertebral body, utilizing the high-speed drill for bony lesions. Then the dural component of the septum is excised so that the two hemicords lie untethered within a single dura tube. The tethered conus must also be released.

Dermal sinus tract

This is a dysraphic state where surface ectoderm persists embedded or rather invaginated within the body and connected to the surface by a cylindrical tract of epithelium. The hallmark of the condition is the opening of the dermal sinus tract in or near the midline. There are often signs of inflammation around the opening and rarely a bead of pus may be expressed. The tract may run either rostral or caudal from its point of entry into the CNS, which occurs anywhere from the external occipital protuberance to the sacrum. The tract may terminate in or on the dura or may penetrate the neuro-axis and extend for a considerable distance within the spinal cord. Radiological evidence of spina bifida around the sinus tract may be possible to detect.

The condition may present with neurological dysfunction from the mass effect of an intradural dermoid cyst caused by the accumulation of desquamated epithelium, or presentation may be from sepsis. The communication with the exterior may lead to otherwise unexplained recurrent bouts of meningitis or a subdural empyema or even spinal cord abscess often extending for a considerable distance within the cord.

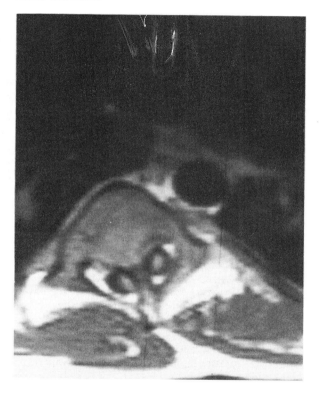

Figure 52.20 Diastematomyelia shown by MRI

A myelogram and CT, or MRI, is necessary for diagnosis. CSF is sampled if meningism is present.

Infection, if present, is controlled with parenteral antibiotics and when the dermal sinus tract is confirmed the exterior opening is excised and the tract followed to its termination. The surgeon must be prepared to open dura and follow the tract even within the cord. There is often considerable arachnoidal scarring. A sinus tract must never be probed and a silogram is absolutely contraindicated. Once detected the condition must be completely eradicated.

Syringomyelia

Spinal cord cysts may occur in association with intrinsic cord tumours, previous spinal trauma, arachnoid adhesions, the Chiari malformation or, rarely, idiopathically. Cord cavitation is thought to develop due to disturbance of CSF hydrodynamics across the craniocervical junction, and the Chiari malformation is the commonest cause encountered clinically.

Three subtypes exist. Type 1 describes descent of the cerebellar tonsils through the foramen magnum. Type 2 describes tonsillar and vermian descent as well as descent and malformation of the entire brain stem and fourth ventricle. This is the type encountered in myelomeningocele, and structural abnormalities of the entire neuro-axis abound in such cases. Type 3 is rare and describes a dysraphic state with a cervical spina bifida containing herniated cerebellar and brain stem tissue.

The cord cavity produces damage by mechanically compressing and dissecting between spinal cord fibre tracts. The features of this disease are a central cord syndrome with dissociated sensory loss. Dorsal column modalities of fine touch and kinaesthesia are preserved, whereas interruption of central, crossing spinothalamic tract fibres causes loss of pain and temperature sensation. The syrinx is usually most capacious in the cervical cord and the sensory loss is said to be yoke (or cape) like. The motor deficit produces weakness and atrophy, particularly of a distal upper limb musculature. As the disease progresses, upper motor neuron disturbances affect the lower limbs. Congenital anomalies such as the Chiari malformation usually produce a scoliosis as well. Thus a diagnosis of 'idiopathic' scoliosis is made once an MRI has excluded cord pathology such as syringomyelia, tumour or diastematomyelia.

Treatment varies. Foramen magnum decompression combined with high cervical laminectomy is probably the most rational treatment because it treats the primary abnormality. There is no evidence that plugging of the obex confers any further benefit to the operation. Syrinx shunting (either into the subarachnoid space, pleural or peritonal cavities) is also frequently performed, but is intuitively the treatment of choice only for post-traumatic syrinxes in the absence of craniovertebral junction pathology. Persistent hydrocephalus will require shunting.

Overall, approximately one-third of patients improve, one-third stabilize and one-third continue to deteriorate with treatment even when MRI demonstrates diminution of the syrinx volume. MRI and clinical evaluation must persist postoperatively and allow complete surveillance.

Vascular disorder

Primary vascular anomalies of the spinal cord are rare. They present with haemorrhage or progressive cord dysfunction. Haemorrhage may either be extradural, subarachnoid or intramedullary (within the cord).

Extradural haemorrhage is associated with an angioma or vertebral haemangioma in most cases. It may also occur in patients with a bleeding disorder such as polycythaemia, haemophilia or uncontrolled anti-coagulation treatment. It does not occur after trauma other than in patients with ankylosing spondylitis.

A subarachnoid haemorrhage is usually due to an intramedullary arteriovenous malformation, and may occasionally occur in tumours such as haemangioblastoma.

Arteriovenous malformation

Arteriovenous malformations are rare, having a ratio to spinal cord tumours of 1:20. They affect males two and a half times more frequently than females, and occur most commonly in the thoracolumbar region. They may present at any age, but usually do so in the 30–60-year-old group.

There are three basic types. An extradural AVM is usually due to one primary feeding vessel entering the spinal canal along a nerve root dural sheath. This single vessel drains intradurally into draining veins. Intradural extramedullary AVMs are still separate from the spinal cord, although the major component is lying between the cord and the dura. Intramedullary AVMs arise from the anterior circulation and pass through the spinal cord. Cord dysfunction is due to compression, a 'steal' phenomenon, disruption by haematoma, thrombosis or elevated spinal venous pressure.

Younger patients tend to have cervical intramedullary malformations, whereas older patients have thoracolumbar extradural malformations. Cord dysfunction may either be acute, progressive or progressive with acute exacerbations. These recurring exacerbations present with the same clinical picture, thereby differentiating this condition from multiple sclerosis.

MRI and myelography in the supine position are useful to diagnose the presence of a spinal vascular malformation. Diagnosis is then confirmed with spinal angiography which localizes the supplying arteries. Digital subtraction angiography will give even clearer images.

Extradural vascular malformations are obliterated by coagulating or excising the supplying artery which is usually located in close proximity to the dural root sleeve. The distended vein linking the malformation to the spinal cord may also be interrupted. Large posterior intradural juxtamedullary components can be removed and there is usually a good plane between the mass and the underlying cord. Surgery for intramedullary vascular malformations is very complicated, with significant risk of neurological morbidity. The approach is still via the posterior aspect of the cord and results are improved with the increasing use of the laser.

Vascular malformations may also be embolized,

provided that all the feeding vessels can be identified and treated. If not, then the malformation will recur.

Vertebral haemangioma

This condition is a hamartomatous malformation that is commonly found at post mortem but very rarely causes symptoms. It resides in the vertebral body and there may be associated haemangiomas in other organs.

Enlargement of the haemangioma causes enlargement of the vertebral body, pedicles and laminae, thereby narrowing the spinal canal. Cord compression may also occur due to spread of the angioma into the extradural space. This enlargement typically develops during pregnancy, with the condition resolving after delivery of the baby.

Diagnosis may be made on plain X-ray showing the characteristic change of the vertebral body with loss of height and increasing of width in both planes (Figure 52.21). Angiography will identify the feeding vessel. MRI scan provides an alternative to plain X-rays, particularly during pregnancy.

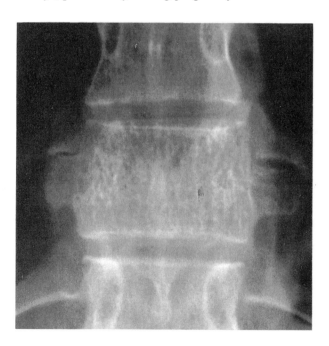

Figure 52.21 The typical honeycomb appearance of a vertebral haemangioma, with loss of height and increase of width of the vertebral body

Should the patient develop cord dysfunction, surgery is indicated and may be complicated because of the very vascular nature of these tumours. Preoperative embolization is being used to reduce haemorrhage. Radiotherapy may be given for chronic symptoms or following surgery, although in an acute exacerbation it can make matters worse by causing swelling.

Functional spinal surgery

The correction of neurological dysfunction resulting from intrinsic spinal cord pathology (other than relieving the mass or ischaemic effect of neoplasm and vascular lesions) is often beyond the realms of surgery. Advances in our knowledge of neurotransmitters and neural circuitry allow modulation of some pain states, cases of spasticity and sphincter dysfunction.

Pain

Pain may be treated in several ways. Assessment in a multidisciplinary pain clinic is useful for patient selection. Pain in the lower half of the body due to malignant disease may be effectively treated by indwelling intrathecal drug delivery systems consisting of a subcutaneous reservoir and pump attached to a fine-bore catheter which is tunnelled into the spinal subarachnoid space. The efficacy of intrathecal narcotics is established by a test dose administered by a lumbar puncture. The necessary amount of infused narcotic is then titrated by manipulating a programmable pump or altering the concentration of narcotic injected into the reservoir percutaneously. The expense of these systems is relatively prohibitive. Pain in the upper half of the body may be similarly managed by a catheter introduced into the ventricular system of the brain.

Midline myelotomy of the caudal spinal cord to divide the crossing spinothalamic fibres which subserve pain is an open procedure, rarely performed, and has the potential hazard of neurological dysfunction as a sequel.

Percutaneous high cervical cordotomy is a straightforward procedure designed to ablate the spinothalamic tract for relief of the pain of malignant disease when life expectancy is short. Bilateral high cervical cordotomies for relief of bilateral pain run the risk of respiratory paralysis.

Deafferentation pain (phantom limb pain) has been successfully managed over the past 10–15 years by radiofrequency operated dorsal root entry zone (DREZ) lesions. The spinal cord is exposed at laminectomy, and using a fine electrode meticulously placed at short intervals in the DREZ of the affected nerve roots (continuously from one segmental level below to two levels above the deafferentated region), the pain conducting circuitry of the spinal cord is selectively ablated by heating to 70°C for a specific duration.

Pain-conducting pathways may be modulated by means of epidural placement of stimulating electrodes. The electrodes are connected to a subcutaneous receiver which is activated by a transmitter optimally programmed by the patient and used transcutaneously as desired. The basic physiology was originally believed to be related to the gate control of pain. This technique of dorsal column stimulation is often used to relieve the pain of the so-called 'failed back syndrome'.

Spasticity

Patients with multiple sclerosis affected by spasticity may be effectively managed by an indwelling intrathecal drug delivery system which infuses baclofen.

The spasticity of cerebral palsy can be modified by selective posterior rhizotomy under electrophysiological monitoring, to attempt to identify pathological reflexes for obliteration in order to improve ambulation.

There is probably little indication for the crudely destructive procedure of cordectomy following complete or near complete spinal cord injury complicated by mass flexion reactions.

Sphincter dysfunction

When spinal cord injury occurs rostral to the lumbosacral enlargement, thus preserving the reflex arcs of the conus and nerves S2–S4, continence may be improved or restored by the selective intradural placement of electrodes around the sacral nerve roots. Thin electrodes are connected via wires that exit the dura to a subcutaneous receiver which is activated by a patient-operated programmable transcutaneous stimulator which is manipulated to provide the best bladder emptying with the least far-field effects of lower limb movement. These implants are costly and demand a well-motivated and reasonably intelligent patient.

Further reading

General

Dickson, R. A. (ed.) (1990) *Spinal Surgery – Science and Practice*, Butterworths, London

Rothman, R. H. and Simeone F. A. (1982) *The Spine*, W. B. Saunders, Philadelphia

Specific

Adendorff, J. J., Boeke, E. J. and Lacarus, C. (1987) Tuberculosis of the spine: results of management of 300 patients. *J. Roy. Col. Surg. Edinb.*, **32**, 152–155

Bohlman, H. H. (1979) Acute fractures and dislocations of the cervical spine. *J. Bone Joint Surg.*, **61A**, 1119–1143

Bracken, M. B., Shepard, M. J., Collins, W. F. *et al.* (1990) A randomized controlled trial of methylprednisolone or naloxone in the treatment of acute spinal cord injury. *New Engl. J. Med.*, **322**, 1405–1411

Crockard, H. A. *et al.* (1986) Transoral decompression and posterior fusion for rheumatoid atlanto-axial subluxation. *J. Bone Joint Surg.*, **68B**, 350–356

Deacon, P. and Dickson, R. A. (1990) Congenital abnormalities. In *Spinal Surgery* (ed. R. A. Dickson), Butterworths, London, pp. 337–353

Ducker, T. B. *et al.* (1978) Experimental spinal cord trauma III: therapeutic effect of immobilization and pharmacological agents. *Surg. Neurol.*, **10**, 71–76

Evans, D. K. (1987) Editorial: Stabilization of the cervical spine. *J. Bone Joint Surg.*, **69B**, 1–2

Findlay, G. F. G. (1987) The role of vertebral collapse in the management of malignant spinal cord compression. *J. Neurol. Neurosurg. Psychiat.*, **50**, 151–154

Findlay, G. F. G. (1987) Common malformations of the nervous system. In *Northfield's Surgery of the Central Nervous System* (ed. J. D. Miller), Blackwells, Oxford, pp. 574–596

Hoffmann, H. J. *et al.* (1985) Management of lipomyelomeningoceles. *J. Neurosurg.*, **62**, 1–8

Hood, R. W. *et al.* (1980) Diastematomyelia and structural spinal deformities. *J. Bone Joint. Surg.*, **62A**, 520–528

Hulme, A. (1960) The surgical approach to thoracic intervertebral disc protrusions. *J. Neurol. Neurosurg. Psychiat.*, **23**, 133–137

Lorber, J. (1971) Results of treatment of myelomeningocele: an analysis of 524 unselected cases, with special reference to possible selection for treatment. *Dev. Med. Child. Neurol.*, **13**, 279–303

Medical Research Council Working Party on Tuberculosis of the Spine (1982) A ten year assessment of a controlled trial comparing debridement and anterior spinal fusion in patients on standard chemotherapy in Hong Kong. *J. Bone Joint Surg.*, **64**, 393–398

O'Laoire, S. A. and Thomas, D. G. T. (1982) Surgery in incomplete spinal cord injury. *Surg. Neurol.*, **17**, 12–15

Shepperd, J. A. N. *et al.* (1989) Percutaneous disc surgery. *Clin. Orthop.*, **238**, 43–49

Torrens, M. J. (1990) Spinal microneurosurgery. In *Spinal Surgery* (ed. R. A. Dickson), Butterworths, London, pp. 209–216

Williams, B. and Page, N. (1987) Surgical treatment of syringomyelia with syringopleural shunting. *Br. J. Neurosurg.*, **1**, 63–80

Young, S. *et al.* (1988) Relief of lumbar canal stenosis using multilevel subarticular fenestration as an alternative to wide laminectomy. *Neurosurgery*, **23**, 626–663

Gynaecology and neonatal surgery

53

Gynaecology and the general surgeon

D. McCoy

This chapter has been written for the general surgeon. No attempt has been made to describe specialized gynaecological techniques, but the routine operations that the general surgeon may need to undertake have been illustrated and detailed. Emphasis has been placed on the indications, complications and diagnostic difficulties that may be encountered. Details of material pre- and postoperative management have been given only if differing from accepted surgical techniques.

Minor gynaecological operations

Dilatation of the cervix and curettage of the uterus

1. Dilatation of the cervix

It is not usually necessary or desirable to dilate the cervix to more than 8 Hegar. A sound should always be passed prior to passing the cervical dilators in order to ensure that the dilators themselves are passed in the curvature of the cervical canal.

INDICATIONS

(a) Prior to curettage.
(b) Prior to insertion of radium.
(c) In cases of cervical stenosis.
(d) Occasionally to treat dysmenorrhoea – excess dilatation should be avoided for fear of causing cervical incompetence in the nulliparous patient.

2. Curettage

INDICATIONS

(a) Dysfunctional uterine haemorrhage – this occasionally helps the symptoms but is more useful in checking the pathology of the uterine curettings.
(b) Bleeding occurring 6 months or more after the cessation of regular menstruation at the menopause.
(c) To exclude intra-uterine pathology at any age.

It is not necessary to illustrate the operation but the surgeon should be careful to:

(i) Complete a proper bimanual examination and assess the size and position of the uterus accurately before passing any instruments.

(ii) Sound the uterus and confirm the size of the cavity and its direction.
(iii) Having dilated the cervix, to introduce small intra-uterine polyp forceps before doing the curettage.
(iv) Send any material obtained for pathological studies.

Evacuation of the uterus

Indications

1. Incomplete abortion.
2. Missed abortion.
3. Hydatidiform mole.
4. Secondary postpartum haemorrhage.

Once again there should be a careful bimanual assessment of the size and position of the uterus. If the uterus is over 12 weeks in size, evacuation should be digital in the case of retained products, or carried out by other means in the case of hydatidiform mole or missed abortion. Three points may be noted:

(a) Ergometrine 0.5 mg intravenously can be given before the onset of cervical dilatation as this in no way impedes dilatation of the uterine cervix but helps to make the uterus contract, thus decreasing the chances of perforation and minimizing blood loss.
(b) The uterus is first evacuated either digitally, with sponge-holding forceps or suction curette.
(c) Evacuation is then completed with a sharp curette. It is not necessary to use only blunt curettage as there is no greater risk of perforation with a sharp curette used intelligently.

Cautery of the cervix

Indications

1. Cervical erosion causing symptoms, e.g. recurrent or excessive vaginal discharge.
2. Large cervical erosions.
3. Chronic cervicitis.
4. Cervical dysplasia up to CIN III.

The cervix is cauterized either with a heated ball or loop under general anaesthesia. Alternative methods are to use a triangular 'cheese-cutting' wire to perform a diathermy conization. Smaller erosions can be treated by cryosurgery, as an outpatient procedure.

When using cautery, care should be taken to avoid any preparation containing surgical spirit during the preoperative toilet of the vagina. This avoids the risk of severe burning should the spirit become ignited by the cauterization.

Shirodkar-type suture

Cervical incompetence may occur following forceful dilatation of the cervix during a previous operation. Many cases would now seem to follow previous vaginal termination of pregnancy.

The typical history of cervical incompetence is of either mid-trimester abortion or premature labour, and in both cases the labour starts with spontaneous rupture of the membranes in the absence of either bleeding or uterine contractions. Cervical suture will not cure premature labour, or recurrent miscarriages for other reasons, and selection of cases is therefore of the greatest importance.

The operation is best performed at about 14–16 weeks' gestation when the pregnancy is relatively stable, and after the 'at risk' period for spontaneous abortion.

Technique

This should be as simple and atraumatic as possible. A braided nylon tape is inserted with quadrantic bites at 12, 3, 6, 9 and 12 o'clock by means of a trocar pointed needle with a large eye, at the level of the internal cervical os. The tape is tied tightly with the knot anteriorly and both ends of the tape are left long. There would seem to be no need to reflect the bladder or incise the vaginal epithelium as such. The patient remains in bed for 48 h postoperatively. She is then allowed home. The suture is removed at 38 weeks.

Conization of the uterine cervix

In this operation the squamocolumnar junction of the cervix is removed in a cone of cervical tissue.

Indications

1. As a diagnostic procedure in the presence of a positive smear to confirm or exclude carcinoma in situ.
2. Used by some surgeons as a definitive treatment of carcinoma in situ.
3. Excision of lesion not accessible to colposcopic view.

It must be stressed that conization of the cervix is not without its risks, mainly from haemorrhage at the time of the operation or secondary haemorrhage about the 10th day. Postoperatively further permanent damage may result with cervical stenosis leading to difficulties in subsequent labour. It is for this reason that the practice of colposcopy and limited punch biopsy of the cervix has grown in popularity.

Cone biopsy is not necessary or desirable in frank carcinoma of the cervix when a wedge biopsy is adequate.

Procedure

1. Dilatation of the cervix should not be performed prior to cone biopsy as this may remove the endocervical epithelium and destroy the evidence of carcinoma in situ.
2. The cervix is marked with a suture to help in orientation of the specimen.
3. The cervix is stained with Lugol's iodine – dysplastic squamous epithelium fails to stain, demonstrating the area for excision.
4. Using a sharp scalpel (no. 11 blade), a cone of cervix is removed to include the squamocolumnar junction and the lower third of the endocervical canal.
5. A dilatation and curettage is performed after this procedure.
6. Haemostasis may be obtained either with quadrantic catgut sutures or by diathermy.

Marsupialization of Bartholin's cyst or abscess

Either a cyst or abscess of Bartholin's gland may be treated by this method. Marsupialization has the advantage of being a relatively minor operation, and avoids the risk of haemorrhage or scarring with subsequent dyspareunia which may attend excision of a Bartholin's gland. Furthermore, as the cyst or abscess is usually in the duct of the gland, after marsupialization the gland can continue its normal secretory function.

The operation

The swelling is opened by a cruciate incision placed so that resulting stoma will open on the inner aspect of the labium and at the posterior aspect of the introitus. The flaps between the limbs of the incision are removed leaving an opening into the cyst, preferably big enough to take the tip of a finger. The walls of the cyst are identified and sutured to the skin edges of the incision with a few fine 3/0 catgut sutures. The roof of the swelling has therefore been removed like the top of an egg, but the floor of the swelling remains. A ribbon gauze pad soaked in proflavine emulsion is inserted into the cavity and removed the next day.

Operations on the tubes, ovaries and round ligaments

The Fallopian tubes

The general surgeon is often confronted with a diagnosis between a general surgical emergency or a gynaecological emergency. The commonest problem is probably to differentiate between acute salpingitis, ruptured ovarian cyst, appendicitis or ectopic pregnancy. Many of these difficulties can be aided by the use of laparoscopy when the pelvic viscera can be inspected directly, and the general surgeon should be encouraged to use this relatively simple technique. On clinical grounds it is worth remembering that:

1. Salpingitis is usually bilateral and accompanied by a higher temperature and tachycardia than appendicitis. There may be a history of sexual contact, vaginal discharge or surgical interference.
2. In appendicitis the pain is usually localized to one side, there is a history of gastrointestinal disturbance, the temperature is usually not grossly elevated and the patient has a fetor.
3. Pregnancy tests using specific antibodies to human chorionic gonadotrophin (HCG) are now accurate and reliable. A negative result can be used to exclude an ongoing pregnancy in the tube. If any doubt remains, laparoscopy should be performed.

Ectopic pregnancy

While resuscitation by blood transfusion is vital, the surgeon should not delay laparotomy. Once the bleeding points have been clamped, the patient's general condition will often improve rapidly.

Examination under anaesthetic is not reliable. An ectopic pregnancy may not only be missed but ruptured during the course of the examination, with disastrous results in the patient who is lying unconscious in the recovery room.

Once the peritoneal cavity has been opened, the uterus and both tubes should be visualized. The affected tube is mobilized, and provided that the other Fallopian tube is present the portion of the tube containing the ectopic is excised. Both severed ends are ligated and thus may be amenable to reanastamosis at a later date. The ovary of the affected side is normally preserved if possible. Occasionally if the Fallopian tube of the opposite side is missing, or if the ectopic is sitting in the fimbriated end of the tube, the ectopic can be milked out and the tube preserved. It should be remembered that ectopic pregnancies tend to occur in diseased tubes and the value of such tubes is debatable unless the circumstances are exceptional.

Should the ectopic pregnancy involve both the tube and ovary, difficulty may be experienced with haemostasis. In such cases a salpingo-oophorectomy should be performed, provided that the presence of an ovary on the opposite side has been confirmed. The peritoneal cavity should be cleared of excess blood clot but not drained.

Bilateral salpingectomy

This may be done for:

1. Chronic salpingitis causing severe symptoms in patients who have failed to respond to repeated courses of antibiotics and in whom the tubes are clearly grossly diseased.
2. Rare conditions, e.g. torsion of the tube.
3. A method of sterilization.

The ovaries

Oophorectomy

REMOVAL OF THE OVARY

1. The indications to remove one ovary may be multiple provided that the other ovary is healthy, for example a large benign ovarian cyst in which the cyst has completely destroyed all normal ovarian tissue. If a significant part of healthy ovarian tissue remains, the cyst alone may be dissected from the remaining tissue – ovarian cystectomy.
2. As part of another operation, for example hysterectomy, when better haemostasis may be assured.

Bilateral oophorectomy, while technically simple, is a much more serious operation and the indications may be:

3. Routinely with hysterectomy on all post-menopausal women, or women over the age of 50 to exclude the small risk of a carcinoma developing in a remaining ovary.
4. As an adjunct to treatment for advanced malignant disease, e.g. carcinoma of the breast.
5. For ovarian carcinoma – any tumour showing obvious signs of malignancy. Clinically this may be suggested by:

(a) Large bilateral tumours.
(b) Where the capsule is perforated by tumour.
(c) Any tumour associated with ascites or obvious deposits in the pouch of Douglas.
(d) Grossly irregular multilocular tumours with large dilated vessels.

Such cases are best treated by hysterectomy and bilateral salpingo-oophorectomy. Difficulties may arise in a younger woman of reproductive age, and sadly it is not unknown for both ovaries to be removed for completely benign ovarian cysts. In doubtful cases, if facilities are not available for frozen section, the surgeon is best advised to remove the offending ovary and then be prepared to operate at a later date after paraffin sections have been taken which confirm the diagnosis, and after having had a chance to explain the situation to both the patient and her relatives. If both ovaries are removed in premenopausal women, hormone replacement therapy should be considered.

Wedge resection of the ovary

In this operation wedges of ovarian tissue are

removed from the antimesenteric border in order to reduce the ovarian mass by about one-third. After haemostasis has been secured the ovary is reconstructed with a continuous catgut suture on a trocar pointed needle. The operation is used in cases of Stein–Leventhal syndrome, which is usually found in patients complaining of infertility. The mechanism by which the operation is effective seems uncertain, but with the greater use of drugs to stimulate ovulation its use may become less frequent.

The round ligaments

Ventrosuspension of the uterus

Retroversion of the uterus is not uncommon, but is often blamed for many symptoms from backache to infertility. It may be:

1. Secondary to some other condition – the treatment is then of that condition.
2. Primary – the uterus is otherwise healthy and mobile.

Surgical correction should only rarely be undertaken as a primary operation for deep dyspareunia and very occasionally for low backache. Before subjecting the patient to surgery it is wise to antevert the uterus with a Hodge pessary, as a temporary measure, to show that once the retroversion is corrected the symptom disappears.

Plication of the round ligaments by means of an over-and-over stitch of silk or some other unabsorbable suture is effective. When the ends of the stitch are tied the uterus is anteverted by the concertina-like effect of the round ligament.

This procedure can also be performed laparoscopically.

Sterilization

Interruption of the patency of the Fallopian tubes is becoming an increasingly popular operation as a form of contraception. It is important that:

1. The patient realizes that the operation is, from a practical point of view, always irreversible.
2. The patient and her husband consent.
3. Any material removed is sent for histology.

The operation may be performed either through a laparoscope, vaginally or abdominally.

Through a laparoscope

This is an increasingly popular method in that there is minimal scarring of the abdomen and the patient's stay in hospital is usually no more than 48 h. Readers are referred to standard textbooks for operative details. With the aid of the laparoscope, the Fallopian tubes are identified and occluded with small plastic clips. The disadvantages of the technique are: that

damage to other viscera may occur from the trocar or diathermy point, failure of the operation due to poor visualization of the Fallopian tubes and cardiac arrhythmia due to the pneumoperitoneum induced with carbon dioxide.

Vaginal sterilization

This is done through the posterior vaginal fornix with the patient in the lithotomy position. The pouch of Douglas is opened, the tubes divided and tied. The advantage is that abdominal scarring is avoided; the disadvantage would seem to be the difficulty of access, operating through a potentially infected passage. The patient cannot have sexual intercourse for some 6 weeks until the vaginal scar has successfully healed.

The abdominal approach

There are numerous ways of sterilizing the patient through the open abdomen which is the method of choice in the puerperal patient.

All would seem to have a failure rate of 0.5–1% and there would seem to be no better results from complicated techniques, such as burying the tubes. The most simple and popular is the Pomeroy method in which the tubes are picked up and a segment is isolated between clamps. The segment is removed and the ends tied and left as widely separated as possible. The tubes are then returned to the peritoneal cavity.

Tubal reconstruction

As the demand for sterilization grows, so does the demand for tubal reconstruction. Techniques employed are very refined and do not fall within the scope of this book.

Abdominal hysterectomy and its modifications

It is intended to describe total hysterectomy in detail and to explain the differences between the various operations, illustrating the main operational points.

Total abdominal hysterectomy

This involves removal of the body and cervix of the uterus.

Indications

Indications are: symptomatic benign uterine disease, preferably after child-bearing has been completed, e.g. uterine myomas, dysfunctional uterine bleeding, chronic pelvic sepsis, endometriosis, carcinoma in situ, and increasingly when sterilization has been requested in the presence of menorrhagia.

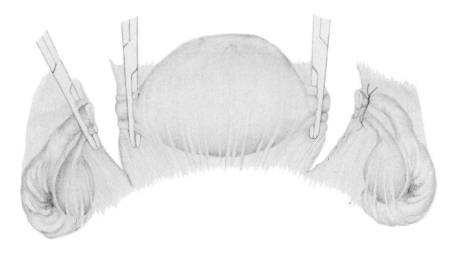

Figure 53.1 Abdominal hysterectomy. Division of broad ligaments

Operative details

A Pfannenstiel incision is usually used but if diffi-culties are expected owing to the size of the uterus, previous adhesions or obesity, a lower midline in-cision may be wiser. The bladder should always be emptied preoperatively.

1. DIVISION OF BROAD LIGAMENTS (Figure 53.1)

Parallel haemostatic clamps are applied across the broad ligaments to include the round and ovarian ligaments with the Fallopian tubes. The tissues are divided and the lateral pedicle transfixed and doubly ligated.

2. MOBILIZATION OF THE BLADDER

The peritoneum is picked up at its reflection from the bladder to the uterus and divided transversely with scissors, enabling the bladder to be pushed down from the anterior wall of the uterus and cervix, taking the ureters with it. The bladder and ureters are mobilized until the longitudinal fibres of the anterior vaginal wall are clearly identified, and the bladder and ureters are free of them.

3. DIVISION AND LIGATION OF THE UTERINE ARTERIES

The uterine vessels now exposed are secured by either straight or curved hysterectomy clamps. The tip of the clamp should reach some halfway down the cervix and be applied as closely to the cervix as possible. The tissue medial to the clamp is divided and the pedicle ligated and doubly tied.

4. SECURING OF THE VAGINAL ANGLE AND UTEROSACRAL LIGAMENTS (Figure 53.2)

Angled Kocher's forceps are now applied to include the vaginal angle and uterosacral ligaments in their grasp. The tip of the instrument should reach just below the cervix. The tissues medial to the clamp are divided and the pedicle tied. The ligature is left long and used as a second tie around the uterine pedicle, thus doubly securing this vessel and preventing any bleeding from the vessels between the vaginal angle and the uterine artery.

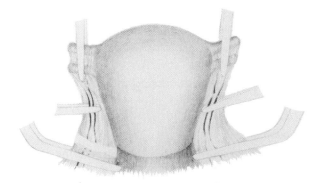

Figure 53.2 Abdominal hysterectomy. Clamping of uterine arter-ies and uterosacral ligaments prior to division

5. OPENING THE VAGINA

The vagina will have been entered with the last incision. The incision is continued transversely across the anterior vaginal wall to expose the cervix which is grasped with volsellum forceps, the posterior vaginal wall is divided transversely and the uterus removed.

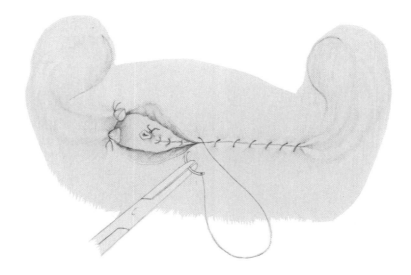

Figure 53.3 Abdominal hysterectomy. The peritoneum is reconstituted over the previously sutured and closed vaginal vault

6. CLOSURE OF THE VAGINAL VAULT

The vaginal vault is now closed either by a continuous suture uniting anterior and posterior walls or by interrupted mattress sutures.

7. CLOSURE OF PERITONEUM (Figure 53.3)

Starting at either side, the anterior peritoneum is picked up, then the round ligament, ovarian ligament and posterior peritoneum. This suture is tied to invert the ovarian pedicle within the peritoneum leaving the ovary free within the abdominal cavity. The long end of the suture is used as a continuous stitch to close the peritoneum until the pedicle on the opposite side is dealt with in the same way. Recent work may suggest that the peritoneum is left open in order to reduce the risk of adhesions.

Subtotal hysterectomy

The body of the uterus is removed leaving the cervix intact.

Indications

The principal indication is benign uterine disease where removal of the cervix may be technically too difficult or lead to damage of the bladder or ureters.

Operative details

The operation is similar to total hysterectomy until division of the uterine arteries. The incision is continued between the two uterine clamps to transect the cervix. The cervical remnant is then sutured with a trocar pointed needle and interrupted figure-of-eight sutures to secure haemostasis.

Total hysterectomy and bilateral salpingo-oophorectomy

Indications

The operation is indicated where the ovaries themselves are the site of malignancy which is operable, in cases of endometrial carcinoma, and in menopausal patients in whom any doubt of ovarian abnormality exists. Every attempt should be made to conserve ovaries in young women.

Operative details

DIVISION OF THE BROAD LIGAMENT

The round ligament and the infundibulo-pelvic ligament are clamped and divided lateral to the fimbriated outer end of the Fallopian tube and ovary. Care is taken not to damage the ureter on the side wall of the pelvis.

Extended and Wertheim's hysterectomy

Total hysterectomy with the removal of a vaginal cuff is usually reserved for cases of malignancy where the vaginal vault is a common site of recurrence. In order to remove a reasonable vaginal cuff, the bladder and ureters must be further mobilized to prevent their damage. This requires the division of the uterine artery lateral to the ureters so this may be best achieved – an extended hysterectomy. Should this procedure be combined with dissection of the lymphatic nodes from the obturator fossa, around the iliac and presacral vessels and all lymphatic tissue as far as the pelvic brim, the operation is termed a 'Wertheim's hysterectomy'.

Indications

Wertheim's hysterectomy is indicated for carcinoma of the cervix either as a sole treatment or in conjunction with pre- or postoperative radiotherapy. Its use is now usually confined to stage Ib or early stage IIa carcinoma of the cervix.

Pelvic floor repair operations

Fothergill operation (Manchester repair)

In this operation the uterine cervix is amputated in order to expose the cardinal ligaments so that they may be used to support the vaginal vault. The uterus is left *in situ*. The bladder (cystocele) and rectum (rectocele) are also supported. Any enterocele is sought for and repaired. The perineal body is also refashioned (perineorrhaphy). A posterior repair is usually required as this helps to support the anterior wall, unless the patient is very young or there is a risk of excessive narrowing of the vagina.

Indications

Fothergill repair has to some degree been replaced by vaginal hysterectomy and repair. Its place would seem to be:

1. Where the uterus is enlarged, is held in the abdomen by adhesions, or is itself asymptomatic.
2. Where the uterus does not descend sufficiently for vaginal hysterectomy to be a safe operation.
3. In a young woman with a prolapse who wishes to retain the ability to have children.

Operative details

1. THE INCISION

The site of incision is infiltrated with 1:400 000 adrenaline solution. A dilatation and curettage should be done to exclude any uterine disease. The urethra is marked with tissue forceps and the cervix grasped with downward traction by volsellum forceps. The incision may be either a vertical midline incision from the volsellum to the tissue forceps, or a diamond incision using the urethra as its apex to a point laterally either side of the cervix, and joined by a transverse incision across the posterior aspect of the cervix at the level of the internal os.

Starting at the apex of the incision the skin is removed to expose the bladder, either aided by blunt gauze dissection or a few deft strokes of a scalpel. The bladder is then pushed up to expose the anterior aspect of the cervix and the lower extremity of the cardinal and uterosacral ligaments (Figure 53.4)

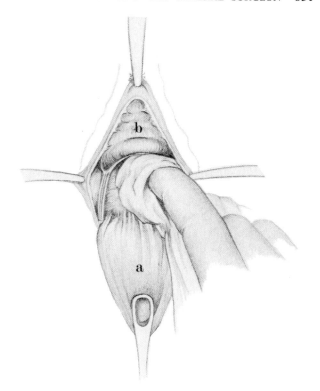

Figure 53.4 Manchester repair. The skin flap (a) is pulled posteriorly and the bladder (b) brushed forwards anteriorly away from the cervix which is beneath the swab

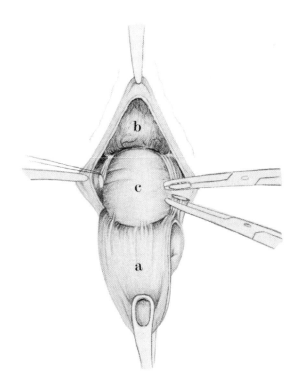

Figure 53.5 Manchester repair. Following separation of the bladder (b) from the vagina and cervix (c) the combined cardinal and uterosacral ligaments are clamped, divided and transfixed

2. DIVISION OF COMBINED CARDINAL AND UTEROSACRAL LIGAMENTS (Figure 53.5)

The ligaments are then clamped, divided and transfixed, the ends of the suture being left long.

3. SEARCH FOR ENTEROCELE

Opportunity is taken at this stage to open the pouch of Douglas and to search for any hernial sac which should be excised, the defect being corrected by uniting the uterosacral ligaments.

4. AMPUTATION OF THE CERVIX (Figure 53.6)

The cervix is now amputated at the level of the division of the cardinal ligaments.

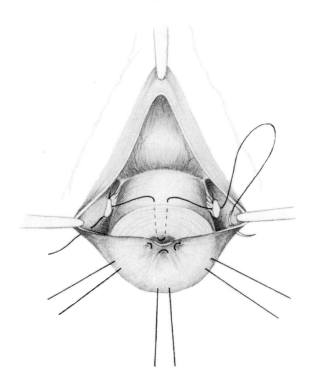

Figure 53.6 Manchester repair. The cervix is amputated and its stump is covered with vaginal skin

5. RE-EPITHELIALIZATION OF THE CERVICAL STUMP

The cervical stump is covered with vaginal skin.

(a) Posteriorly – by the Sturmdorf suture. The centre of the posterior skin incision is transfixed and the suture tied at its midpoint. Both ends are introduced on a trocar pointed needle consecutively down the cervical canal and out through the posterior aspect of the cervix and the skin flap, each slightly on opposing sides of the midline. The posterior skin flap is pulled into the canal covering the posterior aspect of the amputated cervix with skin. The stitch is tied.

(b) Anteriorly – the Fothergill stitch picks up the vaginal edge, cardinal ligament, enters and exits the canal to pick up the identical structures on the other side. Tying the suture apposes the cardinal ligaments and covers the anterior aspect of the cervix with skin.

6. ANTERIOR COLPORRHAPHY

Following excision of redundant vaginal skin the incision anterior to the cervix is now closed either by continuous or interrupted sutures, care being taken to pick up both skin and pubovesical fascia.

7. POSTERIOR COLPOPERINEORRHAPHY

A triangular area is marked out in the vaginal skin over the rectum, the apex being as near the cervix as possible and the base marked by two tissue clamps applied to the lower extremities of the labia minora at the vaginal introitus.

8. REMOVAL OF THE TRIANGLE (Figure 53.7)

A transverse incision is made at the base of the triangle and the vaginal skin is dissected from the rectum, using both blunt and sharp dissection to the apex of the triangle. The redundant vaginal skin of each flap is excised, care being taken not to remove too much skin and overtighten the vagina.

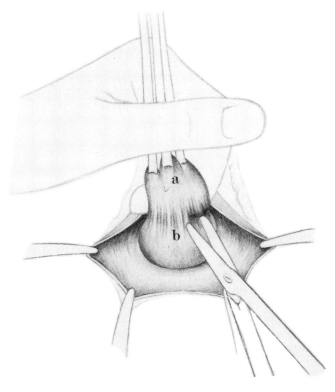

Figure 53.7 Manchester repair. The vaginal skin (a) is separated from the anterior aspect of the rectum (b) and the redundant vaginal skin of each flap is excised

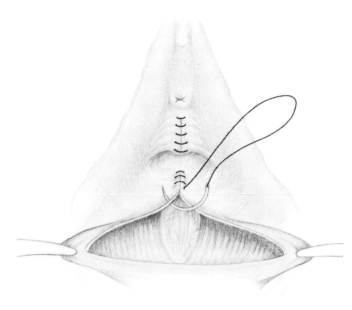

Figure 53.8 Manchester repair. The vaginal epithelium is repaired. Before completing the posterior vaginal epithelial repair, sutures are placed to approximate at the medial edges of the levator ani muscles

9. REPAIR OF THE VAGINAL EPITHELIUM (Figure 53.8)

The trimmed edges are approximated with a continuous suture working from the apex downwards.

10. INSERTION OF THE LEVATOR ANI SUTURES

Before completing the posterior vaginal epithelial repair, sutures are placed to approximate the medial edges of the levator ani muscles. Two or three interrupted sutures usually suffice.

11. REPAIR OF PERINEAL BODY

Once the vaginal skin has been repaired, the resulting defect in the perineal body is closed with two or three deep sutures and similarly two or three sutures close the skin.

12. POSTOPERATIVELY

A vaginal pack is inserted and removed after 24 h. The bladder may be drained, either by urethral or suprapubic catheters, from between 2 and 5 days until the urethral oedema has settled.

Vaginal hysterectomy

This entails removal of the uterus per vaginam.

Indications

1. Vaginal vault prolapse with or without a malfunctioning uterus.

2. Surgical preference rather than a Manchester repair.

This operation is usually combined with the repair of a vaginal prolapse. For the sake of brevity the details of the repair will be omitted and reference should be made to the section on Fothergill repair. Contraindications for vaginal hysterectomy are dealt with in that section.

Operative details

The operation is similar to the Manchester repair until subsection 2. At this stage the pouch of Douglas should be opened.

1. A finger is now passed up behind the uterus and introduced over the fundus to help demonstrate the uterovesical pouch of the peritoneum which is opened transversely, care having been taken to ensure that the bladder has been pushed upwards, well clear both in the midline and laterally.

2. DIVISION OF THE UTERINE VESSELS (Figures 53.9 and 53.10)

Once the combined uterosacral and cardinal ligaments have been divided, a finger is passed up behind the broad ligament and the uterine vessels identified. These are either transfixed or clamped and the pedicle divided medial to the clamp. The pedicle is then transfixed and doubly tied, the ligature being cut.

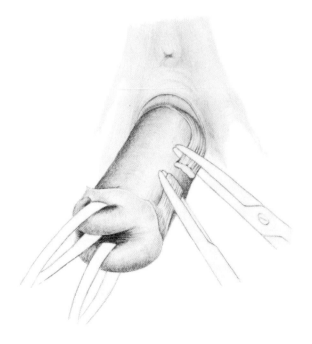

Figure 53.9 Vaginal hysterectomy. After opening the pouch of Douglas, the cervix is drawn down with volsellum forceps, exposing the cardinal ligaments which may then be clamped, divided and ligated

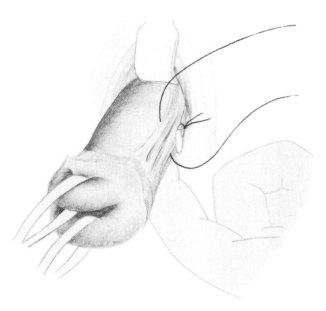

Figure 53.10 Vaginal hysterectomy. After division of the cardinal ligaments, the uterine vessels may be mobilized, ligated and divided

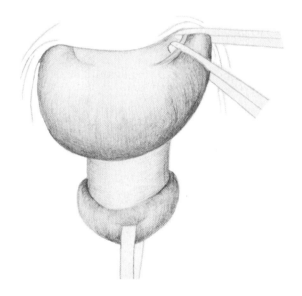

Figure 53.11 Vaginal hysterectomy. With further traction on the cervix, the Fallopian tubes, round ligaments and ovarian ligaments will be brought into view, when they may be clamped, divided and ligated

3. DIVISION OF THE FALLOPIAN TUBES, ROUND LIGAMENTS AND OVARIAN LIGAMENTS (Figure 53.11)

If there is gross descent, traction on the uterus will now demonstrate these structures and they can readily be secured by a strong clamp. Should there be difficulty, a finger should be introduced behind the uterus before applying the clamp to ensure that no

other viscus is included in the clamp. The pedicle is divided, transfixed and doubly tied, both ends of the ligature being left long and clamped to the drapes. Following this procedure on the opposite side, the uterus is removed and haemostasis carefully checked.

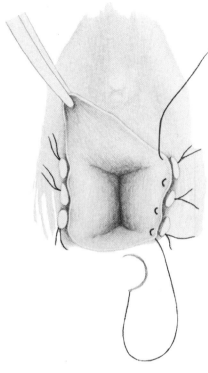

Figure 53.12 Vaginal hysterectomy. After removing the uterus, the peritoneum is carefully closed, following which the pedicles of the cardinal ligaments and the uterosacral ligaments are brought together in the midline and sutured

4. CLOSURE OF THE PERITONEUM (Figure 53.12)

Starting on one side the three pedicles are demonstrated and the peritoneum closed and tied to exteriorize these pedicles. The suture continues transversely across the vault and ends by a similar closure on the other side.

5. APPROXIMATION OF PEDICLES AND THE UTEROSACRAL LIGAMENTS

The two lowest pedicles (cardinal) are tied together in the midline and one suture on either side left long. The upper pedicles are also tied together and both ends of the suture left long. Any potential gap between the uterosacral ligaments which may allow enterocele formation is now obliterated with interrupted sutures.

6. FIXATION OF THE VAGINAL VAULT

The sutures used to tie the uterosacral ligaments are

now used to transfix the middle of the skin flap made when the skin was divided on the posterior aspect of the cervix. When tied, these obliterate the dead space and help support the new vaginal vault. Similarly, both ends of the suture used to tie the combined tubo-ovarian pedicles are used to transfix the vaginal skin edge of the same side at the point marking the base of the original diamond incision. This obliterates dead space but also helps to support and widen the new vaginal vault. The repair of the bladder and rectum now continues as described under Manchester Repair.

Operations for incontinence of urine

It is important before attempting any surgical correction of urinary symptoms to obtain an accurate history. Stress incontinence can be cured by operations which are designed to:

1. Elongate the urethra, and restore it to its place behind the pubic symphysis.
2. Restore the posterior vesical urethral angle.
3. Support the bladder and urethra with the anterior vaginal walls and associated fascial tissues.

Many patients may complain of symptoms of urge incontinence or of urinary infection. These are not cured by surgery and may even be made worse.

Urge incontinence is relatively common compared to stress incontinence and must account for many of the so-called failures of surgical repair for stress incontinence. It is wise, therefore, before contemplating any repair to ensure that the symptoms are amenable to surgery by bladder pressure studies and to make sure the urine itself is sterile.

There are many operations for stress incontinence but two types are commonly performed – the vaginal repair and the abdominal repair.

The vaginal repair (Kelly type) (Figure 53.13)

1. The incision is as for an anterior colporrhaphy.
2. The bladder and urethra are carefully identified and mobilized from any adhesions. Attention is paid to freeing the bladder neck.
3. The tissues on either side of the bladder and the urethra are approximated below the urethra and bladder neck by interrupted sutures placed about 1 cm apart from below upwards.

The nature of the tissues used by this method varies according to how far laterally they are sought. Usually the pubovesical fascia is used as a buttress, but if a very wide dissection is performed laterally the anterior border of the levator ani may be drawn across.

Any redundant vaginal skin is trimmed away and the vaginal wall closed with interrupted sutures. A pack is inserted for 48 h and the bladder drained either with a urethral catheter for 5 days or a small

suprapubic catheter which allows the patients to void urine spontaneously when they are able.

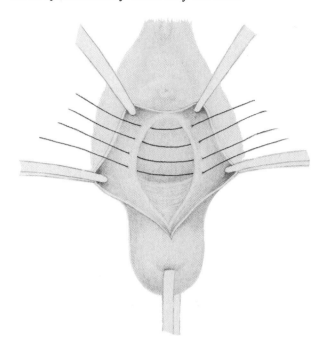

Figure 53.13 Stress incontinence. Vaginal repair (Kelly operation). Following removal of vaginal skin, the deep fascia is secured with interrupted catgut sutures which, when tied, raise and thrust forwards the bladder neck

The abdominal repair (Marshall–Marchetti–Krantz) (Figure 53.14)

The patient is placed supine with the legs slightly apart and the head tipped downwards. A 30 ml Foley catheter is placed in the bladder and the balloon distended. A tape is tied over the end of the side tube and runs down between the patient's legs to hang over the end of the table. When pulled on, this helps to identify the vesico-urethral junction by the site of the balloon in the bladder.

1. The abdomen is opened through a transverse incision.
2. The peritoneum is not opened but the retropubic space is opened by blunt dissection with either a swab on a holder or the surgeon's fingers. The bladder neck and the urethra are identified. Any large veins that might bleed are diathermized.
3. Non-absorbable black silk sutures are placed on either side of the vesico-urethral junction and urethra on a no.4 J-shaped needle carrying 2/0 silk. The sutures are placed as low as possible and run from the para-urethral and paravesical tissues through the periosteum on the back of the pubic symphysis. The sutures are left long until they have all been inserted and then tied starting with the lowest on each side and working upwards. If much bleeding is evident, the retropubic space should be drained. The wound is closed. The catheter is left in for 5 days, the patient

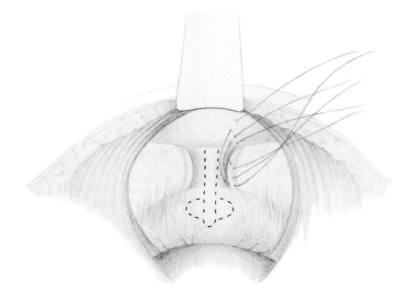

Figure 53.14 Stress incontinence. Abdominal approach (Marshall–Marchetti–Krantz). Retropubic space is dissected via a transverse incision. Non-absorbable silk sutures are placed on either side of the vesico-urethral junction and the urethra. The sutures are placed as low as possible and run from the para-urethral and paravesical tissues through the periosteum on the back of the pubic symphysis. When these sutures are tied, the bladder neck is drawn upwards and forwards

being placed on a suitable antibiotic while the catheter is *in situ*.

Burch colposuspension

Many gynaecologists would now prefer to perform a Burch colposuspension. The position, draping and incision are the same as the Marshall–Marchetti–Krantz procedure.

1. The rectopubic space is opened; the bladder and urethra separated from the pubic symphysis.

2. Either the surgeon or assistant will do a vaginal examination and exert pressure upwards to identify the lateral fornix of the vagina.

3. Through the abdominal incision the bladder is reflexed medially to expose the paravaginal tissues, and either 2 or 3 sutures of usually non-absorbable material inserted from above downwards towards the bladder neck parallel to the bladder as indicated by the assistant's finger.

4. The other end of the suture is then inserted into the pectineal part of the inguinal ligament and the sutures tied from below upwards, tying the pairs of sutures on either side at the same time.

5. The space should be drained by a vacuum suction drain. The bladder is drained by suprapubic catheterization.

Vulvectomy

Simple vulvectomy is removal of the vulva itself.

Radical vulvectomy includes removal of the vulva with its lymphatic drainage, i.e. the superficial and deep inguinal and femoral lymph nodes.

Simple vulvectomy

Indications

1. Non-malignant lesions of the vulva causing severe symptoms, usually itching, when conservative treatment has failed, i.e. leucoplakia, lichen sclerosis.

2. Pre-invasive changes in the above lesion, i.e. excision biopsy.

3. Carcinoma of the vulva when the patient is too unfit to stand more radical surgery. This may be combined with radiotherapy to regional lymph nodes or excision of lymph nodes at a later date when the patient has recovered from the vulvectomy.

Operative details

The patient is placed in lithotomy and catheterized. Either a diathermy cutting needle or a scalpel may be used to incise the skin.

1. VAGINAL INCISION

The incision runs anterior to the urethra around the introitus on both sides to the posterior fourchette.

2. VULVAL INCISION

The incision runs on both sides from the pubic symphysis downwards along the line of the junction between the thigh and the vulva. The incisions meet on the perineum just anterior to the anus. The primary incision is deepened to demonstrate the deep fascia.

3. REMOVAL OF THE VULVA

The vulva is now removed by a diathermy cutting needle, care being taken to keep in the plane of the deep fascia. It is wise to identify the crura of the clitoris and electively clamp this with transfixation of the pedicle to secure haemostasis. The whole area is very vascular and careful haemostasis with fine catgut sutures and diathermy coagulation is of prime importance. Constant care must be taken not to damage the urethra anteriorly.

4. CLOSURE OF THE INCISION

Primary closure should usually be possible with fine 0/0 catgut on a cutting needle to the vaginal/skin edge. Black silk sutures should be used to close the skin edges anterior to the urethra.

5. POSTOPERATIVELY

It is advisable to leave a self-retaining Foley catheter *in situ* with continuous drainage of 48 h until acute discomfort has passed. A sterile gauze dressing should be applied to the area and held in place with a T-bandage.

Radical vulvectomy

Indications

1. Carcinoma of the vulva.
2. Other malignant conditions of the vulva, e.g. melanoma.
3. Adenocarcinoma of Bartholin's gland.

The operation

Dissection of the lymphatic glands is carried out with the patient in the dorsal position and the legs slightly separated. Preferably two surgical teams work synchronously, one on either side for the lymphatic dissection, and once the groin incisions have been closed, as far as is practicable, the area is covered with sterile towels and the patient placed in the modified lithotomy position while vulvectomy is performed as previously described.

1. MARKING OUT THE SKIN FLAPS

Postoperative morbidity is a greater risk to the patient than the operation. It is important that primary skin closure is achieved without tension on the suture line if at all possible, so that early mobilization of the patient may be achieved. Bearing this in mind, it is wise to plan the skin incision very carefully before starting the operation, and it is sometimes helpful to draw these on the skin of the anaesthetized patient with methylene blue on a cottonwool bud.

2. THE INCISION (Figure 53.15)

A curved incision runs from one anterior superior iliac spine to the opposite side, reaching the upper border of the pubic symphysis in the midline. A second incision on either side runs from the anterior superior iliac spine along the lower border of the inguinal ligament with a triangular extension over the femoral triangle running medially to join the proposed vulval incision.

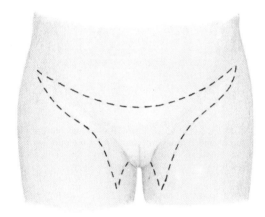

Figure 53.15 Incision for radical vulvectomy

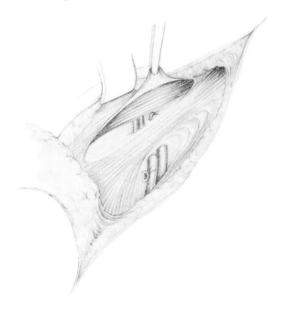

Figure 53.16 Radical vulvectomy. Block dissection of inguinal nodes

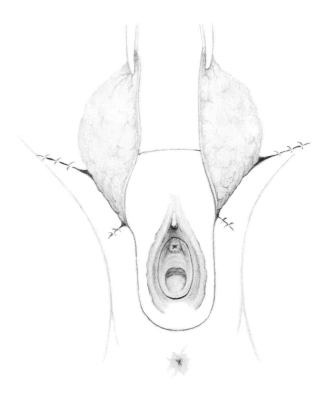

Figure 53.17 Radical vulvectomy. Following clearing of nodes in both inguinal and femoral regions, the mons pubis is cleared and the whole block of tissue turned forwards. The inguinal and femoral skin incisions are closed at this stage

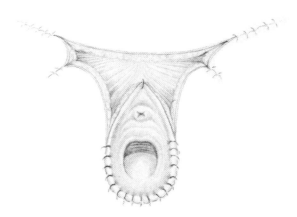

Figure 53.18 Radical vulvectomy. The skin of the perineum is now sutured directly into the vagina

3. DISSECTION OF THE INGUINAL AND FEMORAL LYMPH NODES (Figures 53.16–53.18)

Starting laterally, the incision is deepened to show the aponeurosis of the external oblique and the inguinal ligament. The skin, fat and lymph nodes are now reflected medially to uncover these structures. Over the femoral triangle the borders of the triangle are defined, i.e. the sartorius laterally and the pectineus

medially. The long saphenous vein is isolated at the apex of the triangle, clamped and tied. The vein is now followed until it turns down to join the femoral vein. It is carefully isolated, clamped and divided at this junction. The vein is doubly tied, care being taken not to stenose the femoral vein.

Further venous tributaries, i.e. the superficial external pudendal and the superficial circumflex iliac veins, are demonstrated, clamped and tied at the extremities of the incision.

The whole block of glands, fat and vessels is now removed from the femoral triangle, clearing the femoral vessels up to the inguinal ring. The gland of Cloquet is removed from the femoral canal medial to the femoral vein.

If there is clinical or pathological (frozen section) evidence to believe that these glands are involved in neoplastic disease, the surgeon may choose to remove the external iliac lymph nodes by opening the inguinal canal from external to internal ring, dividing the internal oblique and transversus abdominis muscles in the line of the incision, and by peritoneal retraction exposing the lymph nodes around the external iliac vessels. These nodes and those in the canal can now be removed, the defect being closed by interrupted sutures.

Once the nodes have been cleared in the inguinal and femoral region of both sides, the mons pubis is cleared and the whole block of tissue turned downwards. The inguinal skin incisions are now closed along with their femoral extensions by black silk sutures. It will not be possible to close the medial part of the incision until the vulvectomy has been performed.

Great attention is paid to haemostasis but it is useful to insert suction drainage tubes under the skin of the groin incisions, the area then being covered with sterile towels and the patient placed in lithotomy for completion of the vulvectomy.

Postoperative care

The area is dressed with tulle gras and cottonwool. The groin incisions can be dressed separately from the vulval incision. The drains are left until all drainage has ceased. Great attention is paid to mobilization of the patient. The silk sutures are removed on the 10th day. The bladder is drained for 5 days with an indwelling catheter.

Caesarean section

There are two methods of performing Caesarean section:

1. Incising the lower segment of the uterus.
2. Incising the upper segment of the uterus.

Lower segment Caesarean section is the more commonly performed.

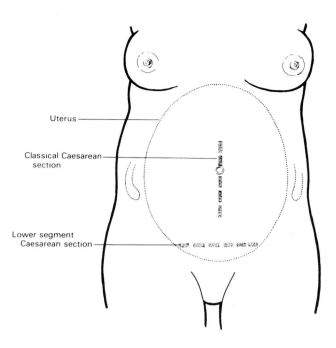

Figure 53.19 Incisions for classic and for lower segment Caesarean section

Lower segment Caesarean section

Indications (Figure 53.19)

These are many and varied. Caesarean section should be considered for good clinical reasons only, as it carries an increased risk to the mother, not only at the time but in future pregnancies. Greater awareness of fetal wellbeing has, however, increased recourse to Caesarean section in place of either difficult labour or difficult instrumental delivery.

1. Placenta praevia – in all but the most minor forms of placenta praevia.
2. Cephalopelvic disproportion – either in absolute disproportion on erect lateral pelvimetry, or after a failed trial of labour.
3. Failure to progress in labour judged by:
   (a) Descent of fetal head in relationship to maternal pelvic spines.
   (b) Failure of the cervix to dilate.
   (c) Excessive caput and moulding of the fetal skull.
4. Fetal distress diagnosed by:
   (a) Clinical grounds.
   (b) Changes in the fetal heart trace.
   (c) Changes in the pH of a sample of fetal scalp blood.

A combination of fetal blood sampling combined with use of the fetal heart trace can do much to lower an increasingly high Caesarean section rate for apparent fetal distress.

5. Malpresentation – brow or shoulder presentation. Caesarean section is used increasingly in the delivery of breech presentations.
6. Prolapse of umbilical cord.

Other indications finding increasing favour are severe pre-eclampsia and eclampsia.

The operation

This may be undertaken under general anaesthesia or epidural anaesthesia. The advantages of epidural anaesthesia as regards more rapid maternal recovery and the experience of instant bonding are self-evident.

1. The patient is placed as for any abdominal operation with a diathermy pad *in situ* and the bladder draining freely from an indwelling catheter.
2. The abdominal incision may be transverse (Pfannenstiel) or vertical (midline or paramedian) depending on the speed of the operation or surgeon's performance.
3. The rectus muscles are separated and the peritoneum opened longitudinally. The paracolic gutter may be packed to absorb spilled liquor or blood. The uterus is corrected for rotation and deviation to the right.
4. The reflection of peritoneum from the bladder to the uterus is identified and the peritoneum divided transversely just above it.
5. The lower flap of peritoneum is pushed downwards with a gauze swab exposing the lower uterine segment. A Doyen retractor is used to keep the bladder clear of the operating site.
6. The lower segment is incised transversely and the incision extended either with the fingers or by surgical incision to make an opening big enough to deliver the baby – care must be taken not to extend the incision too far, or tearing may occur into the uterine vessels.
7. The baby's head is delivered either with a hand inside the uterus or with Wrigley's forceps. Fundal pressure by the assistant will help to deliver the body of the baby.
8. Once the baby is delivered the cord is clamped, the baby handed to an assistant and the placenta and membranes delivered through the incision by cord traction. Digital exploration is used to confirm that the uterine cavity is empty.

Note: Should the transverse incision be found to be too small or inappropriate, the incision should be extended from one extremity converting it into an 'L' not a 'T' incision (Figure 53.20).

9. Following delivery of the placenta and membranes the lower segment is repaired with two layers of continuous catgut (no. 1). The first layer is haemostatic and the second varying the first layer and restoring the constitution of the myometrium. Great attention must be paid to this as the safety of future pregnancies depends on this reconstruction of the uterine wall.
10. The peritoneum is closed on the uterine incision, the packs removed, the paracolic gutters

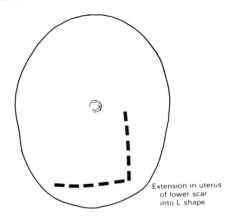

Extension in uterus
of lower scar
into L shape

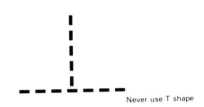

Never use T shape

Figure 53.20 Lower segment Caesarean section. If found to be too small or inappropriate, the transverse incision should be extended into an 'L' shape, not a 'T' shape

cleaned and the abdomen closed in the usual way.

11. The vagina should also be swabbed out to ensure that there is no excessive vaginal bleeding.

Classic Caesarean section

This operation is seldom done as the risk of the scar rupturing in subsequent pregnancies is 10 times greater than that of lower segment Caesarean section. It is a much easier operation, however. The incision is vertical on the anterior wall of the uterus and the bladder is undisturbed.

The indications would seem to be:

1. The completely inexperienced surgeon performing a Caesarean section for the first time with little skill in delivery of the baby in order to avoid the hazards of the lower segment Caesarean section operation.
2. Where the lower segment is inaccessible due to large pelvic veins, fibroids or previous bladder surgery.
3. When the baby could not be delivered through a lower segment, e.g. transverse lie with prolapsed arm.
4. In extreme haste, e.g. postmortem Caesarean section.

54

Surgery of the newborn

J. D. Atwell

Introduction and general principles

The scope of paediatric surgery is wide and the needs vary depending on the age of the neonate, infant or child. In the neonatal period the successful outcome of surgery depends on many factors such as surgical techniques, expert paediatric anaesthesia, nursing skills and staffing on intensive care units, the availability of micro-methods for haematological and biochemical investigations, full paediatric radiological services and specialized equipment.

It has been shown that one of the most important results of the concentration of such cases in neonatal units is a fall in the operative mortality from 72% to 24% (Rickham, 1952; Forshall and Rickham, 1960). In recent years, with the improvements in neonatal resuscitation and the use of expensive monitoring equipment together with advances in surgical technique and total parenteral nutrition, the average mortality has decreased to about 10%. Therefore only if these services are available can neonatal surgery be safely undertaken and achieve results that are acceptable.

The nature of neonatal surgery has changed over the past 15 years. Factors such as the policy of treating neonates with spina bifida and hydrocephalus, intensive care of the premature infant and antenatal diagnosis by cytology, biochemical estimations and ultrasonography have brought about these changes. The decrease in the number of admissions with spina bifida is partly due to the estimation of alpha-fetoprotein in maternal serum and amniotic fluid and to a decrease in its true incidence. A comparison of the admission to the author's unit of 1970/1971 and 1983/1984 and 1989/1990 reflects these changes (Table 54.1).

1. Antenatal diagnosis

In recent years, 25% of perinatal deaths are due to fetal malformations. Many of these congenital malformations can be detected by antenatal screening. Ultrasonography in the second and third trimester is used in the detection of such anomalies, but may be associated with false-positive and false-negative diagnoses which may cause difficulties in management. Renal anomalies, exomphalos and gastroschisis, congenital diaphragmatic hernia, intestinal atresias, tumours, spina bifida, anencephaly, hydrocephalus and encephalocele are among the commoner conditions

diagnosed by these methods. The antenatal diagnosis of severe congenital anomalies may pose problems to obstetricians: Should the pregnancy be terminated? Would an elective early delivery improve the prognosis? Should mothers be transferred for delivery in an obstetric unit adjacent to a paediatric surgical unit? There is no doubt that a multidisciplinary approach is required with close cooperation between obstetricians, paediatric surgeons, paediatricians, geneticists and radiologists for the careful monitoring of such cases which can only lead to an improvement in their management (Northern Regional Health Authority Foetal Abnormality Survey, 1988).

Table 54.1 Neonatal surgical admissions 1970/71, 1983/84 and 1989/1990

Diagnosis	1970	1971	1983	1984	1989	1990
Spina bifida	51	44	12	8	8	11
Oesophageal atresia	6	13	6	5	7	11
Diaphragmatic hernia	4	6	5	8	8	2
Necrotizing enterocolitis	–	–	8	14	8	15
GU system	6	7	13	13	11	9

2. Anaesthesia

The advances in neonatal anaesthesia have largely been responsible for the progress of neonatal surgery. First, in the neonate the surface area available for gaseous exchange is reduced in relation to body weight compared to the adult. Therefore any loss of functioning pulmonary tissue, e.g. diaphragmatic hernia or increased oxygen requirement due to cooling, will produce a pulmonary deficiency in an infant with minimal pulmonary reserves. Secondly, the small calibre of the airway passages means that the airway resistance will become critical with the accumulation of any secretions, especially as in the neonate the cough reflex is depressed. These factors may cause hypoventilation and the risks of aspiration pneumonia are increased. The newborn is also prone to other pulmonary disorders often related to prematurity and the need to establish a separate existence following birth. The respiratory distress syndrome, apnoeic attacks, aspiration of meconium and pulmonary and ventricular haemorrhage are such examples which may complicate the pre- and postoperative course of the surgical neonate.

Principles of management

Analgesics are avoided preoperatively. In recent times there has been a tendency to recommend the use of opioid derivatives for relief of postoperative pain in the newborn. This change of policy is not without risk, especially in the premature infant. Difficulties exist with dosage, aspiration of secretions and depression of respiration which have a morbidity and even a mortality. In order to prevent such complications the patient requires close observation, including monitoring respiration, cardiovascular parameters and if necessary blood gases. Unless these facilities are available in an intensive care situation, it would be safer to avoid the use of opioids in full-term and premature infants.

Atropine is the only premedication used and is given intramuscularly at a dosage of 0.2 mg. Postoperatively the humidity in the incubator is kept at maximal levels and may be increased by the use of an ultrasonic nebulizer. All the nurses are instructed in routine chest physiotherapy. Aspirations may be reduced by aspirating the pharynx at regular intervals and keeping the stomach empty by nasogastric aspiration until evidence that peristalsis and adequate gastric emptying are occurring (absence of bile in the aspirates). Death resulting from aspiration of vomit or from secretions should be considered as avoidable. The nursery should be fully equipped for resuscitation. Following the repair of a diaphragmatic hernia or exomphalos, it may be necessary to maintain the newborn on positive-pressure ventilation.

3. Nursing care

The successful outcome of neonatal surgery is dependent on constant nursing supervision by nurses skilled and experienced in neonatal care throughout the 24 h of each day. Failure of this provision will result in unnecessary deaths. Unfortunately due to the shortage of nurses such ideals are not always fulfilled. Expensive monitoring equipment may assist in recording the vital parameters of the sick neonate, but these should be considered as an aid to nursing rather than a replacement of nursing skills.

Principles of management

As stated above, the nursing care is the most vital aspect in the management of the surgical neonate. The observations made on such an infant are many (Appendix 1), but probably the most important are the care of the airway and prevention of the aspiration of vomit. Nasogastric aspiration is used routinely following surgical procedures on the gastrointestinal tract. It is essential to use an adequate sized tube (no. 10 Fr. gauge) with 1- or $\frac{1}{2}$-hourly aspirations with free drainage into a receptacle between aspi-

rations. Oral feeding is not started until the aspirates are clear, i.e. non-bile stained. Oral feeding is always introduced gradually, and in the full-term infant with 5% dextrose at 5.0 ml/h and then with increasing volumes and a change to half and finally full strength feeds. This transitional period may take several days or even weeks in infants with prolonged gastrointestinal problems, e.g. after the repair of a gastroschisis, or surgery for necrotizing enterocolitis, and may have to be combined with total parenteral nutrition.

4. Temperature control and regulation

The surface area of the infant per total body mass is greater than that of an adult; therefore the infant is more prone to heat loss than the adult. In the premature infant the heat losses are correspondingly greater due to the lack of subcutaneous tissue. Exposure to cold results in heat production and an increased oxygen consumption which may be harmful to the infant if it is already under stress. Sclerema neonatorum is a condition seen in neonates and premature infants where the subcutaneous tissue and skin undergo a change resulting in a very characteristic 'hardened' feel to the tissues, especially in the extremities. It is related to cooling and infection and is commoner in the premature infant. The incidence may be reduced by careful measures to prevent heat loss during transport, investigation, operation and postoperative care of the infant.

PREVENTION OF HEAT LOSS

The infant requiring surgery is transported in a suitable portable incubator. In patients with a condition such as gastroschisis, when the heat loss may be severe, it can be reduced by wrapping the infant in aluminium foil. 'Cling' foil is an alternative which has the added advantage that the intestine is visible and any impairment of its blood supply is immediately apparent. On arrival in the neonatal surgical unit the infant is nursed in an incubator preheated to the correct temperature. Exposure of the infant for radiological investigation, collection of blood and intravenous infusion is kept to a minimum and any exposed areas should be wrapped in warm padded gauze. Heat loss at the time of induction of general anaesthesia may be rapid and can be reduced by the use of water blankets and additional overhead heating. Similarly during the operation the temperature in the theatre is kept higher than in the normal operating theatre. The neonate's temperature is monitored throughout these procedures with an electrical thermometer with either a skin electrode or with oesophageal or rectal probes. Every attempt is made to maintain the body temperature between 36°C and 37°C as oxygen consumption is minimal at this level. In the sick neonate it is important to record simultaneously the central (core) temperature as well as the

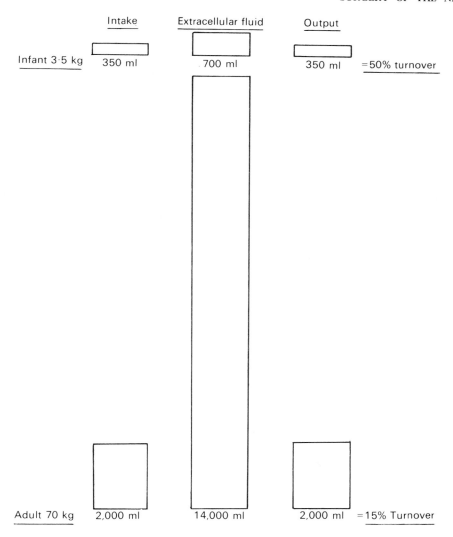

Intake   Extracellular fluid   Output

Infant 3·5 kg   350 ml   700 ml   350 ml   =50% turnover

Adult 70 kg   2,000 ml   14,000 ml   2,000 ml   =15% Turnover

Figure 54.1 Fluid transfers in a 3.5 kg infant compared with a 70 kg adult. Note how increased losses or decreased intake have a more marked effect on the homeostasis of the infant

peripheral temperature, as diverging temperatures are indicative of a reduction in peripheral blood flow.

5. Homeostasis

(a) Fluid and electrolytes

BASIC DATA

The total body water of the neonate is higher than that of the adult (80:60%); the distribution between the intracellular and extracellular spaces is 35% and 45%, respectively, in the infant and 40% and 20% in the adult. Changes of fluid balance with increased losses or decreased intake therefore have a greater effect in the neonate compared to the adult (Figure 54.1). A comparison of the daily gastrointestinal fluid turnover in a 70 kg adult and a 3.5 kg neonate is seen in Figure 54.2.

PRINCIPLES OF MANAGEMENT

Maintenance fluid. A neonate requires 150 ml/kg/day if being fed orally. In the premature infant this is increased to 200 ml/kg/day. Following intestinal surgery, when fluid is given intravenously and the bowel is aspirated regularly, the transfers shown in Figure 54.2 are reduced; therefore the maintenance intravenous fluid requirements are less. In such circumstances the infant needs 70 ml/kg/day unless there is jaundice or urinary complications such as obstruction.

The newborn infant in the 1st week of life requires even less fluid and this can be administered on a regimen of 10 ml/kg/day in the 1st day of life, increasing to the full 70 ml/kg/day by the 7th and subsequent days. The maintenance fluid should be isotonic and N/5 saline in 4.3% dextrose is suitable.

DAILY GASTRO-INTESTINAL TURNOVER

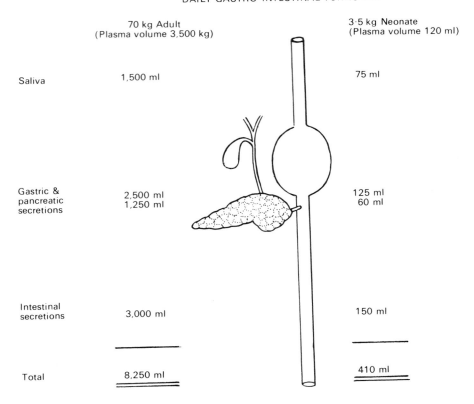

	70 kg Adult (Plasma volume 3,500 kg)	3·5 kg Neonate (Plasma volume 120 ml)
Saliva	1,500 ml	75 ml
Gastric & pancreatic secretions	2,500 ml 1,250 ml	125 ml 60 ml
Intestinal secretions	3,000 ml	150 ml
Total	8,250 ml	410 ml

Figure 54.2   Daily gastrointestinal fluid turnover of a 3.5 kg infant compared with a 70 kg adult

Replacement of fluid losses. Initial assessment of fluid losses in an infant is difficult but depends on the degree of dehydration as assessed by the loss of weight (difference between birth weight and weight on admission), loss of skin elasticity, depression of the anterior fontanelle, pulse rate and results of biochemical estimations. Later losses following surgical procedures are usually easier to estimate as they are recorded accurately on an hourly basis, e.g. nasogastric aspiration. The composition of intestinal aspirates in the newborn averages 100–120 mmol/litre of sodium, 5–15 mmol/litre of potassium and 100–120 mmol/litre of chloride (Young, 1966, 1968). Therefore, the ideal solution for replacement purposes is N saline given on a volume-for-volume basis.

Correction of acid base balance

(i) Acidosis. A metabolic acidosis is the commonest acid base disturbance found either due to disturbance of gastrointestinal or renal physiology or due to cardiorespiratory arrest. In the first instance it may be corrected by the intravenous administration of 1/6th molar lactate solution; correction is slow due to the need to metabolize the lactate in the liver, which may take up to 2 h (3.0 ml/kg 1/6 M lactate raise the HCO_3 1 mmol). Immediate correction of acidosis can be achieved with intravenous 8.4% sodium bicarbonate (1.0 ml/kg $NaHCO_3$ raises the HCO_3 1 mmol).

(ii) Alkalosis. This occurs when the obstruction is proximal to the opening of the bile ducts such as in some patients with duodenal atresia and congenital hypertrophic pyloric stenosis. The alkalosis can be corrected by the intravenous administration of N saline (3.0 ml/kg N saline will lower the HCO_3 1 mmol). Only in very exceptional circumstances is the use of ammonium chloride needed.

(iii) Potassium. Intravenous replacement of potassium losses is restricted for the first 24 h following the birth of the infant or surgery. The neonate requires 3–5 mmol potassium per day. The easiest way to administer this is to add 1 g potassium chloride (13.4 mmol) to the maintenance and replacement fluids, i.e. the potassium is diluted in 500 ml units; the patient then receives the appropriate aliquot of potassium.

(b) Blood transfusion

BASIC DATA

The normal haemoglobin of a neonate is 190 g/litre and falls to a level of 110 g/litre at 3 months of age. This fall is due to the fetal haemoglobin being replaced by adult haemoglobin.

The normal white blood cell count in a neonate is 12 000, with a predominance of lymphocytes (70%). These values fall to normal adult levels by 1 year of age.

PRINCIPLES OF MANAGEMENT

A sample of the infant's and mother's blood is required for grouping and cross-matching. In assessing the need for a blood transfusion it must be realized that the blood volume for a neonate varies between 70 ml/kg (full-term infant) and 85 ml/kg (premature infant). For example, an 8.5 ml blood loss in a 1 kg premature infant represents a 10% loss and requires a replacement transfusion; similarly a blood loss of 28 ml in a 4 kg infant represents a 10% loss and requires replacement.

In view of the significance of small losses of blood in neonatal surgery, careful measurements of these losses is essential: this is achieved by accurate weighing of the swabs in the operating theatre.

(c) Total parenteral nutrition

BASIC DATA

The full-term infant requires 100 cal/kg/day, rising to 150 cal/kg/day in the premature infant. Intravenous feeding may be given by either a peripheral or a central vein.

PRINCIPLES OF MANAGEMENT

(i) Peripheral intravenous feeding. A suitable regimen includes the consecutive administration of three solutions changing at hourly intervals, i.e. Vamin, Intralipid and 10% dextrose. These may be administered at the rate of 6.0 ml/h for a 1 kg infant, 12 ml/h for a 2 kg infant and 18 ml/h for a 3 kg infant (Puri *et al.*, 1975).

(ii) Central intravenous feeding. This requires a central line with the tip of the catheter in the right atrium. The internal jugular vein is usually used and the catheter is led subcutaneously to a distal site either on the anterior chest wall or above and behind the ear: the former is the preferred site. As hypertonic parenteral solutions can cause tissue damage unless given directly into large veins with a high flow, it is important to check the position of the catheters by radiological methods before treatment starts. The solution should be made up daily in the pharmacy under strict aseptic conditions. The composition of a suitable solution is calculated from the electrolyte and calorie requirements of the infant.

(iii) Monitoring of parenteral nutrition. Regular estimations are needed for haemoglobin, plasma pro-teins, urea and electrolytes, calcium, magnesium and phosphate and screening of the plasma to check that the intralipid has been cleared. The infants are weighed daily.

(d) Specific metabolic problems

I. JAUNDICE

All newborn babies have a rising level of bilirubin in the serum for the first 3 days of life. Jaundice which persists and becomes more severe requires full investigation and treatment in order to prevent brain damage due to kernicterus. Premature and infected infants are more susceptible to jaundice. Haemolytic disease of the newborn is suspected if the mother is rhesus negative with detectable rhesus antibodies. Careful monitoring of the level of bilirubin in the serum is therefore required to prevent brain damage and rising levels will require treatment with either phototherapy or an exchange transfusion.

II. HAEMORRHAGIC DISEASE OF THE NEWBORN

The liver in the newborn is immature and may be inefficient 'at synthesizing blood-clotting factors. In order to prevent bleeding, all infants are given an intramuscular injection of vitamin K_1 prior to operation. In the majority of paediatric medical and obstetric units this drug will have been given routinely in order to prevent this complication.

III. HYPOCALCAEMIA

The level of calcium may fall after birth and is related to immaturity of the parathyroid glands. It is particularly prone to occur in premature infants, the infants of diabetic mothers and infants fed on cows' milk with the increased phosphate content which interferes with absorption of calcium. Operations in the neonatal period and infection increase the risk of this condition. Treatment is by the intravenous administration of 5–10 ml calcium gluconate. This may be given orally diluted in 100 ml per day to prevent further signs of hypocalcaemia.

IV. HYPOMAGNESAEMIA

This diagnosis should be confirmed when fits occur in the absence of hypoglycaemia and hypocalcaemia (Atwell, 1966). Treatment consists of magnesium acetate 2.5 mmol intravenously, to be followed by a daily oral intake of 5.0 mmol of magnesium chloride.

V. HYPOGLYCAEMIA

Hypoglycaemia is often found in the neonatal period. At risk are premature and dysmature infants, infants of diabetic and prediabetic mothers, twins and infants of mothers with toxaemia of pregnancy. Other factors which increase the risks are infection, anoxia, birth and surgical trauma. The level considered important is 1.6 mmol/litre in the neonate. Levels below this require treatment, although symptoms are usually delayed until the level falls below 1.0 mmol/litre. Hypoglycaemia may be prevented by early oral feeding, but this is often impossible in infants following an operation in the neonatal period. The incidence of hypoglycaemia is reduced by using N/5 saline in 4.3% dextrose as the standard maintenance intravenous fluid and monitoring of blood levels with the Dextrostix (Ames) at 4-hourly intervals. Hypoglycaemia can be treated by the intravenous administration of 5.0 ml/kg of 20% dextrose or 10–20 ml 10% dextrose.

(e) Zinc and copper deficiencies

In infants on parenteral nutrition the plasma level of zinc begins to fall within 2 weeks and increases with time. Supplements of 40 µg/kg/day prevent this fall in full-term infants, but high levels are required in premature babies and infants with increased losses with an enterostomy. In these patients the requirement is increased up to 300 µg/kg/day. Copper losses through faecal fistulas occur after 4 weeks of parenteral nutrition. Careful monitoring of zinc and copper levels in infants on parenteral nutrition and with enterostomies is required with adequate replacement in order to prevent deficiencies occurring (Suita *et al.*, 1984).

6. Infection

After and during delivery the newborn is exposed to the risks of infection. The immune response of the newborn infant is low and is further reduced if breast feeding is not established. This is due to the failure to transfer maternal antibodies which are present in high concentrations in the colostrum and breast milk. The incidence of infection has an adverse effect on surgical results and increases neonatal morbidity and mortality.

Principles of management

Prevention of infection and cross-infection is the keynote of success and depends on strict nursing techniques. Neonatal units should have a controlled environment for temperature and humidity and ideally a positive-pressure system as recommended for operating theatre suites. The infant is nursed in an incubator with its own positive pressure system and barrier nursing techniques are used. The routine care of the umbilicus with spirit swabbing and powdering is essential. Bacteriological screening of infants in the unit is done on admission and at regular intervals with umbilical, nose, throat, skin, stool and rectal swabs. Blood culture, urine culture and lumbar puncture are carried out if infection is suspected. Administration of antibiotics is usually required in neonates undergoing surgical corrective procedures because of the possible complications related to the primary condition, e.g. aspiration pneumonia with oesophageal atresia, septicaemia with necrotizing enterocolitis.

7. Equipment

A neonatal surgical unit is an intensive care unit and as such must be equipped accordingly with specialized instruments, e.g. incubators, apnoea alarm blankets, oxygen monitors, temperature, pulse and respiratory rate monitors, etc. Essential items which are required for equipping a neonatal surgical unit are listed in Appendix II.

8. Results

In any infant with a severe congenital anomaly there is an increased incidence of other congenital defects. There is the well-known example of the association of rectal atresia with oesophageal atresia and duodenal obstruction with Down's syndrome. Renal and vertebral anomalies may coexist. These associated defects will have an adverse effect on the management of any congenital anomaly requiring surgery, thus increasing the operative mortality. Similarly the mortality of any operative procedure in the neonatal period is dependent on the maturity of the neonate, the full-term infant withstanding surgery better than the premature infant.

These factors are important when assessing the results of surgical treatment and have been incorporated into a classification used routinely by most neonatal surgical centres. Grade A infants have a birth weight above 2.5 kg and there are no associated congenital defects. In Grade B infants the birth weight may range between 1.8 and 2.5 kg or higher and there is a second moderately severe associated congenital defect. In Grade C infants the birth weight is less than 1.8 kg or higher and there is a second severe associated congenital defect, e.g. oesophageal atresia and congenital heart disease such as the tetralogy of Fallot.

Congenital defects of the anterior abdominal wall

Surgical embryology

Closure of the omphalocele in the fetus with the return of the midgut contents to the true abdominal cavity (Figure 54.3) will allow the normal development of the anterior abdominal wall. Initially the membrane of the omphalocele is thin and transparent but at a later stage it becomes invaded by the ventro-lateral portion of the myotomes and dermatomes. These structures differentiate to form the abdominal musculature. A strip of muscle is found in the free ventral edge which will become the rectus abdominis

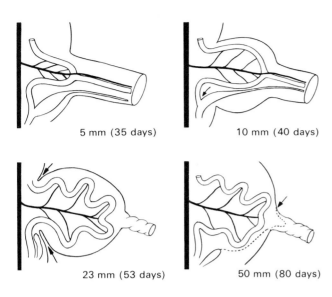

Figure 54.3 Embryology of the anterior abdominal wall

5 mm (35 days)

10 mm (40 days)

23 mm (53 days)

50 mm (80 days)

(Figure 54.4). Fusion of these free edges in the mid-line closes the abdominal cavity. Fusion first occurs in the upper abdomen, then in the suprapubic region and finally in the umbilical region (Duhamel, 1963). Development of the anterior abdominal wall is complete by the 80th day of intra-uterine life (50 mm embryo). Failure of the closure of the abdominal folds will result in a series of different congenital defects. If the proximal fold is deficient a syndrome of ectopia cordis, diaphragmatic hernia and exomphalos results (Cantrell *et al.*, 1958). Failure of the mid-lateral folds results in a defect at the umbilicus. i.e. an exomphalos. Failure of fusion of the distal folds will result in the formation of either an exomphalos or ectopia vesicae and more rarely, when associated with absence of the hindgut, a vesico-intestinal fissure (Rickham, 1960). Failure of the ribbon of muscle in the free edge of the lateral folds on one side will allow a normal insertion of the umbilical vessels but with a defect adjacent to the umbilical ring. This, together with loss of the covering membrane, will result in a gastroschisis (Bernstein, 1940).

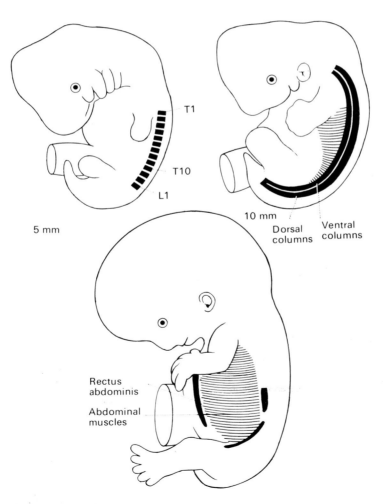

T1

T10

L1

5 mm

10 mm

Dorsal columns

Ventral columns

Rectus abdominis

Abdominal muscles

Figure 54.4 Development of the abdominal wall musculature from the myotomes

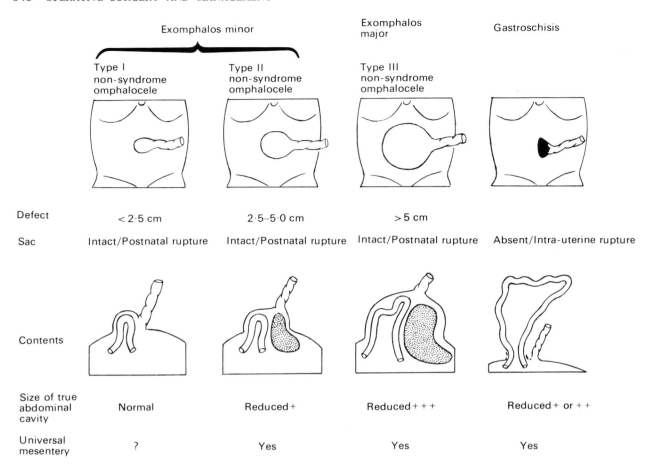

Figure 54.5 Classification of the common types of congenital anterior abdominal wall defects

Surgical anatomy and pathology

There are differing classifications in use for the description of abdominal wall defects; these depend on the size and position of the defect at the umbilicus and the presence or absence of the covering membrane (Figure 54.5).

If the defect is less than 2.5 cm in diameter at the umbilicus it can be called either a 'hernia into the cord' (Figure 54.5) or a 'type I non-syndrome omphalocele'. If the defect is between 2.5 and 5.0 cm it is called an 'exomphalos minor' or a 'type II non-syndrome omphalocele'. These defects are often grouped together as exomphalos minor as the surgical treatment of such defects is very similar. If the defect at the umbilicus is larger than 5.0 cm it is called 'exomphalos major' (Figure 54.5) or 'type III non-syndrome omphalocele' (Shuster, 1967).

The high incidence of associated anomalies with exomphalos allows certain ones to be classified as 'syndrome omphaloceles': namely the 'upper midline syndrome' with sternal, diaphragmatic pericardial and cardiac defects; the 'lower midline syndrome' with bladder exstrophy and vesico-intestinal fissure;

and the 'Beckwith–Wiedemann syndrome' with macroglossia and gigantism.

In 'gastroschisis' (Figure 54.5) the defect is usually small, i.e. less than 2.5 cm, and is to the right of the normal insertion of the umbilical vessels. The sac is absent and the abdominal viscera have protruded through the defect to lie on the anterior abdominal wall. They are usually swollen and oedematous, having been bathed in the amniotic fluid prior to delivery. This swelling may be extreme to produce apparent shortening of intestinal length. Occasionally larger defects are found in association with gastroschisis (2.5–5.0 cm and greater than 5.0 cm), but these are extremely rare.

The incidence of associated anomalies with gastroschisis is low and is usually confined to anomalies of the gastrointestinal tract, such as an intestinal atresia and malrotation.

A universal mesentery and anomalies of intestinal rotation are common to both gastroschisis and exomphalos. Prematurity is not often found in infants with exomphalos, but there is a statistically significant difference in the birth weights of infants with exomphalos and gastroschisis, the latter usually being less than 2.25 kg compared to birth weights of over 3.0 kg (Moore, 1977).

The size of the defect and rupture or absence of the sac will determine the timing and type of any surgical repair. In large defects the true abdominal cavity is small (Figure 54.6) and immediate closure with its resultant increase in intra-abdominal pressure results in interference with venous return to the heart and limits respiratory movements. This combination of complications in the past has often resulted in a cardiorespiratory death.

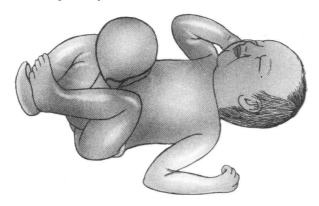

Figure 54.6 Exomphalos major. Note the umbilical cord insertion to the left and inferiorly. The contents of the sac will include the liver and the small bowel on a universal mesentery

Surgical management

Clinical features

Diagnosis is immediate and visual and treatment is determined by the size of the defect or whether the sac is intact or has ruptured.

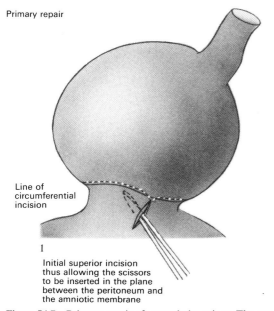

Primary repair

Line of circumferential incision

1

Initial superior incision thus allowing the scissors to be inserted in the plane between the peritoneum and the amniotic membrane

Preoperative care

The immediate management is to cover the defect with 'cling film' in order to prevent drying of the sac. Loss of body temperature in infants with a ruptured sac or gastroschisis can be minimized by wrapping the infant in aluminium foil or 'cling film' and transferring in a portable incubator to a neonatal surgical unit. The infant is nursed on his back with the bowel resting on the anterior abdominal wall, thus preventing ischaemic changes which may occur if the bowel falls to the side.

Radiographs of the chest and abdomen are taken to exclude any associated cardiac and diaphragmatic defects and atresia of the intestine. Maternal and infant blood is sent for grouping and cross-matching. A nasogastric tube is passed and aspirated at hourly intervals and left on free drainage. If primary closure is considered impossible without a dangerous rise of intra-abdominal pressure, a catheter should be passed into the inferior vena cava to monitor the pressure during the operation.

Operative repair of exomphalos

1. PRIMARY CLOSURE

This is only suitable for small defects, i.e. less than 5.0 cm diameter. The incision is made at the junction of the skin with the amniotic membrane and continued circumferentially around the defect. Entering the correct plane may be easier with an incision at right angles to the skin margin which will allow curved dissecting scissors to be passed under the skin edges (Figure 54.7).

The peritoneum is then opened and incised around the neck of the sac. The umbilical vein is ligated

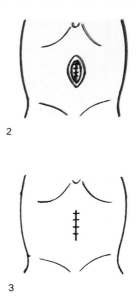

2

3

Figure 54.7 Primary repair of exomphalos minor. The contents are easily reduced in such patients as the true abdominal cavity contains the liver and is relatively normal in size. Vitello-intestinal remnants should be checked for carefully at operation and divided. Similarly the umbilical arteries and the urachus are divided between ligatures.

In small defects a formal laparotomy is not undertaken, but in larger defects an associated malrotation may require treatment. A Meckel's diverticulum with or without a band passing to the umbilicus should always be looked for and removed if present. In the larger defects the liver may be adherent to the wall of the sac. The contents of the sac are then returned to the abdominal cavity.

The repair of the defect is then completed with interrupted non-absorbable sutures to approximate the free edges, the skin is closed with interrupted sutures (Figure 54.7).

2. STAGED REPAIR OF EXOMPHALOS MAJOR

(a) The 'Gross' operation (Gross, 1948). The aim of this operation is to convert the intact exomphalos sac into a skin-covered ventral hernia which can be repaired at a second-stage operation when the infant is older.

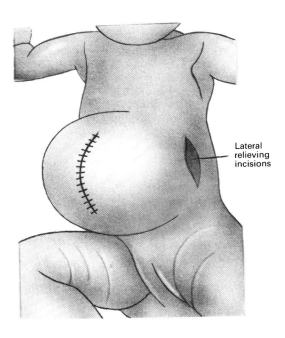

Lateral relieving incisions

Figure 54.8 Repair of exomphalos major by the Gross technique. Note the lateral relieving incisions to allow the skin to cover the defect and to be sutured in the midline

At operation the umbilical vessels are ligated and divided as close to the wall of the sac as possible. The skin is mobilized in a similar manner as described for primary closure. The incision is in the midline at the upper margin of the defect and at right angles to the junction of skin and the coverings of the sac. The skin is then undermined and mobilized except at or above the costal margin, thus preventing later herniation

and moulding of the liver within the sac. The skin is then closed with interrupted sutures over the convexity of the exomphalos. Lateral relieving incisions may be required to allow sufficient freeing of the skin to cover the defect (Figure 54.8). The repair of the ventral hernia thus formed is delayed until the abdominal cavity can safely accommodate the visceral contents of the sac.

(b) Silastic 'bag' or 'silo' (Shuster, 1967). This operation is the treatment of choice and is suitable for exomphalos major and gastroschisis if primary skin closure is impossible. It has resulted in an improvement in the operative mortality as it allows a staged reduction of the contents of the sac over a period of 2–3 weeks and removes the need for a second-stage repair of the ventral hernia which follows other forms of operative treatment.

The principles of the operative technique are similar whether used for repair of a gastroschisis or exomphalos major. A Silastic pouch is fashioned and sutured to the free edges of the defect with a continuous 2/0 silk suture (Figure 54.9). The two halves are then sutured in the midline superiorly and inferiorly to form a bag which contains the contents of the sac. Finally, the bag is closed by a continuous suture.

In patients with a gastroschisis no attempt is made to cleanse the surface of the oedematous bowel as this may well prolong any recovery period and lead to a localized perforation and peritonitis. It is important to exclude an intestinal atresia in neonates with gastroschisis and to correct any malrotation and atresia in neonates with an exomphalos. Care must be taken when freeing the liver from the sac as the bare area is adherent to it. Elongation of the inferior vena cava to the level of the wound margin is also found and it may kink on returning the liver to the abdomen, thus interfering with venous return. Over succeeding days, usually at 48–72-hourly intervals, it is possible to reduce the size of the Silastic pouch. This should be done under a general anaesthetic. This procedure is repeated until final closure can be achieved. Closure within two weeks is the aim as infection and separation of the Silastic at the margins of the defect may become troublesome.

(c) The 'Grob' technique (Grob, 1963). In exomphalos major, skin is often seen growing onto the surface of the sac; the extent is variable. If the surface of the sac can be kept clean the skin will grow over the sac by secondary intention, converting it into a skin-covered ventral hernia. This healing can be assisted by the use of 2% mercurochrome or antibiotic sprays to reduce the incidence of infection. Unfortunately this method of treatment is lengthy and a large defect may take 3–4 months for epithelialization. Mercury poisoning has been described as a complication of this treatment and therefore its use has been discontinued and has largely been replaced by the use of a Silastic prosthesis for staged repair of this defect.

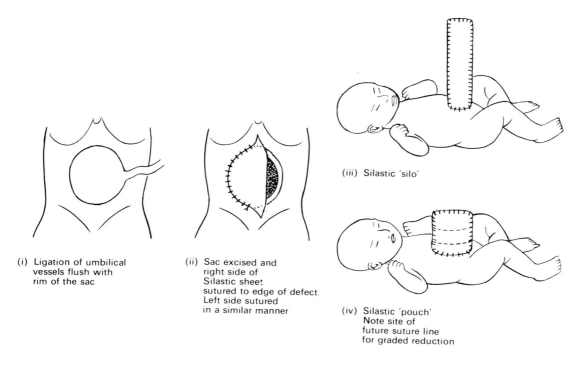

(i) Ligation of umbilical
    vessels flush with
    rim of the sac

(ii) Sac excised and
    right side of
    Silastic sheet
    sutured to edge of defect.
    Left side sutured
    in a similar manner

(iii) Silastic 'silo'

(iv) Silastic 'pouch'
    Note site of
    future suture line
    for graded reduction

Figure 54.9 Staged repair of exomphalos major and for gastroschisis using a Silastic sheet to fashion either a 'silo' or a 'pouch'. Reduction in the size of these is then performed every 48–72 h, thus allowing skin closure by the 10th–14th postoperative day

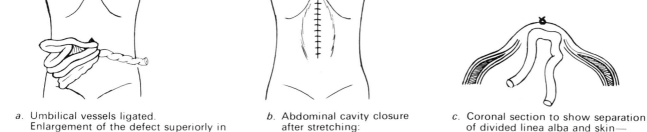

a. Umbilical vessels ligated.
    Enlargement of the defect superiorly in
    the midline up to the xiphisternum

b. Abdominal cavity closure
    after stretching:
    skin closure only

c. Coronal section to show separation
    of divided linea alba and skin—
    covered ventral hernia

Figure 54.10 Repair of gastroschisis. Defect enlarged by dividing skin and linea alba in the midline superiorly to the xiphisternum. Abdominal cavity enlarged by inserting the fingers under the margins of the defect and stretching the abdominal muscles. Skin closure only with interrupted sutures. Resultant residual ventral hernia is repaired at a later date

Operative repair of gastroschisis

1. PRIMARY CLOSURE

'One-stage' repair operations are possible in approximately 50% of patients, especially when combined with the use of mechanical ventilation in the postoperative period. However, care must be taken that the rise in intra-abdominal pressure by such a closure does not interfere with venous return to the heart.

2. TWO-STAGE REPAIR

At operation the bowel is inspected carefully to exclude an associated intestinal atresia. The defect is then extended in the midline to the xiphisternum (Figure 54.10). The abdominal wall is then stretched by inserting fingers under the free edge of the defect in order to increase the capacity of the abdomen. Skin closure over the abdominal contents is all that is required. This leaves a small ventral defect which may require repair at a second-stage operation (Thomas and Atwell, 1976).

3. SILASTIC SAC

This operation, described under the repair of exom-

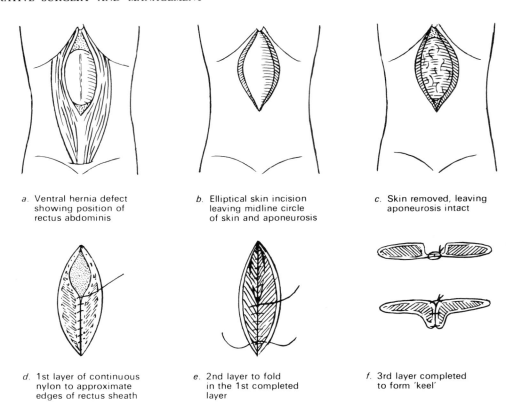

a. Ventral hernia defect showing position of rectus abdominis

b. Elliptical skin incision leaving midline circle of skin and aponeurosis

c. Skin removed, leaving aponeurosis intact

d. 1st layer of continuous nylon to approximate edges of rectus sheath

e. 2nd layer to fold in the 1st completed layer

f. 3rd layer completed to form 'keel'

Note extraperitoneal principle of the operation, thus reducing incidence of postoperative distension

Figure 54.11 Maingot 'keel' operation for the secondary repair of the ventral hernia following successful repair of a gastroschisis

phalos major, is only rarely required in gastroschisis. Its use should be limited to those patients in whom skin closure would result in a need for mechanical ventilation. A pouch or silo may be fashioned (see Figure 54.9). In deciding on management, an order of priorities is useful: namely, skin is better than Silastic, Silastic is better than mechanical ventilation.

Operative repair of the secondary ventral hernia

This may be necessary after the operative repair of either exomphalos major or gastroschisis. The operation of choice is the extraperitoneal 'keel' operation of Maingot (Maingot, 1961).

The margins of the defect are incised to leave an ellipse of skin (Figure 54.11). The skin is then dissected free from the underlying fibroperitoneal layer which is left intact. This extraperitoneal approach avoids the complication of an ileus leading to a rise in the intra-abdominal pressure which interferes with wound healing. The edges of the sheath covering the rectus abdominis muscle are seen and closed with a continuous monofilament nylon suture. This is repeated until closure of the defect is obtained by the formation of a midline keel. The skin is closed with

interrupted non-absorbable sutures or subcuticular Vicryl, leaving a suction drain subcutaneously (Redivac).

Postoperative care

The standard nursing care has been described in the section on general principles. The main aims of treatment are to prevent respiratory failure, to feed the infant and to prevent infection. Thus the success of postoperative care depends on the efficient management of assisted ventilation, if required, parenteral nutrition, which may be prolonged for a number of weeks in patients with gastroschisis, and the use of antibiotics.

Complications

EARLY

Associated anomalies. These have already been described, but malrotation, intestinal atresia, diaphragmatic hernia and cardiac defects may cause problems in the postoperative period.

Prematurity. Low birth weight is well recognized in

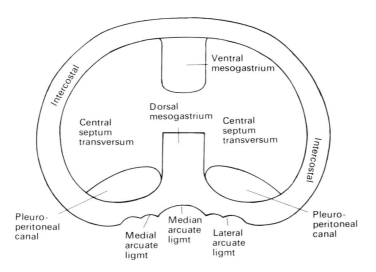

Figure 54.12 Embryological development and origins of the diaphragm

association with gastroschisis, but is less common in exomphalos unless associated with chromosomal defects. Whether the low birth weight is due to premature delivery, intra-uterine growth retardation or a combination of such defects is uncertain. Pre-term infants tolerate surgery poorly and develop complications due to their respiratory immaturity or relative immunological enzymatic and haematological insufficiency. Mature but 'small for dates' babies are particularly prone to hypoglycaemia.

Respiratory failure. Increase in intra-abdominal pressure following operative repair interferes with respiratory exchange and assisted ventilation may be required for a period postoperatively. Superadded complications may be the respiratory distress syndrome in a premature infant and congenital heart disease.

Infection. Prophylactic broad-spectrum antibiotic cover is an essential adjunct to surgery in these infants as septicaemia is now the second most common cause of death.

Prolonged ileus. The duration of the postoperative ileus in infants with gastroschisis is related to the rate of resolution of the pre-existing inflammatory changes. The reduction in length of the bowel is secondary to inflammatory thickening and is not a primary anomaly. Subsequent operations and radiological studies (Touloukian and Spackman, 1971) have shown a normal length and mucosal pattern of the bowel, thus confirming that the changes seen in the bowel at birth are reversible.

LATE

Growth and development. The growth and develop-

ment in infants with exomphalos and gastroschisis have been normal in the majority of patients (Thomas and Atwell, 1976).

Ventral hernia. A ventral hernia following repair of exomphalos or gastroschisis may be planned or unplanned. The repair of such defects has been described: the extraperitoneal 'keel' operation (Maingot, 1961) is the operation of choice.

Inguinal hernia. Subsequent development of inguinal hernias is not uncommon and is probably related to a pre-existing peritoneal sac and the raised intra-abdominal pressure following repair of the umbilical defect.

Congenital diaphragmatic hernia

Surgical embryology

The development of the diaphragm is completed by the 10th week of intra-uterine life, thus dividing the coelomic cavity into its abdominal and thoracic compartments. The diaphragm is formed by a fusion of mesoderm from different origins (Figure 54.12). The peripheral part develops from the intercostal muscle and the central part from the septum transversum and the dorsal and ventral mesogastrium. The posterolateral spaces are then closed by the pleuroperitoneal folds. This latter component is initially membranous, but later muscle fibres grow between these layers to complete the formation of the diaphragm.

The development of the right side of the diaphragm is completed before the left, which may account for the high incidence of left-sided defects. The pleuroperitoneal folds in the posterolateral position (foramen of Bochdalek) are the last to form which may account for the high incidence of defects at this site.

Failure of fusion of the central and lateral portions of the diaphragm may result in a defect in the antero-lateral portion of the diaphragm (foramen of Morgagni). Central defects are extremely rare and may be associated with other serious congenital malformation such as congenital aplasia of the spleen and congenital heart disease. Aplasia of the diaphragm may be found in association with any of the defects, resulting in the partial or complete absence of the hemidiaphragm.

The midgut is developing at the same time as the diaphragm with an increase in length followed by the closure of the omphalocele with return of its contents to the abdominal cavity. The intestine then undergoes rotation and fixation to take up its adult anatomical position. Early return of the midgut or a delay in the development of the diaphragm may be contributory factors in the aetiology of diaphragmatic hernia. This is reflected in the very high incidence of a universal mesentery and malrotation of the intestine in these patients.

Associated malformations of the lungs are a common finding in diaphragmatic hernia and include extralobar sequestration (Berman, 1958), aplasia and hypoplasia of the lungs (Sabga *et al.*, 1961). The causation of these associated malformations is obscure, but if the intestine entered the pleural cavity between the 75th and 90th days of intra-uterine life causing compression of the lung, it would coincide with the stage of development of the airways within the lung (Kitagawa *et al.*, 1971). A reduction in the airway number and alveolar counts has been reported in pathological studies on one infant dying with a diaphragmatic hernia. The alveolar numbers were almost normal when related to the number of terminal bronchioli in the lung.

After operative correction of a diaphragmatic hernia, many lungs which appear small and hypoplastic will expand and fill the pleural cavity. The method of postnatal growth of a hypoplastic lung is debatable; it is unlikely that any new airways or new arterial branches would develop in this region (Kitagawa *et al.*, 1971). Alveolar multiplication, together with intra-acinar multiplication, would be expected but whether this would proceed until the normal total alveolar number is reached is unlikely. The most likely result would be multiplication to give the normal alveolar number supplied by each terminal bronchiolus. As the lung expands to fill the pleural cavity there will be compensatory emphysema.

The association of congenital heart disease with diaphragmatic hernia is common and the main contributory cause of death. In our series of 44 patients 18 died and 11 of these were found to have congenital heart disease. The most common finding was a widely patent ductus arteriosus (10), coarctation of the aorta (2), hypoplastic left heart and aorta (1), ventricular septal defect (1), right-sided aortic arch (1) and a single ventricle (1). The high incidence of a widely patent and high flow ductus may be related to the severe hypoxia and raised pulmonary vascular resistance leading to persistence of the fetal type of circulation (Collins *et al.*, 1977). The mesonephros also contributes to the closure of the diaphragm and renal ectopia has been recorded with diaphragmatic hernia (Bulgrin and Holmes, 1955). Other congenital defects found in association with diaphragmatic hernia include congenital absence of the spleen, pericardial defects, ectopia cordis, exomphalos, undescended testes, de Lange syndrome, vertebral and musculo-skeletal anomalies, spina bifida cystica and inguinal hernias.

Surgical anatomy

1. Types of defect

A. POSTEROLATERAL DEFECT (FORAMEN OF BOCHDALEK)

This is the commonest defect found in the neonatal

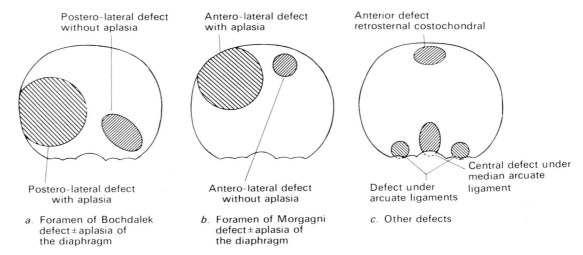

Postero-lateral defect without aplasia

Antero-lateral defect with aplasia

Anterior defect retrosternal costochondral

Postero-lateral defect with aplasia

Antero-lateral defect without aplasia

Defect under arcuate ligaments

Central defect under median arcuate ligament

a. Foramen of Bochdalek defect ± aplasia of the diaphragm

b. Foramen of Morgagni defect ± aplasia of the diaphragm

c. Other defects

Figure 54.13 Types of congenital diaphragmatic hernia

period (over 75%). The defects can be subdivided into two subgroups (Harrington, 1948): those with the defect confined to the pleuroperitoneal canal and those with an additional aplasia of part of the adjacent diaphragm (Figure 54.13). The aplasia of the diaphragm may involve one-half of the whole diaphragm or more commonly is partial to produce a hemi-absence of one side of the diaphragm.

B. ANTEROLATERAL DEFECT (FORAMEN OF MORGAGNI)

This is a rarer defect in the newborn, but in a similar manner to posterolateral defects aplasia of the diaphragm may be found in association with it to produce a larger defect (Figure 54.13).

C. OTHER DEFECTS

These are rare and often found in association with multiple congenital defects (Figure 54.13). Two such patients have been seen in our series of 44 and in both it was impossible to reduce the contents and repair the defect; both patients died. In one of our two patients the defect was bilateral and associated with the syndrome of congenital absence of the spleen, multiple congenital heart defects, a midline liver with anomalous portal venous return and a midline stomach. The second patient was associated with a thoracic meningocele. Occasionally a true anterior or retrosternal costochondral defect is found.

2. Side of defect

Left-sided defects (60%) are more common than right-sided defects. Whether this is related to the later closure of the left side of the diaphragm or to the liver protecting the right side remains unanswered. Central defects are very rare and in our experience are impossible to repair. Bilateral diaphragmatic hernias are extremely rare and in 1965 a search of the surgical literature yielded only nine such patients (Fitchett and Tavarez, 1965).

3. Hernial sac

In the majority of defects the hernial sac is absent (65%). Diaphragmatic hernia with a hernial sac must be differentiated from eventration of the diaphragm. In the former there is no muscle tissue between the folds of the pleura and peritoneum, whereas in eventration muscle and fibrous tissue are found between the layers.

Surgical management

Clinical features

The diagnosis of a congenital diaphragmatic hernia must be suspected in any newborn with respiratory difficulties, an apparent dextrocardia due to a shift of the mediastinum and a scaphoid abdomen.

Preoperative care

The diagnosis is confirmed by a single radiograph of the chest and abdomen. This shows displacement of the mediastinum by gas-filled loops of intestine in the chest. It is important to include the abdomen on the film, as confirmatory evidence of the diagnosis will be provided by an abnormal gas pattern below the diaphragm. Occasionally the hernial sac, if present, can be seen on the radiograph.

In the differential diagnosis, multiple staphylococcal lung cysts and congenital cystic adenomatoid malformation of the lung have caused mistakes and in some patients unnecessary operations. In these conditions the gas pattern below the diaphragm is normal, thus providing the most helpful diagnostic sign. There is *no* need for the use of contrast studies which may be harmful.

Administration of oxygen by a face mask is *harmful* as this will merely increase the gaseous content of the bowel in the chest, leading to a further shift of the mediastinum and compression of the contralateral lung. The oxygen content of the incubator may be increased, but if there is no improvement an endotracheal tube is passed and positive-pressure respiration established. Arrangements are made for an anaesthetist or doctor experienced in endotracheal intubation of a neonate to accompany the infant on transfer to a neonatal surgical unit.

A nasogastric tube (no. 10 Fr. gauge) is passed into the stomach and aspirated. The tube is left open on free drainage into a gallipot and is aspirated at half-hourly intervals.

The infant is nursed in an incubator, lying on the side of the defect and with the head slightly elevated. These measures may improve the expansion of the lung on the contralateral side.

Samples of the mother's and infant's blood are sent for grouping and cross-matching and an intravenous drip is established. Levels of electrolytes in the serum and blood gases are determined.

In the past, the successful management of a congenital diaphragmatic hernia depended upon early operation, i.e. as an emergency. In recent times the operation is delayed to allow resuscitation, correction of acid base disturbances and ventilatory support. Only when the neonate is in a stable condition is operative repair undertaken which may be several days later. The results of this change in policy have now been evaluated: the mortality remains high in patients with symptoms and signs developing in the first 6 h following delivery (Bloss *et al.*, 1980; Bohn *et al.*, 1983; Vacanti *et al.*, 1984) and some die before undergoing operative closure of the defect.

In the preoperative period a tension pneumothorax may require urgent treatment. Insertion of a needle through an intercostal space allows the air to escape:

the needle is then connected to an underwater-seal drainage bottle.

Operation

An abdominal approach is preferred as it is easier to reduce the contents and treat the associated universal mesentery and malrotation. The infant is placed flat on its back and a curved subcostal incision is made 2.0 cm below the costal margin (Figure 54.14). The abdomen is opened and the defect is inspected. The stomach and loops of small and large bowel are seen entering the pleural cavity (Figure 54.14). The spleen, lobes of the liver and kidney may also be contents of the hernial sac.

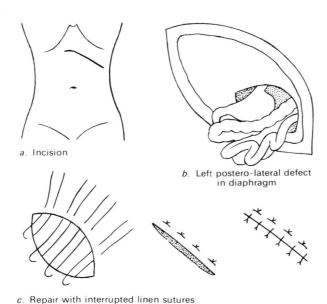

a. Incision

b. Left postero-lateral defect in diaphragm

c. Repair with interrupted linen sutures

Figure 54.14 Operative repair of a posterolateral diaphragmatic hernia

The contents are gently reduced into the abdominal cavity. Close inspection is necessary to find if a hernial sac is present. This can easily be missed as it is thin walled and subject to the negative intrathoracic pressure and covers the chest wall and the unexpanded lung. If a sac is present it is excised from the free margin of the defect in the diaphragm, taking extreme care about haemostasis. This manoeuvre is made easier if the sac is opened at one point to reduce the negative intrathoracic pressure. The sac is then easily pulled into the abdominal cavity.

The lung is inspected. It is often small and hypoplastic. The anaesthetist should be dissuaded from attempting to inflate it. An underwater pleural drain is then inserted through a lower intercostal space in the posterior axillary line.

The defect in the diaphragm is then repaired (Figure 54.14). In small hernias the edges are approximated with a layer of 2/0 or 3/0 non-absorbable interrupted mattress sutures. These are tied and the free edge is then sutured with a row of interrupted 2/0 or 3/0 sutures. In larger defects, especially if the posterior rim of diaphragmatic muscle is absent, the repair is more difficult. Under these circumstances the anterior free edge of the diaphragm may be sutured to the intercostal muscles or to the periosteum of the ribs or even to the posterior layer of perirenal fascia. In extreme cases either a Silastic prosthesis is tailored and sutured into the defect or a reverse latissimus dorsi flap is used (Bianchi *et al.*, 1983).

Attention is then turned to the abdomen and any associated malrotation is corrected by dividing Ladd's band and mobilizing the bowel to leave the small intestine on the right, and the large bowel on the left side of the abdomen (Ladd's operation).

The closure of the abdomen is often the most difficult part of the operation due to the small size of the true abdominal cavity. The range of alternative procedures used to ease this stage of the operation is as follows:

1. Normal closure in layers.
2. Stretching of the abdominal wall with the fingers inserted under the free edge of the wound.
3. Skin closure only leaving a planned ventral hernia which will require a secondary repair at a later date.
4. Insertion of a Silastic patch into the wound with or without skin cover. This is then repaired within the first 2 postoperative weeks (cf. repair of exomphalos, page 850).
5. The use of a respirator in the postoperative period to maintain a satisfactory respiratory exchange until the abdominal cavity enlarges sufficiently so that normal respiration may be established.

In patients who have presented within the first 24 hours of life it is advisable to insert an underwater drain to the contralateral pleural cavity. This will prevent any mortality due to the contralateral lung developing a tension pneumothorax in the immediate postoperative period (Young, 1968). Hypoplasia of the lung and assisted ventilation may be predisposing factors for the development of this complication.

Postoperative care

NURSING CARE

This is intensive and the infant is 'specialled'. Observations of pulse and respiratory rate are constantly monitored or measured at regular intervals. Temperature is monitored or measured at hourly intervals. Peripheral circulation is checked by pressure on the finger pulp space and the time taken for the return of the colour is measured and recorded. The head is kept slightly elevated within the incubator. Hypoglycaemia is checked for by Dextrostix tests at 4-hourly intervals, or more frequently if the infant is premature. Care of the mouth and frequent aspiration of any secretions are essential.

The pleural drains are watched carefully and clamped at any time before moving the infant. Physiotherapy and suction are performed hourly.

The nasogastric tube is aspirated at half-hourly intervals for 12 h and then at hourly intervals, and in between aspirations is left on free drainage. Abdominal girth measurements are recorded 4-hourly. Oral feeds are not introduced until the aspirates are minimal and non-bile stained, meconium has been passed and the abdomen is soft.

Routine nursing care is given to the wound and to the care of the umbilicus. Intake and output charts are accurately kept and intravenous drips are maintained on a standard regimen.

Many of these infants will be maintained on a ventilator postoperatively for a variable time and require the intensive management that such a regimen needs.

Antibiotic cover is given as a routine because of the risks of infection and because of the poor immunological response of the newborn.

Complications

EARLY

Tension pneumothorax. This complication should be prevented by the routine insertion of bilateral underwater chest drains.

Pulmonary hypoplasia. In some infants it is impossible to achieve a satisfactory pulmonary exchange. The hypoxia may be the cause of the persistence of the fetal circulation with widely patent high-flow ductus arteriosus which is so often found at a postmortem examination.

Infection. This should be minimized by strict barrier nursing, intensive physiotherapy and antibiotic care.

Associated malformations. Congenital heart disease and other malformations are often found in infants with a diaphragmatic hernia and increase the mortality.

Gestational age. Prematurity and 'small for dates infants' have specific complications such as hypoglycaemia, hypocalcaemia and hypomagnesaemia which require careful monitoring and treatment.

LATE

Recurrence. Whether this is due to the difficulties in achieving a satisfactory repair, or the poor expansion of the lung on the affected side, or to raised intra-abdominal pressure due to difficulties in closing the abdomen, is open to conjecture.

Ventral hernia/inguinal hernia. The factors listed above predispose to the development of these complications.

Undescended testis. This associated defect is probably related to the primary defect and will require surgical treatment at a later date.

EVENTRATION OF THE DIAPHRAGM

Only rarely does this condition present in the neonatal period. Whether it is due to a failure of migration of muscle fibres into the developing diaphragm, atrophy or hypoplasia of part of the diaphragm is uncertain. The presenting features are similar to those of a diaphragmatic hernia, but in the older infant or child there is often a history of recurrent chest infections. Treatment is surgical with plication of the diaphragm.

Oesophageal atresia and tracheo-oesophageal fistula

Surgical embryology

The oesophagus and trachea develop from the primitive foregut and their differentiation is completed between the 3rd and 5th weeks of intra-uterine life. The ingrowth of the ventral ridges of the foregut (laryngotracheal sulcus) starts at 21–23 days and has finished by 27–32 days of intra-uterine life (3–8 mm embryo). This process starts caudally and eventually with fusion of the lateral ridges the oesophagus becomes separated from the developing tracheo-oesophageal tree (Figure 54.15). Failure of fusion of the tracheo-oesophageal septum at some point will lead to the formation of a tracheo-oesophageal fistula.

The causation of oesophageal atresia is more obscure and remains unknown. Many theories have been suggested such as inflammation and ulceration, deficiency of material where the lung primordium uses up the common material available, relative pressure changes either from an enlarged cardiac primordium or from external pressure, malposition of the large vessels, vascular insufficiency or compression of the oesophagus due to external pressure of the developing pneumo-enteric processes (Rickham and Johnston, 1969). The development of oesophageal atresia could be due to other factors related to segmentation of the embryo. The segmentation of para-axial mesoderm on each side of the notochord and the formation of the sclerotomes and myotomes and formation of the membranous vertebras on an intersegmental plane occurs at a similar time. As the upper oesophagus contains striated muscle, the foregut may be susceptible to vascular changes caused by segmentation, and this may be important in the causation of oesophageal atresia (Bond-Taylor *et al.*, 1973). The high incidence of vertebral and other associated

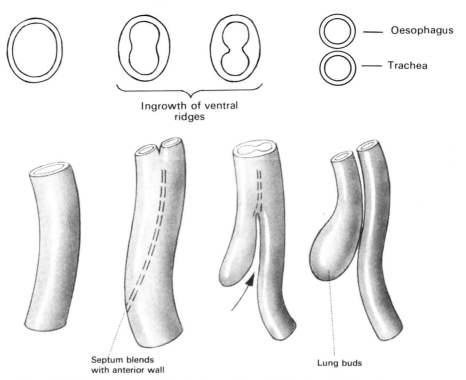

Figure 54.15 Development of the trachea and bronchial tree from the foregut

anomalies with oesophageal atresia lends support to this hypothesis. Similarities occur in anorectal malformations where there is a high incidence of vertebral and associated anomalies; striated muscle is present and the vertebral column is in close approximation to the developing bowel.

Surgical pathology and anatomy

Oesophageal atresia occurs in a variety of differing forms, but can be conveniently subdivided into three basic types: oesophageal atresia with and without a tracheo-oesophageal fistula and tracheo-oesophageal fistula without an oesophageal atresia (Figure 54.16). These basic types account for 95% of the patients. The other 5% of patients with congenital anomalies of the oesophagus have additional fistula and other defects superimposed on this basic pattern.

The blood supply of the oseophagus is poor when related to other parts of the alimentary tract. The upper oesophagus receives its supply from the inferior thyroid arteries, the middle third of the oesophagus from the intercostal and bronchial arteries and by branches from the aorta and the lower third from the left gastric and phrenic arteries. The middle third of the oesophagus therefore has the poorest blood supply and this may have been one of the causes of anastomotic leaks and operative failure in the past.

In oesophageal atresia there is usually a wide disparity in size between the upper hypertrophied pouch and the lower distal oesophageal segment which is thin walled and has a narrow lumen. The blood supply to the lower oesophageal segment is poor when compared to the rich blood supply of the hypertrophied upper oesophageal segment. Variations occur in the degree of separation of the blind upper pouch of the oesophagus and the distal lower segment whether associated or unassociated with a tracheo-oesophageal fistula. In the latter group of patients there is usually wide separation which makes any primary repair using the oesophagus impracticable. In patients with a tracheo-oesophageal fistula the segments may overlap or be separated by up to 4 cm. Prematurity is a complicating factor in oesophageal atresia, particularly in the patients without a tracheo-oesophageal fistula.

Associated anomalies are found in 50% of infants with oesophageal atresia and tracheo-oesophageal fistula. These range from vertebral and musculoskeletal (40%), genito-urinary (30%), gastrointestinal (25%), cardiovascular (20%) and other miscellaneous defects (5%). The associated anomalies are often life threatening and may modify surgical treatment in addition to altering the morbidity and mortality of the primary condition.

Surgical management

Clinical features

A history of hydramnios should alert the clinician to the possible diagnosis of oesophageal atresia as it is

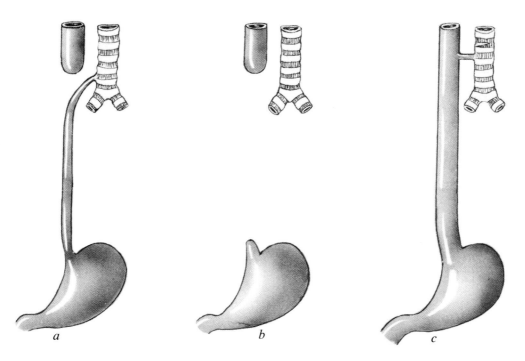

Figure 54.16 Types of congenital oesophageal atresia and tracheo-oesophageal fistula. *a*, Oesophageal atresia *with* tracheo-oesophageal fistula (86%). *b*, Oesophageal atresia *without* tracheo-oesophageal fistula (6%). *c*, Tracheo-oesophageal fistula *without* oesophageal atresia (3%)

found in half of the cases. The inability to swallow saliva results in aspiration into the tracheobronchial tree and may interfere with respiration and lead to pneumonia. Early diagnosis at this stage will reduce the risks of these complications. Reflux of acid juices from the stomach through a tracheo-oesophageal fistula causes a serious and often fatal pneumonitis.

The diagnosis of oesophageal atresia is confirmed by passing a radio-opaque no. 10 catheter which is held up 10 cm from the lip margins. Lateral and posteroanterior radiographs of the chest and abdomen are taken; the presence or absence of gas below the diaphragm thus differentiates the patients into those with or without a tracheo-oesophageal fistula.

The diagnosis of a tracheo-oesophageal fistula without an oesophageal atresia should be suspected in any infant who has difficulties in feeding – in particular, cyanotic attacks with the feed or recurrent chest infections affecting the right upper lobe. In some infants air passes from the tracheobronchial tract into the gastrointestinal tract to cause abdominal distension similar to that found in Hirschsprung's disease. The diagnosis is confirmed by demonstrating the fistula with contrast material on cine radiology. In some cases the fistula may be seen and cannulated with a ureteric catheter during oesophagoscopy or bronchoscopy. If the infant is oesophagoscoped and intubated, anaesthetic gases can be detected passing through the fistula and into the eye of the examiner!

Preoperative care

The infants are nursed level in an incubator. Additional oxygen and humidity are often required. Periodic aspiration of the upper oesophageal pouch at half-hourly intervals will reduce the incidence of an aspiration pneumonia. Antibiotics are given and blood is sent to the laboratory for estimations of haemoglobin and urea and electrolytes in the serum and grouping and cross-matching.

Choice of operation

1. OESOPHAGEAL ATRESIA AND TRACHEO-OESOPHAGEAL FISTULA

(a) Fit full-term infant. Primary anastomosis is the operation of choice, with either a gastrostomy or transanastomotic tube for feeding in the postoperative phase. A gastrostomy is safer. Recent observations have shown that a gastrostomy induces gastro-oesophageal reflux (Jolley *et al.*, 1986). However, if the gastrostomy is left on free drainage, a build-up of intragastric pressure is prevented and reflux is less likely to occur.

(b) Premature infant. Staging of the procedures may improve the operative results. Various operations and sequences of operation are possible:

(i) Gastrostomy and suction of the upper pouch with a Replogle tube, followed at a later date by primary anastomosis. An alternative to gastrostomy is parenteral nutrition.
(ii) Ligation and division of fistula and gastrostomy followed by primary anastomosis at a later date.

(c) Widely separated upper and lower oesophageal segments. Either (i) ligation of tracheo-oesophageal fistula, gastrostomy and cervical oesophagostomy, or (ii) ligation of tracheo-oesophageal fistula, gastrostomy and continuous suction of the upper oesophageal pouch. This second procedure, if successful, may avoid the need for oesophageal reconstruction as a delayed primary anastomosis may be possible.

(d) Infant with severe pulmonary complications. In these infants treatment should be delayed or staged until the chest condition improves.

(e) Infant with multiple congenital anomalies. Careful staging of the various operations is vital for a successful outcome.

2. OESOPHAGEAL ATRESIA WITHOUT TRACHEO-OESOPHAGEAL FISTULA

(a) Fit full-term infant. Either (i) gastrostomy and cervical oesophagostomy and later oesophageal reconstruction, or (ii) a primary oesophageogastrostomy (Ivor Lewis operation) (Atwell and Harrison, 1980) or colonic replacement of the oesophagus (Sherman and Waterson, 1957).

(b) Premature infant. Either suction of the upper segment or a cervical oesophagostomy. This can be combined with either a gastrostomy or total parenteral nutrition until the infant reaches a weight suitable for either staged operations and early or late oesophageal reconstruction.

3. TRACHEO-OESOPHAGEAL FISTULA WITHOUT OESOPHAGEAL ATRESIA

Ligation of the tracheo-oesophageal fistula is performed through a left cervical approach, cf. cervical oesophagostomy. Preoperative oesophagoscopy and cannulation of the fistula with a ureteric catheter will make the identification of the fistula much easier at the operation.

Gastrostomy (Figure 54.17)

A transverse left upper abdominal muscle-cutting incision is made. The body of the stomach is delivered into the wound by placing Babcock tissue forceps onto the greater curvature, taking care to avoid any injury to the gastro-epiploic vessels.

A seromuscular purse-string suture is then inserted at the site of the proposed gastrostomy which is well

up into the body of the stomach. The stomach is opened with the cutting diathermy and a no. 12 latex Malecot catheter is introduced and the purse-string suture of 3/0 chromic catgut is tied. A second purse-string is then inserted and tied. The catheter end is then passed out through a second stab incision 1 cm above the wound. Four non-absorbable silk sutures (3/0 silk) are then placed in position in the N., S., E. and W. positions. These seromuscular and peritoneal sutures, when tied, hold the anterior wall of the stomach firmly against the abdominal wall, thus reducing the risk of leakage. The wound is then closed in layers.

The use of a percutaneous gastrostomy has now replaced the standard Stamm gastrostomy in many centres.

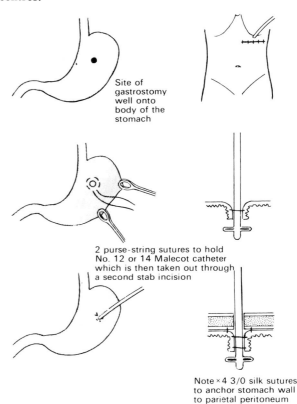

Site of gastrostomy well onto body of the stomach

2 purse-string sutures to hold No. 12 or 14 Malecot catheter which is then taken out through a second stab incision

Note × 4 3/0 silk sutures to anchor stomach wall to parietal peritoneum

Figure 54.17 Operative technique for fashioning a Stamm gastrostomy in the newborn

Ligation of tracheo-oesophageal fistula and primary anastomosis (Figure 54.18)

1. TRANSPLEURAL ROUTE

The patient is positioned on the table as shown. The vertical incision is anterior to the midaxillary line and extends from the axilla to the 8th rib. The serratus anterior is incised down to the rib cage and the shoulder girdle is displaced posteriorly. Care is taken to preserve the nerve supply of the serratus anterior. Anteriorly the pectoral muscles are freed from the rib cage with the cutting diathermy to the line of the nipple. Superiorly care must be taken as the incision extends to the floor of the axilla. The chest is then opened through the 4th intercostal space using cutting diathermy to divide the muscles down to the pleura. As the lung collapses the incision is extended anteriorly to the nipple line and posteriorly to the angle of the rib. Straight and curved mastoid retractors are suitable in the newborn period to keep the chest open. The edges of the curved retractor are placed under the rib margins and then a straight retractor is used to separate the skin margins.

REPAIR of oesophageal atresia: primary anastomosis

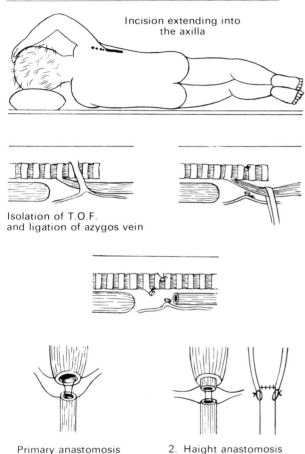

Figure 54.18 Transpleural method of primary anastomosis of oesophageal atresia after ligation of tracheo-oesophageal fistula

The lung is then retracted inferiorly and anteriorly to expose the mediastinal surface of the right pleural cavity. The azygos vein is identified and divided between ligatures. The vagus and phrenic nerves are identified. The tracheo-oesophageal fistula is seen passing upwards and merging with the posterior wall of the trachea and is closely related to the vagus nerve. The fistula is isolated with a sling, taking care to preserve the small blood vessels supplying the

lower segment of the oesophagus. The fistula is then transfixed and ligated with 3/0 silk as close to the tracheal wall as possible. If a gastrostomy is not established it is important to pass a fine tube into the stomach to deflate it. This reduces the risks of forceful regurgitation of gastric contents in the early post-operative period, leading to possible breakdown of the anastomosis.

The upper pouch is identified. It may be seen in relationship to the posterior wall of the trachea and may overlap the site of the previously ligated tracheo-oesophageal fistula. Often the upper pouch is widely separated and identification is difficult. This is simplified by asking the anaesthetist to pass a no. 10 catheter into the pouch. A no. 2 polyvinyl tube has previously been passed into the no. 10 catheter. Once identified the upper pouch is mobilized, held with a stay suture and its fundus is opened.

Interrupted silk sutures (4/0) are used for the anastomosis. On completion of the posterior layer of the anastomosis the catheter in the upper pouch is gently advanced into view; the end of this tube is then cut off and the inner polyvinyl tube is pulled into the chest and the anaesthetist withdraws the outer catheter. The polyvinyl tube is passed into the lower oesophageal segment and on into the stomach. The anterior portion of the anastomosis is then completed over the tube. If a gastrostomy has been performed the polyvinyl tube is passed into the lower segment, to facilitate the completion of the anastomosis, but it is then withdrawn.

An underwater pleural drain is inserted (no. 12 latex Malecot catheter with the limbs cut off). The open end of the catheter is left as near as possible to the anastomosis.

The chest is closed in layers. Three chromic catgut (3/0) rib sutures are inserted and used to approximate the ribs. The intercostal muscles are closed with continuous 3/0 absorbable sutures. The serratus anterior is closed with interrupted 2/0 or 3/0 chromic catgut. The skin is closed with a 3/0 subcuticular nylon suture and held with beads and aliminium stops at each end.

Specific problems

(a) Disparity in size: The disparity in size of the upper and lower oesophageal segments may make the anastomosis difficult.

(b) Avascularity of lower segment: This should be avoidable by taking extreme care in handling the tissues and keeping mobilization of the lower segment to a minimum.

(c) Aberrant right subclavian artery: This anomaly is often found in association with oesophageal atresia and may increase the technical difficulty of the anastomosis.

(d) Tension on the anastomosis: If the ends of the upper and lower oesophageal segments are widely separated, primary anastomosis may be impossible.

In some patients the anastomosis is completed under increased tension with a much higher risk of breakdown and an increased mortality. Careful judgement is required in making the decision of whether to complete the anastomosis or to ligate the fistula and leave the upper pouch for either repeated aspiration and stretching or performing a cervical oesophagostomy.

Two other procedures are useful in overcoming the technical problem of widely separated oesophageal segments (Figure 54.19):

(i) Circular myotomy (Livaditis operation):
 Circular myotomy of the upper pouch down to the submucosal layer may increase length and allow completion of the anastomosis.
(ii) Anterior flap (Gough operation):
 An anterior flap may be fashioned from the wide upper oesophageal segment and folded down, thus providing additional length. The anastomosis is completed without tension.

Oesophageal atresia: Modifications of primary anastomosis

a. Circular myotomy
(Livaditis opn)

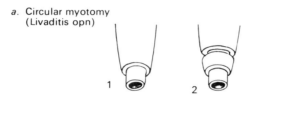

b. Anterior flap
(Gough opn)

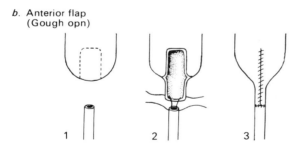

Figure 54.19 Operative procedures to assist in achieving a primary anastomosis with widely separated upper and lower oesophageal segments

2. EXTRAPLEURAL ROUTE (Holder, 1964)

Stages in this operation are similar to the primary repair and ligation of the tracheo-oesophageal fistula. Technically it is more difficult and time consuming and the pleural cavity is often opened inadvertently. The advantage of the extrapleural route is that if an anastomotic leak occurs it can be treated successfully by conservative measures.

Cervical oesophagostomy

This operation allows saliva to escape onto the surface of the neck and thus reduce the incidence of pneumonia. It can be used as a preliminary procedure or following complications of a primary repair. The incision is made in a skin crease along the left clavicle, extending from the sternal head of the sternomastoid to the midpoint of the clavicle. The clavicular head of sternomastoid is divided with cutting diathermy. The sternal head is left attached but may be divided at its periosteal attachment and reflected upwards. The omohyoid muscle is divided and the great vessels in the neck are retracted laterally. The lateral wall of the oesophagus and trachea are seen. The lateral lobes of the thyroid are retracted anteriorly. The oesophagus is then identified and mobilized, care being taken to avoid damaging the left recurrent laryngeal nerve. The fundus of the oesophagus is then opened and sutured to the skin with interrupted silk sutures. If the sternal head of sternomastoid was divided it is then sutured to its periosteal attachment.

Ligation of isolated tracheo-oesophageal fistula

The incision is above the left clavicle extending from the midline of the neck to the mid-clavicular line. The clavicular head of sternomastoid is then identified and divided with cutting diathermy. The sternal head can be divided at its periosteal attachment and reflected upwards to expose the omohyoid and the great vessels in the carotid sheath. The belly of omohyoid is divided.

The oesophagus can be approached from either behind or in front of the great vessels, the latter being the method of choice. The oesophagus and trachea are identified together with the left recurrent laryngeal nerve. The fistula is identified. Slings placed around the oesophagus above and below the fistula often make its identification easier. The fistula is transfixed on the tracheal side with a 3/0 silk suture and divided. The oesophageal side of the fistula is repaired with 3/0 non-absorbable sutures. The wound is closed in layers with an infant Redivac drain down to the site of the fistula.

Postoperative care

NURSING

Observations for the routine postoperative care of the newborn are as previously described. The infant is nursed level.

UNDERWATER PLEURAL DRAIN

This is left *in situ* for 5–10 days, i.e. until the infant has been fed orally for the first time.

GASTROSTOMY

The gastrostomy is left on free drainage into a gallipot at the level of the infant. This reduces intragastric pressure and decreases the possibility of gastro-oesophageal reflux which can cause disruption of the anastomosis.

The gastrostomy tube is aspirated at hourly intervals. Dextrose followed by milk feeds can be introduced any time after 4–5 days until the critical initial healing phase is over.

If the gastrostomy tube becomes dislodged in the first 10 days postoperatively, the infant must be taken to the operating theatre for reintroduction of the tube. This may be done without an anaesthetic, but during this early phase it is possible to push the stomach off the anterior abdominal wall on reintroducing the catheter resulting in peritonitis. After the first 10 days it is usually safe to replace the gastrostomy tube on the ward: delay is to be avoided as the opening can close very quickly. When the infant is on full oral feeds the gastrostomy tube is removed.

PREVENTION OF INFECTION

Chest physiotherapy and antibiotics are used to reduce pulmonary complications.

PARENTERAL FLUID AND CALORIES

Intravenous fluid is administered to maintain the internal homeostasis of the infant. Parenteral nutrition is not used initially but reserved for use in the complicated patient.

VENTILATORY SUPPORT

It is advisable to maintain the neonate on positive-pressure respiration if the anastomosis is considered to be under tension. This additional method of postoperative support appears to reduce the incidence of an anastomotic leak.

Complications

EARLY

Anastomotic leak. This is the most dangerous complication, especially when it occurs between the 3rd and 5th day. It is heralded by the appearance of saliva or bile-stained fluid in the tubing of the underwater pleural drain. If disruption occurs early the chest is reopened and either a second repair is attempted or the lower segment is transfixed and ligated and a cervical oesophagostomy is established. A gastrostomy is required for feeding if not already established at the primary operation.

Anastomotic leaks which occur later than 7 days can usually be treated conservatively with antibiotics and suction. Oral feeding is delayed until healing is complete. Any leak from the anastomosis predisposes to stricture formation and the development of a recurrent tracheo-oesophageal fistula.

Pneumonia. This complication affects the mortality

of the primary treatment. It is not possible to differentiate whether this is a postoperative complication or a continuation of preoperative aspiration problems but is largely preventable by early diagnosis. Physiotherapy, antibiotics and aspiration of secretions are all that is usually required. Other patients will need assisted ventilation and possibly a tracheostomy.

Prematurity. The association of oesophageal atresia with prematurity is accompanied by an increased mortality and in such patients staging of operations is necessary to ensure a successful outcome (Koop and Hamilton, 1965).

Associated anomalies. The high incidence of associated malformations may complicate the management of oesophageal atresia. Often congenital heart disease may become apparent in the postoperative period and be a cause of late death. An intravenous pyelogram is performed before discharge in all patients to exclude associated renal anomalies (Atwell and Beard, 1974).

Tracheomalacia. This complication, although rare, can cause severe respiratory problems and as tracheostomy may be required. It should be differentiated from subglottic stenosis which may be an associated congenital defect.

LATE

The late complications are stricture, recurrent fistula, hiatus hernia and dysmotility of the oesophagus. All of these complications may present in a similar manner with respiratory and feeding difficulties.

A barium swallow will exclude stricture and hiatus hernia with reflux. Recurrent fistula and dysmotility of the oesophagus are difficult to demonstrate without cine radiology.

Congenital hypertrophic pyloric stenosis

Surgical pathology and anatomy

Congenital pyloric stenosis is a relatively common condition of early infancy; males are more often affected than females (sex ratio 5:1). The aetiology remains unknown but genetic factors are important as the incidence is increased in siblings of affected persons (× 15) and in the offspring of affected persons (affected father: risk 1 in 10; affected mother: risk 1 in 4). Thus it appears that a mother may transmit the condition more strongly to the next generation, although the condition is commoner in the male.

Although called 'congenital' this is not strictly true as it has never been reported in a stillborn infant. Similarly the stomach has been noted to be normal at a laparotomy performed for vomiting; in such an infant at a later laparotomy for persistence of symp-

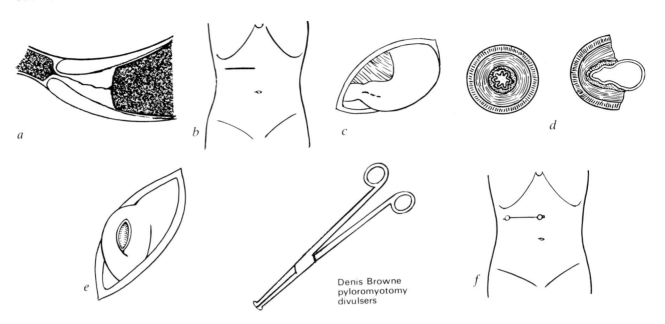

Figure 54.20 Congenital hypertrophic pyloric stenosis. *a*, The shaded area shows the 'rat tail' sign of congenital pyloric stenosis. In later stages the 'tail' disappears leaving a gap consisting of hypertrophied muscle and redundant mucosa and submucosa. *b*, Skin crease transverse incision and rectus split. *c*, Incision through the pylorus down to the submucosa which bulges out. *d*, Release of mucosa and submucosa shown schematically following division of the pyloric sphincter thus increasing the size of the lumen. *e*, The incision in the pylorus changes direction at a right angle as the duodenal fornix is approached. When this change of direction is seen the distal incision is adequate. *f*, Skin closure with a continuous subcuticular nylon with beads and stops

toms a classic pyloric tumour has been found and treated by pyloromyotomy. Current investigations have suggested that the gastrointestinal hormones such as gastrin (Janik *et al.*, 1978) and secretin are involved, but whether this is cause or effect remains uncertain. It seems likely that the cause of congenital hypertrophic pyloric stenosis is multifactorial (Carter, 1961). One possible explanation is that hypertrophy of the pylorus occurs in everyone after birth, but only in a few are the changes severe enough to cause symptoms.

There is hypertrophy of all of the muscle layers which is maximal in the region of the pylorus; this hypertrophy may be severe enough to produce a duodenal fornix. The obstruction is also aggravated by the pyloric mucosa and submucosa which become oedematous and appear as an obstructive element proximal to the sphincter (Figure 54.20).

Surgical management

Clinical features

The onset of symptoms is usually gradual in an infant who has given no previous cause for concern. The majority of patients present at 3–5 weeks of age, although this can range between 1 week and 5 months. Vomiting of feeds occurs, initially small amounts but later the vomit becomes forceful and projectile; the vomit is never bile stained. The infant

fails to gain weight. As the vomiting increases in amount, the baby becomes dehydrated and alkalotic. The diagnosis is confirmed by palpating the pyloric tumour during a test feed and by noting visible peristalsis from left to right across the upper abdomen. Constipation and rarely jaundice may be additional signs. Radiological confirmation of the diagnosis demonstrates separation of contrast in the duodenal cap from that in the stomach – the 'gap' or 'rat tail' sign (Figure 54.20).

Preoperative care

The degree of dehydration and metabolic alkalosis is assessed and corrected by an intravenous infusion of normal saline with added potassium. A urinary infection as the cause of symptoms should be excluded by routine bacteriological examination of a clean-catch specimen of the urine. One or two gastric washouts with normal saline are used to remove retained curds from the stomach and for treatment of the associated gastritis. Time spent in adequate preparation of the infant prior to surgery reduces the morbidity and mortality. Congenital hypertrophic pyloric stenosis is no longer an emergency needing immediate surgery.

Operation: Rammstedt's pyloromyotomy
(Figure 54.20)

General anaesthesia is usually used, although if

expert anaesthesia is not available local anaesthesia is satisfactory. A transverse incision is made in a skin crease midway between the umbilicus and costal margin and overlies the full width of the right rectus abdominis muscle. The skin edges are undermined to expose the anterior rectus sheath which is then incised vertically to expose the muscle fibres of the rectus abdominis; these are then split to expose the peritoneum. The peritoneum is then opened and four artery forceps are left on the lateral, upper and lower margins of the peritoneum. The liver is usually seen first and is displaced upwards with a finger and then the tumour is palpated. A moist gauze swab opened out into a single layer is helpful in holding the body of the stomach and makes the delivery of the pyloric tumour easier. The gastroduodenal junction is identified and the line of the proposed incision into the pylorus is planned. The tumour is then incised through the longitudinal and circular muscle fibres down to the submucosa taking care not to open this layer. Denis Browne pyloromyotomy divulsers are used to push through the last innermost layer of circular muscle, then rotated through 90° and opened. The muscle separates proximally onto the antrum and distally towards the pylorus. Sufficient separation is achieved when it is noted that the line of splitting begins to change direction at a right angle to the incision at the gastroduodenal junction. Care must be taken to ensure that the mucosa has not been opened inadvertently at the duodenal fornix; if opened, it must be closed with a horizontal mattress suture of 3/0 chromic catgut. The pylorus is returned to the abdomen and the wound closed in layers using continuous 3/0 chromic catgut for the peritoneum and interrupted for the anterior rectus sheath. The skin is closed with a subcuticular nylon suture with beads and aluminium stops.

Postoperative care

A variety of feeding regimens is used following a Rammstedt's operation (Wheeler *et al.*, 1990). The usual principle is for the infant to be given one or two small dextrose feeds, but feeding is then regraded rapidly over 24–48 h, especially if breast fed. The infant is discharged home on the 3rd or 4th postoperative day. If vomiting persists postoperatively the regrading of feeds may have to be slower and further gastric washouts may be required. The postoperative vomiting may be due to an oesophagitis secondary to the gastric outlet obstruction.

Complications

EARLY

Peritonitis due to failure to recognize that the mucosa was opened at the time of pyloromyotomy. Wound infection and wound dehiscence occasionally occur. Persistent vomiting due to an inadequate pyloromyo-

tomy, gastritis or oesophagitis may require treatment. Rarely a second operation is required.

LATE

Intestinal obstruction due to adhesions may be a late complication, especially if peritonitis was a complication of the initial operation.

Neonatal intestinal obstruction

Surgical embryology

The development of the intestine and its fixation in the peritoneal cavity is completed by the 10th week of intra-uterine life. Initially, the vitello-intestinal duct is the main part of the midgut. Up to the 5th week of intra-uterine life the primitive intestine consists of a hollow tube. This is followed by an active phase of proliferation of the intestinal mucosa which fills the lumen of the developing intestine. The midgut then increases in length and vacuolization of the epithelium is said to occur thus restoring the lumen of the bowel. It has been suggested that failure of the vacuolization (Tandler, 1902) would cause an intestinal atresia (Tandler theory). Other workers have shown by serial sectioning of the fetal intestine that a lumen always persists. This phase of development occurs before the closure of the omphalocele and obliteration of the vitello-intestinal duct.

The development of the duodenum, pancreas, fixation of the intestine and the development of the midgut occur at about the same time.

Duodenum and pancreas

The liver and pancreas develop as two large extramural glands from the duodenum. The combined hepatopancreatic bud grows ventrally and the pancreatic bud dorsally into the mesoduodenum (Figure 54.21). The dorsal outgrowth is proximal to the ventral outgrowth and forms the body and tail of the pancreas with its own duct (Santorini). The ventral outgrowth subdivides into an hepatic component and a pancreatic component which forms the head of the pancreas with its own duct (Wirsung). The duodenum then rotates on its long axis so that the ventral outgrowth lies in the region of the dorsal mesoduodenum. The mechanism causing this rotation remains obscure. As both components continue to grow they fuse to form the adult type of pancreas. A communicating duct joins the two outgrowths, although separate openings of both outgrowths may persist (Figure 54.21)

Fixation of intestine

Closure of the omphalocele with disappearance of the vitello-intestinal duct is complete by the 80th day

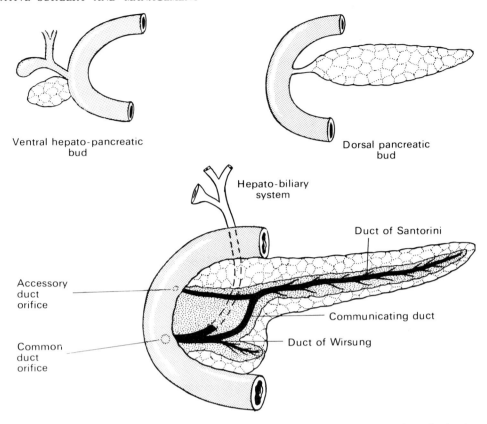

Ventral hepato-pancreatic bud

Dorsal pancreatic bud

Hepato-biliary system

Duct of Santorini

Accessory duct orifice

Communicating duct

Common duct orifice

Duct of Wirsung

Figure 54.21   Development of the pancreas from dorsal and ventral outgrowths from the duodenum

of intra-uterine life. Before this, the true abdominal cavity enlarges to accommodate the returning midgut. Rotation of this gut occurs so that the intestine comes to lie in the adult position. This U-shaped limb of the midgut does not return as an upper and lower limb but as a left (distal) and right (proximal) limb (Figure 54.22a). This may be due to the rapid development of the liver which forces the duodenum inferiorly. The return of the intestine occurs in an orderly manner and rotation of the gut occurs in an anticlockwise direction. This is associated with descent of the caecum (Figure 54.22b,c) and the zygosis of the visceral and parietal peritoneum of the ascending and descending colon; the colon then becomes fixed to the posterior abdominal wall by zygosis of adjacent layers of peritoneum.

Rectum and anal canal

The hindgut comes down to join the proctodeum. The allantoic diverticulum joins the hindgut to form a common cloaca at the junction of the endoderm and ectoderm (Figure 54.23). The cloaca consists of a narrow strip of cells in the anteroposterior plane (Figure 54.23). The separation of the anterior urogenital structures from the posterior hindgut proceeds by the downgrowth of the mesodermal urogenital septum (Figure 54.23). This downgrowth divides the

Table 54.2   Causes of intestinal obstruction in the newborn

I. *Duodenal*	
	Atresia: stenosis
	Annular pancreas
	Malrotation ± volvulus
II. *Jejuno-ileal*	
Inguinal hernia	
Meckel's	Atresia: stenosis
diverticulum	Meconium ileus
Congenital bands	Volvulus neonatorum
III. *Colorectal*	
	Hirschsprung's disease
	Atresia: stenosis
	Anorectal anomalies
IV. *Idiopathic intestinal obstruction*	
	Meconium plug
	Milk plug
	Faecal plug
	CNS
	Hypothyroidism
	Necrotizing enterocolitis
	Exchange transfusion
	Infection
	Pseudo-Hirschsprung's
	Hypoganglionosis
	Hypoplastic left colon
	Drugs
	Cooling

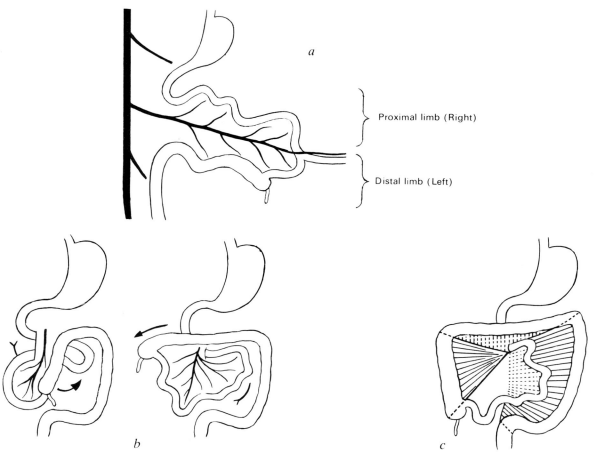

Figure 54.22 Stages in the rotation and fixation of the intestine. *a*, The midgut lengthens on the axis of the superior mesenteric artery into a proximal and distal limb. *b*, Anticlockwise rotation and descent of the caecum. *c*, Fixation of the ascending and descending colon to the posterior abdominal wall by zygosis of adjacent layers of peritoneum

cloacal membrane into two parts, anteriorly the urogenital orifice and posteriorly the anus. Failure of this downgrowth results in a congenital fistula between the anterior and posterior components, i.e. either a recto-urethral fistula, as in the male, or a high recto-vaginal fistula in the female.

Classification

The various forms of neonatal intestinal obstruction are suitably subdivided on a positional basis (Table 54.2). Other rare causes of intestinal obstruction in the neonatal period such as Meckel's diverticulum, intussusception and congenital bands are excluded in this account, also the more common inguinal hernias which may cause neonatal obstruction in the neonatal period, especially in the premature infant.

General principles of surgical management

Clinical features

The classic signs and symptoms of intestinal obstruction are either primary, such as abdominal pain,

vomiting and absolute constipation, or secondary (Figure 54.24). Variations in the pattern of presentation occur depending on whether the obstruction is either complete or incomplete and the level of obstruction within the alimentary tract (Atwell, 1971).

GROUP I

In duodenal atresia the obstruction may be either proximal or distal to the opening of the bile ducts and in some patients bile may enter above and below by the persistence of an accessory duct. The absence of bile in the vomit in duodenal atresia proximal to the bile ducts may cause delay in diagnosis (Young, 1966), but vomiting is usually within the first 48 h. In high intestinal obstruction a history of hydramnios is often obtained and some of the patients are jaundiced. Abdominal distension and visible peristalsis are confined to the upper abdomen and diagnosis is confirmed by a straight radiograph demonstrating a double bubble. Associated anomalies such as congenital heart disease, Down's syndrome and other defects are often found in this group of patients. In

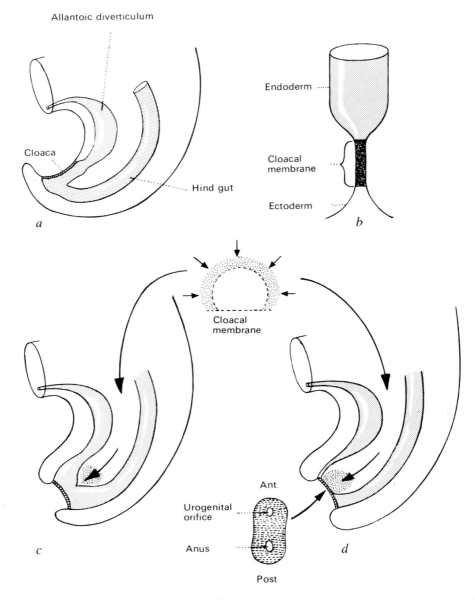

Figure 54.23 Development of the rectum and anal canal. *a*, Cloaca joining allantoic diverticulum with the hind gut. *b*, Cloacal membrane in the anteroposterior plane joining ectoderm and endoderm. *c,d*, Urogenital septum separating the cloacal membrane into anterior and posterior portions (urogenital and anal orifices)

patients with partial duodenal obstruction, such as an annular pancreas, malrotation or volvulus, the clinical presentation is different. The vomiting in these patients may be intermittent and bile or non-bile stained. Distension of the abdomen with volvulus of the small bowel is extremely rare. Blood in the stool is an important sign of impending gangrene of the intestine. The intermittent nature of these signs and symptoms causes difficulty in diagnosis and if associated with volvulus there is an increase in the morbidity and mortality. Straight radiographs of the abdomen show malposition of loops of intestine, a double bubble with some air in the bowel distally

or a homogeneous area in the centre of the film which represents the base of the volvulus.

GROUP II

There is seldom any delay in the diagnosis of jejuno-ileal atresia or meconium ileus. In jejuno-ileal atresia bile-stained vomiting, abdominal distension and fluid levels on a straight radiograph confirm the diagnosis. In incomplete obstruction, such as a jejuno-ileal stenosis, such signs are often masked with minimal vomiting and distension. This is particularly so in ileal stenosis where alterations in the bacterial flora and

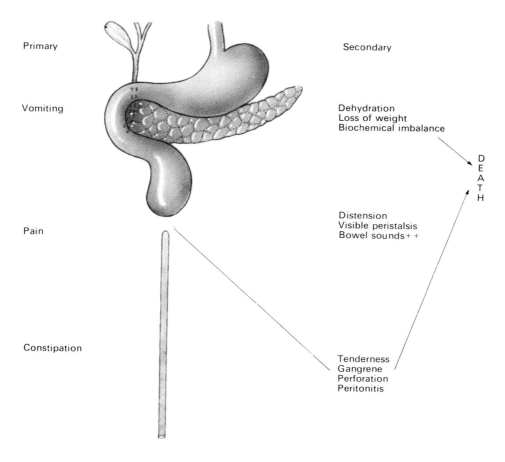

Primary

Vomiting

Pain

Constipation

Secondary

Dehydration
Loss of weight
Biochemical imbalance

D
E
A
T
H

Distension
Visible peristalsis
Bowel sounds+ +

Tenderness
Gangrene
Perforation
Peritonitis

Figure 54.24 Signs and symptoms of intestinal obstruction

transport of water and electrolytes may cause the neonate to present with gastroenteritis. Fortunately an isolated stenosis at this level of the intestine is a rare finding.

In patients with meconium ileus and with meconium peritonitis delay in the diagnosis is extremely rare. Abdominal distension is a striking finding and occurs early and may even cause obstructed labour. The vomiting is often minimal in meconium ileus which contrasts markedly with the degree of distension. Volvulus of the bowel may occur pre- or post-natally in approximately 60% of patients and evidence for this may be found in repeated radiographs. On rectal examination the rectum is empty and tight (cf. Hirschsprung's disease). In some infants there is a family history of fibrocystic disease. Confirmation of the clinical diagnosis is made by finding an elevated level of sodium in the sweat obtained by iontophoresis.

GROUP III

In this group the diagnosis is either simple or extremely difficult. In the newborn with an anorectal malformation the diagnosis is confirmed by inspection and a rectal examination; thus there is no excuse for delay in diagnosis. There are difficulties, however, in differentiating the different types of anorectal malformation which may be found. In infants with Hirschsprung's disease subacute intestinal obstruction is the commonest method of presentation and vomiting occurs within 48 h of delivery in 75% of patients. Abdominal distension, delay in the passage of meconium, a tight and empty rectum on rectal examination and explosive decompression of the bowel on removal of the finger occurs in over 50% of patients. Diagnosis is difficult in some patients due to the intermittent nature of the symptoms, which may be related to difficulty in evacuating meconium or to changes in the consistency of the stool, i.e. because of being breast fed or bottle fed. The subacute obstruction of Hirschsprung's disease may cause diarrhoea, especially after the age of 7 days. Perforation of the caecum causing a pneumoperitoneum and faecal peritonitis is a rare presentation but is accompanied by a high mortality and usually occurs in the first 2 days of life. Diagnosis and management are more difficult in this group.

GROUP IV

Diagnosis and management is more difficult in this group due to the multiplicity of causes, the high incidence of prematurity and the dangers and complications of perforation of the intestine with a resultant pneumoperitoneum and faecal peritonitis. There is often a sequence of events which may assist in diagnosis. Prenatal factors such as a complicated pregnancy and delivery, e.g. multiple births, prematurity, early rupture of the membranes and difficulties with resuscitation are common. Perinatal factors are also important, e.g. exchange transfusion (Corkery *et al.*, 1968), cooling, infection and composition of the feeds. These factors all interact to produce an infant with signs of subacute intestinal obstruction with vomiting, abdominal distension, visible peristalsis, tenderness, loose stools often containing blood or constipation. Later perforation may lead to gross abdominal distension with a pneumoperitoneum. Radiographs show distended loops of bowel with fluid levels, and either evidence of a gradient from the level of the obstruction or the presence of intramural air or air within the portal system, a diagnostic feature of necrotizing enterocolitis. Serial radiographs at 6- or 12-hourly or daily intervals are invaluable in assessing the progress of the condition, and increasing dilatation of isolated loops of bowel (toxic dilatation) is a sign of impending gangrene and perforation.

Preoperative care: general

The principles of preoperative management are the same irrespective of the cause or level of the obstruction. The prevention of the aspiration of vomit is of paramount importance. A no. 10 Fr. gauge nasogastric tube is passed into the stomach and then aspirated at $\frac{1}{2}$–1-hourly intervals. It is left on free open drainage in between aspirations. The degree of dehydration is assessed and intravenous replacement of fluid and electrolytes is started with careful monitoring of the biochemical state of the infant. Samples of the infant's and of the maternal blood are sent for grouping and cross-matching. Radiological examination with straight radiographs of the abdomen in the erect supine and erect lateral position are taken. On rare occasions contrast studies are required such as a barium meal to demonstrate duodenal obstruction of an incomplete type or a barium enema to demonstrate the transitional area in Hirschsprung's disease or malposition of the caecum in malrotation.

Duodenal atresia: stenosis: annular pancreas

Surgical pathology

Atresia, stenosis and annular pancreas may cause an intrinsic obstruction of the duodenum either proximal (25%) or distal to the opening of the bile ducts (75%). Extrinsic factors are significant in some patients with evidence of intra-uterine volvulus or extrinsic bands. The high incidence of associated anomalies (Table 54.3) in this group suggests that in the majority of patients the obstruction occurred in early intra-uterine life.

The level of obstruction is usually found in the second part of the duodenum in close relation to the ampulla of Vater. The bowel above and below the obstruction is often in continuity, especially in patients with a duodenal diaphragm producing a windsock type of deformity. In annular pancreas a constricting ring of pancreatic tissue is found surrounding the duodenum to produce a stenosis or complete obstruction (Figure 54.25).

Table 54.3 Associated anomalies in 40 patients with duodenal atresia and stenosis

I. Trisomy 21		14
II. Gastrointestinal tract		17
Malrotation	6	
Oesophageal atresia and tracheo-oesophageal fistula	3	
Anorectal atresia	1	
Jejuno-ileal atresia	2	
Meckel's diverticulum	2	
Meconium peritonitis	1	
Ectopic pancreas	1	
Congenital bands	1	
III. Congenital cardiovascular disease		3
IV. Vertebral anomalies		6

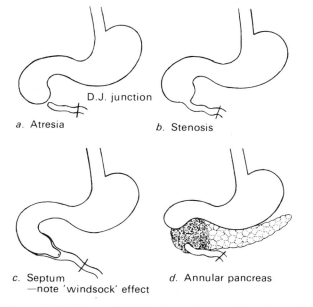

Figure 54.25 Types of duodenal atresia, stenosis and annular pancreas

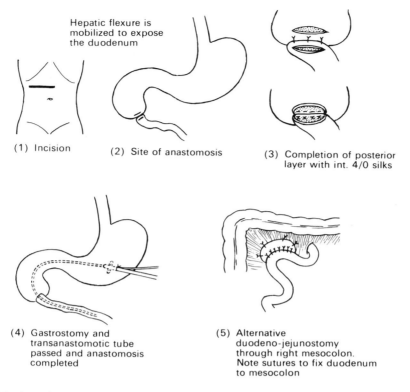

Hepatic flexure is
mobilized to expose
the duodenum

(1) Incision

(2) Site of anastomosis

(3) Completion of posterior
layer with int. 4/0 silks

(4) Gastrostomy and
transanastomotic tube
passed and anastomosis
completed

(5) Alternative
duodeno-jejunostomy
through right mesocolon.
Note sutures to fix duodenum
to mesocolon

Figure 54.26 Operative repair of a duodenal atresia, stenosis or annular pancreas by duodenoduo-denostomy, gastrostomy and transanastomotic feeding tube. Alternative duodenojejunostomy

Surgical management

The operation

The operation of choice is a duodenoduodenostomy, thus restoring continuity. A gastrostomy and trans-anastomotic feeding tube are useful additions and aid the postoperative care. In some patients a duodeno-jejunostomy (retrocolic), gastrostomy and transanas-tomotic feeding tube are easier but less satisfactory. Gastroenterostomy should be avoided.

The abdomen is opened through a transverse supra-umbilical muscle-cutting incision (Figure 54.26). The hepatic flexure is mobilized to expose the duodenum and the site of the intrinsic obstruction is inspected. The bowel proximal and distal to the obstruction is approximated with several seromuscu-lar sutures which are then tied (Figure 54.26). The bowel is opened with cutting diathermy on the hyper-trophied proximal bowel and with iridectomy scissors on the collapsed distal bowel. The posterior part of the anastomosis is completed using interrupted mat-tress sutures of 4/0 silk and each corner is turned in using a Connell suture (Figure 54.26).

The anastomosis is then left at this stage and a gastrostomy is established (cf. oesophageal atresia). In this operation it is essential to pass the transanas-tomotic feeding tube (no. 2 polyvinyl tubing or a no.

3.5 Fr. gauge umbilical vein catheter) through the gastrostomy opening before inserting the Malecot catheter and tying the purse-string suture. The feed-ing tube is then pulled through the pylorus and into the wound at the site of the partially completed duodenoduodenostomy. Then 15 cm of this feeding tube are passed into the upper jejunum. This is difficult and while doing this it is essential to keep the position of the tube constant at the anastomosis. The anterior part of the anastomosis is completed with interrupted Connell sutures of 4/0 silk. On com-pletion of the anastomosis the colon is replaced into the normal anatomical position and the wound is closed in layers.

If a duodenojejunostomy is preferred, a window is made in the transverse mesocolon between the right and middle colic arteries and the dilated duodenum is pulled into view. The anastomosis, gastrostomy and transanastomotic feeding tube are completed in an exactly similar way. The proximal duodenum is sutured to the mesocolon to prevent invagination of the jejunum at this point (Figure 54.26). In patients with a duodenal diaphragm the duodenum is exposed and opened longitudinally.

The diaphragm with its central aperture is often found prolapsed distally. The diaphragm is then excised, either by using cutting diathermy or by over-running the cut edges with a continuous 4/0 catgut suture. The duodenum is closed transversely with interrupted silk sutures.

Postoperative care

The gastrostomy is left on free drainage and aspirated at hourly intervals. The volume of aspirate is usually 100–150 ml per day, and gradually decreases as the anastomosis opens up. Initially these aspirates are replaced by an equal volume of normal saline intravenously. After 24–28 h, however, the aspirates may be injected slowly down the transanastomotic feeding tube at a maximum rate of 1 ml/min. Similarly milk feeds can be started down the feeding tube and are increased until the infant is on full oral requirements. After a time the quantity of gastric aspirate decreases and the catheter may then be spigoted. If this is successful the transanastomotic feed can be reduced in 5.0 ml stages, and instead is given orally. Then, when the infant can manage full oral feeds without vomiting, the gastrostomy and transanastomotic tubes are removed. The transition from tube to full oral feeds may take several days.

Complications

EARLY

An anastomotic breakdown is unusual but may result in a localized or subphrenic abscess. Duodenal ileus may occur due to the gross dilatation and hypertrophy proximal to the atresia. This delay at the anastomosis may persist for a long time postoperatively. Adhesions can form and cause subacute obstruction with vomiting or, combined with duodenal ileus, cause diarrhoea and secondary disaccharide intolerance. The complications of the gastrostomy are listed (see page 860) under 'Oesophageal atresia'. The management of the transanastomotic feeding tube is difficult. The tube may become displaced back into the stomach and if this occurs intravenous fluids or parenteral nutrition are required until full oral feeds can be tolerated. Perforation of the intestine may occur if the tubing is not polyvinyl, or if the feeds are given too rapidly, i.e. maximum rate 1 ml/min.

LATE

Blind loop syndrome. Chronic obstruction at the anastomosis may lead to progressive dilatation and the development of a blind loop syndrome. In these infants there is an iron deficiency anaemia, failure of normal growth and complete loss of appetite. Contrast studies are used for diagnosis and a further laparotomy and either refashioning or excision of the anastomosis is required.

Associated anomalies. Congenital heart disease, Down's syndrome and other gastrointestinal malformations may complicate the initial and late management of duodenal obstruction. Radiological investigations are undertaken to exclude associated renal and vertebral anomalies, e.g. radiograph of the spine and an intravenous pyelogram.

Malrotation: volvulus neonatorum

Surgical pathology

'Malrotation' is the term used to cover a variety of conditions in which there is a failure of the normal rotation of the midgut on returning from the omphalocele to the true abdominal cavity. In many cases there is an associated volvulus. If the caecum lies high and to the left a condensation of parietal peritoneum (Ladd's band) may cross the duodenum and cause obstruction (Figure 54.27). In our experience this component of the obstruction is relatively rare: a much more common finding is volvulus due to the narrow pedicle formed by the attachment of the mesentery. Such a volvulus may endanger the blood supply of the small bowel. In some patients the duodenum and colon may be normal in position but the whole of the small intestine has undergone a volvulus (volvulus neonatorum).

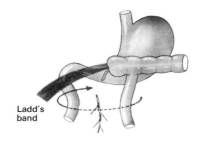

Figure 54.27 Note the narrow base for the attachment of the mesentery of the small bowel thus predisposing to a volvulus. Ladd's band crossing the duodenum may be a cause of obstruction

Other predisposing factors to abnormalities of intestinal rotation are exomphalos, gastroschisis, intrinsic duodenal obstruction, congenital diaphragmatic hernia, duplications of the intestine and abdominal masses such as pelvi-ureteric hydronephrosis or renal tumour (Figure 54.28).

Surgical management

Operation

The abdomen is opened through a supra-umbilical transverse muscle-cutting incision. The intestines are delivered into the wound and inspected carefully. The intestine must be delivered completely into the wound otherwise it will be impossible to recognize the variety of the malrotation that is present. The volvulus, if present (usually clockwise), is untwisted, which will immediately improve the blood supply to the intestine if it had been threatened. Ladd's band is divided and the duodenum mobilized with the proximal small intestine being left to the right. The adhesions to the caecum are divided to widen the base of the pedicle; the caecum is placed to the left with the large bowel, thus the bowel is left in the primitive non-rotated position. No attempt is made to fix the intestine. In patients with a normally fixed intestine and volvulus neonatorum, simple untwisting of the volvulus is insufficient. The duodenum and caecum must be mobilized to produce the non-rotation situation in order to prevent a recurrent volvulus.

Appendicectomy should not be performed, but the parents must be told of the abnormal position of the appendix in order to prevent confusion if an acute abdomen develops at a later date.

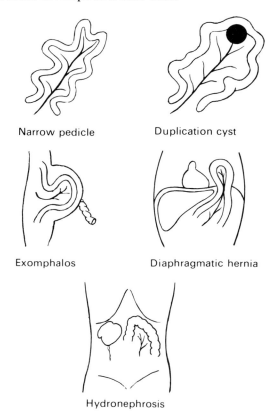

Figure 54.28 Congenital defects which affect the normal rotation and fixation of the intestines during intra-uterine life

In some patients the intestine is gangrenous and a resection and end-to-end anastomosis are performed. Rarely the whole of the midgut is considered non-viable and intestinal resection in such cases is associated with a high mortality and morbidity. In such patients a second look 48 h after a Ladd's operation may allow a more limited resection.

Postoperative care

Duodenal ileus may require nasogastric aspiration and intravenous fluid and calorie replacement until full oral feeds can be tolerated.

Complications

Recurrent volvulus rarely occurs unless one has inadequately treated a volvulus neonatorum. Adhesions causing an intestinal obstruction at a subsequent date may occur in up to 10% of cases and are associated with a mortality. Malabsorption and failure to thrive often follow a massive intestinal resection. This 'short gut' syndrome will need careful monitoring of the biochemical state and replacement of fluid, electrolytes and calories. An anastomotic leak may occur if a resection has been necessary, especially if large lengths of bowel are ischaemic and there has been an attempt to preserve intestinal length.

Jenuno-ileal atresia: stenosis

Surgical pathology

There are two main theories for the pathogenesis of intestinal atresia. In the first (Tandler, 1902) there is a failure of recanalization of the bowel following the proliferation of the intestinal epithelium which occurs in the 6–7 mm embryo. This theory does not explain the findings in patients with absence of part of the bowel and in some of these lanugo, epithelial squames and bile may be detected in the meconium distal to a complete atresia. These findings led to the 'vascular accident theory' for the causation of intestinal atresias.

In this second theory it is suggested that intestinal ischaemia during intra-uterine life will lead to resorption of the affected intestine (Figure 54.29) if it is empty, to produce a septum (type I), fibrous cord (type II) or a complete gap (type III). If the bowel lumen was full of meconium at the site of an intra-uterine perforation it will cause a chemical peritonitis resulting in a meconium peritonitis. Calcification seen on preoperative plain radiographs allows early diagnosis of this complication. In patients with intestinal atresias the pathologist can often establish evidence of meconium peritonitis on microscopical examination of the resected specimen.

The vascular accident theory has been subjected to experimental proof in studies with pregnant bitches (Louw and Barnard, 1955; Louw, 1959). Between the 45th and the 55th day of their pregnancy the uterus was opened and the fetal abdomen of the puppy explored. The blood supply to a segment of intestine was interrupted and the bowel replaced in the abdomen. Finally the maternal uterus was closed and the bitch allowed to go to term. A normal delivery was

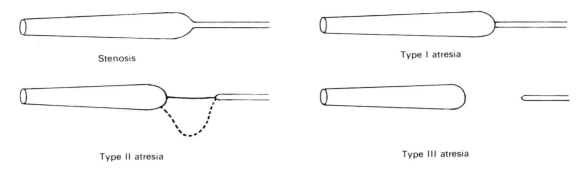

Stenosis

Type I atresia

Type II atresia

Type III atresia

Multiple/Single

Figure 54.29 Types of jejuno-ileal stenosis and atresia

obtained in 38 animals and in those puppies born 12–14 days after an intra-uterine operation lesions were found similar to those found in the human. Thus for jejuno-ileal atresias the vascular accident theory has more support than the failure of vacuolization proposed by Tandler in 1902. Further evidence in support of this conclusion is the low incidence of other congenital malformations in infants with jejuno-ileal atresia.

Surgical management

Operation

1. RESECTION: END-TO-BACK ANASTOMOSIS (Nixon)

The abdomen is opened through a transverse supra-umbilical muscle-cutting incision. The site of the atresia, which may be single or multiple, is identified and any predisposing factor such as volvulus or bands is corrected. The grossly dilated and hypertrophied bowel proximal to the atresia is resected and an end-to-back anastomosis using interrupted 4/0 silk sutures is used to restore continuity (Figure 54.30). Prior to the anastomosis the patency of the collapsed distal bowel is confirmed by injecting normal saline into the bowel lumen and watching the fluid content pass down to the ileocaecal valve. Colonic atresias are so rare that it is not necessary to check for the patency of the colon in these patients.

2. LIMITED RESECTION: GASTROSTOMY: TRANSANASTOMOTIC FEEDING TUBE

In some patients with a high jejunal atresia it is impossible to resect the grossly dilated bowel proximal to the atresia. It is therefore safer to restore continuity and to establish a gastrostomy and transanastomotic feeding tube (cf. duodenal atresia).

3. REFASHIONING OF JEJUNUM (JEJUNAL TAPERING)

An alternative operation in high jejunal atresia is to reduce the calibre of the jejunum proximal to the atresia by refashioning (Figure 54.31) and then to restore continuity by end-to-end anastomosis.

Postoperative care

Prolonged nasogastric aspiration, replacement of fluid and electrolytes and parenteral nutrition are required until full oral feeding can be tolerated.

Complications

EARLY

Aspiration pneumonia should be avoidable by efficient nasogastric aspiration and nursing care. An anastomotic breakdown may be due to the disparity in size between the proximal and distal bowel which

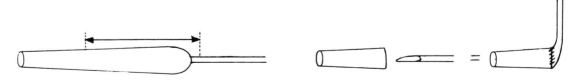

Nixon end-to-back anastomosis

Figure 54.30 End-to-back anastomosis (Nixon) for restoring continuity in jejuno-ileal atresia. Single-layer anastomosis with 4/0 silk sutures

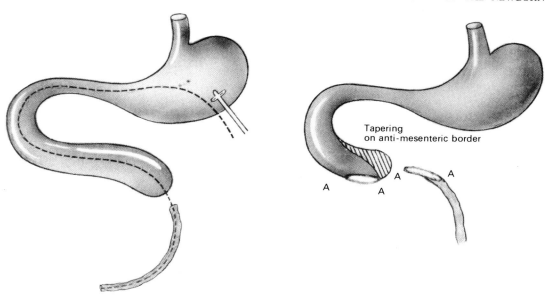

Figure 54.31   Tapering jejunoplasty used for restoring continuity in high jejunal atresia when resection of the proximally dilated bowel is impracticable

increases the technical difficulty of the anastomosis. At re-exploration the anastomosis can be either refashioned or oversewn. Metabolic complications are common and are related to the initial dehydration and prolonged therapy in the postoperative period. Hypokalaemia, hypocalcaemia and hypomagnesaemia may require urgent treatment.

LATE

Malabsorption may be due either to loss of intestinal length or to the development of a secondary disaccharide intolerance. Adhesions can cause an acute intestinal obstruction or be a contributory factor in the causation of malabsorption. Failure to thrive may cause delayed growth and development in these patients. Growth often returns to normal by 1–2 years of age as compensation for loss of intestinal length occurs.

Meconium ileus

Surgical pathology

Fibrocystic disease of the pancreas is genetically determined by an autosomal recessive gene with a recurrence risk in future pregnancies of 1 in 4. In 10–15% of such patients the abnormal viscid meconium and deficient pancreatic secretions cause a bolus type of intestinal obstruction in the neonatal period. The level of the obstruction is usually in the distal ileum but may occur at jejunal and colonic levels. Proximally the bowel is distended and hypertrophied. Dis-

tally the bowel is small and collapsed to produce a 'microcolon' effect. Volvulus and perforation of the distended loop of intestine may occur prenatally or postnatally, leading to meconium peritonitis, intestinal atresia or bacterial peritonitis (Figure 54.32).

Surgical management

Operation

The abdomen is opened through a transverse supraumbilical muscle-cutting incision. The findings are as described above and only rarely is there any difficulty in diagnosing the condition. The operation of choice is the Bishop–Koop ileostomy (Bishop and Koop, 1957) (Figure 54.33). The bowel is inspected and any volvulus is untwisted. The grossly distended bowel is resected proximal to the apex of the obstruction caused by the rabbit-type pellets of abnormal meconium. The distal end of the bowel is brought out as an ileostomy in the right iliac fossa after anastomosing the end of the proximal bowel to the side of the distal ileum. No attempt is made to clear the intestinal content from the bowel lumen except immediately adjacent to the line of the resection.

An alternative method of surgical treatment is to correct the volvulus, resect any gangrenous and/or dilated bowel, to wash out the inspissated meconium with acetyl cysteine and then restore continuity with an end-to-end anastomosis. This procedure does mean a considerable amount of handling of the intestine which may be associated with a protracted postoperative course. Total parenteral nutrition is necessary in some patients with meconium ileus and meconium peritonitis.

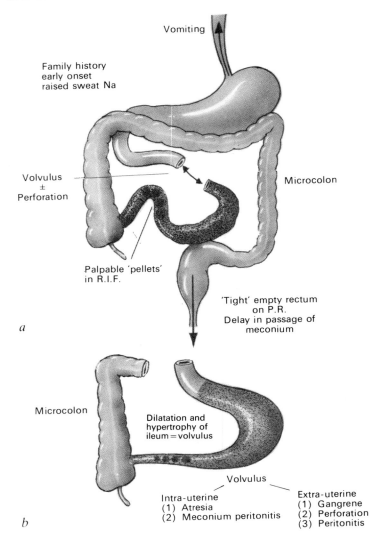

a

b

Figure 54.32   *a*, Clinical features of meconium ileus. *b*, Pathological findings in meconium ileus

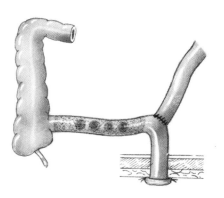

Figure 54.33   Bishop–Koop ileostomy

Conservative treatment is possible in some patients, as the obstruction can be relieved by the hygroscopic effect of a Gastrografin enema. It is not suitable in patients with a volvulus and it is unfortunate that this complication is so common (60%).

Postoperative care

Postoperatively the infant is on intermittent nasogastric aspiration and replacement and maintenance intravenous fluids. Oral Pancrex (pancreatin) (125 mg in 5 ml N saline) is given 4-hourly after aspirating the stomach. Similarly, Pancrex is instilled into the ileostomy stoma using a syringe and a short soft catheter. Initially this is started 24 h after the operation and given at 2-hourly intervals. Within 48–72 h the meconium distal to the stoma liquefies and is passed per rectum. Oral feeding is then started using 5% dextrose and followed by half- and full-strength milk feeds. Specially prepared predigested feeds are well tolerated in such infants (Pregestimil). By the 7th–10th postoperative day the stools should be normal and the fluid losses from the ileostomy will decrease: this now acts as a mucous fistula.

Intraperitoneal closure of the ileostomy is undertaken at a second-stage operation prior to discharge home. Final confirmation of the diagnosis is made either by measuring the tryptic activity of duodenal juice or by measuring the sodium content of a sample of sweat obtained by iontophoresis.

Complications

EARLY

Anastomotic leak may occur as the blood supply to the bowel is reduced in some patients and exploration with further intestinal resection may be required. Failure to thrive is due to multiple factors related to the primary pathology, operation and infective complications.

LATE

Pulmonary complications eventually result in the majority of these patients becoming respiratory cripples. The patients often die in childhood or early adult life from the sequelae of their fibrocystic disease, including complications such as intestinal malabsorption, portal hypertension and liver failure.

Hirchsprung's disease

Surgical pathology

Hirchsprung's disease is due to the congenital absence of ganglion cells (Figure 54.34) from the myenteric (Auerbach's) and submucosal (Meissner's) plexus of the bowel wall. The aganglionosis is always distal, involving the sphincter zone, and extends proximally: the length of this proximal extension varies from patient to patient. If the disease is confined to the bowel distal to the apex of the sigmoid loop, it is known as 'short-segment' disease (65% of patients). Extension of the disease proximal to this point is called 'long-segment' disease (35% of patients). Occasionally the disease extends upwards to involve the small bowel and in rare cases up as high as the stomach. 'Ultra-short segment' disease is used as a subdivision of short-segment disease, the segment between the normal and aganglionic bowel (transitional zone) lying below the reflection of the pelvic peritoneum. Skip lesions have been reported but must be extremely rare and should not be considered in the day-to-day management of an infant with Hirschsprung's disease. The innervation of the bowel is from neuroblasts which migrate down the vagal trunk; this embryological feature may therefore account for the rarity of skip lesions.

In the affected intestine the characteristic histological and histochemical findings are absent ganglion cells, an increase in the number of abnormal medullated nerve fibres and an excess of cholinesterase. Inflating a balloon in the rectum of a normal subject causes relaxation of the anal sphincter. In the patient with Hirschsprung's disease the response is different as

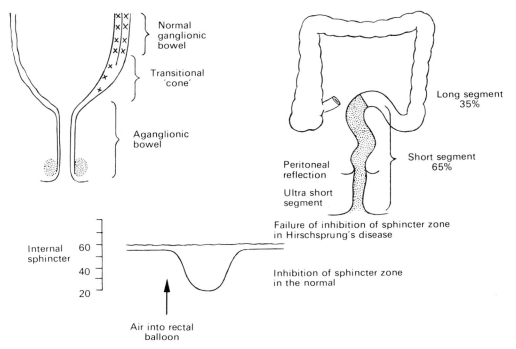

Figure 54.34 Surgical pathology of Hirchsprung's disease

there is no recordable inhibition or relaxation of the sphincter. It has been possible to use these differences of anorectal physiological response for the clinical diagnosis of Hirschsprung's disease (Figure 54.34).

Surgical management

Clinical features

The incidence of Hirschsprung's disease varies between 1 in 2000 to 1 in 5000 live births. It is more common in boys (M:F, 5:1) but in long-segment disease the sex ratio is equal. Genetic factors are important in the aetiology of the disease as a family history may be elucidated in up to 20% of patients. There is a higher incidence of Down's syndrome and urinary tract disorders in patients with Hirschsprung's disease.

It is essential to establish an early diagnosis if the lethal complications of the disease are to be avoided. The commonest method of presentation is with subacute intestinal obstruction in the neonatal period (75%); there is vomiting, abdominal distension and rectal signs such as delay in the passage of meconium and a tight and empty rectum on digital examination and explosive decompression of the bowel on removal of the finger. Diarrhoea commonly occurs after the 1st week of life (25%) and may become severe with its own associated mortality. Distension, leading to perforation of the caecum, is an unusual presentation and is probably associated with competence of the ileocaecal valve. The classic presentation described of the infant with severe constipation and a megarectum is unusual in modern paediatric practice with the emphasis on early diagnosis. Only in this way can the mortality be reduced.

Operations

POLICY

Intestinal decompression with a colostomy or enterostomy is the treatment of choice and if performed in the 1st week of life reduces the incidence of enterocolitis. Histological confirmation of the diagnosis can be obtained by combining this operation with intestinal biopsy above and below the cone or transitional zone. Definitive surgery should never be undertaken until histological confirmation of the diagnosis has been obtained, either by rectal or intestinal biopsy.

Radiological examination with straight films and contrast studies may assist in establishing a diagnosis. Care must be taken in interpreting the results of barium enema examinations to demonstrate the transitional zone (cone), as false positives and false negatives may be obtained. Measurement of the alterations in anorectal physiology with pressure transducers and recorders can assist in diagnosis.

In some patients it is possible to perform the definitive operation as a primary procedure, after suitable preparation with rectal washouts and correction of dehydration and infection. More commonly, and often safer, is careful staging of the surgical operations, i.e. preliminary colostomy or enterostomy. The definitive operation is then delayed until the infant weighs at least 5 kg. In some patients the colostomy closure is performed at this time, but in others it is closed as a third stage. There are three standard definitive operations for the surgical treatment of Hirschsprung's disease: an abdominoperineal pull-through (Swenson), a double-barrelled pull-through using the enterotome (Duhamel) and the mucosal stripping operation, leaving a muscular tunnel through which normal bowel is pulled and anastomosed (Soave) (Figure 54.35).

1. TRANSVERSE COLOSTOMY: ENTEROSTOMY (Figure 54.36)

It is vital to choose the correct site for the colostomy or enterostomy. First it must be in normal ganglionic bowel. Secondly, the positioning of the colostomy depends on the length of aganglionic intestine, e.g. in short-segment disease a right transverse colostomy will allow resection of the aganglionic segment without disturbing the colostomy, i.e. it protects the distal anastomosis following the definitive corrective surgery. In long-segment disease the colostomy should always be positioned in normal bowel immediately adjacent to the cone, thus preserving intestinal length for use at the definitive operation.

A transverse supra-umbilical incision either to the left or right of the midline is used. Inspection of the bowel reveals dilatation and hypertrophy proximal to the transitional zone, the bowel distal being collapsed and of normal calibre. The intestine is then biopsied above and below the cone and the site for the colostomy is selected.

The colostomy is usually sited to the right of the middle colic artery, as the bowel will depend on this blood vessel after excision of the aganglionic intestine. The flimsy greater omentum is dissected free from its attachment to the area chosen for the colostomy. A catheter sling is then passed through the mesocolon and the wound is closed around the loop of transverse colon.

Six non-absorbable sutures are used to anchor the colostomy, being seromuscular on the bowel wall and peritoneal on the abdominal wall side. This is important in order to prevent prolapse of the colostomy, which is one of the commoner complications. The incidence of this complication can be reduced by making the colostomy extremely 'tight' at the time it is established.

The colostomy is opened with cutting diathermy and sutured to the skin with interrupted mucocutaneous non-absorbable sutures. The ends of the rubber catheter acting as the spur are then folded on themselves and tied. This prevents the spur slipping out, but these ends should be sutured to the skin to

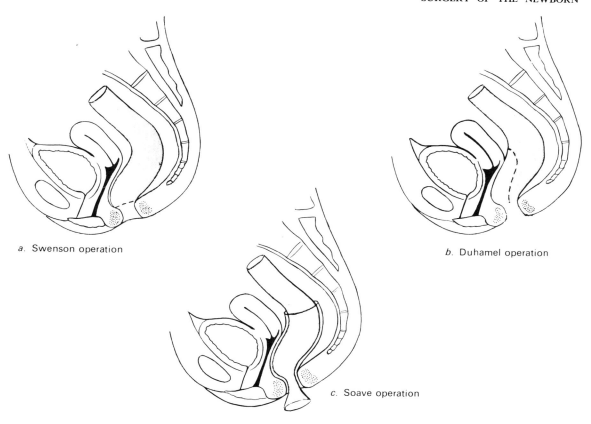

a. Swenson operation

b. Duhamel operation

c. Soave operation

Figure 54.35 Schematic representation of the three basic definitive operations used for the surgical treatment of Hirschsprung's disease

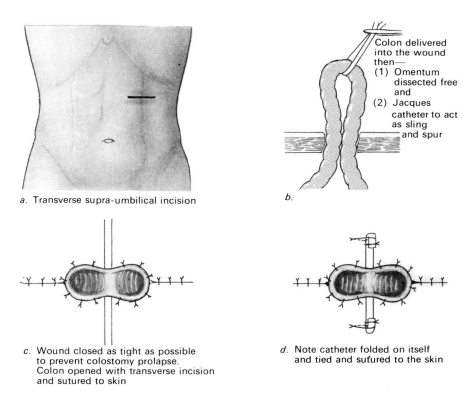

a. Transverse supra-umbilical incision

b.

Colon delivered
into the wound
then—
(1) Omentum
dissected free
and
(2) Jacques
catheter to act
as sling
and spur

c. Wound closed as tight as possible
to prevent colostomy prolapse.
Colon opened with transverse incision
and sutured to skin

d. Note catheter folded on itself
and tied and sutured to the skin

Figure 54.36 Transverse colostomy: operative technique

Intestinal Biopsy

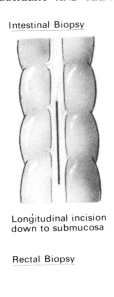 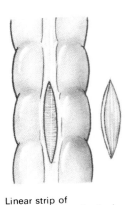 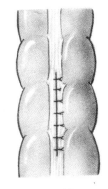

Longitudinal incision
down to submucosa

Linear strip of
circular and longitudinal
muscle removed

Closure with
int. silk sutures

Rectal Biopsy

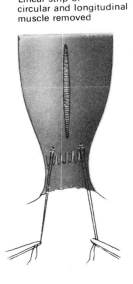

Mucosa and submucosal
biopsy through anus in the
midline posteriorly.
Note stay sutures and
retractors will aid exposure.
Linear incision closed
with continuous 3/0 chromic

Figure 54.37   Diagnosis of Hirschsprung's disease by intestinal and rectal biopsy

prevent rotation of the spur, which is likely to occur in an active infant. A full-thickness piece of colon from the colostomy is sent for histology to confirm the presence of ganglion cells.

2. CLOSURE OF THE COLOSTOMY

A full intraperitoneal closure is required. The skin is incised circumferentially around the stoma and extended along the line of the previous incision. The muscle of the abdominal wall is then separated from the bowel wall and mesocolon by careful dissection and with upward traction the afferent and efferent limbs of the colostomy are delivered into the wound. In the infant it is then necessary to excise the stoma and restore continuity with end-to-end anastomosis using a single layer of interrupted silk sutures. The wound is then closed in layers leaving a fine sliver of a corrugated drain down to the site of the anastomosis.

3. BIOPSY OF THE INTESTINE AND RECTUM (Figure 54.37)

This may be done as an elective operation, e.g. rectal biopsy, or as part of a laparotomy to relieve intestinal obstruction from Hirschsprung's disease, i.e. intestinal biopsy.

Intestinal biopsy.   The site for the biopsy is selected and is linear along the taenia coli. The bowel is held between the finger and thumb to compress the linea, leaving the taenia uppermost. Then using iridectomy scissors the seromuscular layer is excised in a strip. With care and practice the mucosa and submucosa are left intact. The edges of the seromuscular wound are then closed with interrupted silk sutures. It is usually necessary to biopsy the bowel above and below the cone, thus confirming the diagnosis and delineating the extent of the disease.

Rectal biopsy.   The methods are available using

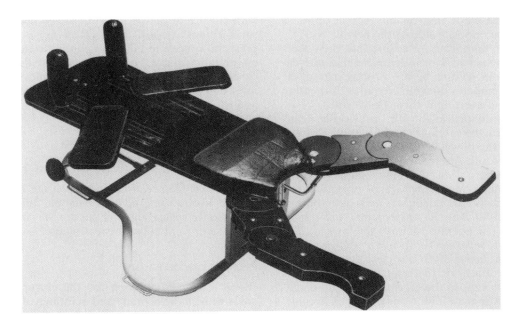

Figure 54.38 Stephens' table for operation on infants in the Trendelenburg–lithotomy position

either a suction biopsy technique or a linear strip of mucosa and submucosa from the posterior wall of the rectum. The former of these methods is better as it avoids tearing of the mucosa, which may occur at the time of the definitive procedure. Both methods require careful histological examination by a pathologist experienced in this type of work; serial sections and specific histochemical techniques are helpful in most patients in confirming the diagnosis.

4. SWENSON'S OPERATION (Figure 54.35a)

The infant is positioned in the extended Trendelenburg–lithotomy position using a special table (Stephens') which is strapped in position on the normal adult operating table (Figure 54.38). The abdomen is opened through a long left paramedian incision from the costal margin to the pubic symphysis. Any adhesions are divided and the small intestine is packed away into the right upper abdomen. The colon is inspected and the 'cone' identified by the marker sutures at the site of the previous intestinal biopsies. The splenic flexure, descending colon and sigmoid colon are mobilized onto their own mesentery by dividing their peritoneal attachments.

The rectum and sigmoid are pulled upwards and initially to the right, in order to incise the peritoneum just medial to the left ureter; this incision is carried forwards in a curve anteriorly to the posterior wall of the bladder. It is important to display the whole course of the left ureter. Similarly with the rectum and sigmoid pulled upwards and to the left, the peritoneum is incised medial to the right ureter and

extended anteriorly to meet the opposite incision on the surface of the bladder. The incision in the right mesocolon is extended upwards towards the third part of the duodenum exposing the inferior mesenteric artery and vein which are ligated and divided. This leaves the left side of the colon dependent on the blood supply through the marginal artery from the middle colic artery.

The posterior pelvic dissection is started by identifying the presacral nerve and freeing the superior pedicle from the lower aorta and down to the sacral promontory. The presacral space is entered with the finger in the midline and the rectum is separated from the sacrum down to the level of the coccyx.

Anteriorly the posterior surface of the bladder is identified together with the vasa and seminal vesicles, which are held anteriorly with a malleable copper blade retractor of the appropriate size. Gentle dissection with pledgets on straight forceps is used to separate the anterior structures from the rectum. It is important at this stage to stay as close to the rectal wall as possible.

In the female the anterior dissection can be made easier by suturing the uterus to the wound edges with stay sutures. The plane between the rectum and posterior vaginal wall is incised with scissors and opened by blunt dissection with a pledget on straight forceps: this plane between the rectum and the posterior wall of the vagina is opened down to the floor of the pelvis.

Finally the lateral ligaments on each side are identified and as these contain the middle haemorrhoidal artery it may either be divided between ligatures or diathermized, keeping close to the rectal wall. The ligaments can be made taut on the rectum upwards and towards the opposite side of the pelvis.

It is extremely important to ensure that the dissection down to the pelvic floor is complete circumferentially around the rectum before proceeding to the final stage of the operation which requires transection of the bowel and everting it through the anus.

The bowel is divided at the level previously determined and a straight vascular clamp is applied proximally. Distally the bowel is invaginated and is closed with interrupted silk sutures. Care at this stage must be taken to ensure that the blood supply to the normal ganglionic bowel, which will be brought down for the anastomosis, is adequate, and that there is sufficient length so that the anastomosis will not be under tension. The operator goes to the lower end of the table with a separate scrub nurse and assistant, the first assistant being left to complete the abdominal part of the operation. At the lower end the buttocks are separated to expose the anus (Joll's thyroid self-retaining retractor is useful for this purpose). Sponge-holding forceps are inserted into the anus and passed upwards into the rectum, being guided by the abdominal operator. The forceps are opened and closed in order to grasp the invaginated end of bowel just below the level of the transection. The distal rectum and anal canal can be evaginated by gentle traction and left hanging freely. Inspection of the everted bowel mucosa should reveal the anal valves in the anterior, lateral and posterior position, thus confirming that the pelvic dissection was adequate.

The everted bowel is divided longitudinally in the anterior position to expose and open the rectal wall; this is extended to 1 cm from the anal valves. Curved ductus arteriosus forceps are passed through this opened bowel to grasp the prepared ganglionic bowel. It is important to ensure that the vascular pedicle is lying posteriorly and that the bowel is not twisted. This proximal bowel is pulled and guided from above so that it appears below through the incised everted rectum and anal canal.

The anastomosis is now completed. Initially the bowel is sutured with a single non-absorbable suture in the anterior position, which is used as a stay suture. The everted rectum is pulled laterally and is divided with cutting diathermy to just beyond the left lateral position and a further stay suture is inserted. The procedure is then repeated for insertion of the right lateral stay suture. The everted rectum is now left attached posteriorly and the bowel anastomosis is held by the anterior and lateral sutures. The final part of the bowel is then divided and the proximal and distal bowel are held by inserting a posterior stay suture. The anastomosis is now completed by placing interrupted sutures between adjacent stay sutures. When the anastomosis is complete the stay sutures are divided but left long; the anastomosis is pushed gently through the anus with a finger to take up its normal position.

The abdominal part of the operation is completed with closure of the peritoneum of the pelvic floor. A small infant suction drain (Redivac) is left in the presacral space and taken out lateral to the wound by an extraperitoneal route. The pelvic floor is then closed with a continuous 3/0 chromic suture. The intestines are then replaced into their normal position and the wound is closed.

Specific pre- and postoperative care

PRELIMINARY ENTEROSTOMY: COLOSTOMY

The specific feature after this procedure is that nasogastric aspiration and intravenous fluids may be required for several days as the stoma is made tight in order to prevent subsequent prolapse.

CLOSURE OF COLOSTOMY

Blood is always required for the closure of a loop colostomy in the neonate and in infancy. Preoperative bowel preparation with neomycin or cephradine and metronidazole is advisable.

RECTAL BIOPSY

Careful observation must be made postoperatively for evidence of continuing hidden haemorrhage. This can usually be prevented by closing a posterior linear biopsy with a continuous chromic catgut suture. This complication is less likely to occur if a suction biopsy technique is used. Similarly the incidence of pelvic cellulitis and peritonitis is reduced by this technique.

SWENSON'S OPERATION

Preliminary washouts of the bowel distal to the colostomy are used to prepare the bowel. In long-segment disease mechanical preparation of the intestine with 'Golytely' (a polyethylene glycol electrolyte solution produced by Braintree Laboratories Inc., Braintree Mass., USA) is very effective and safe in neonates and young infants (Wheeler *et al.*, 1991). Broad-spectrum antibiotic cover is also given pre- and postoperatively. The bladder is catheterized and emptied immediately prior to surgery. This catheter is not required postoperatively as micturition in the infant is reflex and retention of urine is not seen as a complication. A presacral suction drain (Redivac: infant) is left *in situ* and removed after 48 h.

Complications

PRELIMINARY ENTEROSTOMY: COLOSTOMY

The persistence of the pre-existing enterocolitis may be life threatening. Prolapse of the colostomy is not uncommon and occasionally a cutaneous fistula is seen at the site of one of the seromuscular and peritoneal sutures. Wound infection is common.

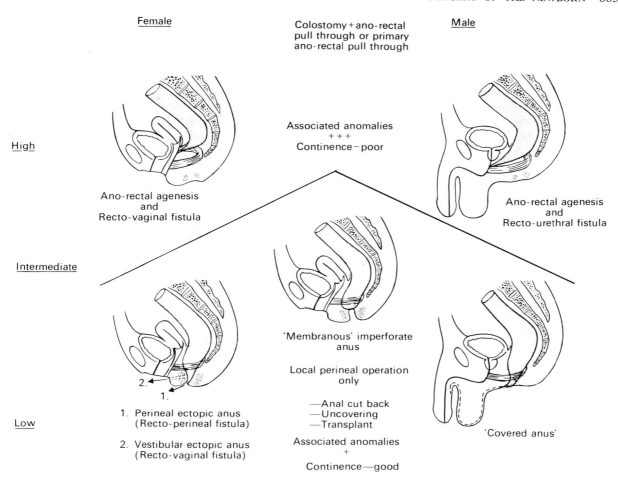

Figure 54.39 Schematic representation of the different types of congenital anorectal malformations. The classification depends on the relationship of the anomaly to the level of the pelvic floor (levator ani)

CLOSURE OF COLOSTOMY

Nasogastric aspiration and intravenous fluids are required until the anastomosis opens up. An anastomotic leak is rare. Wound infection is common.

RECTAL: INTESTINAL BIOPSY

Haemorrhage which may be hidden. A localized intraperitoneal abscess or peritonitis may complicate an intestinal biopsy, especially if the mucosa and submucosa were opened. In some patients this complication may follow a local perforation from enterocolitis.

SWENSON'S OPERATION

An anastomotic leak is the most serious complication and needs a defunctioning colostomy or enterostomy to control the pelvic cellulitis: stricture as a sequelae is often seen. Haemorrhage into the presacral space also acts as a focus for infection. Wound infection and postoperative ileus are not uncommon. Errors in assessing the length of aganglionic intestine should not occur if adequate intestinal biopsies have been obtained and carefully examined. Damage to the autonomic nerves during the pelvic dissection may cause urinary incontinence and impotence as a late sequelae. These complications are avoidable by a meticulous surgical technique.

Anorectal malformations

Surgical pathology

Congenital anorectal anomalies are subdivided into two main groups (Santulli *et al.*, 1970). In high anomalies the rectum ends above the level of the pelvic floor and usually has a fistulous communication with the viscus lying anteriorly, i.e. the posterior urethra in the male and the vagina in the female. In low anomalies the rectum has passed through the pelvic floor and opens onto the surface in an abnormal position which is usually anterior to the normal anus, e.g. vestibular ectopic anus in the female, 'covered' anus in the male (Figure 54.39). A very rare intermediate type of anomaly is caused by a membranous obstruction at the junction of the developing proctodeum and hindgut. In classifying anorectal malformations a plea is made for the use of descriptive terminology rather than the use of numerical classifications, also to avoid the term 'imperforate anus' unless used to describe the rare intermediate type.

Congenital anomalies are often found in association with anorectal malformations such as vertebral anomalies, urinary tract malformations, gastrointestinal and cardiovascular defects. These associated defects are often serious and adversely alter the prognosis for the infant (Stephens, 1963).

Surgical management

Clinical features

The diagnosis of a congenital anorectal malformation is easy; it is all too apparent, provided the anus has been inspected and examined as an essential part of the routine examination of the newborn. There can be no excuse for delay in diagnosis.

Differentiation between the different types of anorectal malformation is more difficult and is dependent on experience and further investigation. It is vitally important to determine whether the lesion is a high or low one as the surgical treatment and results, particularly concerning continence, are largely dependent on this fact.

The standard method used to establish the diagnosis is to take a straight lateral radiograph of the infant upside down centred on the greater trochanter (Wangensteen method) and with a radio-opaque marker on the anus. A line is then drawn between the symphysis pubis and the tip of the sacrum (Stephens' pubococcygeal line). If a shadow of gas in the rectum is seen above the pubococcygeal line the anomaly is a low one; if below, the anomaly is a high one (Figure 54.40). False positives and false negatives may occur with this simple investigation; variations may occur due to the age of the patient (unreliable under 24 hours of age), sacral anomalies and the viscosity of the meconium. Despite these reservations the technique is easy and reliable for diagnosis in the majority of patients.

Another method used to differentiate the type of anomaly requires the use of contrast material. The perineum is explored with a needle and syringe; if air or meconium is obtained, some radio-opaque contrast is injected into the space (20% Hypaque) and lateral views taken to determine the relationship of the viscus to the pelvic floor.

Air in the bladder or meconium on the tip of the penis are indicative of high defects with a recto-urethral fistula. Similarly in the covered anus in the male white or green meconium may be seen anterior to the anus which is covered with an inverted V fold of skin which merges with the median raphe on the scrotum. In the female a careful search must be made for any ectopic opening in the vulvar, vestibular or perineal regions.

Operations

POLICY

The correct surgical treatment requires accurate diagnosis. High anomalies are treated with a temporary colostomy, followed by a definitive operation which includes either an abdomino-anorectal pull-through or a posterior sagittal anoplasty. The colostomy is closed as a third-stage procedure. Argument exists about the optimum time and type of operation for the definitive operation, but early operation in the first few months of life is recommended. In selected patients a primary single-stage abdomino-anorectal pull-through operation is satisfactory. In patients with low anomalies a colostomy is not required as surgical treatment with a local perineal operation gives excellent results in the majority of patients.

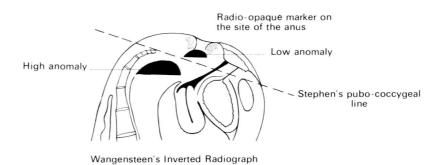

Figure 54.40 Diagnosis of high and low anorectal anomalies by observing the position of gas in the distal bowel when the infant is radiographed in the inverted position. A lateral radiograph is taken centred on the greater trochanter

TRANSVERSE COLOSTOMY

With high anorectal anomalies a left transverse colostomy is the standard treatment. Operative details have already been described (see page 878).

ABDOMINOPERINEAL ANORECTAL PULL-THROUGH

This operation is either performed in the neonatal period as a primary procedure or is deferred until the infant is 1 year of age if a preliminary colostomy has been used. The principle of the operation is to ligate the fistula and to pull the bowel through the pelvic floor into the perineum to form a new anus. The success of the operation depends on the bowel being pulled through anterior to the puborectalis sling which is closely wrapped around the posterior urethra at the site of the fistula. Failure to achieve this will impair results as continence in the high anomalies is largely dependent on an efficient anorectal angle due to the sling effect of the puborectalis muscle.

The infant is placed in position in the Trendelenburg–lithotomy position using a special table designed for the purpose (see Figure 54.38). The bladder is catheterized and an efficient scalp vein infusion is established. The incision is a left long paramedian. The bladder is mobilized by dividing the urachus and applying traction. In the female the uterus may be pulled forwards by stay sutures between the skin edge and around the Fallopian tube. These manoeuvres will allow adequate visualization of the pelvis and in the male will help to lift up the prostatic urethra.

The abdominal phase starts with an incision in the peritoneum medial to the course of the right and left ureters. These incisions meet anteriorly on the posterior part of the bladder. The presacral space is entered by blunt dissection, taking care to leave the pelvic autonomics either in the mesentery of the rectum or laterally, so that the bladder innervation is not jeopardized.

The fistula to the posterior urethra or vagina is identified and ligated after transfixation. It is important to ligate the fistula as close to the urethra as possible without damaging or narrowing the urethra. This is facilitated by passing a metal bougie into the bladder before transfixing the fistula.

The rectum is mobilized so that there is sufficient length to bring the bowel down to the perineum without any tension.

The perineal dissection starts with the excision of an ellipse of skin (or a cruciate incision) over the site of the anus. The external sphincter is identified in the subcutaneous tissues and is split in the midline. A metal bougie is passed into the urethra which acts as a guide in making the tract from the anus upwards to the site of the ligated fistula. Curved artery forceps or divulsors are passed along this tract which can then be gently stretched with graduated Hegar's dilators. The bowel can then be grasped and pulled through

this tract and down to the perineum. The rectum is sutured to the pelvic floor with chromic catgut sutures in the midline and laterally. The rectal mucosa is sutured to the skin edges using interrupted silk sutures.

The abdominal wound is closed leaving an infant suction drain into the presacral space (Redivac).

POSTERIOR SAGITTAL ANORECTOPLASTY

A preliminary colostomy is established. A course of preoperative irrigations distal to the colostomy are given. The bladder is catheterized with a no. 8 Fr. gauge Foley and the site of the anus identified using an electrostimulator. The infant is operated on in the frog position.

The midline skin incision extends from the midsacrum through the site of the anus to the perineum. The sphincteric muscle is identified and the coccyx is split in the sagittal plane. The levator ani is split in the midline and dissected from the smooth longitudinal muscle coat of the rectum. The bowel is then mobilized by sharp and blunt dissection.

The bowel is opened in the midline to identify the associated fistula to the bladder, prostate or bulbar urethra. The submucosal plane is used to identify the fistula which is then transected and closed. The bowel is mobilized to obtain sufficient length to suture it to the site of the anus. The sphincters are repaired and the wound is closed. Occasionally tapering of the distal bowel is required (de Vries and Pena, 1982; Pena and de Vries, 1982).

ANAL CUTBACK

This operation is suitable for low anomalies in the female, e.g. ectopic anus, rectovestibular fistula or rectoperineal fistula.

The newborn is held in the lithotomy position and a sound is passed into the ectopic opening to ascertain its direction and size. The blade of straight scissors is then inserted and a cut is made in the midline posteriorly to enlarge the opening. The mucosa and skin margins of the enlarged opening are sutured with interrupted silk sutures.

'LAYING OPEN' A COVERED ANUS

This operation is a minor modification of the anal cutback procedure. The fistulous tract on the scrotum is identified and a probe passed backwards along the tract to pass through the anus and into the rectum. The ridge of skin with the apex lying anteriorly covers the normal site of the anus. This is excised using straight scissors in the horizontal plane, thus exposing the normal anus with its identifiable anal columns and valves. The anus is dilated up to a no. 12 or 14 Hegar and mucocutaneous silk sutures are inserted.

Postoperative care

TRANSVERSE COLOSTOMY

See under Hirschsprung's disease (page 877).

ABDOMINO-ANORECTAL PULL-THROUGH

Blood transfusion may have been required at the time of operation; further loss should be watched for by regular inspection of the infant Redivac drainage bottle. Nasogastric aspiration and intravenous replacement are continued until the aspirates are non-bile stained, abdominal distension is absent and bowel sounds have returned. Oral feeding can start after the first colostomy action or bowel action. Antibiotics are used for the first 7 postoperative days.

Dilation of the new anus and rectum are started after the 10th postoperative day and continued daily or at regular intervals until the healing is complete and the anus is supple; this may take several months.

ANAL CUTBACK

Apart from the anal dilatations no specific treatment is required.

'LAYING OPEN' A COVERED ANUS

Regular dilatations are required after the 7th postoperative day. Following this and after discharge home these are continued by the mother who has received careful instruction in performing this procedure.

Complications

In all anorectal malformations close supervision is required for some years because some children will develop a secondary megarectum as a late complication. This complication is preventable if adequate long-term follow-up care and assessment are undertaken.

TRANSVERSE COLOSTOMY

See under Hirschsprung's disease (page 878); see also page 885.

ABDOMINO-ANORECTAL PULL-THROUGH

Early: Retraction of the bowel may be due to inadequate mobilization of the bowel and is therefore preventable. Peritonitis due to contamination can cause postoperative ileus, localized abscess formation and adhesions. Stricture may be ischaemic in origin or due to inadequate preparation of the pathway for the bowel through the pelvic floor.

Late: Stenosis occurs at the mucocutaneous junction and may require dilatations or operative correction by an anoplasty. Mucosal prolapse and bleeding require similar treatment. Incontinence is the main problem as the results of this operation are disappointing in at least 50% of the patients. The degree of continence is dependent on accurate technique, which results in the bowel being pulled through anterior to the puborectalis sling. If the puborectalis sling is palpated anterior to the pulled-through rectum some improvement may be obtained by a secondary pull-through operation. In some patients the best results are obtained with a terminal left iliac colostomy. Calculi can form in a small pocket at the site of the recto-urethral fistula. Rarely an abscess forms at this site and may rupture intraperitoneally.

ANAL CUTBACK

Either stricture or stenosis may occur if the cutback has been inadequate. Occasionally the levator ani may be damaged if the cutback has been too radical. Secondary megarectum due to inefficient defaecation can be prevented in most patients by careful supervision, regular rectal examinations and with the help of a sensible and cooperative mother. Aesthetic complications occur in adolescence due to the appearance of the perineum. The 'shotgun' perineum described by Sir Denis Browne is aesthetically displeasing but functionally adequate. Further surgery in such patients should be resisted as bowel control may suffer.

'LAYING OPEN' A COVERED ANUS

Either stenosis or secondary megarectum may occur. Both are preventable and bowel control in these patients is normal.

'Idiopathic' neonatal intestinal obstruction

Surgical pathology

A newborn infant presenting with subacute intestinal obstruction may mark the onset of further complications such as gangrene and perforation of the bowel secondary to ischaemia or inflammation. Advances and changes in obstetric and paediatric care and resuscitation of premature infants may account for the increased incidence of such cases in recent years.

The pathological findings in these infants (Figure 54.41) depend on many factors including the timing of exploration laparotomy. Simple necrosis leading to perforation with little inflammatory response is seen in some patients; in others the necrosis is associated with inflammation in the bowel wall immediately adjacent to the site of the perforation. Necrosis, inflammation and widespread haemorrhagic exudate maximal in the submucosa and mucosa may be seen in others with more widespread changes (disseminated intravascular coagulation). In the final sub-

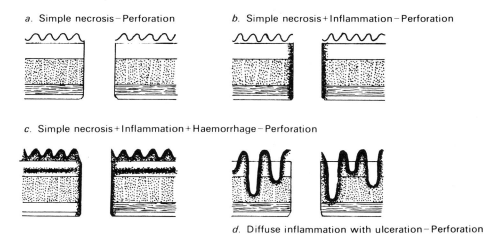

Figure 54.41 Surgical pathology of necrotizing enterocolitis

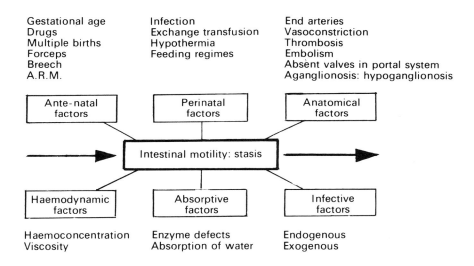

Figure 54.42 Factors of aetiological significance in necrotizing enterocolitis

group similar findings are associated with diffuse acute inflammatory changes and pneumatosis of the bowel wall (necrotizing enterocolitis).

These pathological changes may result in gangrene and perforation of the bowel, localized abscesses or generalized peritonitis. Septicaemia is common and accounts for the high mortality. Active medical and surgical treatment can result in full recovery, but in others the recovery is complicated by subacute or acute intestinal obstruction secondary to adhesions and stricture formation. The operative findings resemble the different types of intestinal atresia found in the newborn (see Figure 54.29), thus suggesting that ischaemia is a significant factor in their causation. At operation the bowel is found to be gangrenous with patent pulsatile vessels up to the margin of the intestine. Thus it appears that the changes seen are secondary to alteration in blood flow through the intrinsic intramural vessels lying in the submucosa of

the bowel. Severe anoxia and other stressful factors may cause intense vasoconstriction of these intramural vessels ('diving reflex'). Many factors may initiate this physiological response in the newborn which leads to mucosal damage, stasis, infection and their sequelae (Figure 54.42). Breast feeding has been shown to provide a protective effect in the experimental animal, but necrotizing enterocolitis is sometimes found in the breast-fed and full-term infant.

Surgical management

Clinical features

Different antenatal and perinatal factors are important in these infants, e.g. prematurity, anoxia, multiple births, cold injury, exchange transfusion, alteration in feeding regimens (milk plug syndrome: Cook and

Rickhan, 1969; faecal plug syndrome: Zachary, 1957), stercoral ulceration, infection, particularly with *Clostridium difficile*, drugs, hypothyroidism, hypoplastic left colon syndrome, abnormal meconium (meconium plug syndrome), the use of intra-arterial cannulas and leaching of polymers from such catheters. Similarly it can be seen as a complication secondary to stasis, cf. Hirschsprung's disease and congenital anal stenosis. Stasis or hypomotility of the bowel is therefore an important common denominator and the infection found in some of these patients is endogenous rather than exogenous in origin (Figure 54.42).

There is often a prodromal phase: the onset of such changes may be marked by jaundice, apnoea and cyanotic attacks in premature infants during the first 2 days of life. Then signs of subacute intestinal obstruction develop with abdominal distension and vomiting of bile. The signs at this stage will be intermittent and resemble those seen in patients with Hirschsprung's disease. It is very rare to find a premature infant with Hirschsprung's disease. Later, as signs advance, the obstruction becomes more obvious as the distention increases. The umbilicus may become everted and inflamed with a red flare radiating from it. Tenderness on palpation and abdominal masses may develop. Diarrhoea and blood in the stool become apparent and are serious signs. Perforation of the bowel with a dramatic increase in the size of the abdomen due to a pneumoperitoneum is not uncommon; finally, faecal peritonitis and abscess formation occur.

A straight X-ray of the abdomen may show a pneumoperitoneum with air under the diaphragm, evidence of intestinal obstruction with fluid levels and distended loops, gas in the bowel wall or even within the portal system. The latter sign is of serious prognostic significance.

Treatment

POLICY

The clinical problem in the management of these patients is to decide whether they need an operation or whether they can be safely treated by conservative measures. It is better to resect gangrenous bowel before perforation occurs rather than to find faecal peritonitis on exploratory laparotomy. Faecal peritonitis in the premature infant is associated with complications which may adversely affect the morbidity of the condition and severely limit the choice of operative procedures.

CONSERVATIVE TREATMENT

The principles of management are to rest the bowel, treat the infection, maintain the internal environment, feed the infant and monitor carefully the changes which herald perforation of the intestine.

All oral feeding is stopped and a nasogastric tube is passed (no. 8 Fr. or no. 10 Fr. gauge), aspirated at regular intervals and left on free drainage. The aspirates are replaced intravenously with an equal volume of normal saline.

Antibiotics are given intravenously: either cephalosporins or gentamicin and Pyopen (carbenicillin) and metronidazole. Oral antibiotics are given to reduce the bacterial flora in the lumen of the bowel.

Replacement infusions of fresh blood and plasma are required in severe cases. Low molecular weight Rheomacrodex (dextran) can be used to improve the blood flow in the small vessels in the wall of the intestine (10–20% of the blood volume may be administered over 2 h).

Observations of central or core temperature and peripheral temperature, pulse and respiratory rate are monitored and also regular measurements of the abdominal girth are recorded (see Appendix I).

Serial straight radiographs of the abdomen are taken and repeated at 12 h, 24 h or longer intervals, depending on the clinical response of the patient. Careful note is taken of distended loops, fluid levels, faecal content and intramural gas and any alterations seen on repeated radiographs. Progressive dilatation of the same loop of intestine suggests toxic dilatation and impending gangrene and perforation. Pneumoperitoneum with gross abdominal distension producing respiratory embarrassment is an absolute indication for surgery. Localized perforations may become walled off by adjacent loops of bowel and are not absolute indications for surgery, but at a later date adhesions, strictures and abscesses may require surgical treatment.

Conservative measures can be performed for long periods with the aid of parenteral nutrition, thus allowing reparative healing to occur. In some patients oral feeding can be re-established, in others subacute obstruction persists due to structure formation, and is associated with failure to thrive which is a further indication for surgery.

OPERATIONS

Operation is reserved for patients in whom conservative treatment has failed or when complications develop.

Laparotomy. The abdomen is opened through a transverse supra-umbilical muscle-cutting incision. It is important to examine carefully the length of the gastrointestinal tract, looking for areas of gangrene, focal areas of necrosis, haemorrhages and perforation. The bowel wall is like wet tissue paper and great care in handling is necessary.

Intestinal resection and primary anastomosis. Nonviable bowel is resected and continuity restored by primary anastomosis. Resections may be single or multiple and involve jejunum, ileum and colon.

Intestinal resection and exteriorization. Resection and primary anastomosis are not always possible due to the extent of the disease, the degree of peritoneal soiling and doubts about the viability of the bowel. In such patients a proximal stoma is established (ileostomy, colostomy), the bowel is resected and the distal bowel is brought out as a mucous fistula through a separate stab incision. At a second-stage operation continuity can often be restored.

Colostomy: ileostomy. In some patients the bowel is considered to be viable, but doubts may exist about the precise diagnosis, e.g. Hirschsprung's disease. It is then necessary to biopsy the wall of the intestine and rectum and defunction the bowel by a proximal stoma. After recovery and if the biopsy is normal the stoma is closed at a second-stage operation when the infant is thriving and weighing about 5 kg.

Drainage of intraperitoneal abscess. Occasionally, localized abscesses in the right iliac fossa or subphrenic space may require treatment and drainage.

'Second-look' operations. In some patients the length of bowel involvement is so extensive that surgical resection is incompatible with survival. Under such circumstances the abdomen is closed and intensive conservative measures are indicated. After an interval of 2–4 days the abdomen can be explored and a more limited resection may be possible in some patients. The average length of the intestine for the duodenojejunal junction to ileocaecal valve in the neonate is 200 cm. Loss of intestinal length of up to two-thirds of this can still result in survival and reasonable growth and development.

Postoperative care

The principles of postoperative care are the same as for the preoperative conservative management of such patients and have been outlined in this section and in the introduction.

Complications

EARLY

Septicaemia and overwhelming infection may cause death of the patient early in the course of the disease. Clostridial infections are found in this group of patients and gas in the biliary tree on the straight radiograph is a serious prognostic sign but is not invariably fatal as was originally thought. Peritonitis and abscess formation occur. Wound infection and dehiscence and faecal fistula secondary to a breakdown of an intestinal anastomosis or a further perforation are not unusual.

LATE

Adhesions and strictures producing subacute obstruc-

tion, failure to thrive and secondary disaccharide intolerances are seen. Later acute intestinal obstruction from bands is seen. Loss of intestinal length (short gut syndrome) may interfere with growth and development.

APPENDIX I
Routine nursing observations of the surgical newborn
Either: (1) Nurse in a warm room temperature (27°C)
Or: (2) Nurse in an incubator, temperature 30–33°C or overhead heated cot.

Temperature recorded at 1-hourly intervals.
Pulse rate observation at $\frac{1}{2}$–1-hourly intervals by listening to apex beat.
Respiratory rate at $\frac{1}{2}$–1-hourly intervals.

Inspection of i.v. site at 1-hourly intervals.
Measurement of abdominal girth at 2–4-hourly intervals.
Nasogastric aspiration at $\frac{1}{2}$–1-hourly intervals and to be left on free drainage in between. Check position of end of catheter at 2-hourly intervals.

Change position of newborn at 2-hourly intervals.
Care of the mouth 2–4 hourly.
Care of eyes 2–4 hourly.
Restraining mittens to be checked every 4 h to prevent a cotton thread causing a ring constriction gangrene.
Care of the wounds and dressing.
Observations of urine stream, volume and frequency.
Meconium passed is saved for inspection and recorded.
Daily weighing.
Measurements of skull circumference (occipito-frontal) at weekly intervals.
Testing for phenylketonuria with the Guthrie test before discharge home.
The neonate should have been on normal feeds for 8 days before testing.
Regular cleansing with cottonwool when in incubator and daily bath when in cot.

Chest physiotherapy 1-hourly. Careful suction of mouth and nasopharynx.

Care of chest drains, gastrostomy tubes and transanastomotic feeding tubes.

Nursing care of a neonate on a ventilator
1. Infant is specialled throughout the 24 h.
2. Nurse flat with head extended.
3. Careful fixation of ventilator tubes.
4. Prevention of blockage of endotracheal tube by:

   (a) Instil 0.5 ml normal saline $\frac{1}{2}$–hourly and immediately after endotracheal aspiration. The nurse wears sterile gloves for the procedure. Disposable catheter used once only.
   (b) Any rise in ventilator pressure is indicative of blocking or kinking.
   (c) Emergency trolley for reintubation should be immediately available.

5. Care to eyes and mouth.
6. Use special care chart to record:

(a) Infant's TPR on a graph.
(b) Incubator temperature.
(c) Room temperature.
(d) Oxygen concentration.
(e) Peripheral circulation.
(f) Position of infant.

7. Observations of the ventilator:
(a) Rate.
(b) Inspiratory pressure.
(c) Expiratory pressure.
(d) Blow-off valve.
(e) Oxygen concentration.
(f) Oxygen and air (litres/min).

APPENDIX II
Essential equipment for a neonatal surgical unit
Respirators (Vickers Neovent).
Apnoea alarms (Vickers Mk III).
Oxygen monitor (Hudson).
Roberts' pumps.
Paediatric (90 ml) underwater pleural drainage sets.
Cardiorators (Hewlett Packard).
Incubators: overhead heaters (Ohio): Bassinets.
Intravenous infusion pumps (Ivac Corporation).
Chest vibrator (Pifco).
Electric thermometers.
Oxygen and CO_2 cutaneous monitor (Radiometer).
Oxygen cutaneous monitor (Kontron).
Phototherapy unit (Vickers).
Handley constant infusion pumps.
Doppler blood pressure equipment (Sonicaid).
Electric heating blankets.
Infant inflating bags (Penlon Cardiff).
Electronic nebulizers (Mistogen Equipment).
Portable oxygen cyclinders for incubators (BOC).
Anaesthetic resuscitation equipment.
Blood gas analyser.
Bilirubinometer.
Osmometer.
Blood glucose analyser (Ames).

References

Atwell, J. D. (1966) Magnesium deficiency following neonatal surgical procedures. *J. Pediatr. Surg.*, **1**, 427–440

Atwell, J. D. (1968) The early diagnosis and surgical treatment of Hirschsprung's disease in infancy. *Proc. R. Soc. Med.* **61**, 339–340

Atwell, J. D. (1971) Pitfalls in the diagnosis of intestinal obstruction in the newborn. *Proc. R. Soc. Med.*, **64**, 374–377

Atwell, J. D. and Beard, R. C. (1974) Congenital anomalies of the upper urinary tract associated with oesophageal atresia and tracheo-oesophageal fistula. *J. Pediatr. Surg.*, **9**, 825–831

Atwell, J. D. and Harrison, G. S. M. (1980) Observations on the role of oesophagogastrotomy in infancy and childhood with particular reference to the long-term results and operative mortality. *J. Pediatr. Surg.*, **15**, 303–309

Berman, E. J. (1958) Extralobar (diaphragmatic) sequestration of the lung. *Arch. Surg.*, **76**, 724–731

Bernstein, P. (1940) Gastroschisis, a rare teratological condition in the newborn. *Arch. Pediatr.*, **57**, 503–505

Bianchi, A., Doig, C. M. and Cohen, S. J. (1983) The reverse latissimus dorsi flap for congenital diaphragmatic hernia repair. *J. Pediatr. Surg.*, **18**, 560–563

Bishop, H. C. and Koop, C. E. (1957) Management of meconium ileus: resection. Roux-en-Y anastomosis and ileostomy irrigation with pancreatic enzymes. *Ann. Surg.*, **145**, 410–414

Bloss, R. S., Turmen, T. and Beardmore, H. E. (1980) Tolazoline therapy for persistent pulmonary hypertension after diaphragmatic repair. *J. Pediatr.*, **97**, 984–988

Bohn, D. J., Filler, J. R. M., Ein, S. H. *et al.* (1983) The relationship between $PaCO_2$, and ventilation parameters in predicting survival in congenital diaphragmatic hernia. *J. Pediatr. Surg.*, **18**, 666–671

Bond-Taylor, W., Starer, F. and Atwell, J. D. (1973) Vertebral anomalies associated with oesophageal atresia and tracheo-oesophageal fistula with particular reference to the initial operative mortality. *J. Pediatr. Surg.*, **8**, 9–13

Bulgrin, J. G. and Holmes, F. H. (1955) Eventration of diaphragm with high renal ectopia: case report. *Radiology*, **64**, 249–251

Cantrell, J. R., Haller, J. A. and Ravitch, M. M. (1958) A syndrome of congenital defects involving the abdominal wall, sternum, diaphragm, pericardium and heart. *Surg. Gynecol. Obstet.*, **107**, 602

Carter, C. O. (1961) Genetic factors in pyloric stenosis. *Proc. R. Soc. Med.*, **54**, 453–454

Collins, D. L., Pomerance, J. J., Travis, K. W. *et al.* (1977) A new approach to congenital postero-lateral diaphragmatic hernia. *J. Pediatr. Surg.*, **12**, 149–155

Cook, R. C. M. and Rickham, P. P. (1969) Neonatal intestinal obstruction due to milk curds. *J. Pediatr. Surg.*, **4**, 599–605

Corkery, J. J., Dubowitz, V., Lister J. *et al.* (1968) Colonic perforation after exchange transfusion. *Br. Med. J.*, **4**, 345–349

de Vries, P. and Pena, A. (1982) Posterior sagittal anorectoplasty. *J. Pediatr. Surg.*, **17**, 638–643

Duhamel, B. (1963) Embryology of exomphalos and allied malformations. *Arch. Dis. Child.*, **38**, 142–147

Fitchett, C. W. and Tavarez, V. (1965) Bilateral congenital diaphragmatic herniation: case report. *Surgery*, **57**, 305–308

Forshall, I. and Rickham, P. P. (1960) Experience of a neonatal surgical unit. *Lancet*, **ii**, 751–754

Freeman, N. V. (1974) Hirschsprung's disease. *Update*, 177–190

Grob, M. (1963) Conservative treatment of exomphalos. *Arch. Dis. Child.*, **38**, 148–150

Gross, R. E. (1948) New method for surgical treatment of large omphaloceles. *Surgery*, **24**, 277–292

Harrington, S. W. (1948) Various types of diaphragmatic hernia treated surgically; report of 430 cases. *Surg. Gynecol. Obstet.*, **86**, 735–755

Holder, T. M. (1964) Transpleural versus retropleural approach for repair of tracheo-oesophageal fistula. *Surg. Clin. North Am.*, **44**, 1433–1439

Janik, J. S., Akbar, A. M., Burrington, J. D. *et al.* (1978) The role of gastrin in congenital hypertrophic pyloric stenosis. *J. Pediatr. Surg.*, **13**, 151–154

Jolley, S. G., Tunell, W. P., Hoelzer, D. J., Thomas, S. and

Smith, E. I. (1986) Lower oesophageal pressure changes with the tube gastrostomy: a causative factor of gastroesophageal reflux in children. *J. Pediatr. Surg.*, **21**, 624–627

Kitagawa, M., Hislop, A., Boyden, E. A. *et al.* (1971) Lung hypoplasia in congenital diaphragmatic hernia. *Br. J. Surg.*, **58**, 342–346

Koop, C. E. and Hamilton, J. P. (1965) Atresia of the oesophagus. Increased survival with staged procedures in the poor-risk infant. *Ann. Surg.*, **162**, 389–401

Louw, J. H. (1959) Congenital intestinal atresia and stenosis in the newborn. Observations on its pathogenesis and treatment. *Ann. R. Coll. Surg. Engl.*, **25**, 209–234

Louw, J. H. and Barnard, C. N. (1955) Congenital intestinal atresia: observations on its origin. *Lancet*, **ii**, 1065–1067

Maingot, R. (1961) Operations for sliding herniae and for large incisional herniae. *Br. J. Clin. Pract.*, **15**, 993–996

Moore, T. C. (1977) Gastroschisis and omphalocele: clinical differences. *Surgery*, **82**, 561–568

Pena, A. and de Vries, P. (1982) Posterior sagittal anorectoplasty: important technical consideration and new applications. *J. Pediatr. Surg.*, **17**, 796–811

Puri, P., Guiney, E. J. and O'Donnell, B. (1975) Total parenteral feeding in infants using peripheral veins. *Arch. Dis. Child.*, **50**, 133–136

Replogle, R. L. (1963) Esophageal atresia: plastic sump catheter for drainage of the proximal pouch. *Surgery*, **54**, 296–297

Rickham, P. P. (1952) Neonatal surgery: early treatment of congenital malformations. *Lancet*, **i**, 332–339

Rickham, P. P. (1960) Vesico-intestinal fistula. *Arch. Dis. Child.*, **35**, 97–102

Rickham, P. P. and Johnston, J. H. (1969) *Neonatal Surgery*, Butterworths, London, p. 201

Sabga, G. A., Neville, W. E. and Del Guercio, L. R. M. (1961) Anomalies of the lung associated with congenital diaphragmatic hernia. *Surgery*, **50**, 547–554

Santulli, T. V., Kiesewetter, W. B. and Bill, A. H., Jr (1970) Ano-rectal anomalies: a suggested international classification. *J. Pediatr. Surg.*, **5**, 281–287

Sherman C. D. and Waterston, D. (1957) Oesophageal reconstruction in children using intrathoracic colon. *Arch. Dis. Child.*, **32**, 11–16

Shuster S. R. (1967) A new method for the staged repair of large omphaloceles. *Surg. Gynecol. Obstet.*, **125**, 837–850

Soave, F. (1977) Megacolon: long-term results of surgical treatment. In *Progress in Pediatric Surgery*, Vol. 10, (eds P. P. Rickham, W. Ch. Hecker and J. Prévot), Urban and Schwarzenberg, Munich, pp. 141–149

Stephens, F. D. (ed.) (1963) *Congenital Malformations of the Rectum, Anus and Genito-urinary Tracts*, Churchill Livingstone, Edinburgh

Suita, S., Ikeda, K., Hayashida, Y. *et al.* (1984) Zinc and copper requirements during parenteral nutrition in the newborn. *J. Pediatr. Surg.*, **19**, 126–130

Tandler, J. (1902) Zur Entwicklung des menschlichen Duodenums im fruehen Embryonalstadium. *Morphol. Jahrb.*, **29**, 187–216

Thomas, D. F. M. and Atwell, J. D. (1976) The embryology and the surgical management of gastroschisis. *Br. J. Surg.*, **63**, 893–897

Touloukian, R. J. and Spackman, T. J. (1971) Gastrointestinal function and radiographic appearance following gastroschisis repair. *J. Pediatr. Surg.*, **6**, 427–433

Vacanti, J. P., Crone, R. K., Murphy, J. D. *et al.* (1984) The pulmonary hemodynamic response to perioperative anaesthesia in the treatment of high risk infants with congenital diaphragmatic hernia. *J. Pediatr. Surg.*, **19**, 672–679

Venugopal, S., Zachary, R. B. and Spitz, L. (1976) Exomphalos and gastroschisis: a 10 year review. *Br. J. Surg.*, **63**, 523–525

Wheeler, R. A., Davies, N., Griffiths, D. M. and Burge, D. M. (1991) The use of Golytely for bowel cleansing in the first three months of life (personal communication)

Wheeler, R. A., Najmaldin, A. S., Stoodley, N., Griffiths, D. M., Burge, D. M. and Atwell, J. D. (1990) Feeding regimes after pyloromyotomy. *Br. J. Surg.*, **77**, 1018–1019

Young, D. G. (1966) Neonatal acid-base disturbances. *Arch. Dis. Child*, **41**, 201–203

Young, D. G. (1968) Contralateral pneumothorax with congenital diaphragmatic hernia. *Br. Med. J.*, **4**, 433–434

Young, W. F. (1964) Practical management of the newborn in regard to their water and electrolyte needs. *Maandschr. Kindergeneesk.*, **32**, 316–334

Zachary, R. B. (1957) Meconium and faecal plugs in the newborn. *Arch. Dis. Child.*, **32**, 22

Transplantation surgery

55

Renal transplantation

T. W. J. Lennard

Renal transplantation is well-established therapy for patients with end-stage renal failure, offers the best quality of life and remains the ultimate aim for the majority of patients on long-term dialysis.

Close cooperation between the medical and surgical staff treating the patient with end-stage renal failure is vital. This enables satisfactory preparation of the potential recipient, and collaborative postoperative surveillance is greatly facilitated when all medical personnel involved work as a team.

Preoperative

In the preoperative preparation for patients awaiting transplantation, care must be taken to ensure that when a kidney becomes available the patient is in the best possible condition for surgery and its associated immunosuppression. Assessment can be divided into general, lower urinary tract and vascular components.

General

Patients must be free from infection (either acute or chronic) and this includes renal tuberculosis, dental sepsis, chronic pyelonephritis, chronic ambulatory peritoneal dialysis (CAPD) peritonitis or catheter exit-site infection, recent chest infections and infection with potentially lethal viruses such as hepatitis B or the human immunodeficiency virus. If the patient is haemodialysed, then good dialysis should be obtained with satisfactory urea, creatinine and electrolyte levels. Where the haemoglobin is less than 6 g/dl, anaemia should be corrected with blood transfusion or recombinant erythropoietin. Care must be taken to control hypertension and the control of any diabetes must be optimal.

Urinary tract and vascular

The potential site of the transplant should be assessed and removal of very large polycystic kidneys, correction of bladder neck obstruction and formation of an ileal conduit after urodynamic investigations should be carried out as required. Angiography may be needed if there is evidence of significant vascular disease, either to assess the coronary or the peripheral vascular tree.

Pre-transplant blood transfusion has been shown to confer a graft survival advantage and in some centres it is advised, therefore, that patients should undergo third-party blood transfusion prior to transplantation. Although this observation was first made in 1973, mechanisms to explain the effect have yet to be defined and more effective immunosuppressive drugs such as cyclosporin A may lessen the transfusion benefit.

The patient's tissue type, blood group and antibody status will be held on a central database and the donor tissue type, blood group and details will be entered into the database, allowing the best possible match between donor and recipient. There is little doubt that transplants with five or six HLA antigen matches have a much improved graft survival compared with less well-matched ones and this provides the strongest possible case for organ sharing. In addition, patients with a high percentage of pre-formed circulating cytotoxic antibodies due to previous transplants, blood transfusions or pregnancy should be given priority for a given kidney if they do not show any evidence of reactivity against that kidney. Patients doing badly on dialysis, for whatever reason, should be given priority for transplantation. Where possible the cytomegalovirus (CMV) status of the patient should be known and only CMV-compatible kidneys used (i.e. CMV-positive kidney transplanted to CMV-positive recipient). Failing this, appropriate prophylaxis with antiviral agents or gamma globulin should be administered if the CMV barrier is crossed.

Operative details

Host nephrectomy

The indications for host nephrectomy include large polycystic kidneys, chronic infection within a kidney, bleeding from a kidney, uncontrollable hypertension or neoplasia. The usual surgical approach is through the bed of the 12th rib, maintaining an extrapleural and extraperitoneal plane of dissection. The patient is placed in the lateral position over the break in the table (with maximum break) and an incision is made from the line of the 12th rib towards the umbilicus. The incision is deepened down through the body-wall muscles, and Gerota's fascia is easily identified once the peritoneum has been reflected anteriorly. The kidney can be palpated through its fatpad and although there is usually a good plane between fat and the capsule of the kidney in health, this is not always the case with chronic infection of the kidney where the fat can often be adherent to the kidney capsule and the kidney small and difficult to feel. This fat must be dissected off the kidney and the renal vessels identified individually and if possible ligated in continuity or cross-clamped, divided and then secured with absorbable ties. The use of non-absorbable ties on the renal artery or vein can result in a persistent sinus which can be both difficult and dangerous to deal with. The ureter is identified and traced as far distally as possible towards the bladder. After mobilization, it is cross-clamped, divided and the distal stump secured using an absorbable tie.

There is nearly always some oozing from the renal bed and it is advisable therefore to place a closed suction drain down to the area of dissection, particularly if the patient is on haemodialysis and is likely to be heparinized in the postoperative period.

The wound is closed with absorbable sutures in layers, using materials such as braided polyglactin for the muscle layers and polydioxanone for the external oblique aponeurosis.

The live donor

The potential living donor must have normal renal function equally divided between both kidneys assessed by isotope renogram or intravenous pyelogram. Tissue typing, cytotoxic cross-match testing and blood group testing will have confirmed the compatibility of the match pair, and angiography is required to define the vascular anatomy and ureters in the donor. Live donor transplants should only be performed between consenting and fully informed adults who are related genetically or by marriage.

Living donor nephrectomy is performed in a similar way to host nephrectomy, except that the plane of dissection between the fat and the kidney capsule is well defined as there is no renal parenchymal disease. The donor operation is carried out in the same or an adjacent theatre, in synchrony with the recipient operation. As much length as possible of the renal artery and vein should be obtained to facilitate the implantation of the kidney in the recipient. On the left side it is necessary to ligate and divide the left adrenal vein as it enters the left renal vein superiorly and the left gonadal vein as it enters inferiorly. The ureter together with the periureteric vessels are dissected and divided as far distally as possible. The donor kidney is removed after cross-clamping the vessels of supply and perfused (Figure 55.1) with cold washout solution. If the pleura is inadvertently opened during the nephrectomy it can be closed with a continuous 3/0 absorbable suture after maximum inflation of the lung by the anaesthetist. A closed suction drain can be left down to the bed of the kidney if required and the wound is closed in layers with absorbable sutures as for host nephrectomy.

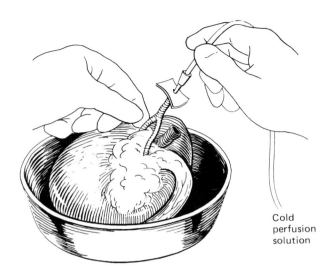

Cold perfusion solution

Figure 55.1 Donor kidney – irrigation of renal artery with cold perfusion solution

Cadaveric donors

The majority of donors will be maintained on a ventilator and all will have a confirmatory diagnosis of brainstem death made by practitioners independent of the transplant team. Cadaveric donor nephrectomy is frequently part of a multiple organ donation which might include removal of the heart, lungs, liver, pancreas and corneas. After the relatives have been counselled and consent has been obtained, the donor is usually given intravenous fluids (to include blood if necessary) and inotropes as required.

Donors who have received a head injury may have diabetes insipidus and in all cases careful attention to fluid balance is important to prevent unexpected cardiac arrest. It may be necessary to use vasopressin to reduce polyuria. The donor must be free of infection and will have been shown to have a normal or, after rehydration, an improving urea and creatinine level and to be seronegative for transmissible diseases, such as hepatitis B and human immunodeficiency virus. In addition, all potential donors should be free of transplantable carcinoma, tuberculosis and long-standing hypertension. Systemic steroids are often given prior to the organs being removed, as is intravenous heparin, to prevent sludging within the capillaries of the organs. The operation of cadaveric donor nephrectomy is carried out in exactly the same way as any general surgical operation and with the same care and precautions. Strict asepsis is observed and the procedure should be carried out in an operating theatre with attendant anaesthetic and nursing staff.

A long midline incision from xiphisternum to pubic symphysis is used and frequently combined with a median sternotomy for removal of other organs. In some cases access is improved by a cruciate abdominal incision. After laparotomy to exclude any unexpected pathology and confirm the presence of healthy kidneys, the right colon and then the left colon are raised onto their primitive mesenteries by dividing the lateral peritoneal attachments of both. Both kidneys in their fatpads will then be exposed and the vessels of supply to the kidneys can be defined, as are the ureters. Division of the right gonadal vein and the embryological attachment of the small bowel mesentery allows the right colon and small bowel to be reflected towards the head of the table, thus exposing the inferior vena cava and aorta as far rostrally as the renal vessels and the superior mesenteric artery.

Perfusion *in situ* of the organs is preferred to removal and subsequent perfusion, as the former minimizes any warm ischaemia. Organs which do not need to be perfused for the purposes of transplantation should have their vascular supply interrupted by ligation in continuity. This will include, in the majority of cases, the superior mesenteric artery passing over the left renal vein, the coeliac axis and the inferior mesenteric artery. A segment of the infrarenal aorta and cava can then be cannulated with vascular perfusion cannulae and these are secured in place with a purse-string suture around these vessels. Into the aortic perfusion cannula will be introduced icecold perfusion fluid, either of intracellular or extracellular composition. The recently described perfusion fluid from the University of Wisconsin (UW solution) can be used in an attempt to prolong cold storage times of the removed organs. The cannula into the infrarenal inferior vena cava is attached to a suction bottle, so that once perfusion has begun immediate removal of unwanted blood and perfusate can be carried out, preventing venous hypertension of perfused organs. Immediately before perfusion, the aorta above the renal arteries at the level of the diaphragm is cross-clamped (Figure 55.2). Once the organs have been perfused and cooled *in situ* they can be removed. Ventilation can be discontinued once perfusion has begun.

In multi-organ retrievals, the order of removal is heart and lungs, liver and finally kidneys. The kidneys are removed one at a time, beginning with dissection of the great vessels. The cava is opened in the midline anteriorly to well above the level of the kidneys. Inspection of the interior of the cava will identify any venous anomalies, as the orifices of aberrant veins will be clearly seen. The midline of the posterior cava is then divided, taking care to protect the underlying right renal artery. The renal veins and their caval patches are then separated from the suprarenal cava and retracted to reveal the arterial anatomy. A similar dissection of the aorta will demonstrate any aberrant vessels which can be included on the aortic patch, making the recipient operation easier and avoiding the potentially disastrous consequences of damaging a lower pole artery which may supply the ureter.

Donor lymph nodes and spleen are removed at the end of retrieval and packaged with the kidneys to enable further tissue typing to be carried out, and a final cytotoxic cross-match between recipient serum

and donor lymphocytes. It is advisable to take lengths of the common or external iliac artery and vein so that in cases where the renal artery or vein may not be long enough, jump grafts can be constructed, to facilitate the transplant. Each kidney (together with the extra lengths of artery and vein from the iliac system) is placed into perfusion fluid in a sterile plastic bag which in turn is placed into a second plastic bag and secured. The bags are then deposited each in a separate insulated box, appropriately labelled (R. and L.) containing ice and are ready for transport to the recipient centre (Figure 55.3).

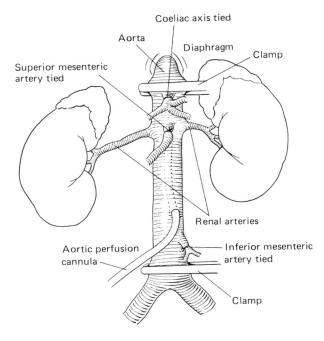

Figure 55.2 Position of clamps, cannula and ligated branches at the time of aortic perfusion

Static cold preservation is satisfactory for up to 48 h, particularly if the kidneys have been removed without warm ischaemia as a result of *in situ* perfusion. It is a legal requirement to complete the donor operation form, which should accompany the donor organ with full details of the donor kidney, its preservation and anatomy and the names of the surgeons involved in the donor nephrectomy.

The organization of cadaveric donor nephrectomy is greatly facilitated by the transplant coordinator. This post is often filled by a senior nurse who is able to help in counselling of the bereaved family and also advising the donor hospital what is involved and required, since the donor hospital may be unfamiliar with the procedure of cadaveric donor nephrectomy.

Recipient operation

Where possible, the tissue type of the donor will have been obtained from peripheral blood analysis prior to organ removal. A shortlist of potential recipients will have been drawn up and these patients will have been assessed for fitness to undergo transplantation at the recipient centre. Early involvement of the anaesthetic staff is important and, where necessary, preoperative dialysis should be carried out promptly to reduce cold storage time of the donor organ to an absolute minimum.

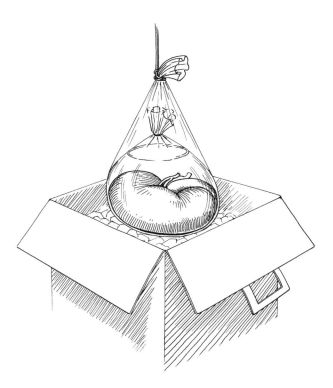

Figure 55.3 Donor kidney – enclosure in two sterile plastic bags and preservation in unsterile ice

Once the final cytotoxic cross-match test has shown no reaction between recipient serum and donor lymphocytes, the recipient should be informed of the result of the test and counselled with regard to the likely outcome following transplantation. Two fears are commonly present in the minds of the recipient: (a) lack of immediate function, and (b) rejection. Recipients should be advised that immediate function does not always occur although, in the majority, transplant function occurs promptly, obviating the need for subsequent dialysis. Delayed primary function, however, should not be a cause for undue concern in the recipient, and if he or she is warned of this preoperatively, anxiety is much reduced.

The majority of transplant recipients will exhibit some degree of rejection and it is advisable to warn them of this. Many transplant centres provide their dialysis patients with a booklet outlining what happens at the time of transplantation and this is helpful in the preparation of potential recipients. Recipients

should be told that rejection can usually be rapidly and promptly diagnosed and reversed and that acute rejection does not necessarily mean loss of the kidney. A full discussion of the varied immunosuppressive regimens available is beyond the scope of this text, but these drugs are usually begun prior to, or at time of, operation, as are broad-spectrum prophylactic antibiotics.

The recipient will be placed supine on the operating table, and after preparation with a suitable antiseptic an extraperitoneal incision is made in the chosen iliac fossa. Either groin can be used for the right or left kidney, so the choice of side will depend on previous transplants, local factors (CAPD exit site, conduit) and coexistent vascular disease in the recipient. A curved suprainguinal incision running between the anterior superior iliac spine and the pubic tubercle is used. After division of the fat and subcutaneous tissues, the external oblique muscle aponeurosis will be divided in the line of its fibres and the internal oblique and transversus abdominus muscles divided, usually with cutting diathermy. Great care should be taken with haemostasis, especially if the patient is on haemodialysis and is to be heparinized for dialysis in the early postoperative period. After division of the body wall muscles, the inferior epigastric vessels will be seen running superiorly and somewhat laterally and these should be cross-clamped, divided and secured with absorbable ties. In the male, the spermatic cord will be seen and in the female the round ligament. The former should be taped and protected and the latter can be divided to facilitate access to the iliac vessels. The peritoneum can be reflected off the external iliac vessels with a combination of sharp and blunt dissection. In patients who have had CAPD peritonitis, this can be a difficult plane and care should be taken not to open the peritoneum as this can make subsequent CAPD difficult if not impossible in the early postoperative period. Any peritoneal opening should be immediately closed with a continuous absorbable suture. The peritoneum and its contents should be reflected off the external iliac vessels as far as the origin of the internal iliac artery. Exposure is maintained by a variety of retractors. Perhaps the most useful is the Omnitract retractor (CLS Medical Ltd), which allows a number of blades to be inserted to facilitate exposure of the vessels and the bladder for transplantation.

Lymphatics coursing over the external iliac artery and vein are secured with small metal clips or fine 4/0 non-absorbable ties to minimize the risk of postoperative lymphocele. Tapes should be passed around the external iliac artery and vein and these vessels fully mobilized. While there are usually no branches of the external artery, the vein not infrequently has small stumpy posterior branches running directly backwards and care must be taken to identify these before traction is placed on the vein or forceps passed around the vein to mobilize it. The external iliac artery should be palpated to assess any atheromatous plaques and where possible the internal iliac artery should be exposed and palpated.

Several factors will influence the choice of the arterial vessel to be used. Haemodynamically, an end-to-end anastomosis between the internal iliac artery and the recipient renal artery is preferable. This is only possible where there is a satisfactory length of internal iliac artery, no extensive atheroma present and where there is a single artery on the donor kidney (Figure 55.4). Care must be taken when mobilizing the internal iliac artery and dividing its early

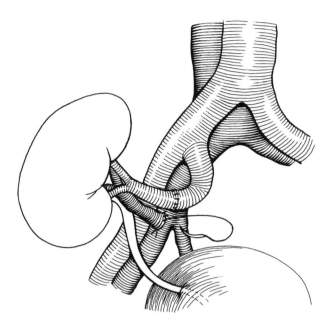

Figure 55.4 Recipient operation – the renal artery may be united end to end with the internal iliac artery. Inset shows stay suture facilitating accurate visualization of vascular anastomosis

branches, since the corresponding vein lies very close to the artery and can be damaged. The internal iliac artery should not be used bilaterally when there has been a previous transplant in a man because of the risk of impotence. Multiple donor arteries need to be anastomosed onto the external iliac artery, preferably with a patch of aorta, or if they are disparate some bench surgery may be required to anastomose the smaller renal vessels end to side to the major donor artery using interrupted 6/0 prolene. If the external and the internal iliac vessels appear small (particularly in children or women), the anastomosis should be made more proximally and the common iliac artery or aorta used. The external iliac vein generally will be the vein of choice, but the common iliac or the inferior vena cava can also be used if a more proximal artery is used.

Once the artery of supply has been identified, the area where the arteriotomy will be made should be confirmed, taking care to avoid any obvious atheromatous patches. Before beginning the transplant,

ensure the ureter of the donor kidney is positioned inferiorly and the kidney is wrapped in ice-cold saline-soaked swabs to reduce warming. It is customary to make the venous anastomosis first and the vessel receiving the renal vein (usually the external iliac) will be controlled with a side-biting atraumatic venous clamp. The venotomy is made using a no. 11 blade, avoiding the same horizontal plane as the arteriotomy so that the venous and arterial anastomoses do not overlap (Figure 55.5). Stay sutures of 5/0 prolene are then placed either side of the venotomy after flushing the vein with heparinized saline. The venotomy should be made a few millimetres smaller than the diameter of the donor renal vein to prevent any purse-stringing or stenosis of this low-pressure system. The donor artery and vein should be trimmed in length to avoid kinking when the kidney is placed in its final position at the end of the operation. The venous anastomosis is then completed using continuous 5/0 prolene. It is conventional to use a separate suture for each side of the anastomosis to prevent purse-stringing. The chosen recipient artery is clamped opened and flushed with heparinized saline. Stay sutures can then be placed and the anastomosis performed either with interrupted or continuous 5/0 prolene sutures in the same way as the vein.

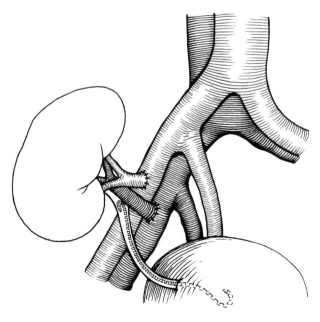

Figure 55.5 Recipient operation – end-to-side anastomosis of renal artery and renal vein to external iliac artery and external iliac vein with anastomosis of donor ureter to the mucosa of the bladder and placement of a double 'J' stent

The anastomosis time for the artery and vein is noted, since a prolonged second warm ischaemia time may result in increased primary non-function. Once the two vascular anastomoses have been completed, the venous clamp is removed first, followed by the distal clamp on the arterial system and then the proximal arterial clamp. It is not unusual for some bleeding to occur from the suture lines, but avoid the temptation to place sutures immediately to control this since it often stops with gentle swab packing and time. The hasty placement of additional sutures in the presence of a blood-filled field can cause more damage than good. If, after a couple of minutes, there continues to be obvious bleeding from a defect in either anastomosis this can usually be reinforced with a single suture. In addition, some small hilar vessels may be identified which are bleeding and these can be controlled with diathermy, small sutures or metal clips. Exceptionally it may be necessary to reclamp the donor vessels and repeat one of the anastomoses if, on the initial reperfusion, there is an obvious defect such as arterial stenosis, an intimal flap or uncontrollable bleeding.

During the anastomosis, it is usual for the anaesthetist to give the recipient 500 mg of methyl prednisolone and in some centres 200 ml of 20% mannitol is given to help induce a diuresis.

Once the vascular anastomoses are completed, attention is turned to the ureteroneocystotomy. The bladder can usually be identified easily in the midline, just behind the symphysis pubis, and it often has several large veins coursing over it. These veins should be controlled with diathermy and the bladder opened for 6 cm between tissue forceps or stay sutures. The bladder is a very vascular organ and it is helpful to incise it with cutting diathermy and secure all bleeding points before attempting to implant the ureter. If the bladder is small and contracted following a long period of anuria, then preoperative placement of a urinary catheter may assist in its accurate identification.

Once opened, the bladder can be checked visually and microbiological swabs of any urine present sent for culture and sensitivity. A tunnel is made in the side of the bladder using a suitable curved artery forceps, extending into the submucosal plane of the bladder for approximately 2 cm, and the ureter is then introduced along this tunnel. Once it is inside the bladder, the end of the ureter can be trimmed to produce a fishmouth or spatulated end. Interrupted 3/0 catgut sutures are then used to anastomose the full thickness of the ureter to the mucosa of the bladder. The small vessels of supply which run along the ureter should be secured with a fine 3/0 catgut tie. This will reduce the risk of postoperative haematuria and clot retention. A temporary stent can be left in the ureter if required as a splint (see Figure 55.5).

Once the ureter has been secured with three or four interrupted catgut sutures, the bladder is lavaged with heparinized saline, all the clots are removed and it is closed in two layers of continuous absorbable suture material. As an alternative to opening the bladder and performing the anastomosis from within, the onlay technique can be used. The ureter is then sutured directly onto a small opening in the bladder using a series of 3/0 absorbable sutures, and no formal cystotomy is required. A final check is made of the anastomoses and the hilum of the kidney to ensure that these are not bleeding and two extraperitoneal closed suction drains are then placed down to the anastomoses and the bladder. The wound is then closed with interrupted absorbable sutures to the muscle layers and continuous nylon or polydioxanone to the external oblique aponeurosis. After the abdominal wound has been closed a urinary catheter is inserted into the bladder and connected to a urinometer. Patients are returned to a specialist area, which might be either an intensive care unit or a dedicated organ grafting unit for the immediate postoperative period, so that monitoring of fluid input and output can be carried out, along with regular estimations of urea, creatinine and electrolyte levels.

Postoperative complications

Postoperative complications can be minimized and often anticipated as a result of careful clinical monitoring, regular biochemical and haematological checks and routine scans. Palpation of the transplant site should take place twice a day, noting any change in the size of the graft or any tenderness. The general condition of the patient is observed, looking particularly for evidence of fever, general malaise or fluid retention. In addition, regular monitoring of the blood level of immunosuppressive agents where possible and assessment of creatinine clearance will provide valuable information on the continuing progress of the transplant and the adequacy or otherwise of immunosuppression. Maintenance preventive anti-rejection drugs include azathioprine, cyclosporin A, FK 506 and low-dosage prednisolone, and in the treatment of acute rejection episodes high-dose prednisolone, antilymphocyte globulin and monoclonal anti-T-cell antibodies can be used.

Imaging the kidney with radioisotopes will give valuable information on perfusion of the graft and ultrasound scans will provide an accurate assessment of dilatation of the urinary tract. It is not uncommon with rejection to see a moderate degree of dilatation of the calyces and this is usually readily distinguished from more distal ureteric obstruction by ultrasound. Core biopsy is the gold standard for the diagnosis of rejection and in some centres fine-needle aspiration cytology and intrarenal manometry are equally good at distinguishing rejection from other causes of transplant malfunction.

Complications can be categorized into those which are immunological and those which are non-immunological.

Immunological

Immunological complications should include infection but, following the use of cyclosporin A, wound and other local infections, which used to occur when large doses of steroids and azathioprine were used, are now rarely seen. Problems with systemic infection can occur when multiple immunosuppressive agents are used to control severe rejection. These include *Pneumocystis carinii*, cytomegalovirus infection and systemic bacterial infection from indwelling dialysis lines, CAPD or bladder catheters.

Rejection, although classically presenting with a tender enlarged kidney associated with fever and diminished urine output, can present as a wide spectrum of clinical syndromes, ranging from virtually no systemic features or local clues (the so-called smouldering and silent rejection) to a fulminant acute picture with collapse and deranged blood clotting, hypertension and severe systemic toxicity. In the majority of instances acute rejection can be reversed (see above) but on occasions, if the patient is systemically unwell or if there has been an associated split in the kidney due to oedema and swelling, then transplant nephrectomy may be required. One of the most important and sometimes difficult decisions to make is when to abandon further immunosuppressive therapy and remove a transplanted kidney. There is often the temptation to continue additional immunosuppressives to salvage a graft when perhaps the better option would be to remove the severely damaged and rejected kidney and allow the patient to recover for a subsequent transplant. Transplant nephrectomy is a difficult operation, often with considerable blood loss, and the transplanted kidney is usually oedematous, soft and friable. Because of the associated swelling, it can be difficult to identify the vessels of supply to the kidney and care must be taken not to damage the external iliac vessels when the renal artery and vein are cross-clamped.

Wherever possible, all donor tissue should be removed, including arterial and venous patches, and if necessary a vein patch should be taken from the recipient's saphenous vein and used to prevent stenosis of the external iliac artery after its closure. For this reason the ipsilateral groin should always be prepared and accessible at the time of transplant nephrectomy. If, however, the transplant has been *in situ* for a long period of time, it can be difficult if not impossible to identify accurately the renal artery and figure of 90% 1-year survival should be achieved in patients who are receiving their first cadaveric transat the hilum is preferable.

Non-immunological failures

Non-immunological failures include arterial or venous occlusion, leading to infarction of the kidney. In most series these vascular accidents account for around 3% of transplant losses. In the case of arterial thrombosis, renal function deteriorates rapidly and may not be associated with any pain. In a venous infarct there is again rapid deterioration of transplant function, but the kidney becomes acutely oedematous and swollen and it can be difficult to differentiate this from acute rejection. An isotope perfusion scan will usually help in this differential diagnosis.

Bleeding can occur rarely from the arterial anastomoses or from small vessels in the hilum of the kidney, and any swelling occurring suddenly in a graft, particularly around the time of haemodialysis, should raise the suspicion of haemorrhage. Urgent exploration of the transplant is required to control the bleeding. Later vascular sequelae include renal arterial stenosis. This may present as hypertension, which is difficult to control, or deteriorating renal function. Angiography with balloon dilatation of the stenosis is a common first-line treatment. If this fails, it can be followed by corrective surgery for the stenotic vessel. Ureteric problems include leakage of urine in the early post-transplant period which is usually manifested by painful swelling in the region of the kidney in the face of continued reasonable function and biochemical evidence of urine in the drains or coming from the wound. Urinary leaks can present late after transplant when there has been primary non-function and only become apparent when the kidney produces urine.

Urinary fistulas in transplanted individuals on immunosuppression rarely obey the laws of fistulas applicable elsewhere in general surgery and do not tend to close spontaneously. Early exploration is therefore advised and the usual source of the leak is at the neo-ureterocystotomy. Reimplantation of the ureter or additional sutures to secure it to the bladder are required. Occasionally, the ureter will have infarcted and in these instances it must be judged whether it is possible to anastomose the bladder onto the pelvis of the kidney if this is still viable. If the bladder cannot be mobilized to permit this, then it may be possible to anastomose the pelvis of the kidney to the native host ureter.

Ureteric stenosis can also occur in the postoperative period, presenting as an acute diminution in renal function with ultrasound evidence of a dilated collecting system. This is best treated by antegrade percutaneous nephrostomy. A nephrostogram can be performed giving an outline of the collecting system and identifying the site of the obstruction. Once transplant function has been stabilized through the percutaneous nephrostomy, it may be possible to place a stent across the stenosis, again by the percutaneous route, or it may be necessary to carry out corrective open surgery to relieve the cause of the obstruction.

It is difficult to quote an overall success rate for the operation of renal transplantation because there are many different circumstances which may increase or decrease the likelihood of successful engraftment. A figure of 90% 1-year survival should be achieved in patients who are receiving their first cadaveric transplant with a reasonable HLA match. The majority of transplant failures occur within the first 3 months after operation due to acute rejection. There is a much slower attrition rate thereafter due largely to chronic rejection, an as yet poorly understood phenomenon.

56

Transplantation of the liver and pancreas

Sir Roy Calne

Liver transplantation

Liver transplantation was first performed in man by Starzl *et al.* (1963). The operation was slow to develop because it is a formidable assault in patients who are by definition in the last phase of terminal liver disease and there is nothing equivalent to dialysis in patients with kidney disease. The operation is technically difficult, but the success rate is steadily improving and there are now approximately 70 centres practising liver grafting in North America and a similar number in Europe.

The first experimental and some of the early clinical trials of liver transplantation were concerned with accessory liver grafting to save the sick patient from dangerous removal of their own diseased liver. Unfortunately it is technically difficult to fit the irregular mass of the liver into the abdomen without compromising the vascular anastomoses by twisting or kinking and even when surgery is satisfactory, there is marked competition between the transplant and the patient's own liver, so an accessory liver is only likely to work when the patient's own liver function is severely compromised. This excludes an interesting category of patients with enzyme deficiencies who might otherwise be treated by an accessory liver graft or even grafting of hepatocytes.

In malignant disease a recipient hepatectomy is, of course, part of the operation but in non-malignant cirrhotic disease, if the diseased liver is left intact, it is likely to develop malignancy. Therefore, in this chapter I will be discussing only the orthotopic operation which is commonly performed.

Surgical experiments leading to application to man were pioneered by Moore *et al.* (1959) at the Peter Bent Brigham Hospital and at the same time by Starzl *et al.* (1959) in Denver. Clamping of the portal vein and vena cava led usually to death from reduced venous return to the heart and to congestion in the territory drained by the portal vein. Survival could only be achieved by shunting blood from the inferior vena cava and portal venous systems to the superior vena cava. Following Starzl's first human transplant in 1963, the early results were extremely dismal; very sick people were submitted to surgery with a high operative and perioperative mortality. Nevertheless, some patients did do well and Starzl found that shunting of blood from the portal and caval systems was usually not necessary in man. The Cambridge/King's College Hospital liver transplant programme began in 1968 and for 10 years there was little interest outside of Denver and Cambridge. In 1984, however, there were a number of long-term survivors and the whole subject was discussed at a consensus meeting in

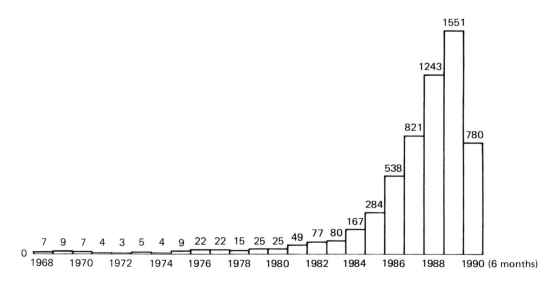

Figure 56.1 Evolution of liver transplantation – 1968–90 (Courtesy of the European Liver Transplant Registry)

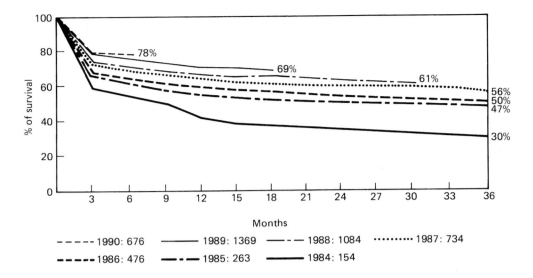

Figure 56.2   Evolution of survival of liver transplants (Courtesy of the European Liver Transplant Registry)

Washington. It was concluded that liver transplantation was the treatment of choice for certain end-stage liver diseases. There has been a steady increase in the number of liver grafts throughout the world; European Liver Transplant Registry results are shown in Figures 56.1 and 56.2.

Indications

1. *Chronic liver disease* due to cirrhosis caused by primary biliary cirrhosis, chronic active hepatitis and alcohol. In children, biliary atresia and α_1-antitrypsin deficiency are the commonest indications.

2. *Acute liver failure* due to viral hepatitis, idiosyncratic reaction to drugs and poisoning. Often these patients are children and there is great difficulty in timing the surgery since approximately 60% of patients will recover if given appropriate specialist intensive care. Those who die tend to deteriorate rapidly. However, by means of widespread collaboration between those interested in liver grafting, a donor can now usually be found in time to save these patients before irreversible brain damage has occurred. Another cause of acute fulminating liver failure is when a liver allograft ceases functioning or when it never starts to function, so called 'primary non-function', and grafts that have failed due to acute irreversible rejection or blockage of a major blood vessel. The same degree of urgency arises as in other cases. Also in this category are a very small number of acute liver trauma cases where the damage to the liver is so great that total hepatectomy is necessary.

3. *Primary malignancy of the liver* with or without underlying cirrhosis. Patients who have no cirrhosis are good candidates for surgery, whereas those with cirrhosis, particularly if they have Australia antigenaemia, have a high recurrence rate of viral infection

following operation. The results of liver transplantation for secondary tumour are extremely bad and it is likely that immunosuppressive drugs speed the growth of microscopic malignant deposits. For all types of primary malignancy of the liver, of which the most common diseases are hepatoma and cholangiocarcinoma, the recurrence rate after surgery even in apparently well-screened suitable cases is very high, approximately 60% within a year.

4. *Inborn errors of metabolism* with or without underlying liver disease. α_1-antitrypsin deficiency and Wilson's disease are the commonest indications with liver disease. Without liver disease, primary oxalosis and haemophilia are examples. In oxalosis, it is usually necessary to transplant the kidney together with a liver, and the patient's liver looks quite normal and all its functions are normal apart from the enzyme deficiency.

5. *Multiple organ transplants* have been performed for a number of indications, the commonest being the kidney and pancreas for diabetic renal failure. The liver can also be transplanted with other organs, and when this has been done the allograft reactions appear to be milder and more easily controlled than when the organs are transplanted without the liver; for example, kidney, pancreas or heart have all been transplanted with the liver. One of our patients had heart, lungs and liver transplanted from the same donor and she is well 7 years after operation. These observations in the clinic are consistent with much experimental work, especially in our laboratories, showing liver allografts are less severely rejected than grafts of other organs or tissues, and a liver allograft will often permit acceptance of other tissues from the same donor source. In certain experimental circumstances, operational tolerance can be produced in the pig and the rat with mature immune systems without

any immunosuppressive agents being given (Calne *et al.*, 1969; Zimmerman *et al.*, 1979).

Patient assessment

There are three phases of assessment as described below.

1. Medical/hepatological

The patient has disease of the liver for which no other treatment is available and where the outcome is inexorably fatal, and where the disease has reached the right stage for a transplant operation. In cases of parenchymatous non-malignant liver disease, it is important to determine the patient's quality of life. In primary biliary cirrhosis, the prognosis can be related with some confidence to deterioration of liver function tests. In other cirrhotic processes there is a tendency for the progression to vary in its pace. However, a patient who develops severe encephalopathy or who repeatedly bleeds from varices may require a transplant when there is some residual liver function. If the patient is able to lead an independent existence, operation is not indicated; likewise, a patient who is in deep coma and septic is too late to be a good candidate.

When the liver disease prevents the patient from normal activity, for example, work, running a house or shopping, then very often the patient will opt for an operation and this is probably a right decision because once the nutritional state has deteriorated the complications after operation are likely to be severe.

Each disease requires a separate assessment; for example in Budd–Chiari syndrome, a cavagram is necessary to determine the state of the vena cava. In all cases the portal vein must be checked for patency; this can be done by ultrasound. In patients with malignant disease, the diagnosis should be established by needle biopsy, and CT and bone scanning are important to check that obvious tumour has not spread outside the liver. An adenocarcinoma may be primary or secondary; in such cases, it is necessary to investigate the whole of the gastrointestinal tract, pancreas and the renal tract to make sure that there is no small occult primary.

In acute liver failure, assessment is particularly difficult. Deterioration is usually manifested by increasingly severe coma which eventually becomes irreversible with cerebral swelling and coning. The time available to do a transplant in such cases may be very short, but by active cooperation between centres a donor organ may be found before irreversible damage has occurred.

2. Surgical

Viewing the assessment from the surgical point of view, if the patient has had extensive intraperitoneal surgery the operation will not only be more tedious but also much more dangerous, as a cirrhotic liver with portal hypertension usually results in intense vascular adhesions.

An extremely important and difficult part of the surgical assessment is to attempt to gauge the size of the donor liver that could be transplanted into the patient. This is especially the case with children. Although there is a vogue for reducing the size of livers to fit into children, a total liver transplant is a simpler procedure and probably more satisfactory. Very small children have an extremely small space between the anterior abdominal wall and the posterior limits of the peritoneum. If there is a large disparity of size, even a lobe of a large liver may not fit into the anterior–posterior diameter.

Adults with end-stage cirrhosis often have small shrunken livers but a large peritoneal cavity due to ascites. Complicating factors such as a thrombosed portal vein or inferior vena cava can greatly increase surgical risks.

3. Anaesthetic

It is essential that an anaesthetist who is familiar with all aspects of liver transplantation assesses the patient to ensure that respiratory, cardiovascular and renal functions are sufficient to withstand this huge operation. Patients with serious cardiac or renal impairment will be designated for elective bypass during the operation if they are accepted for surgery. Another important factor is whether the muscle wasting is too severe to permit the patient to breathe and aerate the lungs after surgery.

Having gone through these three different assessment procedures, the patient will then be placed on the waiting list. Although various categories of urgency have been suggested, it seems from a practical point of view that since all patients are by definition in a serious state, the only special category should be the hyper-urgent patient with fulminating hepatic necrosis, acute allograft failure or the patient who has had his liver removed, for example, because of liver trauma and has been kept alive in an intensive care unit with a portal-caval shunt and haemofiltration.

Donor operation

The liver is removed from the donor with brain-stem death, mechanically ventilated with circulation intact. The cerebral catastrophe is usually the result of head injury or intracranial haemorrhage. The selected donor is ABO compatible unless the recipient is in a hyper-urgent category, since the results of transplantation violating the ABO system are bad, for example, in a 'B' liver into an 'O' recipient. The criteria in the donor are similar for all organ donors except that it is especially important to exclude evidence of alcoholism for liver grafting. In children we try to match the CMV status of the donor to that of the recipient, since CMV infection can be very serious in an immunosuppressed child.

The liver is usually removed in combination with other organs and the objective is to complete the dissection without interfering with the circulation and to ensure that the procedure for the removal of each organ will not disturb the anatomy or physiology of any of the other organs to be grafted. We hope that in future a single team will remove all the organs, rather than at the present where there is often chaotic arrangement of teams interested in different organs descending on the donor hospital and disturbing the work of that institution.

A bilateral subcostal incision is made which is extended vertically above the manubrium; the sternum is split with a Gigli saw giving access to the chest and exposure of the upper abdomen. In the laparotomy the structures in the free edge of the lesser omentum are separated from each other; the bile duct is divided close to the duodenum. The hepatic artery is followed to the coeliac and then to the aorta. An accessory left hepatic artery arising from the left gastric is a common abnormality (23%), and if found, the left gastric and this vessel must be preserved. Seventeen per cent of the patients have the main arterial supply to the right lobe of the liver arising from the superior mesenteric artery and passing behind the portal vein. In such cases the abnormal vessel is followed to the superior mesenteric which is taken with the specimen and revascularized, usually by joining it to the stump of the splenic artery. The peritoneal attachments to the liver are then divided, taking care to suture ligate any vessels; the right adrenal vein is divided so that the right lobe of the liver can be lifted from the hepatic fossa.

The kidneys are usually mobilized and if the pancreas is to be used this is also mobilized at this time using the spleen as a handle. If the whole pancreas is removed with the duodenum, then the vascular dissection is somewhat complicated. The liver, being a vital organ, should take preference in its vascular supply, but the whole pancreas will need both the splenic artery and the superior mesenteric and if these cannot be preserved, then appropriate arterial grafts may be necessary using the iliac or femoral vessels of the donor.

When the abdominal dissection is completed, the heart or heart and lungs can be removed; if the heart is removed, it is a very quick procedure. The aorta is cross-clamped in the chest as soon as the heart is removed, then the intra-abdominal organs can be dealt with. If prolonged dissection of the heart and lungs is necessary, the patient can be put on cardiopulmonary bypass, with hypothermia. After full heparinization, cannulae are inserted into the aorta and portal vein to perfuse the liver and to wash out the liver and other intra-abdominal organs with cold preserving solution. There is a danger that in removing the heart the suprahepatic cava will be sacrificed and it is extremely important to ensure that this

does not happen, otherwise the liver cannot be transplanted. A swab inserted between the dome of the liver and the diaphragm helps preserve the suprahepatic cava which is divided within the pericardium. The organs are now removed after dividing the supplying vessels. The liver is then placed in ice-cold preservation fluid; 100 ml is run through the biliary system via an incision in the fundus of the gallbladder which is not mobilized. An additional flush of 100 ml of preserving fluid is passed through the hepatic artery and portal vein.

The suprahepatic vena cava is dissected free from the muscular diaphragm and the three phrenic veins are suture ligated. Further surgery can be performed on the cold organ, the so-called 'back bench' procedure, once back in the operating room.

The University of Wisconsin solution, first used in experimental liver grafting by Jamieson et al. (1989a,b), has transformed the results of liver preservation, so that the organ can now be kept safely for 24 h. Simplifications of this solution by Jamieson result in a cheaper and probably more effective solution with reduced potassium content and no starch, but with the essential lactobionate and raffinose or impermeable molecules (Jamieson et al., 1989a). The recipient operation can now be started early in the morning, to the advantage of the patient who will be operated on by a rested surgical team.

Recipient operation

This is based on the original description by Starzl et al. (1963). The patient is likely to be very weak and ill, and most skilful anaesthesia and monitoring are necessary; pulse, ECG, arterial and central venous pressures are recorded continuously. Large intravenous lines are inserted into the territory of the superior vena cava; usually both the internal jugular veins are cannulated by the anaesthetist. The incision is usually bilateral subcostal, with a vertical extension to the xiphoid. The operation is done entirely through the abdomen. Dissection may be very difficult and tedious due to portal hypertension and coagulopathy. Meticulous suture ligation of all tissue to be cut is the only satisfactory method of managing the bleeding tendency, especially from high-pressure venules. The structures in the free edge of the lesser omentum are separated from each other and controlled. Dissection behind the liver is the last part of this phase of the operation, since bleeding in this area cannot be controlled until the liver is removed.

In very sick patients, especially cirrhotics with renal or cardiac impairment, vena caval clamping may not be tolerated. In such cases and also in patients with severe portal hypertension with coagulation defects, we assist the circulation. Of several techniques used in the past, we now favour simple venovenous bypass *without systemic heparin*, oxygenation or a heat exchanger. We use the Biomedicus centrifugal action pump and heparin-bonded tubing (Figure 56.3).

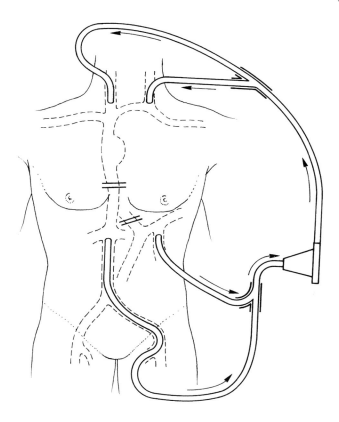

Figure 56.3 Venovenous bypass. Blood is taken from the inferior vena cava via the saphenous or femoral vein and from the portal vein directly. No systemic heparinization; the tubing is bonded with heparin. The Biomedicus pump works by centrifugal action. Blood is returned into the superior vena cava through the left brachial vein. A side arm is used to infuse a low dose of prostacyclin to inhibit platelet aggregation (From Calne, 1985, by permission of Wolfe Medical Publications)

The vena cava is temporarily clamped below the liver. If this severely impairs cardiac function the clamp is removed and bypass is prepared. More blood is transfused and if the heart is capable of withstanding clamping of the vena cava, removal of the liver is proceeded with as quickly as possible. The hepatic artery is ligated and divided, the portal vein clamped and divided and the vena cava similarly dealt with above and below the liver. It is very important that the interval during which the diseased liver is devascularized should be as short as possible, while the organ is still connected to the systemic venous system via the hepatic veins. Manipulation of the liver in this state can lead to massive flooding of the circulation with potassium ions, leading to cardiac arrest. Very rapid transfusion of stored blood should be avoided if possible because this can impair cardiac activity by causing an increase in the serum potassium level and cooling of the heart. The central venous pressure is kept positive to avoid air embolus. The special clamp is applied to the vena cava above the liver. This takes a small cuff of diaphragm and has a clip on it to prevent slipping (Figure 56.4). Following removal of the diseased liver the hepatic fossa is inspected for bleeding and any haemorrhagic points are suture ligated.

The donor liver is then removed from its ice-cold environment and the upper inferior vena caval anastomosis is performed with a 2/0 Mersilene stitch, the posterior wall being sutured from within. The bulk of the donor liver may obscure vision and this anastomosis can be difficult. The portal venous anastomosis is then constructed with a 5/0 prolene stitch. When the posterior layer is completed, a catheter is inserted into the portal vein. Gelfusin, 400 ml at room temperature, is perfused through the portal vein, to wash

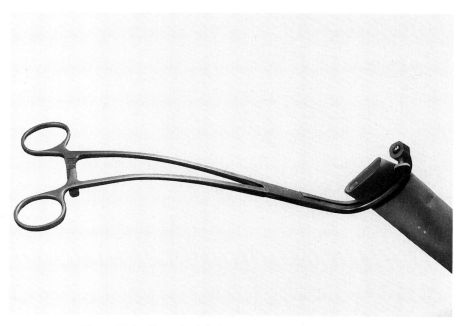

Figure 56.4 Clamp for inferior vena cava above the liver

out potassium ions present in the original cooling fluid and accumulating from anoxia. The effluent runs out of the inferior vena cava below the liver. The portal venous anastomosis is then completed and the cava below the liver is clamped. The suprahepatic IVC clamp is removed. This is a critical moment since, despite administration of bicarbonate and calcium intravenously, potassium from the mesenteric circulation and liver may lead to cardiac irregularities, hypotension and even asystole.

The operation continues with a running 4/0 prolene stitch to anastomose the donor and recipient venae cavae below the liver. The main hepatic and gastroduodenal arteries of the recipient are clamped. An oblique incision is made to include the orifice of the gastroduodenal artery. A Carrel patch of donor aorta containing the coeliac artery is trimmed so as to fit this orifice. The anastomosis is constructed with a running 6/0 prolene stitch.

Biliary drainage is the Achilles heel of liver transplantation. Serious complications have followed with all techniques so far described. There is clearly an advantage in preserving the mechanism of the sphincter of Oddi in preventing ascending cholangitis in immunosuppressed patients. Cholangitis is common in patients where the sphincter of Oddi is bypassed, for example, in children with biliary atresia after a Kasai operation. When a Roux loop is used, it should always be at least 36 cm long to discourage ascending infection. Techniques relying on the cystic duct for drainage of bile are unsatisfactory because this duct is of small calibre. Direct duct-to-duct anastomosis is anatomically and physiologically most appropriate, maintaining the sphincter and providing a normal conduit for bile drainage. Starzl first used this technique with a T-tube inserted into the recipient duct with one limb acting as a stent across the anastomosis. We have obtained good results with this technique, but the stent itself may cause complications, encouraging the deposit of biliary sludge, and the upper limb may ride up into the right or left hepatic duct causing damage or occlusion. For the past 4 years I have obtained satisfactory results with a duct-to-duct anastomosis without a stent, but with decompression of the unmobilized gallbladder with a fine T-tube – the technique described by Wall et al. (1989). Interrupted 5/0 PDS stitches are used for the biliary anastomosis and the T-tube is brought out through a stab incision in the upper part of the abdomen. A cholangiogram is performed at 2 weeks and, if the appearance is satisfactory, the T-tube is clamped and removed after 3 months.

In children with biliary atresia, the gallbladder conduit technique is most commonly used in our institution, anastomosing the donor common duct to the Hartmann's pouch area of the gallbladder and then the fundus of the gallbladder to the Roux loop.

The monitoring used during the operation is continued postoperatively. Urine output and body temperature are recorded. The patient usually requires warming, as the blood transfusions and a long operation reduce the body temperature. If the patient has good lung function, extubation is usually possible in the first 24 h. With severe cirrhotics who often have arteriovenous pulmonary shunts, at least 48 h of ventilation may be necessary before the endotracheal tube is removed.

Drain removal begins on the second day, one drain each day. The patient is given preoperative antibiotics prophylactically and these are continued for 48 h. Cultures are taken from the blood, wound, T-tube, mouth and perineum daily.

The use of bypass

Reference has already been made to this in experimental liver transplantation. In children and most adults, liver transplantation is performed without bypass and we feel that since it is an expensive addition with its own complications, bypass should only be used where it is expected to increase the safety of the patient. The technique we employ is cannulating the IVC via the saphenofemoral junction and the portal vein through the inferior mesenteric. This has the advantages of simplicity and the portal system can be decompressed early in the dissection before directly visualizing the portal vein. Moreover, the use of the anaesthetist's lines for the inflow of blood means that the dissection of upper arm is avoided and the procedure is thereby simplified.

This bypass can be started at any time during the operation and is usually stopped when the liver is revascularized. Flows of between 1 and 2 litres/min can be achieved. When the cannulae are removed, the inferior mesenteric vein is tied and the saphenofemoral junction incision is repaired.

Management of bleeding

Haemorrhage is the main enemy of surgeons and it is a particular worry in liver transplantation because of the extensive dissection required and the fact that the patient is likely to have impaired clotting and increased pressure in the portal venous system. There is no substitute for meticulous careful haemostatic technique, especially suture ligating all vessels that can be seen. Nevertheless, haemorrhage can still occur and in order to combat this, clotting factors must be given together with platelets. A good view is necessary, so there must be powerful suction. We use the Haemonetics cell saver, aspirating and washing shed blood and reinfusing it by a rapid infuser. When all these steps have been taken, the patient may still be oozing from the dissected surface and the wound and even from the anaesthetic line sites. A pitressin infusion is given routinely during the operation according to the London, Ontario technique (Wall et al., 1989) and can be continued in the postoperative phase. However, there is danger that this may cause ischaemia to the liver. Aprotenin has been shown to reduce surgical haemorrhage (Mallett *et al.*, 1990). Our early experience with the use of intraoperative aprotenin has been favourable. It can even push the clotting balance too far and cause vascular thrombosis. Previously, we used to bind the abdomen, especially in cases where there was severe ascites and a large peritoneal cavity. However, recently we have been able to exert external pressure on the abdomen and the legs much more satisfactorily by using a 'G' suit with controlled pressure in the inflatable leggings and corset area. Pressures can be monitored according to the renal output and in our limited experience we have found this to be of value. We usually start with a pressure of approximately 40 mmHg and if bleeding stops and urine output continues satisfactorily, we reduce it by 10 mmHg every 6 h. If the patient, nevertheless, continues bleeding or the abdomen fills up with blood clots, the wound will need to be re-explored. After the removal of vast amounts of clots, it is unusual to find a significant bleeding point. However, the removal of clots itself often stabilizes the patient's condition and seems to be followed by less bleeding afterwards. When clot has been removed, a careful inspection with packing is made in all portions of the peritoneal cavity, particularly the upper quadrants. Then hot packs are applied and left in place for 20 min to see whether there is any significant bleeding. After this 'coffee break', further inspection is made and any bleeding points dealt with and then the wound is reclosed with drainage.

Immunosuppression

We employ a basic triple therapy of azathioprine, steroids and cyclosporine, but because of the vulnerability of the kidneys to nephrotoxicity of cyclosporine we do not start this drug until there is evidence of good renal function with a satisfactory urine flow. In patients who are especially at risk, for instance those receiving second transplants or those who are in renal failure, anti-lymphocyte preparations, either poly- or monoclonal, are given instead of cyclosporine. However, such treatment can only be used effectively for approximately 10 days when the patient will produce antibodies against the foreign protein. In liver grafting there is a high incidence of acute rejection, but this is usually reversible with increased dosage of corticosteroids or anti-lymphocyte preparations if they have not already been given. The diagnosis is confirmed by percutaneous needle biopsy and it is suspected when there is any impairment of liver function, particularly a rise in serum bilirubin and transaminase levels. The standard immunosuppression in Cambridge is shown in Table 56.1.

There has been a great deal of interest recently in a new immunosuppressant, a macrolide chemically related to erythromycin called FK506, developed initially in Japan, and subsequently investigated experimentally by us in Cambridge and then in Pittsburgh. It has been used in clinical practice in Pittsburgh at 1/100th of a dose that is effective in animals. The early reports of clinical experience has been extremely encouraging and multi-centre trials are underway.

Besides rejection following liver transplantation, patients are at risk to bacterial, viral and fungal infections and any patient receiving immunosuppressive treatment is more likely to develop common cancers and especially in danger of developing lymphoma; these risks persist indefinitely. More discreet immunosuppression may soon be available and monoclonal antibodies have already been engineered so as to remove foreign animal protein; the so-called 'humanized' antibodies will soon be assessed for transplantation and should have the advantage of not producing an immune response against themselves, thus permitting long-term treatment.

Table 56.1 Immunosuppression protocol

Intraoperatively
500 mg methyl prednisolone – small adult
1 g methyl prednisolone – large adult
Azathioprine 1.5 mg/kg

Days 1–10
Prednisolone 1 mg/kg
Azathioprine 1.5 mg/kg
Cyclosporine 2–4 mg/kg in divided doses
(*to be given only if good renal function*)

Anti-rejection therapy
Day 1 Hydrocortisone 2 g
Day 2   1 g b.d.
Day 3   1 g b.d.
Day 4   500 mg b.d.
Day 5   500 mg b.d.

or ATG

Tissue typing

Due to the shortage of donors, tissue typing has not been used prospectively in liver transplantation but it has been mentioned that grafting across the ABO barrier gets poor results. An unexpected finding concerning the HLA system in two retrospective analyses was a negative correlation between tissue match and outcome (Donaldson *et al.*, 1987; Markus *et al.*, 1988). This is now being studied prospectively in a European multi-centre trial.

Recurrence of original diseases

This can occur in many liver diseases, for example alcoholism, viral hepatitis, malignancy and autoimmune cirrhosis. It cannot occur with inborn errors of metabolism or biliary atresia. (Results of the European Liver Transplant Registry are shown in Figures 56.1 and 56.2 and our own results are summarized in Figure 56.5.)

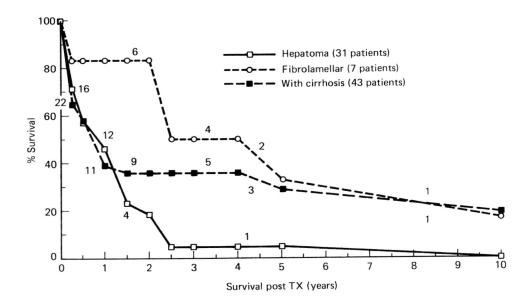

Figure 56.5 Survival after orthotopic liver transplantation for hepatoma, Cambridge/King's College Hospital series 1968–90

With experience, many errors in selection, surgery, anaesthesia and postoperative care have been defined and are now avoided. Patients who have good liver function after a year tend to do well long term and can be fully integrated into society, requiring less maintenance immunosuppression than recipients of other organ grafts. The longest survivor is a patient of Starzl's of 23 years, after transplantation with normal liver function; our longest surviving patient is 19 years and he is still at work. Sport and all kinds of activities including childbirth can be enjoyed after successful liver grafting.

Pancreas transplantation

The most serious complication of diabetes in young patients is renal failure and blindness due to microangiopathy. Uraemic diabetics do badly on dialysis; retinopathy progresses and shunt sites are liable to infection. Kidney transplantation for these patients is also disappointing, mainly due to steroids which aggravate the diabetes and make control more difficult, and diabetic nephropathy can recur in the transplant. For these reasons much experimental work has been devoted to transplantation of insulin-secreting tissue in the hope that this might prevent progress of the microangiopathy.

The history of pancreas grafting is more chequered than that of the liver, and controversy still exists as to when and if the procedure should be used. Surgical complications following pancreas grafting are common, especially those following leakage of pancreatic exocrine secretion. Another important consideration in pancreas grafting is the nature of the diabetic disease. The autoimmune process that initiates most cases of juvenile diabetes may persist for many years, as demonstrated by the recurrence of specific beta cell isletitis in recipients of pancreases from two identical twins and a HLA identical sibling in Minneapolis (Sutherland *et al.*, 1984). The first clinical attempt at grafting the pancreas was in 1967 by Kelly and colleagues in Minneapolis and since then the Minneapolis group has maintained the lead in this field (Kelly *et al.*, 1967). Dr Sutherland has established an up-to-date registry of international reporting of pancreas transplantation (Figures 56.6 and 56.7).

The concept of transplanting separated islets of beta cells has been investigated vigorously. In animals, short-term success has been achieved, especially in rodents (Gray and Morris, 1987), but even with autografts long-term success has not been reported in large animals receiving separated islets (Gray *et al.*, 1986; Sutton *et al.*, 1987). In humans, no long-term function has been reported with allografts despite numerous attempts. It has proved extremely difficult to separate islets from the human pancreas without damaging them, and islets injected into the bloodstream, usually into the portal circulation, tend to lose function after a short period. This may be due to failure of nutrition or metabolic exhaustion. Allografted islets are more susceptible to rejection than the vascularized pancreas.

It has been very difficult to diagnose rejection in the pancreas before the process becomes irreversible; probably this is due to the damaged islets releasing insulin in the course of their death and impairment of glucose haemostasis does not occur, until the rejec-

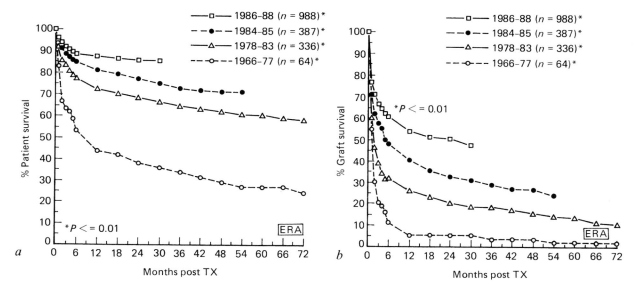

Figure 56.6 *a*, Patient survival rates by world era. *b*, Pancreas graft function survival rates by world era (From Sutherland *et al.*, 1990, by permission)

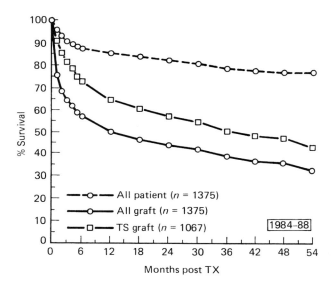

Figure 56.7 Patient survival and pancreas graft function survival rate curves for all and for technically successful 1984–88 cases reported to the Registry as of 18 January 1989 (From Sutherland *et al.*, 1990, by permission)

tion is advanced. However, in a pancreas transplant together with the kidney from the same donor, monitoring of renal function gives a good indication of the nature and timing of the immune response of the recipient against the donor, even though the severity of damage may not be the same in the two organs.

Many techniques have been described for transplanting a vascularized pancreas. The body and tail vascularized by the splenic vessels was popular due to its simplicity, but opinion has swung towards trans-

planting the whole pancreas despite the increased surgical complexity of the donor operation. The whole pancreas provides nearly double the number of islets.

The exocrine secretion may be totally inhibited by injecting polymers into the pancreatic duct system, which causes autolysis and destruction of the exocrine tissue. This approach, pioneered by Dubernard *et al.* (1978), together with the availability of cyclosporine opened the way to a relatively safe transplantation of the pancreas. Alternatively the exocrine secretions can be drained into the gastrointestinal tract or into the renal tract. The blood vessels of the pancreas are usually anastomosed to systemic vessels, but techniques allowing venous drainage into the portal system are preferable on theoretical grounds in providing physiological delivery of insulin to the liver for first passage where it is normally involved in its initial metabolism.

In surgery where there are multiple opinions, the usual conclusion is that there is no consensus and this would be true of pancreas grafting. However, in the past 5 years in North America there has been enthusiasm for transplanting the whole pancreas together with the kidney and drainage of pancreatic juice via a segment of the duodenum into the bladder. This technique, pioneered by Sollinger *et al.* (1984) and modified by Corry *et al.* (1986), allows a simple and safe operation in the recipient, and monitoring of amylase in the urine gives a direct indication of pancreatic function where rejection can be diagnosed by a fall of exocrine secretion in the urine. Surprisingly, few complications have been described from the presence of pancreatic juice in the bladder. Activation of trypsin to produce cystitis and other infectious complications has been unusual and there have so far been no cases of cancer developing either in the bladder or in the grafted specimen. Since surgical opinion is swinging towards accepting this operation as the best available at present, the following is a brief description of the procedure.

Donor operation

In the operation described by Corry (1988) the pancreas removal involves elevation of the spleen and freeing the tail of the pancreas, together with mobilization of the duodenum surrounding the pancreas starting with Kocher's manoeuvre and continuing until the aorta has been reached. The coeliac and superior mesenteric arteries are not separately dissected. The small blood vessels encountered adjacent to the pancreas are ligated. The aorta is approached above the coeliac and below the superior mesenteric. Great care is taken not to damage the pancreas, which is very susceptible to injury from handling, by holding the spleen like a handle rather than the pancreas itself. The pancreas is preserved with University of Wisconsin solution. If the whole of the coeliac artery is not needed for the liver, a Carrel patch is taken at the aorta to include the orifices of the coeliac and superior mesenteric arteries, but taking care not to damage the orifices of the renal arteries.

The order in removing intra-abdominal organs is the liver first, followed by the kidneys and the pancreas last, so that the duodenum is divided only after the other organs are removed. When the liver is removed, its vessels are preserved and the donor common iliac artery with its two branches are used for arterial vascularization of the pancreas, the two branches being anastomosed end to end to the superior mesenteric and splenic arteries. The internal iliac is anastomosed to the splenic, the external to the superior mesenteric; the iliac vein is joined to the portal vein.

The duodenum is clamped, stapled and divided just beyond the pylorus and distally beyond the head of the pancreas. The row of staples is inverted by a seromuscular suture. The intervening portion of the duodenum is opened so that the duodenal contents can be flushed out and the mucosa cooled with 1% neomycin solution.

If the liver is not to be used, a section of the portal vein is taken with the splenic. If the portal vein is needed for the liver, then the iliac vein is used as a graft to the splenic vein.

Recipient operation

The right iliac fossa is preferable to the left. The venous anastomosis is placed distally on the external iliac to avoid producing an acute angle where the portal vein joins the splenic vein. The spleen is removed after the pancreas is vascularized. The

duodenal–bladder anastomosis is performed with the inner layers full thickness with absorbable PDS sutures and the outer seromuscular layer with fine non-absorbable prolene sutures. The pancreas is placed in the iliac fossa with the peritoneum opened widely to permit drainage of any fluids leaked from the pancreas into the peritoneal cavity. The renal transplant is performed via a separate incision on the other side.

Complications

The two commonest complications described after this technique are bleeding from the duodenal segment, with ulceration and metabolic acidosis due to high bicarbonate losses in the urine which can be treated orally by sodium bicarbonate. The acidosis is particularly severe when there is renal impairment. Duodenal ulceration with bleeding may require surgical treatment to remove the affected portion of the duodenum.

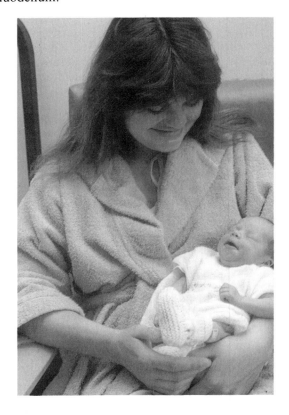

Figure 56.8 Patient J. B. following successful pregnancy 3 years after combined renal and segmental paratopic pancreas transplantation. She is now well 8 years post-operation

Postoperative care and immunosuppression

The postoperative care of the patient with a pancreas and kidney graft is similar to that of kidney graft patients, except that the blood glucose must be watched carefully; function usually returns if the pancreas is vascularized satisfactorily. The diabetic state usually reverses within a few days and the blood sugar levels usually remain within normal limits.

Immunosuppression is similar to that described above under that section in liver transplantation. Cyclosporine is withheld in patients with poor renal function, but if function is good, cyclosporine can be started immediately. Rejection is treated in a similar manner as for the liver, and diagnosis depends on renal function, renal biopsy and urinary amylase levels.

For patients who have done well with pancreas transplantation, the double operation has been excellent therapy, allowing full return to normal society without the burden of repeated dialysis, harsh dietary and fluid control and repeated injections of insulin. Although many patients will have irreversible changes in the retina, progressional retinal disease is usually slow or arrested after pancreas transplantation. Atherosclerotic macroangiopathy may continue to progress, but microangiopathy in the kidney has not been reported. Patients can return to sport and other vigorous activities and childbirth (Figure 56.8).

References

Calne, R. Y. (ed.) (1985) Recipient operation. In *A Colour Atlas of Liver Transplantation*, Wolfe Medical Publications, London

Calne, R. Y. (1987) *Liver Transplantation*, 2nd edn, Grune and Stratton, Orlando, Florida

Calne, R. Y., Sells, R. A., Pena, J. R., Davis, D. R., Millard, P. R., Herbertson, B. M., Binns, R. M. and Davies, D. A. L. (1969) Induction of immunological tolerance by porcine liver allografts. *Nature*, **233**, 472–476

Corry, R. J. (1988) Pancreatic-duodenal transplantation with urinary tract drainage. In *Pancreatic Transplantation* (ed. C. Groth), Grune and Stratton, London

Corry, R. J., Nghiem, D. D., Schulak, J. A., Bentel, W. D. and Gonwa, T. A. (1986) Surgical treatment of diabetic nephropathy with simultaneous pancreatic duodenal and renal transplantation. *Surg. Gynecol. Obstet.*, **162**, 547

Donaldson, P. T., Alexander, G. J. M., O'Grady, J. *et al.* (1987) Evidence for an immune response to HLA class 1 antigens in the vanishing-bile duct syndrome after liver transplantation. *Lancet*, **1**, 945–948

Dubernard, J. M., Traeger, J., Neyra, P., Touraine, J. L., Tranchant, D. and Blanc-Brunat, N. (1978) A new method of preparation of segmental pancreatic grafts for transplantation: trials in dogs and in man. *Surgery*, **84**, 633–640

Gray, D. W. R. and Morris, P. J. (1987) Developments in isolated pancreatic islet transplantation. *Transplantation*, **43**, 321–331

Gray, D. W. R., Warnock, G., Sutton, R., Peters, M., McShane, P. and Morris, P. J. (1986) Successful auto-transplantation of isolated islets of Langerhans in the cynomolgus monkey. *Br. J. Surg.*, **73**, 850

Jamieson, N. V., Lindell, S., Sundburg, R., Southard, J. H. and Belzer, F. O. (1989a) Evaluation of simplified variants of the UW solution using the isolated perfused rabbit liver. *Transplant Proc.*, **21**, 1294–1295

Jamieson, N. V., Sundberg, R., Lindell, S., Claesson, K., Moen, J., Vreugdenhil, P. K., Wight, D. G. D., Southard, J. H. and Belzer, F. O. (1989b). 24–28 hour preservation of the canine liver by simple cold storage using UW lactobionate solution. *Transplant. Proc.*, **21**, 1292–1293

Kelly, W. D., Lillehei, R. C., Merkel, F. K. *et al.* (1967) Allotransplantation of the pancreas and duodenum along with the kidney in diabetic nephropathy. *Surgery*, **61**, 827–837

Mallett, S. V., Cox, D., Burroughs, A. K. and Rolles, K. (1990) Aprotenin and reduction of blood loss and transfusion requirement in orthotopic liver transplantation. *Lancet*, **336**, 886–887

Markus, B. H., Duquesnoy, R. D. *et al.* (1988) Histocompatibility and liver transplant outcome. Does HLA exert a dualistic effect? *Transplantation*, **46**, 372–377

Moore, F. D., Smith, L. L., Burnap, T. K., Dallenbach, F. D., Dammin, G. J., Gruber, U. F., Shoemaker, W. C., Steenburg, R. W., Ball, M. R. and Belko, J. S. (1959) One-stage homotransplantation of the liver following total hepatectomy in dogs. *Transplant. Bull.*, **6**, 103

Sollinger, H. W., Cook, K., Kamps, D., Glass, N. R. and Belzer, F. O. (1984) Clinical and experimental experience with pancreatico-cystostomy for exocrine pancreatic drainage in pancreas transplantation. *Transplant. Proc.*, **16**, 749–751

Starzl, T. E., Berhard, V. M., Cortes, N. and Benvenuto, R. (1959) A technique for one-stage hepatectomy in dogs. *Surgery*, **46**, 880

Starzl, T. E., Marchioro, T. L., Von Kaulla, K. N., Hermann, G., Brittain, R. S. and Waddell, W. R. (1963) Homotransplantation of the liver in humans. *Surg. Gynecol. Obstet.*, **117**, 659

Sutherland, D. E. R., Sibley, R., Zu, X. Z., Michael, A., Srikauta, S., Taub, F., Najarian, J. and Goetz, F. C. (1984) Twin to twin pancreas transplantation: reversal and re-enactment of the pathogenesis of type I diabetes. *Trans. Ass. Am. Phys.*, **XCVII**, 80–87

Sutherland, D. E. R. *et al.* (1990) *Report of the International Pancreas Transplant Registry – 1990*, University of Minnesota

Sutton, R., Gray, D. W. R., McShane, P., Peters, M. and Morris, P. J. (1987) The metabolic efficiency and long-term fate of intraportal islet grafts in the cynomolgus monkey. *Transplant. Proc.*, **19**(5), 3575

Wall, W., Grant, D., Mimeault, R., Girvan, D. and Duff, J. (1989) Biliary tract reconstruction in liver transplantation. *Can. J. Surg.*, **32**(2), 97–100

Zimmerman, F. A., Butcher, G. W., Davies, H. ff. S., Brons, G., Kamada, N. and Turel, O. (1979) Technique for orthotopic liver transplantation in the rat and some studies of the immunological responses to fully allogeneic liver grafts. *Transplant. Proc.*, **11**, 571–577

57

Heart, heart–lung and lung transplantation

J. A. Hutter and J. Wallwork

Introduction

Over the past decade heart and heart–lung transplantation have become established treatments for patients with end-stage cardiac or pulmonary disease. Double and single lung transplantation have continued to evolve as established procedures. Following the introduction of cardiac transplantation by Barnard in 1967 (Barnard, 1967), the operation generated widespread interest and enthusiasm, but the early results were disappointing. However, the success of the current transplantation programmes springs from the pioneering work of Shumway and colleagues at Stanford University Medical Center where the clinical transplant programme has continued uninterrupted since 1968. The successful development of heart–lung transplantation (Reitz *et al.*, 1982) followed the introduction of cyclosporine as the mainstay of immunosuppressant therapy and the development of preservation techniques which allowed distant procurement of organs (Wallwork *et al.*, 1987). Single and double transplantation have become safer following the introduction of the omental wrap to vascularize the bronchial and tracheal anastomosis (Cooper *et al.*, 1987). Most recently, sequential right and left lung transplantation have been introduced.

Recipient selection

Recipients for cardiac transplantation are selected from patients with end-stage cardiac failure from a variety of causes (Figure 57.1) and whom conventional modes of therapy have been exhausted. They will generally have New York Heart Association class IV symptoms and have a life expectancy judged to be measured in months. No absolute upper age limit can be applied, but 60 years of age is generally accepted as the upper limit. Paediatric cardiac transplantation is now routinely undertaken, congenital heart disease and cardiomyopathy being the primary indication (Figure 57.1) in this age group. Recipients for cardiac transplantation should have no other systemic illness or systemic infection; diabetes mellitus is no longer an absolute contraindication to transplantation. The right ventricle of a normal donor heart is unable to sustain the pulmonary circulation when the pulmonary vascular resistance of the recipient is severely elevated, and 5 Wood units is generally considered as the upper limit for orthoptic cardiac transplantation. The introduction of the 'domino' procedure, whereby the heart of a heart–lung transplant recipient is used as a donor organ, has allowed some relaxation of this upper limit, as the right ventricle may have hypertrophied to overcome the elevated pulmonary vascular resistance of the domino organ donor. Theoretically the donor heart will be able to sustain the pulmonary circulation of the recipient who also has an elevated pulmonary vascular resistance, although as experience grows this is not always practical. However, domino transplantation has enabled better use of donor organ resources and the majority of recipients with primary lung disease donate their hearts to heart-transplant recipients.

The indications for combined heart and lung transplantation (Figure 57.2) have widened. Primary pulmonary hypertension and the Eisenmenger syndrome were the common indications in the early years of

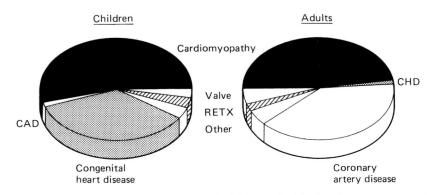

Figure 57.1 Indications for heart transplantation in children and adults (CAD, coronary artery disease; CHD, congenital heart disease; RETX, retransplantation)

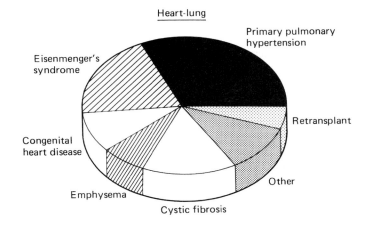

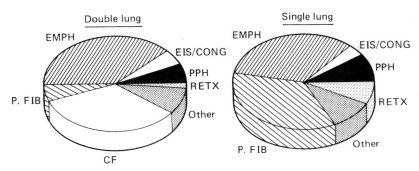

Figure 57.2 Indications for heart–lung and lung transplant procedures (EMPH, emphysema; EIS, Eisenmenger complex; CONG, congenital heart disease; P.FIB, pulmonary fibrosis; PPH, primary pulmonary hypertension; RETX, retransplantion; CF, cystic fibrosis)

heart–lung transplantation, but the use of this technique in patients with cystic fibrosis has recently accelerated (Scott *et al.*, 1988). The initial fears that with cystic fibrosis the inevitable pulmonary infection with resistant bacterial and fungal organisms such as *Pseudomonas* and *Aspergillus* would lead to overwhelming sepsis following transplantation have fortunately not been justified. Currently cystic fibrosis is the most common indication for combined transplantation. Other indications for heart–lung transplantation include pulmonary fibrosis, pulmonary thromboembolic disease, sarcoidosis, histiocytosis X, bronchiectasis, lupus scleroderma, haemosiderosis, lymphangioleiomatosis, acute adult respiratory distress syndrome and leiomyosarcoma of the pulmonary artery.

Single lung transplantation requires a balance between perfusion and ventilation of the transplanted lung and therefore pulmonary fibrosis is physiologically ideal for single lung transplantation (Dark and Cooper, 1987). In these patients the remaining lung is usually free of infection, has a high pulmonary vascular resistance and is less compliant than the transplanted lung. The transplanted lung therefore receives the bulk of both the ventilation and perfusion. The

indications for single and double lung transplantation reported to the International Registry (Kriett and Kaye, 1991) are shown in Figure 57.2.

A stable psychological and social background are also essential requirements to ensure that the patient will overcome the considerable emotional and social stresses that the transplantation will involve.

In order to maximize the benefit that can be obtained from the limited pool of organ donors the choice of recipient should be made giving priority to those most likely to survive and gain maximum benefit (Hutter *et al.*, 1988a). The choice of a moribund recipient with multi-organ failure, often requiring mechanical support of the circulation and having a lower chance of survival, would be considered inappropriate by many surgeons.

Donor selection

The main factor which determines the number of transplantation operations performed is the limited availability of donor organs. Trauma and subarachnoid haemorrhage are the most common causes of brain death in haemodynamically stable patients, and there should be no history of heart disease. A requirement of only minimal inotropic support of the circulation is acceptable. To achieve this may require aggressive fluid replacement and treatment of diabetes insipidus with intramuscular vasopressin. However, over-transfusion of fluid must be avoided, particularly in lung donors, in order to prevent pulmonary oedema. Serum thyroxine, levels have been shown to fall following brain death, and replacement therapy may lessen the need for inotropic agents and will also improve the condition of the donor organ (Novitsky *et al.*, 1987). Lung donors in addition must be free from pulmonary infection and lung contusion and have normal alveolar gas exchange.

Requests to relatives to consider organ transplantation must be handled sensitively and expertly. Although there is as yet no obligation on doctors to discuss organ donation, it should be remembered that more disappointment and distress to relatives may result by doctors denying relatives the opportunity to consider organ donation than by the assumption that the proposal may be declined.

Donor–recipient matching

In contrast to renal transplantation the majority of cardiac transplantation centres do not perform a tissue type cross-match between donor and recipient. The time required for tissue typing is considerable and the limited pool of potential recipients makes tissue typing impractical. The heart donor and recipient should however be of compatible ABO blood group and of similar weight. Occasionally when the recipient has a high reactive antibody titre a direct lymphocyte cross-match should be performed.

Transplantation of lungs with a greater volume than the volume of the recipient's chest cavity will result in areas of atelectasis and subsequent infection, and significant cardiac tamponade may occur when the sternum is closed. Conversely, if the transplanted lungs are too small to fill the recipient's chest cavity hyperinflation may result in air leaks. If a pneumothorax is allowed to persist, a pleural effusion may develop which might become infected. However, if the recipient's chest is hyperinflated as a result of cystic fibrosis, emphysema or other chronic lung disease, then the chest volume may be expected to decrease after transplantation. Under these circumstances, transplantation with slightly smaller lungs may be appropriate. Ideally the chest X-ray of recipient and donor should be directly compared, but when this is not possible an estimate of lung volume can be made from a formula relating lung volume to height. Donors must not carry HIV or hepatitis B virus. The importance of organ-transmitted diseases including cytomegalovirus (CMV) has been demonstrated in both cardiac (Hakim *et al.*, 1985) and heart–lung recipients (Hutter *et al.*, 1989). A significant mortality and morbidity from primary pulmonary CMV has

occurred when the heart and lungs have been transplanted from CMV-positive donors to CMV-negative recipients.

Organ procurement and preservation

Currently a large proportion of organs are procured from multi-organ donors, and this requires close cooperation, collaboration and diplomacy between the various transplant teams. Recent developments in organ preservation now allow distant procurement in all cases, including the organs for heart–lung transplantations (Wallwork *et al.*, 1987). The cardiac donor operation is carried out without cardiopulmonary bypass. Standard median sternotomy is employed and the heart and great vessels are carefully inspected, as this represents the last opportunity for haemodynamic evaluation and anatomical inspection of the graft. The heart and great vessels are dissected and the donor is fully heparinized. Inflow occlusion is achieved by ligation of the superior vena cava and clamping the inferior vena cava. The aorta is cross-clamped near the take-off of the innominate artery. A cold cardioplegic solution is administered via the aortic root, and the superior vena cava and right superior pulmonary vein are immediately incised to eliminate the possibility of distension of either the right or left side of the heart. Topical cold saline is applied concurrently with instillation of cardioplegia. The graft is then removed by transection of the remaining pulmonary veins, and venae cavae. The aorta is transected at the level of the innominate artery and the pulmonary artery is transected at its bifurcation. The graft is then transported in normal saline at 4°C.

Removal of the organs for heart–lung transplantation requires initial mobilization of the great vessels as described above. The right common carotid artery is then divided to improve access to the trachea and the azygous vein is ligated and divided close to the superior vena cava. The lungs are mobilized by division of the inferior pulmonary ligaments. The lungs may be preserved by designated fluids, such as the Papworth solution (Wallwork *et al.*, 1987), infused directly into the pulmonary artery, and the inclusion of prostacycline in this fluid (which is known to be a potent pulmonary vasodilator) ensures even distribution throughout the lungs. Prostacycline may prevent leucocyte sequestration and platelet aggregation in the lungs, and damage to the pulmonary vascular endothelium may also be prevented by its inhibiting complement activation.

Alternatively the whole patient may be cooled prior to removal of the organs following institution of cardiopulmonary bypass, but since this requires transport of a cardiopulmonary bypass machine to the donor's hospital, it is not usually practical.

Following preservation of the organs they are removed as a single heart–lung block. This is achieved

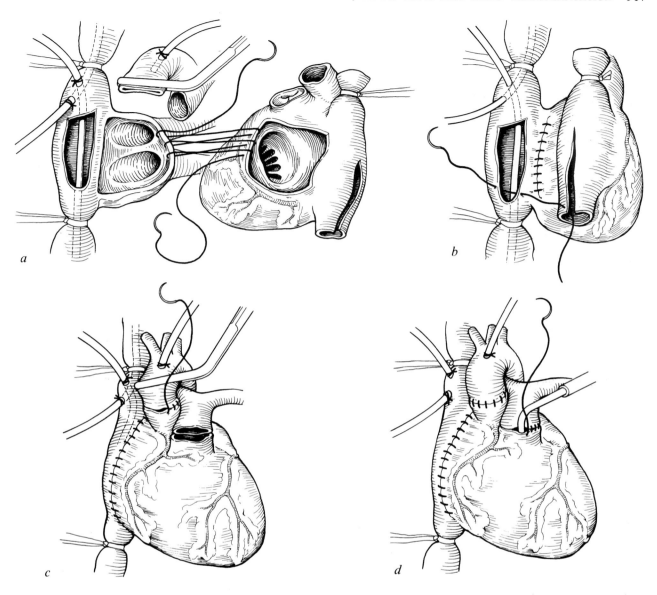

Figure 57.3 Operative technique for human cardiac transplantation: *a*, Cannulation technique is similar to routine cardiac procedures utilizing central cannulation. Tapes have been placed around the superior and inferior venae cavae and the aorta has been cross-clamped to exclude the heart from the circulation.The recipient heart has been excised at the atrioventricular groove. The superior vena cava of the donor heart has been ligated. The left atrial anastomosis has been started. *b*, The left atrial anastomosis has been completed. The incision in the donor right atrium is curved away from the superior vena cava and the adjacent sinoatrial node. The right anastomosis is begun at the inferior border of the atrial septum. *c*, The right atrial anastomosis is completed. A perfusion catheter has been inserted into the left atrium through which cold (4°C) normal saline is infused to further cool the left ventricular cavity as well as to displace air. The aortic anastomosis is being completed. *d*, The aortic cross-clamp has been released following completion of the aortic anastomosis. The perfusion catheter has been removed from the left atrium and the pulmonary anastomosis is completed with the heart fibrillating

by dissection in the plane between trachea and oesophagus, requiring division of the ligamentum arteriosum only. The endotracheal tube is partially withdrawn and the trachea is stapled and divided in the upper mediastinum maintaining lung inflation. The aorta is divided at the level of the right common carotid artery, and having divided the superior and inferior venae cavae the organs are removed and placed in cold saline for transportation at 4°C.

When multi-organ procurement is performed, the abdominal organs are mobilized prior to removal of the thoracic organs, allowing the abdominal organs to be removed rapidly following removal of the thoracic organs. Current preservation techniques of the heart and lungs allow a safe preservation period of between 4 and 6 h, and appropriate transport arrangements are mandatory. In order to minimize the preservation period, careful coordination of the procedures is required to ensure that the recipient is fully prepared for institution of cardiopulmonary bypass immediately the donor organs arrive at the transplant centre.

Recipient surgical technique

Cardiac transplantation

The technique for orthoptic cardiac transplantation varies little from the method described in the report by Lower and Shumway (1960) (Figure 57.3). The recipient operation is carried out via median sternotomy using cardiopulmonary bypass. Cannulation of the aorta is accomplished near the origin of the innominate artery, and cannulation of the venae cavae is performed selectively inserting the cannulae through an adjacent portion of right atrium. Snares are placed around the venae cavae to exclude air. After institution of cardiopulmonary bypass and systemic cooling to 28°C, the aorta is immediately cross-clamped to eliminate the risk of thromboembolic phenomena. The heart is excised commencing in the right atrium, just lateral to the right atrial appendage. This incision is carried inferiorly along the atrio-ventricular groove, through the coronary sinus and across the atrial septum into the left atrium. The aorta and pulmonary artery are then transected at the immediate supravalvular level, and the excision is completed by continuation of the left atrial incision just posterior to the left atrial appendage. The donor heart is then brought into the field and prepared for implantation. The left atrial anastomosis is performed first, beginning in the area of the recipient left superior pulmonary vein and the donor left atrial appendage. The right atrial anastomosis is started at the mid-point of the atrial septum and completed, taking care to avoid any distortion that may result from the different sizes of the donor and recipient atria. An end-to-end anastomosis of the pulmonary artery and aorta are then completed using a continuous monofilament suture. The heart is then perfused with oxygenated blood by removal of the aortic cross-clamp and, following very careful exclusion of air from the cardiac chambers, cardiopulmonary bypass is discontinued. Isoprenaline is often required to increase the sino-atrial node rate of the denervated donor heart. A permanent pacing wire is commonly attached to the apex of the left ventricle to facilitate insertion of a pacing system at a later date if required, and temporary pacing wires may be attached to the surface of the donor atrium.

Heart–lung transplantation

The technical challenge of heart–lung transplantation is considerable. Having instituted cardiopulmonary bypass as described above, the diseased lungs are removed individually (Jamieson *et al.*, 1984), taking great care to achieve haemostasis in the thoracic cavity and posterior mediastinum. This is particularly troublesome when a previous thoracotomy has been performed, or in cyanotic heart diseases where mediastinal blood vessels may become enlarged to provide a collateral circulation. The phrenic nerves must be preserved and the recurrent laryngeal nerve as it passes around the aortic arch is protected by leaving a cuff of pulmonary artery attached to the ligamentum arteriosum. The heart is then removed as described above, with the addition of removing the left atrium, leaving only a cuff of the right atrium. Careful handling and dissection of the trachea is essential to maintain an adequate blood supply to the tracheal anastomosis. Having removed the thoracic organs, very careful haemostasis of the posterior mediastinum is ensured.

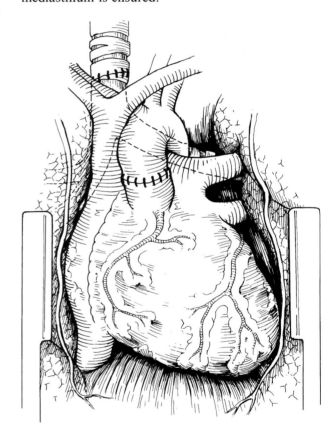

Figure 57.4 Following transplantation of the heart–lung organs, showing suture lines in the aorta and right atrium. The tracheal anastomosis is hidden behind the aorta

Implantation of the heart–lung donor block requires anastomosis of the right atrium, aorta and trachea (Figure 57.4). The bronchial blood supply of the heart–lung transplant donor organs is sufficient to vascularize the remaining segment of the donor trachea. However, following double lung transplantation or single lung transplantation the bronchial or

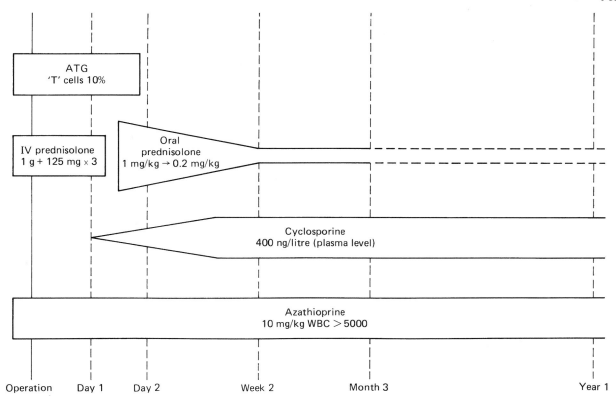

Figure 57.5 Schematic representation of the Papworth regimen for immunosuppression following heart transplantation

tracheal anastomosis may be covered by a pedicle of omentum to ensure adequate vascularity of the anastomosis. Double lung transplantation requires a technically difficulty anastomosis of the donor and recipient left atria, but has the significant advantage of preserving the recipient's own heart. Single lung transplantation is performed by a thoracotomy and does not generally require cardiopulmonary bypass. Care is required to avoid devascularization of the bronchial anastomosis, but despite an omental wrap late stenosis of the bronchial anastomosis is a common problem. Most recently, sequential transplantation of both lungs has been performed successfully, thereby avoiding the need for cardiopulmonary bypass and providing technically easier procedures than a double lung transplant.

Postoperative care and immunosuppression

The early management of heart and heart–lung transplant patients follows those principles which are now well established for conventional cardiac surgery. Early withdrawal of ventilation support is recommended and emphasis placed on rapid return of mobility and early rehabilitation. Immunosuppression is provided by a combination of drugs which include anti-thymocyte globulin (ATG), prednisolone, azathioprine and cyclosporine. Various regimens are currently used, and the Papworth regimen is shown schematically in Figure 57.5.

Cardiac rejection is monitored closely by regular endomyocardial biopsy during the initial hospital period. The bioptone is introduced via the internal jugular vein and several samples of the right side of the interventricular septum are taken. Histological grading (Billingham *et al.*, 1990) determines the need for augmentation of the immunosuppression regimen. Non-invasive techniques, such as echocardiography and pacemaker threshold potentials, are currently being evaluated as an adjunct to endomyocardial biopsy.

Initially it was assumed that cardiac and lung rejection would occur simultaneously, but it is now recognized that rejection of each organ can occur independently (McGregor *et al.*, 1985). Therefore, a technique for recognition of lung rejection in heart–lung transplantation is required. A decline in the respiratory function tests and X-ray changes may occur but are not sufficiently sensitive. Transbronchial biopsy (Higenbottam *et al.*, 1987) has however proved to be a useful technique and can usually differentiate lung rejection from a lung infection. An international histological grading system has recently been introduced (Yousem *et al.*, 1990), based largely on the work of Stewart at Papworth Hospital (Hutter *et al.*, 1988b).

Complications

Following transplantation, early death may occasionally result from organ failure, but acute rejection or overwhelming infection is more common. An episode of rejection occurs in about one-third of patients following cardiac or cardiopulmonary transplantation, but careful management of the patient and early confirmation of the diagnosis when combined with suitable augmentation of the immunosuppressant regimen will abort the rejection episode in the majority of cases. Uncontrollable early rejection is now rare.

A disturbing later complication of clinical cardiac transplantation is that of graft atherosclerosis. More than a third of patients have angiographically demonstrable lesions 3 years after transplantation and the likelihood of this complication appears to be as high among patients undergoing transplantation for cardiomyopathy as coronary artery disease. In view of the denervated state of the heart, angina is not a feature and the problem remains occult, presenting with the insidious onset of congestive cardiac failure or sudden death. The disease is usually diffuse with involvement of distal coronary vessels which precludes coronary artery bypass grafting. When the process is severe, retransplantation must be contemplated.

Following lung transplantation, obliterative bronchiolitis has become the major long-term threat, resulting in a gradual decline in respiratory function. This process may be the result of a chronic rejection process. It is hoped that the earlier recognition of acute rejection episodes aided by such techniques as the transbronchial biopsy will reduce the incidence of obliterative bronchiolitis occurring later in the post-transplant period. Retransplantation remains the only treatment for this condition, but the result is often disappointing.

Results

In 1991, the International Registry of Heart Transplantation (Kriett and Kaye, 1991) contains results on transplantation in over 16 000 patients (Table 57.1). Following cardiac transplantation the registry shows a 1-year survival rate of 81% and a 5-year survival of 69% (Figure 57.6). Although the operative mortality is higher in children there is no difference in late survival related to recipient age. The postoperative causes of death have been similar in children and adults. Rejection has accounted for 30% of deaths and fatal infections have been reported in 20%. Other reported cases of death have included cerebrovascular

accident (4%), malignancy (5%), kidney or liver failure, pulmonary embolism, gastrointestinal complications, trauma and suicide.

Table 57.1 Types of heart and lung transplantation (From the International Registry of Heart Transplantation)

Type of transplant		RETX	Total
Hearts			
Orthotopic	15 942	413	16 355
Heterotopic	321	11	332
Lungs			
Heart–lung	984	41	1 025
Double lung	117	3	120
Single lung	416	31	447

RETX, Retransplant procedure.

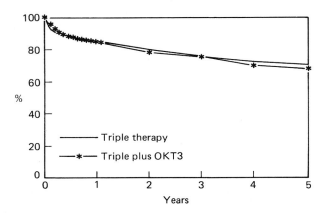

Figure 57.6 Actuarial 5-year survival following heart transplantation (From the International Registry of Heart Transplantation)

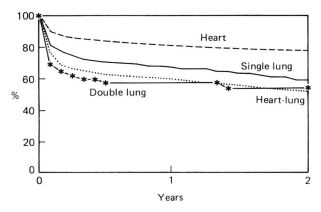

Figure 57.7 Actuarial survival associated with heart, combined heart–lung and single lung transplantation

The causes of death are similar for all forms of lung transplantation. The most common cause of early death has been intraoperative technical complications, including primary graft failure and haemorrhage. Other less frequent causes have included cerebrovascular events, renal and hepatic failure. Infection has been a major factor in mortality, both early and late, with all lung transplantation techniques. The current 1-year actuarial survival is 59% for combined heart–lung, 67% for single lung and 57% for double lung transplantation (Figure 57.7).

It must, however, be emphasized that the quality of life of the survivors is excellent, with many leading a normal active lifestyle.

The future

Cardiomyoventriculoplasty (Acker *et al.*, 1987) is an exciting development that may be suitable for some patients currently suitable only for transplantation. The latissimus dorsi muscle is isolated and following repeated stimulation of the nerve the metabolic composition of the skeletal muscle changes into a 'slow' muscle more akin to cardiac muscle, becoming more resistant to fatigue. The muscle is then wrapped around the ventricle, or aorta; alternatively, a neoventricle is created. Pacemaker stimulation of the muscle is coordinated with cardiac activity, thereby augmenting cardiac function. Progress in xenograft transplantation will await further development in specific depression of the immune system. Mechanical hearts are developing rapidly and have become established treatment in some centres, particularly as a bridge to cardiac transplantation or to maintain a transplant recipient suffering an acute rejection episode until retransplantation becomes possible. Developments of long-term implantable assist devices, driven electrically through a battery system that can be recharged transcutaneously by an electromagnetic induction system, may offer a long-term solution to the needs of a wide variety of patients with end-stage cardiac disease.

References

Acker, M. A., Hammond, R. L., Mannion, J. D., Salmons, S. and Stevenson, L. W. (1987) Skeletal muscle as the potential power source for a cardiovascular pump: assessment *in vivo. Science*, **236**, 324–327

Barnard, C. N. (1967) The operation. *S. Afr. Med. J.*, **41**, 1271

Billingham, M. E., Cary, N. R., Hammand, M. E., Kennitz, J., Marboe, C., McCallister, H. A., Snovar, D. C., Winters, G. L. and Zerbe, A. (1990) A Working Formulation for Standardization of Nomenclature in the Diagnosis of Heart and Lung Rejection: Heart Rejection Study Group. *J. Heart Transplant.*, **9**, 587–593

Cooper, J. D., Pearson, F. G., Patterson, G. A. *et al.* (1987) Technique for successful lung transplantation in humans. *J. Thorac. Cardiovasc. Surg.*, **93**, 173–181

Dark, J. and Cooper, J. D. (1987) Transplantation of the lungs. *J. Hosp. Med.*, **37**, 443–445

Hakim, M., Wreghitt, T. G., English, T. A. H., Stovin, P. G. I., Cory-Pearce, R. and Wallwork, J. (1985) Significance of donor transmitted disease in cardiac transplantation. *J. Heart Transplant.*, **4**, 302–306

Higenbottam, T., Stewart, S., Penketh, A. and Wallwork, J. (1987) The diagnosis of lung rejection and opportunistic infection by transbronchial biopsy. *Transplant. Proc.*, **14**, 3777–3778

Hutter, J. A., Higenbottam, T., Stewart, S. and Wallwork, J. (1988a) Heart lung transplantation. Better use of resources. *Am. J. Med.*, **85**, 4–11

Hutter, J. A., Stewart, S., Higenbottam, T., Scott, J. and Wallwork, J. (1988b) Histologic changes in heart lung transplant recipients during rejection and a routine biopsy. *J. Heart Transplant.*, **7**, 440–444

Hutter, J. A., Wreghitt, T., Scott, J., Higenbottam, T. and Wallwork, J. (1989) The importance of cytomegalovirus in heart lung transplant recipients. *Chest*, **95**, 627–631

Jamieson, S. W., Stinson, E. B., Oyer, P. E., Baldwin, J. C. D. and Shumway, N. E. (1984) Operative techniques for heart lung transplantation. *J. Thorac. Cardiovasc. Surg.*, **87**, 930–935

Kriett, H. H. J. M. and Kaye, M. P. (1991) The Registry of the International Society for Heart Transplantation: Eighth Official Report – 1991. *J. Heart Transplant.*, **10**, 491–498

Lower, R. R. and Shumway, N. E. (1960) Studies on orthoptic transplantation of the canine heart. *Surg. Forum*, **11**, 18

McGregor, C. G. A., Baldwin, J. C., Jamieson, S. W. *et al.* (1985) Isolated pulmonary rejection after combined heart lung transplantation. *J. Thorac. Cardiovasc. Surg.*, **90**, 623–630

Novitsky, D., Cooper, D. K. C. and Reichart, B. (1987) The value of hormonal replacement in improving organ viability in the transplant donor. *Transplant. Proc.*, **19**, 2937–2938

Reitz, B. A., Wallwork, J., Hunt, S. A. *et al.* (1982) Heart lung transplantation: successful therapy for patients with pulmonary vascular disease. *N. Engl. J. Med.*, **306**, 557

Scott, J., Higenbottam, T., Hutter, J. A., Hodson, M., Stewart, S., Penketh, A. and Wallwork, J. (1988) Heart lung transplantation for cystic fibrosis. *Lancet*, **2**, 192–193

Wallwork, J., Jones, K., Cavrocchi, N., Hakim, M. and Higenbottam, T. (1987) Distant procurement of organs for clinical heart lung transplantation using a single flush technique. *Transplantation*, **44**, 654–658

Yousem, S. A., Berry, G. J., Brunt, E. M., Chamberlain, D., Hruban, R. H., Sibley, R. K., Stewart, S. and Tazelaar, H. D. (1990) A Working Formulation for the Standardization of Nomenclature in the Diagnosis of Heart and Lung Rejection: Lung Rejection Study Group. *J. Heart Transplant.*, **9**, 593–601

Perfusion techniques in cardiac surgery

58

Perfusion techniques in cardiac surgery

J. S. Bailey

Special techniques are needed during surgery on the heart and great vessels to maintain tissue viability, to avoid massive blood loss and to prevent air embolism. These techniques involve the extracorporeal maintenance of a circulation, artificial oxygenation of blood and modification of tissue metabolism by chemical and physical means.

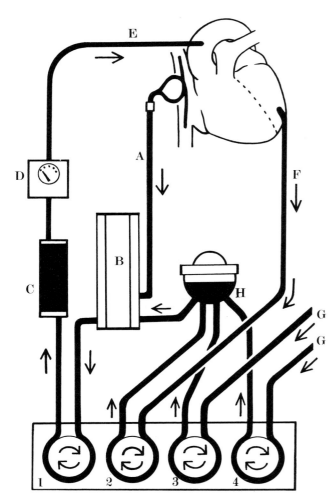

Figure 58.1 Diagram of standard extracorporeal circulation for cardiac surgery. Blood draining from the venae cavae siphons (A) into an oxygenator (B) when it is taken by a roller pump through a heat exchanger (C) and a filter on the arterial line (D). It is then returned to the ascending aorta (E). Left ventricular vented blood (F) and cardiotomy sucker blood (G) are returned to the cardiotomy and debubbling reservoir (H) by roller pumps and then passed to the oxygenator for further recirculation. The heat exchanger is frequently incorporated with the disposable oxygenator

Extracorporeal circulation (Figure 58.1)

If, for anatomical reasons, the heart must be excluded from the circulation during surgery, tissue viability can be maintained by providing an artificial circulation. This circulation must provide blood of good quality and sufficient quantity to all organs for the duration of surgery. No absolute parameters of quality and quantity exist. Individual tissues vary in their needs and further modification of need can be obtained by interfering with metabolic activity chemically or by lowering the temperature.

Cardiopulmonary bypass

Blood is removed either from the right atrium or the superior and inferior venae cavae, artificially oxygenated and returned at physiological pressure to the arterial tree. In addition, shed blood is harvested and returned to the extracorporeal circulation.

Cardiotomy suckers

Once the patient has been anticoagulated any blood shed can be returned to the extracorporeal circuit. Roller pumps are used to provide suction and return the blood to a cardiotomy reservoir from which it flows through a filter into the oxygenator. Many alternative sucker ends have been designed to minimize the trauma to the blood caused by the sudden acceleration of a blood and air mixture into the suction end. Haemolysis is produced by this suction, however applied, and it should therefore be kept to a minimum.

Constituent parts of the extracorporeal circuit

Pumps

Twin roller pumps are almost universally used to provide perfusion and suction for extracorporeal circulation. Haemolysis is minimized if the rollers are set to be just non-occlusive on the Silastic tubing on which they run.

Oxygenators

These work on many different principles of gas-to-blood interface, but three are commonly used: bubble oxygenators, rotating disc oxygenators and membrane oxygenators.

Heat exchangers

Reusable heat exchangers of many different designs exist. The important properties are low priming volume, low blood flow resistance and removal of any danger of contamination of the blood path by the water. Currently they may be included in the oxygenator or are available as disposable equipment. Tubing and flexible reservoirs are made of polyvinyl chloride. Rigid reservoirs and tube connections are made of polycarbonate. The gradual introduction of completely disposable equipment has been promoted because of the need for and difficulty of adequate removal of all protein from reusable equipment.

Priming fluids

The extracorporeal circulation can be filled with as simple a solution as 5% dextrose or as complicated a substance as whole blood. The lowered viscosity generated by blood dilution minimizes blood damage. This dilution can be safely performed to a lowest packed cell volume of 20% calculated from the patient's circulating volume and the priming volume of the extracorporeal circulation used. While recognizing enormous individual preferences among users, it is usual to include a mixture of crystalloid and colloid. Table 58.1 is an example.

Table 58.1

25% of volume	Plasma or plasma substitute (Haemaccel)
75% of volume	Balanced electrolyte solution (Plasmalyte) Corrected to approximately pH 7.4 with 8.4% $NaHCO_3$

Preparation for bypass

1. Monitoring

After induction of anaesthesia and endotracheal intubation, preparation is made for measurement of:

1. Arterial blood pressure.
2. Venous blood pressure.
3. Temperature.
4. Urine output.
5. ECG.

Since these monitoring sites will be maintained for 24 hours or longer, scrupulous sterility must be maintained in placing cannulas and catheters and fixation of dressings must be planned to maintain their sterility. It is a convenient practice to undertake full skin preparation of operating site and monitoring sites at the same time.

2. Position on operating table

Most open heart surgery is undertaken through a midline sternum-splitting incision. The patient lies supine on the operating table. If temperature regulation is to be undertaken, a water blanket is placed under the patient. It is of particular importance in open heart surgery to protect pressure points. The length of time taken and pathological circulation during bypass make skin necrosis more likely. In the supine position, the back of the head, scapulas, posterior ischial spines, sacrum and heels take most pressure. Morbidity from foot drop is also a recognized hazard from the weight of the feet producing plantar flexion.

3. Skin preparation and draping

Skin preparation begins 48 hours before surgery with chlorhexidine baths. Povidone-iodine is a good skin preparation. Towelling the operation site will vary with the needs of the theatre team. A proprietary sterile adhesive polythene sheet is often used to cover the residual skin after draping is completed.

Operation

The skin is incised from the suprasternal notch to 3 cm below the xiphoid process, in the midline. The incision is deepened with diathermy down to and through the periosteum of the sternum (Figures 58.2 and 58.3).

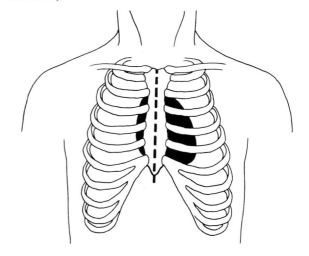

Figure 58.2 Median sternotomy

The two halves of the rectus abdominis muscles are separated by diathermy of the linea alba and a plane developed behind the xiphoid process which is divided in the midline by heavy scissors. This separates the xiphoid slips of the diaphragm so that a finger can be introduced behind the lower part of the sternum into the mediastinum.

The skin is retracted at the top corner and the deep fascia incised to expose the clavicular heads of the sternomastoid and the deep aspect of the sternum and sternothyroid muscles. These are separated in the midline after dividing the interclavicular ligament,

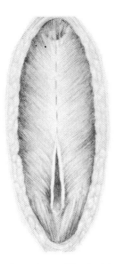

Figure 58.3 Median sternotomy. The incision is marked out on the sternum and the linea alba is opened prior to sternotomy

and the finger can then be passed into the anterior mediastinum behind the upper part of the manubrium.

The sternum is now divided using a pneumatic or electric-powered saw. Should neither of these be available, the Gigli saw is very useful (Figure 58.4). During division of the sternum, the anaesthetist holds the lungs still in aspiration to avoid entering the pleura.

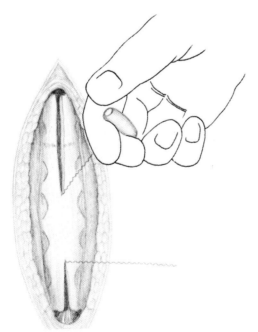

Figure 58.4 Median sternotomy using the Gigli saw

The sternal edges are held back by a self-retaining sternal spreader, revealing the deep thoracic fascia overlying the medial extensions of the pleura and the

pericardium, and splitting to invest the thymus or its adult remnants in the upper part of the mediastinum.

The loose connective tissue forming the fascial layer is swept off the pericardium. Over the thymus it is more condensed and formal division of the superficial and deep layers is needed to mobilize the thymus, especially in children. Care at this stage will prevent injury to the innominate vein which crosses the upper part of this dissection receiving short thymic veins. The level of the innominate vein varies, being lower in patients with short necks.

The pericardium is now opened by a vertical incision in the midline. At the lower end it fuses with the diaphragm and the peritoneum as a single sheet. With care the layers can be separated and the incision continued down through pericardium and diaphragm leaving the peritoneum intact. This manoeuvre provides considerably increased exposure of the diaphragmatic part of the heart from the inferior vena cava towards the left ventricular apex.

The edges of the pericardium are picked up in 'stay sutures' and fixed to the edges of the incision in the chest wall or to the sternal spreader, according to preference.

Cannulation (Figure 58.5)

Blood is returned from the extracorporeal circulation to the ascending aorta, femoral artery or external iliac artery. Of these, the ascending aorta is generally preferred.

Collection of venous blood is most simply undertaken from the right atrium direct. To be complete, retrieval must be through a large-bore cannula (12.5 mm ID) and from an undistorted atrium. In addition, the cardiac incisions made must be confined to the systemic side of the heart in the absence of abnormal communication between left- and right-sided chambers.

If cardiac surgery demands retraction of the heart to distort the right atrium, separate cannulas must be passed from the right atrium retrograde into superior and inferior venae cavae. If, in addition, the right atrium or ventricle is to be incised, or communication exists between right- and left-sided chambers, in addition to separate caval cannulation occlusive tapes must be placed around the cavae to stop blood loss or air entrainment after cardiotomy. This anatomical situation allows collection of all venous return except that from the coronary sinus, which must be collected by a separate atraumatic suction apparatus.

Before cannulation, the patient must be heparinized, using 3 mg heparin/kg body weight, initially and reinforced during surgery.

Air removal

While the chest is opened, the perfusionist will be priming and de-airing the extracorporeal circulation. Bubbles tend to adhere to the plastic components of

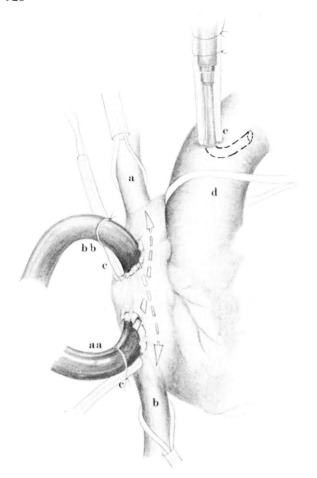

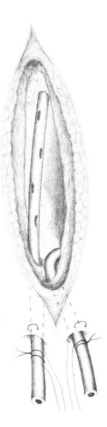

Figure 58.6 Median sternotomy, closure. Pericardial and anterior mediastinal drains are inserted

Figure 58.5 Cannulation for cardiopulmonary bypass. The superior (a) and inferior venae cavae (b) are snared and cannulated individually (aa and bb). The cannulas are secured by the snares (c). The ascending aorta (d) is cannulated; the aortic cannula (e) must point away from the aortic valve and care is taken that it does not enter the innominate or internal carotid artery

the apparatus and can be removed by percussion during a high-flow internal circulation.

After introduction of the aortic cannula, the clamp which is in place is removed slowly and blood allowed to fill the cannula, and its connecting tube. Slow air displacement prevents frothing. Connection must then be made between the extracorporeal circulation and the cannula in such a manner that bubbles are not enclosed.

Finally the tubing is placed where it will not interfere with surgery and fixed to the drapes. At this stage, it is vital to check free communication between the lumen of the aorta and the extracorporeal tubing. This is indicated by a free swing of the pressure gauge in the arterial line of the pump circuit.

Closure (Figures 58.6 and 58.7)

At least two drains must be left in the mediastinum. These are introduced through separate stab incisions

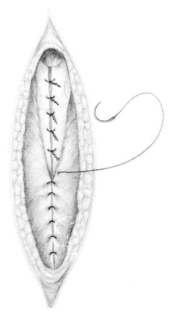

Figure 58.7 Median sternotomy, closure. The sternum is wired with interrupted sutures and the superficial tissues are carefully closed

each side of the midline below the costal margin. One will lie within the pericardium to the left of the inferior vena cava between the curve in the diaphragm and the ventricle to end in the posterior part of the pericardial space.

The second, which must have multiple side-holes, lies the full length of the anterior mediastinum from the suprasternal notch, deep to the sternum and superficial to the pericardium. The pericardium may be closed and the sternal edges brought together with interrupted wire sutures. The deep fascia is then securely closed. The linea alba is closed with non-absorbable sutures and care is necessary for incisional hernia is a well-known complication of this exposure.

Myocardial preservation

Aortic valve replacement demands aortic cross-clamping and dissection close to the coronary ostia. Under these circumstances no coronary arterial flow can occur. Various methods of myocardial preservation have been adopted at different times by different surgeons.

1. Warm ischaemia

Surgery is undertaken as swiftly as possible during the ischaemic cardiac arrest. Like all tissue, the myocardium will tolerate a period of ischaemia with progressive damage as time extends. At 37°C this is not recommended for longer than 10 minutes.

2. Cold ischaemia

When the temperature of the myocardium is lowered, ischaemia can be tolerated for longer periods. Clearly experimental work in humans cannot be used to decide absolute levels. Increasing clinical experience suggests that 1 hour can be tolerated at 20°C and 2 hours at 15°C. Various methods of obtaining myocardial cooling are used by cold coronary perfusion, by epicardial cooling, by endocardial cooling or combinations of these three. Whatever method is used, it is vital that the method described by the original proponent is used in detail rather than a personal approximation. Whole body cooling will inevitably produce myocardial cooling, but direct measurement of the myocardial temperature must be included to ensure adequate cooling of heart muscle.

3. Chemical cardioplegia

In asystole the myocardium is resistant to ischaemia for longer than when rhythmic contraction or ventricular fibrillation is occurring. This can be produced by anti-arrhythmic drugs such as lignocaine or procaine and by high concentrations of potassium ions. Many recipes have been successfully used, and argument continues about the added value of steroids and

mannitol and other ions such as calcium. The combination of chemical cardioplegia with cold is commonly used in modern practice.

The solution, as given in Table 58.2, is infused into the coronary arteries at a perfusion pressure of approximately 100 mmHg measured at the aortic root.

Table 58.2

Cardioplegic solution				
1000 ml Plasmalyte 148 (Baxter)				
Sodium	140	mmol		
Potassium	5	mmol		
Magnesium	1.5	mmol		
Chloride	98	mmol		
Acetate	27	mmol		
Gluconate	23	mmol		
Plus additives:				
Potassium chloride	20	mmol	in 10 ml	
Sodium bicarbonate	17	mmol	in 17 ml	
Methyl prednisolone	500	mg	in	8 ml
Dextrose 50%	50	ml		
This solution is stored and used at 4°C.				

When the aortic valve is competent the solution can be perfused through a wide-bore needle into the ascending aorta after the aorta has been clamped. When the aortic valve is incompetent the aorta must be opened after clamping and the solution instilled directly into the coronary ostia by hand-held coronary cannulas, 600 ml into the left and 400 ml into the right. If ischaemia of longer than 1 hour is needed, further infusions should be performed at the end of each hour. Properly applied, this technique produces rapid onset of electrical silence. At the end of the procedure, when air has been removed from the heart, the aorta is unclamped. Usually slow sinus rhythm returns within a minute. In a heart with severe preoperative myocardial decompensation, activity may return as ventricular fibrillation requiring electrical defibrillation.

4. Selective coronary perfusion (now rarely used)

This method of myocardial preservation during aortic valve replacement was popular for many years among surgeons, and proved very successful. However, it is now more or less universally accepted that the myocardial preservation provided by cold cardioplegia is superior to that offered by coronary artery perfusion. When surgery is undertaken with a closed aorta coronary perfusion continues, and the heart beats. If the whole venous return is captured by the venous drainage, no ejection occurs. However, cardiac movement may impede accurate surgery and myocardial tone will demand traumatic retraction for exposure. Similar conditions can be obtained with the aorta open and the coronary ostia individually cannulated. If myocardial contraction embarrasses surgery electrical fibrillation may be added.

Decompression of the heart

Distension of the left ventricle may produce irreversible myocardial damage and must be prevented. Damage to the lungs is produced by persistent elevation of the left atrial pressure. For these two reasons, the left ventricle should usually be vented during cardiopulmonary bypass.

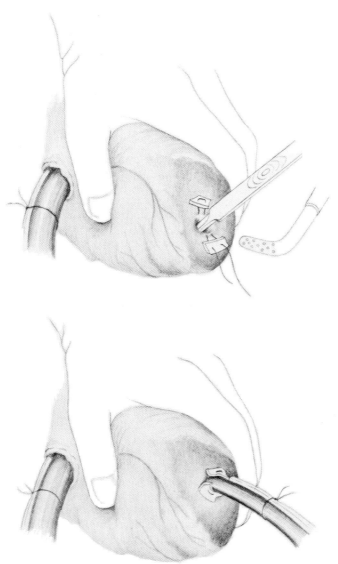

Figure 58.8 Left ventricular venting

1. Apical venting of the left ventricle (Figure 58.8)

The most convenient method of introduction of a

vent involves placing a square stitch in the left ventricle, making a stab incision at its centre, dilating this and introducing a suitable multiple side-holed vent.

2. Transatrial venting of the left ventricle (Figure 58.9)

If the apex is inaccessible, because of preoperative adhesions or in the presence of severe left ventricular hypertrophy, apical venting may be difficult or dangerous; the vent can be introduced through a pursestring placed in the anterior wall of the right superior pulmonary vein and advanced to enter the left ventricle across the mitral valve.

Blood from the vent is returned to the extracorporeal circulation after filtration, and the option of gravity drainage or active suction by a roller pump must be offered.

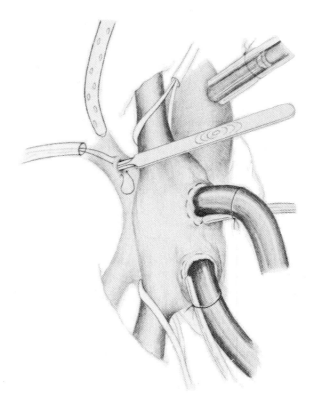

Figure 58.9 Transatrial venting of the left ventricle

Surgery during circulatory standstill without cardiopulmonary bypass

If the superior and inferior venae cavae are occluded as they enter the right atrium there will be complete inflow occlusion of the heart, which will empty with cessation of cardiac output. The venous pressure will rise and arterial pressure fall, and the heart will continue to contract.

The brain will survive 3 minutes of inflow occlusion at 37°C and during this time pulmonary commissurotomy and removal of large pulmonary emboli can be undertaken.

Longer periods of circulatory standstill can be tolerated at lower temperatures. Cooling to 30°C can be safely done by surface cooling but this method is obsolete in cardiac surgery, as at this temperature only 10 minutes of cerebral ischaemia is tolerated. If longer periods of arrest are required, lower temperatures are demanded and must be produced by core cooling on bypass. This technique is of special value in small children.

Profound hypothermia for circulatory standstill

Using conventional cardiopulmonary bypass with a heat exchanger in the circuit allows progressive cooling of the perfusate and consequent cooling of the patient. The brain temperature can be indirectly assessed by a temperature probe either in the nasopharynx adjacent to the basisphenoid or in the external auditory canal where it must be insulated by wax from the ambient air. When the predetermined 'brain' temperature is reached, the pumps are stopped, cardiac inflow prevented by occlusion of the venae cavae and clamping of the aorta and main pulmonary artery, and the heart is emptied through the atrial cannula which is then removed.

During 'suspended animation' thus produced, sur-gery can be undertaken in a totally relaxed, bloodless heart unencumbered by cannulas.

Total circulatory standstill can be survived for 45 minutes at 20°C and 90 minutes at 15°C measured in the nasopharynx or external ear.

At the end of surgery, air is evacuated from the heart which is filled with blood or crystalloid solution, the cannulas are replaced, the extracorporeal circulation restored and rewarming undertaken by gradual warming of the circulating blood. Once rewarming is complete and normal, cardiac activity is restored, the bypass is discontinued and the heart decannulated.

Profound hypothermia with autogenous oxygenation (Drew technique) (Figure 58.10)

This method of inducing profound hypothermia using the patient's lungs for autogenous oxygenation was introduced in 1959. With this technique the patient may be cooled to 15°C at which temperature circulatory arrest is instituted by ceasing perfusion and occluding the superior and inferior venae cavae. At this temperature surgical procedures may be undertaken for maximum periods of 90 minutes. This technique has proved of immense value in cardiac surgical procedures on infants and children and did, in fact, anticipate the technique of profound hypothermia using an oxygenator. There is little doubt that the use of profound hypothermia with circulatory standstill is a most useful method in the cardiac

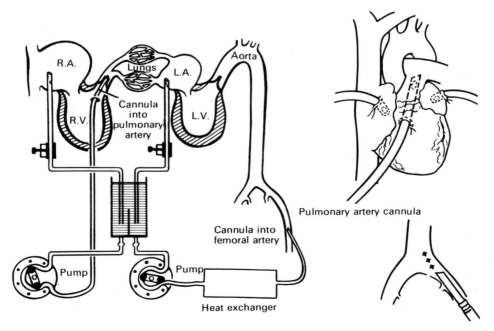

Figure 58.10 Profound hypothermia with autogenous oxygenation (the Drew technique). In addition to right atrial drainage and systemic arterial return, it is necessary to cannulate separately the main pulmonary artery and the left atrial appendage in order to perfuse the lungs which will oxygenate blood during total bypass

surgery of infants and children, but with the advent of high-quality membrane oxygenators profound hypothermia with autogenous oxygenation is used by few surgeons. For coronary artery surgery this technique can be used with continuing bypass without cooling.

Intra-aortic balloon counter-pulsation

Low cardiac output may follow open heart surgery or myocardial infarction. Improvement in left ventricular function can be gained by diastolic pressure augmentation which alters the pressure/time relationship in the aortic route in such a way that there is an opportunity to maximize diastolic coronary flow.

Diastolic pressure augmentation

A balloon in the descending aorta immediately distal to the left subclavian artery is alternately inflated and deflated by a pump triggered by the ECG. The controls of the device allow the precise timing of this action so that the inflation and deflation times and intervals can be varied.

Diastolic augmentation is achieved by deflating the balloon in systole, creating a volume equal to the balloon volume into which the LV can eject unhindered, followed by diastolic inflation which augments the diastolic filling of the aorta by the volume in the balloon with an inevitable increase in pressure.

Equipment

One of several available dedicated consoles is used to activate the pump to pump air in a primary circuit which compresses a balloon in a rigid cylinder. The balloon in the cylinder is connected by a catheter to the intra-aortic balloon and this secondary system is filled with CO_2 or helium. The low viscosity of the latter allows the use of finer catheters and will allow the pump to follow the ECG at faster heart rates. Balloons are made as single- or twin-chamber devices.

Methods of balloon introduction

Conventionally the balloon is introduced from the common femoral artery either at open operation or by a percutaneous Seldinger technique. When peripheral arterial or lower aortic disease impedes the balloon during advancement from the femoral artery a single chamber balloon is introduced from the ascending aorta. This technique is obviously only of use when counter-pulsation is to be used following thoracotomy.

Femoral artery introduction

The common femoral artery is exposed through a vertical skin incision immediately inferior to the inguinal ligament, by incision of the roof of the sub-sartorial canal. The balloon and catheter are laid from the patient's left midclavicular point to the

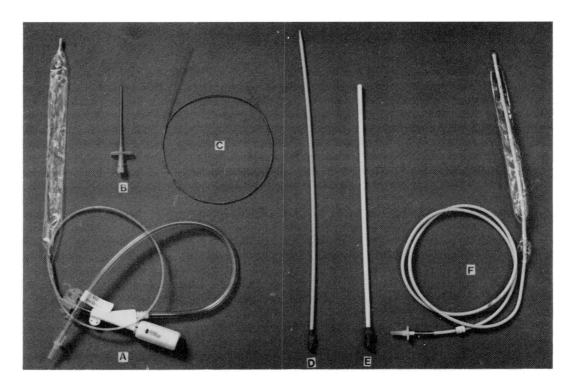

Figure 58.11 Balloons and introducers for percutaneous introduction of intra-aortic balloon

inguinal ligament and a ligature used to mark this length for introduction. The common femoral, superficial femoral and deep femoral arteries are isolated with slings and clamped.

An 8 mm vascular graft is threaded over the balloon and catheter. The common femoral artery is incised longitudinally and the balloon inserted up to the marking ligature and the common femoral sling tightened. Balloon pumping can now begin.

The vascular graft is sutured to the arteriotomy with two continuous 5/0 prolene sutures. Corded tape tied tightly around the vascular graft prevents leakage and the vascular clamps and slings are removed. The graft is buried by closing the skin and the catheter allowed to emerge from the lower end of the incision.

Following completion of counter-pulsation the incision is reopened and the balloon removed. The femoral artery is cleared proximally and distally by femoral embolectomy procedures. The graft is trimmed to leave a flap which is closed to create a patch angioplasty.

Percutaneous femoral introduction (Figure 58.11)

This is undertaken by first measuring the catheter and balloon length and marking as before. The balloon is introduced through an intra-arterial sheath which is itself introduced over a guide wire after dilatation of the arterial puncture site by a cannulated tapering dilator introduced over the guide wire.

When counter-pulsation is no longer required the balloon is removed and firm pressure over the arterial puncture for 10 minutes usually controls bleeding.

Ascending aorta introduction

This is used when the support is required following surgery and the balloon cannot be passed up the aorta because of aorto-iliac atheroma.

Two concentric purse-string sutures are applied to the ascending aorta. The ends are drawn through 5 mm polythene tubing to act as tourniquets. The single-chamber balloon is introduced through the centre of these and directed round the aortic arch. The purse-strings are tightened and secured with heavy ligature clips.

The skin only is closed leaving the balloon catheter emerging from the lower end of the incision. The incision is covered with a sterile adhesive 'drape'.

When counter-pulsation is no longer needed the chest is opened, the balloon removed, the aorta closed by tying the purse-string and the chest is closed formally.

Further reading

Drew, C. E. and Anderson, I. M. (1959) Profound hypothermia in cardiac surgery. *Lancet*, **i**, 748

Drew, C. E., Keen, G. and Benazon, D. B. (1959) Profound hypothermia. *Lancet*, **i**, 745

Gibbon, J. H. (1954) Application of mechanical heart and lung apparatus to cardiac surgery. *Minn. Med.*, **37**, 171

Lillehei, C. W., Cohen, M., Warden, H. E. *et al.* (1955) The direct vision intracardiac correction of congenital anomalies by controlled cross circulation. *Surgery*, **38**, 11

Amputations and prostheses

59

Amputations and prostheses

K. P. Robinson

An amputation is an operation which results in the severance of part of the body from the patient and is therefore considered to be a mutilating procedure with an inevitable loss of function. However, it is important to accept the philosophy that the production of a satisfactory amputation stump together with a well-designed prosthesis is a method of treatment which may save the patient's life and which may restore or even improve the function of the diseased extremity. Therefore the surgical technique and management of a patient having amputation surgery are of the greatest importance for that patient's future existence. The formation of an amputation stump is an operation to be performed with care, precision and considerable experience if the patient is to have the best result.

Indications

The indications for amputation may be considered as absolute indications to save life or relative indications to improve function. In trauma, amputation may be life saving if the patient is entrapped by immovable debris when an amputation may be required to release him. This is the only situation in which a guillotine amputation is acceptable. Amputation in trauma may also be required to prevent the crush syndrome and where traumatic gangrene has occurred or is threatened and cannot be averted. In severe burns the limb may be so destroyed that an amputation is required. When gas gangrene occurs amputation may be required despite hyperbaric oxygen and penicillin and may be life saving. Although considerable progress has been made in the treatment of neoplasms by radiotherapy and more recently by chemotherapy, there is still a place for amputation when a sarcoma recurs despite these measures. Marjolin's ulcer and Kaposi's sarcoma may also require amputation if other methods of treatment are not successful.

Acute embolism or intravascular thrombosis may produce peripheral gangrene, although embolectomy should be successful in the majority of patients. Atheroma is principally responsible for chronic occlusion of large vessels to and in the lower limb and the commonest cause of rest pain, ischaemic ulcers and peripheral gangrene which are the indications for amputation if they cannot be relieved by vascular surgery, by sympathectomy or by sympathetic block.

Atheroma is encountered prematurely and severely in diabetic patients, but in these patients the additional factors of diabetic neuropathy, diminished resistance to staphylococcal invasion and the diffuse microangiopathy must be treated before any decision is taken concerning amputation. In diabetics it is particularly important to control the diabetic state, to counter infection by antibiotics and surgical drainage of deep sepsis. This may involve local resection of osteomyelitis or excision of septic arthroses, usually achieved by ray amputations in the foot; however, without an adequate major arterial blood supply such local procedures are destined to increase the area of local gangrene and precipitate the need for a major amputation. Debridement confined to dead tissue does not involve this rule, but a preliminary local amputation without sutures may be preferred, accepting this as the initial procedure to allow sepsis to resolve before the major amputation is performed.

In the field of vascular surgery established ischaemic gangrene will require amputation and it is not often realized that rest pain is extremely severe and the deterioration which it will produce in an elderly patient will lead to bronchopneumonia and death in a remarkably short space of time if the painful extremity is not removed. In diabetic patients septic gangrene is the precursor of life-threatening septicaemia and amputation cannot be avoided. When combined with ischaemia the level must reach full vascularized tissue, otherwise a local amputation will be adequate. In Buerger's disease amputation is frequently required, as the scattered nature of the arterial blocks rarely gives the opportunity for vascular surgery.

However, it is where the relative indications are concerned that considerable judgement is required in the decision to make an amputation. The indication is to relieve pain, restore health and restore function. In general it is the informed comparison of the function of the proposed stump and available prosthesis with the existing function that the patient has prior to operation, and it is probably wise for the decision for an elective amputation for relative indications to always be made by more than one surgeon, and where possible with the informed cooperation of the patient who has had the opportunity of meeting other patients in the same situation and can assess their quality of life. Probably in no field is this more difficult than in patients with congenital disorders in whom pressure from parents and the lack of informed decision by the patients, too young to be aware of the full implications of their deformity, put the heaviest responsibility on the medical advisers. In general, an extremely conservative approach using orthoses to a maximum will be the general principle. The indications for amputation where massive trauma to a limb has resulted in infection or gangrene or obvious inability to heal are easy to discern; but there are many limbs damaged by trauma in which non-union or malunion of fractures and joint instability or fixation and extensive soft-tissue damage may lead to long-term morbidity and ultimate impairment of function, which at an early stage may be avoided by a well-chosen amputation. Similarly the long-term morbidity of osteomyelitis, fungal infections of the deep tissues of the foot, leprosy and diabetes may all require an amputation procedure at a carefully judged time.

The occasional large benign tumour and the very rare secondary tumour may be an indication for amputation. While arterial ischaemia with rest pain is a clear-cut indication for an amputation, venous ulceration and gangrene due to arteriovenous fistulas may again require considerable judgement, and perhaps in no situation is the decision more difficult than in patients with a neurological deficit after injury or disease to the brachial or sciatic plexus.

Selection of level for amputation

In congenital disorders the level of amputation can only be determined by a careful study of the individual case. However, in trauma the level of amputation is determined by the most distal level at which sound healing of a well-functioning stump can be obtained. If a guillotine amputation has been required, then amputation at a more proximal level will in general be necessary. But where a formal amputation can be performed preservation of all satisfactory tissue should be obtained and no functioning joint should be sacrificed. In neoplastic disease the consideration is the adequate clearance of malignant tissue. Skin tumours should be widely cleared. Soft-tissue sarcomas should include the whole of the muscle group in which the tumour is situated and where neurofibrosarcomas are concerned, frozen sections should be taken of the nerve proximally to ensure adequate clearance. Bone tumours in general require the whole length of the affected bone to be resected, as intramedullary spread is not uncommon. In vascular disease there is some controversy in the selection of level; in a non-diabetic patient healing can be assured if the level of amputation is immediately below the most distal palpable arterial pulsation (Taylor, 1967). However, this results in a preponderance of above-knee levels of amputation in elderly patients who may well later become bilateral amputees (Kihn et al., 1972) with a much diminished chance of rehabilitation, although Hall and Shucksmith (1971) report 75% able to walk.

Therefore the level of amputation is often selected at a lower level with an increased risk of delayed wound healing and the need for reamputation.

Many methods of determination of the site of adequate perfusion for healing of the amputation stump have been used; the Doppler ultrasound ankle systolic pressure should exceed 40 mmHg if a below-knee amputation is to succeed and the transcutaneous oxymetry reading in the skin at the amputation site should exceed a partial pressure of oxygen also of 40 mmHg. Isotope clearance studies are of value as are other arterial pressure studies, wave form analysis and dye injection methods but these all have difficulties in routine application.

The author's own preference is for amputation at the below-knee level (Hunter-Craig et al., 1970), provided that there is adequate bleeding from the skin and soft tissue at the time of operation. Others recommend through-knee amputation (Howard et al., 1969; Chilvers et al., 1971; Green et al., 1972; Newcombe and Marcuson, 1972), Gritti–Stokes (Martin et al., 1967) and supracondylar (Weale, 1969) amputations as a compromise giving good wound healing and a longer stump. It is rare for foot and distal amputations to be successful in severe vascular disorders with the exception of patients in whom the blood flow is restored by surgery and in diabetes where the factors of infection, peripheral neuropathy, microangiopathy and bacterial invasion may cause limited wet gangrene regardless of the state of the major arteries. Where amputation has to be performed for clostridial myositis or gangrene due to gas-forming organisms, the level of amputation must be selected above the involved group of muscles.

Management

Once the decision for amputation has been taken with the informed consent of the patient and the knowledge of the patient's doctor, close relatives and sometimes employer, the patient requires a full physical examination taking into account respiratory and cardiac function and the state of the musculoskeletal system. Ideally at this stage the patient should be examined by a limb-fitting surgeon, a physical medicine specialist and, in the elderly, a geriatric specialist. At this stage the social workers and occupational therapist should be informed of the situation. If there is time in the preoperative period a visit to the limb-fitting centre, with a chance to observe other patients in their rehabilitation and to obtain the interest of the prosthetic surgeon, is most helpful. The physiotherapist, who will deal with the patient after operation, should be responsible for the preoperative training. There is much advantage in the admission of the patient to a specialist unit or at least referral to an experienced team in amputation management.

A particular hazard in lower limb amputations is

the development of gas gangrene, usually due to auto-infection from bowel organisms, and prophylaxis should begin before operation with culture of a rectal swab. An enema or suppository is given before the operation and thick coverage of the perineum with cotton wool is provided to filter any flatus passed during the operation. In addition systemic penicillin should begin after the operation and continue for 5 days afterwards. The skin of the limb to be amputated should be doubly sterilized with a povidone solution and kept covered with a sterile towel until it is finally exposed in the operating theatre. Where there is an infected extremity, enclosing this in an airtight plastic bag before entry to the operating theatre may limit the chances of contamination of the amputation wound.

Anaesthesia

Where possible the operation is performed under general anaesthetic as most amputations involve the cutting of bone and despite ear plugs or headphones with music in the conscious patient, the noise can be distressing, but otherwise there is no contra-indication to a regional anaesthetic, and in the lower limb a spinal anaesthetic or epidural anaesthetic provides a highly satisfactory surgical field. In the very frail elderly patient a through-knee amputation is especially suitable for use with a regional anaesthetic as it is silent, speedy and is relatively atraumatic. Where an amputation has to be performed at the site of an accident, a nerve block is most suitable and can be introduced while the patient is inhaling a nitrous oxide–oxygen mixture.

Moderate hypotension with careful blood volume control is advisable for the proximal amputations, and provision of a central venous pressure monitor and of urine output measurement via a catheter is required. Blood should be available for transfusion; 4 units for fore- and hindquarter amputations.

Surgical principles involved in amputation

Where an amputation is performed for sepsis, either existing or threatened due to contamination of a traumatized extremity, primary suture should be avoided. A guillotine operation in which all the tissues are incised at the same level will inevitably result in retraction of the skin and muscles and protrusion of the bone end even if skin traction is applied after the operation, and should be reserved for the release of trapped victims. A modification of this in which the skin is cut distal to the bone as a sleeve is more acceptable but will inevitably lead to a cicatrized terminal scar adherent to the bone with retraction of muscles from the vicinity of the bone end. Both these types of amputation should be used only if the need for a reamputation procedure is accepted. In battle-

field amputations the simplest and most distal amputation is accepted but the formation of short equal flaps including muscle closed with delayed primary suture after 5–6 days is very much preferable and on many occasions may avoid the need for a further amputation procedure.

For the elective amputations, whether of the upper or lower limb, it is important that the procedure is conducted as a precision operation with delicate handling of all tissues with adequate assistance to support the limb in the most favourable position. Where ischaemic disease is present a tourniquet is avoided as this may crush a segment of atheroma and precipitate a thrombosis proximal to the stump, but for all other amputations a pneumatic tourniquet should be routinely applied proximal to the amputation site – with safeguards to prevent its inflation to too high a pressure, or for too long a period and with safeguards to avoid it being overlooked at the end of the operation.

The level of amputation should always be carefully measured from the bony landmarks with a rule and the proposed skin incision marked with Bonney's blue dye or other indelible marker and the line of section through the other soft tissues should be repeatedly checked with the rule as the skin will usually retract. The skin flaps are cut and the incision deepened through the fat to the deep fascia. Diathermy is used for haemostasis of the smallest vessels and fine catgut sutures for the remaining vessels. The smallest amount of dead tissue should be retained in the stump and there seems little advantage in using heavy surgical materials. A skin hook should be used to handle the skin rather than dissecting or other forceps. Muscles should be cut cleanly with a scalpel and where a myoplasty is to be performed, that is, the suture of opposing muscles across the bone end to retain their function, then a sufficient length of muscle should be retained from the distal part of the limb to enable this suturing to be effected under natural tension.

An alternative procedure to myoplasty is myodesis – the fixation of muscle to the bone end – and this involves drilling of the bone in order to fix the sutures to the bone end. Where an osteomyoplasty is performed, part of the bone is incorporated in the muscle rearrangement; an example is the fibular bridge which can be employed in the osteomyoplasty of a below-knee amputation. Where muscle is sutured 0 or 1/0 chromic catgut sutures are required. It is important, if muscles are to function within the stump, that their blood supply and innervation are preserved. The presence of active muscles in the stump will ensure that the muscle pump aids venous return, the muscle mass will not waste and the function of the muscle concerned will be preserved. An amputation stump with an adequate myoplasty or myodesis will at rest lie in a natural position as there is no unopposed muscle function to produce a deformity.

The treatment of blood vessels is important. Mass

ligature of arteries, veins and nerves should be avoided and the veins should be ligated with fine catgut. If thrombosis is noted within the veins this is an indication to excise more of the muscle mass and to give prophylactic heparin following the operation. Ligature of the veins and arteries together is avoided as arteriovenous fistulas have been described from this technique. The arteries require a fine double catgut ligature and where the arteries are occluded it is sometimes useful to perform a catheter thrombectomy using a Fogarty catheter to increase the blood supply to the stump. The nerves require particular attention and these should be freed from any pressure or ligature and drawn down to be cut transversely with a sharp scalpel so that they will retract 2–3 cm above the scar area; this is important not only for the named major nerve trunks but also for cutaneous nerves and small branches. The formation of neuroma at the amputation site is inevitable, but unless it is in an area of friction or high pressure should not be responsible for symptoms. It is likely that mismanagement of the nerve trunk is responsible for much postoperative and long-term pain in amputation stumps.

The bone requires particular attention. The periosteum should be elevated for the minimum distance and the site of amputation should, if possible, avoid the nutrient vessels to the medullary cavity. The value of leaving a flap of periosteum to cover the open end of the medullary cavity of a bone is of debatable value, but it has been stated that an open medullary cavity prejudices the whole haemodynamic pattern of the shaft of a long bone. A flap of periosteum may be conserved to suture over the open medullary cavity. The bone may be cut with a hand or power saw; the latter allowing for more precise shaping of the bone end. However, the saw cut is always jagged with sharp spicules and careful rounding of all surfaces by a bone rasp and file is required. This process may take 10–15 minutes and is of the greatest importance as the bone end should be able to float atraumatically in the soft tissues within the socket of any prosthesis that is provided.

The general technique should result in a supple stump in which the bone end is covered with an adequate thickness of soft tissue with functioning muscles. The fascia, fat and skin should be mobile over the bone end. The scar should be linear and not attached to the deep tissues. It seems that with modern prosthetic fitting a terminal scar over the bone end is of no disadvantage provided the other criteria are satisfactory. The general shape of the stump should be a cylinder with a hemi-spherical extremity and the diameter of the cylinder should not be wider than the diameter of the contralateral limb. Haematoma deep infection and muscle necrosis should be carefully avoided by good surgical technique and established infection with a ring sequestrum at the site of bone section should not be encountered. There should be a minimum of foreign material in the stump. The skin and muscles should have a normal vascular supply. Unexplained postoperative pain in the early period is a sign of ischaemic musculature and an unsatisfactory stump.

Following operation the amputation stump is usually covered with a dressing, although in upper limb amputations this is not essential. An absorbent cotton gauze fluffed appears to be the best material and if this is covered with a 10 cm crepe bandage, applied in a lazy S spiral, it is possible to provide uniform support to the whole stump without producing the proximal constriction which is inevitable in the conventional way of bandaging an amputation stump in which loops of bandage are restrained by a tight proximal turn. However, if the bandage is wider than 10 cm the spiral cannot be made to conform with the stump. There is great controversy about the best way in which an amputation wound should be dressed, with an increasing tendency to avoid anything but the softest net bandage.

There is a natural tendency of a terminal wound to become oedematous and pressure is applied to avoid this, but in many cases a badly applied bandage will itself produce distal oedema due to proximal constriction. A plaster-of-Paris shell applied to the amputation stump will protect it from inadvertent trauma or outside infection and will prevent muscle spasms. This is ideal if it can be rapidly changed should there be any anxiety about the underlying wound, but it may conceal pressure necrosis, ischaemia and infection. A compromise is a wholly split plaster shell retained with bandage.

To avoid these problems intermittent pressure applied in a plastic sleeve with a valvular seal at the top has been used in the technique of the controlled environment chamber, but this apparatus is rather cumbersome and only likely to be available at special centres. A pneumatic sleeve has been applied on the operating table and retained as a dressing with some success. The immediate preoperative fitting of a prosthesis has been successfully used in many centres, a plaster socket being fitted at the completion of the operation to which is applied an upper limb prosthesis or a lower limb foot and extension piece, so that the upper limb patient can use the prosthesis from the moment he or she wakes up and the lower limb patient can make ground contact after 48 hours and partially weight-bear at 1 week. It is essential that if a plaster socket is used there are facilities for its immediate removal and replacement if there is any anxiety about the underlying stump, and this is the main limitation to its general usage.

An alternative to plaster is a low-temperature, heat-labile plastic mesh which can be moulded to the stump at operation or shortly after and used as either a rigid dressing or a temporary socket. However, in upper limb amputations immediate prosthetic fitting maintains the cortical representation of the arm which is otherwise very quickly lost, with the result that the patient becomes one-handed and may subsequently reject a prosthesis as cumbersome and of doubtful improvement over a one-handed existence.

In the early postoperative period the nursing care is directed to preventing pressure sores on the sacrum and heels. The lower limb amputee should spend two periods of half an hour in the day lying prone to prevent hip flexing and arm movements should be encouraged in the upper limb amputee from an early stage. As soon as the patient has recovered from the operation, a physiotherapy programme encourages active and passive mobility of the remaining joints and limbs and correction of any postural defect. Lower limb amputees are taught to use a wheelchair from the 2nd postoperative day and should be competent in transfer from bed to chair, chair to toilet by 1 week from the operation. In a limb with normal vascularity, soft-tissue healing should be complete by 10–14 days, at which time the skin sutures should be removed, but in the lower limb, especially if the amputation has been for ischaemic disease, sutures should be retained for 21 days and for this reason the most satisfactory suture material is either nylon or prolene, which elicits no inflammatory reaction.

Prosthetic management

Where a plaster socket has been provided on the operating table, function can begin within days of the surgical operation, but only partial weight-bearing is permitted in a lower limb amputation until the 7th to 10th day and then the degree of weight-bearing is progressively increased to full function by 3 weeks. The patient can be taught to grade the pressure using a bathroom scale or pressure-activated biosensor. This represents a great advance over the previous management in which the patient was confined to bed and a wheelchair until his prosthesis was prescribed, sometimes months after the amputation.

The use of an early walking aid pioneered by Devas has considerably reduced this period of delay. The first walking aids were modified pylons, essentially an ischial-bearing device with side-irons, a rocker or foot and a knee hinge with a slide lock. A patient with an amputation at below-knee, through-knee or above-knee level can use one of these from the 10th day after operation and is usually able to walk between parallel bars or with sticks or with a walking frame by the 3rd or 4th postoperative week. Many patients have taken aids of this type home while awaiting their definitive prosthesis.

A considerable advance in early walking aids has come with the pneumatic aid, devised by Little, and modified by Redhead – essentially a pneumatic splint enclosed in a frame with a foot piece. This can be worn from the 7th postoperative day. The patient can wear the appliance for 2 hours at a time, inflated to a pressure of 40 mmHg. It is infinitely adjustable to patients of varying size and can be held in any physiotherapy department in readiness for each new patient. The patient can walk with this aid under supervision until a definitive prosthesis is provided.

In the early weeks after operation the stump is more bulky due to oedema than it will be later on, and the process of shrinkage means that a socket which will fit perfectly on the 14th postoperative day will be much too loose by the 21st, and therefore it is rarely practical to provide a definitive socket until after the 21st postoperative day. The process of shrinkage is much enhanced by the use of a pneumatic prosthesis and slightly delayed by the use of a walking aid in which the stump is not supported. The routine bandaging of an amputation stump is not essential and the traditional method is particularly likely to result in a tourniquet proximal constriction which may cause swelling and breakdown at the suture line. An elastic net sock is much preferred to hold a light fluffed gauze in place. It is unlikely that any amputation stump is fully mature in less than 3 months and it is usual for the first prosthesis to be replaced in this period. Therefore the first definitive prosthesis is usually of a simple type and for manufacturing reasons is often in the nature of a pylon which will allow the patients normal function and the ability to resume their normal environment.

A patient with a lower limb amputation from trauma should be able to return home 4 weeks from the operation and a lower limb amputee for ischaemic disease, even in the geriatric age group, should be able to return home 6–8 weeks after the operation. Upper limb amputees can leave hospital in 10–14 days but will need to attend an arm training school for a much longer period to obtain full rehabilitation.

It is important that before discharge from hospital a home visit has been made to supply special aids, such as hand rails and ramps in the home, to educate the relatives to the needs of the amputee and in the case of employees their employment should be adapted to their ability and this may involve the arrangement of a retraining programme. It is important for the geriatric patient that a geriatrician advises on the best accommodation and the management of the patient after discharge.

Stump complications

These may be seen in both upper and lower limb amputations and can be considered as follows:

1. Delayed healing may be attributed to local problems particularly ischaemia due to an inadequate arterial supply. In infection, whether auto-infection or cross-infection, what is particularly significant is the lack of cooperation of the patient who may contaminate the wound or traumatize the healing stump or maintain the limb in an unsuitable position applying pressure to the suture line. Delayed healing may also be encountered with intercurrent disease, such as diabetes in elderly patients, those with uraemia, malnutrition, anaemia and infection at other sites, and these factors should be carefully corrected.

2. An amputation stump may be painful in the early postoperative period and may cause pain throughout the patient's lifetime. In the early postoperative period the most important cause of pain is ischaemia, particularly of the muscles, whether due to pre-existing arterial disease or to compression of the muscles due to poor operative technique. Deep vein thrombosis may occur in the amputation stump leading to swelling and pain which may not be recognized. Infection is usually apparent by redness, induration and tenderness and osteomyelitis may show by the erosion of the transected bone end. Later pain may be due to incorporation of a nerve trunk in the fibrous scar of the neuroma fortuitously developing in an area exposed to friction or pressure.

If these problems can be excluded it is likely that there is a psychiatric overlay to the problem and depression is frequently encountered. Causalgic pain is sometimes seen in patients who are afraid to use the stump, regarding the phantom sensations, which are an entirely normal phenomenon, as distressing. Psychiatric help may be required in this situation.

3. The scar may be adherent to the bone end and therefore be submitted to tension while the stump is in use, and retrimming is sometimes indicated to free the adherent soft tissue to improve the shape of the bone end.

4. There may be tension of the soft tissues over a prominent bone end. This is a particular problem when an amputation is through a growing bone when the unimpeded epiphyseal lengthening proximal to the amputation causes a conical stump with considerable pain and deformity. The bone end may be prominent due to a poorly judged amputation with tight soft tissues and a badly shaped bone end which may result in osteophyte formation with bony spurs, with sometimes more extensive myositis ossificans. These complications may necessitate a refashioning of the amputation stump.

5. The skin may become thickened and lymphoedematous; sometimes eczema develops due to poor ventilation of the socket and in pressure areas sebaceous cysts may form.

6. Sometimes adventitious bursas are a problem and frequently at the ischium a poorly fitting socket will push a roll of fatty flesh above the socket and cause discomfort. Pressure of the socket in this region may eventually produce arterial and venous thrombosis, although this is often a slow process and usually does not cause any problem in the stump.

7. Otherwise the principal complications of the amputation stump are deformity of the proximal joints progressing to fixation of the proximal joints usually in a flexed position with corresponding loss of function. Flexion deformities may be extremely difficult to treat and prophylaxis is an essential part of the early management of every amputee.

Arm amputations

Forequarter amputation

Forequarter amputation consists of extirpation of the shoulder girdle including the scapula and most of the clavicle and all the structures of the arm (Figure 59.1). The patient is left with a smooth contour to the rib cage and no projection on which to support a prosthesis. The operation can be performed with the dissection starting either from the front or from behind. In both cases the patient is laid on his or her side with the arm to be amputated upwards and fully towelled. A racquet type of incision is used with the handle of the racquet along the clavicle (Figure 59.1). If the dissection is started from the front the clavicle is divided with a Gigli saw 3 cm from the sternoclavicular joint. The pectoralis major and minor are incised at a distance depending on the pathology and the

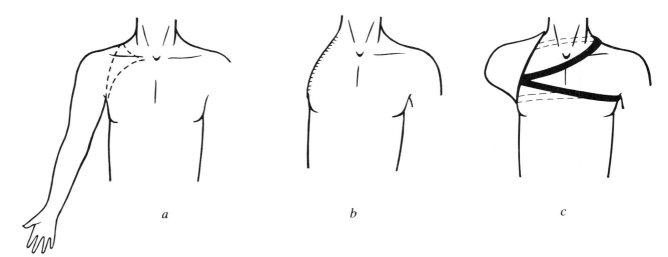

a   *b*   *c*

Figure 59.1 Forequarter amputation. *a*, Skin flaps. *b*, This stump is unsuitable for a prosthesis other than a shoulder pad (*c*)

axillary fascia opened, allowing access to the subclavian vein, the subclavian artery and the trunks of the brachial plexus. These are divided just distal to the tendon of scalenus anterior with double nonabsorbable ligatures with special care to avoid retraction before the ligature is secure, and the arm is lifted to bring the muscular attachments of the scapula into view. The levator scapulae, the serratus anterior, the trapezius and rhomboid muscles are divided and finally the latissimus dorsi, resulting in separation of the upper extremity. The serratus anterior and pectoralis major residue can be sutured together to provide additional cover for the exposed rib cage. An alternative approach is to initiate dissection by dividing the trapezius and latissimus dorsi, posteriorly at the start of the dissection, then incising the serratus anterior, lifting the scapula forwards bringing access to the neurovascular bundle from behind. Advantages are claimed for both techniques.

Following operation few patients are able to use a prosthesis and a light shoulder pad is usually all that is used. A prosthetic arm for cosmetic purposes can be supplied but is not found to be satisfactory by the patients.

Shoulder disarticulation (Figure 59.2)

A racquet or anterior and posterior gap incision is formed at the level of the neck of the humerus and after dissection of the neurovascular bundle the pectoralis major and minor and deltoid are divided close to the humerus. The teres major and minor and the muscles of the rotator cuff are divided, and the anterior capsule with the shoulder joint is incised allowing just the head of the humerus to be dislocated, and incision of the posterior capsule allows the limb to be removed. The pectoralis major, deltoid and rotator cuff muscles are apposed over the glenoid cavity and the skin closed with drainage.

The functional ability of a prosthesis for this amputation is not very satisfactory as despite a large shoulder cap covering the protruding acromion there is some instability and it is difficult to obtain adequate leverage from the opposite shoulder to operate the elbow and the other hand has to be used to lock the prosthesis, either in a flexed or extended position, before shoulder movement can activate a split hook.

Above-elbow amputation (Figure 59.3)

There is no optimum level for amputation measured from the acromion. The most important factor is that sufficient room must be left below the stump to allow an elbow mechanism in the prosthesis. Therefore a clear 10 cm must be allowed above the elbow joint for this purpose. Otherwise the longest lever that can be retained is best for prosthetic function. In practical terms at least three finger-breadths' (4 cm) length of humerus must project below the axillary fold for a socket to use the humerus as a lever; above this level a prosthesis has all the disadvantages of a shoulder disarticulation although the retention of the head of the humerus and amputation through the surgical neck give a better contour to the shoulder. At whichever level is applicable the skin is incised to make equal anterior and posterior flaps and the muscles are cut transversely inclining inwards and upwards to the line of bone section. The bone is rounded with a bone file and the flexor and extensor muscles are sutured together over the bone end to constitute a myoplasty and the deep fascia closed with fine catgut; the skin is closed with fine sutures, nylon or prolene, and with Steristrips. This is the ideal amputation for an immediate preoperative fitting of a prosthesis and if the limb has been measured prior to surgery a normal type of prosthesis can be applied on the operating table.

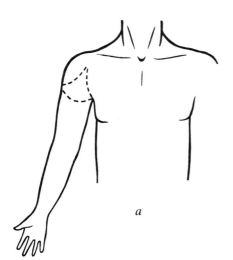

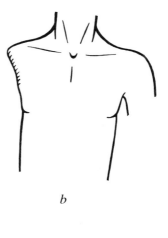

a

b

Figure 59.2 Disarticulation of shoulder. *a*, Skin flaps. *b*, This stump is also unsuitable for a prosthesis

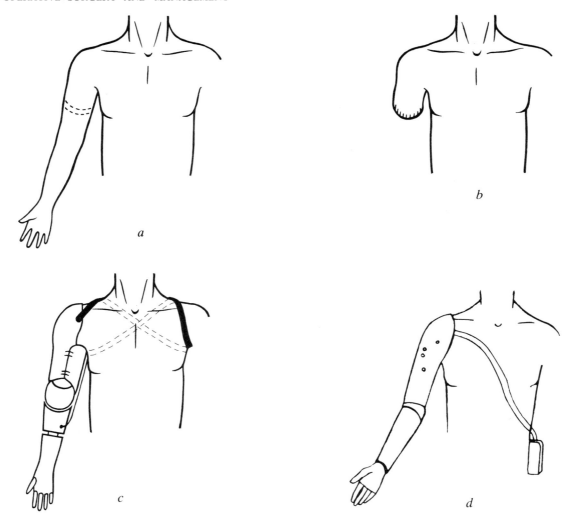

Figure 59.3 Above-elbow amputation. *a*, Skin flaps. *b*, Stump. *c*, Conventional prosthesis. *d*, Swedish myoelectric arm, with battery pack and triggering detectors on upper arm

Elbow disarticulation (Figure 59.4)

If the elbow can be retained, disarticulation at the elbow joint is an acceptable procedure. Anterior and posterior flaps are formed based on the medial and lateral epicondyles. Sufficient length of triceps tendon, biceps and brachialis is retained to allow suture over the articular surface of the humerus and the skin is closed with drainage. The prominence of the epicondyles enables the prosthetic forearm to be retained by a leather and lace suspension. The axis of the elbow joint is anterior to the normal elbow but there is no detriment to function.

Elbow flexion can be operated from the opposite shoulder by a cord which on further movement will operate a splint hook; pronation and supination at mid-forearm are effected by the opposite hand.

Below-elbow amputation (Figure 59.5)

There is no optimal site of amputation below the

elbow but the lever length clear of the biceps tendon should be as long as possible, although sufficient muscle should be available to cover the bone ends to make a myoplastic amputation, and therefore the junction between the lower third and the upper two-thirds of the radius and ulna is ideal. Equal anterior and posterior flaps are formed with suture of the flexor and extensor muscle groups over the transected ulna and radius. At this level an immediate prosthesis can be provided by a plaster socket applied on the operating table carrying a pivot for pronation and supination of either a double hook operated by a cord from the opposite shoulder or a cosmetic hand.

In an attempt to obtain better function at this level Kruckenberg claws have been used, in which the radius and ulna are separated and provided with skin cover, making a lobster claw. This is especially indicated in blind patients and the operation is performed by making an axial incision from four finger-breadths below the elbow joint over the interosseous region on both the anterior and posterior surface of the fore-

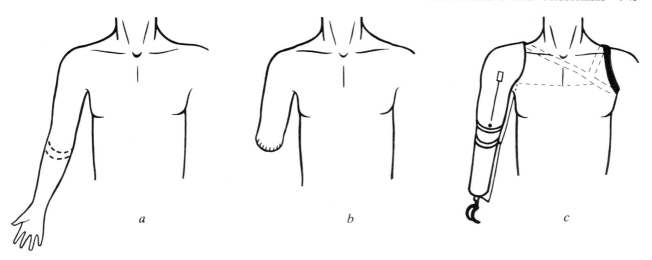

Figure 59.4 Through-elbow amputation. *a*, Skin flaps. *b*, Stump. *c*, Prosthesis which allows elbow flexion to be operated from the opposite shoulder by a cord. Pronation and supination at mid-forearm are effected by the opposite hand.

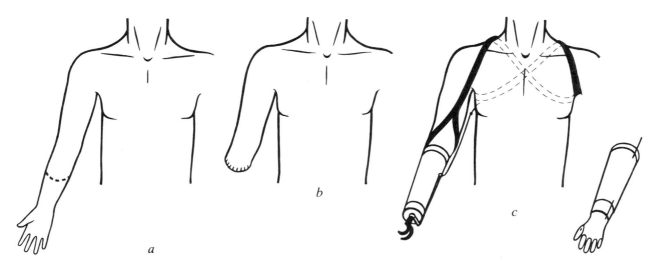

Figure 59.5 Below-elbow amputation. *a*, Skin flaps. *b*. Stump. *c*, Prosthesis which allows double hook or cosmetic hand operated from the opposite shoulder

arm. The flexor digitorum sublimis is split while the profundus and flexor pollicis longus are removed. The interosseous membrane is divided. The median and ulnar nerves are cut distal to the branches supplying the forearm muscles and the interosseous membrane is divided to within 7 cm of the elbow joint. The lateral part of the flexor digitorum sublimis is attached to the flexor carpi radialis and the medial part is sutured to the flexor carpi ulnaris. The ends of the forearm bones are grooved. The radial extensors and flexors are sutured in the radial groove and the ulnar muscles in the ulnar groove. The skin can be closed around the radius but a graft may be placed to close the inner side of the ulnar jaw. The brachioradialis opens the jaws while pronator teres and the forearm flexors close the jaws.

Wrist amputations

The wrist can be disarticulated if there is severe and irretrievable hand injury. As much of the carpal structure as is viable should be retained. The operation is essentially performed through anterior/posterior flaps centred on the ulnar and radial styloid processes which, if no carpal bone is retained, may need to be smoothed flush with the articular surface of the radius. The tendons of the flexor and extensor muscles should be left long enough to allow them to be sutured over the bone end and constitute a myoplasty. A plaster shell can be applied at the completion of the operation and a split hook applied to the plaster for immediate function. It is not possible to utilize the patient's own pronation and supination in the prosthesis and this remains a passive function, while activation of a split hook is achieved by a cord from the opposite shoulder.

Amputations in the hand

This is a particularly difficult problem requiring great experience and should always be managed by a specialist in the field. Part-finger amputations may be unsatisfactory as the release of tendon attachments leads to progressive stiffness and encumbrance due to the rigidity of the remaining portion of the finger. Provided the tendon attachments remain, amputation of the distal phalanx can provide acceptable function, although proximal to this there is a considerable functional deficit, but it is probably always wise to allow the patient to obtain the best use of the remaining digits for a trial period before accepting the need for a more proximal amputation.

Here the problem is whether to leave the patient with an intact metacarpal structure with a wide span across the metacarpophalangeal joints with a strong palm at the expense of a prominent metacarpal head. There is little doubt that heavy manual workers fare best with intact metacarpals, and amputation of a digit should be through the base of the proximal phalanx to preserve the short muscle attachments, but in other patients resection of the metacarpophalangeal joint and part of the metacarpal cut obliquely provides a much more acceptable cosmetic hand. The thumb and index finger are of the greatest practical value and should be preserved if at all possible. The possibility of transference of a digit and its neurovascular connections, as in the procedure of pollicization of an index finger, should be carefully considered before any decision is made to amputate.

A digital amputation can be made either with a racquet incision or by anterior posterior flaps. Considerable care should be taken to avoid ligating the digital nerve. Skin closure with Steristrips and fine 6/0 nylon sutures is recommended.

Where trauma has resulted in extensive digital loss, there should be no attempt to produce any formal amputation, but conservative trimming should aim to produce supple skin cover of smooth bone ends, and provide means of improving function by secondary surgery at a later date.

Power prostheses for upper limb amputees have made considerable progress in the past decade. There is no limit to the mechanical ingenuity that has been expended on this topic but two problems remain – an acceptable power source and sophisticated control mechanisms. Gas power from cylinders is being superseded by battery-powered electric motors, while actuation of the functions can be triggered by myoelectric potentials, or by pressure detectors over functional muscles. Both require considerable education of, and determination by, the patient in order to achieve acceptable results, but the Swedish arm shows how much can be achieved – finger extension and flexion, wrist rotation and elbow flexion and extension.

Amputations at various levels in the lower limb

Translumbar amputation (hemicorporectomy)

Although a dreadful mutilation, amputation at this level has been successfully performed for extensive local tumours in the pelvis and also for extreme trauma to the pelvis and lower limbs (Baker *et al.*, 1970). The amputation is made at the level of the 2nd lumbar vertebra, and the formation of an ileal conduit and the establishment of a left iliac colostomy are necessary. The soft tissues are incised to form two equal anteroposterior flaps, although the best use must be made of the available soft tissue. The aorta and vena cava must be secured at an early stage; while the vena cava may be ligated the aorta is best over-sewn with a continuous arterial suture. The spinal theca should also be closed with a continuous catgut suture and some of the muscle of the posterior flap placed over the end of the vertebral canal.

The patient is nursed flat in the early days after the operation with active physiotherapy to strengthen the arms and shoulders and to ensure adequate ventilation. Once the soft tissues are healed, the patient can be sat up and a chair-like frame constructed to hold the patient securely by the shoulders while allowing free movement of the abdominal wall and arms. A similar truncal socket can be incorporated in an electric wheelchair with hand controls to provide the patient with mobility.

Hindquarter amputation

This procedure, which was established by Sir Gordon Gordon Taylor at a time when any major operation carried a considerable hazard, has now developed into a safe elective procedure (Westbury, 1967), which should be carried out with a hypotensive anaesthetic technique and, where possible, with the use of diathermy to cut across the muscle mass and to secure careful haemostasis throughout.

The patient is positioned on the operating table in a half lateral position with the affected leg fully towelled so that its position can be changed. A urethral catheter should be passed. The anterior skin incision runs just distal to the inguinal ligament and the posterior skin flap incorporates most of the skin of the buttock and some of the muscle fibres of gluteus maximus and medius to carry the blood supply. The anterior incision is deepened to the inguinal ligament which is detached from the anterior superior iliac spine and the abdominal wall muscles are erased from the iliac crest back to the ala of the sacrum. In the extraperitoneal plane the peritoneum is separated from the iliac fossa and access can be obtained by retraction to the back of the pubis, which can then be divided with a Gigli saw. This allows the pelvis to open slightly and exposure can be obtained of the common iliac artery and vein. The iliac artery can be ligated without difficulty but the iliac vein must be carefully dissected to safeguard against the small iliolumbar branches emerging from its concealed posterior aspect. By carefully ligating these, the blood loss from the operation is reduced to a minimum and the iliac vein can then be securely ligated and divided.

The dissection is deepened below the pubis to separate the urethral bulb and muscles from the ischium and the levator ani can be detached from the obturator internus fascia. The ischiorectal fat is separated from the pelvic side-wall and the dissection carried into the greater and lesser sciatic notch. Here the superior and inferior gluteal vessels will be secured and the lumbosacral trunk and elements of the sciatic plexus divided, leaving the ala of the sacrum for division with a Gigli saw before the extremity can be detached. Careful haemostasis is obtained and the skin flaps sutured with suction drainage. The patient can be mobilized a few days after the operation and can learn to walk with crutches at the earliest opportunity.

Once the soft tissues are stable and healed, the patient can be measured for a prosthesis which consists of a large socket for the hemipelvis with shoulder straps for stability and a belt embracing the other side of the pelvis. The underside of the socket is flattened and an anterior hinge suspends the leg, which requires a knee joint locking device. The most popular prosthesis is the Canadian pattern tilting table which will allow these patients to walk with an acceptable gait and to stand and sit with minimal difficulty. Some of these patients are able to walk without the use of any stick or support.

Disarticulation at the hip joint (Figure 59.6)

Through an anterior incision, running just below the inguinal ligament, and a posterior flap performed at the lower part of the buttock skin, the femoral triangle is exposed and the femoral artery and vein can be ligated at the level of the inguinal ligament. The posterior skin flap can incorporate a greater or lesser amount of the gluteal muscle mass according to the reason for the amputation. The anterior muscles are erased from the pelvis until the hip joint is exposed; the capsule and iliofemoral ligaments are divided allowing the head to be dislocated and further dissection reaches the sciatic nerve which is divided with a small ligature to secure only the concomitant artery, and the limb can then be detached. Careful haemostasis is secured and the flaps closed with suction drainage.

Early ambulation with crutches can be achieved and the patient can be fitted with a similar prosthesis to the hindquarter amputation, but weight is carried on the ipsilateral ischial tuberosity and the greater stability of the socket on the bony pelvis enables a better gait to be achieved. The patient may walk well with a swing phase control knee joint but usually a knee lock is provided for greater stability.

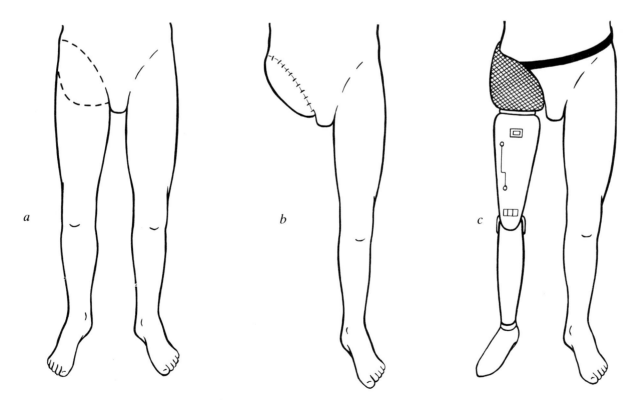

Figure 59.6 Disarticulation of hip. *a*, Skin flaps. *b*, Stump. *c*, Tilting table prosthesis.

Amputation through the upper end of the femur

Through a similar incision to that described for a hip disarticulation, a similar dissection can be performed with the exception that the femur is divided at the junction of the neck and shaft, with the advantage that when the soft tissues cover the bone remnant the stump has a better shape and some weight can be carried by the femoral residue on the ischial tuberosity of the same side. However, with modern cast-resin sockets the prominent femoral remnant may be a disadvantage.

Above-knee level of amputation (Figure 59.7)

The exact level of this amputation is not important, but if a sophisticated knee joint mechanism is to be provided then the lower end of the femur must terminate 13 cm above the axis line of the knee joint before operation. At this level the femoral artery and vein are in the lower part of the subsartorial canal. Two equal flaps (Figure 59.7a) can be based at this level, 13 cm above the knee joint line, skewed to enable the vertical part of the incision to overly the subsartorial canal to provide early and easy access to the femoral vessels, which are individually ligated as the first stage of the dissection. The incision is deepened through the fascia lata, the lower end of the quadriceps and some of the quadriceps expansion is transected just below the line of bone section, and the hamstring muscles are cut a little longer than the bone end. The iliotibial band is cut 5 cm longer than the line of bone section, as are the adductor, gracilis and sartorius tendons. These transected muscles then constitute four groups. The bone is transected and the edges carefully rounded with a bone rasp and file before the drill holes are made. The adductors can be sutured to the iliotibial band across the end of the femur, but unless the bone end is drilled the attached muscles will slip off and the anchoring effect will be lost. The hamstrings are sutured to the quadriceps mass and again the sutures must be stabilized through drill holes in the bone end.

A full myodesis is then obtained. The fascia lata is carefully repaired and the skin closed with fine nylon sutures, suction drainage being provided as a routine. The above-knee amputation heals readily and is usually stable at 14 days (Figure 59.7b). The patient can be supplied with an ischial weight-bearing socket and pylon to facilitate walking training until the stump is sufficiently stable to permit accurate casting for a definitive prosthesis or may use a pneumatic walking aid (Figure 59.7c–e). The myoplastic technique described gives a cylindrical stump which is very suitable for the application of a suction socket which can eliminate the need for any straps or buckles and enables the patient with an above-knee amputation to walk with a nearly normal gait (Figure 59.7e). The myoplastic amputation requires no special postural treatment as it takes a natural position without

hip flexion, although it is advisable for the patient still to lie on his or her face for two periods of half an hour each day to prevent a flexion contracture of the hip developing in the early postoperative period. Physiotherapy is essential to prevent hip flexion, especially prior to the operation.

Supracondylar amputation (Weale, 1969)

Proposed as an alternative to the Gritti–Stokes amputation, the line of bone section is through the lower end of the femur at the level of the adductor tubercle. Equal skin flaps are formed and the popliteal artery and vein secured posteriorly at an early stage in the dissection. The quadriceps expansion and the hamstring tendons are transected 2.5 cm beyond the bone end so that they can be sutured together and attached over the bone end. The bone end, being square and wide, may not need to be drilled to stabilize the attached tendons. The fascia lata and skin are closed with suction drainage if necessary.

The patient can be allowed to stand with crutches and to walk at an early stage with an ischial weight-bearing pylon and socket. When healed and stable, a prosthesis can be supplied with a simple hinge knee joint and lock which is satisfactory but is inferior to a suction socket and sophisticated knee joint mechanism which can be provided for the slightly higher above-knee amputation.

Gritti–Stokes amputation (Figure 59.8)

This amputation, popular in some centres, is performed at the same level as the supracondylar amputation. The adductor tendon remains attached to its tubercle. A long anterior skin flap is fashioned, extending to the tubercle of the tibia, so that the patellar tendon is detached from the tibia and the anterior skin flap and the patella and quadriceps expansion are reflected upwards. A short posterior skin flap is deepened to reach the popliteal nerves and the popliteal vessels. The hamstring muscles are divided at the level of bone section. The patella and quadriceps expansion are pulled upwards to obtain access to the supracondylar region of the femur, which is divided transversely and sharp edges rounded with a file. The saw cut should be higher posteriorly so that muscle tension locks the patella in place. The articular surface of the patella is shaved off with a vertical saw cut while the soft tissues are held in a large swab. The patella is then drilled and drill holes are made through the lower end of the femur so that the patella can be attached to the cut surface of the femur by two strong catgut or nylon sutures. The stump of the patellar tendon is secured to the hamstring muscles providing attachment of the flexor and extensor group. The fascia lata and skin are sutured with small stitches. Suction drainage may be required.

This amputation heals readily and provides a potentially end-bearing stump. Again the patient can

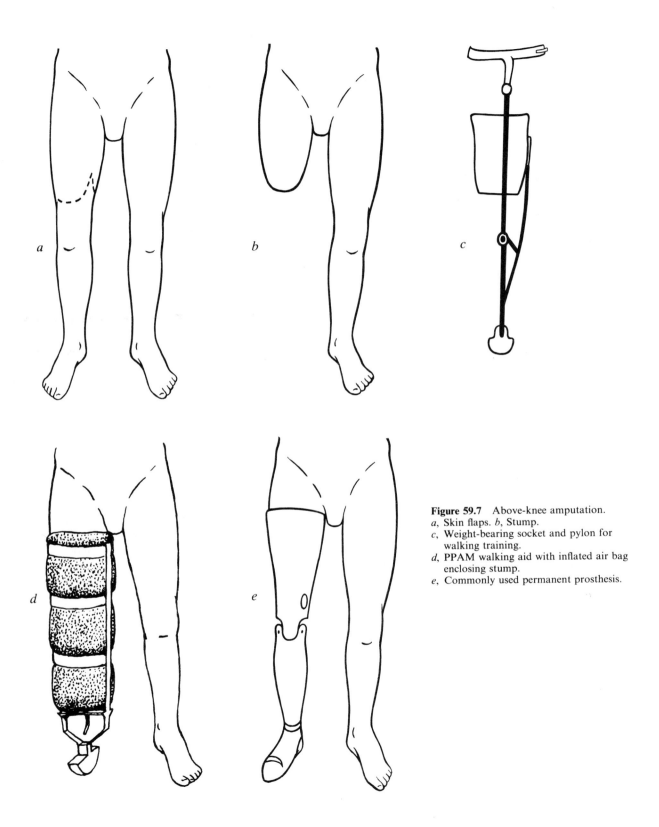

Figure 59.7   Above-knee amputation.
a, Skin flaps. *b*, Stump.
c, Weight-bearing socket and pylon for
   walking training.
d, PPAM walking aid with inflated air bag
   enclosing stump.
e, Commonly used permanent prosthesis.

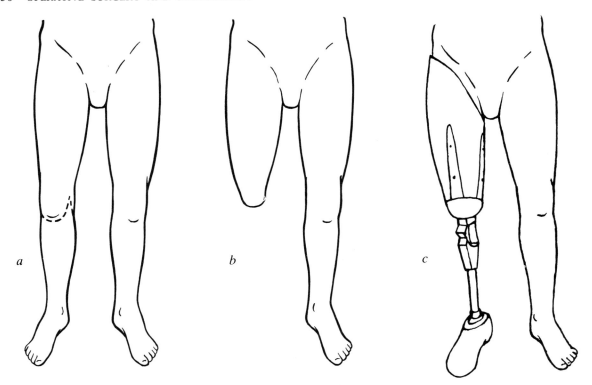

Figure 59.8 Gritti–Stokes amputation. *a*, Skin flaps. *b*, Stump. *c*, Four-bar modular linkage leg in Gritti–Stokes amputation.

have a movable and locking knee joint, but is denied any more sophisticated knee joint mechanism while the tapered stump is not suitable for a suction socket. Nevertheless, the long lever and quick healing characteristics of this amputation make it popular in many quarters. The patient can start walking at an early stage with an ischial-bearing socket and pylon, but many patients continue to use this simple device as detachment and looseness of the patella or avascular necrosis with pain can make end-bearing impossible.

Through-knee amputation (Figure 59.9)

The wide stump, which is capable of end-bearing, that results from this amputation makes it popular with many surgeons. The prosthesis has the disadvantage that the hinged side-irons have to be beside the socket, making it rather wide and cosmetically unacceptable for the younger female patient. However, the stump is durable and painfree and the operation is quick and silent, an advantage in the elderly ischaemic limb, when regional anaesthesia is used. The uncertainties of healing encountered when the conventional anterior flap is used have been avoided by the use of equal lateral skin flaps.

The patient is placed supine on the operating table with the knees hanging over the edge with the end section dropped; some surgeons prefer to lie the patient prone and flex the knee for the anterior dissection. The conventional incision is a long anterior flap extending below the tibial tubercle and a short posterior flap at the level of the knee joint line is made, but the author recommends that equal lateral flaps are formed, from the tibial tubercle descending 4 cm then converging at the joint line posteriorly. Ample skin is needed; the condyles seem very large when the skin is being sutured. With the leg straight the incision is deepened to the tibial periosteum and patellar tendon which is severed from the tibial tubercle and the quadriceps expansion divided so that the knee joint is entered from the front and the patella lifted. With the knee fully flexed the lateral ligaments and the cruciate ligaments may be divided without difficulty. With the leg straight and the foot lifted to flex the hip, the posterior incisions are deepened until the popliteal nerve, the popliteal artery and vein can be individually divided and then the blood vessels ligated. The hamstring tendons are divided 2 cm below the level of the joint line. The patellar tendon is sutured to the cruciate ligaments which are in turn sutured to the hamstring tendons with heavy chromic catgut. It is important that the patella is not drawn down into the intracondylar notch but is allowed to maintain its natural position on the front of the knee joint, where it prevents rotation of the socket on the stump. The skin is closed with fine sutures and Steristrips; a crepe bandage is applied.

Healing is usually rapid and the patient has a firm wide stump capable of end-bearing. Until end-bearing is possible an ischial-bearing pylon can be worn for the purposes of walking training or a pneumatic walking aid, but as soon as the scar is stable a close-

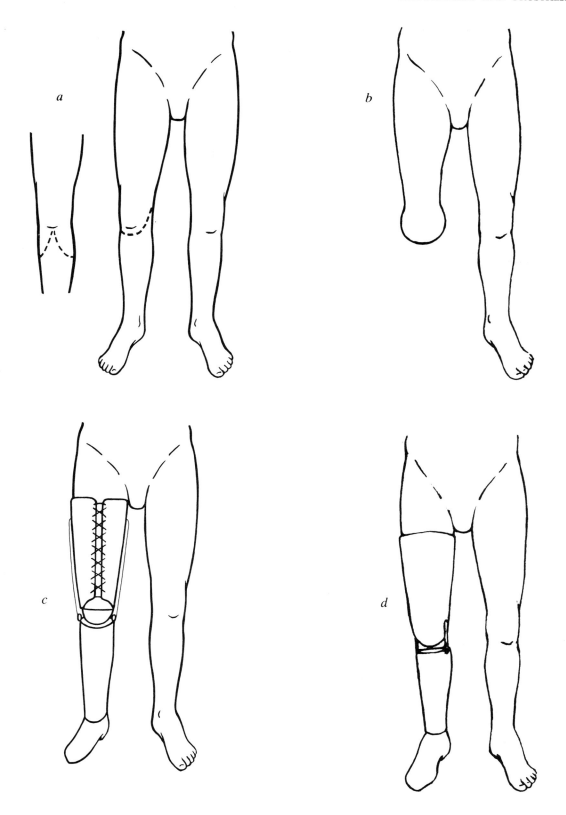

Figure 59.9 Through-knee amputation. *a*, Anteroposterior or lateral flaps may be used. *b*, Stump. *c*, Close-fitting socket prosthesis with locking knee. *d*, Self-suspending socket using shaped liner

fitting socket can be applied. The prosthesis incorporates a simple locking knee joint and the patient is able to walk with an acceptable gait, taking weight on surfaces which normally bear weight.

The through-knee prosthesis has been much improved by the four-bar linkage which puts the joint mechanism below the stump while the axis of movement is in the natural position. The prosthesis is no longer unacceptably wide. An additional development is the use of an inner liner in the through-knee socket which allows the prosthesis to be self-suspending in suitable patients.

Below-knee amputation (Figure 59.10)

Below-knee amputation is frequently used in ischaemic disease when Doppler ultrasound ankle systolic pressure is 40 mmHg or above. The transcutaneous measurement of oxygen diffusion through the skin 10 cm below the knee is a valuable indication of the ability to heal at this level (Burgess *et al.*, 1982); 40 mmHg oxygen tension is the lowest value compatible with safe healing at below-knee level. Below-knee amputation is contraindicated in patients who cannot cooperate to extend the knee. Conventionally performed 14 cm below the knee joint line, the anterior skin flap is two-thirds the diameter of the leg and the posterior skin flap is one-third the diameter of the leg. The muscles, nerves and blood vessels are divided at the level of bone section, the fibula being divided 2 cm above the tibia. The bone ends must be carefully rounded, the skin closed with fine sutures and suction drainage.

In patients with vascular disease, it is recommended that the long anterior skin flap is not used as this is frequently ischaemic (Kendrick, 1956), and instead the anterior skin is divided transversely 12 cm below the knee joint line to 2 cm behind the axis of the limb. A posterior skin flap is fashioned from the posterior skin of the limb, extending down to just above the ankle, the excess in order to allow the flap to be secondarily trimmed (Figure 59.10a) (Burgess *et al.*, 1969; Hunter-Craig *et al.*, 1970). The anterior tibial muscles are divided and the vessels secured. The fibula is divided 2 cm above the line of bone section, 10 cm from the knee joint line. The tibia is divided transversely with a smooth anterior curve cut with a cantilever blade power saw, then carefully rounded with bone file to leave a smooth contour in all planes.

Once the bones are divided, a plane can be entered between the posterior tibial and the gastrocnemius/soleus mass and these muscles are allowed to remain with the posterior flap, while the posterior tibial itself is divided and the peroneal and posterior tibial muscles and nerves individually divided. The Achilles tendon is cut to free the limb before the long posterior flap is trimmed so that a wedge of muscle extends to its distal end, which can then be folded to meet the anterior tibial periosteum where it is sutured to form a myoplasty of the gastrocnemius/soleus mass. Very

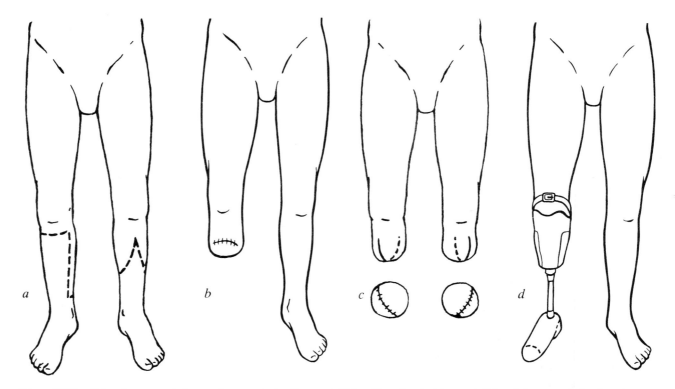

Figure 59.10. Below-knee amputation. *a*, Long posterior flap on right leg. Skew flap incision on left leg. *b*, Long posterior flap stump. *c*, Skewed sagittal flaps stump. *d*, Californian patellar tendon-bearing socket. Modular (without cover).

considerable removal of muscle tissue is needed, especially from the medial and lateral aspects of the flap, if a bulky stump is to be avoided (Figure 59.10b). The posterior skin is trimmed to match the anterior incision and sutured with fine nylon or prolene stitches and Steristrips with suction drainage.

Thermography studies have indicated that skewed sagittal flaps correspond to the distribution of vascular supply better than the long posterior flap, and combined with the gastrocnemius myoplasty produce a stump that requires no secondary shaping and can therefore permit early casting and the supply of prosthesis without any delay (Robinson et al., 1983). The shape which requires no moulding does not require the traditional stump bandage.

This technique often enables healing to occur even when the blood supply is appreciably impaired. The stump is lighty bandaged and the patient may start walking with crutches shortly after the operation and can wear an ischial weight-bearing pylon until the stump is healed and stable or use a pneumatic walking aid (Redhead et al., 1978), until a cast can be taken for a below-knee prosthesis.

A below-knee prosthesis is a nearly total contact socket with a ridge over the patellar tendon, so that the maximum weight-bearing occurs at this point, but is also shared by the flare of the tibial condyles. This socket, the California patellar tendon-bearing socket (Figure 59.10c), is secured by a single strap above the patella and the lower leg prosthesis carries an ankle joint or a flexible foot and enables a normal gait to be achieved; the young patient is quite able to run. To utilize knee flexion 4 cm of stump must project beneath the hamstring tendons of the flexed knee. If the stump is unsatisfactory for a patellar tendon-bearing socket, a thigh corset with side-steels and locking knee hinge will allow the stump to be relieved of all stress in a prosthesis that was the conventional one until 26 years ago.

Syme's amputation (Figure 59.11)

This has been popular with many surgeons as the patient is able in an emergency to stand and walk without a prosthesis. The original level of amputation was through the ankle joint with the medial and lateral malleolus trimmed. The amputation has been modified to divide the tibia and fibula 1 cm above the joint line and an anterior incision is made over the ankle joint, extending to a point just anterior to the malleoli, when the incision is carried down underneath the heel. The ankle joint is entered from the front and the incision carried to the calcaneum which is carefully enucleated from the posterior tissues, safeguarding the calcaneal vessels which carry the blood supply to the heel skin. When the foot is detached the heel skin can be rotated forwards so that the skin can be sutured across the front of the stump. The stump is bulbous transversely and the skin from the back of the heel forms the lower end of the stump (Figure 59.11b).

This heals well, provided the blood supply is not impaired, but it is not recommended where the vascular supply is critical. The bulbous nature of the stump makes it sometimes necessary to fit a 'window' in the socket; alternatively it must be laced throughout its length to enable the stump to be inserted (Figure 59.11c). A flexible foot is provided and the patient may walk with a normal gait provided that the heel pad is not displaced.

Wagner has utilized the Syme's amputation in the treatment of septic diabetic gangrene as a two-stage procedure. First, the foot is removed by disarticulation of the talo-tibiofibular joint and suturing the heel flap while providing irrigating suction drainage to the dead space in the heel flap. Six weeks later through vertical, lateral and medial incisions the malleoli are removed with an osteotome and the soft tissues remodelled. The stump is enclosed in plaster, and weight-bearing can be achieved in 2 weeks. The viability of the heel skin depends on the integrity of the calcaneal branches of the peroneal and posterior tibial arteries. It is essential that these are not damaged in the surgical procedure.

Other amputations can be performed in the region of the ankle joint, although they are infrequently used in this country at the present time. In the Pirogoff amputation, rather than the calcaneum being enucleated from the heel, the calcaneum is cut across so that its posterior 2 cm remain in the heel flap and this is attached to the lower end of the tibia, making a longer stump than in the Syme's amputation. The difficulties in fixation have led to its infrequent use. The Gunther and Le Fort procedures are similar in principle. If the calcaneum and talus are retained and the amputation performed through the talonavicular joint, the Chopart amputation, the unapposed Achilles tendon and peroneal muscles result in flexion and eversion of the heel, which produce an unstable stump. This can be overcome by arthrodesis of the subtalar joint, as in the Spitzi amputation, or tenodesis to stabilize the peroneal and tibial muscles.

Forefoot amputation

The Lisfranc amputation is performed with a short distal flap and a long plantar flap of sole skin with bone section along the base of the metatarsals, preserving the navicular and cuboid bones. This makes a stable amputation if the anterior and posterior tibial tendons are preserved and the only prosthesis required is a surgical boot, filling the space for the absent forefoot. The further anteriorly this amputation can be performed the less the disability and a mid-tarsal amputation can be performed in the same way.

Digital amputation

A single or multiple digital amputation can be performed through a racquet incision or anterior and posterior flaps. Where possible, amputation through

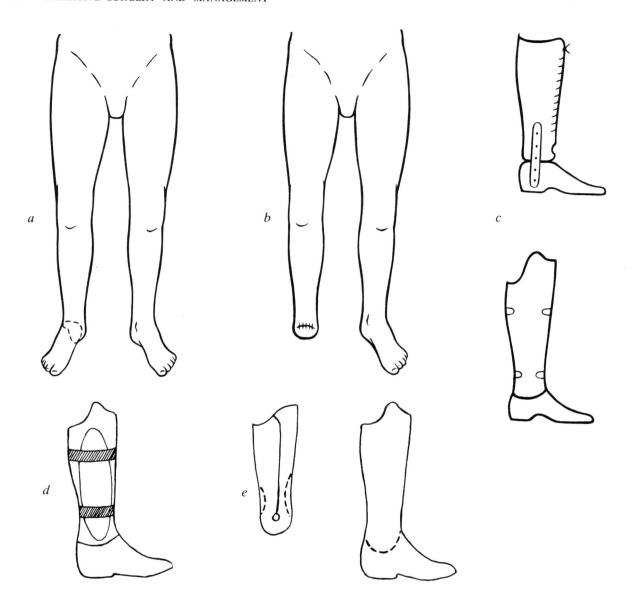

Figure 59.11 Syme's amputation. *a*, Skin flaps. *b*, Stump. *c*, Lace-up prosthesis with flexible foot. *d*, Door in socket to allow entry of stump. *e*, Split liner to accommodate bulbous end.

the base of the phalanx is preferred to disarticulation at a joint, as the joint capsule can be preserved intact and the tendon attachments can be saved. If there is a septic arthrosis of the metatarsophalangeal joint, as is frequently found in infected diabetic gangrene, it is necessary to resect the greater part of the metatarsal, constituting a 'ray' amputation and the skin flaps fall in over the resected bone. Granulation tissue will not cover bare tendon, bone and joint capsules. Therefore enough bone must be resected to give lax skin cover. In the ischaemic foot, sutures should be avoided and Steristrips are very satisfactory.

References

Baker, T. C., Berkowitz, T., Lord, G. B. *et al.* (1970) Hemicorporectomy. *Br. J. Surg.*, **57**, 471–476

Burgess, E. M., Matsen, F., Wyss, C. R. *et al.* (1982) Segmental transcutaneous measurements of PO$_2$ in patients requiring below the knee amputation for peripheral vascular insufficiency. *J. Bone Joint Surg.*, **64A**, 378–382

Burgess, E. M., Romano, R. L. and Zettl, J. H. (1969) *The Management of Lower Extremity Amputations.* 11 TR: 10–6. Prosthetic and Sensory Aids Service, US Veteran Administration

Chilvers, A. S., Briggs, J,., Browse, N. L. *et al.* (1971) Below and through-knee amputation for ischaemic disease. *Br. J. Surg.*, **58**, 824–826

Green, P. W. B., Hawkins, B. S., Irvine, W. T. *et al.* (1972) An assessment of above- and through-knee amputations. *Br. J. Surg.*, **59**, 873–875

Hall, R. and Shucksmith, H. S. (1971) The above-knee amputation for ischaemia. *Br. J. Surg.*, **58**, 656–659

Howard, R. R. S., Chamberlain, J. and Macpherson, A. I. S. (1969) Through-knee amputation in peripheral vascular disease. *Lancet*, **ii**, 240–242

Hunter-Craig, I., Vitali, M. and Robinson, K. P. (1970) Long posterior flap myoplastic below-knee amputation in vascular disease. *Br. J. Surg.*, **57**, 62–65

Kendrick, R. R. (1956) Below-knee amputation in arteriosclerotic gangrene. *Br. J. Surg.*, **44**, 13–17

Kihn, R. B., Warren, R. and Beebe, G. W. (1972) The geriatric amputee. *Ann. Surg.*, **176**, 305–314

Martin, P., Renwick, S. and Maelor Thomas, E. (1967)

Gritti–Stokes amputation in arteriosclerosis: a review of 237 cases. *Br. Med. J.*, **3**, 837–838

Newcombe, J. F. and Marcuson, R. W. (1972) Through-knee amputation. *Br. J. Surg.*, **59**, 260–266

Persson, B. M. (1981) Lower leg amputation with sagittal section in vascular diseases – a study of 692 patients. *Beitr. Orthop. Traumatol.*, **28** (12), 656–663

Redhead, R. G., Davies, B. C., Robinson, K. P. *et al.* (1978) Post-amputation pneumatic walking aid. *Br. J. Surg.*, **65**, 611–612

Robinson, K. P. Hoile, R. and Coddington, T. (1982) Skewflap myoplastic below-knee amputation: a preliminary report. *Br. J. Surg.*, **69**, 554–557

Taylor, G. G. W. (1967) Amputation of the lower limb for ischaemic disease. *Proc. R. Soc. Med.*, **60**. 69–70

Weale, F. E. (1969) The supra-condylar amputation with patellectomy. *Br. J. Surg.*, **56**, 589–593

Westbury, G. (1967) Hindquarter amputation. *Ann. R. Coll. Surg.*, **40**, 226–234

Index